Queenan's Management of High-Risk Pregnancy

Queenan's Management of High-Risk Pregnancy

An Evidence-Based Approach

EDITED BY

CATHERINE Y. SPONG
Professor and Chair
Department of Obstetrics and Gynecology
Paul C. MacDonald Distinguished Chair in Obstetrics and Gynecology
University of Texas Southwestern Medical Center
Dallas, TX, USA
Editor-in-Chief Contemporary OB/GYN

CHARLES J. LOCKWOOD
Dean
Morsani College of Medicine
Executive Vice President
USF Health
Executive Vice President
Tampa General Hospital
Professor of Obstetrics, Gynecology and Public Health
University of South Florida
Tampa, FL, USA

SEVENTH EDITION

WILEY Blackwell

Contents

The color plate section can be found facing p. 226

List of Contributors

Pouya Abhari
Department of Obstetrics, Gynecology and Reproductive Sciences
University of Miami/Jackson Memorial Hospital
Miami, FL, USA

Alfred Abuhamad
Department of Obstetrics and Gynecology
Eastern Virginia Medical School
Norfolk, VA, USA

Richard M.K. Adanu
School of Public Health
University of Ghana
Ghana College of Physicians and Surgeons
Accra, Ghana

Emily H. Adhikari
Department of Obstetrics and Gynecology
University of Texas Southwestern Medical Center
Dallas, TX, USA

Maria Andrikopoulou
Department of Obstetrics and Gynecology
Columbia University Irving Medical Center
Columbia Presbyterian Hospital
New York, NY, USA

Sami Backley
Department of Obstetrics, Gynecology and Reproductive Sciences
McGovern Medical School
The University of Texas Health Sciences Center
Houston, TX, USA

Martina L. Badell
Department of Gynecology and Obstetrics
Emory University School of Medicine
Atlanta, GA, USA

Michal Fishel Bartal
Department of Obstetrics, Gynecology and Reproductive Sciences
McGovern Medical School
The University of Texas Health Science Center
Houston, TX, USA

Department of Obstetrics and Gynecology
Sheba Medical Center
Tel Hashomer
Sackler School of Medicine
Tel Aviv, Israel

Ron Beloosesky
Department of Obstetrics and Gynecology
Ruth and Bruce Rappaport Faculty of Medicine
Technion
Haifa, Israel

Vincenzo Berghella
Department of Obstetrics and Gynecology
Thomas Jefferson University
Philadelphia, PA, USA

Katherine H. Bligard
Department of Obstetrics and Gynecology
Washington University School of Medicine in St. Louis
St. Louis, MO, USA

Angela R. Boyd
Department of Obstetrics and Gynecology
Joe R. and Teresa Lozano Long School of Medicine
San Antonio, TX, USA

Ann M. Bruno
Department of Obstetrics and Gynecology
University of Utah School of Medicine
Salt Lake City, UT, USA

Catalin S. Buhimschi
Department of Obstetrics and Gynecology
University of Illinois College of Medicine
Chicago, IL, USA

Elizabeth O. Buschur
Department of Internal Medicine
The Ohio State University College of Medicine
Columbus, OH, USA

Alison G. Cahill
Department of Women's Health
Dell Medical School
University of Texas at Austin
Austin, TX, USA

Serban Constantinescu
Transplant Pregnancy Registry International
Philadelphia, PA, USA
Department of Medicine
Section of Nephrology, Hypertension and Kidney Transplantation
Lewis Katz School of Medicine at Temple University
Philadelphia, PA, USA

Deborah L. Conway
Department of Obstetrics and Gynecology
Joe R. and Teresa Lozano Long School of Medicine
San Antonio, TX, USA

Lisa A. Coscia
Transplant Pregnancy Registry International
Philadelphia, PA, USA

Mary E. D'Alton
Department of Obstetrics and Gynecology
Columbia University Irving Medical Center
Columbia Presbyterian Hospital
New York, NY, USA

Ronan Daly
Department of Obstetrics and Gynaecology
Royal College of Surgeons in Ireland
Rotunda Hospital
Dublin, Ireland

Cara D. Dolin
Department of Obstetrics and Gynecology
Women's Health Institute
Cleveland Clinic Lerner College of Medicine
Cleveland, OH, USA

Georgios Doulaveris
Department of Obstetrics & Gynecology and Women's Health
Montefiore Medical Center
Albert Einstein College of Medicine
Bronx, NY, USA

Deborah A. Driscoll
Department of Obstetrics and Gynecology
Perelman School of Medicine at the University of Pennsylvania
Philadelphia, PA, USA

Carolynn M. Dude
Department of Gynecology and Obstetrics
Emory University School of Medicine
Atlanta, GA, USA

Lorraine Dugoff
Department of Obstetrics and Gynecology
Perelman School of Medicine at the University of Pennsylvania
Philadelphia, PA, USA

Elaine L. Duryea
Department of Obstetrics and Gynecology
University of Texas Southwestern Medical Center
Dallas, TX, USA

Sarah Rae Easter
Department of Obstetrics and Gynecology
Department of Anesthesiology, Perioperative and Pain Medicine
Brigham and Women's Hospital
Harvard Medical School
Boston, MA, USA

Ann Erickstad
Department of Obstetrics and Gynecology
Texas Tech University Health Sciences Center
Lubbock, TX, USA

Kelly S. Gibson
Department of Reproductive Biology
Case Western Reserve University
MetroHealth Medical Center
Cleveland, OH, USA

Laura Goetzl
Department of Obstetrics, Gynecology and Reproductive Sciences
McGovern Medical School
The University of Texas Health Sciences Center
Houston, TX, USA

Gilbert J. Grant
Department of Anesthesiology, Perioperative Care and Pain Medicine
Grossman School of Medicine
New York University
New York, NY, USA

Christina S. Han
Department of Obstetrics and Gynecology
University of California at Los Angeles
Los Angeles, CA, USA

Lorie M. Harper
Department of Women's Health
Dell Medical School
University of Texas at Austin
Austin, TX, USA

Christina L. Herrera
Department of Obstetrics and Gynecology
University of Texas Southwestern Medical Center
Dallas, TX, USA

G.J. Hofmeyr
Department of Obstetrics and Gynaecology
University of Botswana
Gaborone, Botswana
University of the Witwatersrand
Johannesburg, South Africa
Walter Sisulu University
East London, South Africa

Denise J. Jamieson
Vice President for Medical Affairs and Dean of the Roy J. and
Lucille A. Carver College of Medicine
University of Iowa
Iowa City, IA, USA

Anthony M. Kendle
Department of Obstetrics and Gynecology
Morsani College of Medicine
University of South Florida
Tampa, FL, USA

Michelle A. Kominiarek
Department of Obstetrics and Gynecology
Northwestern University Feinberg School of Medicine
Chicago, IL, USA

Mark B. Landon
Department of Obstetrics and Gynecology
Ohio State University College of Medicine
Columbus, OH, USA

Hanmin Lee
Department of Surgery
University of California, San Francisco
San Francisco, CA, USA

Regan J. Lemley
Department of Neurology
Brigham and Women's Hospital
Harvard Medical School
Boston, MA, USA

Fergal D. Malone
Department of Obstetrics and Gynaecology
Royal College of Surgeons in Ireland
Rotunda Hospital
Dublin, Ireland

Ann McHugh
Department of Obstetrics and Gynecology
Columbia University Irving Medical Center
New York, NY, USA

Brian M. Mercer
Department of Reproductive Biology
Case Western Reserve University
The MetroHealth System
Cleveland, OH, USA

Audrey A. Merriam
Department of Obstetrics, Gynecology and Reproductive Sciences
Yale University School of Medicine
New Haven, CT, USA

Russell S. Miller
Department of Obstetrics and Gynecology
Columbia University Irving Medical
Center
New York, NY, USA

Kenneth J. Moise Jr.
Department of Women's Health
Dell Medical School
University of Texas at Austin
The Comprehensive Fetal Care Center
Dell Children's Medical Center
Austin, TX, USA

Michael J. Moritz
Transplant Pregnancy Registry International
Philadelphia, PA, USA
Deparment of Surgery
Lehigh Valley Health Network
Allentown, PA, USA
Morsani College of Medicine
University of South Florida
Tampa, FL, USA

Andrew Myers
Department of Internal Medicine
USF Health Morsani College of Medicine
Tampa, FL, USA

Michael Nageotte
Miller Children's and Women's Hospital
Long Beach, CA, USA
University of California
Irvine, CA, USA

Jennifer Namazy
Department of Allergy and Immunology
Scripps Clinic
San Diego, CA, USA

M.N. Nassali
Department of Obstetrics and Gynaecology
University of Botswana
Gaborone, Botswana

David B. Nelson
Department of Obstetrics and Gynecology
University of Texas Southwestern Medical Center
Dallas, TX, USA

Anna Hayes Nutter
Department of Obstetrics and Gynecology
Eastern Virginia Medical School
Norfolk, VA, USA

Sarah G. Običan
Department of Obstetrics and Gynecology
University of South Florida
Tampa, FL, USA

Anthony O. Odibo
Department of Obstetrics and Gynecology
Washington University School of Medicine in St. Louis
St. Louis, MO, USA

John Owen
Department of Obstetrics and Gynecology
The University of Alabama at Birmingham
Birmingham, AL, USA

Asa Oxner
Department of Internal Medicine
USF Health Morsani College of Medicine
Tampa, FL, USA

Yinka Oyelese
Obstetric Imaging
Beth Israel Deaconess Medical Center
Harvard Medical School
Boston, MA, USA

Michael J. Paidas
Department of Obstetrics, Gynecology and Reproductive Sciences
Miller School of Medicine
University of Miami
University Health Tower
Jackson Health System
Miami, FL, USA

Shivani Patel
Department of Obstetrics and Gynecology
University of Texas Southwestern Medical School
Dallas, TX, USA

Christian M. Pettker
Department of Obstetrics, Gynecology and Reproductive Sciences
Yale University School of Medicine
New Haven, CT, USA

Michael Richley
Department of Obstetrics and Gynecology
University of California at Los Angeles
Los Angeles, CA, USA

Scott Roberts
Department of Obstetrics and Gynecology
University of Texas Southwestern Medical Center
Dallas, TX, USA

Stephanie T. Ros
Department of Obstetrics and Gynecology
University of South Florida
Tampa, FL, USA

Michael G. Ross
Department of Obstetrics and Gynecology
Geffen School of Medicine
Department of Community Health Sciences
Fielding School of Public Health
University of California at Los Angeles (UCLA)
Harbor-UCLA Medical Center
Torrance, CA, USA

George R. Saade
Department of Obstetrics and Gynecology
Eastern Virginia Medical School
Norfolk, VA, USA

Michael Schatz
Department of Allergy
Kaiser Permanente Medical Center
San Diego, CA, USA

Rachel C. Schell
Department of Obstetrics and Gynecology
University of Texas Southwestern Medical Center
Dallas, TX, USA

Claudio V. Schenone
Department of Obstetrics and Gynecology
University of South Tampa
Tampa, FL, USA

Marisa Eve Schwab
Department of Surgery
University of California, San Francisco
San Francisco, CA, USA

Baha M. Sibai
Department of Obstetrics, Gynecology and Reproductive Sciences
McGovern Medical School
The University of Texas Health Science Center
Houston, TX, USA

Caroline Signore
Eunice Kennedy Shriver National Institute of Child Health and Human Development
Bethesda, MD, USA

Robert M. Silver
Department of Obstetrics and Gynecology
University of Utah School of Medicine
Salt Lake City, UT, USA

Lynn L. Simpson
Department of Obstetrics and Gynecology
Columbia University Irving Medical Center
New York, NY, USA

Rachel Sinkey
Department of Obstetrics and Gynecology
The University of Alabama
Birmingham, AL, USA

Stephen F. Thung
Department of Obstetrics, Gynecology and Reproductive Sciences
Yale School of Medicine
New Haven, CT, USA

P. Emanuela Voinescu
Department of Neurology
Brigham and Women's Hospital
Harvard Medical School
Boston, MA, USA

Michelle E. Whittum
Department of Obstetrics and Gynecology
University of South Florida
Tampa, FL, USA

Edward R. Yeomans
Department of Obstetrics and Gynecology
Texas Tech University Health Sciences Center
Lubbock, TX, USA

Foreword

I am delighted – indeed tickled – to pen this foreword for the Seventh Edition of *Queenan's Management of High-Risk Pregnancy*! The book is now edited by my esteemed colleagues, Dr. Charles J. Lockwood and Dr. Catherine Y. Spong, with whom I have had the good fortune to have worked on prior editions of this textbook as well as our co-edited textbooks *Protocols of High Risk Pregnancy: Evidence Based Management*. We share a common academic lineage as successive editors-in-chief of *Contemporary ObGyn*. I recall the conversations at meetings and at airports with Drs. Lockwood and Spong inviting them to join me as editors in the previous editions, all with the fervent hope that one day they would carry the book forward to future generations. That time has arrived!

Looking back to the origins of this book, in the 1980s I had the good fortune to assemble chapters derived from terrific articles by esteemed authors in *Contemporary ObGyn*. This book was successful because these chapters were succinct, evidence based, up to date, and easy to understand – the perfect management tool for the busy practitioner. They included clinical vignettes to highlight important concepts. I never had difficulty getting the leading authors to participate in this project and I recognize this was because they were also passionate educators, master clinicians, and incredible colleagues with collaborative willingness to work together.

I had always hoped this book would serve all levels of trainees as well as busy practitioners and established colleagues. With ever-changing evidence in obstetrics and maternal fetal medicine, it has been critical to ensure that chapters were up to date and new chapters were added to address topics previously undescribed. For example, this edition includes SARS CoV2 virus, vaping, and various advances in obstetrical management to name a few.

Over the past 40 years plus we have seen extraordinary advances in prenatal screening and diagnosis. The seventh edition, under the leadership of Drs. Lockwood and Spong, upholds the textbook's place as a classic, outlining a practical approach to management for physicians and trainees. I am honored to have my name as part of the title.

John T. Queenan
Professor and Chairman Emeritus of Obstetrics and Gynecology
Georgetown University School of Medicine
Washington, DC

Preface

The seventh edition *of Queenan's Management of High-Risk Pregnancy*, like its predecessors, is directed to all health professionals involved in the care of women with high-risk pregnancies. This book has its origins from a series of articles appearing in *Contemporary OB/GYN* that were the inspiration for the first edition in 1980. *Contemporary OB/GYN*, was in turn, the inspiration of John T. Queenan. Its legacy was carried forward first by Charles J. Lockwood and now by Catherine Y. Spong. As with prior editions, *Queenan's Management of High-Risk Pregnancy* contains clear, concise, practical material presented in an evidence-based manner. Each chapter is followed by an illustrative case report to help put the subject in perspective.

In this new edition we have focused on including topics most critical to providing good care, each written by outstanding authorities on the subject to ensure they are focused, timely, and authoritative. This dynamic process requires adding new chapters as the evidence dictates and eliminating others so that the reader is presented with the most clinically useful contemporary information. We are delighted to ensure John T. Queenan's legacy

continues in this latest edition, as we are committed to his vision and inspiration to have clear, concise protocols that ensure that busy practitioners have needed information at their fingertips.

The seventh edition comes at a time when health care has experienced a pandemic, virtual visits and encounters are increasingly common, and health care settings continue to rapidly evolve. We continue to emphasize evidence-based information and clinical practicality and included chapters addressing timely topics such as infectious diseases in pregnancy, vaping, operative vaginal delivery, postpartum hemorrhage, and pregnancies in women with disabilities. To ensure applicability for health professionals in developing countries we have protocols on maternal anemia, malaria, and HIV infection.

We are committed to bringing the busy practitioner the best possible clinical information. As a reader if you find an area that needs correction or modification or have comments to improve this effort, we welcome your feedback.

Catherine Y. Spong and Charles J. Lockwood

Acknowledgments

We are fortunate to work in cooperation with a superb editorial staff at Wiley Blackwell Publishing under the direction of our publisher. Commissioning editor Sophie Bradwell, managing editor Harini Arumugam, and content refinement specialist Praveen Kumar Bondili have also provided guidance and editorial skills that are evident in this edition.

It is vital that we also acknowledge with great appreciation and admiration our authors, experts with busy schedules who took the time to ensure their protocols are evidence-based, clear, concise, and practical. Their contributions to this book are in the best traditions of academic medicine and we hope that they will be translated into a considerable decrease in morbidity and mortality for mothers and infants.

We also hope that by using this book, you will improve the delivery of care for your patients. Your dedication to women's health has made it a joy to prepare this resource.

Chapter 1
Overview of High-Risk Pregnancy

Catherine Y. Spong[1] and Charles J. Lockwood[2]
[1]Department of Obstetrics and Gynecology, University of Texas Southwestern Medical Center, Dallas, TX, USA
[2]Department of Obstetrics and Gynecology, University of South Florida, Morsani College of Medicine, Tampa, FL, USA

We live in an era of dynamic change, where the accelerating pace of information accretion touches all aspects of our lives. Nowhere is this acceleration of knowledge more dynamic or more critical than in medicine. Obstetrics has seen extraordinary changes in practice with enormous gains in molecular genetics, imaging, and evidence-based management of both common and uncommon conditions. And despite the acquisition of these powerful tools, we live at a time of rising maternal mortality and morbidity, rising rates of preterm birth, a chronic opioid crisis, serial viral pandemics, and the increasing politicization of obstetrical practice. In addition, the business of medicine grows ever more complex, and the amount of non-value-added work is accelerating. All this poses serious challenges for the busy clinician and are the ingredients of professional burnout. In the edition of Queenan's classic textbook, as we have in the prior six editions, we try to simplify the work of busy obstetricians by distilling the latest and most rigorous evidence on the management of high-risk pregnancies.

We provide new insights into the management of maternal substance use, simplify approaches to prenatal screening and diagnosis of fetal genetic abnormalities, provide indications for fetal surgery and cover the range of established perinatal pathogens such as group B beta-hemolytic streptococcus, malaria, hepatitis, and HIV – and emerging infections such as Zika and COVID-19. We also cover the evidence-based management of common obstetrical complications such as preterm birth, preeclampsia, recurrent pregnancy loss, breech presentation, and postpartum hemorrhage. The latest in diagnosis and treatment of serious maternal pre-existing medical conditions including cardiac and renal disease, systemic lupus erythematosus, chronic hypertension, diabetes, thromboembolism, thrombocytopenia, and anemia are described. Indications, risks, and techniques for a full range of obstetrical procedures are also explored from operative vaginal delivery to induction of labor, fetal monitoring, and fetal diagnostic procedures.

We have assembled a very talented team of experts on all these topics who distill volumes of new data leavened with their own extensive clinical experience to provide management pearls and algorithms. All this is in keeping with the philosophy of the founding editor, Dr. John Queenan, a towering figure in American obstetrics and gynecology and a founding father of modern maternal–fetal medicine. Through his textbooks and long-standing editorship of *Contemporary Ob/Gyn*, John focused on the "doctors in the trenches" and sought to enhance their practice while saving them time and effort. We are honored to continue John's legacy in this seventh edition.

Chapter 2
Nutrition in Pregnancy

Cara D. Dolin[1] *and Michelle A. Kominiarek*[2]

[1]Department of Obstetrics and Gynecology, Women's Health Institute, Cleveland Clinic Lerner College of Medicine, Cleveland, OH, USA

[2]Department of Obstetrics and Gynecology, Northwestern University Feinberg School of Medicine, Chicago, IL, USA

The study of nutrition in pregnancy begins with natural experiments during war and famine. Classic studies from Holland and Leningrad during World War II suggest that when caloric intake during pregnancy was acutely restricted to <800 kcal/day, birthweights were reduced [1]. Exposure to famine conditions during the second half of pregnancy had the greatest adverse effect on birthweight and placenta weight whereas birth length, head circumference, and postpartum weight were effected to a lesser extent [2,3]. With the progressive loss of calories, maternal weight was lost until a critical threshold was met. Once maternal weight loss stabilized, the placenta and then fetal weights were reduced. When the rationing to 800 kcal/day stopped, maternal weight was the first to recover, followed by placenta weight and finally birthweight.

Although these studies are used as *prima facie* evidence of a link between nutrition and fetal development, a more discerning examination reveals that many common factors are associated with nutrition and fetal development. Although the onset of food rationing was distinct and the birthweight and other anthropomorphic measurements were recorded reliably, other factors were not identified. For example, menstrual data were notoriously unreliable and accurate gestational dating was challenged by the stress of war. Furthermore, in Holland and Leningrad, the stress of war may have been associated with both preterm delivery and reduced birthweight.

In more recent times, the "fetal origins hypothesis" suggests that nutrition during pregnancy not only is associated with birthweight, but also has lifelong effects on metabolism and risk for chronic disease in adulthood [4]. For example, studies have described associations between birthweight and hypertension, diabetes, and coronary heart disease. These studies were also limited by selection bias and failure to account for factors such as socioeconomic status in the pathway of fetal and adult health [5–8].

Today, social determinants of health, including economic stability, education access and quality, healthcare access, neighborhood and built environment, and social and community contexts are key considerations in the study of pregnancy and nutrition [9]. For example, people may live in an environment with access to food but may have limited access to healthy foods. A person's diet in wartime Europe or the lack of adequate access to healthy food today is challenging to evaluate but likely depends on both the quantity (e.g. total kilocalories) and overall quality. Body mass index (BMI) is used to categorize people according to their height and weight and predict their associated health outcomes [10]. Measures than can complement BMI to determine risk for health outcomes include waist circumference, body fat analysis, and other metabolic markers such as inflammatory status and insulin resistance [11]. In pregnancy, BMI is the anthropomorphic measure that is most readily available. A person's prepregnancy weight or BMI along with their weight changes during pregnancy may estimate nutritional status but are not replacements for measures of diet quantity and quality.

The purpose of this chapter is to review the associations between nutrition and perinatal outcomes. We summarize the basic concepts of fetal growth, the multiple predictors of fetal growth, gestational weight gain, adverse perinatal outcomes related to either inadequate or excessive weight gain, and recommendations for caloric, vitamin, mineral, and other supplements during pregnancy.

Fetal growth

After the first trimester, estimated fetal weight is derived from ultrasound biometry (i.e. head circumference, femur length, abdominal circumference) and referenced to either population or customized growth standards to create a

Queenan's Management of High-Risk Pregnancy: An Evidence-Based Approach, Seventh Edition. Edited by Catherine Y. Spong and Charles J. Lockwood.

weight percentile. The term fetal growth restriction is used to describe a fetus with an ultrasound estimated fetal weight <10th% for gestational age or having an abdominal circumference <10th% as determined by ultrasound [12]. According to birth and death certificates from 2 288 806 births in California from 1970–1976, birthweight was used as a proxy for fetal growth rates whereby the growth peaked at 250 g per week at 33 weeks and then declined to 75 g per week at 40 weeks (Figure 2.1). The comparison of coincidental estimated fetal weight and birthweight reveals a relatively large error; 20% of estimated fetal weights will differ from the actual weight by one standard deviation or more, 400-600 g at term [13].

Twin pregnancies have a proportionally lower rate of growth, reaching a maximum at 175 g per week at 31 weeks (Figure 2.1) [14]. A study of live births of twins delivered between 1990 and 1996 evaluated birthweights according to type of placentation. Between 30 and 40 weeks, twins with dichorionic placentation were heavier than those with a monochorionic placentation [15]. There is still controversy as to whether singleton or separate twin standards should be the comparison reference in multifetal pregnancies. A prospective cohort study of 171 dichorionic twins evaluated the fetal growth trajectory and compared the findings to a singleton growth standard. By 35 weeks of gestation, nearly 40% of twins would be classified as small for gestational age with the use of a singleton, non-Hispanic White reference [16].

It is important to study the extremes of fetal growth as growth restriction is associated with increased risk for stillbirth, acidosis, and neonatal intensive care unit admissions whereas macrosomia (i.e. birthweights greater than 4500 g) is associated with an increased risk for abnormal labor, cesarean delivery, birth injury, >30 minutes of assisted ventilation, and infant mortality [17]. The velocity of fetal growth may inform the mechanisms of abnormal growth [18]. Fetal length peaks earlier than weight, as the fetus stores fat and hepatic glycogen, which contribute to increasing abdominal circumference in the third trimester. When an exposure occurs early in pregnancy, such as with alcohol exposure, severe starvation, smoking, perinatal infection (i.e. cytomegalovirus infection), chromosomal or developmental disorders, or chronic vasculopathies (i.e. diabetes, autoimmune disease, chronic hypertension), the result is a fetus with similarly reduced growth of its length, head circumference, and abdominal circumference [19].

When the exposure occurs after the peak in the velocity of length growth, the result is a disproportionately reduced body-length ratio, with a larger head circumference relative to abdominal circumference. This pattern usually is the result of new onset or developing vasculopathy (i.e. placental thrombosis/infarcts, preeclampsia) or a reduction of the absorptive capacity of the placenta (i.e. postdate pregnancy). Although the classification of symmetrical vs. asymmetrical fetal growth restriction has been referenced to the timing of an exposure and proposed etiologies, more recent studies suggest growth and developmental delay from birth until 4 years of age are similar in symmetrical and asymmetrical growth restriction. Furthermore, ratios of head and abdominal circumferences did not independently predict adverse outcomes [20,21].

Fetal growth requires the transfer of nutrients as building blocks and the transfer of oxygen to support fetal growth and development. Maternal pulmonary, gastrointestinal, and cardiac systems adapt for fetal and placental needs. These adaptations are partially driven through placenta hormones (i.e. human placental lactogen). The central role of the placenta in the production of pregnancy hormones, the transfer of nutrients, and fetal respiration is demonstrated by the fact that 20% of the oxygen supplied to the fetus is diverted to the metabolic activities of the placenta and placental oxygen consumption at term is about 25% higher than the amount consumed by the fetus as a whole. The absorptive surface area of the placenta is strongly associated with fetal growth; the chorionic villus surface area grows from about 5 m^2 at 28–30 weeks to 10 m^2 by term.

The measured energy requirement of pregnancy totals 55 000 kcal for an 11 800 g of weight gain or 4.7 kcal/g of weight gain [22]. This value is considerably less than the 8.0 kcal/g required for weight gain in nonpregnant people. This discrepancy is likely due to the poorly understood relationship between pregnancy hormones (i.e. human placental lactogen, corticosteroids, sex steroids) and the pattern of nutrient distribution. Table 2.1 describes the work as measured by weight that occurs to produce an appropriately grown fetus at term. Weight gain is

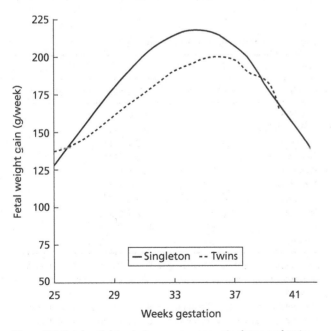

Figure 2.1 Fetal weight gain in grams among singleton and twin pregnancies.

Table 2.1 Sources of weight gain in pregnancy

	Maternal gains		Fetal gains
Blood volume	2 kg (4.4 lb)	Fetus	3.5 kg (7.7 lb)
Uterine size	1 kg (2.2 lb)	Placenta	0.6 kg (0.7 lb)
Breast size	1 kg (2.2 lb)	Amniotic fluid	1.2 kg (2.6 lb)
Fat increase	3 kg (6.6 lb)		
Total (maternal + fetal) weight gain	12.3 kg (27 lb)		

Table 2.2 Factors associated with fetal growth

Factors	Clinical examples
Genetics	Parental anthropometrics
	Chromosomal disorders
	Congenital anomalies
Uterine volume	Müllerian duct abnormalities
	Fibroids
Maternal intake	Eating disorders (anorexia)
	Inadequate or excessive weight gain
	Iron deficiency anemia
	Micronutrient deficiencies (folic acid)
Maternal absorption	Inflammatory bowel disease
	Bariatric surgery
Maternal hyper metabolic states	Hyperthyroidism
	Adolescent pregnancy
	Extreme exercise
Maternal cardiorespiratory function	Cardiac disease
	Sarcoidosis
	Asthma
Uterine blood flow	Hypertension/preeclampsia
	β-adrenergic blockers
	Diabetic vasculopathy
	Autoimmune vasculopathy
	Smoking (nicotine)
	Chronic environmental stress
Placental transfer	Diabetes
	Smoking (carbon monoxide)
Placental absorption	Placental infarcts or thrombosis
Fetal blood flow	Congenital heart disease
	Increased placental resistance
	Polycythemia
Fetal metabolic state	Drug effects (amphetamines)
	Genetic metabolic disease
Reduced fetal cell numbers	Alcohol
	Chromosomal disorders

essentially linear throughout the second and third trimesters of pregnancy [23].

Many factors affect the transfer of nutrients and oxygen to the fetus. Table 2.2 lists factors and clinical examples that can be associated with abnormal fetal growth. Although the etiologies for fetal growth restriction can vary, they often share a final common pathway of suboptimal fetal nutrition and uteroplacental perfusion.

Diet quantity and quality, appropriate absorption and distribution of macro- and micronutrients, cardiorespiratory adaptions, uterine blood flow, placental transfer, placental blood flow, and appropriate fetal metabolism of nutrients and oxygen are among some factors that are associated with fetal growth. Additionally, parental and fetal genetics and uterine characteristics can be associated with fetal growth. Abnormal uterine characteristics such as Müllerian duct abnormalities or large uterine fibroids have also been associated with abnormalities in fetal growth.

Obstetric history reveals a strong tendency to repeat gestational age and birthweight as the result of shared genetic and environmental factors. Bakketeig et al. analyzed almost 500 000 consecutive births in Norway [24]. Table 2.3 depicts the results of their analysis which shows a cumulative risk for outcomes such as small and large for gestational age birthweight suggesting there are intrinsic factors and not necessarily complications during pregnancy or delivery contributing to these perinatal outcomes.

Ultimately, any evaluation of the association between nutrition and perinatal outcomes such as birthweight should control for risk factors (Table 2.2). Most studies of nutrition during pregnancy use the BMI (weight [kg]/(height in meters)^2) or weight gain during pregnancy as a proxy for nutritional status. Integration of diet quality, and supplements are needed to provide details on nutritional states. Most studies rely on self-reported prepregnancy weight to determine the initial weight, calculate a BMI, and approximate risks for adverse perinatal outcomes. A systematic review of the accuracy of self-reported weight suggested the magnitude of error for a

Table 2.3 Obstetric history and birthweight

Incidence of adverse outcome in		
First birth	Second birth	Subsequent birth (relative risk[a])
Term AGA	–	1.4% (1.0)
Preterm low BW	–	13.1% (4.5)
Term SGA	–	8.2% (5.5)
BW >4500 g	–	22.6% (9.0)
Postterm	–	5.3% (2.2)
Term AGA	Term AGA	1.5% (0.5)
Preterm low BW	Preterm low BW	19.7% (6.8)
Term SGA	Term SGA	29% (19.3)
BW >4500 g	BW >4500 g	45.5% (18.2)
Post term	Post term	33.3% (13.9)

AGA, appropriate for gestational age; BW, birthweight; SGA, small for gestational age (2500 g); preterm, 36 weeks and 2500 g; post term, 44 weeks.
[a]The relative risk is the ratio of incidence of "poor" outcomes in the target cohort divided by the incidence of "poor" outcomes in the lowest risk cohort, women in whom all births were normal. Adapted from Hadlock [13].

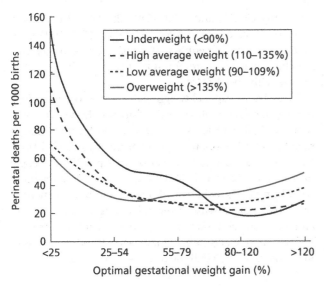

Figure 2.2 Perinatal mortality rates by prepregnancy weight and height (Metropolitan Life Insurance tables) and the percentage of optimal weight gain. Reproduced from Naeye with permission from Elsevier [27].

self-reported weight was small, varied by prepregnancy weight and race or ethnicity but did not largely bias associations with pregnancy outcomes [25]. If a prepregnancy weight is not available or deemed inaccurate, another option is to use a measured weight at the first prenatal visit to calculate BMI [26]. There is added imprecision with the measurement of weight gain, especially if the prepregnancy weight is not known or prenatal care begins after the first trimester. Studies also use different measures of the final pregnancy weight including the last weight at an outpatient prenatal visit vs. a weight upon admission to labor and delivery, thus creating adding inconsistencies to these measurements.

Body mass index, weight gain, and adverse pregnancy outcomes

BMI and weight gain have powerful associations with birthweight and perinatal outcomes. Naeye examined the association between weight gain and perinatal outcomes from the National Collaborative Perinatal Project [27]. About 56 000 people were followed from prenatal enrollment through birth with infants followed through 7 years. They found that progressive increases in prepregnancy weight or weight gain, or both, were significantly associated with increases in birthweight. Prepregnancy weight and weight gain appear to have independent and additive effects. However, increasing prepregnancy weight diminishes the association of weight gain and birthweight. For example, among nonsmokers, the difference in birthweight across weight gains (less than 7.3 kg [16 lb]) vs. more than 15.9 kg [35 lb]) was 556 g (19% difference)

for underweight people, 509 g (16.4% difference) for normal-weight people, and 335 g (10% difference) for overweight people. Similarly, among smokers, the difference in birthweight was 683 g (27%) for underweight people, 480 g (16.4%) for normal-weight people, and 261 g (8%) for overweight people [27].

Perinatal mortality rates in underweight people (<90% of expected pregnancy weight in the Metropolitan weight-for-height charts) are strongly associated with weight gain (Figure 2.2) [27]. Poor weight gain (defined as <30 pounds) in underweight people is associated with a fivefold increase in perinatal mortality.

Data from the 1980 National Natality Survey also provided information on the association between weight gain and birthweight [28]. A probability sample of all live births to people in the United States in 1980 was employed. BMI and weight gain were associated with birthweights less than 2500 g at more than 37 weeks gestation.

These large national studies [27,28] contributed to the first guidelines for weight gain [29]. The impetus for formulating the guidelines was to decrease low birthweight and therefore the emphasis was on gaining enough or eating enough to reduce low birthweight. The weight gain guidelines for people with obesity were imprecise–"at least 15 pounds." However, providers now had information to counsel their patients on appropriate weight gain and its associations with perinatal outcomes. Changes in sociodemographic and anthropometrics in the United States in the subsequent 20 years included increasing maternal age at delivery, increasing pregnancy complications, greater racial and ethnic diversity, increasing gestational weight gain, and increasing BMI of adults [30]. The National Academy of Medicine updated its guidelines for gestational weight gain in 2009 (Table 2.4) [23]. The primary change to the guideline was a specific weight gain recommendation for people with obesity (5–9 kg). Although several studies have since suggested that outcomes such as cesarean delivery improve with weight gain less than these guidelines for people with higher classes of obesity, there is a trade-off of increased risk for SGA infants with lower amounts of weight gain [31–33]. As such, the weight gain goals for people in all obesity classes continues to require additional research and the goals remain the same [34].

The study of BMI, weight gain, and gestational age at delivery is complex [35]. People who deliver preterm have less opportunity to gain weight. Therefore, total weight gain should be adjusted for the gestational age at delivery. Net gain per week of gestation controls for the pregnancy duration. Cnattingius et al. examined infants born in Sweden, Denmark, Norway, Finland, and Iceland from 1992 to 1993 [36]) including 167 750 with singleton births for whom prepregnancy BMI data were available. The results were adjusted for age, parity, education, cigarette smoking, and whether the person was living with a

Table 2.4 Recommended total weight gain during pregnancy

Prepregnancy BMI (kg/m²)	Recommended total weight gain (kg/lb)
Underweight (BMI <18.5)	12.7–18.2 kg (28–40 lb)
Normal (BMI 18.5–24.9)	11.4–15.4 kg (25–35 lb)
Overweight (BMI 25.0–29.9)	6.8–11.4 kg (15–25 lb)
Obese–all classes[a] (BMI ≥30)	5.0–9.1 kg (11–20 lb)

BMI, body mass index.
[a]Class I: BMI 30–34.9, Class II: BMI 35–39.9, Class III: BMI ≥40Adapted from [29].

partner. Prepregnancy BMI of 20 or greater was associated with a decrease in SGA infants (adjusted odds ratio [OR] 0.5–0.7; 95% confidence interval [CI] 0.4–0.8). Weight gain of less than 0.25 kg/wk was associated with an adjusted OR of 3.0 (95% CI 2.5–3.5) for SGA infants. Among people with a BMI less than 24.9kg/m², there was no association with late fetal death or preterm delivery. People with overweight (BMI 25.0–30.0) and obesity (BMI ≥ 30.0) had an increased risk of late fetal death (after 28 weeks completed gestation). The adjusted ORs (95% CI) for fetal death were 1.7 (1.1–2.4) for people with overweight and 2.7 (1.8–4.1) for people with obesity.

Obesity

The prevalence of obesity in the United States in women 20–39 years old is 40%, with 9% having class III obesity (BMI >40 kg/m²).(30) In addition to an increased risk of gestational diabetes, hypertensive disorders of pregnancy, and wound infections, people with obesity are more likely to have spontaneous miscarriage (OR 1.2, 95% CI 1.01–1.46) and stillbirth [37, 38]. The risk of stillbirth increases with increasing severity of obesity from a hazard ratio of 1.71 for those with a prepregnancy BMI of 30.0–34.9 kg/m² to 3.16 for those with a BMI ≥50 kg/m² compared to those without obesity (Table 2.5) [39] A meta-analysis of the risks of obesity and major congenital malformation revealed higher risk of neural tube defects (OR 1.87, 95% CI 1.62–2.15), cardiovascular defects (OR 1.30, 95%

CI 1.12–1.51), cleft lip and palate (OR 1.20, 95% CI 1.03–1.40), and more limb reduction defects (OR 1.34, 95% CI 1.03–0.73) among neonates of people with obesity. Interestingly, gastroschisis was less common (OR 0.17, 95% CI 0.1–0.3) in people with obesity [40].

Excessive gestational weight gain, >20 lb, occurs in 57% of pregnancies complicated by obesity [41]. Excessive gestational weight gain is associated with postpartum weight retention [38]. Importantly, 50% of all people retain >10 lb at 6 months postpartum. At 1 year postpartum 25% of people have still retained >10 lb [42]. Postpartum weight retention contributes to the epidemic of obesity and development of cardiometabolic diseases later in life. Improvement in diet and nutrition habits during pregnancy can not only provide maternal and fetal benefit but may also extend to the rest of the household and continue past the pregnancy.

Nutrition assessment and counseling

Pregnancy is an important opportunity to engage patients about their nutrition and dietary habits. During pregnancy, there is increased contact with health care providers and awareness of healthy behaviors [43]. People are often more receptive to advice and dietary changes, especially if framed to benefit the fetus [44].

At the initial prenatal visit, height and weight should be measured to determine BMI. A complete review of the medical and surgical history should be performed to identify conditions that may affect nutritional status, such as prior bariatric surgery, inflammatory bowel disease, diabetes, chronic infection such as human immunodeficiency virus infection, allergies, autoimmune disease, and renal disease. It is important to ask about past or present history of an eating disorders as pregnancy can trigger a relapse for some patients [45]. Patients with substance use disorders are also at risk of poor nutrition [46]. Specific diets, such as vegetarian or ketogenic should also be investigated. Patients at nutritional risk should be referred to a registered dietitian for a more detailed nutritional assessment and personalized nutrition plans.

	Underweight	Normal weight	Overweight	Obese
Number	29317	442885	137388	19987
Preeclampsia	0.6%	0.88%	1.7%	4.9%
Gestational diabetes	0.6%	0.92%	2.3%	4.5%
Nonelective cesarean	9.3 %	10,6%	11.6%	14.3%
SGA	12.1%	8.4%	8.3%	7.3%
LGA	3.9%	7.1%	9.4%	13.9%
Preterm birth	5.2%	5.3%	8.1%	8.6%
Stillbirth	0.14%	0.16%	0.34%	0.51%
Early neonatal death	0.6%	0.04%	0.04%	0.21%

Table 2.5 The prevalence of adverse pregnancy outcomes associated with meeting Institute of Medicine targets

LGA, large for gestational age; SGA, small for gestational age. Adapted from Yao et al. [39].

A nutrition screening tool to understand overall diet pattern and identify areas for improvement in diet quality as well assess the patient's willingness to make lifestyle changes is useful. A 24-hour dietary recall is another commonly used dietary assessment tool. A patient is asked what food, beverages, and supplements they consumed in the past 24 hours, from midnight to midnight the previous day. Most people have very little variation in their day-to-day dietary patterns [47]. Counseling regarding a healthy diet and appropriate gestational weight gain should occur during the initial prenatal visit and throughout the pregnancy as needed [48].

Food security

Food insecurity, defined as a lack of consistent access to the nutritionally adequate and safe food needed for a healthy life, affected more than 10% in the United States in 2019 [49,50]. Food insecurity disproportionately impacts women, specifically single mothers affecting one third [50]. There is also a significant racial and ethnic disparity with both non-Hispanic Black and Hispanic households more than twice as likely to report food insecurity as compared with White households. Food security is an important social determinant of health and is associated with adverse health outcomes in nonpregnant adults including obesity, diabetes, hypertension, and mental health problems [51,52].

Universally, pregnant people should be screened during pregnancy for food insecurity [53]. The Hunger Vital Sign™ (Box 2.1), is a brief, validated, two-item screen for food insecurity with 97% sensitivity, that allows clinicians to quickly identify almost all patients at risk for food insecurity [54,55]. Those who screen positive can be offered referrals to community-based resources [56].

Energy intake during pregnancy

Energy or caloric needs increase during pregnancy to support fetal growth, as well as the growth of the placenta, uterus, breast tissue, and fat stores. Additionally,

---

Box 2.1 The Hunger Vital Sign: Food security screening questions

1. Within the past 12 months, you worried that your food would run out before you got money to buy more.
2. Within the past 12 months, the food you bought just did not last and you did not have money to get more.

Answer: Never true, sometimes true, often true, patient declined.
A positive screen is an answer of "often true" or "sometimes true" (vs "never true") to either or both statements.

Adapted from Hager et al. [54].

---

physiologic changes during pregnancy, including increased cardiac output, increased work of breathing, and metabolic rate of fetal tissues, lead to an increase in baseline resting energy expenditure of 25–30% [57,58]. During the first trimester, the total daily energy expenditure increases only slightly as compared with prepregnancy [58]. Given this fact, no additional calories are recommended during the first trimester of pregnancy [59]. However, during the second and third trimesters an additional 340 kcal/day and 452 kcal/day are recommended, respectively, in those with a normal prepregnancy weight, to meet the metabolic demands of pregnancy [59]. In people with obesity, there is evidence that lower energy intake is still associated with adequate gestational weight gain by mobilization of existing maternal fat mass rather than increased energy intake [60].

Healthy dietary pattern in pregnancy

Dietary patterns have been studied to understand which support a healthy pregnancy and decrease risk of adverse pregnancy outcomes. A meta-analysis found that diets higher in vegetables, fruits, whole grains, nuts, legumes, fish, and vegetable oils, and lower in meats and refined grains, decreased the risk of hypertensive disorders of pregnancy [63]. This dietary pattern reduced the risk of preeclampsia by 14–29% and reduced the risk of hypertensive disorder of pregnancy by 30–42% [63]. Similarly, diets higher in vegetables, fruits, whole grains, nuts, legumes, and fish, and lower in red and processed meats decreased the risk of gestational diabetes [63]. A diet higher in vegetables, fruits, whole grains, nuts, legumes, seeds, seafood, and lower in red and processed meats and fried foods was associated with lower risk of preterm birth in a meta-analysis including 11 studies [64]. However, almost all studies had cohorts composed mostly of healthy White women with access to healthcare. There is little research on the impact of dietary patterns in a racially and ethnically diverse population or in those of lower socioeconomic status.

Overall, the US Dietary Guidelines for Americans recommend that a healthy dietary pattern during pregnancy for a person of normal weight consist of 3 cup eq/day of a variety of vegetables including dark-green vegetables, red and orange vegetables, beans, peas, lentils, starchy vegetables, and other vegetables; 2 cup eq/day of a variety of fruits; 8 ounce eq/day of grains with at least 50% coming from whole grains; 3 cup eq/day of dairy or fortified soy beverages; and 6 ounces eq/day of protein foods including nuts, seeds, beans, lentils, soy products, poultry, eggs, and meats [59]. Depending on individual caloric goals these amounts may vary. Less than 10% of calories should come from added sugar and less than 10% from saturated fat. Sodium in the diet should be limited to

<2300 mg daily [59]. A general rule for counseling is that half of the food during each meal should come from vegetables and fruits, the other half from whole grains and healthy sources of protein.

Multivitamins

Ideally nutrients should be obtained from whole food sources during pregnancy; however, to ensure adequate micronutrients needed for proper growth and development of the fetus it is recommended that all pregnant people take a daily prenatal multivitamin containing at least 400 mcg of folic acid [65]. In low- and middle-income countries multivitamin supplementation is associated with a reduction in low birthweight and slight reduction in preterm birth [66]. A meta-analysis of 35 studies including almost 99 000 women living in high-income countries found that multivitamin use in pregnancy decreased the risk of small for gestational age neonates as well as decreased the risk of various congenital anomalies [67]. Despite recommendations that all pregnant people should take a prenatal multivitamin, almost one third (30%) of people report not using any dietary supplements during pregnancy [68].

Additional individual micronutrient supplements should be recommended for people at risk of, or with documented, micronutrient deficiencies. Specific populations that may need individual micronutrient supplementation include those who follow a vegan diet (vitamin B_{12}) and those with history of bariatric surgery prior to pregnancy [69,70].

Micronutrients in pregnancy

Iron

Anemia can lead to adverse pregnancy outcomes including low birthweight, preterm delivery, and perinatal mortality [71]. Anemia is defined by a hemoglobin below 11.0, 10.5, and 11.0 g/dL in the first, second, and third trimesters, respectively [72,73]. Nutrition-related causes of anemia include dietary deficiency or malabsorption of key nutrients needed for the production of red blood cells including iron, vitamin B_{12}, or folate [71].

Iron needs increase more than 30% during pregnancy. The recommended daily allowance (RDA) of iron during pregnancy is 27 mg daily compared to 18 mg for nonpregnant people of reproductive potential [59]. Extra needs support expansion of erythrocyte mass by 15–35% (500 mg) and fetal and placental growth (300–350 mg) and prepare for blood loss during delivery (250 mg) [75]. Iron needs decrease to 9 mg daily for those breastfeeding during the first year postpartum and then return to prepregnancy recommendation when menstruation resumes [59].

Iron is found in the diet as heme iron from animal sources, such as lean meat, seafood, and poultry, and non-heme iron from plant sources, such as beans, lentils, nuts, and dark leafy vegetables. Iron is also fortified in many products including bread and cereal which is the source of 50% of dietary iron in the United States. Although heme iron is more easily absorbed, non-heme iron absorption can be enhanced by pairing with foods rich in ascorbic acid such as citrus fruits, strawberries, tomatoes, peppers, and broccoli. Dairy products, coffee, tea, and certain medications, such as levothyroxine, and supplements, such as calcium, can decrease iron absorption. Although iron is readily available from many healthy food sources, most pregnant people do not consume the recommended amount of iron from food sources with a median dietary intake of only 15–17 mg/day [68,71]. It is recommended that all pregnant people begin low-dose iron supplementation in the first trimester [71]. Most prenatal multivitamins contain the RDA for iron during pregnancy. If patients have, or are at risk of, iron deficiency anemia an additional iron supplement is recommend [71]. For patients who cannot tolerate oral iron, do not respond to oral iron therapy, or have severe iron-deficiency anemia in the third trimester, parenteral iron can be considered [71,76].

Folate/folic acid

Folate is an essential nutrient and plays a crucial role in many biochemical pathways in the body. Humans cannot make folate and must obtain it through dietary intake or supplementation. The term folate refers to vitamin B_9, a water-soluble vitamin found in food sources, and folic acid refers to the synthetic form found in supplements and fortified foods. Food folates are in the tetrahydrofolate form and often have additional glutamate residues to make them polyglutamates whereas folic acid is the oxidized monoglutamate form. This is an important distinction because their bioavailability is very different. Folic acid is almost completely bioavailable when consumed on an empty stomach whereas folate must be digested to a monoglutamate form prior to absorption resulting in about 50% bioavailability [77].

During pregnancy there is rapid cellular growth to support the development of the fetus and placenta, thus folate needs are higher during pregnancy. The RDA for folate in pregnancy is 600 mcg dietary folate equivalent (DFE) [59]. Lactating people are recommended to have 500 mcg DFE [59]. One mcg DFE is equal to 1 mcg of food folate, 0.6 mcg of folic acid from fortified foods or supplements when taken with food or 0.5 mcg of folic acid from supplement taken on an empty stomach [78].

Neural tube defects (NTDs), congenital malformations of the cranium or spine that result from failure of normal neural tube closure during early pregnancy, are one of the most common birth defects in the United States [79]. NTDs are thought to be multifactorial with risk factors including genetic predisposition and environmental exposures, including preconception folate deficiency [79]. Preconception folic acid has been shown to decrease the risk of recurrent NTDs with a 3.5-fold protective effect [80,81]. The US Preventive Services Task Force recommends that all people of reproductive potential take a daily supplement of 400–800 mcg of folic acid [82]. Supplementation with 400 mcg of folic acid should begin at least one month prior to conception and continue until 12 weeks gestation [79]. Most prenatal vitamins contain at least 400 micrograms of folic acid. Those with a higher risk of NTD, including prior pregnancy or child affected by NTD, partner with a previously affected pregnancy or child, or personal or partner history of NTD, are recommended to take 4 mg (4000 mcg) of folic acid at least 3 months prior to pregnancy and continue until 12 weeks gestation [79].

Folate is found in a wide variety of foods including vegetables, fruits, nuts, beans, seafood, eggs, meat, and poultry. Some of the highest folate levels are found in spinach, edamame, asparagus, and brussels sprouts. Beginning in 1998 the US Food and Drug Administration required most grain products to be fortified with folic acid to reduce the risk of NTDs. The fortification program has been a great public health success and has been successful in decreasing NTDs in the United States independent of folic acid supplement use [83].

Calcium

Calcium is required for fetal development, specifically for development of the fetal skeleton which requires 30 g of calcium over the course of gestation. Fetal calcium deposition increases throughout pregnancy with a peak of 350 mg/day in the third trimester [84]. During pregnancy, these needs are met through increased absorption of dietary calcium, as well as increased bone turnover [85,86]. One study demonstrated calcium absorption is 57% and 72% in the second and third trimesters respectively [87]. In those with low calcium intake absorption substantial increases to 69% in early pregnancy and 87% in late pregnancy, demonstrating the human body's incredible ability to adapt to the needs of the pregnancy [84] However, there are physiologic limits to these adaptations and those with inadequate calcium consumption during pregnancy may be at risk of adverse pregnancy outcomes. Calcium supplementation may decrease the risk of preeclampsia and preterm birth in women with low calcium diets (<900 mg/day), primarily those living in middle- and low-income countries, and at high risk for preeclampsia [88]. However, there are conflicting studies and more research is needed to evaluate the effectiveness of calcium supplementation in pregnancy to prevent adverse outcomes [89].

The RDA for is 1000 mg, slightly higher for teenagers 14–18 years old at 1300 mg daily [59]. Based on National Health and Nutrition Examination Survey (NHANES) data, the mean intake of calcium during pregnancy from food sources alone is 1093 mg and from food and supplements is 1311 mg [68]. Foods high in calcium include dairy products, fish with bones, and vegetables such as kale, broccoli, and cabbage. In the United States some cereal, tofu, and fruit juices are fortified with calcium. Prenatal multivitamins typically contain 200–300 mg of calcium. Most do not need additional supplements during pregnancy unless consuming lactose intolerance or vegan diet.

Vitamin D

Vitamin D is a fat-soluble vitamin critical in the absorption, distribution, and storage of calcium; it also plays an important role in the normal function of tissues throughout the body, immune health, and inflammation [90]. Ultraviolet rays in sunlight are the major source of vitamin D through dermal synthesis. Ultraviolet light converts 7-dehydrocholesterol to cholecalciferol (vitamin D3) in the skin. Vitamin D3 is then converted to 25-hydroxyvitamin D (25-OH-D) in the liver. 25-OH-D is the major circulating form of vitamin D and is measured in the serum when assessing for vitamin D deficiency. Finally, 25-OH-D is converted in the kidney to 1,25-hydroxyvitamin D (active form) and 24,25-dihydroxyvitamin D (inactive metabolite) [90].

The prevalence of risk of vitamin D deficiency (<30 nmol/L) in pregnant people in the United States is 7%, and the prevalence of risk of insufficiency is 21% (30–49 nmol/L) [91]. Severe vitamin D deficiency in pregnancy has been associated with skeletal abnormalities in the fetus including reduced bone mineralization, congenital rickets, and fractures [92,93]. Although evidence is limited, a 2019 Cochrane review found that vitamin D supplementation during pregnancy may reduce the risk of preeclampsia, gestational diabetes, low birthweight, and severe postpartum hemorrhage [94]. Further studies are needed to explore these associations.

There are relatively few food sources of vitamin D. Vitamin D can be found naturally in fish oil and egg yolks. In the United States, milk and other dairy products, as well as some cereals are fortified with vitamin D. The RDA for vitamin D in both pregnancy and lactation is 600 International Units (IU) or 15 mcg daily [59]. Most prenatal vitamins contain 400 IU [95].

People at risk of vitamin D deficiency include those with limited sun exposure due to northern latitude, cold climate, and/or wearing full clothing while outside, homebound or institutionalized patients, those with lactose intolerance, those with prior bariatric surgery, or those who follow a strictly plant-based diet. It is recommended that these individuals be screened for vitamin D deficiency during pregnancy Although the definition of vitamin D insufficiency and deficiency remains controversial it is generally accepted that 25-OH-D ≤ 30 nmol/L increases risk to bone health outside of pregnancy [96]. The optimal serum 25-OH-D in pregnancy has not yet been determined [95]. Those found to have insufficiency or deficiency in vitamin D in pregnancy should be recommended to take an additional supplementation of 1000–2000 IU daily of vitamin D. If possible, supplementation should be in the form of cholecalciferol (vitamin D3) rather than ergocalciferol (vitamin D2) due to the superior efficiency of cholecalciferol in raising serum vitamin D levels [97].

Iodine

Iodine is critical in the synthesis of both maternal and fetal thyroid hormones [98]. Adequate iodine intake is essential for normal fetal neurodevelopment. Maternal hypothyroidism is associated with adverse pregnancy outcomes including spontaneous abortion, preterm birth, preeclampsia, and stillbirth [98].

The RDA of iodine during pregnancy is 220 mcg daily and during lactation is 290 mcg daily [59]. Iodine can be obtained from food sources including seaweed, seafood, and eggs. Iodine in dairy and other animal products varies according to the type of feed the animals received. Iodine is an important micronutrient to consider in pregnancy because many prenatal multivitamins do not contain iodine and pregnant women are at risk of iodine deficiency. Traditionally, most people obtained adequate amounts through the consumption of iodized table salt and other food sources. However, with changes in food processing practices and the increasing popularity of non-iodized salt, there is a trend toward lower levels of iodine in the US population [99]. Iodine status is assessed through median urinary iodine concentration (mUIC) and in pregnancy an mUIC <150 mcg/L is associated with inadequate iodine intake. Among participants in NHANES 2011–2014, nonpregnant reproductive age women had an mUIC of 110 mcg/L whereas pregnant people participating in NHANES 2007-2014 had an mUIC of 144 mcg/L [100,101].

Vitamin toxicity

Although vitamins and minerals are important, consumption of high amounts of vitamins and minerals can be dangerous. Fortunately, most water-soluble vitamins are relatively safe during pregnancy; excess intake is readily excreted in the urine. High doses of vitamin C can lead to nephrolithiasis through acidification of the urine causing precipitation of cysteine, urate, or oxalate stones [102]. High doses of vitamin B6 have been associated development of peripheral neuropathy [103].

Of greater significance is the toxicity associated with excess intake of fat-soluble vitamins (vitamins A, D, E, K), which are stored in tissue rather than excreted when consumed at high doses. Vitamin A is consumed in two main forms, provitamin A carotenoids and preformed vitamin A. Provitamin A carotenoids includes beta-carotene and is mainly found in plant sources. Preformed vitamin A includes retinol and retinoic acid and is mainly found in animal sources such as liver, kidney, and egg yolk; it is also the form used in many supplements.

Preformed vitamin A is the more active form of vitamin A and is teratogenic to the fetus at doses >10 000 IU/day leading to spontaneous abortion and major congenital anomalies [104]. Most prenatal vitamins contain provitamin A carotenoids, the form of vitamin A that has not been found to be teratogenic [105].

Toxicity associated with excess mineral intake is primarily associated with adverse symptoms. Iron intake >200 mg/day is associated with gastrointestinal symptoms such as heartburn, nausea, abdominal pain, and constipation in a dose-dependent fashion (placebo 13%; 200 mg 25%; 400 mg 40%) [106]. Magnesium sulfate intake >3 g/day is associated with gastrointestinal symptoms and reduced iron absorption. Excessive iodine intake has been associated with fetal goiter and hypothyroidism [107]. Excessive selenium intake is associated with nausea, vomiting, fatigue, and nail changes. Zinc intake >150 mg/day has been associated reduced iron and copper absorption, as well as gastrointestinal symptoms [108].

Caffeine consumption in pregnancy

More than 82% of women report consuming caffeine [111]. During pregnancy, one study found 58% of people consume caffeine during early pregnancy (between 10 and 13 weeks), mostly from soda, coffee, and tea [112]. More women, 76%, report caffeine intake in the second trimester (between 16 and 22 weeks) [112].

It is recommended to limit caffeine consumption during pregnancy to <200–300 mg/day [59,113]. Caffeine in the diet most often comes from soda, coffee, and tea, which contain approximately 40, 96, and 48 mg of caffeine per eight ounces, respectively. At baseline, the mean caffeine intake in nonpregnant reproductive age women is <200 mg/day [111]. During pregnancy < 1% of people report consuming more than 200 mg/day [112].

The recommendation to limit caffeine consumption during pregnancy was developed due to the concern for potential increased risk of spontaneous abortion, preterm birth, and fetal growth restriction [113]. However, most studies have significant limitations with conflicting results [114–117]. Despite these limitations, intake of low to moderate amounts of caffeine (<200 mg/day) does not appear to increase risk of adverse pregnancy outcomes and may even provide beneficial cardiometabolic effects during pregnancy [112,113,118].

Seafood consumption in pregnancy

Seafood contains omega-3 polyunsaturated fatty acids, specifically eicosapentaenoic acid (EPA) and docosahexaenoic acid (DHA), that are important for fetal development and have anti-inflammatory properties [119]. Omega-3 fatty acid intake (both from supplements and food) during pregnancy is associated with a decreased risk of preterm birth at <37 weeks (OR 0.89, 95% CI 0.81–0.97) and <34 weeks (OR 0.58, 95% CI 0.44–0.77) [120]. Although EPA and DHA are important for fetal neurodevelopment, the meta-analysis did not find differences in cognition, IQ, vision, language, behavior, and other neurodevelopment and growth outcomes [120].

Although seafood consumption in pregnancy has health benefits, it is important to limit intake of methylmercury, which can accumulate in the tissue of fish, particularly larger fish such as shark, swordfish, and king mackerel [59,121]. Exposure to methylmercury can lead to adverse neurodevelopmental outcomes [121] (Figure 2.3). Although there is not enough evidence to routinely recommend omega-3 fatty acid supplementation, it is recommended that during pregnancy consumption of 8 to 12 ounces per week of a variety of seafood low in methylmercury is recommended [59].

Multifetal pregnancy

Multifetal pregnancies, 97% of which are twin pregnancies, are associated with increased maternal and fetal risks, including fetal growth restriction [122]. Although a

multifetal pregnancy would be expected to increase the nutritional demand for the mother, there is limited research to guide clinical recommendations. Unfortunately, confounders are more pronounced in multifetal pregnancies, and the nutritional component of adverse pregnancy outcomes is much harder to delineate. The analysis is complicated further by different fetal growth rates related to differences between monozygotic, dizygotic same-sex, and dizygotic mixed-sex twins. Recommendations for gestational weight gain during pregnancy for twin gestations is based on the interquartile range of weight gain in people who gave birth to twins without low birthweight (>2500 gm) [123]. It is recommended that those with normal weight (BMI 18.5–24.9 kg/m^2) gain 37–54 lb, overweight (BMI 25–29.9 kg/m^2) gain 31–50 lb, and those with obesity (BMI ≥ 30 kg/m^2) gain 25–42 lb [123]. Multifetal pregnancies may be at higher risk of micronutrient deficiencies give the increased demand and may require additional supplementation beyond routine prenatal vitamin [124,125].

Nutrition during lactation

A healthy dietary pattern should be continued after delivery, to minimize postpartum weight retention, for long-term maternal health, and for the health of the infant if

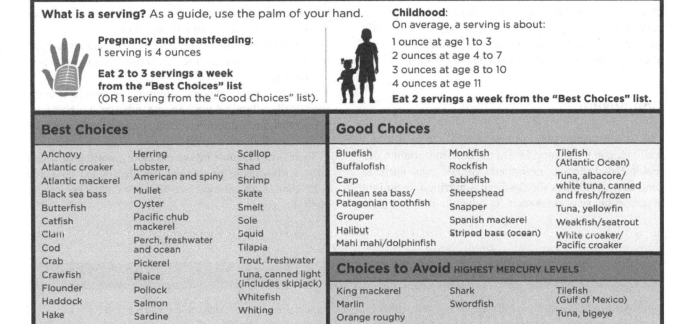

Figure 2.3 Guide for safe seafood consumption during pregnancy from the US Food and Drug Administration.

breastfeeding. Exclusive breastfeeding for the first 6 months of life, followed by continued breastfeeding and complementary foods through the first year of the infant's life, is recommended [126,127]. To meet the metabolic demands of milk production while allowing for loss of gestational weight gain, a normal weight person should increase their daily calorie intake by 330 calories in the first 6 months postpartum and 400 calories 7–12 months postpartum [59]. Macronutrients and micronutrients, including vitamins and minerals, are found in human milk in various concentrations throughout different stages of lactation and infant growth. Some micronutrient concentrations remain stable within human milk, despite maternal intake, instead using maternal stores. For other micronutrients, the concentrations fluctuate with dietary and supplement intake [128]. The RDA for vitamins A, E, and C as well as the B vitamins are increased for lactating people [59]. For this reason it is recommended that a multivitamin is continued through lactation to ensure adequate micronutrient intake. As discussed previously, those at nutritional risk of micronutrient deficiencies should be screened for micronutrient deficiencies and recommended supplementation as needed. The type of fat found in human milk reflects maternal dietary intake. It is recommended people consume 200–300 mg of omega-3 long-chain polyunsaturated fatty acids (DHA) to ensure the appropriate DHA concentrations in milk. This can be achieved by including one to two portions of fish in the diet weekly, continuing to avoid fish high in methylmercury [127]. There is no evidence that avoidance or early exposure to food antigens such as peanuts and milk affects incidence of atopic disease in the infant [129].

Conclusion

Diet and nutrition play an essential role in health and well-being in pregnancy. One of the most important modifiable risk factors is gestational weight gain. Early in pregnancy, clinicians should discuss nutrition, including a comprehensive assessment to identify those at risk.

Contrary to popular opinion, pregnancy is not a time to "eat for two" but rather a time to focus on eating "twice as healthy". General principles for nutrition in pregnancy include:
- Counseling on gestational weight gain goals should be provided early in pregnancy.
- Those of normal weight require an additional 340 kcal/day in the second trimester and 452 kcal/day in the third trimester. During lactation an additional 330 calories is recommended in the first 6 months postpartum and an additional 400 calories 7–12 months postpartum.
- A healthy dietary pattern in pregnancy can be simplified to as half of the food for each meal should come from vegetables and fruits, the other half from whole grains and healthy sources of protein.
- A daily prenatal multivitamin beginning 1 month prior to conception and continue through pregnancy and lactation is recommended.
- Those at nutritional risk, including those with inflammatory bowel disease or prior bariatric surgery, should be screened for micronutrient deficiencies and supplemented as needed.
- Those who follow a plant-based dietary pattern (vegetarian or vegan) should take a vitamin B_{12} supplement.
- Iron needs increase more than 30% in pregnancy and iron-deficiency anemia is common.
- Folic acid is important to reduce the risk of neural tube defects. A prenatal vitamin containing 400–800 mcg of folic acid is recommended 1 month prior to conception for those at low risk of a neural tube defect.
- In middle- and low-income countries, calcium supplementation may decrease the risk of preeclampsia and preterm birth.
- Excessive intake of some vitamins can lead to toxicity, specifically, vitamin A is a known teratogen at high doses.
- Caffeine consumption during pregnancy should be limited to <200–300 mg/day.
- To ensure adequate intake of healthy, polyunsaturated fatty acids during pregnancy, people should consume 8–12 ounces of seafood weekly from choices low in methylmercury.

CASE PRESENTATION

A 32-year-old G0 with type 2 diabetes and obesity (BMI 46) presents for preconception consultation. Her glycated hemoglobin (HbA1c) is 8.6%. She has had diabetes for 6 years and is taking metformin 500 mg twice a day. She works two jobs and doesn't have time to exercise. She is worried about her diabetes and how it may affect a future pregnancy.
You perform a 24-hour food recall:
Breakfast: Bacon, egg, and cheese biscuit sandwich

Lunch: Turkey sandwich, chips, apple
Dinner: Pizza, cookie
Beverages: Juice with breakfast, soda with dinner
- What do you think she can do to optimize her health prior to pregnancy?
  o Answer: Work to optimize her glycemic control, lose weight as able

- What advice would you give her?
  - Answer: Follow healthy dietary pattern, increase physical activity with goal of at least 150 minutes per week, begin taking a prenatal vitamin
- Why is preconception folic acid important? How much folic acid should she take?
  - Folic acid is important to reduce the risk of neural tube defects. A prenatal vitamin containing 400–800 mcg of folic acid is recommended 1 month prior to conception for those at low risk of a neural tube defect.

She presents 1 year later now 8 weeks pregnant. She has worked with her primary care physician to better control her diabetes and her HbA1c is now 6.4%. She reports she is taking a daily prenatal vitamin containing folic acid. She has lost some weight by adding more physical activity into her routine and currently has a BMI of 40. Although she is excited about the pregnancy, she is worried that her pregnancy weight gain will set back her weight loss progress.

- What are your recommendations for gestational weight gain?
  - Gestational weight gain goal is 11 to 20 lb (5–9.0 kg)
- How many extra calories does she need to support the pregnancy?
  - Those with obesity may not need any extra calories to support pregnancy. She should focus on consuming a variety of healthy foods.
- How will you counsel her about a healthy dietary pattern in pregnancy?
  - A healthy dietary pattern during pregnancy consists of a variety of vegetables including dark-green vegetables, red and orange vegetables, beans, peas, lentils, starchy vegetables, a variety of fruits, whole grains, dairy or fortified soy beverages, healthy sources of protein foods including nuts, seeds, beans, lentils, soy products, poultry, eggs, and meats. Less than 10% of calories should come from added sugar and less than 10% from saturated fat. Sodium in the diet should be limited to <2300 mg daily.

References

1. Bergner L, Susser MW. Low birth weight and prenatal nutrition: an interpretative review. Pediatrics. 1970;46(6):946–66.
2. Kyle UG, Pichard C. The Dutch Famine of 1944–1945: a pathophysiological model of long-term consequences of wasting disease. Curr Opin Clin Nutr Metab Care. 2006;9(4):388–94.
3. Stein Z. Famine and human development : the Dutch hunger winter of 1944–1945. New York: Oxford University Press; 1975.
4. Barker DJ, Osmond C, Golding J, Kuh D, Wadsworth ME. Growth in utero, blood pressure in childhood and adult life, and mortality from cardiovascular disease. BMJ. 1989;298(6673):564–7.
5. Frankel S, Elwood P, Sweetnam P, Yarnell J, Smith GD. Birthweight, body-mass index in middle age, and incident coronary heart disease. Lancet. 1996;348(9040):1478–80.
6. Rich-Edwards JW, Stampfer MJ, Manson JE, Rosner B, Hankinson SE, Colditz GA, et al. Birth weight and risk of cardiovascular disease in a cohort of women followed up since 1976. BMJ. 1997;315(7105):396–400.
7. Huxley RR, Shiell AW, Law CM. The role of size at birth and postnatal catch-up growth in determining systolic blood pressure: a systematic review of the literature. J Hypertens. 2000;18(7):815–31.
8. Law CM, Egger P, Dada O, Delgado H, Kylberg E, Lavin P, et al. Body size at birth and blood pressure among children in developing countries. Int J Epidemiol. 2001;30(1):52–7.
9. ACOG Committee Opinion No. 729 Summary: importance of social determinants of health and cultural awareness in the delivery of reproductive health care. Obstet Gynecol. 2018;131(1):198–9.
10. Guidelines (2013) for managing overweight and obesity in adults. Preface to the Expert Panel Report (comprehensive version which includes systematic evidence review, evidence statements, and recommendations). Obesity (Silver Spring). 2014;22 Suppl 2:S40.
11. Corrales P, Vidal-Puig A, Medina-Gomez G. Obesity and pregnancy, the perfect metabolic storm. Eur J Clin Nutr. 2021;75(12):1723–34.
12. Society for Maternal-Fetal Medicine. Martins JG, Biggio JR, Abuhamad A. Society for Maternal-Fetal Medicine Consult Series #52: Diagnosis and management of fetal growth restriction: (Replaces Clinical Guideline Number 3, April 2012). Am J Obstet Gynecol. 2020;223(4):B2–B17.
13. Hadlock FP, Deter RL, Harrist RB, Park SK. Estimating fetal age: computer-assisted analysis of multiple fetal growth parameters. Radiology. 1984;152(2):497–501.
14. Luke B. Nutritional influences on fetal growth. Clin Obstet Gynecol. 1994;37(3):538–49.
15. Ananth CV, Vintzileos AM, Shen-Schwarz S, Smulian JC, Lai YL. Standards of birth weight in twin gestations stratified by placental chorionicity. Obstet Gynecol. 1998;91(6):917–24.
16. Grantz KL, Grewal J, Albert PS, Wapner R, D'Alton ME, Sciscione A, et al. Dichorionic twin trajectories: the NICHD Fetal Growth Studies. Am J Obstet Gynecol. 2016;215(2):221 e1–e16.
17. Boulet SL, Alexander GR, Salihu HM, Pass M. Macrosomic births in the United States: determinants, outcomes, and proposed grades of risk. American journal of obstetrics and gynecology. 2003;188(5):1372–8.
18. Owen P, Donnet ML, Ogston SA, Christie AD, Howie PW, Patel NB. Standards for ultrasound fetal growth velocity. Br J Obstet Gynaecol. 1996;103(1):60–9.
19. Lubchenco LO. Assessment of gestational age and development of birth. Pediatr Clin North Am. 1970;17(1):125–45.
20. Bocca-Tjeertes I, Bos A, Kerstjens J, de Winter A, Reijneveld S. Symmetrical and asymmetrical growth restriction in preterm-born children. Pediatrics. 2014;133(3):e650–6.
21. David C, Gabrielli S, Pilu G, Bovicelli L. The head-to-abdomen circumference ratio: a reappraisal. Ultrasound Obstet Gynecol. 1995;5(4):256–9.

22. Durnin JV. Energy requirements of pregnancy: an integration of the longitudinal data from the five-country study. Lancet. 1987;2(8568):1131–3.
23. Institute of Medicine and National Research Council. Weight gain during pregnancy: reexamining the guidelines. Washington, DC, National Academies Press; 2009.
24. Bakketeig LS, Hoffman HJ, Harley EE. The tendency to repeat gestational age and birth weight in successive births. Am J Obstet Gynecol. 1979;135(8):1086–103.
25. Headen I, Cohen AK, Mujahid M, Abrams B. The accuracy of self-reported pregnancy-related weight: a systematic review. Obes Rev. 2017;18(3):350–69.
26. ACOG Practice Bulletin No 156: obesity in pregnancy. Obstet Gynecol. 2015;126(6):e112–e26.
27. Naeye RL. Weight gain and the outcome of pregnancy. Am J Obstet Gynecol. 1979;135(1):3–9.
28. Taffel SM. Maternal weight gain and the outcome of pregnancy. Vital Health Stat 21. 1986(44):1–25.
29. Institute of Medicine. Nutrition during Pregnancy. Washington, DC, National Academies Press; 1990.
30. Hales CM, Carroll MD, Fryar CD, Ogden CL. Prevalence of obesity and severe obesity among adults: United States, 2017–2018. NCHS Data Brief. 2020(360):1–8.
31. Faucher MA, Barger MK. Gestational weight gain in obese women by class of obesity and select maternal/newborn outcomes: a systematic review. Women Birth. 2015;28(3):e70–9.
32. Blomberg M. Maternal and neonatal outcomes among obese women with weight gain below the new Institute of Medicine recommendations. Obstet Gynecol. 2011;117(5):1065–70.
33. Bodnar LM, Siminerio LL, Himes KP, Hutcheon JA, Lash TL, Parisi SM, et al. Maternal obesity and gestational weight gain are risk factors for infant death. Obesity (Silver Spring). 2016;24(2):490–8.
34. Siega-Riz AM, Bodnar LM, Stotland NE, Stang J. The current understanding of gestational weight gain among women with obesity and the need for future research. NAM Perspect. 2020;2020.
35. Hutcheon JA, Bodnar LM, Joseph KS, Abrams B, Simhan HN, Platt RW. The bias in current measures of gestational weight gain. Paediatr Perinat Epidemiol. 2012;26(2):109–16.
36. Cnattingius S, Bergström R, Lipworth L, Kramer MS. Prepregnancy weight and the risk of adverse pregnancy outcomes. N Engl J Med. 1998;338(3):147–52.
37. Lashen H, Fear K, Sturdee DW. Obesity is associated with increased risk of first trimester and recurrent miscarriage: matched case-control study. Hum Reprod. 2004;19(7):1644–6.
38. ACOG Practice Bulletin No. 230: obesity in pregnancy. Obstet Gynecol. 2021;137(6):e128–e44.
39. Yao R, Ananth CV, Park BY, Pereira L, Plante LA. Obesity and the risk of stillbirth: a population-based cohort study. Am J Obstet Gynecol. 2014;210(5):457.e1–9.
40. Stothard KJ, Tennant PW, Bell R, Rankin J. Maternal overweight and obesity and the risk of congenital anomalies: a systematic review and meta-analysis. JAMA. 2009;301(6):636–50.
41. Goldstein RF, Abell SK, Ranasinha S, Misso M, Boyle JA, Black MH, et al. Association of gestational weight gain with maternal and infant outcomes: a systematic review and meta-analysis. JAMA. 2017;317(21):2207–25.
42. Michel S, Raab R, Drabsch T, Günther J, Stecher L, Hauner H. Do lifestyle interventions during pregnancy have the potential to reduce long-term postpartum weight retention? A systematic review and meta-analysis. Obes Rev. 2019;20(4):527–42.
43. Yee LM, Simon MA, Grobman WA, Rajan PV. Pregnancy as a "golden opportunity" for patient activation and engagement. Am J Obstet Gynecol. 2021;224(1):116–8.
44. Forbes LE, Graham JE, Berglund C, Bell RC. Dietary change during pregnancy and women's reasons for change. Nutrients. 2018;10(8).
45. Kimmel MC, Ferguson EH, Zerwas S, Bulik CM, Meltzer-Brody S. Obstetric and gynecologic problems associated with eating disorders. Int J Eat Disord. 2016;49(3):260–75.
46. Committee Opinion No. 711: opioid use and opioid use disorder in pregnancy. Obstet Gynecol. 2017;130(2):e81–e94.
47. Procter-Gray E, Olendzki B, Kane K, Churchill L, Hayes RB, Aguirre A, et al. Comparison of dietary quality assessment using food frequency questionnaire and 24-hour-recalls in older men and women. AIMS Public Health. 2017;4(4):326–46.
48. ACOG Committee Opinion no. 548: weight gain during pregnancy. Obstet Gynecol. 2013;121(1):210–2.
49. US Department of Agriculture. Definitions of food security. [Updated 2022 Oct 17]. Available from: https://www.ers.usda.gov/topics/food-nutrition-assistance/food-security-in-the-u-s/definitions-of-food-security/.
50. Coleman-Jensen A, Rabbitt MP, Gregory CA, Singh A. Household food security in the United States in 2019. Washington, DC: US Department of Agriculture, Economic Research Service; 2020.
51. Seligman HK, Laraia BA, Kushel MB. Food insecurity is associated with chronic disease among low-income NHANES participants. J Nutr. 2010;140(2):304–10.
52. Bruening M, Dinour LM, Chavez JBR. Food insecurity and emotional health in the USA: a systematic narrative review of longitudinal research. Public health nutrition. 2017;20(17):3200–8.
53. ACOG Committee Opinion No. 729: importance of social determinants of health and cultural awareness in the delivery of reproductive health care. Obstet Gynecol. 2018;131(1):e43–e8.
54. Hager ER, Quigg AM, Black MM, Coleman SM, Heeren T, Rose-Jacobs R, et al. Development and validity of a 2-item screen to identify families at risk for food insecurity. Pediatrics. 2010;126(1):e26–32.
55. Gundersen C, Engelhard EE, Crumbaugh AS, Seligman HK. Brief assessment of food insecurity accurately identifies high-risk US adults. Public Health Nutr. 2017;20(8):1367–71.
56. Dolin CD, Compher CC, Oh JK, Durnwald CP. Pregnant and hungry: addressing food insecurity in pregnant women during the COVID-19 pandemic in the United States. Am J Obstet Gynecol MFM. 2021;3(4):100378.
57. Berggren EK, O'Tierney-Ginn P, Lewis S, Presley L, De-Mouzon SH, Catalano PM. Variations in resting energy expenditure: impact on gestational weight gain. Am J Obstet Gynecol. 2017;217(4):445.e1–.e6.
58. Most J, Dervis S, Haman F, Adamo KB, Redman LM. Energy intake requirements in pregnancy. Nutrients. 2019;11(8).
59. US Department of Agriculture and US Department of Health and Human Services. Dietary guidelines for Americans, 2020-2025. 9th ed. December 2020. Available from: DietaryGuidelines.gov.
60. Most J, Amant MS, Hsia DS, Altazan AD, Thomas DM, Gilmore LA, et al. Evidence-based recommendations for energy intake in pregnant women with obesity. J Clin Invest. 2019;129(11):4682–90.

61. Tapsell LC, Neale EP, Satija A, Hu FB. Foods, nutrients, and dietary patterns: interconnections and implications for dietary guidelines. Adv Nutr. 2016;7(3):445–54.

62. Deshmukh-Taskar PR, Radcliffe JD, Liu Y, Nicklas TA. Do breakfast skipping and breakfast type affect energy intake, nutrient intake, nutrient adequacy, and diet quality in young adults? NHANES 1999-2002. J Am Coll Nutr. 2010;29(4):407–18.

63. Raghavan R, Dreibelbis C, Kingshipp BL, Wong YP, Abrams B, Gernand AD, et al. Dietary patterns before and during pregnancy and maternal outcomes: a systematic review. Am J Clin Nutr. 2019;109(Suppl 7):705s–28s.

64. Raghavan R, Dreibelbis C, Kingshipp BL, Wong YP, Abrams B, Gernand AD, et al. Dietary patterns before and during pregnancy and birth outcomes: a systematic review. Am J Clin Nutr. 2019;109(Suppl 7):729s–56s.

65. ACOG Committee Opinion No. 762: prepregnancy counseling. Obstet Gynecol. 2019;133(1):e78–e89.

66. Keats EC, Haider BA, Tam E, Bhutta ZA. Multiple-micronutrient supplementation for women during pregnancy. Cochrane Database Syst Rev. 2019;3(3):Cd004905.

67. Wolf HT, Hegaard HK, Huusom LD, Pinborg AB. Multivitamin use and adverse birth outcomes in high-income countries: a systematic review and meta-analysis. Am J Obstet Gynecol. 2017;217(4):404.e1–.e30.

68. Bailey RL, Pac SG, Fulgoni VL, 3rd, Reidy KC, Catalano PM. Estimation of total usual dietary intakes of pregnant women in the United States. JAMA Netw Open. 2019;2(6):e195967.

69. Herrmann W, Schorr H, Obeid R, Geisel J. Vitamin B-12 status, particularly holotranscobalamin II and methylmalonic acid concentrations, and hyperhomocysteinemia in vegetarians. Am J Clin Nutr. 2003;78(1):131–6.

70. Dolin CD, Chervenak J, Pivo S, Ude Welcome A, Kominiarek MA. Association between time interval from bariatric surgery to pregnancy and maternal weight outcomes. J Matern Fetal Neonatal Med. 2021;34(20):3285–91.

71. ACOG Practice Bulletin No. 233: anemia in pregnancy. Obstet Gynecol. 2021;138(2):e55–e64.

72. Recommendations to prevent and control iron deficiency in the United States. Centers for Disease Control and Prevention. MMWR Recomm Rep. 1998;47(Rr-3):1–29.

73. Zofkie AC, Garner WH, Schell RC, Ragsdale AS, McIntire DD, Roberts SW, et al. An evidence-based definition of anemia for singleton, uncomplicated pregnancies. PloS One. 2022;17(1):e0262436.

74. Mei Z, Cogswell ME, Looker AC, Pfeiffer CM, Cusick SE, Lacher DA, et al. Assessment of iron status in US pregnant women from the National Health and Nutrition Examination Survey (NHANES), 1999-2006. Am J Clin Nutr. 2011;93(6):1312–20.

75. Scholl TO. Maternal iron status: relation to fetal growth, length of gestation, and iron endowment of the neonate. Nutr Rev. 2011;69 Suppl 1(Suppl 1):S23–9.

76. Hamm RF, Wang EY, Levine LD, Speranza RJ, Srinivas SK. Implementation of a protocol for management of antepartum iron deficiency anemia: a prospective cohort study. Am J Obstet Gynecol MFM. 2021;4(2):100533.

77. Gropper SS. Advanced nutrition and human metabolism. 6th ed. Belmont: Wadsworth, Cengage Learning; 2013.

78. Food labeling: revision of the Nutrition and Supplement Facts Labels. Final rule. Fed Regist. 2016;81(103):33741–999.

79. Practice Bulletin No. 187: neural tube defects. Obstet Gynecol. 2017;130(6):e279–e90.

80. Prevention of neural tube defects: results of the Medical Research Council Vitamin Study. MRC Vitamin Study Research Group. Lancet. 1991;338(8760):131–7.

81. Dolin CD, Deierlein AL, Evans MI. Folic acid supplementation to prevent recurrent neural tube defects: 4 milligrams is too much. Fetal Diagn Ther. 2018;44(3):161–5.

82. Bibbins-Domingo K, Grossman DC, Curry SJ, Davidson KW, Epling JW, Jr., García FA, et al. Folic acid supplementation for the prevention of neural tube defects: US Preventive Services Task Force Recommendation Statement. JAMA. 2017;317(2):183–9.

83. Williams J, Mai CT, Mulinare J, Isenburg J, Flood TJ, Ethen M, et al. Updated estimates of neural tube defects prevented by mandatory folic acid fortification – United States, 1995–2011. MMWR Morb Mortal Wkly Rep. 2015;64(1):1–5.

84. Hacker AN, Fung EB, King JC. Role of calcium during pregnancy: maternal and fetal needs. Nutr Rev. 2012;70(7):397–409.

85. Zeni SN, Ortela Soler CR, Lazzari A, López L, Suarez M, Di Gregorio S, et al. Interrelationship between bone turnover markers and dietary calcium intake in pregnant women: a longitudinal study. Bone. 2003;33(4):606–13.

86. Cross NA, Hillman LS, Allen SH, Krause GF, Vieira NE. Calcium homeostasis and bone metabolism during pregnancy, lactation, and postweaning: a longitudinal study. Am J Clin Nutr. 1995;61(3):514–23.

87. Ritchie LD, Fung EB, Halloran BP, Turnlund JR, Van Loan MD, Cann CE, et al. A longitudinal study of calcium homeostasis during human pregnancy and lactation and after resumption of menses. Am J Clin Nutr. 1998;67(4):693–701.

88. Hofmeyr GJ, Lawrie TA, Atallah Á N, Torloni MR. Calcium supplementation during pregnancy for preventing hypertensive disorders and related problems. Cochrane Database Syst Rev. 2018;10(10):Cd001059.

89. Hofmeyr GJ, Betrán AP, Singata-Madliki M, Cormick G, Munjanja SP, Fawcus S, et al. Prepregnancy and early pregnancy calcium supplementation among women at high risk of pre-eclampsia: a multicentre, double-blind, randomised, placebo-controlled trial. Lancet. 2019;393(10169):330–9.

90. Bringhurst FR, Demay MB, Kronenberg HM. Bone and mineral metabolism in health and disease. In: Jameson JL, Fauci AS, Kasper DL, Hauser SL, Longo DL, Loscalzo J, editors. Harrison's principles of internal medicine. 20th ed. New York: McGraw-Hill Education; 2018.

91. Looker AC, Johnson CL, Lacher DA, Pfeiffer CM, Schleicher RL, Sempos CT. Vitamin D status: United States, 2001-2006. NCHS Data Brief. 2011(59):1–8.

92. Pawley N, Bishop NJ. Prenatal and infant predictors of bone health: the influence of vitamin D. Am J Clin Nutr. 2004;80(6 Suppl):1748s–51s.

93. Gale CR, Robinson SM, Harvey NC, Javaid MK, Jiang B, Martyn CN, et al. Maternal vitamin D status during pregnancy and child outcomes. Eur J Clin Nutr. 2008;62(1):68–77.

94. Palacios C, Kostiuk LK, Peña-Rosas JP. Vitamin D supplementation for women during pregnancy. Cochrane Database Syst Rev. 2019;7(7):Cd008873.

95. ACOG Committee Opinion No. 495: vitamin D: screening and supplementation during pregnancy. Obstet Gynecol. 2011;118(1):197–8.

96. Giustina A, Adler RA, Binkley N, Bollerslev J, Bouillon R, Dawson-Hughes B, et al. Consensus statement from 2(nd) International Conference on Controversies in Vitamin D. Rev Endocr Metab Disord. 2020;21(1):89–116.

97. Tripkovic L, Lambert H, Hart K, Smith CP, Bucca G, Penson S, et al. Comparison of vitamin D2 and vitamin D3 supplementation in raising serum 25-hydroxyvitamin D status: a systematic review and meta-analysis. Am J Clin Nutr. 2012;95(6):1357–64.

98. Thyroid disease in pregnancy: ACOG Practice Bulletin, Number 223. Obstet Gynecol. 2020;135(6):e261–e74.

99. Hollowell JG, Staehling NW, Hannon WH, Flanders DW, Gunter EW, Maberly GF, et al. Iodine nutrition in the United States. Trends and public health implications: iodine excretion data from National Health and Nutrition Examination Surveys I and III (1971-1974 and 1988-1994). J Clin Endocrinol Metab. 1998;83(10):3401–8.

100. Herrick KA, Perrine CG, Aoki Y, Caldwell KL. Iodine status and consumption of key iodine sources in the U.S. population with special attention to reproductive age women. Nutrients. 2018;10(7).

101. Perrine CG, Herrick KA, Gupta PM, Caldwell KL. Iodine status of pregnant women and women of reproductive age in the United States. Thyroid. 2019;29(1):153–4.

102. Ferraro PM, Curhan GC, Gambaro G, Taylor EN. Total, dietary, and supplemental vitamin C intake and risk of incident kidney stones. Am J Kidney Dis. 2016;67(3):400–7.

103. van Hunsel F, van de Koppel S, van Puijenbroek E, Kant A. Vitamin B(6) in health supplements and neuropathy: case series assessment of spontaneously reported cases. Drug Saf. 2018;41(9):859–69.

104. Rothman KJ, Moore LL, Singer MR, Nguyen US, Mannino S, Milunsky A. Teratogenicity of high vitamin A intake. N Engl J Med. 1995;333(21):1369–73.

105. Mathews-Roth MM. Lack of genotoxicity with beta-carotene. Toxicol Lett. 1988;41(3):185–91.

106. Hallberg L, Ryttinger L, Sölvell L. Side-effects of oral iron therapy. A double-blind study of different iron compounds in tablet form. Acta Med Scand Suppl. 1966;459:3–10.

107. Connelly KJ, Boston BA, Pearce EN, Sesser D, Snyder D, Braverman LE, et al. Congenital hypothyroidism caused by excess prenatal maternal iodine ingestion. J Pediatr. 2012;161(4):760–2.

108. Fiske DN, McCoy HE, 3rd, Kitchens CS. Zinc-induced sideroblastic anemia: report of a case, review of the literature, and description of the hematologic syndrome. Am J Hematol. 1994;46(2):147–50.

109. Nehlig A, Daval JL, Debry G. Caffeine and the central nervous system: mechanisms of action, biochemical, metabolic and psychostimulant effects. Brain Res Brain Res Rev. 1992;17(2):139–70.

110. Ikeda GJ, Sapienza PP, McGinnis ML, Bragg LE, Walsh JJ, Collins TF. Blood levels of caffeine and results of fetal examination after oral administration of caffeine to pregnant rats. J Appl Toxicol. 1982;2(6):307–14.

111. Fulgoni VL, 3rd, Keast DR, Lieberman HR. Trends in intake and sources of caffeine in the diets of US adults: 2001-2010. Am J Clin Nutr. 2015;101(5):1081–7.

112. Hinkle SN, Gleason JL, Yisahak SF, Zhao SK, Mumford SL, Sundaram R, et al. Assessment of caffeine consumption and maternal cardiometabolic pregnancy complications. JAMA Netw Open. 2021;4(11):e2133401.

113. ACOG Committee Opinion No. 462: moderate caffeine consumption during pregnancy. Obstet Gynecol. 2010;116(2 Pt 1):467–8.

114. Savitz DA, Chan RL, Herring AH, Howards PP, Hartmann KE. Caffeine and miscarriage risk. Epidemiology. 2008; 19(1):55–62.

115. Weng X, Odouli R, Li DK. Maternal caffeine consumption during pregnancy and the risk of miscarriage: a prospective cohort study. Am J Obstet Gynecol. 2008;198(3):279.e1–8.

116. Gleason JL, Tekola-Ayele F, Sundaram R, Hinkle SN, Vafai Y, Buck Louis GM, et al. Association between maternal caffeine consumption and metabolism and neonatal anthropometry: a secondary analysis of the NICHD fetal growth studies-singletons. JAMA Netw Open. 2021;4(3):e213238.

117. Bech BH, Obel C, Henriksen TB, Olsen J. Effect of reducing caffeine intake on birth weight and length of gestation: randomised controlled trial. BMJ. 2007;334(7590):409.

118. Browne ML. Maternal exposure to caffeine and risk of congenital anomalies: a systematic review. Epidemiology. 2006;17(3):324–31.

119. James MJ, Gibson RA, Cleland LG. Dietary polyunsaturated fatty acids and inflammatory mediator production. Am J Clin Nutr. 2000;71(1 Suppl):343s–8s.

120. Middleton P, Gomersall JC, Gould JF, Shepherd E, Olsen SF, Makrides M. Omega-3 fatty acid addition during pregnancy. Cochrane Database Syst Rev. 2018;11(11):Cd003402.

121. Lando AM, Fein SB, Choinière CJ. Awareness of methylmercury in fish and fish consumption among pregnant and postpartum women and women of childbearing age in the United States. Environ Res. 2012;116:85–92.

122. Practice Bulletin No. 169: multifetal gestations: twin, triplet, and higher-order multifetal pregnancies. Obstet Gynecol. 2016;128(4):e131–46.

123. Institute of Medicine. Weight gain during pregnancy: reexamining the guidelines. Rasmussen KM, Yaktine AL, editors. Washington, DC: National Academies Press; 2009.

124. Zgliczynska M, Kosinska-Kaczynska K. Micronutrients in multiple pregnancies-the knowns and unknowns: a systematic review. Nutrients. 2021;13(2).

125. Goodnight W, Newman R. Optimal nutrition for improved twin pregnancy outcome. Obstet Gynecol. 2009;114(5): 1121–34.

126. ACOG Committee Opinion No. 756: optimizing support for breastfeeding as part of obstetric practice. Obstet Gynecol. 2018;132(4):e187–e96.

127. Breastfeeding and the use of human milk. Pediatrics. 2012;129(3):e827–41.

128. Dror DK, Allen LH. Overview of nutrients in human milk. Adv Nutr. 2018;9(Suppl 1):278s–94s.

129. Muraro A, Halken S, Arshad SH, Beyer K, Dubois AE, Du Toit G, et al. EAACI food allergy and anaphylaxis guidelines. Primary prevention of food allergy. Allergy. 2014;69(5):590–601.

Chapter 3
Alcohol and Substance Use Disorder

Anthony M. Kendle and Sarah G. Običan
Department of Obstetrics and Gynecology, University of South Florida, Tampa, FL, USA

Introduction

The implications for substance use and substance use disorder in pregnancy are significant. These conditions not only pose complicated barriers to accessing comprehensive and nondiscriminatory health care, but they contribute to the rising maternal mortality in the United States. Review of death certificate data in the United States from 2010 to 2019 found that drug use accounted for 11.4% of pregnancy-associated deaths–deaths that occurs from any cause during pregnancy or within 12 months after delivery [1]. Unlike death from other common causes of pregnancy-related morbidity (i.e. hemorrhage, hypertension, infection), mortality rates from drug overdose are rapidly increasing. From 2017 to 2020, drug overdose deaths rates among pregnant and postpartum people increased from 6.56 to 11.85 per 100 000, representing an 81% increase over the 4-year period [2]. According to the 2022 mortality and morbidity weekly report, almost 14% of pregnant patients drinking currently and 5% reported binge drinking in the last 30 days [3].

When pregnant people with alcohol use or substance use disorder present for prenatal care, there is opportunity to promote positive change both for the pregnancy and long-term maternal outcomes. There are several clinical and psychosocial nuances to providing prenatal care to patients with substance use disorder, and patients receive the greatest benefit from integrated or co-located care models that incorporate specialties such as obstetrics, maternal–fetal medicine, addiction medicine, psychiatry, behavioral health, and social work. Unfortunately, optimizing clinical care is further challenged by policies toward pregnant people that prioritize criminalization and stigmatization of health behavior rather than achievement of holistic well-being. Available evidence has demonstrated that punitive drug policies toward pregnancy promote avoidance of recommended healthcare services and social support systems while perpetuating negative social determinants of health such as loss of finances, housing, and employment. Despite

expansion of pregnancy-specific drug and alcohol policies in the United States during the past several decades, the result has been an increase in preterm birth, low birth weight, and neonatal abstinence syndrome without any appreciable decrease in alcohol use during pregnancy and an increase in other substance use disorders [4,5].

While the body of literature involving pregnant people with substance use disorder is growing, contemporary data with novel approaches should be incorporated into evidence-based approaches. Maternal outcome data are often based on large epidemiologic studies that lack granularity. Studies reporting neonatal outcomes are often small case series or retrospective studies. These reports are limited by the frequent use of multiple substances, predominant experience with first-trimester exposure only, animal studies that may not reliably predict the human response, retrospective and uncontrolled methodology, patient recall often later during gestation, and selective acceptance by editors of only reports with positive findings. Table 3.1 summarizes fetal, neonatal, and obstetric complications associated with various exposures. In general, separating confounders that are intimately linked to substance use disorder (such as social determinants of health, mental health disorders, and polysubstance use) is an additional research priority that has limited interpretation of previously cited maternal–infant dyad outcomes.

In this chapter, we review general approaches for screening, identification, and management of various substance use disorders during pregnancy including alcohol, opioids, cannabis, stimulants, and benzodiazepines.

Screening and testing for substance use disorder

The American College of Obstetrics and Gynecology (ACOG) recommend that all pregnant people be screened for alcohol and substance use disorder at their initial prenatal visit [6]. History of past and present substance use should address the frequency, amount, and time during

---

Queenan's Management of High-Risk Pregnancy: An Evidence-Based Approach, Seventh Edition. Edited by Catherine Y. Spong and Charles J. Lockwood.

Table 3.1 Specific substances and their associations with fetal, neonatal, and obstetric complications

Complications	Associated fetal/neonatal effects	Associated obstetric complications
Alcohol	Microcephaly; growth deficiency; CNS dysfunction including mental retardation and behavioral abnormalities; craniofacial abnormalities (i.e. short palpebral fissures, hypoplastic philtrum, flattened maxilla); behavioral abnormalities	Spontaneous abortion, possible other poor pregnancy outcomes*
Cigarettes	No anomalies; reduced birthweight (200 g lighter); facial clefting; attention deficit hyperactivity disorder	Spontaneous abortion Preterm birth Placenta previa Placental abruption Reduced risk of preeclampsia
Cannabis Marijuana THC Hashish	No anomalies; corresponding decrease in birth weight; subtle behavioral alterations (reduced executive functioning)	Reduction of gestation 0.8 wk
CNS sedatives Barbiturates Diazepam Flurazepam Meprobamate Methaqualone	No pattern of anomalies; depression of interactive behavior; impaired "executive function" behavioral	
CNS stimulants Antiobesity drugs Cocaine Methylphenidate Methamphetamines Phenmetrazine	No clear association with malformations; excess activity in utero; congenital anomalies (heart, biliary atresia); depression of interactive behavior; urinary tract defects; symmetric growth restriction; placental abruption; cerebral infarction; brain lesions; fetal death; neonatal necrotizing enterocolitis	Spontaneous abortion Premature birth Placental abruption
Hallucinogens LSD Ketamine Mescaline Dimethyltryptamine Phencyclidine (PCP)	No anomalies; chromosomal breakage (LSD); dysmorphic face; behavioral problems	Spontaneous abortions
Opiates/codeine/heroin Hydromorphone Hydrocodone Meperidine Methadone Morphine Opium Pentazocine (and tripelennamine)	No anomalies; intrauterine withdrawal with increased fetal activity; depressed breathing movements; fetal growth restriction; perinatal mortality; neonatal withdrawal	Preterm delivery Preterm rupture of the membranes Meconium-stained amniotic fluid
Inhalants Gasoline Glue Hairspray Paint	Similar to the fetal alcohol and fetal hydantoin syndromes; growth restriction; increased risk of leukemia in children; impaired heme synthesis	Preterm labor

CNS, central nervous system; THC, tetrahydrocannabinol.
*Fetal growth restriction, stillbirth.
Adapted from [35].

gestation of a specific substance in a nonjudgmental way. Despite these recommendations, this remains an area for improvement. For example, a recent survey by the Centers for Disease Control and Prevention (CDC) found that approximately 80% of pregnant people were asked about alcohol use at their last health care visit. Of those who screened positive, only 28.8% were counseled about risks to their health and 16.1% were advised to reduce intake [7]. Furthermore, another survey of 800 ACOG fellows found that 28% did not feel prepared to screen their patients, 58% did not use a validated screening tool, and 22% of providers did not recommend abstinence [8]. There are several validated screening tools to assess patients at-risk for alcohol and other substance use disorder (Box 3.1). Patients

Box 3.1 Validated screening tools to assess alcohol and substance use

TACE[a]

T Tolerance: How many drinks does it take to make you feel high?
>2 drinks = 2 points
A Annoyed: Have people annoyed you by criticizing your drinking?
Yes = 1 point

C Cut down: Have you ever felt you ought to cut down on your drinking?
Yes = 1 point
E Eye opener: Have you ever had a drink first thing in the morning to steady your nerves or get rid of a hangover?
Yes = 1 point

Scoring: ≥ 2 points, positive screening for at-risk drinking

Alcohol Screening Questionnaire (USAUDIT)[b]

Points	0	1	2	3	4	5	6	Score
How often do you have a drink containing alcohol?	Never	Less than monthly	Monthly	Weekly	2–3x per week	4–6x per week	daily	
How many drinks containing alcohol do you have on a given day you are drinking?	1 drink	2 drinks	3 drinks	4 drinks	5–6 drinks	7–9 drinks	10 or more drinks	
How often do you have 4 or more drinks on one occasion?	Never	Less than monthly	Monthly	Weekly	2–3 times a week	4–6 times a week	Daily	

Scoring: **Pregnant:** any use | **Nonpregnant:** ≥7 pts

Alcohol quantity and drinking questions[c]

1. In a typical week, how many drinks do you have that contain alcohol?
   Positive for at risk drinking >7 drinks.
2. In the past 90 days, how many times have you had more than 3 drinks on any one occasion?
   Positive for at risk drinking if more than one time.

4 Ps Plus Questionnaire[d]

Parents: Did any of your parents have a problem with alcohol or other drug use?
Partner: Does your partner have a problem with alcohol or drug use?
Past: In the past, have you had difficulties in your life because of alcohol or other drugs, including prescription medications?
Present: In the past month have you drunk any alcohol or used other drugs?
Scoring: Answering "yes" to any of these questions should prompt further questioning.

[a]Sokol RJ, Martier SS, Ager JW. The T-ACE questions: practical prenatal detection of risk-drinking. Am J Obstet Gynecol. 1989;160:863–8.
[b]Adapted from Centers for Disease Control and Prevention. Planning and implementing screening and brief intervention for risky alcohol use: a step-by-step guide for primary care practices. Atlanta, GA: CDC, National Center on Birth Defects and Developmental Disabilities; 2014.
[c]National Institute on Alcohol Abuse and Alcoholism. Helping patients who drink too much: a clinician's guide. Updated 2005 edition. Bethesda (MD): NIAAA; 2005.
[d]Chasnoff IJ, Wells AM, McGourty RF, Bailey LK. Validation of the 4P's Plus screen for substance use in pregnancy validation of the 4P's Plus. J Perinatol. 2007 Dec;27(12):744–8. doi: 10.1038/sj.jp.7211823. Epub 2007 Sep 6. PMID: 17805340.

may present to prenatal care or labor and delivery with obstetric and medical conditions that are associated with substance use disorder; however, many of these conditions lack specificity (Table 3.2).

There are two important considerations prior to screening patients. First, physicians should be aware of state-mandated reporting requirements when substance use during pregnancy is identified. Even when reporting is mandatory, the physician–patient relationship should uphold autonomy, confidentiality, and informed consent within the limits of legal requirements [6]. Second, physicians should be prepared to obtain consent to offer treatment and offer additional resources and interventions for

their patients. The Screening, Brief Intervention and Referral to Treatment (SBIRT) is an evidence-based, comprehensive, and integrated tool to guide management of patients at risk for or with active substance use disorder [9]. SBIRT can be performed in any health care setting with the goal of linking patients to medical and other community-based resources to address substance use behavior.

• **Screening**: Using validated screening tools (as described), providers can rapidly assess the presence and severity of substance use.

• **Brief Intervention**: In patients identified as moderate risk for substance use problems, providers engage in a directed, motivational, and nonjudgmental conversation

Table 3.2 Examples of patient presentation associated with underlying alcohol or substance use disorders in pregnancy

Obstetric	Medical
Abruptio placentae	Anemia
Birth outside hospital	Arrhythmias
Congenital anomalies	Bacterial endocarditis
Fetal alcohol spectrum disorder	Cellulitis or phlebitis
Fetal distress	Cerebrovascular accident
Fetal growth restriction	Drug overdose or endocarditis
Neonatal abstinence syndrome	Hepatitis B and C
Prenatal care–none, sporadic, or late prenatal care	HIV seropositivity
	Infective endocarditis
Preterm labor and delivery	Lymphedema
Preterm rupture of the membranes	Myocardial ischemia or infarction
Spontaneous abortion	Pancreatitis
Stillbirth	Poor dental hygiene
Sudden infant death syndrome	Poor nutritional status
	Sepsis
	Sexually transmitted infections
	Tuberculosis

Note that these presentations are not exclusive to alcohol and substance use disorder in pregnancy. Although these should remain on the differential, alternative etiologies should also be worked up.

with the patient regarding substance use behavior. The goal of brief intervention is to increase patient insight into substance use behavior and assess readiness for change.

• **Referral to Treatment:** Providers facilitate seamless transition to specialty services to continue to address substance use behavior, which may include addiction medicine, mental health providers, and recovery programs. Reluctant patients should be continually engaged at future visits, and community resources should be leveraged to overcome burdens that may prevent patients from receiving treatment (e.g. transportation).

It is important to distinguish screening for substance use disorder from drug testing. As with mandatory reporting guidelines, some states have outlined requirements for perinatal drug testing, and providers should be familiar with these policies [6]. However, there are commonly no policies to guide perinatal drug testing. In pregnancy, two techniques for urine toxicology are available: screening immunoassays–quick, inexpensive, with high false-positive rates–and confirmatory chromatography-mass spectrometry testing–more specific tests that should be used to confirm all screening immunoassays. There are several flaws with urine drug testing. Principally, the inherent nature of urine toxicology detects drug metabolites in a biologic compartment at a single time point, and as such, a positive drug test does not indicate the dose, frequency, temporality, or habit of use [10]. As such, a positive urine toxicology does not indicate active drug use or abuse nor does a negative

urine toxicology preclude these. Owing to this limitation, urine drug toxicology is not part of the diagnosis of substance use disorder. A recent study highlights the limitations and potential consequences of perinatal drug testing. Among a cohort of 33 maternal-infant dyads who had neuraxial analgesia with fentanyl during labor, 62% of mothers tested positive for fentanyl by immunoassay and 90.5% were positive by mass spectrometry after delivery. Of neonatal urine tested by mass spectrometry, 76.9% were positive for fentanyl despite 100% intrapartum exposure [11].

A second fallacy to consider is that a positive urine drug toxicology can have serious implications for families. A positive urine drug screen is considered child abuse in 23 of the 50 United States and can result in referral to child protective services, criminal action, and loss of parental rights regardless of substance use history or frequency [12]. The linking of a diagnostic medical test to legal ramifications is troubling. In an already vulnerable patient population, this type of response to an aspect of their health care dismantles patient–provider trust and perpetuates avoidance of additional health care services [5]. Furthermore, these policies exacerbate disparities in health care and social justice. Despite substance use in pregnancy occurring among all sociodemographic groups, Black and Hispanic women were 4.26 to 5.75 times more likely to undergo urine drug testing compared to their White counterparts for an indication other than self-reported substance use [13].

There is certainly a role for urine toxicology during pregnancy, as it can be an important component of measuring adherence and determining need for additional support in patients actively receiving treatment for substance use disorders. However, as with any diagnostic test ordered for a patient, the ordering provider should have a clear plan for addressing this test result and the results of said test should be important to guide additional *medical* management of the patient.

Alcohol

Maternal effects

Societally, the use of alcohol is considered an accepted and enjoyable form of celebration and human interconnectedness. However, at-risk alcohol use has been associated with numerous adverse medical health outcomes including increased mortality and cancer risk (breast, liver, rectum, mouth) [14,15]. Additionally, alcohol use is associated with an increased risk for unplanned pregnancies, sexually transmitted diseases, physical injury, and seizures. At-risk alcohol use also increases psychosocial problems including depression, suicide, domestic violence, sexual assault, loss of support relationships and child custody [16].

Effects on the fetus

Virtually all chemicals cross the placenta easily because of their lipid solubility, low molecular weight, lower pKa, and lack of protein binding. Unlike prescription or non-prescription drugs, alcohol and substances of abuse are more likely to be intentionally or inadvertently taken at toxic doses. Consuming many drinks per occasion (i.e. binge drinking, > five drinks) may be more harmful to the developing fetus than the same amount spread over several days because of higher peak blood alcohol content [17]. Moreover, the common practice of using multiple substances (including smoking) make it difficult to ascribe specific fetal effects and perinatal outcomes to any one certain substance. Nonjudgmental and accurate evaluation of exposure, including dosage and timing are encouraged but may be inaccurate due to stigma.

Teratogenic effects on the fetus depend on the developmental stage. Through a simplified model, different gestational ages increase the risk of varied poor pregnancy outcomes: from fertilization to implantation (miscarriage), from second through eighth weeks (fetal anomalies), and from ninth week to birth (shortened gestation, restricted growth, neurobehavior impairment).

Pregnancy outcomes: Miscarriage, growth, preterm birth, and stillbirth

Data on pregnancy outcomes are still conflicting, but overall, the literature supports that alcohol use in pregnancy increases the risk of poor pregnancy outcomes. Miscarriages occur at twice the background rate in women exposed to >1 oz of alcohol, two times per week [18,19]. Drinking more than five alcoholic beverages per week in the first trimester has also been associated with spontaneous abortion [20]. Another study noted second-trimester alcohol exposure carries an increased risk of still birth to 8.83/1000 births (from 1.37/1000 nondrinking pregnant population) [21]. Still, the literature is controversial as another prospective study noted that low/moderate alcohol intake (defined as ≤ 12 g of alcohol) was not associated with spontaneous abortion or stillbirth [22]. Fetal and postnatal growth can be affected by alcohol consumption. One study found that consuming > three alcoholic beverages/week was associated with both fetal growth restriction and low birth weight. The magnitude of this effect on growth was increased when patients used cigarettes as well [21–23].

Fetal anomalies

In 1968, Paul Lemoine first described fetal effect of prenatal alcohol exposure. Established in 1973 by Drs. Ken Jones and David Smith, the term fetal alcohol syndrome (FAS) identified a common pattern of malformations, growth deficits and dysmorphic features proposing a diagnostic criterion for the disorder. FAS encompasses the criteria for the dysmorphic features and FAS and falls under the larger group of individuals with fetal alcohol spectrum disorder (FASD), which includes those who may have cognitive and behavioral differences without the physically recognizable features of FAS. In the United States it is estimated that as many as 1 in 20 school-aged children are affected by fetal alcohol spectrum disorder [24].

The dysmorphic features of FAS were initially thought to occur in >30% of exposed fetuses but in somewhat more recent literature, the prevalence is thought to be around 4% among heavy daily users [25,26]. However, with trained professionals, the dysmorphic features are considered specific enough for establishing a diagnosis in patients (Table 3.3) though the assessment for these dysmorphic features of FAS requires a careful physical examination by trained physicians to differentiate from genetic conditions or other exposures. Earlier literature has implicated alcohol exposure to be associated with fetal congenital heart defects, but a more recent National Birth Defects Prevention Study did not show an increased risk of congenital heart disease [27]. Exposure to alcohol has since been removed from indications for fetal echocardiography. Prenatal anatomic screening by ultrasound is still indicated though apart from fetal growth, many of the FAS dysmorphic features may be difficult to identify on prenatal ultrasound [28].

Cognitive and behavioral outcomes

The long-term impact of prenatal alcohol and other substances on infant and child development presents other challenges. Although animal studies have shown that alcohol and drugs reduce the density of cortical neurons and change dendritic connections, the significance to human development is unclear [29]. Studies of behaviors in animals have shown long-term changes, and abnormal neurobehavioral findings in the newborn raise concerns about how those conditions may affect subsequent development. It has been suggested that consumption of less than one alcoholic drink per day early in the pregnancy does not impair cognitive abilities when measured in offspring at age 14 years [30]. Another study evaluating

Table 3.3 Potential phenotype of fetal alcohol syndrome

- Abnormalities in prenatal and postnatal growth
- Facial features: short palpebral fissures, smooth/longer philtrum, thin vermillion
- Midface hypoplasia
- hypertelorism
- Anteverted nose
- Ptosis
- Epicanthal folds
- Abnormally shaped ears
- Digit abnormalities including camptodactyly (limited extension) and clinodactyly
- Abnormal hand creases

self-report of alcohol intake of two beverages per day was associated with a seven-point decrease in IQ of the offspring [31]. Another consideration about effects on the human fetus is the number of drinks consumed per occasion by the mother, not just the number of drinks per day or week. Maternal binge drinking may lead to the eventual childhood finding of more social disinhibition and defects in numerical and language skills [32]. Binge drinking was also associated with a 1–3-month lag in reading and arithmetic levels in first grade [33].

Prenatal treatment

Prenatal pharmacotherapy can be an option for patients during pregnancy and outweighs the risks of treatment. If pharmacotherapy is initiated, it should be co-managed with an addiction specialist. Fetal monitoring should be done during the treatment. In cases of acute intoxication, it should be noted that after last intake, withdrawal may occur 6–24 hours and delirium tremens 72–96 hours after. A benzodiazepine taper may be used in the transition. Although there is little published evidence on treatment in pregnancy and with variable outcomes, disulfiram, acamprosate, and naltrexone have been successfully used in treatment of alcohol use disorder in pregnancy [34].

Opioids

Opioids are any natural, synthetic, or semisynthetic compound that interact with the three primary opioid receptors. The term opiate specifically refers to naturally occurring compounds derived from plant material such as the opium poppy, such as morphine, codeine, and thebaine, and therefore "opioid" is a more appropriate term when referring to this drug class. Opioids are prescribed in clinical settings for treatment of acute and chronic pain mediated through binding of mu opioid receptors located throughout the nervous system. Commonly prescribed opioids include oxycodone, hydromorphone, hydrocodone, meperidine, codeine, morphine, and fentanyl. In addition to reduction of pain signaling, these compounds also produce a rewarding or euphoric effect. This property increases the propensity for nonmedical and illicit use of opioid agonists.

Opioid-related overdose deaths began to rise in the United States in the 1990s. Although the epidemic was first driven by prescription opioids, heroin-related deaths began to rise in 2010. In 2013, government agencies began to implicate synthetic opioids such as fentanyl as the cause of overdose deaths at an alarming rate. Since 2016, synthetic opioids continue to be the leading cause of overdose death [36]. The national trends of opioid use have followed similar patterns in the sphere of pregnancy. Between 2000 and 2007, 22.8% of pregnant patients insured by Medicaid filled a prescription for opioids [37].

Moreover, in labor more than 75% of pregnant people receive either parenteral or neuraxial opioids for pain management. Furthermore, one third of births in the United States occur by cesarean delivery, necessitating a substantial amount of postpartum opioid prescriptions. In this sense, opioid exposure is nearly ubiquitous in pregnancy.

Maternal effects

Continued use of opioids leads to tolerance (the need for higher subsequent doses to achieve the desired effect), physical dependence, and ultimately disordered use [38]. Opioid use disorder is a diagnosis based on specific criteria outlined in the *Diagnostic and Statistical Manual of Mental Disorders, Fifth Edition*. Withdrawal from opioids is characterized by a constellation of signs and symptoms including tachycardia, diaphoresis, restlessness and irritation, pupillary constriction, joint pain, rhinorrhea, vomiting, diarrhea, and yawning. Although opioid withdrawal is nonfatal, efforts to avoid withdrawal may result in the patient engaging in high-risk or criminal behavior.

Injection of opioids is associated with an increased morbidity before and during pregnancy, including injection site cellulitis and abscess formation, sepsis, bacterial endocarditis, septic emboli, venous thromboembolism, osteomyelitis, septic arthritis, and an increased risk of blood borne pathogens such as HIV, hepatitis B, and hepatitis C [39]. In 2019, intravenous drug use accounted for 16% of new HIV diagnoses among women [40].

Opioid overdose classically presents as a combination of altered mental status, respiratory depression, and mydriasis. It is associated with high rates of maternal mortality. From 2017 to 2019, mental health conditions—including overdose and substance use disorder—accounted for 22.7% of deaths during pregnancy or within the first 12 months postpartum [41]. Increasing trends of pregnancy-related overdose mortality is largely attributed to fentanyl and other synthetic opioids with most of these deaths occurring in the late postpartum period [2]. Prompt recognition and treatment of overdose are paramount. However, even for patients with opioid use disorder who are stable on treatment, the risk for relapse and overdose is highest during months 7–12 postpartum [42]. As such, continued engagement with health care and support services are a vital component in reducing maternal mortality.

Effects on the fetus

Reports on teratogenicity from opioid exposure are limited by co-exposure to multiple substances, predominant experience with first-trimester exposure only, retrospective and uncontrolled methodology, patient recall often later during gestation, and publication bias. Pregnancy data are available for many of the commonly prescribed opioids. In the Norwegian Mother and Child Cohort

Study of 2666 pregnancies with codeine exposure, there was no difference in congenital malformations compared to control (adjusted odds ratio [aOR] 0.9, 95% confidence interval [CI] 0.8–1.1) [43]. Other smaller retrospective studies of first-trimester codeine use found inconsistent associations with respiratory tract malformations, pyloric stenosis, inguinal hernia, cardiac defects, cleft lip, and neural tube defects [44–47]. Cohort studies and case series of hydrocodone and oxycodone exposure did not demonstrate an increased risk of congenital anomalies [44].

However, public health advisories on pregnancy have cited increased risk of neural tube defects, congenital heart defects, and gastroschisis associated with opioid pain medication. These associations stem primarily from maternal interviews from the National Birth Defects Prevention Study (1997–2005) [48]. Although they found modestly increased odds of specific birth defects, the study was significantly limited by recall bias (up to 3 years after exposure) and did not consider dose, duration, or frequency of the opioid exposure.

Additional population-based studies have cited a 30% increase in preterm birth and a 60% increase in stillbirth to pregnancies exposed to opioids [49]. In sensitivity analyses, the preterm birth rate was driven by first- and second-trimester exposure to codeine, morphine, and oxycodone. The stillbirth rate was driven by first-trimester codeine exposure, but the low incidence of this outcome limits the precision of this outcome. Notably, many of these studies excluded patients with opioid use disorder. Exposure data of heroin and fentanyl have never described an associated birth defect syndrome. Heroin, however, has been associated with preterm delivery, fetal growth restriction, meconium-stained amniotic fluid, and perinatal death [50–53].

Concern neonatal effects from opioid exposure during pregnancy has not only shaped the treatment of maternal opioid use disorder, but it has also generated significant social stigma for this patient population. Neonatal opioid withdrawal syndrome (NOWS) is subtype of neonatal abstinence syndrome that is characterized by irritability, hypertonia, tremors, poor feeding, and gastrointestinal dysfunction. There is no relationship between the severity of NOWS and the dose of maternal medication for opioid use disorder (MOUD) prior to delivery [54], thus maternal dose of MOUD should never be discontinued or weaned prior to delivery. In fact, methadone regimens emphasizing frequent dose adjustments and multiple daily doses were associated with reduced need for neonatal abstinence syndrome treatment [55].

The mainstays of treatment for NOWS include pharmacologic treatment with opioids and nonpharmacologic interventions. Modern approaches to NOWS treatment that emphasize rooming in, caregiver presence, skin-to-skin contact, optimal feeding, and frequent consolation have dramatically reduced infant length of stay after birth and need for opioids to control symptoms [56,57]. Initial reports of long-term childhood outcomes described increased developmental delay, behavioral concerns, and lower IQ. These early studies, however, failed to control for social determinants of health and did not account for parental mood disorders, polysubstance use, trauma history, or parenting practices. Contemporary literature has not found any negative neurodevelopmental outcomes in the first 3 years of life among children born with NOWS [58,59]. The MOTHER study–a randomized trial comparing buprenorphine- and methadone-exposed infants–found that buprenorphine treatment during pregnancy was associated with reduced need for treatment of neonatal abstinence syndrome as well as shorter neonatal lengths of stay [54]. Recently, a large population-based cohort study comparing methadone and buprenorphine for treatment of OUD during pregnancy confirmed previous findings of less severe neonatal abstinence syndrome in the buprenorphine group as well as lower rates of preterm birth and small for gestational age infants without any difference in adverse maternal outcome [60].

Patients with opioid use disorder should be encouraged to breastfeed if they have been stabilized on MOUD. Methadone and buprenorphine are transferred to human milk in low concentrations [61–63]. Breastfeeding has been shown to reduce the severity of NOWS, reduce need for neonatal opioid treatment, and decrease hospital length of stay without any evidence of neonatal morbidity [64,65]. The American Academy of Pediatrics recommends breastfeeding in mothers who are taking methadone or buprenorphine [66]. Patients who are taking buprenorphine-naloxone combination product should not be discouraged from breastfeeding as the infant oral bioavailability from naloxone in breastmilk is negligible. Patients with opioid use disorder should be discouraged from breastfeeding if they continue to have substance use or experience a return to use postpartum, or if they have an additional contraindication to breastfeeding such as HIV [67].

Prenatal treatment

Many people with OUD receive no or limited prenatal care. Barriers to care in this population include fear of legal consequences from illicit drug use, financial instability, challenges with transportation or childcare, fear of losing custody of other children, general stigma and label avoidance, or prior negative experiences with healthcare systems [68]. In addition to routine prenatal care, the following are some unique considerations for patients with opioid use disorder:

• Screen for other substances and exposures using validated tools (as previously)
• Check state Prescription Drug Monitoring Program (PDMP) databases to review prescribing providers,

especially for patients taking opioids for management of chronic pain
• Prescription and education should be provided for naloxone
• Laboratory testing for sexually transmitted infections including chlamydia, gonorrhea, syphilis, hepatitis B, hepatitis C, and HIV
• Metabolic panel to assess liver function and preexisting renal disease [69]
• Conder echocardiogram and cardiology consultation in patients with history of bacterial endocarditis or prior valvular heart disease
• Assessment of fetal growth in the third trimester between 30 and 32 weeks gestation
• Antenatal testing starting at 32 weeks gestation is indicated only in the setting of polysubstance use (including nicotine) [69].

The approach to management of patients with OUD is determined through shared decision making. For motivated patients, transitioning to MOUD with long-acting opioid therapy is gold standard treatment in pregnancy and is associated with low rates of return to substance use and overdose.

Methadone

Methadone is a long-acting opioid receptor agonist with a half-life ranging from 10.4 to 51.2 hours [70]. It has high oral bioavailability; however, blood concentrations and elimination are highly variable among different individuals receiving the same dose [71]. Methadone is primarily metabolized by the liver by CYP3A4, and thus, its metabolism can be affected when co-administered with other inducers or inhibitors of the cytochrome P450 [72]. Specific drug-drug interactions that deserve attention include but are not limited to benzodiazepines, ethanol, antidepressants (specifically amitriptyline and fluoxetine), and several antiretroviral drugs. It is therefore important for providers to carefully record all drugs and substances a patient is taking before prescribing methadone [73]. In 2006, the Food and Drug Administration placed a black boxed warning on methadone due to its association with cardiac arrhythmia. Systematic review of available literature determined this association to be based on data from case reports of torsades de pointes, largely in patients using high doses of methadone or those with existing QT interval prolongation [74]. The American Heart Association recommends obtaining a baseline ECG for all patients initiating methadone upon presentation to a treatment program [75].

Methadone induction is usually initiated 18 to 24 hours after the patient's last opioid use or when the patient has clinical features of moderate withdrawal. Starting doses of methadone range from 10 to 30 mg. Additional doses of 5–10 mg can be given every 4 to 6 hours during induction to address persistent symptoms of withdrawal, usually targeting a total daily dose of 80–120 mg (although higher doses may be appropriate). Caution should be employed when increasing methadone doses given the risk of respiratory depression and overdose. Patients should be informed prior to methadone induction that stabilization can take several days to weeks. With few exceptions, methadone for treatment of OUD must be dispensed (usually on a daily basis) at a federally certified facility, which can be a barrier for some patients.

The physiologic and pharmacokinetic changes that occur during pregnancy influence methadone maintenance therapy. Dose increases are frequently required as pregnancy progresses, particularly in the third trimester. Additionally, because of more rapid clearance of methadone during pregnancy, some patients may benefit from split dosing: dividing the total daily dose into twice daily dosing to avoid withdrawal symptoms and cravings occurring later in the day [76]. It is imperative that patients do not attempt to decrease or taper their dose of methadone prior to delivery as this is associated with increased drug craving and risk of return to substance use without any change in incidence or severity of NOWS [9].

Buprenorphine

Buprenorphine is a partial opioid receptor agonist. This unique property imparts a less potent opioid response compared to full agonists (the ceiling effect) and thus a more favorable safety profile [77]. Buprenorphine has low oral bioavailability owing to extensive first-pass metabolism by CYP3A4 [78] and is administered in a sublingual formulation. Unlike methadone, buprenorphine can be prescribed. This medication is available in the United States as a mono-product tablet (Subutex) or as a sublingual film of buprenorphine-naloxone 4 mg/1 mg (Suboxone). The inclusion of naloxone in the combination product is meant to discourage diversion through intravenous administration. Prior clinical practice avoided the administration of buprenorphine-naloxone in pregnancy because of concern for potential adverse fetal effects from naloxone. Meta-analysis of 1875 maternal–infant dyads concluded that pregnant people treated with buprenorphine-naloxone do not have significantly different outcomes compared to those treated with other forms of MOUD [79].

Buprenorphine's partial agonism requires special consideration during medication induction because of its potential to rapidly precipitate severe withdrawal in patients with recent opioid exposure. As such, initial doses of buprenorphine should not be started until the patient has moderate symptoms of withdrawal or more than 24 hours has elapsed since last opioid use. This is particularly challenging in patients abusing long-acting opioids or fentanyl and may require longer periods of abstinence and lower starting doses. Buprenorphine is typically started at doses of 4 mg and increased every

2–4 hours by 4 mg increments to address withdrawal symptoms. The average total daily dose of buprenorphine for OUD in pregnancy is 16 mg/day. Twice daily dosing is often used in pregnancy. Similar to methadone, it is common that a patient requires dose increases of buprenorphine after stabilization as pregnancy progresses [80].

Naltrexone

Naltrexone is an opioid receptor antagonist and is currently available as an oral and an injectable extended-release formulation (Vivitrol). There are several potential benefits to naltrexone therapy owing to its complete blockade of the opioid receptor: it does not produce euphoric effects, there is no risk for abuse or development of tolerance, and it is not associated with neonatal abstinence syndrome [81]. However, transitioning to naltrexone requires 7–10 days of complete abstinence from opioids, during which time the risk for return to opioid use, shown to be as high as 72% in nonpregnant populations [82]. Additionally, the rapid plasma clearance of the drug that occurs during pregnancy increases the risk of relapse if doses are missed. In a recent, large cohort of 121 pregnant patients receiving naltrexone therapy, 81 continued treatment to delivery, and no patients experienced relapse during the 7-day abstinence period [83]. Still, there is currently insufficient evidence to recommend its use during pregnancy [84]. Patients have previously been managed successfully on these medications may continue treatment during pregnancy. Investigations of maternal and fetal outcomes are ongoing.

Medically supervised withdrawal

Patients who are motivated to discontinue opioid use and either decline or do not have access to MOUD programs may be candidates for supervised withdrawal. Patients should be thoroughly counseled about the benefits of MOUD, specifically discussing that medically supervised withdrawal is associated with higher rates of maternal relapse, overdose, participation in risky behavior, and worse engagement in prenatal care without any benefit to the neonate [67].

Harm reduction strategies

Pregnancy is an opportunity for many people to engage with the healthcare system and receive treatment for OUD. Some pregnant people, however, are unwilling or unable to participate in pharmacotherapy or behavioral therapy for treatment of OUD. In these cases, it is important that the provider remains supportive and redirect care to emphasize harm reduction strategies [85].

All patients with OUD should have a prescription and receive education for naloxone, regardless of whether they are on MOUD treatment. Family members and loved ones should also be encouraged to carry naloxone with them. Naloxone is an opioid agonist that is available as an injection or as a packaged nasal spray. It is indicated for the rapid reversal of opioid overdose. A population-based study of opioid-overdose emergency department visits demonstrated that pregnant women were less likely to receive naloxone than pregnant women (aOR 0.16 [0.12–0.23]) [86].

Needle exchange programs or syringe services programs are an effective, community-based service for harm reduction. These programs are associated with significant reduction in HIV and hepatis C transmission [87,88]. In addition to providing blood-borne pathogen screening, these programs often offer connection to MOUD services, resulting in higher uptake of participation in drug treatment programs [89].

Intrapartum and postpartum care

The labor and delivery process can be especially distressing for people with OUD. Patients may be afraid about inadequate pain control, may worry about facing judgment and stigma from health care providers, and face uncertainty about newborn withdrawal. For patients who are stabilized on MOUD it is important to continue their maintenance medication during the entire hospitalization. Although many patients with MOUD are motivated to avoid parenteral opioids during labor, these are not contraindicated. However, mixed agonist-antagonists such as nalbuphine and butorphanol should not be administered during labor as these medications can precipitate acute withdrawal for those taking MOUD. Epidural is the preferred method for optimizing pain control for vaginal birth. If cesarean is necessary, neuraxial analgesia with epidural or spinal is also preferred. In cases where neuraxial analgesia is contraindicated, a transversus abdominus plane block should be considered after the surgery to provide long-lasting pain relief. After delivery, pain control should be multimodal with emphasis on nonopioid analgesics such as acetaminophen and nonsteroidal anti-inflammatory drugs (NSAIDs). Consultation with anesthesia or pain management specialists may be beneficial to minimize postpartum opioid use.

Pain medication requirements after cesarean delivery is variable. Prior studies have estimated that post-cesarean opioid requirements for people on MOUD were 60–80% higher compared to those without opioid dependent [90,91]. In a secondary analysis of the MOTHER trial, however, patients on MOUD did not have significantly different NSAID analgesic requirements after vaginal or cesarean delivery, and the use of opioid agonist analgesia after cesarean was higher in the comparison group compared to patients maintained on MOUD [92]. As such, both in-hospital postpartum pain management and decision to prescribe opioid analgesia on discharge should be individualized, balancing goals of adequate postoperative pain control and risk of return to opioid use.

In addition to routine postpartum care, patients with OUD should maintain close postpartum follow up with addiction medicine providers and begin to transfer care to a primary care physician for continued health surveillance.

Cannabis

Cannabis is harvested from the hemp plant and is consumed either through ingestion, vaping, or smoking. Delta-9-tetrahydrocannabinol (THC) binds to cannabinoid receptors in the central and peripheral nervous system to produce effects of euphoria and relaxation. It is a commonly used substance in pregnancy. Prevalence of use during pregnancy ranges from 2% to 28%, with increasing prevalence especially among patients <25 years old [93], in part owing to an increasing number of states legalizing medical and recreational use in the United States. Many pregnant people self-medicate with cannabis to treat common ailments of pregnancy, especially nausea, vomiting, and pain [94]. Additionally, TCH-containing products are often used to address mood disorders. Pregnant people with depression are over three times more likely to use cannabis compared to their counterparts without a diagnosis [95].

There is no screening tool for cannabis use in pregnancy, but providers should ask about its use at the first prenatal visit. Cannabinoid metabolites are detected in urine anywhere from 1 to 30 days after use [96], and thus a positive urine drug screen for cannabis does not reliably indicate active use or frequency of use.

Immediate maternal effects of cannabis use include altered cognition and motor function. There are no data, however, specifically addressing how the use of cannabis in pregnancy interacts with existing mood disorder and postpartum depression. Although rare, cannabinoid hyperemesis syndrome has been described in the literature and may overlap with traditional nausea and vomiting of pregnancy [97]. Improvement of symptoms with hot baths or showers is a hallmark feature of this condition. Treatment in pregnancy remains supportive, with symptoms typically resolving within 48 hours of cannabis discontinuation.

Although cannabinoids cross the placenta, to date there is no literature to suggest a birth defect syndrome related to cannabis exposure [98]. Cannabis exposure has been associated with birth outcomes of low birth weight, preterm birth, and stillbirth in systematic review and meta-analysis with conflicting results. These associations may be more representative for patients with "heavy use," but are further limited by observational study designs and confounding by co-exposure to tobacco [99,100].

There are no pharmacologic interventions to treat cannabis use or cannabis use disorder in pregnancy. Patients should receive counseling about potential adverse health outcomes of continued cannabis use during pregnancy in addition to motivational interviewing encouraging discontinuation of cannabis. Alternative first-line treatments for symptoms of nausea and vomiting of pregnancy, mood disorders, and/or pain should be discussed with patients who are self-treating with cannabis during pregnancy. Breastfeeding should be discouraged in patients who continue to use cannabis postpartum, although there are insufficient data from infants exposed to cannabis through breastmilk [101].

Stimulants

The drug class of stimulants includes cocaine and amphetamines. Nationwide, stimulants represent the second most used and abused substance; stimulant use in the pregnant population is increasing, mirroring trends in the general population [102]. These drugs exert their effect in the central nervous system by increasing synaptic concentrations of dopamine by blocking reuptake. Methamphetamine further exerts its effects by stimulating additional release of neurotransmitters. Stimulant use is increasingly common, and many pregnant people may use these drugs to lose weight, to regulate schedules for shift work, or to treat symptoms of attention deficit disorder. In addition to the rapid onset of euphoric effects and increased wakefulness, these drugs increase sympathetic tone and results in widespread vasoconstriction. Metabolites of methamphetamine and cocaine are detectable in maternal urine for 48 hours and for 2–4 days after use, respectively [96].

Maternal effects of both cocaine and amphetamines in pregnancy include increased risk of severe hypertension, myocardial infarction, and transmission of blood borne pathogens [102]. Cocaine is additionally associated with cases of maternal renal failure, hepatic rupture, and stroke. Methamphetamine is comparatively more cardiotoxic, able to produce a methamphetamine-associated cardiomyopathy through direct and indirect myocardial damage [103]. Pregnant people with history of stimulant use should be carefully evaluated for existing cardiovascular conditions. It is important to distinguish side effects from stimulant use from other obstetric complications such as preeclampsia and peripartum cardiomyopathy. Furthermore, in patients presenting with hypertension suspected to be secondary from cocaine use, beta blockers such as labetalol must be avoided so as not to precipitate an unopposed alpha-adrenergic response [104].

As with other substances, the teratogenic and neonatal effects of stimulant use during pregnancy are limited to observational data and often confounded by other substance co-exposures and social determinants of health. There is insufficient evidence to clearly associate stimulant use with a defined birth defect syndrome.

An increased incidence of genitourinary defects, intestinal atresia, and limb defects have been reported with cocaine exposure [105]. Methamphetamine exposure is not consistently linked to specific birth defects aside from cleft palate [106]. However, the neurotoxic effect of methamphetamine may extend to fetal brain development and affect long-term neurodevelopment [107]. Stimulant use disorder during pregnancy has been associated with fetal growth restriction, small for gestational age, preterm birth, and stillbirth [108–111]. In a population-based study comparing pregnancy hospitalizations to patients with cocaine vs. methamphetamine use, cocaine use was associated with higher prevalence of neonatal morbidity, including preterm delivery, chorioamnionitis, and poor fetal growth, whereas methamphetamine was associated with greater maternal hypertensive morbidity [112]. Breastfeeding is contraindicated in patients with active stimulant use in the postpartum period [113].

There is no pharmacologic treatment for stimulant use disorder in pregnancy. Psychosocial interventions are the mainstay of treatment, including SBIRT, intensive residential treatment programs, and behavioral therapy [114]. Contingency management–providing incentives to patients who demonstrate abstinence or participation in clinical treatment–has proven an effective strategy to reduce stimulant use [115].

Vaping (E-cigarettes)

Tobacco products are known to be harmful to pregnant patients by increasing poor pregnancy outcomes such as preterm birth, miscarriage, stillbirth, and sudden infant death [116]. Although part of a far less regulated industry than tobacco and despite containing a multitude of chemicals, vaping is often marketed as a safer alternative for pregnant patients. There is a rise in vaping in the younger population potentially of childbearing age. Pregnant patients who desire to quit smoking have fewer available interventions and reported using vaping to help with smoking cessation [117].

Vaping products have been available for over 10 years. The chemicals such as propylene glycol, nicotine, vegetable glycerin and flavorings (but also acrolein, diacetyl, heavy metals, cadmium, benzene) are heated, created into an aerosol and delivered to a person via inhalation [116]. When compared to the pregnancy and smoking literature, there is a paucity of maternal and fetal outcomes data with vaping exposure. Furthermore, the available literature is difficult to separate from those also exposed to cigarette smoking. The prevalence of vaping has been difficult to establish but the range has been between 1.2% and 7% [118,119]. Although vaping may increase the risk of small for gestational age, one study from maternity hospitals in Ireland found that the birthweight of babies did not differ between mothers who vaped in the third trimester from those who did not smoke or vape. However, those pregnant patients who vaped had babies with significantly higher birthweights than mothers who smoked tobacco [120]. The literature is still unclear if vaping decreases the relapse to smoking and if there are any worsening fetal or maternal outcomes. ACOG and the CDC recommend against vaping in pregnancy [121].

Benzodiazepines

In clinical practice, benzodiazepines are commonly prescribed as short-term treatment for anxiety, panic attacks, seizures, and insomnia. These medications bind to the $GABA_A$ receptor in the central nervous system and enhance the inhibitory effect of the receptor when bound by the GABA neurotransmitter. Benzodiazepine dependence develops rapidly. In one report, half of patients developed dependence after 1 month of use [122]. Withdrawal symptoms from benzodiazepines include flu-like symptoms, anxiety, panic, agitation, and sleep disruption: because many of these symptoms include indications for which patients started taking benzodiazepines in the first place, withdrawal reinforces patients' dependence [123]. Abrupt discontinuation of benzodiazepines can result in seizures and severe, potentially life-threatening withdrawal. As such, benzodiazepines should be tapered over several weeks to months and should be guided by a mental health provider or provider with experience tapering benzodiazepines [124]. In pregnancy, providers must also recognize the potential adverse outcomes that associated with uncontrolled anxiety or sleep disturbance, and as such, offering alternative pharmacotherapy and behavioral therapies to address these patient conditions is an important component of management.

Available evidence does not suggest teratogenic effects of benzodiazepines, although pregnancy is lacking for many of the derivatives used today. Although animal studies and early observational studies of diazepam exposure raised concern for increased association with facial clefts, a 2011 systematic review did not substantiate this association. Observational studies of alprazolam exposure are mixed. A study of 444 exposed infants found a twofold increased odds for cardiac defects; however, there was inadequate adjustment for confounders and other exposures [125]. There are even fewer human data regarding lorazepam exposure. Continued exposure to benzodiazepines throughout pregnancy is associated with neonatal abstinence syndrome, previously termed "floppy infant syndrome" [126]. Neonatal abstinence syndrome resulting from benzodiazepine exposure is generally well tolerated and does not require neonatal pharmacotherapy. However, fetal co-exposure of benzodiazepines and opioids results in a more severe and protracted form of NOWS [127].[7] In patients who continue to use benzodiazepines postpartum, breastfeeding can be safely considered, although patients should monitor infants for excessive drowsiness [128].

Screening for benzodiazepine use should occur during pregnancy and providers should follow SBIRT framework. Benzodiazepines are present in urine toxicology up to 3 days after use for short-acting medications (e.g. lorazepam, alprazolam) and up to 30 days for long-acting medications (e.g. diazepam) [96]. There are no evidence-based pharmacotherapies for treatment of benzodiazepine use disorder in pregnancy.

CASE PRESENTATION

A 32-year-old G1P0 at 24 weeks 0 days gestation was brought to the obstetric triage unit from jail after developing fever and chills. She denies chest pain, but she endorses increased shortness of breath. She is febrile with a temperature of 102.0 °F. The patient relates that she has been incarcerated for the past 2 weeks after failing to comply with a court order for involuntary substance abuse treatment that had been filed by a family member. Prior to incarceration, she admits to injecting fentanyl daily and intermittently snorting cocaine. She is currently enrolled in a drug treatment program through the jail and has been stabilized on buprenorphine 8 mg twice daily. She denies any symptoms of withdrawal or cravings.

She is tachycardic to 132 beats per minute and has a blood pressure of 100/72 mmHg. On physical exam, she is alert and oriented but appears slightly diaphoretic. Chest auscultation demonstrates normal breath sounds. A diastolic heart murmur is appreciated over the left sternal border. Her abdominal exam is unremarkable. Initial laboratory evaluation is notable for a white blood cell count of 19 000/L, platelet count of 96 000/mcL, alanine transaminase 120 U/L, and aspartate transaminase 75 U/L. Her hepatitis C antibody is positive and viral load is elevated. An echocardiogram is obtained demonstrating a 2.3 cm vegetation on the pulmonary valve with moderate to severe pulmonic valve regurgitation. The patient is admitted to the antepartum unit for treatment of infective endocarditis. She is started on intravenous (IV) vancomycin. Blood cultures later return with growth of methicillin-resistant staphylococcus aureus.

Although the patient's condition improves with several doses of IV antibiotics, she is concerned that she is missing her mandated drug treatment program through jail. She is also not able to contact family members to let them know she is hospitalized. The patient tells you that she desperately wants to complete her program so that she does not have to deliver her baby "in jail." She is connected to community resources and a Plan of Safe Care is developed. After evaluation by cardiology and cardiothoracic surgery determines no cardiac interventions are necessary at this time, the patient completes several weeks of IV antibiotics and is discharged back to jail. She later has a vaginal delivery of a 37-week male infant. A Child Protective Services case is opened after birth. The infant experiences minimal symptoms of neonatal opioid withdrawal syndrome and is discharged in the custody of maternal grandmother on day of life 5. The patient enrolls in an intensive inpatient treatment program postpartum and is working toward reunification.

References

1. Margerison CE, Roberts MH, Gemmill A, Goldman-Mellor S. Pregnancy-associated deaths due to drugs, suicide, and homicide in the United States, 2010–2019. Obstet Gynecol. 2022;139(2):172–80.

2. Bruzelius E, Martins SS. US trends in drug overdose mortality among pregnant and postpartum persons, 2017–2020. JAMA. 2022;328(21):2159–61.

3. Gosdin LK DN, Kim SY, Dang EP, Denny CH. Alcohol consumption and binge drinking during pregnancy among adults aged 18-49 Years–United States, 2018–2020. MMWR Morb Mortal Wkly Rep. 2022(71):10–13.

4. Roberts SCM, Thompson TA, Taylor KJ. Dismantling the legacy of failed policy approaches to pregnant people's use of alcohol and drugs. Int Rev Psychiatry. 2021;33(6):502–13.

5. Faherty LJ, Kranz AM, Russell-Fritch J, Patrick SW, Cantor J, Stein BD. Association of punitive and reporting state policies related to substance use in pregnancy with rates of neonatal abstinence syndrome. JAMA Netw Open. 2019;2(11):e1914078.

6. Committee opinion no. 633: alcohol abuse and other substance use disorders: ethical issues in obstetric and gynecologic practice. Obstet Gynecol. 2015;125(6):1529–37.

7. Luong J, Board A, Gosdin L, Dunkley J, Thierry JM, Pitasi M, et al. Alcohol use, screening, and brief intervention among pregnant persons - 24 US jurisdictions, 2017 and 2019. MMWR Morb Mortal Wkly Rep. 2023;72(3):55–62.

8. Anderson BL, Dang EP, Floyd RL, Sokol R, Mahoney J, Schulkin J. Knowledge, opinions, and practice patterns of obstetrician-gynecologists regarding their patients' use of alcohol. J Addict Med. 2010;4(2):114–21.

9. Substance Abuse and Mental Health Services Administration. Clinical guidance for treating pregnant and parenting women with opioid use disorder and their infants. Rockville, MD: SAMHSA; 2018.

10. Terplan M. Test or talk: empiric bias and epistemic injustice. Obstet Gynecol. 2022;140(2):150–2.

11. Siegel MR, Mahowald GK, Uljon SN, James K, Leffert L, Sullivan MW, et al. Fentanyl in the labor epidural impacts the results of intrapartum and postpartum maternal and neonatal toxicology tests. Am J Obstet Gynecol. 2022 Nov 23:S0002-9378(22)02185–8.

12. Kurtz T, Smid MC. Challenges in perinatal drug testing. Obstet Gynecol. 2022;140(2):163–6.

13. Perlman NC, Cantonwine DE, Smith NA. Racial differences in indications for obstetrical toxicology testing and relationship of indications to test results. Am J Obstet Gynecol MFM. 2022;4(1):100453.

14. Alcohol-attributable deaths and years of potential life lost–United States, 2001. MMWR Morb Mortal Wkly Rep. 2004;53(37):866–70.

15. Hamajima N, Hirose K, Tajima K, Rohan T, Calle EE, Heath CW Jr, et al. Alcohol, tobacco and breast cancer–collaborative reanalysis of individual data from 53 epidemiological studies, including 58 515 women with breast cancer and 95 067 women without the disease. Br J Cancer. 2002;87(11):1234–45.

16. Committee opinion no. 496: at-risk drinking and alcohol dependence: obstetric and gynecologic implications. Obstet Gynecol. 2011;118(2 Pt 1):383–8.

17. Bailey BN, Delaney-Black V, Covington CY, Ager J, Janisse J, Hannigan JH, et al. Prenatal exposure to binge drinking and cognitive and behavioral outcomes at age 7 years. Am J Obstet Gynecol. 2004;191(3):1037–43.

18. Kline J, Shrout P, Stein Z, Susser M, Warburton D. Drinking during pregnancy and spontaneous abortion. Lancet. 1980;2(8187):176–80.

19. Windham GC, Fenster L, Swan SH. Moderate maternal and paternal alcohol consumption and the risk of spontaneous abortion. Epidemiology. 1992;3(4):364–70.

20. Kesmodel U, Wisborg K, Olsen SF, Henriksen TB, Secher NJ. Moderate alcohol intake in pregnancy and the risk of spontaneous abortion. Alcohol Alcohol. 2002;37(1):87–92.

21. Kesmodel U, Wisborg K, Olsen SF, Henriksen TB, Secher NJ. Moderate alcohol intake during pregnancy and the risk of stillbirth and death in the first year of life. Am J Epidemiol. 2002;155(4):305–12.

22. Gaskins AJ, Rich-Edwards JW, Williams PL, Toth TL, Missmer SA, Chavarro JE. Prepregnancy low to moderate alcohol intake is not associated with risk of spontaneous abortion or stillbirth. J Nutr. 2015;146(4):799–805.

23. Windham GC, Fenster L, Hopkins B, Swan SH. The association of moderate maternal and paternal alcohol consumption with birthweight and gestational age. Epidemiology. 1995;6(6):591–7.

24. May PA, Chambers CD, Kalberg WO, et al. Prevalence of fetal alcohol spectrum disorders in 4 US communities. JAMA. 2018;319(5):474–82.

25. Jones KL, Smith DW, Streissguth AP, Myrianthopoulos NC. Outcome in offspring of chronic alcoholic women. Lancet. 1974;1(7866):1076–8.

26. Jensen TK, Hjollund NH, Henriksen TB, et al. Does moderate alcohol consumption affect fertility? Follow up study among couples planning first pregnancy. BMJ. 1998;317(7157):505–10.

27. Zhu Y, Romitti PA, Caspers Conway KM, Shen DH, Sun L, Browne ML, et al. Maternal periconceptional alcohol consumption and congenital heart defects. Birth Defects Res A Clin Mol Teratol. 2015;103(7):617–29.

28. AIUM practice parameter for the performance of fetal echocardiography. J Ultrasound Med. 2020;39(1):E5–e16.

29. Sampson PD, Streissguth AP, Bookstein FL, et al. Incidence of fetal alcohol syndrome and prevalence of alcohol-related neurodevelopmental disorder. Teratology. 1997;56(5):317–26.

30. O'Callaghan FV, O'Callaghan M, Najman JM, Williams GM, Bor W. Prenatal alcohol exposure and attention, learning and intellectual ability at 14 years: a prospective longitudinal study. Early Hum Dev. 2007;83(2):115–123.

31. Streissguth AP, Barr HM, Sampson PD. Moderate prenatal alcohol exposure: effects on child IQ and learning problems at age 7 1/2 years. Alcohol Clin Exp Res. 1990;14(5):662–9.

32. Lui S, Terplan M, Smith EJ. Psychosocial interventions for women enrolled in alcohol treatment during pregnancy. Cochrane Database Syst Rev. 2008;(3):Cd006753.

33. Streissguth AP, Barr HM, Olson HC, Sampson PD, Bookstein FL, Burgess DM. Drinking during pregnancy decreases word attack and arithmetic scores on standardized tests: adolescent data from a population-based prospective study. Alcohol Clin Exp Res. 1994;18(2):248–54.

34. Kelty E, Terplan M, Greenland M, Preen D. Pharmacotherapies for the treatment of alcohol use disorders during pregnancy: time to reconsider? Drugs. 2021;81(7):739–48.

35. REPROTOX. The Reproduction Toxicology Center. 2023 [cited 2023 Mar 31]. Available from: https://reprotox.org.

36. Ahmad FB CJ, Rossen LM, Sutton P. Provisional drug overdose death counts. Hyattsville, MD: National Center for Health Statistics; 2023.

37. Desai RJ, Hernandez-Diaz S, Bateman BT, Huybrechts KF. Increase in prescription opioid use during pregnancy among Medicaid-enrolled women. Obstet Gynecol. 2014;123(5):997–1002.

38. Kreek MJ, LaForge KS, Butelman E. Pharmacotherapy of addictions. Nat Rev Drug Discov. 2002;1(9):710–26.

39. Shorter D, Kosten TR. The pharmacology of opioids. In: Miller SC, Fiellin DA, Rosenthal RN, Saitz R, editors. The ASAM principles of addiction medicine. 6th ed. Philadelphia: Wolters Kluwer; 2019. p.136–49.

40. Centers for Disease Control and Prevention. HIV surveillance report, 2019. Vol. 32. 2021 [cited 2023 Mar 31]. Available from: https://www.cdc.gov/hiv/library/reports/hiv-surveillance/vol-32/index.html.

41. Trost SL, Beauregard J, Chandra G, Njie F, Berry J, Harvey A, et al. Pregnancy-related deaths: data from Maternal Mortality Review Committees in 36 US states, 2017-2019. Atlanta, GA: Centers for Disease Control and Prevention, US Department of Health and Human Services; 2022.

42. Schiff DM, Nielsen T, Terplan M, Hood M, Bernson D, Diop H, et al. Fatal and nonfatal overdose among pregnant and postpartum women in Massachusetts. Obstet Gynecol. 2018;132(2):466–74.

43. Nezvalová-Henriksen K, Spigset O, Nordeng H. Effects of codeine on pregnancy outcome: results from a large population-based cohort study. Eur J Clin Pharmacol. 2011;67(12):1253–61.

44. Heinonen OP, Slone D, Shapiro S. Birth defects and drugs in pregnancy. Littleton: Publishing Sciences Group; 1977.

45. Saxén I. Associations between oral clefts and drugs taken during pregnancy. Int J Epidemiol. 1975;4(1):37–44.

46. Rothman KJ, Fyler DC, Goldblatt A, Kreidberg MB. Exogenous hormones and other drug exposures of children with congenital heart disease. Am J Epidemiol. 1979;109(4):433–9.

47. Bracken MB, Holford TR. Exposure to prescribed drugs in pregnancy and association with congenital malformations. Obstet Gynecol. 1981;58(3):336–44.

48. Broussard CS, Rasmussen SA, Reefhuis J, Friedman JM, Jann MW, Riehle-Colarusso T, et al. Maternal treatment with opioid analgesics and risk for birth defects. Am J Obstet Gynecol. 2011;204(4):314.e1–11.

49. Brogly SB, Velez MP, Werler MM, Li W, Camden A, Guttmann A. Prenatal opioid analgesics and the risk of adverse birth outcomes. Epidemiology. 2021;32(3):448–56.

50. Ostrea EM, Chavez CJ. Perinatal problems (excluding neonatal withdrawal) in maternal drug addiction: a study of 830 cases. J Pediatr. 1979;94(2):292–5.

51. Naeye RL, Blanc W, Leblanc W, Khatamee MA. Fetal complications of maternal heroin addiction: abnormal growth, infections, and episodes of stress. J Pediatr. 1973;83(6):1055–61.

52. Little BB, Snell LM, Klein VR, Gilstrap LC, 3rd, Knoll KA, Breckenridge JD. Maternal and fetal effects of heroin addiction during pregnancy. J Reprod Med. 1990;35(2):159–62.

53. Fajemirokun-Odudeyi O, Sinha C, Tutty S, Pairaudeau P, Armstrong D, Phillips T, et al. Pregnancy outcome in women who use opiates. Eur J Obstet Gynecol Reprod Biol. 2006;126(2):170–5.

54. Jones HE, Kaltenbach K, Heil SH, Stine SM, Coyle MG, Arria AM, et al. Neonatal abstinence syndrome after methadone or buprenorphine exposure. N Engl J Med. 2010;363(24):2320–31.

55. McCarthy JJ, Leamon MH, Willits NH, Salo R. The effect of methadone dose regimen on neonatal abstinence syndrome. J Addict Med. 2015;9(2):105–10.

56. Pahl A, Young L, Buus-Frank ME, Marcellus L, Soll R. Non-pharmacological care for opioid withdrawal in newborns. Cochrane Database Syst Rev. 2020;12(12):Cd013217.

57. Grisham LM, Stephen MM, Coykendall MR, Kane MF, Maurer JA, Bader MY. Eat, sleep, console approach: a family-centered model for the treatment of neonatal abstinence syndrome. Adv Neonatal Care. 2019;19(2):138–44.

58. Jones HE, Kaltenbach K, Benjamin T, Wachman EM, O'Grady KE. Prenatal opioid exposure, neonatal abstinence syndrome/neonatal opioid withdrawal syndrome, and later child development research: shortcomings and solutions. J Addict Med. 2019;13(2):90–2.

59. Kaltenbach K, O'Grady KE, Heil SH, Salisbury AL, Coyle MG, Fischer G, et al. Prenatal exposure to methadone or buprenorphine: Early childhood developmental outcomes. Drug Alcohol Depend. 2018;185:40–9.

60. Suarez EA, Huybrechts KF, Straub L, Hernández-Díaz S, Jones HE, Connery HS, et al. Buprenorphine versus methadone for opioid use disorder in pregnancy. N Engl J Med. 2022;387(22):2033–44.

61. Marquet P, Chevrel J, Lavignasse P, Merle L, Lachâtre G. Buprenorphine withdrawal syndrome in a newborn. Clin Pharmacol Ther. 1997;62(5):569–71.

62. McCarthy JJ, Posey BL. Methadone levels in human milk. J Hum Lact. 2000;16(2):115–20.

63. Ilett KF, Hackett LP, Gower S, Doherty DA, Hamilton D, Bartu AE. Estimated dose exposure of the neonate to buprenorphine and its metabolite norbuprenorphine via breastmilk during maternal buprenorphine substitution treatment. Breastfeed Med. 2012;7:269–74.

64. Welle-Strand GK, Skurtveit S, Jansson LM, Bakstad B, Bjarkø L, Ravndal E. Breastfeeding reduces the need for withdrawal treatment in opioid-exposed infants. Acta Paediatr. 2013;102(11):1060–6.

65. Ballard JL. Treatment of neonatal abstinence syndrome with breast milk containing methadone. J Perinat Neonatal Nurs. 2002;15(4):76–85.

66. Sachs HC. The transfer of drugs and therapeutics into human breast milk: an update on selected topics. Pediatrics. 2013;132(3):e796–809.

67. Committee Opinion No. 711: opioid use and opioid use disorder in pregnancy. Obstet Gynecol. 2017;130(2):e81–e94.

68. Howard H. Experiences of opioid-dependent women in their prenatal and postpartum care: Implications for social workers in health care. Soc Work Health Care. 2016;55(1):61–85.

69. ACOG Committee Opinion No. 828: indications for outpatient antenatal fetal surveillance:. Obstet Gynecol. 2021;137(6):e177–97.

70. Meresaar U, Nilsson MI, Holmstrand J, Anggård E. Single dose pharmacokinetics and bioavailability of methadone in man studied with a stable isotope method. Eur J Clin Pharmacol. 1981;20(6):473–8.

71. de Vos JW, Geerlings PJ, van den Brink W, Ufkes JG, van Wilgenburg H. Pharmacokinetics of methadone and its primary metabolite in 20 opiate addicts. Eur J Clin Pharmacol. 1995;48(5):361–6.

72. Beckett AH, Taylor JF, Casy AF, Hassan MM. The biotransformation of methadone in man: synthesis and identification of a major metabolite. J Pharm Pharmacol. 1968;20(10):754–62.

73. Ferrari A, Coccia CP, Bertolini A, Sternieri E. Methadone--metabolism, pharmacokinetics and interactions. Pharmacol Res. 2004;50(6):551–9.

74. Chou R, Weimer MB, Dana T. Methadone overdose and cardiac arrhythmia potential: findings from a review of the evidence for an American Pain Society and College on Problems of Drug Dependence clinical practice guideline. J Pain. 2014;15(4):338–65.

75. Tisdale JE, Chung MK, Campbell KB, Hammadah M, Joglar JA, Leclerc J, et al. Drug-induced arrhythmias: a scientific statement from the American Heart Association. Circulation. 2020;142(15):e214–33.

76. Pond SM, Kreek MJ, Tong TG, Raghunath J, Benowitz NL. Altered methadone pharmacokinetics in methadone-maintained pregnant women. J Pharmacol Exp Ther. 1985;233(1):1–6.

77. Walsh SL, Preston KL, Stitzer ML, Cone EJ, Bigelow GE. Clinical pharmacology of buprenorphine: ceiling effects at high doses. Clin Pharmacol Ther. 1994;55(5):569–80.

78. Iribarne C, Picart D, Dréano Y, Bail JP, Berthou F. Involvement of cytochrome P450 3A4 in N-dealkylation of buprenorphine in human liver microsomes. Life Sci. 1997;60(22):1953–64.

79. Link HM, Jones H, Miller L, Kaltenbach K, Seligman N. Buprenorphine-naloxone use in pregnancy: a systematic review and metaanalysis. Am J Obstet Gynecol MFM. 2020;2(3):100179.

80. Jones HE, Johnson RE, Jasinski DR, Milio L. Randomized controlled study transitioning opioid-dependent pregnant women from short-acting morphine to buprenorphine or methadone. Drug Alcohol Depend. 2005;78(1):33–8.

81. Jones HE, Chisolm MS, Jansson LM, Terplan M. Naltrexone in the treatment of opioid-dependent pregnant women: the case for a considered and measured approach to research. Addiction. 2013;108(2):233–47.

82. Minozzi S, Amato L, Vecchi S, Davoli M, Kirchmayer U, Verster A. Oral naltrexone maintenance treatment for opioid dependence. Cochrane Database Syst Rev. 2011;(2):Cd001333.

83. Towers CV, Katz E, Weitz B, Visconti K. Use of naltrexone in treating opioid use disorder in pregnancy. Am J Obstet Gynecol. 2020;222(1):83.e81–83.e88.

84. Ecker J, Abuhamad A, Hill W, Bailit J, Bateman BT, Berghella V, et al. Substance use disorders in pregnancy: clinical, ethical, and research imperatives of the opioid epidemic: a report of a joint workshop of the Society for Maternal-Fetal Medicine, American College of Obstetricians and Gynecologists, and American Society of Addiction Medicine. Am J Obstet Gynecol. 2019;221(1):B5–B28.

85. Hawk M, Coulter RWS, Egan JE, Fisk S, Friedman MR, Tula M, et al. Harm reduction principles for healthcare settings. Harm Reduct J. 2017;14(1):70.

86. Forbes LA, Canner JK, Milio L, Halscott T, Vaught AJ. Association of patient sex and pregnancy status with naloxone administration during emergency department visits. Obstet Gynecol. 2021;137(5):855–63.

87. Fernandes RM, Cary M, Duarte G, Jesus G, Alarcão J, Torre C, et al. Effectiveness of needle and syringe Programmes in people who inject drugs - An overview of systematic reviews. BMC Public Health. 2017;17(1):309.

88. Platt L, Minozzi S, Reed J, Vickerman P, Hagan H, French C, et al. Needle syringe programmes and opioid substitution therapy for preventing hepatitis C transmission in people who inject drugs. Cochrane Database Syst Rev. 2017;9(9):Cd012021.

89. Des Jarlais DC, Nugent A, Solberg A, Feelemyer J, Mermin J, Holtzman D. Syringe service programs for persons who inject drugs in urban, suburban, and rural areas–United States, 2013. MMWR Morb Mortal Wkly Rep. 2015;64(48):1337–41.

90. Jones HE, O'Grady K, Dahne J, Johnson R, Lemoine L, Milio L, et al. Management of acute postpartum pain in patients maintained on methadone or buprenorphine during pregnancy. Am J Drug Alcohol Abuse. 2009;35(3):151–6.

91. Meyer M, Wagner K, Benvenuto A, Plante D, Howard D. Intrapartum and postpartum analgesia for women maintained on methadone during pregnancy. Obstet Gynecol. 2007;110(2 Pt 1):261–6.

92. Höflich AS, Langer M, Jagsch R, Bäwert, A., Winklbaur, B., Fischer, G. 4,et al. Peripartum pain management in opioid dependent women. Eur J Pain. 2012;16(4):574–84.

93. Brown QL, Sarvet AL, Shmulewitz D, Martins SS, Wall MM, Hasin DS. Trends in marijuana use among pregnant and non-pregnant reproductive-aged women, 2002–2014. JAMA. 2017;317(2):207–9.

94. Retail Marijuana Public Health Advisory Committee. Monitoring health concerns related to marijuana in Colorado: 2016. Changes in marijuana use patterns, systematic literature review, and possible marijuana-related health effects. Glendale: Colorado Department of Public Health & Environment; 2016.

95. Goodwin RD, Zhu J, Heisler Z, Metz TD, Wyka K, Wu M, et al. Cannabis use during pregnancy in the United States: the role of depression. Drug Alcohol Depend. 2020;210:107881.

96. Moeller KE, Kissack JC, Atayee RS, Lee KC. Clinical interpretation of urine drug tests: what clinicians need to know about urine drug screens. Mayo Clin Proc. 2017;92(5):774–96.

97. Sood S, Trasande L, Mehta-Lee SS, Brubaker SG, Ghassabian A, Jacobson MH. Maternal cannabis use in the perinatal period: data from the pregnancy risk assessment monitoring system marijuana supplement, 2016-2018. J Addict Med. 2022;16(4):e225–e233.

98. Metz TD, Borgelt LM. Marijuana use in pregnancy and while breastfeeding. Obstet Gynecol. 2018;132(5):1198–1210.

99. Conner SN, Bedell V, Lipsey K, Macones GA, Cahill AG, Tuuli MG. Maternal marijuana use and adverse neonatal outcomes: a systematic review and meta-analysis. Obstet Gynecol. 2016;128(4):713–23.

100. Gunn JK, Rosales CB, Center KE, et al. Prenatal exposure to cannabis and maternal and child health outcomes: a systematic review and meta-analysis. BMJ Open. 2016;6(4):e009986.

101. Braillon A, Bewley S. Committee Opinion No. 722: marijuana use during pregnancy and lactation. Obstet Gynecol. 2018;131(1):164.

102. Smid MC, Metz TD, Gordon AJ. Stimulant use in pregnancy: an under-recognized epidemic among pregnant women. Clin Obstet Gynecol. 2019;62(1):168–84.

103. Reddy PKV, Ng TMH, Oh EE, Moady G, Elkayam U. Clinical characteristics and management of methamphetamine-associated cardiomyopathy: state-of-the-art review. J Am Heart Assoc. 2020;9(11):e016704.

104. Kuczkowski KM. Anesthetic implications of drug abuse in pregnancy. J Clin Anesth. 2003;15(5):382–94.

105. Hoyme HE, Jones KL, Dixon SD, Jewett T, Hanson JW, Robinson LK, et al. Prenatal cocaine exposure and fetal vascular disruption. Pediatrics. 1990;85(5):743–7.

106. Wright TE, Schuetter R, Tellei J, Sauvage L. Methamphetamines and pregnancy outcomes. J Addict Med. 2015;9(2):111–17.

107. Won L, Bubula N, McCoy H, Heller A. Methamphetamine concentrations in fetal and maternal brain following prenatal exposure. Neurotoxicol Teratol. 2001;23(4):349–54.

108. Gorman MC, Orme KS, Nguyen NT, Kent EJ, 3rd, Caughey AB. Outcomes in pregnancies complicated by methamphetamine use. Am J Obstet Gynecol. 2014;211(4):429.e421–27.

109. Gouin K, Murphy K, Shah PS. Effects of cocaine use during pregnancy on low birthweight and preterm birth: systematic review and metaanalyses. Am J Obstet Gynecol. 2011;204(4):340.e1–12.

110. Kalaitzopoulos DR, Chatzistergiou K, Amylidi AL, Kokkinidis DG, Goulis DG. Effect of methamphetamine hydrochloride on pregnancy outcome: a systematic review and meta-analysis. J Addict Med. 2018;12(3):220–6.

111. Smith LM, LaGasse LL, Derauf C, et al. The infant development, environment, and lifestyle study: effects of prenatal methamphetamine exposure, polydrug exposure, and poverty on intrauterine growth. Pediatrics. 2006;118(3):1149–56.

112. Cox S, Posner SF, Kourtis AP, Jamieson DJ. Hospitalizations with amphetamine abuse among pregnant women. Obstet Gynecol. 2008;111(2 Pt 1):341–7.

113. American Academy of Pediatrics Committee on Drugs. Transfer of drugs and other chemicals into human milk. Pediatrics. 2001;108(3):776–89.

114. Dutra L, Stathopoulou G, Basden SL, Leyro TM, Powers MB, Otto MW. A meta-analytic review of psychosocial interventions for substance use disorders. Am J Psychiatry. 2008;165(2):179–87.

115. Prendergast M, Podus D, Finney J, Greenwell L, Roll J. Contingency management for treatment of substance use disorders: a meta-analysis. Addiction. 2006;101(11):1546–60.

116. Calder R, Gant E, Bauld L, McNeill A, Robson D, Brose LS. Vaping in pregnancy: a systematic review. Nicotine Tob Res. 2021;23(9):1451–8.

117. Nagpal TS, Green CR, Cook JL. Vaping during pregnancy: what are the potential health outcomes and perceptions pregnant women have? J Obstet Gynaecol Can. 2021;43(2):219–26.

118. Hawkins SS, Wylie BJ, Hacker MR. Use of ENDS and cigarettes during pregnancy. Am J Prev Med. 2020;58(1):122–8.

119. Kapaya M, D'Angelo DV, Tong VT, England L, Ruffo N, Cox S, et al. Use of electronic vapor products before, during, and after pregnancy among women with a recent live birth–Oklahoma and Texas, 2015. MMWR Morb Mortal Wkly Rep. 2019;68(8):189–94.

120. McDonnell BP, Dicker P, Regan CL. Electronic cigarettes and obstetric outcomes: a prospective observational study. Bjog. 2020;127(6):750–6.

121. Tobacco and nicotine cessation during pregnancy: ACOG Committee Opinion, Number 807. Obstet Gynecol. 2020;135(5): e221–e229.

122. de las Cuevas C, Sanz E, de la Fuente J. Benzodiazepines: more "behavioural" addiction than dependence. Psychopharmacology (Berl). 2003;167(3):297–303.

123. Soyka M. Treatment of benzodiazepine dependence. N Engl J Med. 2017;376(12):1147–57.

124. Lader M, Tylee A, Donoghue J. Withdrawing benzodiazepines in primary care. CNS Drugs. 2009;23(1):19–34.

125. Källén B, Borg N, Reis M. The use of central nervous system active drugs during pregnancy. Pharmaceuticals (Basel). 2013;6(10):1221–86.

126. Gillberg C. "Floppy infant syndrome" and maternal diazepam. Lancet. 1977;2(8031):244.

127. Sanlorenzo LA, Cooper WO, Dudley JA, Stratton S, Maalouf FI, Patrick SW. Increased severity of neonatal abstinence syndrome associated with concomitant antenatal opioid and benzodiazepine exposure. Hosp Pediatr. 2019;9(8):569–75.

128. Bennett PN, editor. The WHO Working Group: drugs and human lactation. New York: Elsevier; 1988.

Chapter 4
Environmental Agents and Reproductive Risk

Laura Goetzl and Sami Backley

Department of Obstetrics, Gynecology and Reproductive Sciences, McGovern Medical School, The University of Texas Health Sciences Center, Houston, TX, USA

Obstetricians are frequently asked about the reproductive risks of specific environmental, work-related, or dietary exposures. Although few exposures have been associated with a measurable increase in risk of congenital anomaly, fetal death, or growth impairment, ongoing research continues to identify new areas of concern. Research linking low levels of environmental exposures is hampered by the cost and difficulty of prospective cohort studies with accurate ascertainment of exposure to specific agents at various gestational periods. In this chapter, we discuss the principles concerning the evaluation of the developmental toxicity of occupational and environmental exposures in general and review selected agents that have been associated with reproductive toxicity.

Background incidence of adverse outcome

Increased attributable risk of an individual environmental agent must be placed in the context of the background incidence of adverse pregnancy outcome in the general population. Approximately 26% of recognized pregnancies result in miscarriage and 3% result in children with major malformations, defined as a malformation requiring medical or surgical attention or resulting in functional or cosmetic impairment. This high background risk introduces statistical problems in the identification of toxicity. If the increase in adverse outcome is relatively small, it is likely to go undetected unless the study sample size is quite large.

Biologic evidence of toxicity

Two types of evidence are generally employed when evaluating agents for evidence of reproductive toxicity: animal studies and epidemiologic studies in human populations.

Studies with experimental animals offer the advantage of studying varying levels of exposure (from minimal to substantial) at specific key developmental time periods. In addition, outcomes are standardized and typically include measures of fertility, fetal weight, viability, and presence and patterns of malformations. If low doses of a compound produce an increase in malformations, a role for the agent in disrupting embryo development is possible. Limitations of animal testing include species variations in toxicity (i.e. compounds may be toxic to human embryos but not to various animal embryos, and vice versa). In addition, evaluation of functional attributes such as behavior or immunocompetence is not a part of standard testing schemes. Therefore, absence of toxicity in animal protocols provides only limited information on possible adverse effects on human development.

Human epidemiologic studies can be subdivided, in increasing order of scientific merit, into case reports, case-control studies, retrospective cohort studies, and well-designed prospective cohort studies. Often, case reports of malformations or pregnancy loss will emerge first, raising hypotheses that lead to further study. However, case reports alone are insufficient evidence on which to establish the presence or degree of risk. The evaluation of toxicity requires comprehensive assessment of both exposures and outcomes. Accurate occupational and environmental exposures are difficult to measure in humans and it is even more difficult to pinpoint precise exposure at a specific gestational age. Outcome assessment can also be difficult because the identification of abnormalities in children is affected by the age of the child and the thoroughness with which abnormalities are sought. Relying on birth certificates or obstetrician reports, for example, will yield a lower rate of identification of abnormalities than will examination using a standardized assessment protocol.

General principles

Principles of reproductive toxicity apply to environmental agents just as they do to pharmaceuticals and these principles are summarized here. These ideas were popularized by Wilson [1] in the 1950s based on his work with experimental animals, but they remain applicable decades later in a discussion of human risk.

• A large proportion of adverse outcomes are unrelated to exposures. Only 5% of congenital malformations are estimated to be attributable to exposure to a chemical agent or pharmaceutical [2].

• A specific agent may be nontoxic at low doses but toxic at higher doses. For example, X-ray exposures of >50 rad during pregnancy have been associated with microcephaly and developmental disability, but X-ray exposures in the range of most diagnostic procedures (<1 rad) are not associated with an increase in adverse pregnancy outcome.

• Each fetus will respond differently to a given exposure based on their genetic susceptibility and other factors. For a given toxic exposure, responses can range from unaffected to significantly affected.

• The timing of exposure during pregnancy will influence the response. Target tissues will have different sensitivities to toxicity at different times during gestation. Although the first trimester is typically the most sensitive time period for many congenital malformations (e.g. limb and heart defects), there are a number of examples of severe toxicity from exposures at other times in pregnancy. For example, agents that affect fetal growth and neurologic development, such as mercury and ethanol, will continue to be toxic throughout the second and third trimesters.

• Toxicity must occur via a biologically plausible mechanism. Therefore, chemicals that cannot cross the placenta or agents such as microwaves that cannot penetrate into the uterus are unlikely causes of reproductive toxicity.

Specific agents

Research demonstrating adverse reproductive effects of various chemical and environmental agents is continuously evolving. In this section we present a snapshot of the current knowledge. Computerized databases are available and can provide access to regularly updated summaries of chemical exposures (Table 4.1). The American College of Obstetricians and Gynecologists' Committee Opinion No. 832 summarizes some of the important environmental agents with potential reproductive toxicities (Box 4.1; adapted from ACOG). Women at highest risk of occupational exposure include those working in agriculture (pesticides), manufacturing (organic solvents and heavy metals), dry cleaning (solvents), cleaning services (organic solvents), and beauty salons (solvents and phthalates) [3].

Lead

Lead readily crosses the placenta by passive diffusion [4,5]. In women with significant occupational lead exposure (pottery glazes, batteries), rates of stillbirth and miscarriage are increased [6] as well as rates of gestational hypertension, low birthweight, impaired neurodevelopment, premature rupture of membranes, and premature birth [7–9]. Over time, with the reduction in lead alkyl additives in gasoline and the use of lead-based paints, lead levels in women of reproductive age have declined. Surveillance from the 1980s suggested that 9% of White women and 20% of African-American women exceeded blood lead levels of 10 μg/dL [10]. By the 1990s, overall percentages declined to 0.5% [11].

Box 4.1 Potential reproductive effects of common chemicals or pollutants

Chemical or pollutant	Potential reproductive effect
Bisphenol A (BPA), solvents, polybrominated diphenyl ether (PBDE), flame retardants	Infertility and miscarriage
Ambient air pollutants, pesticides, phthalates, PBDEs, perfluorochemicals (PFCs), toluene (solvent)	Preterm birth and low birthweight
Ambient air pollutants, BPA, lead, mercury, pesticides, phthalates, PBDEs, flame retardants, polychlorinated biphenyls (PCBs)	Neurodevelopmental impairment

Table 4.1 Reproductive toxicology sources

Individual source	Web address	Practitioner cost 2022
Reprotox	www.reprotox.org	$199/yr
Teris	http://depts.washington.edu/terisweb/teris/	$257.50/yr
Organization of Teratology Information Specialists (OTIS)	www.otispregnancy.org/ Limited number of fact sheets for download	Free
IRIS (Integrated Risk Information System)	https://iris.epa.gov/AtoZ/?list_type=alpha	Free
LactMed	https://www.ncbi.nlm.nih.gov/books/ NBK501922/?report=classic	Free

Although significant occupational exposures are rare in the United States, lower levels of perinatal lead exposure have been linked to adverse reproductive outcomes. Even mild elevations in maternal lead levels have been associated with significantly increased risks of miscarriage (5–9 µg/dL, odds ratio [OR] 2.8; 10–14 µg/dL, OR 5.4; >15 µg/dL, OR 12.2) [12] preterm birth (>10 µg/dL, OR 3.2), and small for gestational age birthweight (>10 µg/dL, OR 4.2) [13]. Increased maternal bone and blood lead levels have also been associated with a minor-to-moderate increased risk of pregnancy-induced hypertension [14,15]. Cord blood concentrations less than 30 µg/dL, and perhaps as low as 10 µg/dL [16,17], have been linked to measurable deficits in early cognitive development. Although the results are not consistent, elevated maternal lead levels during pregnancy have been associated with lower IQ scores at age 8 [18] and tests of attention and visuoconstruction at ages 15–17 [19], There is some suggestion that male fetuses may be more susceptible to adverse *in utero* effects of lead exposure on subsequent neurodevelopment [20]. Although isolated studies have linked maternal lead exposure to an increased fetal risk of neural tube defects [21] and total anomalous pulmonary venous return [22], these findings have not been consistent. One potential mechanism through which lead may result in adverse developmental effects is the inverse relationship between maternal lead levels and fetal DNA methylation [23].

Sources of lead exposure include lead solders, pipes, storage batteries, construction materials (e.g. lead-based paints), eating food from lead-glazed ceramic pottery, dyes, and wood preservatives. A validated questionnaire for screening pregnant women is underused in practice and does not help to identify those with elevated blood lead levels from those without. Risk factors for maternal lead levels that exceed 10 µg/mL include occupational exposures and house remodeling; however, screening high-risk women still fails to identify approximately 30% of cases [24]. Women at risk of lead exposure should be evaluated prior to pregnancy if possible, including those who work with lead or those living with someone identified as having an elevated blood lead level. Screening is also recommended in newly arrived pregnant refugees/emigrees; women from Mexico, Bangladesh, and Pakistan are among those at highest risk (https://www.cdc.gov/immigrantrefugeehealth/guidelines/lead-guidelines.html). If the blood level is higher than 30 µg/dL, chelation therapy should be considered prior to conception. Women with blood levels of 5 µg/dL or higher during pregnancy should be offered counseling on identifying sources of lead exposure, avoidance of further exposure, nutritional counseling along with confirmatory and follow-up laboratory workup. Levels >45 µg/dL during pregnancy should be managed with clinicians experienced in management of lead toxicity and a maternal–fetal medicine subspecialist. There is no agreement on how to manage women with lower levels of blood lead, although our preference at the time of writing would be to use chelation therapy to reduce blood lead concentrations to 10 µg/dL or less. Pregnancy itself may lead to a mobilization of bone stores of lead, with increased exposure [9,25–27]. Calcium treatment (1000–1200 mg/day) decreases bone mobilization during pregnancy and may provide modest reduction of maternal blood lead levels during pregnancy (–1 µg/dL) [25,28,29]. Current pregnancy is a relative contraindication to chelation therapy as ethylenediaminetetraacetic acid (EDTA) may chelate other key minerals necessary for development and has been linked to malformations in animal models [30]. Chelation therapy during pregnancy should be individualized based on the maternal serum lead level and the gestational age.

Mercury

Methyl mercury, a byproduct of such industries as incineration of solid waste and fossil fuel combustion facilities and cement production, pollutes our oceans and waterways. Methyl mercury crosses the placenta freely and accumulates in fetal tissues at concentrations exceeding maternal levels [31,32]. Elevated levels of mercury are associated with pregnancy complications and infant developmental problems. At high levels, methyl mercury can result in fetal neurotoxicity with microcephaly, cerebral palsy, deafness, and blindness (Minimata Bay, Japan [33,34]), but is not reproducibly associated with congenital malformations. However, most exposure to mercury occurs at low levels from fish consumption (methyl mercury), dental amalgams (mercury vapor), or the vaccine preservative thimerosal (ethyl mercury). Thimerosal has been removed from most vaccines in the United States and is therefore an unlikely potential source of exposure.

Fish consumption remains a modifiable source of fetal and childhood mercury exposure. Several large cohort studies have addressed the effects of low levels of *in utero* mercury exposure from maternal fish consumption on neuropsychologic development. Studies from the Faroe Islands (>1000 mother–infant pairs) and New Zealand (237 pairs) [35,36] found subtle deficits in language, attention, intelligence, and memory in school- aged children. Another, more recent study from the Seychelles (779 mother–infant pairs) did not find an association between *in utero* mercury exposure and outcome at 9 years; however, the final power to detect these outcomes was only 50% [37]. In 2001, based on these findings and a 2000 report from the National Research Council (NRC) [38], the Environmental Protection Agency issued advice urging pregnant women to limit consumption of fish high in mercury. A benchmark blood level of <5.8 µg/L was recommended by the NRC; exposure above this level was associated with a doubling in the risk of adverse neurologic outcomes. Among women of childbearing age in the United States between 1999 and 2002, 4–8% exceeded this benchmark level [39]. More recent iterations of this advice balance concerns over mercury exposure with the known benefits of fish consumption during pregnancy and lactation (https://www.fda.gov/food/consumers/advice-about-eating-fish, Box 4.2). Moderate intake of relatively safer fish should not be discouraged, as increasing fish consumption has been linked with higher measures of infant cognition [40–42].

Mercury exposure from dental amalgams is usually at a low level and is not easily modified. Both placement and removal of dental amalgams are associated with transient increased levels of mercury exposure and should be avoided during pregnancy [43,44]. Dental personnel may also be exposed to inorganic mercury in vapors released from dental amalgams. Although evidence of documented harm in dental personnel is limited, current

studies lack the power to detect subtle neurodevelopmental deficits. Safe levels of mercury during pregnancy have not been established although suggested guidelines are that environments have a mercury vapor concentration less than 0.01 mg/m^3 (one fifth of Occupational Safety and Health Administration limits of 0.05 mg/m^3).

Pesticides and herbicides

A diverse group of agents is used to control pests such as insects and unwanted plants. Although most exposures are agricultural, significant household exposure can occur, especially in the inner city, and the majority of pesticides cross the placenta readily [45]. Methodologically, it is difficult to isolate a single agent in epidemiologic studies; exposure to pesticides has been estimated by maternal recall, proximity to agricultural pesticide use, or maternal pesticide levels. Of concern, many pesticides act as endocrine disruptors including dichloro-diphenyl-trichloroethane (DDT), chlorpyrifos, atrazine, and others. Serum levels of hexachlorobenzene, a fungicide used to treat seed, have been associated with an increased risk of hypospadias in male offspring [46]. Several studies have linked occupational exposure to pesticides with an increased risk of miscarriage [47,48] and birth defects such as musculoskeletal [49,50] and limb reduction abnormalities [51]. No association or weak associations have been found between parental pesticide exposure and adverse pregnancy outcomes including low birthweight [52], preterm delivery, or early neurodevelopmental outcomes [53]. Although several maternal recall case-control studies have linked household pesticide use with an increased risk of childhood cancer [54,55], no association was found when exposure was estimated by proximity to agricultural pesticide use [56]. High levels of prenatal exposure to chlorpyrifos have been associated lower neurodevelopmental scores and a higher incidence of attention-deficit/hyperactivity disorder at age 3 and lower IQ at age 7 [57–58]. Similar effects have been seen in studies of organophosphates [59].

Minimizing occupational pesticide exposure through the use of protective clothing, adequate ventilation, respiratory masks, and hand washing is recommended. Limiting everyday exposure by minimizing household pesticide use (especially aerosolized pesticides), washing fruits and vegetables or buying organic produce is of uncertain benefit, but is easily accomplished.

Polychlorinated biphenyls

Polychlorinated biphenyls (PCBs) are a heterogeneous group of more than 200 lipid-soluble chemicals that were used extensively in industry until 1979, particularly in the manufacture of electrical transformers. Low-level maternal exposure is largely related to meat, dairy, and fish consumption, particularly fish from contaminated areas such as the Great Lakes. PCBs cross the placenta easily (fetal to

---

Box 4.2 Choosing commercially bought fish to eat based on mercury levels

Choices to avoid

King mackerel	Shark	Tilefish (Gulf of Mexico)
Marlin	Swordfish	Tuna (Bigeye)
Orange roughy		

Good choices: Limit to one serving per week (4 ounces)

Bluefish	Halibut	Sheepshead
Buffalofish	Mahi mahi	Snapper
Carp	Monkfish	Tilefish (Atlantic)
Chilean sea bass	Rockfish	Tuna (albacore/white/yellowfin)
Grouper	Sablefish	Weakfish/seatrout
		Croaker (white/Pacific)

Best choices: Eat 2–3 servings per week (8–12 ounces)

Anchovies	Hake	Shad
Atlantic croaker	Herring	Shrimp
Atlantic mackerel	Lobster	Skate
Black sea bass	Mullet	Smelt
Butterfish	Oyster	Sole
Catfish	Pacific chub mackerel	Squid
Clam	Perch, freshwater/ocean	Tilapia
Cod	Pickerel	Canned light tuna
Crab	Plaice	Whitefish
Crawfish	Pollock	Whiting
Flounder	Salmon	
Haddock	Scallop	

For locally caught fish, check local/state advisories at https://fishadvisoryonline.epa.gov/Contacts.aspx.

maternal serum ratios of 0.6:1.1) and also accumulate in human breastmilk (breastmilk to maternal ratios of 0.6:1.8), contributing to postnatal exposure [60]. The overall effect on birthweight appears to be modest (290 g difference between <10th and >90th percentile exposure) [61] in some studies and insignificant in others [62].

Studies of *in utero* exposure to low levels of PCBs and subsequent neurodevelopment have produced various results. Several studies have shown no relationship between maternal serum levels of PCBs and mental and motor development in infancy/early childhood [63] and at school age [64]. In highly exposed children, one US study showed significant reductions in IQ [65] whereas another in Taiwan showed smaller reductions [66]. Other studies have suggested minor deficits in attention, memory, and motor skills in vulnerable populations of children; deficits were not observed in children in more advantageous circumstances or in those who were breastfed [67,68]. PCBs can also act as endocrine disruptors; current animal studies literature suggests that exposure to endocrine-disrupting chemicals can have a wide range of effects on metabolism such altering insulin metabolism and disrupting energy balance; in animal models, a growing body of literature suggests that exposure to endocrine-disrupting chemicals can have a wide range of effects on metabolism such altering insulin metabolism and disrupting energy balance [69]. Although levels of individual PCB compounds are not significant, total PCB load >2.0 µg/L has been linked to increased risks of hypospadias [70].

Polybrominated diphenyl ethers

Polybrominated diphenyl ether (PBDE) exposure largely occurs through contact with products that have been treated with this chemical due to its flame-retardant properties or through consuming contaminated foods, especially foods with high fat content such as fish. Although they were phased out in the early 2000s, they can persist in the environment and in adipose tissue. In California, removing PBDEs resulted in a 65% reduction of levels in pregnant women over 5 years [71]. Although most data are from animal studies, some limited human data suggest a small drop in IQ associated with higher levels of PBDEs (-3.7 IQ points; 95% confidence interval [CI] 6.56–0.83) [72]. Higher levels of PBDEs have also been associated with and increased risk of preterm birth (OR 5.6; 95% CI 2.2–15.2) [73].

Organic solvents

Organic solvents are among the most common occupational exposure. Many women work in industries where they may be exposed to organic solvents, including dry cleaning and manufacturing using solvent-based adhesives, paints, or lacquers. Common organic solvents include toluene, benzene, and xylene. Significant occupational exposure has been associated with the risk of small for gestation related to solvents 3 months before conception and during pregnancy (OR 1.67 [95% CI 1.02–2.73]) [74]. The risk of any major malformation was 10% and the overwhelming majority of malformations occurred in women with symptomatic exposure. Maternal occupational exposure to solvents is also associated with an increase in major malformations (oral clefts, urinary malformations, and male genital malformations) [75], increased rates of hyperactivity [76] and subtle decreases in visual acuity and abnormalities in red/green color vision [77]. An increase in childhood acute lymphoblastic leukemia has also been associated with self-reported occupational exposure to solvents and petroleum in the United Kingdom [78]. Purposeful maternal solvent abuse (sniffing) has been associated with a fetal syndrome similar to fetal alcohol syndrome in 12.5% of cases, as well as major malformations (16.1%) and neonatal hearing loss (10.7%) [79].

Occupational exposure to solvents should be identified and minimized; similarly, women should avoid exposure to solvents at home, especially in poorly ventilated areas. Regarding nonoccupational exposures to paint fumes, the Danish National Birth Cohort Study found an inverse relationship between exposure to paint fumes and low birthweight in a cohort of 19 000 mothers [80].

Perfluorochemicals

Perfluorochemicals (PFCs) are a group of synthetic chemicals engineered to provide water and/or oil repelling surface treatments. They are commonly found in nonstick pans, coating paper and cardboard packaging products, in carpets, and coating textiles. Perfluorooctane sulfonic acid and perfluorooctanoic acid are the most frequently detected PFCs in humans. Production of these compounds has largely been phased out but they may be found in items manufactured before 2010 and may persist in the environment. Studies have been mixed regarding the human effects of PFC exposure in pregnancy, with conflicting results regarding clinically significant effects on low birthweight [81]. Avoiding use of nonstick pans during pregnancy is reasonable although benefits are difficult to quantify.

Video display terminals

Initial concerns regarding the reproductive risks of video display terminals (VDTs) centered on early reports linking occupational exposure with an increased risk of spontaneous pregnancy loss [82]. However, subsequent well-designed studies suggested no increased risk [83,84]. Therefore, patients can be reassured that there are no known fetal risks associated with working at VDTs.

Bisphenol A

BPA is a hormone disrupter with estrogenic effects that is commonly found in hard plastic items such as food storage containers, bottled water, in the lining of some canned goods, in thermal coatings of cash register receipts, and some dental sealants. In general, plastics that are marked with recycle codes 1, 2, 4, and 5 are very unlikely to contain BPA. Some, but not all, plastics that are marked with recycle codes 3, 6, or 7 may contain BPA.

Scientific concern regarding BPA toxicity in fetuses and infants has increased over the years. It has been found in umbilical blood and amniotic fluid, despite its short half-life showing that it can cross the placental barrier [85]. Pregnancy exposure has been associated with a large number of fetal and perinatal adverse effects, including fetal growth restriction, preterm birth, recurrent miscarriages and neurobehavioral problems [86].

The potential adverse effects of BPA on the fetus, largely identified in animal models, include effects on the brain, especially related to sex-related differences, developing endocrine and reproductive organs such as the prostate and breast tissue, and detrimental neurobehavioral effects. There are scant human data regarding maternal blood levels of BPA in the United States. In one study of 40 Michigan mothers, blood levels of BPA ranged from 0.5 to 23 ng/mL [87]. In *ex vivo* placental perfusion models, BPA has been found to cross the human placenta in its active form even when present in low levels [88]. In one study, third-trimester maternal urine BPA levels were not correlated with birthweight [89]. In a prospective study of 249 mother–infant pairs, maternal urine BPA levels at <16 weeks were associated with increased aggressive behavior in 2-year-old girls [90].

In January 2010, the Food and Drug Administration stated that although standardized toxicity tests support the safety of current low levels of human exposure to BPA, subtle human effects were possible [91,92] with no changes in its position in an updated statement in 2014. Therefore, at this time, it is reasonable for pregnant women to avoid the use of products that contain BPA where possible. Fact sheets for pregnant women (https://www.niehs.nih.gov/health/topics/agents/sya-bpa/index.cfm) and new parents (https://www.mass.gov/doc/how-to-protect-your-baby-from-bpa-bisphenol-a-english-0/download) are available.

Phthalates

Phthalates are a class of chemicals that are added to plastics to make them more flexible and as solvents in cosmetic products especially in scented items. Phthalates do not generally bioaccumulate in the body, therefore, exposure must be ongoing during pregnancy to have adverse reproductive effects. In one study, switching to "phthalate-free" personal care products reduced phthalate levels in young women [93]. Phthalates act as endocrine disrupters and have been associated with an increased risk of male reproductive abnormalities such as hypospadias and reduced anogenital distance in some but not all studies [94,95]. A weak association with increased preterm

birth risk has also been reported [96]. One study suggested an association between prenatal phthalate exposure and an increased risk of attention deficits and depression at ages 4–9 [97]; however, overall no clear pattern of neurodevelopment effects has been found [98]. Some resources for consumers to determine if products they use contain phthalates include the Consumer Product Information Database (www.whatsinproducts.com) and the EWG Skin Deep Cosmetics Database (https://www.ewg.org/skindeep).

Air pollutants

Air pollutants are a complex mixture of particulate matter of different sizes (PM 2.5 to 10), carbon dioxide, carbon monoxide, sulfur dioxide, nitrous dioxide, heavy metals, and polycyclic aromatic hydrocarbons. Because of the effect of air pollution on individuals with respiratory conditions, local alerts are now commonly available via notifications or online (https://airnow.gov). Unfortunately, except for avoiding high traffic areas or wearing a mask during high PM conditions, most exposure is determined by a woman's geographic location and is fixed during pregnancy. Particulate matter, nitrogen dioxide, ozone, and carbon monoxide are the most commonly studied markers of ambient air pollution. Due to the complexity of the exposures, heterogeneity in how pollution levels are measured, potential confounders and other factors, studies can be difficult to interpret, especially when effect sizes are small (e.g. OR 1.1). A systematic review reported that fine PM (PM 2.5) was associated with an increased risk of hypertensive disorders of pregnancy (OR 1.57, 95% CI 1.26–1.96 per 5 µg/m^3 increase) [99]. PM 2.5 also appears to be associated with an increased risk of preterm birth; pooled effect estimates 1.24 (95% CI 1.08–1.41) per 10 µg/m^3 increase [100]. Assuming a smaller effect size of 1.15, one study modeled that 3.3% of preterm births in the United States are attributable to PM 2.5 exposure [101]. Several studies have linked third-trimester exposure to increased risks of stillbirth; however, although ORs may be significantly increased (1.12 to 1.42), absolute risk remains low [102,103]. In contrast, a meta-analysis of PM 2.5 and birthweight observed that studies were equally split between those with and without significant effects [104]. It is possible that observed associations between air pollution and low birthweight are largely driven by effects in women with other comorbidities including smoking, obesity, underweight, or low socioeconomic status [105]. Studies have also linked PM 2.5 exposure, specifically in the third trimester to an increased risk of autism (effect size 1.38–1.42) [106]. Although some studies have linked first-trimester exposure to air pollution to an increased risk of spina bifida, risk appears to be confined to low socioeconomic status neighborhoods [107].

CASE PRESENTATION

A 38-year-old G1 presents at 8 weeks gestation for her first prenatal visit. She is concerned about environmental exposures in general and asks for advice to mitigate risk.

Adequately counseling this patient requires a brief review of any specific exposures that she may be at risk for through her occupation or habits. If specific exposures are identified, then counseling should be performed to minimize exposure as possible. This may require accommodations from her employer. If no specific agent can be identified, general risk mitigation strategies can still be useful. Practical recommendations have been developed and these serve as a useful guide for patients (Box 4.3 adapted from ACOG 832 [3]).

Box 4.3 Practical advice for reducing exposure to environmental agents during pregnancy

Food and water

- Eat fresh food and minimize processed and canned foods that contain plastic liners
- Wash all fruits and vegetables and hands thoroughly and eat organic foods, if possible, to minimize exposures to pesticides
- Trim fat from meat and skin from fish to minimize exposure to fat-soluble chemicals

- Store food in glass or stainless steel containers
- Avoid plastic contains labeled #3, #6, or #7 and use BPA-free baby formula bottles and toys
- Avoid heating or microwaving food in plastic containers or plastic bottles
- Avoid nonstick pans

Around the home

- Remove shoes before entering the home
- Clean floors with a wet mop or wet cloth instead of sweeping and creating airborne particulates
- Use nontoxic household cleaning products (ammonia, vinegar (1 cup white vinegar and 1 cup water), baking soda)
- No home pesticides. Use insect baits, not sprays, dusts, or bombs.
- Minimize use of dry cleaning

- Avoid toxic flame retardants.
- Avoid burning trash
- Ask for volatile organic compounds (VOC)-free and water-based materials for home improvements.
- Delay home improvements/renovations that may involve disturbing leaded paint (houses built before 1978)

Personal habits and products

- Use phthalate-free make up and other personal care products (use fragrance free rather than 'unscented')
- Avoid digital paper receipt handling.

- Avoid lead (some lipsticks, azarcon and greta, bali goli, some Ayurvedic treatments)
- Choose foam products labeled "flame retardant free"
- Wash hands frequently instead of relying on hand sanitizers

Air pollution

- Check local air quality if data are available (e.g. https://airnow.gov).
- Exercise away from high traffic areas

- In high particulate matter conditions, wear a mask and/or use a home air purifier (HEPA filter)
- Avoid idling cars and other vehicles

References

1. Wilson JG. Current status of teratology: general principles and mechanisms derived from animal studies. In: Wilson JG, Fraser FC, editors. Handbook of teratology. New York: Plenum; 1977. p.47–74.
2. Czeizel A, Racz J. Evaluation of drug intake during pregnancy in the Hungarian case-control surveillance of congenital anomalies. Teratology. 1990;42:505–12.
3. Reducing prenatal exposure to toxic environmental agents: ACOG Committee Opinion No. 832. American College of Obstetricians and Gynecologists. Obstet Gynecol. 2021; 138:e40–54.
4. McClain RM, Becker BA. Teratogenicity, fetal toxicity, and placental transfer of lead nitrate in rats. Toxicol Appl Pharmacol. 1975;31:72–82.
5. Lanphear BP, Hornung R, Khoury J, Yolton K, Baghurst P, Bellinger DC, et al. Low-level environmental lead exposure and children's intellectual function: an international pooled analysis [published correction appears in Environ Health Perspect. 2019 Sep;127(9):99001]. Environ Health Perspect. 2005;113(7):894–99. doi: 10.1289/ehp.7688.
6. Scanlon JW. Dangers to the human fetus from certain heavy metals in the environment. Rev Environ Health. 1975; 2:39–64.
7. Nogaki K. On action of lead on body of lead refinery workers: particularly conception, pregnancy and parturition in case of females and on vitality of their newborn. Igaku Kenkyu. 1957; 27:1314–38.
8. Fahim MS, Fahim Z, Hall DG. Effects of subtoxic lead levels on pregnant women in the state of Missouri. Res Commun Chem Pathol Pharmacol. 1976;13:309–31.

9. Center for Disease Control and Prevention. Guidelines for the identification and management of lead exposure in pregnant and lactating women. Atlanta, GA: Centers for Disease Control and Prevention; 2010.

10. Crocetti AF, Mushak P, Schwartz J. Determination of numbers of lead-exposed women of childbearing age and pregnant women: an integrated summary of a report to the US Congress on childhood lead poisoning. Environ Health Perspect. 1990;89:121–4.

11. Brody DJ, Pirkle JL, Kramer RA, Flegal KM, Matte TD, Gunter EW, et al. Blood lead levels in the US population. Phase I of the Third National Health and Nutrition Examination Survey (NHANES III). JAMA. 1994;272:277–83.

12. Borja-Aburto VH, Hertz-Picciotto I, Lopez MR, Farias P, Rios C, Blanco J. Blood lead levels measured prospectively and risk of spontaneous abortion. Am J Epidemiol. 1999;150:590–7.

13. Jelliffe-Pawlowski LL, Miles SQ, Courtney JG, Materna B, Charlton V. Effect of magnitude and timing of maternal pregnancy blood lead (Pb) levels on birth outcomes. J Perinatol. 2006;26:154–62.

14. Rothenburg SJ, Kondrashov V, Manalo M, Jiang J, Cuellar R, Garcia M, et al. Increases in hypertension and blood pressure during pregnancy with increased bone lead levels. Am J Epidemiol. 2002;156;1079–87.

15. Yazbeck C, Thiebaugeorges O, Moreau T, Goua V, Debotte G, Sahuquillo J, et al. Maternal blood lead levels and the risk of pregnancy-induced hypertension: the EDEN cohort study. Environ Health Perspect. 2009;117:1526–30.

16. Bellinger D, Leviton A, Waternaux C, Needleman H, Rabinowitz M. Longitudinal analyses of prenatal and postnatal lead exposure and early cognitive development. N Engl J Med. 1987;316:1037–43.

17. Dietrich KN, Krafft KM, Bornschein RL, Hammond PB, Berger O, Succop PA, et al. Low-level fetal lead exposure effect on neurobehavioral development in early infancy. Pediatrics. 1987;80:721–30.

18. Wasserman GA, Liu X, Popovac D, Factor-Litvak P, Kline J, Waternaux C, et al. The Yugoslavia Prospective Lead Study: contributions of prenatal and postnatal lead exposure to early intelligence. Neurotoxicol Teratol. 2000;22:811–18.

19. Ris MD, Dietrich KN, Succop PA, Berger OG, Bornschein RL, et al. Early exposure to lead and neurophyschological outcome in adolescence. J Int Neuropsychol Soc. 2004;10;261–70.

20. Jedrychowski W, Perera F, Jankowski J, Mrozek-Budzyn D, Mroz E, Flak E, et al. Gender specific differences in neurodevelopmental effects of prenatal exposure to very low lead levels: the prospective cohort study in three-year olds. Early Human Dev. 2009;85:503–10.

21. Bound JP, Harvey PW, Francis BJ, Awwad F, Gatrell AC, et al. Involvement of deprivation and environmental lead in neural tube defects: a matched case-control study. Arch Dis Child. 1997;76:107–12.

22. Jackson LW, Correa-Villasenor A, Lees PS, Dominici F, Stewart PA, Breysse PN, et al. Parental lead exposures and total anomalous pulmonary venous return. Birth Defects Res Part A Clin Mol Teratol. 2004;70:185–93.

23. Pilsner JR, Hu H, Ettinger A, Sánchez BN, Wright RO, Cantonwine D, et al. Influence of prenatal lead exposure on genomic methylation of cord blood DNA. Environ Health Perspect. 2009;117:1466–71.

24. Johnson KM, Specht AJ, Hart JM, Salahuddin S, Erlinger AL, Hacker MR, et al. Risk-factor based lead screening and correlation with blood lead levels in pregnancy. Matern Child Health J. 2022 Jan;26(1):185–92. doi: 10.1007/s10995-021-03325-x. Epub 2022 Jan 12.

25. Gulson BL, Mizon KJ, Korsch MR, Palmer JM, Donnelly JB, et al. Mobilization of lead from human bone tissue during pregnancy and lactation: a summary of long-term research. Sci Total Environ. 2003;303:79–104.

26. Gulson BL, Mizon KJ, Palmer JM, Korsch MJ, Taylor AJ, Mahaffey KR, et al. Blood lead changes during pregnancy and postpartum with calcium supplementation. Environ Health Perspect. 2004;112:499–507.

27. Manton WI, Angle CR, Stanek KL, Kuntzelman D, Reese YR, Kuehnemann TJ, et al. Release of lead from bone in pregnancy and lactation. Environ Res. 2003;92:139–51.

28. Hernandez-Avila M, Gonzalez-Cossio T, Hernandez-Avila JE, Romieu I, Peterson KE, Aro A, et al. Dietary calcium supplements to lower blood lead levels in lactating women: a randomized placebo-controlled trial. Epidemiology. 2003; 14:206–12.

29. Ettinger AS, Lamadrid-Figueroa H, Tellez-Rojo MM, Mercado-García A, Peterson, KE, Schwartz J, et al. Effect of calcium supplementation on blood lead levels in pregnancy; a randomized placebo-controlled trial. Environ Health Perspect. 2009;117:26–31.

30. Brownie CF, Brownie C, Noden D, Krook L, Haluska M, Aronson AL. Teratogenic effect of calcium edetate (CaEDTA) in rats and the protective effect of zinc. Toxicol Appl Pharmacol. 1986;82:426443.

31. Tsuchiya H, Mitani K, Kodama K, Nakata T. Placental transfer of heavy metals in normal pregnant Japanese women. Arch Environ Health. 1984;39:11.

32. Bjornberg KA, Vahter M, Berglund B, Niklasson B, Blennow M, Sandborgh-Englund G. Transport of methylmercury and inorganic mercury to the fetus and breast-fed infant. Environ Health Perspect. 2005;113:1381–5.

33. Matsumoto H, Koya G, Takeucki T. Fetal Minimata disease: a neuropathological study of two cases of intrauterine intoxication by a methyl mercury compound. J Neuropathol Exp Neurol. 1965;24:563–74.

34. Muramaki U. The effect of organic mercury on intrauterine life. Acta Exp Biol Med Biol. 1972;27;301–36.

35. Grandjean P, Weihe P, White RF, Debes F, Araki S, Yokoyama K, et al. Cognitive deficit in 7-year old children with prenatal exposure to methylmercury. Neurotoxicol Teratol. 1997; 19:417–28.

36. Crump KS, Kjellstrom T, Shipp AM, Silvers A, Stewart A. Influence of prenatal mercury exposure upon scholastic and psychological test performance: benchmark analysis of a New Zealand cohort. Risk Anal. 1998;18:701–13.

37. Myers GJ, Davidson PW, Cox C, Shamlaye CF, Palumbo D, Cernichiari E, et al. Prenatal methylmercury exposure from ocean fish consumption in the Seychelles child development study. Lancet. 2003;361:1686–92.

38. National Research Council. Toxicological effects of methylmercury. Washington, DC: National Academy Press; 2000.

39. Centers for Disease Control and Prevention. Blood mercury levels in young children and childbearing-aged women, United States, 1999-2002. MMWR. 2004;53:1018–20.

40. Oken E, Wright RO, Kleinman KP, Bellinger D, Amarasiriwardena CJ, Hu H, et al. Maternal fish consumption, hair mercury, and infant cognition in an US cohort. Environ Health Perspect. 2005;113:1376–80.

41. Daniels JL, Longnecker MP, Rowland AS, Golding J, ALSPAC Study Team. Fish intake during pregnancy and early cognitive development of offspring. Epidemiology. 2004;15: 394–402.

42. Docket No. FDA-2009-N-0018. Report of quantitative risk and benefit assessment of commercial fish consumption, focusing on fetal neurodevelopmental effects (measured by verbal development in children) and on coronary heart disease and stroke in the general population, and summary of published research on the beneficial effects of fish consumption and omega-3 fatty acids for certain neurodevelopmental and cardiovascular endpoints. Federal Register. 2009;74:3615–17.

43. Molim M, Bergman B, Marklund SI, Schutz A, Skerfving S. Mercury, selenium and glutathione peroxidase before and after amalgam removal in man. Acta Odontol Scand. 1990; 48:189–202.

44. Razagui IB, Haswell SJ. Mercury and selenium concentrations in maternal and neonatal scalp hair: relationship to amalgam-based dental treatment received during pregnancy. Biol Trace Elem Res. 2001;81:1–19.

45. Whyatt RM, Barr DB, Camann DE, Kinney PL, Barr JR, Andrews HF, et al. Contemporary-use pesticides in personal air samples during pregnancy and blood samples at delivery among urban minority mothers and newborns. Environ Health Perspect. 2003;111:749–56.

46. Giordano F, Abballe A, de Felip E, di Domenico A, Ferro F, Grammatico P, et al. Maternal exposures to endocrine disrupting chemicals and hypospadias in offspring. Birth Defects Res. 2010;88:241–50.

47. Arbuckle TE, Lin Z, Mery LS, Curtis KM. An exploratory analysis of the effect of pesticide exposure on the risk of spontaneous abortion in an Ontario farm population. Environ Health Perspect. 2001;109:851–7.

48. Garry VF, Harkins M, Lybuvimov A, Erickson L, Long L. Reproductive outcomes in the women of the Red River Valley of the North. The spouses of pesticide applicators: pregnancy loss, age at menarche and exposures to pesticides. J Toxicol Environ Health. 2002; 65:769–86.

49. Hemminki K, Mutanen P, Luoma K, Saloniemi I. Congenital malformations by the parental occupation in Finland. Int Arch Occup Environ Health. 1980;46:93–8.

50. Garry VF, Schreinemachers D, Harkins ME, Griffith J. Pesticide appliers, biocides and birth defects in rural Minnesota. Environ Health Perspect. 1996;104:394–9.

51. Engel LS, O'Meara ES, Schwartz SM. Maternal occupation in agriculture and risk of adverse birth outcomes in Washington state, 1980–1991. Am J Epidemiol 2000;26:193–8.

52. Kristensen P, Ingens LM, Andersen A, Bye A, Sundheim L. Gestational age, birth weight, and perinatal death among births to Norwegian farmers, 1967-1991. Am J Epidemiol 1997;146:329–38.

53. Young JG, Eskenazi B, Gladstone EA, Bradman A, Pedersen L, Johnson C, et al. Association between in utero organophosphate pesticide exposure and abnormal reflexes in neonates. Neurotoxicology. 2005;26:199–209.

54. Daniels JL, Olshan AF, Savitz DA. Pesticides and childhood cancers. Environ Health Perspect. 1997;105:1068–77.

55. Zahm SH, Ward MH. Pesticides and childhood cancer. Environ Health Perspect. 1998;106:893–908.

56. Reynolds P, von Behren J, Gunier RB, Goldberg DE, Harnly M, Hertz A. Agricultural pesticide use and childhood cancer in California. Epidemiology. 2005;16:93–100.

57. Rauh V, Arunajadai S, Horton M, Perera F, Hoepner L, Barr DB, et al. Seven-year neurodevelopmental scores and prenatal exposure to chlorpyrifos, a common agricultural pesticide. Environ. Health Perspect. 2011;119:1196–1201.

58. Rauh VA, Garfinkel R, Perera FP, Andrews HF, Hoepner L, Barr DB, et al. Impact of prenatal chlorpyrifos exposure on neurodevelopment in the first 3 years of life among inner-city children. Pediatrics. 2006;188: e1845–59.

59. González-Alzaga B, Lacasaña M, Aguilar-Garduño C, Rodríguez-Barranco M, Ballester F, Rebagliato M, et al. A systematic review of neurodevelopmental effects of prenatal and postnatal organophosphate pesticide exposure. Toxicol Lett. 2014;230:104–21.

60. DeKoning EP, Karmaus W. PCB exposure in utero and via breastmilk: a review. J Expo Anal Environ Epidemiol. 2000;10:285–93.

61. Hertz - Picciotto I, Charles MJ, James RA, Keller JA, Willman E, Teplin S. In utero polychlorinated biphenyl exposure in relation to fetal and early childhood growth. Epidemiolog.y 2005;16:648–56.

62. Longnecker MP, Klebanoff MA, Brock JW, Guo X. Maternal levels of polychlorinated biphenyls in relation to preterm and small for gestational age birth. Epidemiology. 2005; 16: 641–7.

63. Daniels JL, Longnecker MP, Klebanoff MA, Gray KA, Brock JW, Zhou H, et al. Prenatal exposure to low level polychlorinated biphenyls in relation to mental and motor development at 8 months. Am J Epidemiol. 2003;157:485–92.

64. Gray KA, Klebanoff MA, Brock JW, et al. In utero exposure to background levels of polychlorinated biphenyls and cognitive functioning among school age children. Am J Epidemiol. 2005;162:17–26.

65. Jacobson JL, Jacobson SW. Intellectual impairment in children exposed to polychlorinated biphenyls in utero. N Engl J Med. 1996;335:783–9.

66. Chen Y-CJ, Guo Y-L, Hsu C-C, Rogan WJ. Cognitive development of Yu-Cheng ('oil disease') children prenatally exposed to heat-degraded PCBs. JAMA. 1992;268:3213–18.

67. Vreugdenhil HJI, Lanting CI, Mulder PGH, Boersma ER, Weisglas-Kuperus N. Effects of prenatal PCB and dioxin background exposure on cognitive and motor abilities in Dutch children at school age. J Pediatr. 2002;140:48–56.

68. Jacobsen JL, Jacobsen SW. Perinatal exposure to polychlorinated biphenyls and attention at school age. J Pediatr. 2003;143:780–8.

69. Vandenberg LN, Colborn T, Hayes TB, Heindel JJ, Jacobs DR Jr, Lee DH, et al., Hormones and endocrine-disrupting chemicals: low-dose effects and nonmonotonic dose responses. Endocr Rev. 2012;33(3):378–455.

70. McGlynn KA, Guo X, Graubard BI, Brock JW, Klebanoff MA, Longnecker MP. Maternal pregnancy levels of polychlorinated biphenyls and risk of hypospadias and cryptorchidism in male offspring. Environ Health Perspect. 2009;117:1472–6.

71. Zota AR, Geller RJ, Romano LE, Coleman-Phox K, Adler NE, Parry E. Association between persistent endocrine-disrupting

chemicals (PBDEs, OH-PBDEs, PCBs, and PFASs) and biomarkers of inflammation and cellular aging during pregnancy and postpartum. Environ Int. 2018 Jun;115:9–20. doi: 10.1016/j.envint.2018.02.044. Epub 2018 Mar 10.

72. Lam J, Lanphear BP, Bellinger D, Axelrad DA, McPartland J, Sutton P. Developmental PBDE exposure and IQ/ADHD in childhood: a systematic review and meta-analysis. Environ Health Perspect. 2017 Aug 3;125(8):086001.

73. Peltier MR, Koo HC, Getahun D, Menon R. Does exposure to flame retardants increase the risk for preterm birth? J Reprod Immunol. 2015;107:20–5.

74. Ahmed P, Jaakkola JJ. Exposure to organic solvents and adverse pregnancy outcomes. Hum Reprod. 2007 Oct;22(10):2751–7. doi: 10.1093/humrep/dem200. Epub 2007 Aug 28.

75. Gariantezec R, Monfort C, Rouget F, Cordier S. Maternal occupational exposure to solvents and congenital malformations: a prospective study in the general population. Occupat Environ Med. 2009;66:456–63.

76. Laslo-Baker D, Barrera M, Knittel-Keren D, Kozer E, Wolpin J, Khattak S, et al. Child neurodevelopment outcome and maternal occupational exposure to solvents. Arch Pediatr Adolesc Med. 2004;158:956–61.

77. Till C, Westall CA, Koren G, Nulman I, Rovet JF. Vision abnormalities in young children exposed prenatally to organic solvents. Neurotoxicology. 2005;26:599–613.

78. McKinney PA, Raji OY, van Tongeren M, Feltbower RG. The UK Childhood Cancer Study: maternal occupational exposures and childhood leukaemia and lymphoma. Rad Protect Dosimetry. 2008;132:232–40.

79. Scheeres JJ, Chudley AE. Solvent abuse in pregnancy: a perinatal perspective. J Obstet Gynaecol Can. 2002;24:22–6.

80. Sorensen M, Andersen AM, Raaschou-Nielsen O. Nonoccupational exposure to paint fumes during pregnancy and fetal growth in a general population. Environ Res. 2010;110:383–7.

81. Gao X, Ni W, Zhu S, Wu Y, Cui Y, Ma J, et al. Per- and polyfluoroalkyl substances exposure during pregnancy and adverse pregnancy and birth outcomes: a systematic review and meta-analysis. Environ Res. 2021;201:111632.

82. Gold EB, Tomich E. Occupational hazards to fertility and pregnancy outcome. Occup Med (Lond). 1994;9:435–69.

83. Blackwell R, Chang A. Video display terminals and pregnancy: a review. Br J Obstet Gynaecol. 1988;95:446–53.

84. Rothenberg SJ, Manalo M, Jiang J, Khan F, Cuellar R, Reyes S, et al. Maternal blood lead level during pregnancy in South Central Los Angeles. Arch Environ Health. 1999;54:151–7.

85. Pergialiotis V, Kotrogianni P, Christopoulos-Timogiannakis E, Koutaki D, Daskalakis G, Papantoniou N. Bisphenol A and adverse pregnancy outcomes: a systematic review of the literature. J. Matern Neonatal Med. 2017;31:3320–7.

86. Ejaredar M, Lee Y, Roberts DJ, Sauve R, Dewey D. Bisphenol A exposure and children's behavior: a systematic review. J. Expo. Sci. Environ. Epidemiol. 2016;27:175–83.

87. Padmanabhan V, Siefert K, Ransom S, Johnson T, Pinkerton J, Anderson L, et al. Maternal bisphenol-A levels at delivery: a looming problem? J Perinatol. 2008;28:258–63.

88. Balakrishnan B, Henare K, Thorstensen EB, Ponnampalam AP, Mitchell MD. Transfer of bisphenol A across the human placenta. Am J Obstet Gynecol. 2010;202:e1–7.

89. Wolff MS, Engel SM, Berkowitz GS, Ye X, Silva MJ, Zhu C, et al. Prenatal phenol and phthalate exposures and birth outcomes. Environ Health Perspect. 2008; 116:1092–7.

90. Braun JM, Yolton K, Dietrich KN, Hornung R, Ye X, Calafat AM, et al. Prenatal bisphenol A exposure and early childhood behavior. Environ Health Perspect. 2009;117:1945–52.

91. US Food and Drug Administration. Update on bisphenol A for use in food contact applications. 2010 [updated 2014; cited 2023 Jun 3]. Available from: https://www.fda.gov/media/90124/download.

92. Bisphenol A (BPA): use in food contact application. Updated 2014 Nov [cited 2022 Feb 2]. Available from: https://www.fda.gov/food/food-additives-petitions/bisphenol-bpa-use-food-contact-application.

93. Harley KG, Kogut K, Madrigal DS, Cardenas M, Vera IA, Meza-Alfaro G, et al. Reducing phthalate, paraben, and phenol exposure from personal care products in adolescent girls: findings from the HERMOSA intervention study. Environ Health Perspect. 2016;124:1600–7.

94. Bornehag CG, Carlstedt F, Jönsson BA, Lindh CH, Jensen TK, Bodin A, et al. Prenatal phthalate exposures and anogenital distance in Swedish boys. Environ Health Perspect. 2015;123:101–7.

95. Sathyanarayana S, Grady R, Barrett ES, Redmon B, Nguyen RHN, Barthold JS, et al. First trimester phthalate exposure and male newborn genital anomalies. Environ Res. 2016;151:777–82.

96. Zhang Y, Mustieles V, Yland J, Braun JM, Williams PL, Attaman JA, et al. Association of parental preconception exposure to phthalates and phthalate substitutes with preterm birth. JAMA Netw Open. 2020;3:e202159.

97. Engel SM, Miodovnik A, Canfield RL, Zhu C, Silva MJ, Calafat AM, et al. Prenatal phthalate exposure is associated with childhood behavior and executive functioning. Environ Health Perspect. 2010;118:565–71.

98. Radke EG, Braun JM, Nachman RM, Cooper GS. Phthalate exposure and neurodevelopment: a systematic review and meta-analysis of human epidemiological evidence. Environ Int. 2020;137:105408.

99. Pedersen M, Stayner L, Slama R, Sørensen M, Figueras F, Nieuwenhuijsen MJ, et al. Ambient air pollution and pregnancy-induced hypertensive disorders: a systematic review and metaanalysis. Hypertension. 2014;64: 494–500.

100. Klepac P, Locatelli I, Korošec S, Künzli N, Kukec A. Ambient air pollution and pregnancy outcomes: a comprehensive review and identification of environmental public health challenges. Environ Res. 2018;167:144–59.

101. Trasande L, Malecha P, Attina TM. Particulate matter exposure and preterm birth estimates of U.S. attributable burden and economic costs. Environ Health Perspect. 2016; 124:1913–18.

102. DeFranco E, Hall E, Hossain M, Chen A, Haynes EN, Jones D, et al. Air pollution and stillbirth risk: exposure to airborne particulate matter during pregnancy is associated with fetal death. PLoS One. 2015;10:e0120594.

103. Yang S, Tan Y, Mei H, Wang F, Li N, Zhao J, et al. Ambient air pollution the risk of stillbirth: a prospective birth cohort study in Wuhan, China. Int J Hyg Environ Health. 2018;221:502–9.

104. Yuan L, Zhang Y, Gao Y, Tian Y. Maternal fine particulate matter (PM$_{2.5}$) exposure and adverse birth outcomes: an updated systematic review based on cohort studies. Environ Sci Pollut Res Int. 2019;26:13963–83.

105. Westergaard N, Gehring U, Slama R, Pedersen M. Ambient air pollution and low birth weight - are some women more vulnerable than others? Environ Int. 2017;104:146–54.

106. Weisskopf MG, Kioumourtzoglou MA, Roberts AL. Air pollution and autism spectrum disorders: causal or confounded? Curr Environ Health Rep. 2015;2:430–9.

107. Padula AM, Yang W, Carmichael SL, Tager IB, Lurmann F, Hammond SK, et al. Air pollution, neighbourhood socioeconomic factors, and neural tube defects in the San Joaquin Valley of California. Paediatr Perinat Epidemiol. 2015;29:536–45.

Chapter 5
Genetic Screening for Mendelian Disorders

Deborah A. Driscoll and Lorraine Dugoff
Department of Obstetrics and Gynecology, Perelman School of Medicine at the University of Pennsylvania, Philadelphia, PA, USA

Genetic screening to identify couples at risk for having offspring with inherited conditions such as Tay-Sachs disease, sickle cell disease, and cystic fibrosis has been integrated into obstetric practice. The number of genetic conditions for which carrier screening and genetic testing is available continues to increase. The decision to offer population-based genetic screening is complex due to disease prevalence, carrier frequency; nature and severity of the disorder; options for treatment; intervention and prevention; availability of a sensitive and specific screening and diagnostic test; positive predictive value of the test; and cost [1]. Care must be taken to avoid the potential for psychological harm to the patient and the misuse of genetic information and possible discrimination. Successful implementation of genetic screening programs requires educational materials for providers and patients and genetic counseling services. This chapter reviews Mendelian inheritance, indications for genetic screening, and the current carrier screening guidelines for common genetic disorders.

Family history

Genetic screening begins with an accurate family history, which should be a routine part of a patient's complete evaluation. It is useful to summarize this information in a pedigree to demonstrate the family relationships and which relatives are affected. The family history should include three generations; the sex and state of health should be noted. Stillbirths and miscarriage should be recorded. A history of the more common genetic diseases, chromosomal abnormalities, and congenital malformations such as cardiac defects, cleft lip and palate, and neural tube defects should be routinely sought. The history should also include cognitive and behavioral disorders such as intellectual disability, autism, developmental delay, and psychiatric disorders.

Cancer and age at diagnosis should be noted. Genetic diagnoses should be confirmed by review of the medical records whenever possible. Pedigree analysis is important in determining the type of inheritance of a given Mendelian disorder and is important in providing accurate risk estimate.

Mendelian inheritance

Mendelian inheritance refers to genetic disorders that arise as a result of transmission of a pathogenic variant (formerly referred to as a mutation) in a single gene. Most single-gene disorders are uncommon, usually occurring in 1 in 10 000–50 000 births. Over 11 000 single-gene disorders or traits have been described and can be found in the Online Mendelian Inheritance in Man (OMIM) (www.OMIM.org) [2]. Obstetricians should be familiar with the inheritance patterns and some of the common disorders for which carrier screening is available.

There are three basic patterns of Mendelian inheritance:
- autosomal dominant
- autosomal recessive
- X-linked

Genes occur in pairs; one copy is present on each one of a pair of chromosomes. If the effects of an abnormal gene are evident when the gene is present in a single dose, then the gene is said to be dominant. A carrier of an autosomal dominant disorder has a 50% chance of transmitting the disorder to his or her offspring. In general, pedigree analysis shows the disease in every generation with some exceptions. In some families, the disorder may not be expressed in every individual who inherits the gene. This is referred to as incomplete or reduced penetrance. Affected relatives may have a variable phenotype as a result of differences in expression. Modifying genes and/or the environment can influence the phenotype and hence it may be difficult to predict the outcome accurately. Autosomal dominant disorders may also arise as a result of a sporadic or *de novo* pathogenic variant. If this occurs then a couple does not have a 50% risk of having a subsequent affected child unless germline mosaicism exists. Germline mosaicism refers to the existence of a population of cells with the pathogenic variant in the testes or ovary.

For an autosomal recessive disorder to be expressed, both copies of the gene must be abnormal. Carriers of autosomal recessive disorders are detected either through carrier screening or after the birth of an affected child or relative. Pedigree analysis typically shows only siblings to be affected. In general, carriers are healthy although at the cellular level they may demonstrate reduced enzyme levels; this is not sufficient to cause disease. For example, Tay-Sachs carriers have a reduced level of hexosaminidase A. When both parents are carriers there is a 25% chance of having an affected child and a 50% chance of having a child who is a carrier in each pregnancy.

X-linked diseases such as Duchenne muscular dystrophy or hemophilia primarily affect males because they have a single X chromosome. In contrast, female carriers are less likely to be affected because of the presence of two X chromosomes. A female carrier may show manifestations of the disease because of unfavorable lyonization or inactivation of the X chromosome with the normal copy of the gene. A female who carries a gene causing an X-linked recessive condition has a 50% chance of transmitting the gene in each pregnancy; 50% of the male fetuses will be affected and 50% of the females will be carriers. X-linked disorders can also occur as a result of a *de novo* pathogenic variant. The mother of a child with an X-linked condition is not necessarily a carrier. Similar to autosomal dominant disorders, germline mosaicism must also be considered. A male with an X-linked disorder will pass the abnormal gene on his X chromosome to all of his daughters who will be carriers; his sons receive his Y chromosome and hence will be unaffected. X-linked dominant disorders such as incontinentia pigmenti are rare and affect females; they tend to be lethal in males.

It is now recognized that some genetic conditions do not follow simple Mendelian inheritance. Some genes contain a region of trinucleotide repeats (i.e. (CCG)n) that are unstable and may expand during transmission from parent to offspring. When the number of repeats reaches a critical level, the gene becomes methylated and is no longer expressed (e.g. fragile X syndrome). Testing is available to determine if an individual with a positive family history of intellectual disability carries a premutation, which may expand to a full mutation in their offspring. Trinucleotide repeats are also implicated in several neurologic disorders such as Huntington disease and myotonic dystrophy [3].

Carrier screening

Carrier screening refers to the identification of an individual who is heterozygous or has a pathogenic variant in one of two copies of the gene. The screening test may identify an individual with two pathogenic variants who is so mildly affected it has escaped medical attention. Ideally, carrier screening should be offered to patients and their partners prior to conception to provide them with an accurate assessment of their risk of having an affected child and a full range of reproductive options. Most screening takes place during pregnancy and should be performed as early as possible to allow couples an opportunity to have prenatal diagnostic testing. When carrier screening is performed during an ongoing pregnancy, it is ideal to perform screening on both partners simultaneously so that the results can be obtained in a timely manner. When both parents are carriers or if a patient is a carrier of an X-linked condition, genetic counseling is recommended and they are informed of the availability of prenatal diagnostic testing, preimplantation genetic diagnosis, donor gametes (eggs or sperm), and adoption to avoid the risk for having an affected child. It is helpful to explore their attitudes towards prenatal testing and termination of pregnancy. In addition, they may consider contacting their relatives at risk and informing them of the availability of carrier screening.

In the United States, preconception or prenatal genetic screening tests are available for many inherited conditions. Carrier screening was initially used to screen for conditions based on a patient's family history and race or ethnicity. Ethnicity-based screening is limited as many individuals do not have accurate knowledge of their race or ancestry. Furthermore, restriction of carrier screening based on race or ethnicity is inequitable and has been demonstrated to result in failure to identify carriers who are not from the targeted racial or ethnic group [4]. Panethnic screening, in which carrier screening is offered to all individuals regardless of ethnicity, was first offered for cystic fibrosis and spinal muscular atrophy [5]. Recent advances in next-generation-sequencing technology have enabled high throughput identification of sequence variants across many genes simultaneously at a relatively low cost. This testing strategy is known as expanded carrier screening, which is panethnic screening on a large scale. An expanded carrier screening approach has the potential to identify more pregnancies at risk for severe or profound inherited conditions.

Pretest counseling should be provided prior to carrier screening and counseling points are summarized in Box 5.1. Information about specific genetic disorders and testing can be found on GeneReviews® at www.ncbi.nlm.nih.gov/books/NBK1116. For some patients, genetic counseling may assist with the decision-making process. Patients should also be assured that their test results are confidential and protected by the Genetic Information and Non-Discrimination Act of 2008.

Box 5.1 Pretest counseling points for expanded carrier screening

1. Carrier screening is optional. Patients can choose to participate or decline.
2. Expanded carrier screening panels include conditions that may vary in severity. The panels include many conditions that are associated with significant adverse outcomes including decreased life expectancy, cognitive impairment, and the need for medical and/or surgical intervention.
3. A negative test reduces the chance of having an affected child. It does not eliminate the risk (concept of residual risk).
4. It is common to identify carriers for one or more conditions when using expanded screening panels. In most cases, being a carrier has no significant medical consequences for the individual. If two partners are carriers of different autosomal recessive conditions, offspring are not likely to be affected.
5. Accurate knowledge of paternity is necessary to provide accurate information regarding risk. DNA (or blood) from the biological father is necessary in order to provide risk assessments for autosomal recessive conditions.
6. It is possible that carrier screening will determine that an individual has two pathogenic variants for a condition and thus has an autosomal recessive condition that might affect their health. Expanded carrier screening panels that include autosomal dominant and X-linked conditions may detect individuals affected with one of these conditions. In these situations, individuals should be referred for genetic counseling and appropriate medical management.

Adapted from [6,8].

Carrier screening guidelines

The American College of Obstetricians and Gynecologists (ACOG) states that ethnic-specific, panethnic, and expanded carrier screening are all acceptable strategies for carrier screening. ACOG recommends that each obstetrician-gynecologist, other health care provider, or practice should establish a standard approach that is consistently offered to and discussed with each patient, ideally preconception. If a patient requests a screening strategy other than the one used by the practice or health care provider, the requested test should be made available to the patient after counseling, which should include a discussion of the limitations, benefits, and alternatives. ACOG suggests that conditions included on an expanded carrier screening panel have a severe or moderate phenotype with a frequency of 1 in 100 or greater [7]. At a minimum, ACOG recommends panethnic screening for cystic fibrosis and spinal muscular atrophy as well as a complete blood count and screening for hemoglobinopathies. Fragile X premutation carrier screening is recommended for women with a family history of fragile X-related disorders or intellectual disability suggestive of fragile X syndrome or women with a personal history of ovarian insufficiency. ACOG recommends offering additional screening based on ethnicity or family history including screening for a limited number of diseases in individuals of Ashkenazi Jewish ancestry [5]. These disorders are briefly described next and in Table 5.1.

In 2021, The American College of Medical Genetics and Genomics (ACMG) published a recommendation to offer all pregnant patients and those planning a pregnancy carrier screening with a panel of conditions that have a severe or moderate phenotype and a carrier frequency of ≥1/200 in any ethnic group. This panel consists of 97 autosomal recessive conditions and 16 X-linked conditions. ACMG recommends offering panels that include additional less common genes when a pregnancy is the result of a known or possible consanguineous relationship

Table 5.1 Mendelian disorders frequent among individuals of Ashkenazi Jewish ancestry

Disorder	Carrier rate	Clinical features
Tay-Sachs disease	1 in 30	Hypotonia, developmental delay, loss of developmental milestones, mental retardation beginning at 5–6 m, loss of sight at 12–18 m, usually fatal by age 6
Canavan disease	1 in 40	Hypotonia, developmental delay, seizures, blindness, large head, gastrointestinal reflux
Familial dysautonomia	1 in 32	Abnormal suck, feeding difficulties, episodic vomiting, abnormal sweating, pain and temperature instability, labile blood pressure, absent tearing, scoliosis
Cystic fibrosis	1 in 24	Chronic pulmonary infections, malabsorption, failure to thrive, pancreatitis, male infertility because of congenital absence of the vas deferens
Fanconi anemia type C	1 in 89	Limb, cardiac, and genitourinary anomalies, microcephaly, mental retardation, developmental delay, anemia, pancytopenia, and increased risk for leukemia
Niemann-Pick type A	1 in 90	Jaundice and ascites caused by liver disease, pulmonary disease, developmental delay and psychomotor retardation, progressive decline in cognitive ability and speech, dysphagia, seizures, hypotonia, abnormal gait
Bloom syndrome	1 in 100	Prenatal and postnatal growth deficiency, predisposition to malignancies, facial telangiectasias, abnormal skin pigmentation, learning difficulties, mental retardation
Mucolipidosis IV	1 in 127	Growth and severe psychomotor retardation, corneal clouding, progressive retinal degeneration, strabismus
Gaucher disease	1 in 15	Chronic fatigue, anemia, easy bruising, nosebleeds, bleeding gums, menorrhagia, hepatosplenomegaly, osteoporosis, bone and joint pain

Note: carrier rates apply to individuals of Eastern European Jewish ancestry; clinical features may vary in presentation, severity, and age of onset.

defined as second cousins or closer or if this is warranted based on a family or personal medical history [8].

Patients with a family history of a single gene disorder should be referred to a genetics professional. When a family history suggests that a patient or partner may be at increased risk to be a carrier or to have a child with an inherited condition, the first step is to determine if the gene for that disorder has been identified. If the gene is known, the optimal strategy is to test the affected relative. Many disorders are caused by variants unique to a family, and DNA sequencing is required to identify the disease-causing variant. Once the disease-causing variant is confirmed in the affected individual, testing relatives at risk to be carriers is possible.

Carrier screening tests may be helpful when a particular diagnosis is suspected based on ultrasound findings in the pregnancy. The antenatal evaluation of a fetus with a congenital malformation typically includes a thorough ultrasound examination and fetal echocardiogram to look for associated anomalies, as well as a fetal chromosomal microarray. Single-gene disorders are often considered in the differential diagnosis but until recently were not amenable to prenatal testing. Now that the molecular basis and in many cases the disease-causing variants of many of these disorders have been elucidated, either carrier screening of the parents or diagnostic testing of the pregnancy is possible when a particular diagnosis is suspected. For example, carrier screening for Fanconi anemia type C may be considered as part of the evaluation of a fetus with absent radius [9], particularly if the couple are of Ashkenazi Jewish ancestry, because the carrier frequency is 1 in 90 in this population and a single variant accounts for 99% of the disease-causing variants. Testing the parents to determine their carrier status can help establish or exclude a diagnosis in the fetus with an anomaly.

Hemoglobinopathies

The hemoglobinopathies include structural hemoglobin variants and the thalassemias. Sickle cell disease, a severe form of anemia, is an autosomal recessive disorder common among individuals of African origin but also found in Mediterranean, Arab, southern Iranian, and Asian Indian populations. Approximately 1 in 12 African-Americans is a carrier or has sickle cell trait (Hb AS). The underlying abnormality is a single nucleotide substitution (GAG to GTG) in the sixth codon of the β-globin gene. This mutation leads to the substitution of the amino acid valine for glutamic acid. Sickle cell disorders also include other structural variants of β-hemoglobin. Screening is best accomplished by complete blood count (CBC) with red blood cell indices and a hemoglobin electrophoresis.

The thalassemias are a heterogeneous group of hereditary anemias brought about by reduced synthesis of globin chains. α-thalassemia results from the deletion of 2–4 copies of the α-globin gene. The disorder is most common among individuals of Southeast Asian descent. If one or two of the genes are deleted, the individual will have α-thalassemia minor, which is usually asymptomatic. Deletion of three genes results in hemoglobin H disease, which is a more severe anemia, and a fetus with deletions of all four α-chain genes can make only an unstable hemoglobin (Bart hemoglobin) that causes lethal hydrops fetalis and is associated with preeclampsia. α-thalassemia is also common among individuals of African descent but typically does not result in hydrops.

The β-thalassemias are caused by mutations in the β-globin gene that result in defective or absent β-chain synthesis. β-thalassemia is more common in Mediterranean countries, the Middle East, South East Asia, and parts of India and Pakistan. The heterozygous carrier (P-thalassemia minor) is not usually associated with clinical disability, except in periods of stress. Individuals who are homozygous (β-thalassemia major or Cooley anemia) have severe anemia, failure to thrive, hepatosplenomegaly, growth retardation, and bony changes secondary to marrow hypertrophy. The mean corpuscular volume (MCV) is performed as an initial screening test for patients at risk. Individuals with low MCV (<80 μL^3) should undergo hemoglobin electrophoresis; β-thalassemia carriers have an elevated HbA_2 ($>3.5\%$) or HbF. Diagnosis of α-thalassemia trait is by exclusion of iron deficiency and molecular detection of α-globin gene deletions.

Cystic fibrosis

Cystic fibrosis is an autosomal recessive condition that primarily affects the pulmonary and gastrointestinal system. Cystic fibrosis results from pathogenic variants in the cystic fibrosis transmembrane conductance regulator (CFTR) protein. The most common variant is ΔF508, although over 2000 other disease-causing variants have been described [10]. For individuals with a family history of cystic fibrosis, screening with an expanded panel of pathogenic variants or complete analysis of the CFTR gene by sequencing may be indicated if the disease-causing variant has not been previously identified in the affected relative. Patients with a reproductive partner with cystic fibrosis or congenital absence of the vas deferens may also benefit from this approach. Genetic counseling in these situations is usually beneficial. Cystic fibrosis carrier screening may also identify individuals with two disease-causing variants who have not been previously diagnosed as having cystic fibrosis and should be referred to a specialist for further evaluation.

Spinal muscular atrophy

Spinal muscular atrophy is an autosomal recessive disorder characterized by progressive degeneration of motor neurons with resultant atrophy of skeletal muscle and overall weakness. Variants in the survival motor neuron gene (SMN1) cause spinal muscular atrophy. There are several types of spinal muscular atrophy associated with a wide range of severity ranging from a severe form with symptomatic onset before 6 months and death within the first 2 years of life due to respiratory failure to a milder adult-onset form with a normal life expectancy. Genetic testing for spinal muscular atrophy is complex and, in some cases, precise prediction of the phenotype in affected fetuses may not be possible [5,11].

Fragile X syndrome

Fragile X syndrome, inherited in an X-linked dominant fashion, is the most common cause of inherited intellectual disability and the leading monogenic cause of autism. Hallmark physical features include a long face with prominent ears, hyperextensible joints and macroorchidism. Fragile X syndrome is caused by expansion of a repeated trinucleotide segment that leads to altered transcription of the Fragile X mental retardation 1 (FMR1) gene. Transmission of Fragile X syndrome to a fetus depends on the sex of the parent transmitting the mutation, the number of cytosine-guanine-guanine repeats present in the parental gene and the number of AGG interruptions. Repeat expansion rarely occurs in males. Females with a premutation or a full mutation are at greatest risk of transmitting an expanded full mutation fragile X allele to their offspring. All individuals with intermediate results and carriers of a Fragile X premutation or full mutation should receive genetic counseling to discuss the risk to their offspring of inheriting an expanded full-mutation and to discuss fragile X-associated disorders including premature ovarian failure and fragile X tremor/ataxia syndrome which may affect premutation carriers [5,12]

Jewish genetic diseases

There are a number of autosomal recessive conditions that are more common in individuals of Ashkenazi (Eastern European Jewish) descent (Table 5.1). Several are lethal or associated with significant morbidity. Tay-Sachs was the first disorder amenable to carrier screening based on the measurement of serum or leukocyte hexosaminidase A levels. Today, similar detection rates can be achieved with molecular testing [13]. In addition to Tay-Sachs, ACOG recommends carrier testing for Canavan disease, familial dysautonomia, and cystic fibrosis be offered when one or both parents are of Ashkenazi Jewish descent. These disorders share similar prevalence and carrier rates. The sensitivity of these tests is also very high (95% or higher) and thus, a negative result indicates that the risk of having a child with the disorder is very low. Carrier screening should also be considered for other conditions listed in Table 5.1 [5].

Prenatal diagnosis

Invasive prenatal diagnostic testing is available for patients identified through carrier screening to be at increased risk for having an affected offspring (see Chapter 52). Molecular testing for the specific gene variants can be performed on cells obtained through chorionic villus sampling at 10–12 weeks gestation or amniocentesis after 15 weeks gestation.

Newborn screening

Carriers of Mendelian disorders may be identified through state newborn screening programs, identifying newborns with inherited metabolic disorders who would benefit from early detection and treatment. However, advances in genetics and technology have led to expanded screening programs that include testing for hemoglobinopathies, endocrine disorders, hearing loss, and infectious diseases. Newborn screening for most Mendelian disorders is performed by collecting capillary blood from a heel puncture onto a filter paper. Specimens are then sent to a reference laboratory where they are assayed for the specified diseases. Confirmatory testing is necessary because of the high false-positive rate on the initial screen. In addition to the appropriate referral of the infant for treatment, genetic counseling of the couple is recommended to review the recurrence risk and reproductive options.

CASE PRESENTATION

A 26-year-old healthy primigravida presents for prenatal care at 8 weeks gestation. There is no family history of congenital malformations, genetic disorders, intellectual disability, developmental delay, or neurologic or psychiatric conditions. The patient is of Ashkenazi Jewish descent. Her partner is Caucasian of Northern European descent. Recent CBC was normal.

Her health care provider informs the patient that an expanded carrier screening panel is available that includes screening for cystic fibrosis, spinal muscular atrophy, conditions more common in individuals of Ashkenazi Jewish ancestry as well as additional conditions associated with a severe or moderate phenotype. The patient is informed that the decision to proceed with carrier screening is hers and testing is voluntary. The patient is provided with a pamphlet about carrier screening and informed that ideally screening should be performed on both partners simultaneously so that the results can be obtained in a timely manner. The patient and her partner elect to have concurrent expanded carrier screening.

The patient is determined to be a carrier for Bloom syndrome. The patient's partner is a carrier of ΔF508, the most common pathogenic variant found in approximately 70% of cystic fibrosis patients. The obstetrician explains that although the patient and her partner are each carriers of an autosomal recessive disorder, they have a low risk of having a child affected with either disorder since they are not carriers for the same condition. The obstetrician informs the patient and her partner that although the chance of the couple having a child affected with either disorder is very low, it is not zero due to residual risk. Based on this information the patient elects not to have prenatal diagnostic testing.

The patient and her partner are informed that they inherited the variants for the respective conditions from one of their parents so their siblings may also be carriers and that they share this information with them.

References

1. Holtzman NA. Newborn screening for genetic-metabolic diseases: progress, principles and recommendations. Publication No. (HSA) 78-5207. Washington, DC: US Department of Health, Education, and Welfare; 1977.

2. Mendelian Inheritance in Man, OMIM. [updated 2023 Jun 2; cited 2023 Jun 4]. Available from: www.OMIM.org.

3. American College of Obstetricians and Gynecologists. ACOG Technology Assessment in Obstetrics and Gynecology No. 14: modern genetics in obstetrics and gynecology. Obstet Gynecol. 2018;132:e143–68.

4. Lazarin GA, Haque IS, Nazareth S, Iori K, Patterson AS, Jacobson JL, et al. An empirical estimate of carrier frequencies for 400+ causal Mendelian variants: results from an ethnically diverse clinical sample of 23 453 individuals. Genet Med. 2013;15(3):178–86.

5. American College of Obstetricians and Gynecologists. Committee Opinion No. 691: carrier screening for genetic conditions. Obstet Gynecol. 2017;129:e41–55.

6. Edwards JG, Feldman G, Goldberg J, Gregg AR, Norton ME, Rose NC, et al. Expanded carrier screening in reproductive medicine–points to consider. A joint statement of the American College of Medical Genetics and Genomics, American College of Obstetricians and Gynecologists, National Society of Genetic Counselors, Perinatal Quality Foundation, and Society for Maternal-Fetal Medicine. Obstet Gynecol. 2015;125:653–62.

7. American College of Obstetricians and Gynecologists. Committee Opinion No. 690: carrier screening in the age of genomic medicine. Obstet Gynecol. 2017;129:e35–40.

8. Gregg AR, Arabi M, Klugman S, Leach NT, Bashford MT, Goldwaser T, et al. Screening for autosomal recessive and X-linked conditions during pregnancy and preconception: a practice resource of the American College of Medical Genetics and Genomics (ACMG). Genet Med. 2021;23(10):1793–1806. doi: 10.1038/s41436-021- 01203-z.

9. Merrill A, Rosenblum-Vos L, Driscoll DA, Daley K, Treat K. Prenatal diagnosis of Fanconi anemia (Group C) subsequent to abnormal sonographic findings. Prenat Diagn. 2005;25:20–2.

10. De Boeck K. Cystic fibrosis in the year 2020: a disease with a new face. Acta Pediatr. 2020;109:893–9.

11. D'Amico A, Mercuri E, Tiziano F, Bertini E. Spinal muscular atrophy. Orphanet J Rare Dis. 2011;6:71.

12. Mila M, Alvarez-Mora MI, Madrigal I, Rodriguez-Revenga L, Fragile X syndrome: An overview and update of the FMR1 gene. Clin Genet. 2018;93:197–205.

13. Eng CM, Desnick RJ. Experiences in molecular- based screening for Ashkenazi Jewish genetic disease. Adv Genet. 2001;44:275–96.

Chapter 6
Screening for Congenital Heart Disease

Lynn L. Simpson

Department of Obstetrics and Gynecology, Columbia University Irving Medical Center, New York, NY, USA

Introduction

In recent years, the approach to screening for congenital heart disease has expanded with strategies based on risk and gestational age. For the majority of patients at low risk for fetal heart anomalies, a collaborative practice parameter by the American Institute of Ultrasound in Medicine (AIUM), the American College of Radiology (ACR), the American College of Obstetricians and Gynecologists (ACOG), the Society for Maternal-Fetal Medicine (SMFM), and the Society of Radiologists in Ultrasound (SRU) now recommends that at the time of a standard screening ultrasound examination in the midtrimester, the four-chamber view and views of the outflow tracts be evaluated along with the three-vessel and three-vessel trachea views if technically feasible [1].

For patients at high risk of fetal anomalies, early screening may be warranted. A detailed diagnostic obstetric ultrasound between 12 weeks 0 days and 13 weeks 6 days requires an assessment of cardiac position and axis, the four-chamber view without and with color, and the three-vessel and trachea view with color [2]. For patients suspected to have fetal anomalies that require a detailed second- or third-trimester diagnostic obstetric ultrasound examination, additional assessments are advised. Besides the standard cardiac views, an evaluation of situs, the interventricular septum, the superior and inferior venae cavae, the ductal and aortic arches, and the three-vessel and three-vessel and trachea view are required [3].

As outlined in a collaborative guideline from AIUM, ACOG, ACR, American Society of Echocardiography, Fetal Heart Society, International Society of Ultrasound in Obstetrics and Gynecology, SMFM, and SRU, fetal echocardiography with multiple cardiac views and specialized assessments is indicated for all patients at high risk for congenital heart disease [4]. This includes patients with high-risk maternal, familial, environmental, or fetal factors such as a suspected cardiac structural anomaly or functional abnormality identified during a standard or detailed obstetric ultrasound examination [4]. Although fetal echocardiography is commonly performed between 18 and 22 weeks of gestation, it may be performed late in the first trimester or early in the second trimester in highly specialized centers.

Screening low-risk populations

Congenital heart disease is a common condition that warrants prenatal screening of all pregnancies. With a prevalence of 6 per 1000 live births, it is estimated that 10 of every 1000 fetuses scanned in the second trimester will have a heart anomaly and half of these will be major with serious consequences [5,6]. Intrauterine fetal death occurs in 20–30% of cases, neonatal death in 40–60%, and long-term survival rates are low, ranging from 15% to 40% [7]. The presence of extracardiac anomalies and chromosomal abnormalities contributes to the poor outlook. Overall, 25–45% of fetuses with congenital heart disease have other malformations and 15–50% have abnormal karyotypes [8–10]. Other poor prognostic signs include associated fetal arrhythmias, hemodynamic abnormalities, and the presence of hydrops.

Benefits of cardiac screening

Early prenatal diagnosis of major heart defects is important for counseling patients about pregnancy options, therapeutic interventions, changes in obstetric care, and alternative plans for delivery. Studies have shown that when major congenital heart disease is diagnosed in the second trimester of pregnancy, many patients opt for termination [11]. In one survey of 65 women who previously had borne a child with congenital heart

---

disease, 58% said they would elect to terminate a subsequent affected pregnancy [12].

Without universal screening, the prenatal diagnosis of congenital heart disease is often made late in gestation when options are limited. With early screening and detection of congenital heart disease, patients and their families have time to consider the implications of the condition and to make choices that are best for them. Therapeutic interventions and improved neonatal survival are possible when particular heart malformations are detected prenatally and the timing, mode, and location of delivery can be planned [13]. Referral to a tertiary care center where immediate therapeutic and palliative interventions are available can be life saving. Prompt infusion of prostaglandin E_1 or balloon atrial septostomy can significantly improve prognosis for newborns with certain cardiac defects that require postnatal maintenance of fetal flow pathways. Immediate institution of extracorporeal membrane oxygenation can make the difference between life and death in complex cardiac anomalies, particularly when associated with other structural defects such as congenital diaphragmatic hernia. Experienced neonatologists, pediatric cardiologists, and cardiac surgeons may have a significant impact of an infant's condition and ultimate outcome.

Universal screening for major cardiac anomalies in the general population is essential to reduce the long-term morbidity and mortality of this disease. In experienced centers, routine screening can reassure patients that the fetal heart is normal or identify those patients in need of fetal echocardiography.

High-risk populations for fetal echocardiography

The conventional strategy for the prenatal detection of congenital heart disease has been to refer patients identified to be at risk for fetal echocardiography [4] (see Box 6.1). Unfortunately, it is estimated that over half of prenatal detected heart anomalies are found in patients with no preexisting risk factors and that most cardiac malformations would be missed if fetal echocardiography were done based on these factors alone [14,15]. Despite the initial enthusiasm for nuchal translucency as a screening tool for congenital heart disease, its performance in large studies of unselected and low-risk populations has been disappointing [16,17]. However, it is a reasonable marker or risk factor for major heart anomalies and warrants referral for fetal echocardiography.

Interestingly, the factor most predictive of congenital heart disease is an abnormal cardiac examination at the

Box 6.1 Reasons to refer for fetal echocardiography

Maternal indications

- Pregestational diabetes
- Gestational diabetes diagnosed in first or early second trimester
- In vitro fertilization
- Phenylketonuria
- Autoimmune disease with anti-Sjogren syndrome-related antigen A antibodies and with a prior affected fetus
- First-degree relative of a fetus with congenital heart disease
- First- or second-degree relative with disease of Mendelian inheritance and a history of childhood cardiac manifestations
- Retinoid exposure
- First-trimester rubella infection

Consider if

- Selected teratogen exposure (e.g. paroxetine, carbamazepine, lithium, angiotensin-converting enzyme inhibitors)
- Autoimmune disease with Sjogren syndrome-related antigen A positivity and without a prior affected fetus
- Second-degree relative of a fetus with congenital heart disease

Fetal indications

- Suspected cardiac structural anomaly
- Suspected abnormality in cardiac function
- Hydrops fetalis
- Persistent fetal tachycardia
- Persistent fetal bradycardia
- Frequent episode or a persistently irregular cardiac rhythm
- Major extracardiac anomaly
- Nuchal translucency of 3.5 mm or greater or at or above the 99th percentile for gestational age
- Chromosomal abnormality by diagnostic genetic testing or suspected on cell-free fetal DNA screening
- Monochorionic twinning

Consider if

- Systemic venous anomaly (e.g. persistent right umbilical vein, left superior vena cava, absent ductus venosus)
- Nuchal translucency between 3.0 and 3.4 mm

Adapted from [4].

time of prenatal ultrasonography. In one study of fetal echocardiography, only 4% of patients were referred because of an abnormal cardiac screen, yet defects were detected at a rate of 68% in this group, far in excess of the rate for all other risk factors combined [14]. In many centers, an abnormal cardiac screen during routine obstetric ultrasonography has become the most common reason for referral for fetal echocardiography with a high yield for heart defects [15,18].

Normal fetal heart anatomy

Normal fetal heart anatomy can be visualized with confidence as early as 13–14 weeks of gestation by the transvaginal approach in highly specialized centers [7]. Although patients at risk may benefit from early echocardiography, screening for normal fetal heart anatomy at 18–22 weeks of gestation seems ideal for the low-risk patient [1]. For low-risk populations, the four-chamber view, views of the ventricular outflow tracts, and the three-vessel and three-vessel trachea views if technically feasible are now recommended to evaluate the fetal heart [1]. A detailed obstetric ultrasound or fetal echocardiography is an extended examination with multiple views using additional imaging modalities for patients identified as being at increased risk for congenital heart disease, including those with an abnormal cardiac screen at the time of a standard ultrasound [3,4].

Technique

Two-dimensional cross-sectional imaging

The transabdominal approach is most often used for fetal cardiac screening performed beyond the first trimester of pregnancy. The determination of fetal lie and presentation in the uterus is critical for the evaluation of cardiac and abdominal situs. A transverse sweep through the fetus can quickly confirm normal situs with the stomach and apex of the heart on the left side of the fetus (Figure 6.1). During this sweep, the cardiac position in the fetal chest, cardiac axis, and size of the heart can be subjectively evaluated. On transverse imaging of the fetal abdomen, the inferior vena cava can be seen to the right of the fetal spine and the descending aorta to the left and anterior to the fetal spine.

Four-chamber view

The most important image of the fetal heart is obtained on a cross-sectional transverse view through the fetal chest and heart. The horizontal position of the heart in the chest during fetal life makes this plane easy to obtain in most instances. Although the appearance of the four-chamber view will vary depending on fetal lie and presentation, the landmarks remain the same. A transverse view of the fetal chest will be circular with the bony vertebral body posteriorly, the sternum anteriorly, and complete ribs laterally. A simple approach to the four-chamber view includes an evaluation of size, position, anatomy, and function of the fetal heart.

The four-chamber view is obtained on a transverse image of the fetal thorax just above the diaphragm (Plate 6.1). In this transverse plane, the fetal heart occupies about one third of the area of the fetal chest with an axis about 45° to the left. The atrial and ventricular chambers, interventricular septum, foramen ovale, and atrioventricular valves can all be assessed on the four-chamber view. The two atria and two ventricles should be similar in size, with the left atrium closest to the spine and the right ventricle closest to the sternum. In this transverse cross-sectional plane, the pulmonary veins may be seen entering the left atrium and the aorta descending between the left atrium and the spine. The flap of the foramen ovale should project into the left atrium through a patent foramen ovale. The internal surface of the left ventricle is

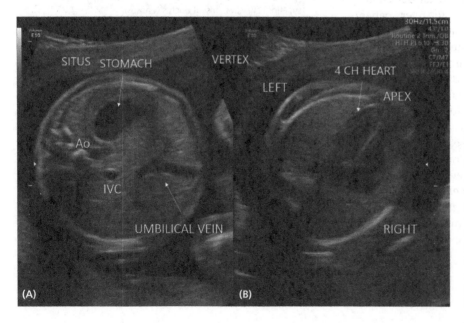

Figure 6.1 (A) Transverse two-dimensional ultrasound of the abdomen of a fetus in vertex presentation with normal left-sided stomach and descending abdominal aorta (Ao) and right-sided inferior vena cava (IVC) with intra-abdominal portion of the umbilical vein (*arrow*) coursing through the right-sided liver. (B) Transverse view of the chest of the same fetus demonstrating normal situs solitus with the fetal heart (*arrow*) in the left chest with its apex pointing leftward.

smooth compared with the trabeculated right ventricle containing the moderator band. The two atrioventricular valves meet at the junction of the interatrial and interventricular septa to form the crux of the heart. The mitral and tricuspid valves should move freely, with the tricuspid valve attached slightly more toward the apex than the mitral valve on the interventricular septum. Ventricular systolic function can be assessed subjectively by observing the ventricular wall movement during systole. The presence of a pericardial effusion also can be identified on the four-chamber view. Systematic evaluation of the four-chamber view can easily be incorporated into a routine 30-minute screening midtrimester ultrasound with adequate visualization in over 95% of fetuses [19].

Ventricular outflow tracts

A major limitation of cardiac screening with the four-chamber view alone is that conotruncal anomalies can easily be missed. Normal four-chamber screening can occur with transposition of the great arteries, tetralogy of Fallot, double-outlet right ventricle, pulmonary and aortic stenosis, and coarctation of the aorta [11]. It is estimated that defects of the great vessels are only associated with an abnormal four-chamber view in about 30% of cases [20]. Consequently, it is now recommended by multiple organizations that views of the aortic and pulmonary outflow tracts be included with an evaluation of the four-chamber view when screening for congenital heart disease [1,4].

With adequate training and experience, it is possible to visualize the four-chamber view and outflow tracts in 90% of pregnant women [21]. The long-axis view of the left ventricular outflow tract and the short-axis view of the right ventricular outflow tract are common images used to evaluate the proximal ventriculoarterial connections (Plates 6.2 and 6.3). The aortic and pulmonary outflow tracts are approximately equal in size in the midtrimester and should be seen to cross as they arise from their respective ventricles during real-time imaging. The aorta arises from the posterior ventricle and has branches originating from its arch that supply the head and upper extremities. The pulmonary artery arises from the anterior ventricle and branches into the ductus arteriosus and pulmonary arteries. The two semilunar valves should be seen to open and close with the pulmonary valve anterior and cranial to the aortic valve.

Three-vessel and three-vessel trachea views

Recent guidelines recommend an assessment of the three-vessel view and three-vessel trachea view when screening for congenital heart disease irrespective of risk [1,3,4]. These views are obtained on transverse images of the upper fetal chest superior to the origins of the great vessels. The information obtained on these two views can aid in the recognition of anomalies of the great vessels and abnormalities of the semilunar valves.

The three-vessel view can include the main pulmonary artery bifurcation or the ductal arch as well as the ascending aorta and superior vena cava [1,4] (see Figure 6.2). An assessment of the size and confluence of the branch pulmonary arteries on this view can be useful for postnatal management planning in cases of congenital heart disease such as tetralogy of Fallot.

The three-vessel trachea view has been used in clinical practice for many years. In this transverse image of the fetal chest just cephalad to the three-vessel view, the ductus arteriosus, transverse aortic arch, superior vena cava and cross-sectional view of the trachea can be evaluated (Plate 6.4). The trachea is often fluid filled and can be identified by its echogenic rings and lack of flow on color imaging. A number of parameters including vessel number, size, alignment, arrangement, direction and nature of flow should be assessed. The ductal arch, transverse aortic arch, and superior vena cava should be aligned left to right, anterior to posterior, and larger to smaller. Flow in the ductus arteriosus and transverse aortic arch should be from anterior to posterior where these two vessels form a "V" as they reach the descending thoracic aorta to the left of the fetal spine.

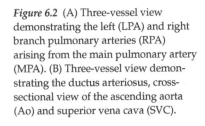

Figure 6.2 (A) Three-vessel view demonstrating the left (LPA) and right branch pulmonary arteries (RPA) arising from the main pulmonary artery (MPA). (B) Three-vessel view demonstrating the ductus arteriosus, cross-sectional view of the ascending aorta (Ao) and superior vena cava (SVC).

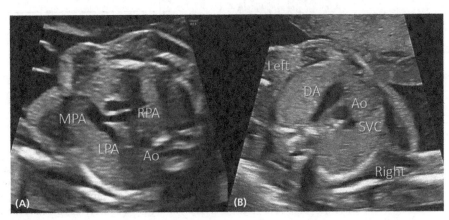

Additional cardiac views

Experts in advanced cardiac imaging and fetal echocardiography extend the examination of the fetal heart beyond the four-chamber view, proximal ventricular outflow tracts, and three-vessel views. A simple stepwise approach to the fetal heart may help to standardize two-dimensional fetal echocardiography [22]. This approach begins with a complete assessment of the four-chamber view followed by serial cephalad transverse planes to assess the great arteries and their connections, the three-vessel view, and the aortic arch (see Figure 6.3). Sweeping cephalad from the four-chamber view displays the five-chamber view, demonstrating the aorta arising from the left ventricle toward the right shoulder of the fetus. Cross-sectional transverse imaging just cephalad to this view shows the pulmonary artery arising from the anterior

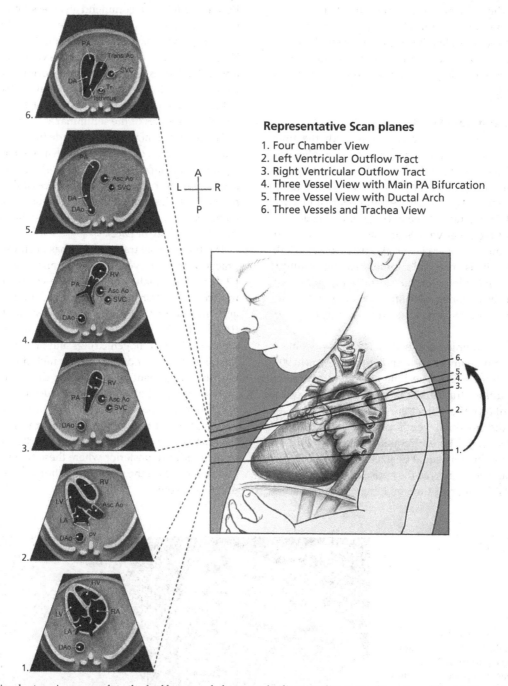

Representative Scan planes

1. Four Chamber View
2. Left Ventricular Outflow Tract
3. Right Ventricular Outflow Tract
4. Three Vessel View with Main PA Bifurcation
5. Three Vessel View with Ductal Arch
6. Three Vessels and Trachea View

Figure 6.3 A simple stepwise approach to the fetal heart can help to standardize two-dimensional imaging of the fetal heart during routine obstetric ultrasound. This approach begins with a complete assessment of the four-chamber view followed by serial cephalad transverse planes to assess the left ventricular outflow tract (LVOT), right ventricular outflow tract (RVOT), their connections, and the three-vessel and three-vessel trachea views [4]/with permission from John Wiley & Sons. PA, pulmonary artery.

right ventricle directed posteriorly to the fetal spine. During this axial sweep toward the fetal head, the left and right ventricular outflow tracts can be observed to cross at their origins with the aortic root located posterior to the main pulmonary trunk. The three-vessel and three-vessel trachea views of the superior vena cava, aorta, and pulmonary artery lie in transverse planes just above the origins of the great arteries and the transverse aortic arch lies just superior to the three-vessel view.

Although the transverse views of the fetal heart are often sufficient to evaluate the normal cardiac anatomy and screen for major anomalies, long-axis and oblique views of the heart may be useful when transverse views are difficult to obtain or when a cardiac defect is suspected. These images may include the short-axis view of the right ventricle and its outflow tract, the long-axis view of the left ventricle and its outflow tract, parasagittal views of the ductal arch and aortic arch, and the inferior vena cava and superior vena cava entering the right atrium (see Figure 6.4). These additional two-dimensional views complete the cross-sectional assessment of the major anatomic structures

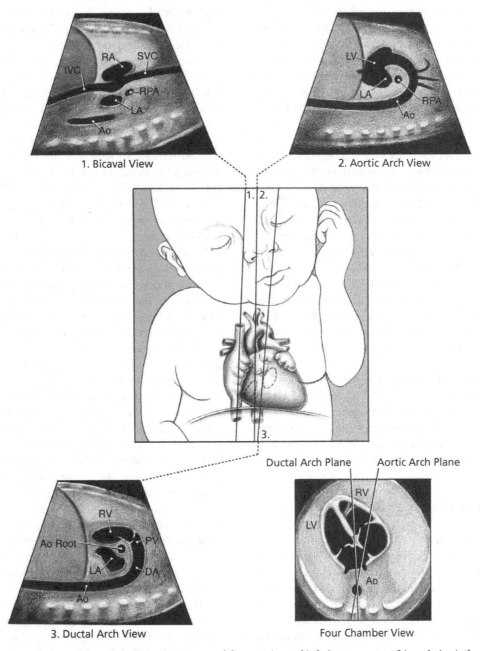

1. Bicaval View

2. Aortic Arch View

3. Ductal Arch View

Four Chamber View

Ductal Arch Plane   Aortic Arch Plane

Figure 6.4 A sagittal sweep from right-to-left allows assessment of the superior and inferior vena cavae (bicaval view), the aortic arch, and the ductal arch [4]/with permission from John Wiley & Sons. Ao, descending thoracic aorta; DA, ductus arteriosus; IVC, inferior vena cava; LA, left atrium; LV, left ventricle; PV, pulmonary valve; RA, right atrium; RPA, right branch pulmonary artery; RV, right ventricle.

of the fetal heart in the transverse and sagittal planes and can be used to confirm normal venoatrial inflows, atrioventricular connections, and ventriculoatrial outflows.

Color Doppler imaging

Color flow mapping of the fetal heart is used by those trained to perform basic cardiac screening as well as those experienced in advanced fetal echocardiography [4]. In general, the cardiac examination is repeated briefly using color Doppler to demonstrate normal directional blood flow through the fetal heart. In addition to confirming normal blood flow patterns, it can identify structures that can be difficult to visualize by two-dimensional ultrasound alone. For example, the small pulmonary veins are often best demonstrated with the use of low velocity color flow mapping. Color Doppler can also be used to identify defects that might be missed on two-dimensional imaging alone. Some ventricular septal defects may be visible only when color Doppler is applied with the ultrasound beam perpendicular to the interventricular septum. Color flow mapping can also identify abnormal flow patterns associated with complex heart defects, valvular stenosis, coarctation, and hemodynamic compromise such as regurgitation and poor contractility. For example, the retrograde aortic flow in hypoplastic left heart syndrome and the reversed ductal flow with pulmonary atresia are easily identified with the use of color Doppler. Turbulent flow or aliasing on color Doppler may be indicative of valvular stenosis or coarctation. In general, color Doppler should be obtained when the ultrasound beam is parallel to the interrogated vessel with less than 20° angle correction.

The addition of color Doppler is now considered an important component of a cardiac screening exam in many centers. Normal flow patterns determined by color flow mapping provide further reassurance to patients and their families that their offspring has no evidence of major structural or functional heart disease.

Expectations from cardiac screening

Four-chamber view

The four-chamber view was introduced as a screening tool for the prenatal detection of heart anomalies in the 1980s [23,24]. Initial reports suggested that the four-chamber view could detect 80–90% of fetuses with congenital heart disease [24,25]. However, the sensitivity of the four-chamber view in detecting cardiac anomalies varied widely in subsequent studies. For example, only 16% of fetuses with heart defects were detected using the four-chamber view in the highly publicized Routine

Antenatal Diagnostic Imaging with Ultrasound (RADIUS) trial of prenatal ultrasonographic screening, and no cardiac malformations were detected before 24 weeks' gestation in facilities other than tertiary-level referral centers [26].

There are many possible explanations for the inconsistent performance of the four-chamber view in screening for congenital heart disease. Different ultrasonographers with varying levels of skill use the four-chamber view under a variety of conditions in clinical practice. Performance is also significantly influenced by factors such as a community setting vs. a tertiary care center, high-risk vs. low-risk patients, level of ascertainment, and availability of outcome information. Screening by skilled sonographers, experienced perinatologists, and expert pediatric cardiologists at teaching hospitals and tertiary reference centers is expected to be superior to that performed in the community. This is reflected in the poor detection rate reported in nontertiary care centers in the RADIUS study [26]. The sensitivity of any screening test also depends on the prevalence of disease in the population being studied. Tertiary care hospitals will see more affected fetuses because they are the facilities to which women with abnormal serum screening, advanced maternal age, and high-risk factors for congenital heart disease are referred for evaluation. The prevalence of congenital heart disease in many tertiary care centers is twice that expected in the general population [27].

The ability to image the fetal heart is also influenced by gestational age, fetal position, amniotic fluid volume, previous abdominal surgery, and maternal body habitus. Even when the four-chamber view is achieved, it is unreasonable to expect that it will identify all cases of congenital heart disease. Certain defects are easily missed on the four-chamber view, such as ventricular septal defects, atrial septal defects, coarctation, tetralogy of Fallot, transposition of the great arteries, double-outlet right ventricle, truncus arteriosus, and total anomalous pulmonary venous return [28]. Prenatal diagnosis of patent foramen ovale and patent ductus arteriosus is precluded by their normal patency in utero. The superior aspect of the interventricular septum tends to be thin, particularly in the apical view, and can be incorrectly diagnosed as a subaortic ventricular septal defect. Small muscular ventricular septal defects are the defects most commonly missed on prenatal ultrasonography. Certain cardiac malformations, such as transposition of the great vessels, double-outlet right ventricle, and tetralogy of Fallot, can be associated with a normal four-chamber view.

Although most congenital heart defects occur during the period of organogenesis, some defects are known to evolve over the course of gestation and may be missed at the time of midtrimester screening. Flow abnormalities such as valvular pulmonic stenosis, aortic stenosis, and coarctation of the aorta are not easy to detect on the four-chamber view. Ventricular hypoplasia has been observed to develop as pregnancy advances and may not be evident on cardiac imaging in the second trimester [29]. Abnormalities of the distal pulmonary arteries and pulmonary veins are not commonly appreciated prenatally due to limited flow and filling of these vessels in utero. Even under optimal conditions, some defects will not be detected at a midtrimester scan by the four-chamber view.

When used as a screening tool in the general population, the four-chamber view can be expected to detect 40–50% of cases of congenital heart disease [24,30]. The four-chamber view should be considered abnormal if there is ventricular or atrial disproportion, myocardial hypertrophy, dilation or hypoplasia of the chambers, septal defects apart from the foramen ovale, or abnormalities of the atrioventricular valves. Congenital heart disease may also be associated with abnormal positioning of the heart in the fetal chest and with axis deviation. Defects expected to be associated with an abnormal four-chamber view include hypoplasia of the right or left ventricle, atrioventricular septal defect, double-inlet ventricle, Ebstein anomaly, single ventricle, and large ventricle septal defect. Screening with the four-chamber view may also identify dextrocardia, situs inversus, ectopia cordis, cardiomyopathies, pericardial effusion, cardiac tumors, valvular atresia, stenosis, and insufficiency. Hypoplastic ventricles and atrioventricular septal defects are the defects most often detected prenatally by the four-chamber view [11,28,30].

Addition of outflow tract views and three-vessel views

Overall, the prenatal detection of cardiac anomalies can be increased from 40–50% with the four-chamber view alone to 60–80% when the ventricular outflow tracts are also assessed [8,31,32]. Although the best detection rates of congenital heart disease have been reported in high-risk populations screened at referral centers, a sensitivity of 66% was observed in a study of primarily low-risk patients screened with views of the four-chamber and outflow tracts [30].

It is clear that multiple cardiac views are crucial for midtrimester screening for many serious congenital heart defects and that the 20–30% increase in detection rate that results from including the outflow tracts along with the four-chamber view can be of clinical importance. Inclusion of the three-vessel and three-vessel trachea views for standard screening in low-risk populations has been reported to further increase the detection rate of outflow tract abnormalities in low-risk populations [33–35]. Detection rates for major heart anomalies can reach over 85%, particularly if color flow mapping is routinely used [33–35]. These views facilitate a detailed evaluation of the main pulmonary artery and its branches, the ductus arteriosus, the ascending aorta and transverse arch, and the superior vena cava along with the trachea. Universal

screening with the four-chamber view, views of the ventricular outflow tracts, and three-vessel and three-vessel trachea views, using two-dimensional ultrasound with color flow mapping, may prove be optimal for midtrimester cardiac assessment of low-risk populations.

Conclusion

Despite the widespread use of obstetric ultrasound, only a third of infants with congenital heart disease born in the United States since the turn of the century have been detected prenatally [13,36,37]. However, recent trends in prenatal detection of major heart malformations are encouraging. A publication from the Society of Thoracic Surgeons congenital heart surgery database of over 30,000 live born infants reported an overall prenatal detection rate of 57% for defects associated with an abnormal four-chamber view such as single ventricle lesions, tricuspid valve disease, congenitally corrected transposition of the great arteries, and complete atrioventricular septal defect and 32% for defects associated with anomalies of the great vessels such as double outlet right ventricle, truncus arteriosus, transposition of the great arteries with an intact interventricular septum, and tetralogy of Fallot [37]. In a recent international study that included stillbirths and terminations as well as live births, at least 50% of critical congenital heart defects were diagnosed prenatally with the highest detection rate for hypoplastic left heart syndrome at 64% [38].

Although these trends are encouraging, there remains room for improvement in the overall detection of congenital heart disease prenatally [37]. One explanation for the low performance of screening is that most infants with heart anomalies are born to low-risk women. Therefore, universal routine screening of all patients is required and using a standard approach may have the best potential to significantly improve the accuracy of prenatal diagnosis of major heart defects [22]. Another explanation for the low antenatal detection rate is that the performance of cardiac screening falls well below expectations (Table 6.1). The four-chamber view should detect 40–50% of defects and the addition of ventricular outflow views and

Table 6.1 Detection of major congenital heart disease

Screening tool	Prenatal detection rate
Preexisting risk factors	<20%
Nuchal translucency	15–50%
Four-chamber view	40–50%
Four-chamber view and ventricular outflow tracts	60–80%
Four-chamber view and three-vessel trachea view	>85%
Fetal echocardiography	>90%

three-vessel views should increase detection to over 85%. Recent studies have shown that an abnormal cardiac screen at the time of routine obstetric ultrasound has become the most common indication for fetal echocardiography. With detection rates consistently over 90% in experienced centers, it might be optimal for all patients to undergo screening fetal echocardiography [39–41]. However, with limited resources, a major goal for providers of obstetric ultrasound must be to improve the quality of cardiac screening so that abnormal fetal hearts are promptly recognized and referred to those skilled in fetal echocardiography.

CASE PRESENTATION

A 26-year-old gravid 3 para 2 presents at 18 weeks gestation for an ultrasound examination. During the fetal survey, the four-chamber view of the fetal heart appears to be normal but the outflow tracts are not well seen. She reports that there was some concern at the time of the first-trimester ultrasound about fluid at the back of the fetal neck but that she was told the likelihood of Down syndrome was low based on her cell-free fetal DNA results. She has no other known risk factors for congenital heart disease. She returns 4 weeks later for a follow-up ultrasound examination and again the outflow tracts are difficult to image but they appear to arise in a parallel fashion from the heart. Upon further evaluation, transposition of the great arteries is diagnosed with the pulmonary artery arising from the posterior left ventricle and the aorta arising from the anterior right ventricle. She is distraught at this news and asks why this was not detected earlier and what should be done now.

The majority of infants with cardiac malformations are born to women with normal pregnancies and no identifiable risk factors for congenital heart disease. However, fetal echocardiography is now recommended when the nuchal translucency is increased at the time of first-trimester screening for aneuploidy. Different cutoff values are used in different centers but an absolute nuchal translucency measurement of >3–3.5mm between 11–13 weeks gestation is a reasonable threshold to flag patients for referral for fetal echocardiography.

Transposition of the great arteries is often associated with a normal four-chamber view and can easily be missed if views of the outflow tracts are not routinely evaluated and seen at the time of the second-trimester anatomic survey of the fetus. One of the clues to this diagnosis is the fact that the outflow tracts do not cross normally as they exit their respective ventricles. Another clue is an abnormal arrangement of the great arteries on the three-vessel view or the visualization of only two vessels, the transverse aortic arch and superior vena cava, on the three-vessel trachea view. A repeat ultrasound or referral for fetal echocardiography is indicated if the fetal heart cannot be adequately visualized as congenital heart disease is the most common of the major anomalies adversely affecting survival. Fortunately, simple transposition of the great vessels has a favorable prognosis but certain steps should be taken when this diagnosis is made. First, a careful examination for additional cardiac and extracardiac anomalies should be performed. The interventricular septum should be carefully examined as those cases with an intact septum should have a timed delivery in a center capable of performing an emergency atrial septostomy. Genetic counseling should be offered and fetal karyotyping considered, particularly if extracardiac anomalies are identified. However, the risk for aneuploidy is low in cases of isolated transposition of the great arteries.

A multidisciplinary team including the obstetrician, maternal–fetal medicine specialist, geneticist, pediatric cardiologist, pediatric cardiothoracic surgeon, and neonatologist should be involved in the counseling of the patient and her family about this condition and its implications. It is only then that the patient can fully understand the diagnosis, her options, and the plan for management, delivery, and neonatal care.

References

1. AIUM-ACR-ACOG-SMFM–SRU practice parameter for the performance of standard diagnostic obstetric ultrasound examinations. J Ultrasound. 2018;37:E13–E24.
2. AIUM practice parameter for the performance of detailed diagnostic obstetric ultrasound examinations between 12 weeks 0 days and 13 weeks 6 days. J Ultrasound Med. 2021;40:E1–E16.
3. AIUM practice parameter for the performance of detailed second- and third-trimester diagnostic obstetric ultrasound examinations. J Ultrasound Med. 2019;38:3093–100.
4. AIUM practice parameter for the performance of fetal echocardiography. J Ultrasound Med. 2020;39:E5–E16.
5. Hoffman JIE, Kaplan S. The incidence of congenital heart disease. J Am Coll Cardiol. 2002;39:1890–900.
6. Buskens E, Steyerberg EW, Hess J, Wladimiroff JW, Grobbee DE. Routine prenatal screening for congenital heart disease: what can be expected? A decision-analytic approach. Am J Public Health. 1997;87:962–7.
7. Johnson B, Simpson LL. Screening for congenital heart disease: a move towards earlier echocardiography. Am J Perinatol. 2007;24:449–56.

8. Bromley B, Estroff JA, Sanders SP, Parad R, Roberts D, Frigoletto FD, Benacerraf BR. Fetal echocardiography: accuracy and limitations in a population at high and low risk for heart defects. Am J Obstet Gynecol. 1992;166:1473–81.

9. Copel JA, Pilu G, Kleinman CS. Congenital heart disease and extracardiac anomalies: associations and indications for fetal echocardiography. Am J Obstet Gynecol. 1986;154:1121–32.

10. Paladini D, Calabro R, Palmieri S, d'Andrea T. Prenatal diagnosis of congenital heart disease and fetal karyotyping. Obstet Gynecol. 1993;81:679–82.

11. Sharland GK, Allan LD. Screening for congenital heart disease prenatally. Results of a 2½-year study in the South East Thames Region. Br J Obstet Gynaecol. 1992;9:220–5.

12. Bjorkhem G, Jorgensen C, Hanseus K. Parental reactions of fetal echocardiography. J Matern Fetal Med. 1997;6:87–92.

13. Friedberg MK, Silverman NH, Moon-Grady AJ, Tong E, Nourse J, Sorenson B, et al. Prenatal detection of congenital heart disease. J Pediatr. 2009;155:26–31.

14. Cooper MJ, Enderlein MA, Dyson DC, Roge CL, Tarnoff H. Fetal echocardiography: retrospective review of clinical experience and an evaluation of indications. Obstet Gynecol. 1995;86:577–82.

15. Simpson LL. Indications for fetal echocardiography from a tertiary care obstetric sonography practice J Clin Ultrasound. 2004;32:123–8.

16. Simpson LL, Malone FD, Bianchi DW, Ball RH, Nyberg DA, Comstock CH, et al. Nuchal translucency and the risk of congenital heart disease. Obstet Gynecol. 2007;109:376–83.

17. Sananes N, Guigue V, Kohler M, Bouffet N, Cancellier M, Hornecker F, et al. Nuchal translucency and cystic hygroma in screening for fetal major congenital heart defects in a series of 12910 euploid pregnancies. Ultrasound Obstet Gynecol. 2010;35:273–9.

18. Friedberg MK, Silverman NH. Changing indications for fetal echocardiography in a university center population. Prenat Diagn. 2004;24:781–6.

19. Tegnander E, Eik-Nes SH, Linker DT. Incorporating the four-chamber view of the fetal heart into the second-trimester routine fetal examination. Ultrasound Obstet Gynecol. 1994;4:24–8.

20. Paladini D, Rustico M, Todros T, Palmieri S, Gaglioti P, Benettoni A, et al. Conotruncal anomalies in prenatal life. Ultrasound Obstet Gynecol. 1996;8:241–6.

21. Devore GR. The aortic and pulmonary outflow tract screening examination in the human fetus. J Ultrasound Med. 1992;11:345–8.

22. Allan L. Technique of fetal echocardiography. Pediatr Cardiol. 2004;25:223–33.

23. Devore GR. The prenatal diagnosis of congenital heart disease: a practical approach for the fetal sonographer. J Clin Ultrasound. 1985;13:229–45.

24. Allan LD, Crawford DC, Chita SK, Tynan MJ. Prenatal screening for congenital heart disease. BMJ. 1986;292:1717–19.

25. Copel JA, Pilu G, Green J, Hobbins JG, Kleinman CS. Fetal echocardiographic screening for congenital heart disease: the importance of the four-chamber view. Am J Obstet Gynecol. 1987;157:648–55.

26. Crane JP, Lefevre ML, Winborn RC, Evans JK, Ewigman BG, Bain RP, et al. A randomized trial of prenatal ultrasonographic screening: impact on the detection, management, and outcome of anomalous fetuses. Am J Obstet Gynecol. 1994;171:392–99.

27. Buskens E, Stewart PA, Hess J, Grobbee DE. Efficacy of fetal echocardiography and yield by risk category. Obstet Gynecol. 1996;87:423–8.

28. Allan LD, Sharland GK, Milburn A, Lockhart SM, Groves AM, Anderson RH, et al. Prospective diagnosis of 1006 consecutive cases of congenital heart disease in the fetus. J Am Coll Cardiol. 1994;23:1452–8.

29. Hornberger LK, Need L, Benacerraf BR. Development of significant left and right ventricular hypoplasia in the second and third trimester fetus. J Ultrasound Med. 1996;15:655–9.

30. Kirk JS, Comstock CH, Lee W, Smith RS, Riggs TW, Weinhouse E. Sonographic screening to detect fetal cardiac anomalies: a 5-year experience with 111 abnormal cases. Obstet Gynecol. 1997;89:227–32.

31. Bronshtein M, Zimmer EZ, Gerlis LM, Lorber A, Drugan A. Early ultrasound diagnosis of fetal congenital heart defects in high-risk and low-risk pregnancies. Obstet Gynecol. 1993;82:225–9.

32. Carvalho JS, Mavrides E, Shinebourne EA, Campbell S, Thilaganathan B. Improving the effectiveness of routine prenatal screening for major congenital heart defects. Heart. 2002;88:387–91.

33. Wong SF, Ward C, Lee-Tannock A, Le S, Chan FY. Pulmonary artery/aorta ratio in simple screening for fetal outflow tract abnormalities during the second trimester. Ultrasound Obstet Gynecol. 2007;30:275–80.

34. Del Bianco A, Russo S, Lacerenza N, Rinaldi M, Rinaldi G, Nappi L, et al. Four chamber view plus three-vessel and trachea view for a complete evaluation of the fetal heart during the second trimester. J Perinat Med. 2006;34:309–12.

35. Edward H, Hamilton R. Single centre audit of early impact of inclusion of the three vessel and trachea view in obstetric screening. Ultrasound. 2018;26:93–100.

36. Acherman RJ, Evans WN, Luna CF, Rollins R, Kip KT, Collazos JC, et al. Prenatal detection of congenital heart disease in southern Nevada. J Ultrasound Med. 2007;26:1715–19.

37. Quartermain MD, Pasquali SK, Hill KD, Goldberg DJ, Huhta JC, Jacobs JP, et al. Variation in prenatal diagnosis of congenital heart disease in infants. Pediatrics. 2015;136:e378–85.

38. Bakker MK, Bergman JEH, Krikov S, Amar E, Cocchi G, Cragan J, et al. Prenatal diagnosis and prevalence of critical congenital heart defects: an international retrospective cohort study. BMJ Open. 2019;9:e028139.

39. Stumpflen I, Stumpflen A, Wimmer M, Bernaschek G. Effect of detailed fetal echocardiography as part of routine prenatal ultrasonographic screening on detection of congenital heart disease. Lance.t 1996;348:854–7.

40. Randall P, Brealey S, Hahn S, Khan KS, Parsons JM. Accuracy of fetal echocardiography in the routine detection of congenital heart disease among unselected and low risk populations: a systematic review. Br J Obstet Gynaecol. 2005;112:22–30.

41. Rakha S, El Marsafawy H. Sensitivity, specificity, and accuracy of fetal echocardiography for high-risk pregnancies in a tertiary care center in Egypt. Arch Pediatr. 2019;26:337–41.

Chapter 7
First- and Second-Trimester Screening for Fetal Aneuploidy and Neural Tube Defects

Ronan Daly and Fergal D. Malone
Department of Obstetrics and Gynaecology, Royal College of Surgeons in Ireland, Rotunda Hospital, Dublin, Ireland

Prenatal screening for Down syndrome (trisomy 21) and other aneuploidies, such as trisomies 13 and 18, has advanced significantly since its advent in the 1980s. Historically, pregnant people 35 years or older were offered prenatal genetic counseling and the option of a diagnostic test such as chorionic villus sampling or amniocentesis. With this screening approach, only 20% of the fetal Down syndrome population are detected antenatally. In the intervening 40 years, the paradigm for prenatal aneuploidy screening has dramatically evolved, with a focus on less invasive testing. Initially, biochemical markers of fetal aneuploidy were identified, such as low levels of the analyte α-fetoprotein (AFP) being associated with an increased risk of fetal Down syndrome. This led to the creation of noninvasive screening tests, with the triple and quadruple tests for aneuploidy being introduced in the mid-1980s.

Further progress was made regarding sonographic markers of aneuploidy, with trisomy 21 strongly associated with an increased nuchal translucency in the first trimester and/or a thickened nuchal fold in the second trimester. Thus, the 1990s saw the creation of the combined test, involving the use of both sonographic and biochemical markers in order to detect aneuploidies and neural tube defects in the first trimester. The introduction of noninvasive prenatal testing (NIPT) revolutionized aneuploidy screening for trisomies 21, 13, and 18. NIPT involves the analysis of cell-free fetal DNA (cffDNA) present in maternal blood to screen for these chromosomal conditions. NIPT has been incorporated by varying degrees into prenatal screening practices worldwide. The evolution and advancement of prenatal diagnosis has enabled it to become available, if requested and after appropriate counseling, to all pregnant people, regardless of maternal age.

First-trimester sonographic screening

The single most powerful sonographic discriminator of Down syndrome from euploid fetuses is first-trimester sonographic measurement of the nuchal translucency space, generally performed between 11 0/7 and 13 6/7 weeks gestation, corresponding with a fetal crown–rump length between 45 and 84 mm [1]. Nuchal translucency (NT) refers to a clearly demarcated fluid-filled or sonolucent space behind the fetal neck. It is present in all fetuses (Figure 7.1). An increased NT measurement is significantly associated with fetal aneuploidy, structural malformations, and adverse pregnancy outcome.

Because the average NT measurement is only 0.5–1.5 mm in thickness, it is absolutely essential that sonographic technique be meticulous, follows an agreed protocol, and is performed only by those with adequate training and experience. An error of only a millimeter can have a significant impact on the Down syndrome risk quoted to an individual patient. Critical components of good NT sonographic technique are demonstrated in Figure 7.1 and include imaging the fetus in a neutral position in the midsagittal plane, including visualization of the palate, mesencephalon and nasal bone, adequate magnification to focus only on the fetal head and upper thorax, discrimination between the nuchal skin and amniotic membrane, and caliper placement on the inner borders of the echolucent space. NT sonography is a more powerful discriminator of Down syndrome fetuses from euploid fetuses at 11 weeks, rather than 13 weeks, and therefore this form of screening should be performed as close to 11 weeks as possible [1].

Several large prospective population screening studies were completed in the United States and Europe, and each confirmed that NT sonography, when performed by

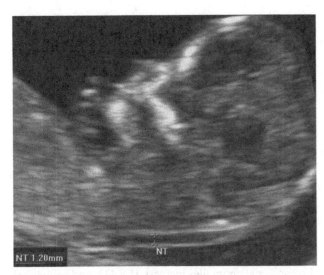

Figure 7.1 Sonographic examination at 12 weeks and 4 days gestation demonstrating measurement of the fetal nuchal translucency (NT).

trained and experienced sonographers, is an effective screening tool for fetal aneuploidy [1–5]. At a 5% false positive rate, NT sonography (combined with maternal age) detects 70% of cases of Down syndrome at 11 weeks but decreases to 64% detection at 13 weeks gestation [1]. In general, NT measurement has limited usefulness as a stand-alone test because of the increased sensitivity and improved positive predictive value achieved with incorporation of other sonographic and maternal serum markers.

Credentialing programs, provided by the US Perinatal Quality Foundation or the UK Fetal Medicine Foundation, ensure that clinicians are adequately trained and certified in obtaining reproducible NT measurements. These programs are highly important for ongoing quality review and evaluation of provider proficiency.

Other sonographic tools that are available for first-trimester screening for fetal aneuploidy include nasal bone sonography, ductus venosus Doppler waveform analysis, and tricuspid regurgitation. The use of nasal bone sonography in the first trimester for general population screening is controversial. A large prospective observational study in a high-risk population [6] described the absence of nasal bone ossification in 73% of fetuses affected by trisomy 21 vs. 0.5% in euploid fetuses. It was estimated that 85% and 93% of trisomy 21 cases would be detected at false-positive rates of 1% and 4%, respectively. The authors concluded that the visualization of the fetal nasal bone would result in a major reduction in the need for invasive testing and a substantial increase in sensitivity. The same investigators suggested a 97% detection rate for Down syndrome with a 5% false-positive rate when combining nasal bone measurements with nuchal translucency and serum markers [7]. In contrast, the FASTER trial [8] did not find that nasal bone assessment is useful in general population screening for Down syndrome as 9 of 11 fetuses with trisomy 21 had nasal bones present. Significant variability has been observed in nasal bone assessment, posing some limitations to its usefulness. Until such time as nasal bone evaluation is subjected to the same rigorous standardization process as nuchal translucency, its application as a screening tool will be likely confined to a second-line assessment once a pregnancy has already been deemed to be at high risk.

The ductus venosus is a fetal blood vessel that carries oxygenated blood from the umbilical vein to the inferior vena cava. A normal first-trimester ductus venosus Doppler waveform is triphasic in appearance, with constant forward flow (Plate 7.1). Reversed flow in the ductus venosus (Plate 7.2) has been associated with both fetal aneuploidy and congenital heart disease [9]. However, the reproducibility of this measurement has been questioned and, like nasal bone sonography, it is likely that this form of first-trimester sonography will remain a second-line screening tool at select expert centers [10].

The presence of significant tricuspid regurgitation at the time of NT sonography is also a useful marker for fetal Down syndrome [11]. A study by Falcon et al. [12] identified tricuspid regurgitation as an independent risk factor for fetal aneuploidy. However, further population screening studies are still needed to validate the role of first-trimester tricuspid regurgitation for this indication.

When considering newer forms of ultrasound evaluation for fetal Down syndrome, a balance needs to be struck between exciting new modalities and robust sonographic techniques that can be easily implemented at a general population level. Just because a new technique may perform well in select expert hands when evaluating high-risk patients does not imply that it will be a useful addition to general population screening.

Combined first-trimester serum and sonographic screening

In Down syndrome pregnancies, first-trimester serum levels of pregnancy-associated plasma protein A (PAPP-A) are decreased compared with euploid pregnancies, and human chorionic gonadotropin (hCG) levels are increased. Because these two serum markers are relatively independent of each other, and of both maternal age and NT measurements, improvements in Down syndrome risk assessment can be achieved by a combined serum and sonographic screening approach. Several large population studies have confirmed that such combined first-trimester screening is significantly better than screening for Down syndrome based on NT sonography alone [1,3]. At a 5% false-positive rate, such combined first-trimester screening detects 87% of cases of Down syndrome at 11 weeks, decreasing to 82% at 13 weeks gestation (compared with 70% and 64% detection rates, respectively, for NT alone) [1]. Looked at differently, to achieve an 85% Down syndrome detection rate at 11 weeks gestation, screening using NT sonography alone would yield a false-positive rate of 20%, whereas combined first-trimester screening would have a false-positive rate of only 3.8% [1].

It is now clear that first-trimester combined screening for fetal Down syndrome should be provided using the combination of NT sonography with appropriate serum markers. The only exception to this may be the presence of a multiple gestation where it can be very difficult to interpret the relative contributions of different placentas to maternal serum marker levels. In this latter situation, it is reasonable to provide a Down syndrome risk assessment based on NT sonography alone.

Another practical problem for the implementation of first-trimester combined screening in the United States is limited access to assays for the free β-subunit of hCG (fβhCG). Both total hCG and fβhCG are very effective discriminators of Down syndrome and euploid pregnancies, but when evaluated as univariate markers, fβhCG is more powerful (15% vs. 28% detection rates, respectively, for a 5% false-positive rate at 11 weeks) [3]. However, in actual clinical practice fβhCG is never used on its own to screen for fetal Down syndrome, but instead will always be used in combination with other serum markers, such as PAPP-A and NT sonography. When the combination of first-trimester NT, PAPP-A, and fβhCG is compared with the combination of NT, PAPP-A, and total hCG, their performance is actually very similar, with Down syndrome detection rates of 83% and 80%, respectively, for a 5% false-positive rate [3]. Therefore, for clinicians in practice, if fβhCG is not available at their local laboratory it would still be possible to achieve similar Down syndrome screening performance using the more widely available total hCG.

First-trimester cystic hygroma

It is clear that there is a subgroup of fetuses with enlarged NT measurements that are at sufficiently high risk for aneuploidy and other adverse outcomes that delaying invasive diagnostic testing until serum markers are available is not necessary. The finding of an increased NT space, extending along the entire length of the fetus, and in which septations are clearly visible, is referred to as septated cystic hygroma, and is an easily identifiable feature during first-trimester sonography (see Plate 7.1). Septated cystic hygroma will be encountered in approximately 1 in every 300 first-trimester sonographic evaluations [13]. Once this diagnosis is made, patients should be counseled regarding a 50% incidence of fetal aneuploidy, with the most common abnormalities being Down syndrome, followed by Turner syndrome and trisomy 18 [13]. Of the remaining euploid fetuses, half will have major structural malformations such as congenital heart defects, diaphragmatic hernia, skeletal dysplasia, or a variety of genetic syndromes. A 2012 review of 944 fetuses diagnosed with a cystic hygroma in the first trimester demonstrated a 39% rate of perinatal loss, with an abnormal outcome occurring in 87% of cases [14]. The study demonstrated that for each increase of 1 mm in the NT measurement the chance of chromosomal anomalies increased by 44% and congenital anomalies by 26%.

The American College of Medical Genetics states that women carrying a fetus with an NT over 4 mm or where a septated cystic hygroma is present should be offered immediate invasive diagnosis using chorionic villus sampling (CVS) as the addition of serum markers would not significantly alter the risk for Down syndrome [15]. Results from the FASTER trial showed that an NT measurement of 3 mm or greater yields a minimum risk of aneuploidy of 1 in 6, and therefore invasive testing should be offered at this cutoff. The American College of Obstetricians and Gynecologists and the Society for Maternal-Fetal Medicine recommend offering genetic counselling and testing in cases with an NT of 3 mm or greater, or above the 99th percentile [16]. Given the association with congenital malformations, fetuses with increased NT or first-trimester cystic hygroma should undergo targeted sonography and/or echocardiography at 18–20 weeks gestation.

Second-trimester sonographic screening

The mainstay for antenatal Down syndrome screening for over 30 years had been second-trimester sonographic evaluation of fetal anatomy, also frequently referred to as the genetic sonogram. Two general approaches have been used in the second trimester: sonographic detection of major structural fetal malformations, and sonographic detection of minor markers for Down syndrome.

The detection of certain major structural malformations that are known to be associated with aneuploidy should always prompt immediate consideration for genetic amniocentesis. The major structural malformations that are associated with Down syndrome include cardiac malformations (atrioventricular [AV] canal defect, ventricular septal defect, tetralogy of Fallot), duodenal atresia, cystic hygroma, or hydrops fetalis. The major malformations associated with trisomy 18 include cardiac malformations (AV canal defect, ventricular septal defect, double-outlet right ventricle), meningomyelocele, omphalocele, esophageal atresia, rocker-bottom feet, cleft lip or palate, cystic hygroma, or hydrops fetalis. Although the genetic sonogram can be performed at any time during the second and third trimesters, the optimal time is likely to be at 17–18 weeks gestation, which is late enough to maximize fetal anatomic evaluation yet early enough to allow for amniocentesis results to be obtained promptly and efficiently. When a major structural malformation is found, such as an AV canal defect or a double-bubble suggestive of duodenal atresia, the risk of Down syndrome in that pregnancy can be increased by approximately 20–30-fold [17]. For almost all patients, such an increase in their background risk for aneuploidy will be sufficiently high to justify immediate genetic amniocentesis.

Second-trimester sonography can also detect a range of minor markers for aneuploidy. The latter are not considered structural abnormalities of the fetus per se but, when noted, may be associated with an increased probability that the fetus is aneuploid. The minor markers that have been commonly linked to Down syndrome include nuchal fold thickening (Figure 7.2), nasal bone absence or hypoplasia, mild ventriculomegaly, short femur or humerus, echogenic bowel, renal pyelectasis, echogenic intracardiac focus, clinodactyly, sandal gap toe, and widened iliac angle [18]. The minor markers that are associated with trisomy 18 include nuchal fold thickening, mild ventriculomegaly, short femur or humerus, echogenic bowel, enlarged cisterna magna, choroid plexus cysts, micrognathia, single umbilical artery, clenched hands, and fetal growth restriction. It should be

noted that almost all data supporting the role of second-trimester sonography for minor markers for aneuploidy are derived from high-risk populations, such as patients of advanced maternal age or with abnormal maternal serum screening results. It is still unclear what the relative contribution of screening for such minor markers will be in lower risk patients from the general population.

To objectively counsel patients following the prenatal diagnosis of a minor sonographic marker, likelihood ratios can be used to create a more precise risk assessment for the patient that her fetus might be affected with Down syndrome. Their use can be easily implemented into clinical practice by simply multiplying the relevant likelihood ratio by the a priori risk. Table 7.1 summarizes the likelihood ratios that can be used to modify a patient's risk for Down syndrome, depending on which minor marker is detected. If no markers are present, the patient's a priori risk can be multiplied by 0.4, effectively reducing her chances of carrying a fetus with Down syndrome by 60% [18]. The likelihood ratio values listed for each marker assume that the marker is an isolated finding. By contrast, when more than one minor marker is noted in the same fetus, different likelihood ratios must be used, with the risk for Down syndrome being increased by a factor of 10 when two minor markers are detected and by a factor of 115 when three or more minor markers are found [18]. It should also be noted that the 95% confidence interval (CI) values for each marker's likelihood ratios are rather wide. These values should therefore be used only as a general guide for counseling patients, and care should be exercised to avoid implying too much precision in the final risk estimates. Accuracy of risk estimates, however, can be maximized by using the best available a priori risk value for a particular patient, such as the

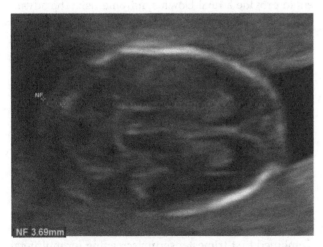

Figure 7.2 Second-trimester sonographic measurement of the fetal nuchal fold (NF) at 15 5/7 weeks gestation. The measurement is taken in the axial plane at the level of the posterior fossa, with calipers placed from the outer skull edge to the outer skin edge.

Table 7.1 Likelihood ratios for Down syndrome when an isolated minor sonographic marker is detected[a]

Minor marker	Likelihood ratio	95% confidence interval
Nuchal fold >5 mm	11	6–22
Echogenic bowel	6.7	3–17
Short humerus	5.1	2–17
Short femur	1.5	0.8–3
Echogenic intracardiac focus	1.8	1–3
Pyelectasis	1.5	0.6–4
Any two minor markers	10	6.6–14
Any three or more minor markers	115	58–229
No markers	0.4	0.3–0.5

[a]The patient's a priori risk is multiplied by the appropriate positive likelihood ratio to yield an individualized posttest risk for fetal Down syndrome.
Reproduced from Nyberg et al. [18] with permission from the American Institute of Ultrasound in Medicine.

results of maternal serum marker screening or first-trimester combined screening, rather than maternal age, when available.

The role of second-trimester genetic sonography after Down syndrome screening has been evaluated in a study of 7842 pregnancies, including 59 with Down syndrome [19]. For a 5% false-positive rate, genetic sonography increased detection rates substantially for combined and quadruple tests, from 81% to 90% respectively.

Second-trimester serum screening

Maternal serum levels of AFP and unconjugated estriol are both approximately 25% lower in pregnancies complicated by Down syndrome compared with euploid pregnancies [20]. By contrast, levels of hCG and inhibin-A are approximately twice as high in pregnancies complicated by Down syndrome [20]. Maternal serum levels of AFP, uE3, and hCG all tend to be decreased in pregnancies complicated by trisomy 18. The combination of AFP, uE3, and hCG, commonly known as the triple screen, can detect 69% of cases of Down syndrome, for a 5% false-positive rate [1]. When inhibin-A is added to this test, commonly known as the quad screen, the Down syndrome detection rate increases to 81%, for a 5% false-positive rate [1, 3]. Notwithstanding this effective performance, given the improved performance of cffDNA as part of noninvasive prenatal testing, second-trimester serum screening has effectively been dropped in most clinical practices.

Combined first- and second-trimester screening

Although first trimester combined screening and second trimester serum screening are separately effective, it has been suggested that screening performance might be further improved by combining screening tests across both trimesters. There are three approaches to combining screening across gestational ages – integrated screening, sequential screening, and contingent screening.

Integrated screening is a two-step screening protocol, with results not being released until all screening steps are completed. Sonographic measurement of NT, together with serum assay for PAPP-A, are obtained between 10 and 13 weeks gestation, followed by a second serum assay for AFP, hCG, uE3, and inhibin-A obtained between 15 and 16 weeks gestation. A single risk assessment is then calculated at 16 weeks gestation. This "fully

integrated" test has a Down syndrome detection rate of 95%, for a 5% false-positive rate [1,3]. A variant of this approach, referred to as the "serum integrated" test, involves blood tests only, including PAPP-A in the first trimester, followed by AFP, hCG, uE3, and inhibin-A in the second trimester. This latter test, which does not require an NT ultrasound assessment, has a Down syndrome detection rate of 86%, for a 5% false-positive rate [1,3].

In contrast to integrated screening, stepwise sequential screening refers to multiple different Down syndrome screening tests being performed, with risk estimates being provided to patients upon completion of each step. A key concept in performing stepwise screening is to ensure that each subsequent screening test that is performed uses the Down syndrome risk from the preceding test as the new a priori risk for later screening or includes all previous marker results in risk calculation. If sequential screening tests are performed independently for Down syndrome without any modification being made for earlier screening results, the positive predictive value of the later tests will inevitably deteriorate, and it is likely that the overall false-positive rate will increase [21].

Contingent screening is a program in which patients have first-trimester screening with NT, PAPP-A, and fβhCG, and only those patients with extremely high-risk results (e.g. >1 in 30) are offered CVS. Patients with extremely low-risk results that are unlikely to be significantly changed by additional later tests (e.g. <1 in 1500) are reassured and are not offered additional Down syndrome screening tests. Finally, borderline risk patients (e.g. those with risks between 1 in 30 and 1 in 1500) return at 15 weeks for quad serum markers and these are combined with the earlier first-trimester markers to provide a final Down syndrome risk. The advantage of this approach is that it may focus the benefits of CVS with the highest risk patients, while significantly reducing the number of second-trimester screening tests performed [22].

Given the improved performance characteristics and simplicity of first trimester cffDNA based noninvasive prenatal testing, these cross-trimester screening programs will unlikely be widely implemented due to their greater complexity and inferior detection rates or false positive rates.

Screening in multiple gestations

Combined first-trimester serum screening for multifetal gestations is less sensitive than in singleton pregnancies. NT measurement in dichorionic twin gestations has comparable detection rates to those in singleton pregnancies [23]. NT measurement in monochorionic gestations is less reliable, however, given the recognition of increased or discordant NT as an early sign for twin-to-twin transfusion syndrome. Maternal serum screening has not been widely used in the setting of multiple gestations because of the potential for discordancy between twins and the impact of different placentas on the various analytes. Options for first-trimester screening for Down syndrome therefore include a fetus-specific risk based on NT alone or providing cffDNA based noninvasive prenatal testing. CffDNA testing in twin pregnancies has been shown to have similar performance rates as testing in singleton pregnancies. Two recent meta-analyses demonstrated detection rates of 95–98.2% and false positive rates of 0.05–0.09% for the detection of Down syndrome, although a higher failure (no-call) rate was noted [24–26]. In a series of 448 twin pregnancies, NT alone yielded an 88% detection rate for a 7% false-positive rate [27]. Another series of 206 twin pregnancies included maternal serum markers and reported a 75% detection rate for a 5% false-positive rate [28].

Currently, the method of choice for screening in multiple gestations is debatable but avoiding serum markers and providing a fetus-specific risk based on NT alone, or cffDNA alone, is a reasonable strategy. Sonographic evaluation of each individual fetus in the second trimester for major structural malformations or minor markers will allow for the calculation of fetus-specific risks for aneuploidy.

Screening for neural tube defects

Screening tests to identify patients at risk for fetal open neural tube defects (NTD), such as open spina bifida and anencephaly, use both maternal biochemical markers and ultrasonography to achieve highest detection rates. Although second-trimester serum screening has been available over the past 2 decades, first-trimester sonographic diagnosis is now available to allow for earlier diagnosis and optimized management options to be offered to the patient, including pregnancy termination. Between 75% and 90% of open NTDs and over 95% of anencephaly can be detected by elevated maternal serum AFP (MSAFP). MSAFP also detects 85% of abdominal wall defects. Serum screening for NTD can be performed between 15 and 22 weeks and optimally between 16 and 18 weeks gestation. Factors influencing MSAFP are multiple gestations, maternal ethnicity, insulin-dependent diabetes mellitus, and a positive family history of open NTD. Cutoff levels for NTD screening are 2.0–2.5 multiples

of the median (MoM) in singleton pregnancies and 4.0–5.0 MoM in twin gestations. These cutoff levels may be laboratory specific [15]. In pregnancies with elevated MSAFP, a targeted ultrasound examination is recommended.

Given that detailed ultrasound survey of fetal anatomy at 20–22 weeks gestation is now an established part of routine clinical practice, the most common form of screening for NTDs is ultrasound assessment of the fetal spine and cranial anatomy. If optimal views of spine, abdominal wall, and intracranial anatomy are not obtained at a targeted ultrasound in patients with elevated MSAFP, consideration may be given to amniocentesis to evaluate for amniotic fluid AFP and acetylcholinesterase levels. Given the association of NTDs with trisomy 18, amniotic fluid should also be sent for genetic evaluation. Sonographic markers observed in most fetuses with NTDs in the second trimester include scalloping of the frontal bones ("lemon" sign) and caudal displacement of the cerebellum ("banana" sign) due to Chiari malformation [29]. Often those fetuses have a small biparietal diameter (BPD) early in the second trimester [30]. Spina bifida can be indicated in the first trimester, between 11 and 13 weeks gestation, by the absence of the intracranial translucency (IT) [31]. The IT represents the fourth cerebral ventricle, which can be visualized on the same midsagittal plane of the fetal face as for measurement of NT and assessment of the nasal bone. The two lines that define the IT are the posterior border of the brainstem anteriorly and the choroid plexus of the fourth ventricle posteriorly. It is unclear, however, what the precise sensitivity and specificity for this marker will be, if used in clinical practice.

Cell-free fetal DNA (cffDNA) screening for fetal aneuploidy

Scientific basis of cffDNA screening

The presence of fetal DNA in the maternal circulation was first described in 1997, with Y-chromosome genetic material found in the blood of mothers carrying male fetuses [32]. Fragments of cffDNA in maternal plasma derive from the apoptosis of placental trophoblasts [33]. The turnover of trophoblastic cells during pregnancy results in the ongoing release of both maternal and fetal cell-free DNA fragments. The quantity of cffDNA rises with gestational age and clears rapidly from the maternal bloodstream following delivery, thereby creating a source of genetic material for genetic screening specific to the active pregnancy [34,35]. CffDNA screening (now known commonly as noninvasive prenatal testing, NIPT) involves analysis of this DNA to determine the probability of certain chromosomal conditions in pregnancy (including trisomies 21, 18, and 13), as well as fetal sex, fetal Rhesus status, and sex chromosome disorders. It has been commercially available since 2011, and its use in over 60 countries has changed the global landscape of first-trimester screening [36]. A number of techniques for screening cffDNA for aneuploidy are used in practice, including whole genome sequencing (massively parallel shotgun sequencing), targeted chromosome sequencing, and analysis of single nucleotide polymorphisms.

Limitations of cffDNA screening

The relative proportion of cffDNA to that of maternal origin in maternal plasma is known as the fetal fraction, and may be a source of testing failure if the fraction is below 4% [37]. Reliable detection of cffDNA can be performed from 9 weeks gestation when the fetal fraction is typically around 10% [38]. Certain factors such as maternal age and body mass index result in an increase in cffDNA of maternal origin, whereas the fetal fraction is lower in multiple pregnancies, IVF pregnancies and some ethnic groups (South-Asian, Afro-Caribbean), which may lead to a higher failure rate [25,39]. In one study, it was shown that 10% of patients weighing 113 kg or greater have a fetal fraction of less than 4%, with this proportion increasing to over 50% at maternal weights of 160kg or greater [40]. The failure rate of NIPT is variously reported as being between 1% and 8% and, in addition to maternal obesity, may also be due to issues with sample collection and assay failures [41–45]. Failed tests due to low fetal fraction are associated with an increased risk of aneuploidy [37,46], with lower fetal fractions demonstrated in pregnancies affected by trisomies 18 and 13 [16]. Genetic counseling for patients who receive a no-call NIPT test result is required, including counseling regarding options for invasive diagnostic testing, repeat screening, or alternate combined testing [47–49].

CffDNA screening performance

A 2015 meta-analysis of 37 studies on the performance of cffDNA testing for aneuploidy screening demonstrated that the test carries a detection rate of 99.2% and a false-positive rate of 0.09% for Down syndrome, higher than those achieved with traditional first trimester combined screening [44]. Gil et al. also found that the sensitivity and specificity of NIPT for Down syndrome were 99.3% and 99.9% respectively, with a positive predictive value of 91% in high-risk populations and 82% in low-risk populations. The 2015 NEXT study assessed cffDNA testing in

screening a population of over 15,000 pregnant people irrespective of their background risk [50]. That study demonstrated that, in regard to Down syndrome screening, the test carries a positive predictive value of 80.9% in all patients studied, and 76% in pregnant people under 35 years of age.

Gil et al. found that the detection rates for trisomies 18 and 13 to be lower than for Down syndrome, 96.3% and 91.0% respectively. False positive rates for both trisomies were 0.13%, with positive predictive values of 87% for trisomy 13 and 84% for trisomy 18 in high-risk patients [44]. However, the positive predictive values of cffDNA testing in low-risk populations in screening for trisomies 18 and 13 were only 37% and 49% respectively. Wang et al. demonstrated a true positive rate of 64% for trisomy 18 and 44% for trisomy 13 in a review of 109 cases of positive cffDNA screening tests in which patients went on to have cytogenetic testing [51]. The positive predictive value is influenced by the prevalence of the condition being tested for, in addition to the sensitivity and specificity of the test. Rarer conditions have a lower positive predictive value than more common conditions, such as Down syndrome, leading to more false-positive results in low-risk patients. High-risk results on cffDNA screening should therefore be confirmed by further diagnostic testing. A 2014 study of over 30000 pregnant people found that 6% of those with a high-risk cffDNA test for chromosomal abnormality terminated their pregnancy without a further confirmatory test [52]. Therefore, it is crucial to counsel patients with individualized positive predictive values for each fetal chromosomal abnormality to counsel them effectively in this regard [16].

Implementation of cffDNA testing in clinical practice

CffDNA screening faces some major challenges to its implementation into clinical practice, including a substantially higher cost than other screening methods, and no-call results which require counselling and potential further testing [33]. However, the American College of Obstetricians and Gynecologists and the Society for Maternal Fetal Medicine have recommended that prenatal genetic screening (using either traditional aneuploidy screening or cffDNA screening) should be offered to all pregnant people regardless of age or background risk of chromosomal anomaly [16]. Other international organizations, however, have recommended that, given the high potential costs of offering primary cffDNA screening, it should instead be offered only in cases of positive conventional screening where invasive diagnostic testing is not desired [53].

CASE PRESENTATION 1

A healthy 40-year-old para 1 attends at 10 weeks gestation for noninvasive prenatal testing. They are appropriately counseled regarding cffDNA screening and the patient undergoes the test. An ultrasound is performed at the time of screening which shows no abnormalities and a fetal crown–rump length of 42 mm. An insufficient fetal fraction of 2.4% is reported, and it was noted that the patient's weight was 75 kg. The patient is counselled regarding the possibility of invasive testing or re-testing. Another blood draw for repeat cffDNA testing at 12 weeks gestation is taken which again demonstrates an insufficient fetal fraction of 2.8%. The patient is offered invasive testing by means of chorionic villus sampling (CVS) but declines due to concerns regarding pregnancy loss. Instead, a detailed fetal ultrasound assessment is performed at 17 weeks gestation, which demonstrates a ventricular septal defect, clenched fists, and a growth-restricted fetus. An amniocentesis is performed and the resultant karyotype shows a nondisjunctional trisomy 18 (47, XY+18). Following counseling, the patient elects to undergo termination of the pregnancy.

CASE PRESENTATION 2

A 32-year-old para 1 is referred from the early pregnancy assessment unit with an increased NT. She attends the prenatal diagnosis clinic at 11 0/7 weeks gestation and a septated cystic hygroma is identified (see Plate 7.1). Following careful counseling regarding the associated risks of aneuploidy and congenital structural abnormalities, the patient agrees to proceed with a transabdominal CVS. Genetic evaluation reveals a normal male karyotype. She attends again at 18 0/7 and 23 4/7 weeks gestation. The first-trimester cystic hygroma has entirely resolved and genetic sonography and echocardiogram reveal no abnormalities. Her pregnancy progresses without complications and she delivers a healthy male infant by vacuum delivery at 40 5/7 weeks gestation, weighing 4500 g.

References

1. Malone FD, Canick JA, Ball RH, Nyberg DA, Comstock CH, Bukowski R, et al. First-trimester or second-trimester screening, or both, for Down's syndrome. N Engl J Med. 2005; 353:2001–11.
2. Snijders RL, Noble P, Sebire N, Souka A, Nicolaides KH. UK multicenter project on assessment of risk of trisomy 21 by maternal age and fetal nuchal-translucency thickness at 10–14 weeks of gestation. Lancet. 1998;351:343–6.
3. Wald NJ, Rodeck C, Hackshaw AK, Walters J, Chitty L, Mackinson AM. First and second trimester antenatal screening for Down's syndrome: the results of the Serum, Urine and Ultrasound Screening Study (SURUSS). Health Technol Assess. 2003;7:1–77.
4. Wapner R, Thom E, Simpson JL, Pergament E, Silver R, Filkins K, et al. First-trimester screening for trisomies 21 and 18. N Engl J Med. 2003;349:1405–13.
5. Malone FD, d'Alton MD, for the Society for Maternal-Fetal Medicine. First trimester sonographic screening for Down syndrome. Obstet Gynecol. 2003;102:1066–79.
6. Cicero S, Curcio P, Papageorghiou A, Sonek J, Nicolaides KH. Absence of nasal bone in fetuses with trisomy 21 at 11-14 weeks of gestation: an observational study. Lancet. 2001;358:1665–7.
7. Cicero S, Rembouskos G, Vandecruys H, Hogg M, Nicolaides KH. Likelihood ratio for trisomy 21 in fetuses with absent nasal bone at the 11-14-week scan. Ultrasound Obstet Gynecol. 2004;23:218–23.
8. Malone FD, Ball RH, Nyberg DA, Comstock CH, Saade G, Berkowitz RL, et al. First trimester nasal bone evaluation for aneuploidy in the general population: results from the FASTER Trial. Obstet Gynecol. 2004,104.1222–8.
9. Matias A, Gomes C, Flack N, Montenegro N, Nicolaides KH. Screening for chromosomal abnormalities at 10-14 weeks: the role of ductus venosus blood flow. Ultrasound Obstet Gynecol. 1998;12:380–4.
10. Hecher K. Assessment of ductus venosus flow during the first and early second trimesters: what can we expect? Ultrasound Obstet Gynecol. 2001;17:285–7.
11. Faiola S, Tsoi E, Huggon IC, Allan LD, Nicolaides KH. Likelihood ratio for trisomy 21 in fetuses with tricuspid regurgitation at the 11 to 13+6 week scan. Ultrasound Obstet Gynecol. 2005;26:22–7.

12. Falcon O, Auer M, Gerovassili A, Spencer K, Nicolaides KH. Screening for trisomy 21 by fetal tricuspid regurgitation, nuchal translucency and maternal serum free beta-hCG and PAPP-A at 11+0 to 13+6 weeks. Ultrasound Obstet Gynecol. 2006;27:151–5.

13. Malone FD, Ball RH, Nyberg DA et al. First trimester septated cystic hygroma: prevalence, natural history, and pediatric outcome. Obstet Gynecol. 2005;106:288–94.

14. Scholl J, Durfee SM, Russell MA, Heard AJ, Iyer C, Alammari R, et al. First-trimester cystic hygroma: relationship of nuchal translucency thickness and outcomes. Obstet Gynecol. 2012;120:551–9.

15. Driscoll DA, Gross SJ for the Professional Practice Guidelines Committee. Screening for fetal aneuploidy and neural tube defects. Genet Med. 2009;11(11):818–21.

16. American College of Obstetricians and Gynecologists. Screening for fetal chromosomal abnormalities. Obstet Gynecol. 2020;136(4):48–69.

17. Nyberg DA, Luthy DA, Resta RG, Nyberg BC, Williams MA. Age-adjusted ultrasound risk assessment for fetal Down's syndrome during the second trimester: description of the method and analysis of 142 cases. Ultrasound Obstet Gynecol. 1998;12:8–14.

18. Nyberg DA, Souter VL, El-Bastawissi A, Young S, Luthhardt F, Luthy DA. Isolated sonographic markers for detection of fetal Down syndrome in the second trimester of pregnancy. J Ultrasound Med. 2001;20:1053–63.

19. Aagaard-Tillery KM, Malone FD, Nyberg DA, Porter TF, Cuckle HS, Fuchs K, et al. Role of second-trimester genetic sonography after Down syndrome screening. Obstet Gynecol. 2009;114(6):1189–96.

20. Wald NJ, Kennard A, Hackshaw A, McGuire A. Antenatal screening for Down's syndrome. J Med Screening. 1994; 4:181–246.

21. Platt LD, Greene N, Johnson A, Zachary J, Thom E, Krantz D, et al. Sequential pathways of testing after first-trimester screening for trisomy 21. Obstet Gynecol. 2004;104:661–6.

22. Cuckle HS, Malone FD, Wright D, Porter TF, Nyberg DA, Comstock CH, et al. Contingent screening for Down syndrome–results from the FASTER trial. Prenat Diagn. 2008; 28:89–94.

23. Sebire NJ, Snijders RJM, Hughes K, Sepulveda W, Nicolaides KH. Screening for trisomy 21 in twin pregnancies by maternal age and fetal nuchal translucency thickness at 10-14 weeks of gestation. Br J Obstet Gynaecol. 1996;103:999–1003.

24. Khalil A, Archer R, Hutchinson V, Mousa H, Johnstone E, Cameron M, et al. Noninvasive prenatal screening in twin pregnancies with cell-free DNA using the IONA test: a prospective multicenter study. Am J Obstet Gynecol. 2021;225(1):79. e1–13.

25. Galeva S, Gil MM, Konstantinidou L, Akolekar R, Nicolaides K. First-trimester screening for trisomies by cfDNA testing of maternal blood in singleton and twin pregnancies: factors affecting test failure. Ultrasound Obstet Gynecol. 2019; 53(6):804–9.

26. Gil MM, Galeva S, Jani J, Konstantinidou L, Akolekar R, Plana MN, Nicolaides KH. Screening for trisomies by cfDNA testing of maternal blood in twin pregnancy: update of The Fetal Medicine Foundation results and meta-analysis. Ultrasound Obstet Gynecol. 2019 Jun;53(6):734–42.

27. Sebire NJ, Souka A, Skentou H et al. Early prediction of severe twin-to-twin transfusion syndrome. Hum Reprod. 2000; 15:2008–10.

28. Spencer K, Nicolaides KH. Screening for trisomy 21 in twins using first trimester ultrasound and maternal serum biochemistry in a one stop clinic: a review of three years experience. Br J Obstet Gynaecol. 2003;110:276–80.

29. Nicolaides KH, Campbell S, Gabbe SG, Guidetti R. Ultrasound screening for spina bifida: cranial and cerebellar signs. Lancet. 1986;8498:72–4.

30. Wald NJ. Prenatal screening for open neural tube defects and Down syndrome: three decades of progress. Prenat Diagn. 2010;30:619–21.

31. Chaoui R, Nicolaides KH. From nuchal translucency to intracranial translucency: towards the early detection of spina bifida. Ultrasound Obstet Gynecol. 2010;35:133–8.

32. Lo Y, Corbetta N, Chamberlain P, Rai V, Sargent I, Redman C, et al. Presence of fetal DNA in maternal plasma and serum. Lancet. 1997;350(9076):485–7.

33. Carbone L, Cariati F, Sarno L, Conforti A, Bagnulo F, Strina I, et al. Non-invasive prenatal testing: current perspectives and future challenges. Genes. 2020;12(1):15.

34. Shaw J, Scotchman E, Chandler N, Chitty L. Preimplantation genetic testing: non-invasive prenatal testing for aneuploidy, copy-number variants and single-gene disorders. Reproduction. 2020;160(5):A1–A11.

35. Galbiati S, Smid M, Gambini D, Ferrari A, Restagno G, Viora E, et al. Fetal DNA detection in maternal plasma throughout gestation. Hum Genet. 2005;117(2-3):243–8.

36. van Schendel R, van El C, Pajkrt E, Henneman L, Cornel M. Implementing non-invasive prenatal testing for aneuploidy in a national healthcare system: global challenges and national solutions. BMC Health Serv Res. 2017;17(1):670.

37. Norton M, Brar H, Weiss J, Karimi A, Laurent L, Caughey A, et al. Non-invasive chromosomal evaluation (NICE) Study: results of a multicenter prospective cohort study for detection of fetal trisomy 21 and trisomy 18. Am J Obstet Gynecol. 2012;207(2):137.e1–8.

38. Wang E, Batey A, Struble C, Musci T, Song K, Oliphant A. Gestational age and maternal weight effects on fetal cell-free DNA in maternal plasma. Prenat Diagn. 2013; 33(7):662–6.

39. Galeva S, Gil M, Konstantinidou L, Akolekar R, Nicolaides K. First-trimester screening for trisomies by cfDNA testing of maternal blood in singleton and twin pregnancies: factors affecting test failure. Ultrasound Obstet Gynecol. 2019; 53:804–9.

40. Ashoor G, Syngelaki A, Poon L, Rezende J, Nicolaides K. Fetal fraction in maternal plasma cell-free DNA at 11-13 weeks' gestation: relation to maternal and fetal characteristics. Ultrasound Obstet Gynecol. 2012;41(1):26–32.

41. Yaron Y. The implications of non-invasive prenatal testing failures: a review of an under-discussed phenomenon. Prenat Diagn. 2016;36(5):391–6.

42. Bianchi D, Sehnert A, Rava R. Genome-wide fetal aneuploidy detection by maternal plasma DNA sequencing. Obstet Gynecol. 2012;119(6):1270–1.

43. Palomaki G, Kloza E, Lambert-Messerlian G, Haddow J, Neveux L, Ehrich M, et al. DNA sequencing of maternal plasma to detect Down syndrome: An international clinical validation study. Genet Med. 2011;13(11):913–20.

44. Gil M, Quezada M, Revello R, Akolekar R, Nicolaides K. Analysis of cell-free DNA in maternal blood in screening for fetal aneuploidies: updated meta-analysis. Ultrasound Obstet Gynecol. 2015;45(3):249–66.

45. Quezada M, Gil M, Francisco C, Oròsz G, Nicolaides K. Screening for trisomies 21, 18 and 13 by cell-free DNA analysis of maternal blood at 10-11 weeks' gestation and the combined test at 11-13 weeks. Ultrasound Obstet Gynecol. 2014;45(1):36–41.

46. Pergament E, Cuckle H, Zimmermann B, Banjevic M, Sigurjonsson S, Ryan A, et al. Single-nucleotide polymorphism-based noninvasive prenatal screening in a high-risk and low-risk cohort. Obstet Gynecol. 2014;124(2):210–18.

47. Rava R, Srinivasan A, Sehnert A, Bianchi D. Circulating fetal cell-free DNA fractions differ in autosomal aneuploidies and monosomy X. Clin Chem. 2014;60(1):243–50.

48. HGSA/RANZCOG Joint Committee on Prenatal Diagnosis and Screening. Prenatal Screening and Diagnostic Testing for Fetal Chromosomal and Genetic Conditions. Melbourne: RANZCOG; 2018 [cited 2023 Jun 4]. Available from: https:// ranzcog.edu.au/wp-content/uploads/2022/05/Prenatal-Screening-and-Diagnostic-Testing-for-Fetal-Chromosomal-and-Genetic-Conditions.pdf.

49. Society for Maternal-Fetal Medicine (SMFM) Publications Committee. #36: Prenatal aneuploidy screening using cell-free DNA. Am J Obstet Gynecol. 2015;212(6):711–16.

50. Norton M, Jacobsson B, Swamy G, Laurent L, Ranzini A, Brar H, et al. Cell-free DNA analysis for noninvasive examination of trisomy. Obstet Gynecol Surv. 2015;70(8):483–4.

51. Wang J, Sahoo T, Schonberg S, Kopita K, Ross L, Patek K, et al. Discordant noninvasive prenatal testing and cytogenetic results: a study of 109 consecutive cases. Genet Med. 2015; 17(3):234–6.

52. Dar P, Curnow K, Gross S, Hall M, Stosic M, Demko Z, et al. Clinical experience and follow-up with large scale single-nucleotide polymorphism-based noninvasive prenatal aneuploidy testing. Am J Obstet Gynecol. 2014;211(5):527. e1–17.

53. Audibert F, De Bie I, Johnson J, Okun N, Wilson R, Armour C, et al. No. 348-Joint SOGC-CCMG Guideline: update on prenatal screening for fetal aneuploidy, fetal anomalies, and adverse pregnancy outcomes. J Obstet Gynaecol Can. 2017; 39(9):805–17.

Chapter 8
Sonographic Dating and Standard Fetal Biometry

Anna Hayes Nutter and Alfred Abuhamad
Department of Obstetrics and Gynecology, Eastern Virginia Medical School, Norfolk, VA, USA

Pregnancy dating

Accurate pregnancy dating is critical, essential for prenatal management and in particular fetal growth restriction. Although uterine size, as measured by fundal height, provides a subjective assessment of fetal size, ultrasound has a far more precise role in confirming gestational age [1].

Overestimation of gestational age based on menstrual dates is responsible for a preponderance of misdated pregnancies and results from delayed ovulation in the conception cycle. For instance, overestimation of true gestational age by the menstrual history results in an underestimate of the rate of preterm delivery [2] and an overestimate of postdated pregnancies. In a retrospective review of a routinely scan-dated population, Gardosi et al. [3] found that 72% of inductions for post-term pregnancy (>294 days) by menstrual dates were not post term according to ultrasound dating.

Ultrasound has an integral role in confirming gestational age, with a high accuracy when performed in the first or second trimester of pregnancy. A study involving in vitro fertilization (IVF) pregnancy has shown that ultrasound has an accuracy in pregnancy dating of 3–4 days when performed between 14 and 22 weeks gestation [1]. Dating during the third trimester is less predictive because of heterogeneity in fetal growth rates and should be avoided.

First trimester

Before 6 weeks gestation, dating can be carried out by measurement and observation of the gestational sac [4]. The gestational sac is visible as early as 4 weeks and should always be visible by 5 weeks of menstrual age.

The size of the gestational sac can be correlated with gestational age [5]. Because the mean sac diameter (MSD) grows at a rate of 1 mm/day, gestational age can be estimated by the formula:

$$\text{Gestational age (days)} = 30\,\text{MSD (mm) [6]}.$$

Among all fetal biometry measurements, determination of the maximum embryonic length (crown–rump length [CRL]) up to 14 weeks gestation is the most accurate for determining gestational age. The random error is in the range of 4–8 days at the 95th percentile [7–12].

Second and third trimesters

When the CRL is above 60 mm, other biometric parameters are more useful pregnancy dating [13]. Standardized measurements include the biparietal diameter (BPD), head circumference (HC), femur length (FL), humeral length (HL), and abdominal circumference (AC). These grow in a predictable way and so can be correlated with gestational age. Virtually any other bone or organ can be measured and compared with gestational age.

In a study of IVF pregnancies, the HC was the most predictive parameter of gestational age between 14 and 22 weeks gestation as it predicts gestational age within 3.4 days [1]. Other parameters such as the BPD, AC, and FL also have good accuracy. Combining various biometric parameters improves the prediction of gestational age slightly over the use of HC alone [1].

The AC is a measure of fetal girth. It includes soft tissues of the abdominal wall as well as a measure of internal organs, primarily the liver. Unlike other commonly used fetal measurements, it is not influenced by bone growth or morphology. At term, 95% of newborns

Queenan's Management of High-Risk Pregnancy: An Evidence-Based Approach, Seventh Edition. Edited by Catherine Y. Spong and Charles J. Lockwood.

are found to be within 20% of an expected length of 50 cm (20 in), whereas infant weight may vary by 100% or more. Therefore, differences in weight must be explained primarily by variations in girth and, not surprisingly, the AC is among the least predictive measures of fetal age but the most predictive of fetal growth [14–16].

Estimation of fetal weight

The best overall measure of fetal size is obtained by estimating fetal weight. Numerous formulas have been described and used [17–19]. Formulas based on three or four fetal biometric indices are more accurate than those based on one or two indices [20]. Using standard biometry, some use head measurements and AC, others use long bone measurements and AC, and others use all these measurements. The AC is included in all commonly used formulas of estimated fetal weight (EFW), and it also strongly influences fetal weight estimates [21]. Weight estimates based on AC alone have also been reported [22,23].

Hadlock [17], Dudley [18], Combs et al. [19], Rose and McCallum [24], and Medchill et al. [25] provide estimations of weight formulas, which include BPD, HC, AC, and FL, resulting in a mean absolute error of approximately 10% [26,27]. Some formulas for estimating fetal weight are volume based and would be expected to be more accurate in predicting fetal weight; however, these volume-based equations have not been shown to be consistently more accurate and some studies have resulted in large systematic errors [28].

In experienced hands, nearly 80% of estimated weights are within 10% of the actual birthweights and most of the remaining are within 20% of birthweights. However, accuracy decreases when less experienced sonographers perform exams [29]. Measures shown to improve fetal weight estimation include improvement in image quality, averaging of multiple measurements, and uniform calibration of equipment [30]. A number of studies have documented that prediction of fetal weight by ultrasound is limited. In one study, Baum et al. [29] found that sonographic estimation of fetal weight was no better than clinical or patient estimates at term.

Macrosomia

The term "large for gestational age" (LGA) describes neonates with a birthweight ≥ 90th percentile for a given gestational age. Macrosomia refers to growth beyond an absolute birthweight, historically 4000 or 4500 g, regardless of gestational age, and can be diagnosed only postnatally. Excessive fetal growth is associated with maternal obesity, excessive gestational weight gain, diabetes, and post-term pregnancy.

Prenatal prediction of birthweight is imprecise and no formula is more accurate than others in the detection of fetal weight [31]. Ultrasound accuracy decreases with increasing fetal weight beyond 4000 g. For suspected macrosomia, clinical measurement and ultrasound are no more precise than the estimate of a parous patient [32].

Fetal growth restriction

Definition

The term "small for gestational age" (SGA) describes newborns with birthweight <10th percentile for gestational age, representing a heterogeneous group of both constitutionally small but "normal" and pathologically growth-restricted neonates. Low birthweight is defined by the World Health Organization as weight at birth less than 2500 g and is the result of preterm birth, fetal growth restriction, or both [33].

Antenatally, small estimated fetal size is referred to as "fetal growth restriction" (FGR). The definition that is most commonly used in clinical practice and adopted by the current Society for Maternal-Fetal Medicine (SMFM) guidelines is an estimated fetal weight or abdominal circumference at <10th percentile for gestational age [34]. At this diagnostic threshold, approximately 70% of "affected" fetuses will be constitutionally small and have no significant increase in perinatal morbidity or mortality [35,36]. An EFW less than the third percentile has been associated with a significantly increased risk of perinatal morbidity and mortality and therefore represents a more severe form of FGR [37,38].

It should be clear that estimated weights and weight percentiles only evaluate fetal size and cannot distinguish growth-restricted potentially compromised fetuses from otherwise healthy fetuses that are constitutionally small and also does not detect fetuses that fail to meet their growth potential. Therefore, estimates of fetal size are considered with other correlates of fetal health, including amniotic fluid, Doppler flow studies, and fetal activity, which may be indicators of reduced uteroplacental blood flow, hypoxemia, or malnutrition. Serial ultrasound evaluation of fetal growth is recommended after the diagnosis of FGR. The optimal interval to balance clinical utility with technical and intra and interobserver variability is 3 to 4 weeks and consider every 2 weeks in severe cases [34,39,40].

The AC is the most sensitive indicator for fetal growth restriction. Compared to ultrasonographic EFW <10th percentile, AC <10th percentile has been shown to predict SGA with similar sensitivity and specificity [41–43]. The growth profile of the AC should therefore be monitored closely in fetuses at risk for growth abnormalities.

Customized growth curves have been developed that account for genetic factors that affect fetal growth such as maternal height, maternal weight, parity, ethnic origin, and fetal gender. Studies [33,44,45] identified racial/ethnic differences in fetal growth, but these custom formulas have not resulted in improved detection or outcomes of FGR [46,47]. Use of population-based fetal growth references (such as Hadlock) is recommended for prediction of neonatal morbidity [47,48].

Symmetric versus asymmetric

"Symmetric" FGR has been used to describe the growth pattern when all biometric measurements are affected, whereas "asymmetric" FGR has been used to characterize a smaller AC compared with other growth parameters. Asymmetric FGR would then show abnormal ratios such as the HC:AC or FL:AC ratio [49].

This classification was thought to reflect the etiology and prognosis of FGR. Symmetric FGR was suggested to reflect underlying fetal condition including aneuploidy, whereas asymmetric FGR reflected uterine–placental vascular dysfunction. However, these assumptions have proved to be largely false, as recent data shows similar growth and developmental delay during the first 4 years of life for both symmetric and asymmetric FGR [50]. Asymmetric FGR was more likely to be associated with a major fetal anomaly in one study [51] and severe uteroplacental vascular insufficiency can initially present as symmetric FGR [52]. Fetuses with symmetric and asymmetric FGR also show a similar degree of acid–base impairment [53]. Given the lack of clinical utility, classifying FGR as symmetric or asymmetric is not currently recommended.

Timing of diagnosis

FGR is classified as early or late based on the gestational age at the time of ultrasound diagnosis, prior to 32 vs. at or after 32 weeks gestation respectively. Early FGR tends to be more severe, is often associated with maternal hypertensive disorders, and follows a characteristic trend of deterioration with abnormalities in the umbilical artery Doppler followed by ductus venosus and finally abnormal biophysical parameters [54–58]. Late FGR accounts for 70–80% of FGR cases, is typically less severe, and less likely to be associated with maternal hypertension or diffuse histopathologic signs of placental underperfusion [59–61].

Risk factors

The most common associations of FGR are with maternal hypertension and/or a history of FGR (Box 8.1). Patients with early FGR should have close monitoring for development of pregnancy-induced hypertensive disorders [62]. Conversely, a history of a prior SGA newborn is a risk factor for preeclampsia [63].

Underlying uterine–placental dysfunction is a commonly cited cause for otherwise unexplained FGR. Uterine–placental dysfunction has been correlated with a

---

Box 8.1 Causes of and associations with fetal growth restriction

Maternal

- Pregnancy-induced hypertension/preeclampsia
- Severe chronic hypertension
- Severe maternal diabetes mellitus
- Collagen vascular disease
- Heart disease
- Smoking
- Poor nutrition
- Renal disease
- Lung disease/hypoxia
- Environmental agents
- Endocrine disorders
- Previous history of fetal growth restriction

Uterine–placental

- Uterine–placental dysfunction
- Placental infarct
- Chronic abruption
- Multiple gestation/twin transfusion syndrome
- Confined placental mosaicism

Fetal

- Chromosome abnormalities
- Anomalies
- Skeletal dysplasias
- Multiple anomaly syndromes (see Box 8.2)
- Infection
- Teratogens

---

range of pathologic findings including failure of physiologic transformation of uterine spiral arteries, smaller placentas, increase in the thickness of tertiary stem villi vessel wall, and decrease in lumen circumference of spiral arterioles. Also, confined placental mosaicism has been found to carry a higher risk of FGR and adverse outcome, including fetal death [64]. Uterine–placental dysfunction produces fetal hypoxemia, which results in subnormal growth, oligohydramnios, and alterations in blood flow [65].

Chromosome abnormalities, including those confined to the placenta (confined placental mosaicism), may exhibit delayed growth as a prominent feature. Abnormal growth and development have also been associated with disturbed genomic imprinting (expression of genes depending on whether they are located on the maternal or the paternal chromosome). This has led to the suggestion that genomic imprinting has evolved as a mechanism to regulate embryonic and fetal growth [66]. Many fetuses with chromosomal anomalies or other genetic syndromes may exhibit growth delay as a dominant feature (Box 8.2). It may be the primary or in some cases the only sonographic evidence of underlying fetal anomalies. Early FGR is a common manifestation of

---

Box 8.2 Genetic syndromes that include fetal growth restriction

- **Aarskog syndrome**. X-linked. Associated with brachydactyly, shawl scrotum, hypertelorism, vertebral anomalies, and moderate short stature. DNA testing is available.
- **Ataxia-telangiectasia syndrome**. Autosomal recessive. Associated with growth deficiency sometimes evident prenatally, ataxia, telangiectasias, and immunodeficiency. DNA testing is available.
- **Bloom syndrome**. Autosomal recessive. More common in Ashkenazi Jewish population. Associated with prenatal growth deficiency, butterfly telangiectasia of the face, microcephaly, mild mental retardation in some cases, and occasional syndactyly and/or polydactyly. DNA analysis is available.
- **Cornelia de Lange/Brachman syndrome**. Autosomal dominant, often *de novo*. Associated with prenatal growth deficiency, micromelia, mental retardation, and synophrys. DNA testing is available.
- **CHARGE syndrome**, characterized by coloboma, heart disease, choanal atresia, retarded growth (typically postnatal onset) or development, central nervous system abnormalities, genital anomalies, and ear anomalies and/or deafness. DNA testing is available.
- **Coffin–Siris syndrome**. Autosomal recessive. Characterized by prenatal growth deficiency, mental retardation, coarse facies, absence of terminal phalanges, and hypoplastic to absent fingernails and toenails. DNA testing is not currently available.
- **Dubowitz syndrome**. Autosomal recessive. Characterized by microcephaly, prenatal growth deficiency, mental retardation, dysmorphic facies, 2,3 toe syndactyly, and eczema. DNA testing is not currently available.
- **Fanconi anemia**. Autosomal recessive. Characterized by radial ray defects including aplasia of the thumbs or supernumerary thumbs, short stature often of prenatal onset, pancytopenia, renal or other urinary tract abnormalities, cardiac defects, and gastrointestinal abnormalities. DNA testing is available.
- **Johanson–Blizzard syndrome**. Autosomal recessive. Rare syndrome associated with prenatal growth deficiency, hypoplastic alae nasi, mental retardation, hydronephrosis, and pancreatic insufficiency. DNA testing is not currently available.
- **Neu–Laxova syndrome**. Autosomal recessive. Rare syndrome associated with severe prenatal growth deficiency, microcephaly, exophthalmos, subcutaneous edema, micrognathia, sloping forehead, syndactyly, contractures, often with pterygia, polyhydramnios, small placenta, and short umbilical cord. Majority of patients are stillborn. DNA testing is not available.
- **Noonan syndrome**. Autosomal dominant. Associated with pulmonic stenosis, other congenital heart defects, webbed neck/increased nuchal translucency, short stature typically of postnatal onset, dysmorphic facies, pectus excavatum, and vertebral anomalies. DNA analysis is available.
- **Pena–Shokier phenotype**. Autosomal recessive in some families. Characterized by prenatal growth deficiency, arthrogryposis, clubfoot, rocker-bottom feet, micrognathia, pulmonary hypoplasia, polyhydramnios, abnormal placenta, and short umbilical cord. DNA testing is not available.
- **Roberts syndrome/Roberts phocomelia**. Autosomal recessive with variable expression. Characterized by thalidomide-type limb reduction defects often more severe in the upper limbs, microcephaly, severe prenatal growth deficiency, mental retardation, cleft lip and/or palate. DNA testing is not available.
- **Seckel syndrome**. Autosomal recessive. Characterized by severe prenatal growth deficiency, mental retardation, microcephaly, prominent nose, micrognathia, and missing ribs. DNA analysis is not available.
- **Silver–Russell syndrome**. Typically sporadic but has been associated with maternal uniparental disomy of chromosome 7 in about 10% of cases. Characterized by prenatal growth deficiency, asymmetry of the limbs, triangular facies, relative microcephaly, and small and/or curved fifth finger. Uniparental disomy testing is available.
- **Smith–Lemli–Opitz syndrome**. Autosomal recessive. Characterized by failure to thrive, microcephaly, 2,3 toe syndactyly, genital abnormalities, polydactyly, and congenital heart defects. Affected fetuses may have low unconjugated estriol MoM on maternal serum screening. Diagnostic testing available.
- **Williams syndrome**. Autosomal dominant microdeletion syndrome caused by a deletion of 7p11.23. Characterized by mild prenatal growth deficiency, congenital heart defect particularly supravalvular aortic stenosis, mental retardation, dysmorphic features, contractures, abnormal curvature of the spine, and renal anomalies. Diagnostic testing available by fluorescence in situ hybridization analysis.

---

major chromosome abnormalities, particularly trisomies 18 and 13, and triploidy [67,68]. SMFM guidelines recommend detailed obstetrical ultrasound examination with early FGR because up to 20% of cases can be associated with fetal or chromosomal abnormalities [69–72]. Further, unexplained isolated early FGR or diagnosis of a fetal malformation or polyhydramnios in the setting of FGR should prompt consideration of fetal diagnostic testing, including chromosomal microarray.

Among other variables, smaller fetal size tends to reflect both maternal and paternal birthweights. Magnus et al. [73] found the mean maternal birthweight was significantly less among those who had experienced two SGA births compared with those with no SGA births (3127 ± 54 g vs. 3424 ± 22 g). Interestingly, the mean paternal birthweight was also lower (3497 ± 88 g vs. 3665 ± 24 g) from affected pregnancies with two previous SGA births.

Outcome

Management of FGR is based on early diagnosis, fetal surveillance, and delivery to optimize outcomes. Infants born SGA recognized as FGR antenatally with appropriate surveillance and delivery planning have a four- to fivefold reduction in morbidity and mortality [74]. Stillbirth rate at all gestational ages with weight below the 10th percentile and below the fifth percentile may be as high as 1.5% and 2.5%, respectively [75–77]. Furthermore, failure to recognize FGR may result in a stillbirth rate two to nine times that of infants diagnosed as SGA at birth [74,78,79]. In addition to an increased risk of perinatal mortality, when compared with appropriately grown fetuses matched for gestational age, FGR fetuses have an increased risk of perinatal morbidity, including severe acidosis at delivery, low Apgar scores, and neonatal intensive care unit admissions [80,81].

Long-term follow-up studies have shown an increased incidence of physical handicap and neurodevelopmental delay in growth-restricted fetuses [82,83]. The presence of chronic metabolic acidemia in utero, rather than birthweight, appears to be the best predictor of long-term neurodevelopmental delay, with rates as high as 20–40% by school age [84,85]. Progression of fetal hypoxemia to acidemia is an important antecedent to adverse short- and long-term outcomes. Therefore, antenatal surveillance aims to detect fetal responses that accompany such deterioration [86]. In contrast, early delivery can result in significant neonatal complications secondary to prematurity [87].

Results of both randomized and observational studies suggest that gestational age is the major contributor to adverse perinatal outcome in deliveries prior to 30–32 weeks gestation [62,87,88]. with a two- to fivefold increased rate of perinatal death among preterm FGR fetuses compared to term [89]. Although there is evidence of increased morbidity with late preterm birth, it should be noted that these findings may not be applicable to fetuses with suboptimal growth and abnormal fetal surveillance [90–92]. Therefore, in pregnancies with growth-restricted fetuses, timing of the delivery is the most critical step in clinical management. Balancing the risk of prematurity with the risk of long-term neurodevelopmental delay is a serious challenge. In addition, FGR fetuses may face long-term adverse adult health outcomes including accelerated atherosclerotic vascular disease, hypertension, and diabetes.

Management

Management relies on cardiotocography for fetal surveillance, evaluating heart rate variability as a sign of fetal well-being. Heart rate variability is the result of the rhythmic integrated activity of autonomic neurons generated by organized cardiorespiratory reflexes [93]. In growth-restricted fetuses, higher baseline rates, decreased long- and short-term variability, and delayed maturation of reactivity are seen [94,95]. Unaided visual analyses of fetal heart rate records have limited reliability and reproducibility [96,97], and overtly abnormal tracings represent late signs of fetal deterioration [98,99].

Doppler ultrasound can help differentiate the growth-restricted fetus from the constitutionally small fetus and improves outcome in high-risk pregnancies [100]. Studies highlight the fetal cardiovascular adaptation to hypoxemia and the progressive stages of such adaptation [101–106].

Fetal arterial Doppler

Umbilical circulation

The umbilical arterial circulation is normally a low-impedance circulation, with an increase in the amount of end-diastolic flow with advancing gestation (Figure 8.1) [108]. Umbilical arterial Doppler waveforms reflect the status of the placental circulation, and the increase in end-diastolic flow that is seen with advancing gestation is a direct result of an increase in the number of tertiary stem villi with placental maturation [109]. Diseases that obliterate small muscular arteries in placental tertiary stem villi result in a progressive decrease in end-diastolic flow in the umbilical arterial Doppler waveforms until absent and then

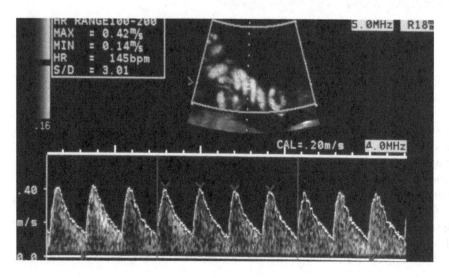

Figure 8.1 Normal Doppler waveforms obtained from the umbilical artery in the third trimester. In the third trimester of pregnancy, the umbilical circulation is a low-impedance circulation. Note the increased amount of flow at end diastole (*white arrow*). Reproduced from Abuhamad [107] with permission from Thieme Medical Publishing.

reverse flow during diastole is noted (Figure 8.2) [110]. Reversed diastolic flow in the umbilical arterial circulation represents an advanced stage of placental compromise and is associated with obliteration of more than 70% of placental tertiary villi arteries [111,112]. The presence of absent or reversed end-diastolic flow in the umbilical artery is commonly associated with severe FGR, oligohydramnios and high perinatal mortality [113].

Doppler waveforms of the umbilical arteries can be obtained from any segment along the umbilical cord. Waveforms obtained from the placental end of the cord show more end-diastolic flow than those obtained from the abdominal cord insertion [114]. Differences in Doppler indices of arterial waveforms obtained from different anatomic locations of the same umbilical cord are generally minor and have no significance in clinical practice [108].

Umbilical artery Doppler waveforms are assessed using the pulsatility index (PI), resistance index (RI), or systolic-to-diastolic (S/D) ratio with abnormal values defined as those greater than the 95th percentile for gestational age or diagnosis of absent or reversed end-diastolic velocity (AEDV or REDV). Umbilical artery decreased diastolic flow may progressively deteriorate to AEDV/REDV over days to weeks and worsening findings may be seen intermittently prior to becoming constant [115]. The recommended frequency for surveillance is dependent on the severity of growth restriction as well as

presence and severity of umbilical artery Doppler abnormalities. In general, umbilical artery Doppler assessment every 1–2 weeks for FGR with EFW 3rd–10th percentile and weekly for FGR <3rd percentile with normal umbilical artery Doppler flow [34]. After a period of stability and in the absence of severe growth restriction, UA Doppler assessment may be performed every 2–4 weeks [34]. Abnormal UA Doppler findings warrant more frequent surveillance: weekly for decreased flow and two to three times weekly for AEDV. Inpatient admission is recommended in the setting of umbilical artery REDV as it is associated with extensive placental degeneration and high risk of perinatal mortality [34,116].

Middle cerebral circulation

The cerebral circulation is normally a high-impedance circulation with continuous forward flow throughout the cardiac cycle [117]. The middle cerebral artery is the cerebral vessel most accessible to ultrasound imaging in the fetus and it carries more than 80% of cerebral blood flow [118]. In the presence of fetal hypoxemia, central redistribution of blood flow occurs, resulting in an increased blood flow to the brain, heart, and adrenals and a reduction in flow to the peripheral and placental circulations. This blood flow redistribution is known as the brain-sparing reflex and has a major role in fetal adaptation to oxygen deprivation [117,119].

The right and left middle cerebral arteries are major branches of the circle of Willis in the fetal brain. The circle of Willis is imaged with color flow Doppler ultrasound in a transverse plane of the fetal head obtained at the base of the skull where the proximal and distal middle cerebral arteries are seen in their longitudinal view, with their course almost parallel to the ultrasound beam (Figure 8.3). Middle cerebral artery Doppler waveforms, obtained from the proximal portion of the

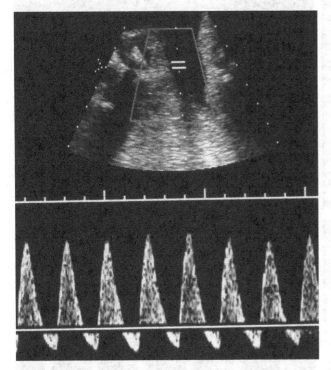

Figure 8.2 Reversed end-diastolic velocity is noted in the umbilical circulation when downstream impedance is increased. These Doppler waveforms are associated with significant fetal compromise. Reproduced from Abuhamad [107] with permission from Thieme Medical Publishing.

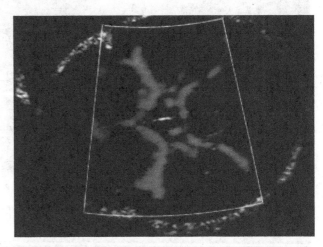

Figure 8.3 Axial view of the fetal head in the second trimester with color Doppler showing the circulation at the level of the circle of Willis. Note the course of the middle cerebral arteries, almost parallel to the ultrasound beam. Reproduced from Abuhamad [107] with permission from Thieme Medical Publishing.

vessel, immediately after its origin from the circle of Willis, have the best reproducibility [120].

Arterial Doppler and fetal growth restriction

Central redistribution of blood flow to the brain, known as the brain-sparing reflex, represents an early stage in fetal adaptation to hypoxemia [103–106] and follows the lag in fetal growth [121]. At this early stage, the brain-sparing reflex is clinically evident by increased end-diastolic flow in the middle cerebral artery (lower middle cerebral artery pulsatility or resistance index) and decreased end-diastolic flow in the umbilical artery (higher umbilical artery resistance index or S/D ratio).

Middle cerebral artery Doppler has not been shown to predict outcome in early FGR and should not be used to guide management; however, the cerebroplacental ratio, derived by dividing the cerebral PI by the umbilical PI, defines the brain-sparing reflex and may have future utility in guiding management in late FGR, though more clinical trials are needed [122,123].

Venous Doppler and fetal growth restriction

Chronic fetal hypoxemia results in decreased preload, decreased cardiac compliance, and elevated end-diastolic pressure in the right ventricle [102,124–127]. These changes are evident by an elevated central venous pressure in the chronically hypoxemic fetus, which is manifested by an increased reverse flow in Doppler waveforms of the ductus venosus (Figure 8.4) and the inferior vena cava (Figure 8.5) during late diastole. Changes in the fetal central venous circulation are associated with an advanced stage of fetal hypoxemia and increased perinatal morbidity and mortality [57,69,128,129]. At this late stage of fetal adaptation to hypoxemia, cardiac decompensation is often noted with myocardial dysfunction [126]. Furthermore, fetal metabolic acidemia is often present in association with Doppler waveform abnormalities of the inferior vena cava and ductus venosus [98,102,103]. Ductus venosus Doppler abnormalities with normal umbilical artery Doppler may be related to fetal vascular, cardiac, or genetic abnormalities rather than a consequence of placental pathology.

Most pregnancies are delivered for other fetal or maternal indications prior to development of absent or reversed A-wave of the ductus venosus, as such findings represent advanced fetal compromise only seen in 11% of fetuses with umbilical artery AEDV/REDV after 32 weeks and are preceded by abnormal cardiotocography findings [130,131]. At <34 weeks gestation, absent or reversed A-wave of the ductus venosus is associated with a 20% and 46% risk of stillbirth [116].

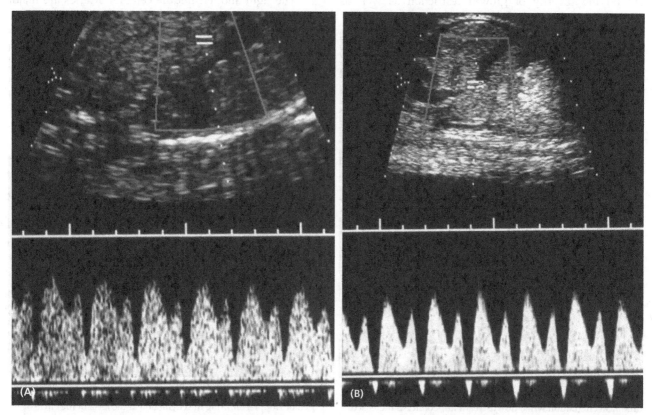

Figure 8.4 Doppler velocity waveforms of the ductus venosus in a normal fetus (A) and a severely compromised fetus (B) in the third trimester of pregnancy. Note the presence of reverse flow during late diastole in the severely compromised fetus (B). Reproduced from Abuhamad [107] with permission from Thieme Medical Publishing.

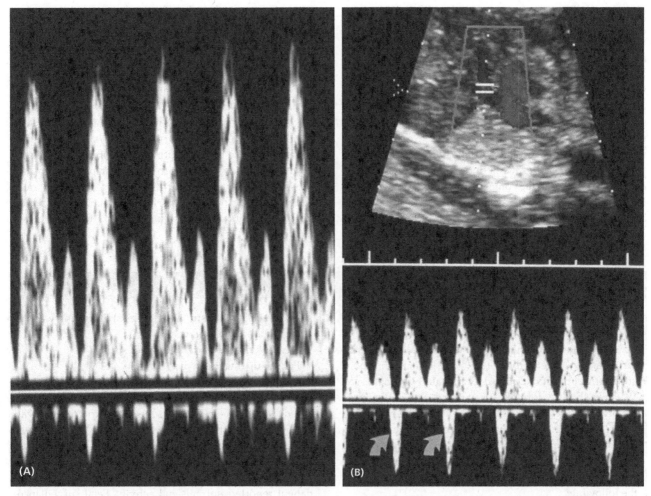

Figure 8.5 Doppler velocity waveforms of the inferior vena cava (IVC) in a normal fetus (A) and a severely compromised fetus (B) in the third trimester of pregnancy. The IVC Doppler waveforms have reverse flow during late diastole (atrial kick) in the normal fetus. Note the increase in reverse flow during late diastole in the severely compromised fetus (B) (*white arrowhead*). (A) Reproduced from Abuhamad [133] with permission from Elsevier; (B) Reproduced from Abuhamad [107] with permission from Thieme Medical Publishing.

The Trial of Randomized Umbilical and Fetal Flow in Europe (TRUFFLE) standardized management of early FGR with umbilical artery Doppler decreased end-diastolic flow based on ductus venosus Doppler or computerized cardiotocography (cCTG) short-term variability monitoring up to 32 weeks gestation with improvement in overall mortality and severe morbidity to 5% and 25% [62]. TRUFFLE reported an increased number of neurologically intact survivors in the group with absent or negative ductus venosus A-wave (95%) compared to the cCTG group (85%); however, these results are not generalizable to health systems that use visual interpretation of CTG and ductus venosus Doppler is not currently recommended for routine surveillance in early FGR in the United States [34,62].

Clinical application

In clinical practice, accurate pregnancy dating is essential for appropriate diagnosis of fetal growth abnormalities. Population-based fetal biometry measurements can be used to diagnose fetal growth restriction in the second and third trimesters of pregnancy. Detailed ultrasound should be performed with early FGR and fetal diagnostic testing should be offered when FGR is detected with a fetal malformation or polyhydramnios at any gestational age [34]. Serial ultrasound examination should be performed for interval fetal growth every 3–4 weeks for FGR and as frequently as every 2 weeks for severe FGR [34].

Doppler ultrasound provides important information on the extent of fetal compromise and guides timing of delivery for FGR fetuses. Umbilical artery Doppler abnormalities present early warning signs and warrant close surveillance.

Serial umbilical artery Doppler evaluation is recommended weekly for pregnancies affected by severe growth restriction or umbilical artery Doppler decreased end-diastolic velocity. Weekly CTG is recommended after viability for FGR without AEDV/REDV. Delivery is recommended at 37 weeks of gestation in FGR with umbilical artery decreased end-diastolic flow or severe FGR. In the setting of FGR with normal umbilical artery

Doppler, delivery is recommended at 38 to 39 weeks gestation.

Umbilical AEDV is associated with increased potential for decompensation and Doppler assessment is recommended two to three times per week [34]. The presence of reversed diastolic flow in the umbilical arteries is a sign of advanced fetal compromise, and strong consideration should be given to delivery except in cases of extreme prematurity. With umbilical artery REDV, management recommendations include hospitalization, antenatal corticosteroids, CTG at least 1–2 times per day, and consideration of delivery in the context of the clinical picture [34]. Delivery is recommended at 30 to 32 weeks for REDV and 33 to 34 weeks for AEDV, with consideration of cesarean delivery based on the clinical picture with AEDV/REDV.

The role for use of cerebroplacental ratio, middle cerebral artery Doppler, and ductus venosus Doppler in pregnancies with FGR is not recommended for routine management [34].

Fetal growth restriction is a complex disorder involving multiple fetal organs and systems [132]. Although fetal biometry and arterial Doppler provide information on the early compensatory phase of this disorder, venous Doppler, fetal heart rate analysis, and the biophysical profile provide information on the later stages, commonly associated with fetal cardiovascular collapse. It is hoped that future studies will shed more light on the pathophysiology of this disease and on the various interactions of diagnostic tools in fetal surveillance.

CASE PRESENTATION

A 40-year-old G3 P2002 has a pregnancy resulting from assisted reproduction with IVF. Prenatal care was pertinent for an abnormal quad screen with elevated maternal serum analyte α-fetoprotein (AFP) and human chorionic gonadotropin (hCG). Detailed ultrasound examination at 19 weeks showed normal fetal anatomy. At a routine prenatal visit at 29 weeks gestation the fundal height measured 26 cm and the patient was referred for an obstetric ultrasound examination. The patient reported good fetal movements, and vital signs were within normal limits with no proteinuria. Ultrasound examination revealed the following:

- Cephalic presentation
- Normal amniotic fluid volume
- BPD and HC at the 26th percentile for gestational age
- AC at the fifth percentile for gestational age
- Estimated fetal weight at the seventh percentile for gestational age
- When the biometric data were reported to the obstetrician, Doppler studies were ordered. Umbilical artery Doppler studies revealed S:D = 8.0 (abnormal for 29 weeks).

In view of the presence of FGR with abnormal arterial Doppler waveforms, plan was made for outpatient management to include:

- Twice-weekly nonstress tests (NSTs), including weekly amniotic fluid assessment
- Weekly umbilical artery Doppler studies
- Follow-up fetal growth in 3 weeks.

At 31 weeks gestation, 3 weeks from diagnosis, absent end-diastolic velocity (AEDV) in the umbilical artery was noted. Fetal biometry showed less than expected interval fetal growth, with estimated fetal weight at the fourth percentile and decreased amniotic fluid volume. The patient was admitted to the hospital for daily testing, a course of steroids, and twice-weekly Doppler studies. The patient reported normal fetal activity. Fetal surveillance studies on admission showed the following.

- Absent end-diastolic velocity with intermittent reversed end-diastolic velocity noted in the umbilical artery.
- NST with normal reactivity.

On the second day of hospitalization, the patient reported decreased fetal movements, NST showed spontaneous decelerations, and Doppler studies showed persistent reversed end-diastolic velocity in the umbilical artery. Biophysical profile scored 4/8. The patient had a cesarean delivery of a male infant, weighing 1150 g with Apgar scores of 4 and 7 at 1 and 5 minutes, respectively. Arterial pH was 7.10 with base excess of −11. Both patients did well with no major complications.

References

1. Chervenak FA, Skupski DW, Romero R, Myers MK, Smith-Levitin M, Rosenwaks Z, et al. How accurate is fetal biometry in the assessment of fetal age? Am J Obstet Gynecol. 1998;178(4):678–87.
2. Bartels DB, Kreienbrock L, Dammann O, Wenzlaff P, Poets CF. Population based study on the outcome of small for gestational age newborns. Arch Dis Child Fetal Neonatal Ed. 2005; 90(1):F53–9.
3. Gardosi J, Vanner T, Francis A. Gestational age and induction of labour for prolonged pregnancy. Br J Obstet Gynaecol. 1997;104(7):792–7.
4. Warren WB, Timor-Tritsch I, Peisner DB, Raju S, Rosen MG. Dating the early pregnancy by sequential appearance of embryonic structures. Am J Obstet Gynecol. 1989; 161(3):747–53.
5. Daya S. Accuracy of gestational age estimation by means of fetal crown-rump length measurement. Am J Obstet Gynecol. 1993;168(3, Part 1):903–8.

6. Nyberg DA, Mack LA, Laing FC, Patten RM. Distinguishing normal from abnormal gestational sac growth in early pregnancy. J Ultrasound Med. 1987;6(1):23–7.

7. Drumm JE, Clinch J, Mackenzie G. The ultrasonic measurement of fetal crown-rump length as a method of assessing gestational age. Br J Obstet Gynaecol. 1976;83(6):417–21.

8. Robinson HP, Fleming JEE. A critical evaluation of sonar "crown-rump length" measurements. Br J Obstet Gynaecol. 1975;82(9):702–10.

9. Daya S, Woods S, Ward S, Lappalainen R, Caco C. Early pregnancy assessment with transvaginal ultrasound scanning. CMAJ. 1991;144(4):441–6.

10. Grange G, Pannier E, Goffinet F, Cabrol D, Zorn JR. Dating biometry during the first trimester: accuracy of an everyday practice. Eur J Obstet Gynecol Reprod Biol. 2000;88(1):61–4.

11. MacGregor SN, Tamura RK, Sabbagha RE, Minogue JP, Gibson ME, Hoffman DI. Underestimation of gestational age by conventional crown-rump length dating curves. Obstet Gynecol. 1987;70(3 Pt 1):344–8.

12. Wisser J, Dirschedl P, Krone S. Estimation of gestational age by transvaginal sonographic measurement of greatest embryonic length in dated human embryos. Ultrasound Obstet Gynecol. 1994;4(6):457–62.

13. Hadlock FP. Sonographic estimation of fetal age and weight. Radiol Clin North Am. 1990;28(1):39–50.

14. Kurjak A, Kirkinen P, Latin V. Biometric and dynamic ultrasound assessment of small-for-dates infants: report of 260 cases. Obstet Gynecol. 1980;56(3):281–4.

15. Landon MB, Mintz MC, Gabbe SG. Sonographic evaluation of fetal abdominal growth: Predictor of the large-for-gestational-age infant in pregnancies complicated by diabetes mellitus. Am J Obstet Gynecol. 1989;160(1):115–21.

16. Basel D, Lederer R, Diamant YZ. Longitudinal ultrasonic biometry of various parameters in fetuses with abnormal growth rate. Acta Obstet Gynecol Scand. 1987;66(2):143–9.

17. Hadlock F. Callen PW, editors. Ultrasonography in obstetrics and gynecology. 3rd ed. Philadelphia: W.B. Saunders; 1994.

18. Dudley NJ. Selection of appropriate ultrasound methods for the estimation of fetal weight. Br J Radiol. 1995;68(808):385–8.

19. Combs CA, Jaekle RK, Rosenn B, Pope M, Miodovnik M, Siddiqi TA. Sonographic estimation of fetal weight based on a model of fetal volume. Obstet Gynecol. 1993;82(3):365–70.

20. Melamed N, Yogev Y, Meizner I, Mashiach R, Bardin R, Ben Haroush A. Sonographic fetal weight estimation. J Ultrasound Med. 2009;28(5):617–29.

21. Hadlock FP, Harrist RB, Carpenter RJ, Deter RL, Park SK. Sonographic estimation of fetal weight. The value of femur length in addition to head and abdomen measurements. Radiology. 1984;150(2):535–40.

22. Smith GCS, Smith MFS, McNay MB, Fleming JEE. The relation between fetal abdominal circumference and birthweight: findings in 3512 pregnancies. Br J Obstet Gynaecol. 1997;104(2):186–90.

23. Gore D, Williams M, O'Brien W, Gilby J. Fetal abdominal circumference for prediction of intrauterine growth restriction. Obstet Gynecol. 2000;(95):S78–9.

24. Rose BI, McCallum WD. A simplified method for estimating fetal weight using ultrasound measurements. Obstet Gynecol. 1987;(69):671–5.

25. Medchill MT PCGJ. Prediction of estimated fetal weight in extremely low birth weight neonates (500-1000 g). Obstet Gynecol. 1991;(78):286–90.

26. Robson SC, Gallivan S, Walkinshaw SA, Vaughan J, Rodeck CH. Ultrasonic estimation of fetal weight: use of targeted formulas in small for gestational age fetuses. Obstet Gynecol. 1993;82(3):359–64.

27. Sabbagha RE, Minogue J, Tamura RK, Hungerford SA. Estimation of birth weight by use of ultrasonographic formulas targeted to large-, appropriate-, and small-for gestational-age fetuses. Am J Obstet Gynecol. 1989;160:854–62.

28. Edwards A, Goff J, Baker L. Accuracy and modifying factors of the sonographic estimation of fetal weight. Aust N Z J Obstet Gynaecol. 2001;41:187–90.

29. Baum JD, Gussman D, Wirth JC. Clinical and patient estimation of fetal weight vs. ultrasound estimation. J Reprod Med. 2002;47(3):194–8.

30. Dudley NJ. A systematic review of the ultrasound estimation of fetal weight. Ultrasound Obstet Gynecol. 2005;25(1):80–9.

31. Hoopmann M, Abele H, Wagner N, Wallwiener D, Kagan KO. Performance of 36 Different weight estimation formulae in fetuses with macrosomia. Fetal Diagn Ther. 2010;27(4):204–13.

32. Chauhan SP, Meydrech EF, Washburne JF, Hudson JL, Martin RW, Morrison JC. Clinical estimate of birth-weight in labour: factors influencing its accuracy. Aust N Z J Obstet Gynaecol. 1993;33(4):371–3.

33. Kiserud T, Piaggio G, Carroli G, et al. The World Health Organization fetal growth charts: a multinational longitudinal study of ultrasound biometric measurements and estimated fetal weight. PLoS Medicine. 2017;14(1):e1002220–e1002220.

34. Society for Maternal-Fetal Medicine; Martins JG, Biggio JR, Abuhamad A. Society for Maternal-Fetal Medicine Consult Series # 52 : diagnosis and management of fetal growth restriction. Am J Obstet Gynecol. 2020;223(4):B2–B17.

35. Ott WJ. The diagnosis of altered fetal growth. Obstet Gynecol Clin North Am. 1988;(15):237–63.

36. McCowan LM, Figueras F, Anderson NH. Evidence-based national guidelines for the management of suspected fetal growth restriction: comparison, consensus, and controversy. Am J Obstet Gynecol. 2018;218(2, Suppl):S855–68.

37. Savchev S, Figueras F, Cruz-Martinez R, Illa M, Botet F, Gratacos E. Estimated weight centile as a predictor of perinatal outcome in small-for-gestational-age pregnancies with normal fetal and maternal Doppler indices. Ultrasound Obstet Gynecol. 2012;39(3):299–303.

38. Pilliod RA, Cheng YW, Snowden JM, Doss AE, Caughey AB. The risk of intrauterine fetal death in the small-for-gestational-age fetus. Am J Obstet Gynecol. 2012;207(4):318.e1–6.

39. Mongelli M, Condous G. Advances in mathematical models of fetal growth: implications for ultrasound practice. Australas J Ultrasound Med. 2014;17(3):93–5.

40. Mongelli M, Ek S, Tambyrajia R. Screening for fetal growth restriction: a mathematical model of the effect of time interval and ultrasound error. Obstet Gynecol. 1998;92(6):908–12.

41. David C, Tagliavini G, Pilu G, Rudenholz A, Bovicelli L. Receiver-operator characteristic curves for the ultrasonographic prediction of small-for-gestational-age fetuses in low-risk pregnancies. Am J Obstet Gynecol. 1996;174(3):1037–42.

42. Blue NR, Yordan JMP, Holbrook BD, Nirgudkar PA, Mozurkewich EL. Abdominal circumference alone versus

estimated fetal weight after 24 weeks to predict small or large for gestational age at birth: a meta-analysis. Am J Perinatol. 2017;34(11):1115–24.

43. Caradeux J, Martinez-Portilla RJ, Peguero A, Sotiriadis A, Figueras F. Diagnostic performance of third-trimester ultrasound for the prediction of late-onset fetal growth restriction: a systematic review and meta-analysis. Am J Obstet Gynecol. 2019;220(5):449–459.e19.

44. Buck Louis GM, Grewal J, Albert PS, Sciscione A, Wing DA, Grobman WA, et al. Racial/ethnic standards for fetal growth: the NICHD Fetal Growth Studies. Am J Obstet Gynecol. 2015;213(4):449.e1–41.

45. Kiserud T, Benachi A, Hecher K, Perez RG, Carvalho J, Piaggio G, et al. The World Health Organization fetal growth charts: concept, findings, interpretation, and application. Am J Obstet Gynecol. 2017;218(2S):S619–29.

46. Blue NR, Savabi M, Beddow ME, Katukuri VR, Fritts CM, Izquierdo LA, et al. The Hadlock method is superior to newer methods for the prediction of the birth weight percentile. J Ultrasound Med. 2019;38(3):587–96.

47. Blue NR, Beddow ME, Savabi M, Katukuri VR, Chao CR. Comparing the Hadlock fetal growth standard to the Eunice Kennedy Shriver National Institute of Child Health and Human Development racial/ethnic standard for the prediction of neonatal morbidity and small for gestational age. Am J Obstet Gynecol. 2018;219(5):474.e1–12.

48. Hammami A, Mazer Zumaeta A, Syngelaki A, Akolekar R, Nicolaides KH. Ultrasonographic estimation of fetal weight: development of new model and assessment of performance of previous models. Ultrasound Obstet Gynecol. 2018;52(1):35–43.

49. David C, Gabrielli S, Pilu G, Bovicelli L. The head-to-abdomen circumference ratio: a reappraisal. Ultrasound Obstet Gynecol. 1995;5(4):256–9.

50. Bocca-Tjeertes I, Bos A, Kerstjens J, de Winter A, Reijneveld S. Symmetrical and asymmetrical growth restriction in preterm-born children. Pediatrics. 2014;133(3):e650–56.

51. Dashe JS, McIntire DD, Lucas MJ, Leveno KJ. Effects of symmetric and asymmetric fetal growth on pregnancy outcomes. Obstet Gynecol. 2000;96(3):321–7.

52. Vik T, Vatten L, Jacobsen G, Bakketeig LS. Prenatal growth in symmetric and asymmetric small-for-gestational-age infants. Early Hum Dev. 1997;48:167–76.

53. Blackwell SC, Moldenhauer J, Redman M, Hassan SS, Wolfe HM, Berry SM. Relationship between the sonographic pattern of intrauterine growth restriction and acid-base status at the time of cordocentesis. Arch Gynecol Obstet. 2001;264(4):191–3.

54. Figueras F, Gratacos E. Stage-based approach to the management of fetal growth restriction. Prenat Diagn. 2014;34(7):655–9.

55. Platz E, Newman R. Diagnosis of IUGR: traditional biometry. Semin Perinatol. 2008;32(3):140–7.

56. Savchev S, Figueras F, Sanz-Cortes M, Cruz-Lemini M, Triunfo S, Botet F, et al. Evaluation of an optimal gestational age cut-off for the definition of early- and late-onset fetal growth restriction. Fetal Diagn Ther. 2014;36(2):99–105.

57. Dall'Asta A, Brunelli V, Prefumo F, Frusca T, Lees CC. Early onset fetal growth restriction. Matern Health Neonatol Perinatol. 2017;3:2.

58. Figueras F, Caradeux J, Crispi F, Eixarch E, Peguero A, Gratacos E. Diagnosis and surveillance of late-onset fetal growth restriction. Am J Obstet Gynecol. 2018;218(2, Suppl):S790–S802.e1.

59. Parra-Saavedra M, Crovetto F, Triunfo S, Savchev S, Peguero A, Nadal A, et al. Neurodevelopmental outcomes of near-term small-for-gestational-age infants with and without signs of placental underperfusion. Placenta. 2014;35(4):269–74.

60. Burton GJ, Jauniaux E. Pathophysiology of placental-derived fetal growth restriction. Am J Obstet Gynecol. 2018;218(2, Suppl):S745–61.

61. Sultana Z, Maiti K, Dedman L, Smith R. Is there a role for placental senescence in the genesis of obstetric complications and fetal growth restriction? Am J Obstet Gynecol. 2018;218(2, Suppl):S762–73.

62. Lees C, Marlow N, Arabin B, Bilardo CM, Brezinka C, Derks JB, et al. Perinatal morbidity and mortality in early-onset fetal growth restriction: cohort outcomes of the trial of randomized umbilical and fetal flow in Europe (TRUFFLE). Ultrasound Obstet Gynecol. 2013;42(4):400–8.

63. Rasmussen S, Irgens LM, Albrechtsen S, Dalaker K. Predicting preeclampsia in the second pregnancy from low birth weight in the first pregnancy. Obstet Gynecol. 2000;96(5 Pt 1):699–700.

64. Stipoljev F, Latin V, Kos M, Miskovic B, Kurjak A. Correlation of confined placental mosaicism with fetal intrauterine growth retardation: a case–control study of placentas at delivery. Fetal Diagn Ther. 2001;16:4–9.

65. Mitra SC, Seshan S v, Riachi LE. Placental vessel morphometry in growth retardation and increased resistance of the umbilical artery doppler flow. J Matern Fetal Med. 2000;9(5):282–6.

66. Devriendt K. Genetic control of intra-uterine growth. Eur J Obstet Gynecol Reprod Biol. 2000;92:29–34.

67. Snijders RJM, Sherrod C, Gosden CM, Nicolaides KH. Fetal growth retardation: Associated malformations and chromosomal abnormalities. Am J Obstet Gynecol 1993;168(2):547–55.

68. Dicke JM, Crane JP. Sonographic recognition of major malformations and aberrant fetal growth in trisomic fetuses. J Ultrasound Med. 1991;10(8):433–8.

69. Bamfo JEAK, Odibo AO. Diagnosis and management of fetal growth restriction. J Pregnancy. 2011;2011:640715.

70. Resnik R. Intrauterine growth restriction. Obstet Gynecol. 2002;99(3):490–6. doi: 10.1016/s0029-7844(01)01780-x.

71. Hendrix N, Berghella V. Non-placental causes of intrauterine growth restriction. Semin Perinatol. 2008;32(3):161–5.

72. Maulik D. Fetal growth restriction: the etiology. Clin Obstet Gynecol. 2006;49(2):228–35.

73. Magnus P, Bakketeig LS, Hoffman H. Birth weight of relatives by maternal tendency to repeat small-for-gestational-age (SGA) births in successive pregnancies. Acta Obstet Gynecol Scand. 1997;165:35–8.

74. Lindqvist PG, Molin J. Does antenatal identification of small-for-gestational age fetuses significantly improve their outcome? Ultrasound Obstet Gynecol. 2005;25(3):258–64.

75. Ego A, Subtil D, Grange G, Thiebaugeorges O, Senat MV, Vayssiere C, et al. Customized versus population-based birth weight standards for identifying growth restricted infants: a French multicenter study. Am J Obstet Gynecol. 2006;194(4):1042–9.

76. Getahun D, Ananth CV, Kinzler WL. Risk factors for antepartum and intrapartum stillbirth: a population-based study. Am J Obstet Gynecol. 2007;196(6):499–507.

77. Pedersen NG, Figueras F, Wøjdemann KR, Tabor A, Gardosi J. Early fetal size and growth as predictors of adverse outcome. Obstet Gynecol. 2008;112(4):765–71.

78. Gardosi J, Madurasinghe V, Williams M, Malik A, Francis A. Maternal and fetal risk factors for stillbirth: population based study. BMJ. 2013;346:f108.

79. Stacey T, Thompson JMD, Mitchell EA, Zuccollo JM, Ekeroma AJ, McCowan LME. Antenatal care, identification of suboptimal fetal growth and risk of late stillbirth: Findings from the Auckland Stillbirth Study. Aust N Z J Obstet Gynaecol. 2012;52(3):242–7.

80. Madden J v, Flatley CJ, Kumar S. Term small-for-gestational-age infants from low-risk women are at significantly greater risk of adverse neonatal outcomes. Am J Obstet Gynecol. 2018;218(5):525.e1–9.

81. Bernstein IM, Horbar JD, Badger GJ, Ohlsson A, Golan A. Morbidity and mortality among very-low-birth-weight neonates with intrauterine growth restriction. Am J Obstet Gynecol. 2000;182(1):198–206.

82. Kok JH, den Ouden AL, Verloove-Vanhorick SP, Brand R. Outcome of very preterm small for gestational age infants: the first nine years of life. Br J Obstet Gynaecol. 1998;105(2):162–8.

83. Fattal-Valevski A, Leitner Y, Kutai M, Tal-Posener E, Tomer A, Lieberman D, et al. Neurodevelopmental outcome in children with intrauterine growth retardation: a 3-year follow-up. J Child Neurol. 1999;14(11):724–7.

84. Leitner Y, Fattal-Valevski A, Geva R, Eshel R, Toledano-Alhadef H, Rotstein M, et al. Neurodevelopmental outcome of children with intrauterine growth retardation: a longitudinal, 10-year prospective study. J Child Neurol. 2007;22(5):580–7.

85. Soothill PW, Ajayi RA, Campbell S, Ross EM, Candy DC, Snijders RM, et al. Relationship between fetal acidemia at cordocentesis and subsequent neurodevelopment. Ultrasound Obstet Gynecol. 1992;2(2):80–3.

86. Frøen JF, Gardosi JO, Thurmann A, Francis A, Stray-Pedersen B. Restricted fetal growth in sudden intrauterine unexplained death. Acta Obstet Gynecol Scand. 2004;83(9):801–7.

87. Turan S, Miller J, Baschat AA. Integrated testing and management in fetal growth restriction. Semin Perinatol. 2008;32(3):194–200.

88. GRIT Study Group. A randomised trial of timed delivery for the compromised preterm fetus: short term outcomes and Bayesian interpretation. Br J Obstet Gynaecol. 2003;110(1):27–32.

89. Pallotto EK, Kilbride HW. Perinatal outcome and later implications of intrauterine growth restriction. Clin Obstet Gynecol. 2006;49(2):257–69.

90. Baschat AA, Cosmi E, Bilardo CM, Wolf H, Berg C, Rigano S, et al. Predictors of neonatal outcome in early-onset placental dysfunction. Obstet Gynecol. 2007;109(2 Pt 1):253–61.

91. Lubow JM, How HY, Habli M, Maxwell R, Sibai BM. Indications for delivery and short-term neonatal outcomes in late preterm as compared with term births. Am J Obstet Gynecol. 2009;200(5):e30–3.

92. Cheng YW, Nicholson JM, Nakagawa S, Bruckner TA, Washington AE, Caughey AB. Perinatal outcomes in low-risk term pregnancies: do they differ by week of gestation? Am J Obstet Gynecol. 2008;199(4):370.e1–7.

93. Hanna BD, Nelson MN, White-Traut RC, et al. Heart rate variability in preterm brain-injured and very-low-birth-weight infants. Neonatology. 2000;77(3):147–55. doi:10.1159/000014209.

94. Nijhuis IJM, ten Hof J, Mulder EJH, Nijhuis JG, Narayan H, Taylor DJ, et al. Fetal heart rate in relation to its variation in normal and growth retarded fetuses. Eur J Obstet Gynecol Reprod Biol. 2000;89(1):27–33.

95. Vindla S, James D, Sahota D. Computerised analysis of unstimulated and stimulated behaviour in fetuses with intrauterine growth restriction. Eur J Obstet Gynecol Reprod Biol. 1999;83(1):37–45.

96. Devoe L, Golde S, Kilman Y, Morton D, Shea K, Waller J. A comparison of visual analyses of intrapartum fetal heart rate tracings according to the new national institute of child health and human development guidelines with computer analyses by an automated fetal heart rate monitoring system. Am J Obstet Gynecol. 2000;183(2):361–6.

97. Bracero LA, Roshanfekr D, Byrne DW. Analysis of antepartum fetal heart rate tracing by physician and computer. J Matern Fetal Med. 2000;9(3):181–5.

98. Hecher K, Hackelöer BJ. Cardiotocogram compared to Doppler investigation of the fetal circulation in the premature growth-retarded fetus: longitudinal observations. Ultrasound Obstet Gynecol. 1997;9(3):152–61.

99. Ribbert LSM, Visser GHA, Mulder EJH, Zonneveld MF, Morssink LP. Changes with time in fetal heart rate variation, movement incidences and haemodynamics in intrauterine growth retarded fetuses: a longitudinal approach to the assessment of fetal well being. Early Hum Dev. 1993;31(3):195–208.

100. Alfirevic Z, Neilson JP. Doppler ultrasonography in high-risk pregnancies: Systematic review with meta-analysis. Am J Obstet Gynecol. 1995;172(5):1379–87.

101. Bahado-Singh RO, Kovanci E, Jeffres A, Jeffres A, Oz U, Deren O, et al. The Doppler cerebroplacental ratio and perinatal outcome in intrauterine growth restriction. Am J Obstet Gynecol. 1999;180(3):750–6.

102. Rizzo G, Capponi A, Talone PE, Arduini D, Romanini C. Doppler indices from inferior vena cava and ductus venosus in predicting pH and oxygen tension in umbilical blood at cordocentesis in growth-retarded fetuses. Ultrasound Obstet Gynecol. 1996;7(6):401–10.

103. Baschat AA, Gembruch U, Reiss I, Gortner L, Weiner CP, Harman CR. Relationship between arterial and venous Doppler and perinatal outcome in fetal growth restriction. Ultrasound Obstet Gynecol. 2000;16(5):407–13.

104. Baschat AA, Gembruch U, Harman CR. The sequence of changes in Doppler and biophysical parameters as severe fetal growth restriction worsens. Ultrasound Obstet Gynecol. 2001;18(6):571–7.

105. Hecher K, Bilardo CM, Stigter RH, Ville Y, Hackelöer BJ, Kok HJ, et al. Monitoring of fetuses with intrauterine growth restriction: a longitudinal study. Ultrasound Obstet Gynecol. 2001;18(6):564–70.

106. Ferrazzi E, Bozzo M, Rigano S, Bellotti M, Morabito A, Pardi G, et al. Temporal sequence of abnormal Doppler changes in the peripheral and central circulatory systems of the severely growth-restricted fetus. Ultrasound Obstet Gynecol. 2002;19(2):140–6.

107. Abuhamad A. Uterine size less than dates: a clinical dilemma. In: Bluth EI, Benson CB, Ralls PW, Siegel MJ, editors. Ultrasound: practical approach to clinical problems. 2nd ed. New York: Thieme Medical Publishing; 2006. p.56–60.

108. Fleischer A, Schulman H, Farmakides G, Bracero L, Blattner P, Randolph G. Umbilical artery velocity waveforms and

intrauterine growth retardation. Am J Obstet Gynecol. 1985;151(4):502–5.

109. Giles WB, Trudinger BJ, Baird PJ. Fetal umbilical artery flow velocity waveforms and placental resistance: pathological correlation. Br J Obstet Gynaecol. 1987;157:900–2.

110. Trudinger BJ, Stevens D, Connelly A, Hales JR, Alexander G, Bradley L, et al. Umbilical artery flow velocity waveforms and placental resistance: the effects of embolization of the umbilical circulation. Am J Obstet Gynecol. 1987;157(6):1443–8.

111. Kingdom JC, Burrell SJ, Kaufmann P. Pathology and clinical implications of abnormal umbilical artery Doppler waveforms. Ultrasound Obstet Gynecol. 1997;9(4):271–86.

112. Morrow RJ, Adamson SL, Bull SB, Knox Ritchie JW. Effect of placental embolization on the umbilical arterial velocity waveform in fetal sheep. Am J Obstet Gynecol. 1989;161(4):1055–60.

113. Copel JA, Reed KL. Doppler ultrasound in obstetrics and gynecology. New York: Raven Press; 1995.

114. Trudinger BJ. Doppler ultrasonography and fetal well being. In:Reeca EA, Hobbins JC, Mahoney M, Petrie RH, editors. Medicine of the fetus and mother. Philadelphia: JB Lippincott; 1992. p.701–23.

115. Rosner J, Rochelson B, Rosen L, Roman A, Vohra N, Tam Tam H. Intermittent absent end diastolic velocity of the umbilical artery: antenatal and neonatal characteristics and indications for delivery. J Matern Fetal Med. 2014;27(1):94–7.

116. Caradeux J, Martinez-Portilla RJ, Basuki TR, Kiserud T, Figueras F. Risk of fetal death in growth-restricted fetuses with umbilical and/or ductus venosus absent or reversed end-diastolic velocities before 34 weeks of gestation: a systematic review and meta-analysis. Am J Obstet Gynecol. 2018;218(2, Suppl):S774–S782.e21.

117. Mari G, Deter RL. Middle cerebral artery flow velocity waveforms in normal and small-for-gestational-age fetuses. Am J Obstet Gynecol. 1992;166(4):1262–70.

118. Veille JC, Hanson R, Tatum K. Longitudinal quantitation of middle cerebral artery blood flow in normal human fetuses. Am J Obstet Gynecol. 1993;169(6):1393–8.

119. Berman RE, Less MH, Peterson EN, Delannoy CW. Distribution of the circulation in the normal and asphyxiated fetal primate. Am J Obstet Gynecol. 1970;108:956–69.

120. Mari G, Abuhamad AZ, Brumfield J, Ferguson JE III. Doppler ultrasonography of the middle cerebral artery peak systolic velocity in the fetus: reproducibility of measurement. Am J Obstet Gynecol. 2001;185:S261.

121. Harrington K, Thompson MO, Carpenter RG, Nguyen M, Campbell S. Doppler fetal circulation in pregnancies complicated by pre-eclampsia or delivery of a small for gestational age baby: 2. Longitudinal analysis. Br J Obstet Gynaecol. 1999;106(5):453–66.

122. Morris RK, Say R, Robson SC, Kleijnen J, Khan KS. Systematic review and meta-analysis of middle cerebral artery Doppler to predict perinatal wellbeing. Eur J Obstet Gynecol Reprod Biol. 2012;165(2):141–55.

123. Meher S, Hernandez-Andrade E, Basheer SN, Lees C. Impact of cerebral redistribution on neurodevelopmental outcome in small-for-gestational-age or growth-restricted babies: a systematic review. Ultrasound Obstet Gynecol. 2015;46(4):398–404.

124. Rizzo G, Arduini D. Fetal cardiac function in intrauterine growth retardation. Am J Obstet Gynecol. 1991;165(4, Pt 1):876–82.

125. Chang CH, Chang FM, Yu CH, Liang RI, Ko HC, Chen HY. Systemic assessment of fetal hemodynamics by Doppler ultrasound. Ultrasound Med Biol. 2000;26(5):777–85.

126. Mäkikallio K, Vuolteenaho O, Jouppila P, Räsänen J. Ultrasonographic and biochemical markers of human fetal cardiac dysfunction in placental insufficiency. Am J Obstet Gynecol. 2001;185(6, Suppl):S98.

127. Tsyvian P, Malkin K, Wladimiroff JW. Assessment of mitral A-wave transit time to cardiac outflow tract and isovolumic relaxation time of left ventricle in the appropriate and small-for-gestational-age human fetus. Ultrasound Med Biol. 1997;23(2):187–90.

128. Ganzevoort W, Mensing Van Charante N, Thilaganathan B, Prefumo F, Arabin B, et al. How to monitor pregnancies complicated by fetal growth restriction and delivery before 32 weeks: post-hoc analysis of TRUFFLE study. Ultrasound Obstet Gynecol. 2017;49(6):769–77.

129. Frauenschuh I, Frambach T, Karl S, Dietl J, Müller T. Ductus venosus blood flow prior to intrauterine foetal death in severe placental insufficiency can be unaffected as shown by doppler sonography. Z Geburtshilfe Neonatol. 2014;218(5):218–22.

130. Baschat AA, Gembruch U, Weiner CP, Harman CR. Qualitative venous Doppler waveform analysis improves prediction of critical perinatal outcomes in premature growth-restricted fetuses. Ultrasound Obstet Gynecol. 2003;22(3):240–5.

131. Schwarze A, Gembruch U, Krapp M, Katalinic A, Germer U, Axt-Fliedner R. Qualitative venous Doppler flow waveform analysis in preterm intrauterine growth-restricted fetuses with ARED flow in the umbilical artery–correlation with short-term outcome. Ultrasound Obstet Gynecol. 2005;25(6):573–9.

132. Romero R, Kalache KD, Kadar N. Timing the delivery of the preterm severely growth-restricted fetus: venous Doppler, cardiotocography or the biophysical profile? Ultrasound Obstet Gynecol. 2002;19(2):118–21.

133. Abuhamad A. Doppler ultrasound in obstetrics. Ultrasound Clin.2006;1(2):293–301.

Chapter 9
Antepartum Fetal Monitoring

Michael Nageotte

Miller Children's and Women's Hospital, Long Beach, California, University of California, Irvine, USA

Antenatal fetal surveillance testing is performed in an effort to decrease stillbirth resulting from certain fetal or maternal conditions which are associated with an increase risk of adverse pregnancy outcomes. Such surveillance, in whatever format, ideally should identify accurately those pregnancies for which delivery is indicated as well as to provide appropriate reassurance when delivery is not indicated. Optimal timing of delivery should both reduce stillbirth and optimize outcome as well as avoid clinically unindicated interventions such as cesarean delivery with their attendant sequelae.

Although widely accepted as the standard of care for specific conditions complicating pregnancy, fetal surveillance testing has consistently been reported to be associated with a decrease frequency of stillbirth in tested high-risk patients. However, the factors that lead to an increased risk of stillbirth are often unknown and fetal surveillance testing have not necessarily been shown to be associated with a decrease in adverse perinatal outcomes for all conditions associated with stillbirth [1]. Consequently, it is neither generally agreed as to what specific pregnancy conditions fetal surveillance testing is indicated nor what specific time such testing should be initiated, what specific form of test should be used, or what should be frequency of testing performed. Although there are publications suggesting associations between testing protocols for specific indications and with a decreased incidence of stillbirth, there are not now–nor will there likely ever be–prospective randomized trials in high-risk pregnancies assessing specific types and frequency of testing in comparison with an equally high-risk population without antepartum surveillance testing that proves efficacy of outpatient antenatal fetal surveillance [2–5].

The American College of Obstetricians and Gynecologists (ACOG) along with the Society for Maternal-Fetal Medicine (SMFM) recommend "surveillance for conditions for which stillbirth is reported to occur more frequently than 0.8 per 1000 (the false-negative rate of a biophysical profile or modified biophysical profile) and that are associated with a relative risk (RR) or odds ratio for stillbirth of more than 2.0 compared with pregnancies without the condition" [6]. This publication further states "that the guidance offered in this Committee Opinion should be construed only as suggestions; this guidance should not be construed as mandates or as all encompassing. Ultimately, individualization about if and when to offer antenatal fetal surveillance is advised."

From both an historic and to some extent a geographic perspective, different forms of antenatal fetal surveillance have been proposed and reported. This review is limited specifically to those tests which are most commonly in use. These are the nonstress test (NST), the modified biophysical profile (NST/amniotic fluid volume assessment), the biophysical profile (BPP), and Doppler velocimetry of the fetal umbilical artery.

Nonstress test

The NST is obtained with the patient in the semi-Fowler position with a left tilt of her abdomen. An external recording of both the fetal heart rate (FHR) and uterine activity is obtained using and electronic FHR monitor. A reactive or normal NST is one in which there is a normal baseline FHR (110–160 beats per minute) with two or more accelerations peaking at least 15 beats per minute above baseline with a duration ot at least 15 seconds within a 30-minute window of recording. A reactive NST means the fetus is neither acidotic nor hypoxic. The absence of accelerations may be the result of several

Queenan's Management of High-Risk Pregnancy: An Evidence-Based Approach, Seventh Edition. Edited by Catherine Y. Spong and Charles J. Lockwood.

factors including gestational age, medication, illicit drug exposure, smoking, and fetal sleep [7].

A persistently nonreactive NST after 40 minutes of monitoring may be concerning for fetal compromise. However, there is a high rate of false positive testing with the NST alone. In addition, gestational age must be considered since as many as 50% of healthy fetuses between 24 and 28 weeks of gestation may have a nonreactive NST [8]. In a setting of an apparently nonreactive NST or simply in an effort to shorten the duration of the test, vibroacoustic stimulation (VAS) may be safely and reliably used to attempt to elicit an acceleration of the FHR. Indeed, VAS may be used up to three times, each stimulation being separated by at least 60 seconds and with a duration of no longer than three seconds without compromising test reliability [9].

In a setting of a persistent nonreactive NST and with the knowledge that such a result has a false positive rate of up to 50% (as defined by fetal survival for at least 1 week following a nonreactive NST), backup testing is recommended if delivery is not otherwise indicated. This currently is with the use of a biophysical profile (BPP). Further, it is important to note that the false negative rate of a reactive NST (fetal death within a week of a reactive NST) is between 1.9 and 5.0 per 1000 live births [10].

Biophysical profile

The BPP is a commonly used form of both primary and back-up antepartum fetal assessment. The BPP combines both fetal heart rate testing and real time ultrasound with the composite measurement of five different fetal variables in an effort to assess for the presence of either acute or chronic fetal hypoxia. These five variables are the NST, fetal breathing, tone, movement, and amniotic fluid. Ultrasound assesses acute variable including fetal breathing (more than one episode of more than 30 seconds), muscle tone (active extension/flexion of limb, trunk or hand), and fetal movement (three or more discrete body/limb movements within 30 minutes. In addition, a chronic or long-term variable of amniotic fluid volume is measured.

Fetal urine production is the predominant source of amniotic fluid volume and is directly dependent upon fetal renal perfusion. In response to sustained fetal hypoxemia, there is a long-term adaptive response mediated by chemoreceptors located in the aortic arch and carotid arteries of the fetus. This results in chemoreceptor-mediated centralization of fetal blood flow by differential channeling of blood to vital organs in the fetus (brain, heart, adrenal glands) at the expense of nonessential organs (lungs, kidneys) by means of peripheral vasoconstriction. In cases of prolonged or repetitive episodes of fetal hypoxemia, there is a persistent decrease in blood flow to the lungs and kidneys resulting in a reduction of urine excretion and amniotic fluid production ultimately resulting in oligohydramnios.

Oligohydramnios is defined either as an amniotic fluid index less than 5.0 cm or, preferably, as a single deepest vertical pocket of amniotic fluid less than 2.0 cm in two vertical ultrasound transducer planes. Amniotic fluid volume, therefore, is a reflection of a chronic fetal condition. On average, it takes approximately 3 days for a fetus to progress from a normal to an abnormal amniotic fluid volume.

As stated, the BPP can be used for either primary surveillance or as a back-up to either the NST or modified biophysical profile (MBPP). Generally, a BPP result is scored with a 0 or a 2 for each of the 5 variables assessed and a composite score or 8 or 10 is considered a negative BPP. Certain findings may indicate further consideration for delivery (e.g. oligohydramnios at term) but in general a value of 6 out of 10 is considered equivocal and needs repeating in less than 24 hours or consideration of delivery. Lesser values than six with the BPP require individualization but generally delivery is indicated unless there is a marked clinical improvement and with the documentation of a repeat BPP test score as being normal. The perinatal mortality significantly increases with a BPP score of 6 or less [11].

In the presence of progressive hypoxemia, studies have confirmed that reactivity in the NST is the first biophysical variable to disappear. This is generally followed by the loss of fetal breathing and subsequently by the loss of fetal movement. Fetal tone is the last variable to be lost in the situation of ongoing in utero hypoxemia of the fetus. This sequence of changes needs to be considered in the interpretation of the BPP.

Modified biophysical profile (NST/amniotic fluid volume)

The MBPP uses the assessment of risk of short-term hypoxia with the use of the NST along with the assessment of long term placental function by evaluation of the amniotic fluid volume. The amniotic fluid assessment can be either with a composite amniotic fluid index (AFI) using real time ultrasound to measure the deepest fluid pocket in all four uterine quadrants or with the more specific diagnosis of oligohydramnios as defined by the deepest vertical pocket of fluid being equal to or greater than 2.0 cm. The MBPP has a lower false negative rate than the NST but has a similar false positive rate [2] Again, using the BPP as a back-up test is recommended for modified BPP tests with a nonreactive NST, significant variable or late decelerations or oligohydramnios. Currently, the MBPP appears to be the most frequent form of antenatal fetal surveillance testing with a common testing protocol being once a week MBPP with an NST 3 to 4 days later [12].

Table 9.1 Orders for fetal diagnostic testing

	ORDERS FOR FETAL DIAGNOSTIC TESTING		
	Miller Children's Hospital Center for Women- Fetal Diagnostic Unit		
Patient Name:		DOB:	
EDC:	First date for testing:		Time:
G: P: Tab: Sab:		L:	
PRENATAL RECORDS REQUIRED ON ALL PATIENTS!		(circle) PNR PNR w/PT	
2021 ACOG-MFM recommendations, type and frequency for diagnostic testing. Please contact the FDU if testing indication is not on this list.			
√	**Factor-FETAL**	**INITIATE**	**TEST & FREQUENCY**
	Fetal Growth Restriction (FGR-formerly IUGR)	At diagnosis	Bi-weekly Mod BPP / Alternating NST
	Twins: uncomplicated dichorionic	36 0/7 weeks	Weekly Mod BPP
	Twins: mono chorionic /di-amniotic	32 0/7	Weekly Mod BPP
	Twins: dichorionic w/other maternal/fetal conditions	At diagnosis	Bi-weekly Mod BPP / Alternating NST
	Decreased fetal movement	When identified	MBPP X 1, unless otherwise indicated
	Factor-MATERNAL	**INITIATE**	**TEST & FREQUENCY**
	HTN: chronic-controlled w/or w-out meds	32	Weekly Mod BPP
	HTN: chronic poor control &/or concurrent conditions	At diagnosis	Bi-weekly Mod BPP / Alternating NST
	HTN: Gest./Pre-E no severe features	At diagnosis	Bi-weekly Mod BPP / Alternating NST
	Diabetes: Gest. Controlled and no other conditions	32 0/7	Bi-weekly Mod BPP / Alternating NST
	Diabetes: Gest, poor control	32 0/7	Bi-weekly Mod BPP / Alternating NST
	Diabetes: Pre-gestational	32 0/7	Bi-weekly Mod BPP / Alternating NST
	Autoimmune Disorders no other conditions	32 0/7	weekly Mod BPP
	Autoimmune Disorders w/other conditions	32 0/7	Bi-weekly Mod BPP / Alternating NST
	Antiphospholipid Syndrome	By 32 0/7 weeks	Bi-weekly Mod BPP / Alternating NST
	Sickle cell-uncomplicated	32 0/7	Bi-weekly Mod BPP / Alternating NST
	Sickle cell -w/other conditions	At diagnosis	Bi-weekly Mod BPP / Alternating NST
	Hemoglobinopathies other than Hb SS disease	Individualized	Individualized
	Renal Disease (Cr> 1.4mg/dl)	32 0/7	Bi-weekly Mod BPP / Alternating NST
	Maternal Age of 40 years or greater	37	Bi-weekly
	IVF	36 0/7	weekly Mod BPP
	Factor-OBSTETRIC	**INITIATE**	**TEST & FREQUENCY**
	Prior **IUFD**@/after 32 weeks	32 0/7	Bi-weekly Mod BPP / Alternating NST
	Prior **IUFD** before 32 weeks	Individualized	Individualized
	Cholestasis	At diagnosis	Bi-weekly Mod BPP / Alternating NST
	Late Term	41 0/7	Bi-weekly Mod BPP / Alternating NST
	Factor-PLACENTAL	**INITIATE**	**TEST & FREQUENCY**
	Chronic placental abruption	At diagnosis	Bi-weekly Mod BPP / Alternating NST
	Isolated **Oligohydramnios**: Deepest verticle pocket (DVP) ≤2cm	At diagnosis	Bi-weekly Mod BPP / Alternating NST
	Polyhydramnios: DVP ≥12cm or AFI≥30cm	32-34 0/7	Bi-weekly Mod BPP / Alternating NST
	Other:		
√	Discontinue testing when / if condition for testing is resolved		
√	**Back up testing for all Non-Reactive or Equivocal Tracings (variable or late decel present, indeterminent baseline) is BPP.**		
ADDITIONAL ORDERS / SPECIAL CONSIDERATIONS:			
Physician Signature:		Date:	Time:
Telephone Order taken by RN: MD:		Date:	Time:
Physician / Physician Group:			

Doppler velocimetry

Doppler velocimetry of the fetal umbilical artery in a fetus with suspected fetal growth restriction (FGR) is a primary mean of surveillance along with fetal heart rate testing [13]. Once FGR is diagnosed, weekly umbilical artery Doppler assessment is performed to evaluate placental resistance in addition to fetal heart rate monitoring [13]. Doppler assessment of the ductus venosus, middle cerebral artery, or uterine artery is not recommended to be used for routine clinical management of early- or late-onset FGR [13]. Umbilical artery Doppler waveforms progress from normal, to elevated S/D ratio, to absent end-diastolic flow, to reversal of diastolic flow. Finding absent or reversed end-diastolic Doppler wave forms in the umbilical artery typically makes delivery indicated as such findings are associated with an increased risk of stillbirth in patients with suspected FGR.

Again, individualization of care is indicated with management decisions needing to be made with additional consideration for gestational age along with the findings of other means of fetal surveillance, such as a BPP or continuous FHR monitoring. Inpatient management and identification of other possible comorbidities (e.g. preeclampsia, hypertension) are often indicated. Management of fetal growth restriction is covered in Chapter 45.

Listed in Table 9.1 are the current antenatal testing guidelines for Miller Children's and Women's Hospital, Long Beach, California. These are consistent with the recent recommendations from ACOG and SMFM, are not mandated, and allow for physicians in discussion with their patients to request such testing for indications that may not be listed and/or to initiate testing at a different gestational age, a different frequency of testing, or a different primary means of surveillance.

CASE PRESENTATION

Patient is a 29-year-old gravida 1 at 38 weeks gestation presenting to Fetal Testing for her scheduled nonstress test. She has had routine prenatal care and is being tested because of concerns for fetal growth restriction (FGR). She has noted significant decrease to absence of fetal movement for the past day and has noted back pain and pelvic pressure for the past 6 hours. She denies membrane rupture or vaginal bleeding.

The nurse is concerned with the initial tracing and calls the physician stating that the FHR is not reactive with frequent contractions and she is possibly observing late decelerations of the fetal heart. The physician orders continued fetal heart monitoring and instructs the nurse to obtain a biophysical profile. He also asks the nurse to do a

pelvic examination on the patient. The examination reveals a cervix that is 1–2 cm dilated, 70% effaced, and with a vertex presentation at -2 station. There is no evidence of membrane rupture or bleeding. The biophysical profile is 2 out of 10 (for amniotic fluid). The patient is directly admitted to the hospital and prepared for delivery.

This tracing is that of a nonreactive NST in a patient with complaints of absent fetal movement. As the patient was term and in very early latent labor, the correct decision was to immediately effect delivery. A depressed, severely growth restricted newborn was delivered by emergency C-section.

Initial tracing in labor and delivery

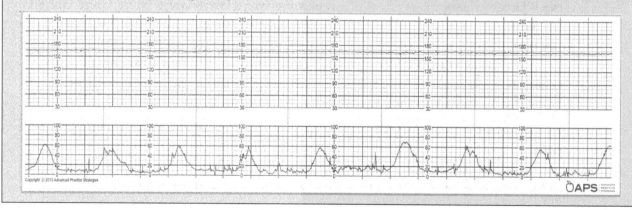

References

1. Johnson GJ, Clark SL, Turrentine MA. Antepartum testing for the prevention of stillbirth: where do we go from here? Obstet Gynecol. 2018;132(6):1407–11.

2. Nageotte MP, Towers CV, Asrat T, Freeman RK. Perinatal outcome with the modified biophysical profile. Am J Obstet Gynecol. 1994;170: 1672–6.

3. Miller DA, Rabello YA, Paul RH. The modified biophysical profile: antepartum testing in the 1990s. Am J Obstet Gynecol. 1996;174:812–17.

4. Signore C, Freeman RK, Spong CY. Antenatal testing – a reevaluation: executive summary of a Eunice Kennedy Shriver National Institute of Child Health and Human Development Workshop. Obstet Gynecol. 2009;113:687–701.

5. Association between stillbirth and risk factors known at pregnancy confirmation. Stillbirth Collaborative Research Network Writing Group. JAMA. 2011;306: 2469–79.

6. American College of Obstetricians and Gynecologists. ACOG Committee Opinion No. 828: Indications for outpatient antenatal fetal surveillance. Obstet Gynecol. 2021;137:e177–97.

7. Oncken C, Kranzler H, O'Malley P. The effect of cigarette smoking on fetal heart rate characteristics. Obstet Gynecol. 2002;99:751–5.

8. Druzin ML, Fox A, Kogut E, Carlson C. The relationship of the nonstress test to gestational age. Am J Obstet Gynecol. 1985;153:386–9.

9. Zimmer EZ, Divon MY. Fetal vibroacoustic stimulation. Obstet Gynecol. 1993;81:451–7.

10. Freeman RK, Anderson G, Dorchester W. A prospective multi-institutional study of antepartum fetal heart rate monitoring. Risk of perinatal mortality and morbidity according to antepartum fetal heart rate results. Am J Obstet Gynecol. 1982;143:771–7.

11. Manning FA, Morrison I, Lange IR, Harman CR, Chamberlain PF. Fetal assessment based on fetal biophysical profile scoring: experience in 12 620 referred high-risk pregnancies. I. Perinatal mortality by frequency and etiology. Am J Obstet Gynecol. 1985;151:343–50.

12. Nageotte MP, Towers CV, Asrat T, Freeman RK, Dorchester W. The value of a negative antepartum test: CST and modified BPP. Obstet Gynecol. 1994;84:231–4.

13. Martins JG, Biggio JR, Abuhamad A. Society for Maternal-Fetal Medicine Consult Series #52: diagnosis and management of fetal growth restriction (replaces Clinical Guideline No. 3, April 2012). Am J Obstet Gynecol. 2020;223: B2–17.

Chapter 10
Interpreting Intrapartum Fetal Heart Tracings

Lorie M. Harper and Alison G. Cahill

Division of Maternal-Fetal Medicine, Department of Women's Health, Dell Medical School, University of Texas at Austin, Austin, TX, USA

Intrapartum electronic fetal monitoring (EFM) was introduced in the 1960s with the goal of diagnosing fetal acidemia [1], a major risk factor for mortality, neonatal encephalopathy, and cerebral palsy [2]. Despite lack of evidence on its utility, EFM was the obstetric procedure reported most frequently in 2003, used in 85.4% of approximately 3.8 million births [3]. Studies of EFM have been poor quality and do not consistently demonstrate decreases in neonatal death or cerebral palsy, although operative deliveries are consistently increased [4–8]. A recent Cochrane meta-analysis demonstrated a decreased risk of neonatal seizures; however, all studies included in the review were at high risk of bias.

In 2008, the National Institute of Child Health and Human Development, the American College of Obstetricians and Gynecologists (ACOG), and the Society for Maternal–Fetal Medicine collaborated on a statement to standardize the definitions and interpretations of fetal heart rate (FHR) monitoring [9]. This statement identified the basic components of a complete description of an EFM tracing and classifies EFM tracings into three categories based on those components.

Components of EFM documentation

Baseline FHR

The mean rate rounded in increments of 5 beats per minute (bpm) over a 10-minute segment, excluding periodic or episodic changes, periods of marked variability. At least 2 minutes of identifiable baseline segments must occur in a 10-minute window. Normal FHR is 110–160 bpm, bradycardia is <110 bpm, and tachycardia is >160 bpm.

Baseline FHR variability

Defined as visually quantifiable fluctuations from the baseline FHR that are irregular in amplitude and frequency. FHR variability is either absent (no discernable variation), minimal (amplitude range from peak to trough ≤5 bpm), moderate (amplitude range >5–25 bpm), or marked (amplitude range >25 bpm).

Accelerations

An abrupt (<30 seconds) increase from baseline to peak of ≥15 bpm lasting 15–120 seconds. When <32 weeks, an acceleration is defined as increases ≥10 bpm above baseline lasting ≥10 seconds.

Decelerations

Documentation of decelerations should include a description of type (e.g. late, early, variable), depth (defined by the nadir of the deceleration), frequency (recurrent if they occur with ≥50% of contractions and intermittent if they occur with <50% of contractions), and length (prolonged is defined as a decrease in the FHR of ≥15 bpm lasting for >2 minutes but <10 minutes before return to baseline).
- *Late deceleration:* a gradual (onset to nadir of ≥30 seconds) decrease of baseline FHR associated with a contraction and lasting ≥30 seconds with return to baseline. The nadir of a late deceleration occurs after the contraction peak.
- *Early deceleration:* a gradual (onset to nadir of ≥30 seconds) decrease and return to baseline of the FHR associated with a contraction. The nadir of an early deceleration occurs with the peak of the uterine contraction and mirrors the onset, peak, and ending of the contraction.
- *Variable deceleration:* a sudden, rapid decrease of the FHR (onset to nadir <30 seconds). The decrease must be ≥15 bpm lasting ≥15 seconds with return to baseline in <2 minutes.

Uterine contractions

Uterine contractions are quantified as the number of contractions present in a 10-minute window, averaged over 30 minutes. Description should include duration, intensity, and relaxation time. Normal uterine contractions are ≤5 contractions in 10 minutes; tachysystole is >5 contractions in 10 minutes. Tachysystole should be described as either with or without FHR decelerations.

Changes and trends in FHR over time

FHR patterns are dynamic and transient, requiring frequent assessment in labor. FHR tracings may move from one category to another over time.

Interpretation of EFM

Category I

Category I tracings have a normal baseline, moderate variability, and no variable or late decelerations. Accelerations are not required for a category I tracing and early decelerations may be present. While it is rare for FHR to remain category I through the entirety of labor, a category I tracing is strongly predictive of a normal fetal acid-base status. The presence of any acceleration (spontaneous or induced), is independently associated with a normal cord pH [10].

Category III

Category III tracings are characterized by absent baseline FHR variability with at least one of the following: recurrent late decelerations, recurrent variable decelerations, or bradycardia. A sinusoidal pattern (defined as having a visually apparent, smooth, sine-wave like undulating pattern with a cycle frequency of 3–5 per minute that persists for ≥20 minutes) is also a category III tracing. Any 10-minute period of a category III tracing in the 2 hours prior to delivery is associated with a 10-fold increase in the risk of fetal acidemia. However, a category III tracing is rare (0.2%) and may still be associated with a normal cord gas [10].

Category II

An FHR tracing is classified as category II if it is neither category I nor category III; this is a broad category and the majority of FHR tracings will be classified as category II at some point in labor. Tracings may be placed in Category II if the baseline is <110 or >160, variability is absent, minimal or marked, variable or late decelerations occur, or fetal stimulation fails to produce an acceleration. An FHR that is classified as category II for the entire last 2 hours of labor has been associated with fetal acidemia in 2–3% of cases, similar to a fetus with a 10-minute period of category III tracing [10].

Management of FHR abnormalities in labor

Although category I tracings are reassuring against fetal acidemia, particularly in the presence of accelerations, these tracings are rare throughout labor and management strategies for category II and III tracings must be developed. As the positive predictive value of category II and III tracings is low, the management of these tracings should not rely solely on operative interventions but should focus on identifying and correcting the cause of the abnormal FHR tracing (tachysystole, maternal hypotension, maternal hypoxia), intrauterine resuscitative measures, and obtaining additional reassurance against fetal acidemia with fetal stimulation. We review several common causes of fetal rate tracing abnormality and commonly used intrauterine resuscitation measures.

Placement of internal monitors (intrauterine pressure catheter, fetal scalp electrode)

Although no studies demonstrate the efficacy of an intrauterine pressure catheter (IUPC) on labor management, placement of an IUPC and fetal scalp electrode (FSE) (when ruptured and with no contraindications) can aid in FHR interpretation and clarification of the timing of decelerations in relation to contractions. Additionally, the FSE typically provides an improved assessment of variability (decreasing artifact from the Doppler-based external monitor) and eliminates issues of discontinuous tracings.

Tachysystole with fetal heart rate changes

When tachysystole occurs, particularly when associated with fetal heart rate changes, several measures should be taken to decrease the number of contractions, thereby improving uteroplacental blood flow and fetal oxygenation. First, the oxytocin infusion should be decreased or stopped. A tocolytic agent (typically a beta-mimetic agent, e.g. terbutaline) should be given if contractions continue in spite of no oxytocin. Betamimetic therapy appears to reduce the number of FHR abnormalities, although it has not been demonstrated to reduce fetal acidemia [11].

Maternal hypotension

Maternal hypotension may occur during labor, particularly immediately after regional anesthesia placement or dosing. Intravenous fluid boluses are frequently given in these settings. Additionally, correction of maternal hypotension with phenylephrine or ephedrine can restore a normal FHR tracing.

Maternal repositioning

Maternal repositioning has the theoretical benefits of improved uteroplacental blood flow with decreased aortocaval compression and reduced cord compression.

Although not systematically studied with demonstrable benefits, this is a simple, readily available intervention with essentially no risk of maternal harm.

Intravenous fluid bolus

An intravenous fluid bolus is frequently given in the setting of a category II–III fetal heart tracing even in the absence of maternal hypotension, with the goal of improving uteroplacental blood flow through volume expansion. However, this intervention has not been well studied and there are no demonstrated benefits to this technique [12]. This strategy should be used with caution in women with preexisting cardiac disease or risk factors for pulmonary edema.

Maternal hyperoxygenation

Maternal oxygen supplementation has been used to improve fetal oxygenation and thus alleviate category II–III tracings. However, this strategy has never been proven beneficial [13], and recent studies demonstrate that it does not hasten the resolution of category II tracings [14] and may worsen neonatal outcomes in acidemia [15]. Therefore, ACOG no longer recommends the use of oxygen supplementation for fetal intrauterine resuscitation in the setting of normal maternal oxygenation [16].

Amnioinfusion

Amnioinfusion uses an IUPC to place fluid (typically normal saline) around the fetus, thereby relieving cord compression. Randomized control trials have demonstrated reduction in variable decelerations and reduced cesarean delivery, although no improvement in neonatal acidemia has been demonstrated [17,18]. Furthermore, amnioinfusion has been shown to be most beneficial if the amniotic fluid volume is low prior to initiation [19].

Fetal stimulation

The most reliable marker of adequate fetal oxygenation and normal acid–base status is the presence of FHR accelerations. The ability to produce a FHR acceleration demonstrates the absence of fetal acidemia [9]. Accelerations can be produced by vibrouacoustic stimulation, transabdominal halogen light, or direct fetal scalp stimulation. Therefore, reassurance in the setting of a category II or III tracing can be obtained every 15 minutes by stimulating an acceleration. If fetal accelerations cannot be produced, this does not predict acidemia. The remainder of the clinical scenario should be considered to direct care, although expeditious delivery in the setting of a category III tracing with no accelerations in response to fetal stimulation is recommended.

Future directions

Given the ubiquitous use of electronic FHR monitoring in labor, much investigation is still needed to better understand the predictive ability of patterns for meaningful clinical outcomes. Category II, which encompasses a wide range of patterns, is seen most frequently during labor and requires further study to better understand their clinical meaning.

CASE PRESENTATION

The patient is a 25-year-old G2P1001 at 38 weeks gestation being induced for preeclampsia. After artificial rupture of membranes is performed with clear amniotic fluid, her fetal heart rate changes from Category I to a Category II pattern (Figure 10.1, panel 1). An IUPC is placed and an amnioinfusion is started, with return to Category I pattern. Her labor pattern progresses normally, and at 8 cm her tracing returns to a Category II pattern. An FSE is placed; subsequently, a Category III tracing is noted (absent variability, recurrent late decelerations, Figure 10.2). She is repositioned and fetal scalp stimulation is performed with a subsequent acceleration, at which time she is 9 cm. Fetal stimulation is performed every 15-minutes with successful stimulation of an acceleration. She progressed to 10 cm and had severe variable decelerations while pushing with minimal variability between contractions. Forceps-assisted vaginal delivery was performed from +3 station. Apgars of 8,9 at 1 and 5 minutes, cord pH 7.23.

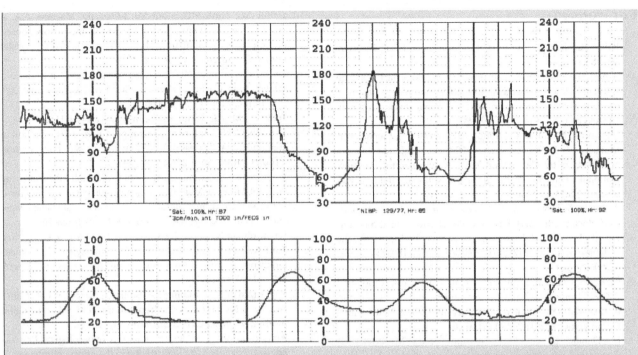

Figure 10.1 The patient progressed to 10 cm and had severe variable decelerations while pushing with minimal variability between contractions.

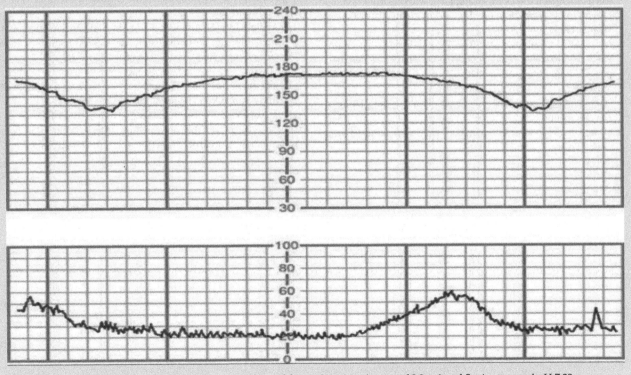

Figure 10.2 Forceps-assisted vaginal delivery was performed from +3 station. Apgars of 8,9 at 1 and 5 minutes, cord pH 7.23.

References

1. Bailey RE. Intrapartum fetal monitoring. Am Fam Physician. 2009;80(12):1388–96.

2. American College of Obstetrics and Gynecology Task Force on Neonatal Encephalopathy. Executive summary: neonatal encephalopathy and neurologic outcome, second edition. Obstet Gynecol. 2014;123(4):896–901.

3. Martin JA, Hamilton BE, Sutton PD, Ventura SJ, Menacker F, Munson ML. Births: final data for 2003. National vital statistics reports: from the Centers for Disease Control and Prevention, National Center for Health Statistics, National Vital Statistics System. Natl Vital Stat Rep. 2005;54(2):1–116.

4. Alfirevic Z, Devane D, Gyte GM, Cuthbert A. Continuous cardiotocography (CTG) as a form of electronic fetal monitoring (EFM) for fetal assessment during labour. Cochrane Database Syst Rev. 2017;2(2):CD006066. doi: 10.1002/14651858. CD006066.pub3.

5. Chen HY, Chauhan SP, Ananth CV, Vintzileos AM, Abuhamad AZ. Electronic fetal heart rate monitoring and its relationship to neonatal and infant mortality in the United States. Am J Obstet Gynecol. 2011;204(6):491.e1–10.

6. MacDonald D, Grant A, Sheridan-Pereira M, Boylan P, Chalmers I. The Dublin randomized controlled trial of intrapartum fetal heart rate monitoring. Am J Obstet Gynecol. 1985;152(5):524–39.

7. McCusker J, Harris DR, Hosmer DW, Jr. Association of electronic fetal monitoring during labor with cesarean section rate and with neonatal morbidity and mortality. Am J Public Health. 1988;78(9):1170–4.

8. Nelson KB, Dambrosia JM, Ting TY, Grether JK. Uncertain value of electronic fetal monitoring in predicting cerebral palsy. N Engl J Med. 1996;334(10):613–8.

9. Macones GA, Hankins GD, Spong CY, Hauth J, Moore T. The 2008 National Institute of Child Health and Human Development workshop report on electronic fetal monitoring: update on definitions, interpretation, and research guidelines. Obstet Gynecol. 2008;112(3):661–6.

10. Cahill AG, Tuuli MG, Stout MJ, López JD, Macones GA. A prospective cohort study of fetal heart rate monitoring: deceleration area is predictive of fetal acidemia. Am J Obstet Gynecol. 2018;218(5):523.e1–12.

11. Kulier R, Hofmeyr GJ. Tocolytics for suspected intrapartum fetal distress. Cochrane Database Syst Rev. 2000(2): CD000035. doi: 10.1002/14651858.CD000037.

12. Bullens LM, van Runnard Heimel PJ, van der Hout-van der Jagt MB, Oei SG. Interventions for intrauterine resuscitation in suspected fetal distress during term labor: a systematic review. Obstet Gynecol Surv. 2015;70(8):524–39.

13. Raghuraman N, Temming LA, Doering MM, Stoll CR, Palanisamy A, Stout MJ, et al. Maternal oxygen supplementation compared with room air for intrauterine resuscitation: a systematic review and meta-analysis. JAMA Pediatrics. 2021;175(4):368–76.

14. Raghuraman N, López JD, Carter EB, Stout MJ, Macones GA, Tuuli MG, et al. The effect of intrapartum oxygen supplementation on category II fetal monitoring. Am J Obstet Gynecol. 2020;223(6):905.e1–7.

15. Raghuraman N, Temming LA, Stout MJ, Macones GA, Cahill AG, Tuuli MG. Intrauterine hyperoxemia and risk of neonatal morbidity. Obstet Gynecol. 2017;129(4):676–82.

16. American College of Obstetricians and Gynecologists. Practice advisory: oxygen supplementation in the setting of category II or III fetal heart rate tracings. 2022 [updated January 2022; cited 2023 Jun 4]. Available from: https://www.acog.org/clinical/clinical-guidance/practice-advisory/articles/2022/01/oxygen-supplementation-in-the-setting-of-category-ii-or-iii-fetal-heart-tracings.

17. Abdel-Aleem H, Amin AF, Shokry M, Radwan RA. Therapeutic amnioinfusion for intrapartum fetal distress using a pediatric feeding tube. Int J Gynaecol Obstet. 2005;90(2):94–8.

18. Miyazaki FS, Nevarez F. Saline amnioinfusion for relief of repetitive variable decelerations: a prospective randomized study. Am J Obstet Gynecol. 1985;153(3):301–6.

19. Spong CY, McKindsey F, Ross MG. Amniotic fluid index predicts the relief of variable decelerations after amnioinfusion bolus. American Journal of Obstet Gynecol. 1996;175(4):1066–70.

Chapter 11
Sickle Cell Anemia

Scott Roberts

Department of Obstetrics and Gynecology, University of Texas Southwestern Medical Center, Dallas, TX, USA

Sickle cell disease (SSD) affects approximately 100 000 Americans. It occurs in about 1 out of every 365 Black or African American births and about 1 out of every 16 300 Hispanic-American births. About 1 in 12 to 1 in 13 Black or African American babies is born with sickle cell trait (SCT) [1]. Hemoglobinopathies, which result from quantitative defects in hemoglobin (Hb) (the thalassemias) and Hb structural variants, are prevalent in malaria-endemic regions (the Mediterranean, Asia, and sub-Saharan Africa) owing to natural selection [2]. Population migration has spread these genotypes making SCD a global health problem The clinically significant hemoglobinopathies include α- and β-thalassemia, SCD, HbE disease, and HbC disease [3, 4]. Globally it is estimated that more than 330 000 affected births occur annually, mainly with SCD (83%) and the thalassemias (17%) [3]. Our focus is on sickle cell disease and its variants.

SSD is a member of a family of genetic disorders involving abnormal hemoglobin. Each hemoglobin molecule is made up of two α-globin (141 amino acids) and two β-globin chains (146 amino acids). These chains conform to facilitate solubility, oxygen affinity and transport, and a stable biconcave structure in the red blood cell (RBC). Solubility and reversible oxygen binding are the key properties which are deranged in hemoglobinopathies. Sickle hemoglobin (S) results from the substitution of glutamic acid by valine in the β-globin chain at position 6, and hemoglobin C from substitution of the same amino acid but by lysine. The β-globin genes are expressed codominantly so that homozygous SS or the compound heterozygote SC must be expressed for clinical morbidity to be significant. In contrast, the β-thalassemia variant of the β-globin gene causes the production of normal hemoglobin A to be absent or reduced.

The most prevalent hemoglobinopathy is sickle cell anemia resulting from the homozygous SS genotype. One of every 12 African Americans is a carrier for the hemoglobin S gene and hence ($1/12 \times 1/12 \times 1/4 = 1/576$) approximately 1 in 600 African American newborns have sickle cell anemia [5]. The prevalence of the hemoglobin C allele is approximately 1 in 40 and the β-thalassemia gene approximately 1 in 40 to 1 in 50 in this population [6]. These disorders are associated with increased maternal and perinatal morbidity and mortality.

Red blood cells with hemoglobin S undergo sickling under conditions of decreased oxygen tension. This results in hemolysis, increased viscosity, and vaso-occlusion (VOC), and leads to further decreased oxygenation. This VOC leads to local infarction in all major organ systems, surviving adults with sickle cell anemia have undergone autosplenectomy after multiple episodes of VOC and infarction. The bone pain, so typical of sickle cell crises, represents VOC in the bone marrow. Other chronic and acute changes from sickling include bony abnormalities such as osteonecrosis of the femoral and humeral heads, renal medullary damage, hepatomegaly, ventricular hypertrophy, pulmonary infarctions, pulmonary hypertension, cerebrovascular accidents, leg ulcers, and a susceptibility to infection and sepsis [7–9].

Because of hemolysis of defective RBCs, most patients with sickle cell anemia have hemoglobin values of approximately 7–8 g/dL. Iron therapy will not treat their anemia and may worsen their condition due to iron overload. Folic acid requirements, however, are considerable (4 mg/day) as there is intense hematopoiesis occurring to compensate for the markedly shortened RBC lifespan [10]. Patients with sickle cell/Hemoglobin C Disease (SCD) are usually less anemic, with hemoglobin levels near 10 g/dL, and painful crises occur less frequently. Manifestations of S/β-thalassemia disease are quite variable but can present similarly to severe SS disease. In either SCD disease or S/β-thalassemia, iron studies should be performed and iron supplemented if indicated.

Pregnancy is a serious burden to women with sickle hemoglobinopathies, especially those with hemoglobin SS disease. Pregnancy usually results in an increased frequency of sickle cell crises (VOC events). Infections and pulmonary complications are common. Maternal

Table 11.1 Pregnancy outcomes in women with and without sickle cell disease adjusted for baseline characteristics

	SS Disease N = 4262 (%)	No SS Disease N = 8 817 059 (%)	Adjusted OR 95% CI
Maternal			
Maternal death	0.16	0.01	9.03 (3.79–21.98)
Preeclampsia	9.55	3.25	2.92 (2.46–3.46)
Eclampsia	0.68	0.09	5.87 (3.44–10.04)
Gestational hypertension	2.60	2.90	0.67 (0.45–1.00)
Venous thromboembolism	1.15	0.08	16.64 (11.33–24.45)
Cardiomyopathy	0.16	0.01	10.02 (4.28–23.46)
Cesarean section	36.03	27.65	1.31 (1.16–1.48)
Placental abruption	1.62	1.09	0.72 (0.43–1.18)
PPROM	3.21	3.82	0.48 (0.33–0.72)
Fetal			
IUGR	5.28	1.73	2.36 (1.86–2.99)
IUFD	1.20	0.43	1.79 (1.08–2.95)
Fetal distress	18.51	12.60	0.87 (0.74–1.02)

Adapted from [11].
CI, confidence interval; IUGR, intrauterine growth restriction; IUFD, intrauterine fetal demise; OR, odds ratio; PPROM, preterm premature rupture of membranes; SS disease.

mortality has decreased dramatically over the years because of improvements in medical care but remains high. A population-based, retrospective cohort study on all births in the Healthcare Cost and Utilization Project National Inpatient Sample from 1999 to 2008 provides adjusted effects of risk factors and outcomes for maternal patients with and without sickle cell disease (Table 11.1).

Hemoglobin SCD

In nonpregnant women, morbidity and mortality from sickle cell/hemoglobin C disease are much lower than those seen with SS homozygous disease. Fewer than half of the women with SCD have ever been symptomatic prior to pregnancy. However, during pregnancy and the puerperium, attacks of severe bone pain and episodes of pulmonary infarction and embolization become more common [12].

A particularly worrisome complication is *acute chest syndrome* seen in both SS and SC disease related to embolization of necrotic fat and cellular bone marrow, and VOC sickling, with resultant respiratory insufficiency. This syndrome is characterized by a noninfectious pulmonary infiltrate with fever, leading to hypoxemia and acidosis, and, infrequently, death. Acute chest syndrome is the leading cause of death among patients with sickle cell disease [13]. Odds ratios for morbidity and mortality between Hb SS and Hb SCD disease are listed in Table 11.2.

Table 11.2 Pregnancy morbidity with hemoglobin SS and SC disease

	Odds ratio	
Outcome	Hb SS	Hb SC
Preeclampsia	2–3.1	2
Stillbirth	6.5	3.2
Preterm delivery	2–2.7	1.5
Growth restriction	2.8–3.9	1.5
Maternal mortality	11–23	11

Adapted from [14], p. 1082.
Hb, hemoglobin; SCD, sickle cell disease.

Hemoglobin S/β-thalassemia disease

This heterozygous condition usually is much milder than either SS or SC disease. Variable amounts of hemoglobin A are produced depending on the variant of the β-thalassemia allele inherited. Hemoglobin F is made in abundance with extramedullary hematopoiesis to make up for abnormally low hemoglobin A. In its most usual form, a level of A2 above 3.5% on hemoglobin electrophoresis is diagnostic. In the most severe form of S/β-thalassemia disease (β-thalassemia^0), no hemoglobin F is made, and the resulting phenotypic expression is of severe SS disease.

Either of the sickle cell variants can have symptoms as bad as or worse than any particular SS patient. Particularly unnerving and dangerous is the previously asymptomatic SC or S/β-thalassemia patient who presents with acute chest syndrome in pregnancy.

Management during pregnancy

Close observation is mandatory during pregnancy. Pregnant people are at increased risk for infection, which in turn can aggravate sickling crises. With the increased RBC mass typically required during pregnancy, folate supplementation is important. Any strain that impairs erythropoiesis or increases RBC destruction aggravates the anemia. Clinical presentations that cause anemia and pain may be overlooked (e.g. placental abruption, ectopic pregnancy, appendicitis, and pyelonephritis). The diagnosis of sickle cell crisis should be reserved until other possible causes are ruled out.

Covert bacteriuria and acute pyelonephritis are increased. Frequent (monthly or every trimester) screening urine cultures to discover asymptomatic bacteriuria and treat before symptomatic. Acute pyelonephritis can result in the release of endotoxin, which lyses sickle cells and suppresses hematopoiesis, resulting in severe anemia and sickle crises. Pneumonia is common, caused by *Streptococcus pneumoniae*, and the polyvalent pneumococcal vaccine is recommended. Annual inactivated influenza vaccine should be administered. Hepatitis B vaccination is recommended. For patients who have undergone autosplenectomy, vaccination against *Haemophilus influenzae* type B and *meningococcus* is recommended. If prophylactic penicillin has been used in these patients prior to pregnancy it may be continued.

Crises are hallmarked by intense pain, usually from involved bone marrow. Dehydration, hypoxia, acidosis, infection, and cold may precipitate an acute pain event; therefore, these conditions should be avoided, if possible.

As many as 40% of sickle cell patients have acute chest syndrome [15]. Episodes can develop acutely and do so more often late in pregnancy. Intravenous hydration along with opioid analgesics should be given. Oxygen by nasal cannula will decrease the sickling at the capillary level and improve symptoms. Any focus of infection should be treated as it may be responsible for the crisis. The risks of low birthweight, fetal growth restriction, pre-term delivery, and preeclampsia are increased.

Cardiac dysfunction is prevalent in SS Disease. After years of pulmonary infarction, restrictive airway disease can lead to ventricular hypertrophy and pulmonary hypertension [16]. There is increased preload and decreased afterload with a normal ejection fraction. This condition is augmented by the increasing volume of pregnancy. Chronic hypertension can aggravate the pre-existing cardiac dysfunction. Severe preeclampsia, sepsis, or secondary pulmonary hypertension can lead to heart failure. A multidisciplinary approach should be used involving obstetrician specialists and subspecialists (e.g. cardiology, pulmonary, and hematology) focusing on current end organ effects [17].

Acute pain

In the acute care setting immediate relief for VOC episodes with analgesics (usually parenteral narcotics) is recommended within 1 hour of arrival. Frequent reassessments should be done every 30–60 minutes to optimize pain control. This includes hydration with intravenous fluids and administration of supplemental oxygen. [18]

Chronic pain

Mild chronic pain can be treated with acetaminophen, moderate pain with oral narcotics such as hydrocodone with or without acetaminophen. Also, for mild and moderate pain nonmedicinal strategies (massage, warm heating pads, mind-body techniques) may hasten recovery and may be sufficient to manage pain in some cases. It cannot be stressed enough that the care of these patients should be multidisciplinary involving hematology, psychiatry, and social services.

Pain causes significant morbidity for those living with SS Disease. It is estimated that 30–40 % of adolescents and adults suffer from chronic pain with detrimental effects on health-related quality of life [18]. Unfortunately, there is a paucity of clinical SS Disease pain research and limited understanding of the complex biological differences between acute and chronic pain. Further, there is evidence that clinicians and nursing staff often ascribe pain episodes to instances of opioid use disorder. The consequence of this systematic bias is the undertreatment of pain with SS Disease [19].

Prophylactic red blood cell transfusions

Some use prophylactic RBC transfusions. Managed correctly, sickle crises can be held to a minimum. Hematocrit and hemoglobin electrophoresis are monitored monthly and transfusion effected to keep the hematocrit above 25% and the S fraction of hemoglobin no greater than 60%. Prophylactic transfusions will not modify an existing sickle crisis. However, exchange transfusion in the face of crisis, acute chest syndrome, stroke, and infection can be valuable.

Transfusion is not without its complications. Transfusion-related lung injury occurs in approximately 1 in 5000 units of blood products transfused [20]. Delayed hemolytic transfusion reactions are reported in as many as 10% of patients [21]. The rate of viral infection from transfusion is exceedingly low with modern pretransfusion blood screening techniques. Progressive implementation of nucleic acid–amplification technology screening for HIV, hepatitis C virus, and hepatitis B virus has reduced the residual risk of infectious-window-period donations, such that per unit risks are <1 in 1 000 000 in the United States [22]. The rate of alloimmunization has been reported at 3% per unit in the sickle disease population [23]. Because of these concerns and the need for repeated transfusions in this population, all blood should be typed and crossed and leukocyte reduced. One randomized trial reports there is no benefit in maternal or perinatal mortality from the use of prophylactic transfusions [24]. A meta-analysis from 2015 reports a reduction in maternal and perinatal morbidity and mortality [25].

Much of the decrease in perinatal and maternal morbidity and mortality is ascribed to improved perinatal care in the sickle disease population. Managing without prophylactic transfusions, however, can involve multiple long and painful hospitalizations [12,24].

In our institution, SSD patients are managed conservatively, reserving prophylactic blood transfusions, if at all, for unique situations in which perinatal morbidity seems to be the highest: low hemoglobin F concentration, frequent pain crises, history of acute chest syndrome or severe anemia. Worsening anemia, painful crisis or chest syndrome may benefit from exchange transfusion [26].

Other treatments

Hydroxyurea augments Hb F production and reduces the number of sickling episodes. However, it has been found to be teratogenic in animals and is contraindicated in pregnancy [10]. Allogeneic hematopoietic stem cell transplantation is currently the only curative option for treatment of SSD; however, its availability remains limited and transplant decisions are generally based on a patient's benefit vs. risk and donor availability. Certainly, this has a long way to go and would not be useful in the antenatal population [27,28].

Fetal assessment

Pregnancies in women with sickle cell disease are at increased risk for spontaneous abortion, preterm labor, fetal growth restriction, and stillbirth [29]. Frequent assessment for the detection of fetal growth restriction, oligohydramnios, and assurance of fetal activity is important. Formal antepartum surveillance may be used to augment fetal assessment (e.g. biophysical profile, umbilical artery Doppler in the presence of fetal growth restriction). Published data concerning antepartum surveillance in pregnancies complicated by sickle cell disease are limited.

Labor and delivery

Management should take into account the degree of underlying cardiac dysfunction. Preparatory consultation with an anesthesiologist is helpful. Route of delivery otherwise should be based solely on obstetric indications. Epidural anesthesia is ideal. If a difficult vaginal or cesarean delivery is foreseen, and the patient's hematocrit is less than 20%, packed RBCs should be administered. Blood should be typed and crossed and readily available. Fluid administration should be conservative to avoid circulatory overload and pulmonary edema.

Genetic evaluation

Referral to a genetic counselor is a good idea for couples with mothers affected with SSD. Use of donor sperm or donor egg without hemoglobinopathy can be used insuring heterozygote offspring. Also, preimplantation diagnoses can ensure the fetus will not be affected with SCD. The latter involves in vitro fertilization [30].

Prenatal genetic evaluation is possible for the sickle hemoglobinopathies. Maternal and paternal electrophoresis will elucidate the potential genotypes. When there is reasonable suspicion and probability, amniocentesis or chorionic villus sampling should be offered, and polymerase chain reaction (PCR) used to detect abnormal fetal genotypes.

Efforts to identify fetal SSD with noninvasive techniques using cell free DNA, followed by PCR and massively parallel sequencing assay-based estimation of fetal fraction are ongoing. This technique does not require DNA sampling from fathers or siblings. It does not yet have the accuracy and performance parameters as for other genetic disorders (e.g. trisomy 21) but is expected to be available for SSD in the relatively near future, as further technological advances are made.

CASE PRESENTATION

Patient A presented at 7 weeks gestation. She is a 35-year-old G4P3 (LC 1) with one previous cesarean (last delivery) and stwo spontaneous vaginal deliveries. Her first spontaneous vaginal delivery was a term fetal demise (2008). This was followed by a preterm delivery with placental insufficiency, also a fetal demise (2011). Her last delivery was in 2013 by cesarean section, again preterm after spontaneous labor with an unstable lie. She is Hispanic and diagnosed with Hb S/β-thalassemia⁰ disease. The father of the babies was negative for any allele consistent with hemoglobinopathy.

Her medical history is complicated by many of the conditions associated with SSD: In 1995, she underwent splenectomy and cholecystectomy. Since then, she has remained current on pneumococcal, meningococcal, hepatitis B, influenza, and COVID vaccinations. Painful crises are infrequent except in pregnancy. When not pregnant she is managed with hydroxyurea. In 2008 she had a pulmonary embolism while admitted for sickle cell crisis.

She has long-standing pulmonary hypertension from sickle cell/β-thalassemia⁰ disease (probable multiple pulmonary embolisms from VOC) identified in 2011. Chronic transaminitis was documented in 2007.

She developed nephrolithiasis in 2013 and was hospitalized for infected stones and urosepsis in 2014 requiring pressors in the medical intensive care unit. She had two subsequent episodes of urosepsis prior to this current pregnancy. Percutaneous nephrostomies and ureteral stents were employed. By then she had suffered two intrauterine fetal demises. She was diagnosed with renal tubular acidosis type I. During the last decade she was diagnosed with congestive hepatopathy and sickle cell nephropathy. Her baseline hemoglobin is about 21 and she has had relatively few painful crises when not pregnant.

She has a history of 10 blood transfusions and discovered to have alloimmunization with anti-Jka (too low to titer). She has not required chelation therapy. Hematology recommends during this pregnancy prophylactic transfusions to keep her hemoglobin > 9. She normally takes lisinopril and spironolactone to alleviate symptoms of dyspnea and fatigue from pulmonary hypertension. She is taken off lisinopril and spironolactone and hydroxyurea with her current pregnancy and placed on Lasix. She currently receives lovenox 40 mg sc q day.

Her creatinine is between 0.45 and 0.60 mg %. B-type natriuretic peptide is 588 pg/mL. She has transaminitis with aspartate transaminase of 202 U/L. She continues with proteinuria and has a 24-hour total urine protein of 397 mg/24 hours. Maternal echocardiogram in the first trimester reveals an ejection fraction of 57%. There is a moderately dilated left atrium and mildly dilated right atrium. She has stable cardiomegaly and mild pulmonary hypertension. There is mild bilateral renal caliectasis on renal ultrasound but no stones.

She was admitted with painful crisis involving her back and neck. This was controlled with oral oxycodone (she declined patient-controlled analgesia morphine), supplemental oxygen, and fluids. In consultation with hematology and cardiology she was transfused 2 units with a goal of Hb > 9. After 3 days her condition stabilized and she was dismissed with oral narcotics. Lasix was continued to address her cardiac overload. Progressive hepatopathy is felt possibly due to autoimmune hepatitis but steroids were not started. Fibroscan reveals chronic liver disease and cirrhosis. Esophagogastroduodenoscopy is scheduled in the second trimester to rule out esophageal varices. With a history of provoked PE in 2010, she is placed on lovenox prophylaxis.

She was readmitted at 19 weeks due to hyperbilirubinemia and found to have abdominal pain and altered mental status (AMS). She had bacteremia with *Salmonella* and *Staphylococcus aureus*. The patient completed a course of nafcillin and ceftriaxone. Plasmapheresis was started in the setting of AMS, multiorgan failure, and sepsis but was discontinued after her AMS resolved. Her hospital course was further complicated by acute hypoxic respiratory failure secondary to aspiration pneumonia requiring intubation. She was extubated with resolution but 3 weeks later (while still in the hospital) went into labor and had spontaneous vaginal delivery of a baby girl, Apgars 5/9, 1140 g.

She continued to have medical complications including sepsis and seizures but clinically improved and was discharged with close follow-up on postpartum day 23.

This case highlights some of the significant and not atypical problems with sickle cell and sickle cell/β-thalassemia^0 disease in pregnancy. Many organ systems are showing the results of long-term vaso-occlusive disease. It should be emphasized that some of the worst morbidity occurs in SSD and sickle cell/β-thalassemia^0 disease and that evaluation and management should be similar to those of the SS patient. Clearly these and similar cases require a multidisciplinary team to achieve good perinatal results.

References

1. Centers for Disease Control and Prevention. Sickle cell disease: data and statistics. [last reviewed 2022 May 2; cited 2023 Jun 4]. Available from: https://www.cdc.gov/ncbddd/sicklecell/data.html
2. Taylor SM, Parobek CM, Fairhurst RM. Haemoglobinopathies and the clinical epidemiology of malaria: a systematic review and meta-analysis. Lancet Infect Dis. 2012;12:457–68.
3. Modell B, Darlison M. Global epidemiology of hemoglobin disorders and derived service indicators. Bull. World Health Organ. 2008;86:480–7.
4. Murray CJ, Vos T, Lozano R, Naghavi M, Flaxman AD, Michaud C, et al. Disability-adjusted life years (DALYs) for 291 diseases and injuries in 21 regions, 1990–2010: a systematic analysis for the Global Burden of Disease Study 2010. Lancet 2013;380:2197–223.
5. Angastiniotis M, Modell B. Global epidemiology of hemoglobin disorders. Ann N Y Acad Sci. 1998;850:251–69.
6. Motulsky AG. Frequency of sickling disorders in US Blacks. N Engl J Med. 1973;288:31–3.
7. Powars DR, Sandhu M, Niland-Weiss J, Johnson C, Bruce S, Manning PR. Pregnancy in sickle cell disease. Obstet Gynecol. 1986;67:217–28.
8. Poddar D, Maude GH, Plant MJ, Scorer H, Serjeant GR. Pregnancy in Jamaican women with homozygous sickle cell disease: fetal and maternal outcome. Br J Obstet Gynaecol. 1986;93:927–32.
9. Chakravarty EF, Khanna D, Chung L. Pregnancy outcomes in systemic sclerosis, pulmonary hypertension, and sickle cell disease. Obstet Gynecol. 2008;111:927–34.
10. American College of Obstetricians and Gynecologists. ACOG Practice Bulletin No. 78: Hemoglobinopathies in pregnancy. Obstet Gynecol. 2007;109:229–37. PMID 17197616.
11. Alayed N, Kezouh A, Oddy L, Abenheim AA. Sickle cell disease and pregnancy outcomes: population-based study on 8.8 million births. J Perinat Med. 2014;42(4):487–92.
12. Cunningham FG, Pritchard JA, Mason R. Pregnancy and sickle hemoglobinopathy: results with and without prophylactic transfusions. Obstet Gynecol. 1983;62:419–24.
13. Vichinsky EP, Neumayr LD, Earles AN, Williams R, Lennette ET, Dean D, et al. Causes and outcomes of the acute chest syndrome in sickle cell disease. N Engl J Med. 2000;342:1855–65.
14. Cunningham FG, Leveno KJ, Bloom SL, Dashe JS, Hoffman BL, Casey BM, et al. Williams obstetrics. 25th ed. New York: McGraw-Hill Education; 2018.
15. Chakravarty EF, Khanna D, Chung L. Pregnancy outcomes in systemic sclerosis, pulmonary hypertension, and sickle cell disease. Obstet Gynecol. 2008;111:927–34.
16. Powars D, Weidman JA, Odom-Maryon T, Niland JC, Johnson C. Sickle cell chronic lung disease: prior morbidity and the risk of pulmonary failure. Medicine (Baltimore). 1988;67:66–76.

17. Rees DC, Olujohungbe AD, Parker NE, Stephens AD, Telfer P, Wright J. Guidelines for the management of the acute painful crisis in sickle cell disease. British Committee for Standards in Haematology General Haematology Task Force by the Sickle Cell Working Party. Br J Haematol. 2003;120:744–52.

18. Brandow AM, Carroll CP, Creary S, Edwards-Elliott R, Glassberg J, Hurley RW, et al. American Society of Hematology guidelines for sickle cell disease: management of acute and chronic pain. Blood Adv. 2020;4(12):2656–701.

19. Al Zahrani O, Hanafy E, Mukhtar O, Sanad A, Yassin W. Outcome of multidisciplinary team interventions in the management of sickle cell disease patients with opioid use disorders: a retrospective study. Saudi Med J. 2020;41(10):1104-10.

20. Silliman CC, Boshkov LK, Mehdizadehkashi Z, Elzi DJ, Dickey WO, Podlosky L, et al. Transfusion-related acute lung injury: epidemiology and a prospective analysis of etiologic factors. Blood. 2003;101:454–62.

21. Garratty G. Severe reactions associated with transfusion of patients with sickle cell disease. Transfusion. 1997;37:357–61.

22. Chidambaram V, Jones JM, Lokhandwala PM, Bloch EM, Lanzkron S, Stewart R, et al. Low rates of transfusion-transmitted infection screening in chronically transfused adults with sickle cell disease. Transfusion. 2021;61(8):2421–9.

23. Cox JV, Steane E, Cunningham G, Frenkel EP. Risk of alloimmunization and delayed hemolytic transfusion reactions in patients with sickle cell disease. Arch Intern Med. 1988;148:2485–89.

24. Koshy M, Burd L, Wallace D, Moawad A, Baron J. Prophylactic red-cell transfusions in pregnant patients with sickle cell disease: a randomized cooperative study. N Engl J Med. 1988;319:1447–52.

25. Malinowski AK, Shehata N, D'Souza R, Kuo KH, Ward R, Shah PS, et al: Prophylactic transfusion for pregnant women with sickle cell disease: a systematic review and meta-analysis. Blood. 2015;126(21):2424.

26. National Institutes of Health, National Heart, Lung, and Blood Institute, and Division of Blood Diseases and Resources. The management of sickle cell disease. NIH publication No. 02–2117. Bethesda, MD: National Institutes of Health; 2002.

27. Meir ER, Dioguardi J, Kamani N. Current attitudes of parents and patients toward hematopoietic stem cell transplantation for sickle cell anemia. Pediatr Blood Cancer. 2015 Jul;62(7):1277–84.

28. Meier ER, Abraham A, Fasano RM, editors. Sickle cell disease and hematopoietic stem cell transplantation. Cham: Springer International Publishing; 2018.

29. Serjeant GR, Loy LL, Crowther M, Hambleton IR, Thame M. Outcome of pregnancy in homozygous sickle cell disease. Obstet Gynecol. 2004;103:1278–85.

30. Vrettou C. Kakourou G, Mamas T, Traeger-Synodinnos J. Prenatal and preimplantation diagnosis of hemoglobinopathies. Int J Lab Hematol. 2018 May;40 Suppl 1:74–82.

Chapter 12
Anemia

Elaine L. Duryea and Rachel C. Schell

Division of Maternal-Fetal Medicine, Department of Obstetrics and Gynecology, University of Texas Southwestern Medical Center, Dallas, TX, USA

During a singleton gestation, plasma volume increases approximately 1000 mL and red blood cell (RBC) volume increases by 25% (300–450mL). This lag in RBC production behind plasma expansion results in a physiologic dilutional anemia of pregnancy, which reaches a nadir during the late second to early third trimester (Table 12.1) [1]. The Centers for Disease Control and Prevention define anemia as a hemoglobin (Hb) below the fifth centile for a healthy, iron-supplemented population [2,3]. This translates to a threshold of Hb less than 11 g/dL in the first and third trimesters, and less than 10.5 during the second trimester [1]. Historically rates of anemia in pregnancy have been found to vary widely between different populations and socioeconomic classes [4–6]. However, one recent study examining two cohorts of women receiving prenatal care at a large county vs. private hospital in the same city found no difference in the fifth percentile between the two populations, which was 11g/dL in the first, 10.3g/dL in the second, and 10.0 in the third trimester for either cohort [7]. This confirms that a uniform definition for anemia is appropriate for all women with adequate access to prenatal care. Furthermore, other retrospective data examining the impact of varying standards for the definition of anemia between pregnant mothers of different races may be harmful to Black women and should be avoided [8].

Consequences

In developed countries, maternal anemia has been associated with increased risk of preterm birth and low birth-weight infants, as well as neonatal and perinatal death [9–12]. In addition, maternal complications associated with anemia include preeclampsia, cesarean delivery, postpartum depression, and an increased likelihood for transfusion either intrapartum or postpartum despite equivalent blood loss [13–15]. Women with anemia are asymptomatic or describe vague symptoms such as fatigue and palpitations though their anemia may significantly increase their risk of adverse outcomes as detailed previously. Therefore, screening for anemia during pregnancy is recommended regardless of symptoms.

Causes of anemia in pregnancy

Anemia may be the result of any of the acquired or inherited causes that may be seen outside of pregnancy. The majority of acquired anemias during pregnancy are the result of iron deficiency, though other deficiencies such as vitamin B_{12} and folate may occur, especially in women at increased risk for malabsorption such as those having undergone bariatric surgery [16]. Anemia associated with chronic disease should be considered in the setting of medical comorbidities such as renal, liver, or autoimmune disorders or in patients with chronic health conditions such as HIV. Diagnosis of inherited causes of anemia such as thalassemia or hemoglobinopathy are often known prior to pregnancy but may not be established in women who are largely asymptomatic and have not had consistent access to medical care. The American College of Obstetricians and Gynecologists recommends universal screening of pregnant women with complete blood count with RBC indices, with the addition of a hemoglobin electrophoresis offered in addition to women at high risk based upon ethnicity [17]. In certain geographic locations, malaria is a significant cause of anemia during pregnancy, and this diagnosis should always be considered when caring for women with recent travel to endemic areas [18].

Diagnostic workup and treatment

Causes of anemia may be classified by pathophysiology, such as comparing acquired vs. inherited causes, or mechanisms of anemia such as decreased RBC production vs. increased destruction. In clinical practice, more

---

Queenan's Management of High-Risk Pregnancy: An Evidence-Based Approach, Seventh Edition. Edited by Catherine Y. Spong and Charles J. Lockwood.

Table 12.1 Changes in laboratory hematologic indices in pregnancy

	Nonpregnant	Pregnant
Hemoglobin (g/dL)	12–16	11–14
Hematocrit	36–46%	33–44%
RBC count ($\times 10^6$/mL)	4.8	4.0
MCV (fL)	80–100	unchanged
MCHC	31–36%	unchanged
Reticulocytes ($\times 10^9$/L)	50–150	unchanged
Ferritin (ng/mL)	>25	>20
RDW (red cell distribution width)	11–15%	unchanged

Adapted from ACOG Practice Bulletin No. 107: induction of labor. Obstet Gynecol. 2009 Aug;114(2 Pt 1):386–97.
MCHC, mean corpuscular hemoglobin concentration; MCV, mean corpuscular volume.

often the evaluation of maternal anemia starts with the mean corpuscular volume (MCV), based on which anemias are defined as microcytic (less than 80 fL), normocytic (80–100 fL) or macrocytic (greater than 100 fL), Figure 12.1.

Macrocytic anemia

Appropriate workup of macrocytic anemia (MCV >100 fL) should begin with assessment of serum folate and vitamin B_{12} levels. Some common causes of macrocytic anemia are shown in Figure 12.1.

Vitamin B_{12} deficiency is rare, as most healthy individuals have 2–3 years' storage available in the liver. However, vitamin B_{12} deficiency can be encountered in individuals who have undergone bariatric surgery with partial gastric resection and are noncompliant with recommended vitamin B_{12} supplementation (350 mcg/day sublingually plus 1000 mcg IM every 3 months if needed), in individuals with pernicious anemia (an extremely uncommon autoimmune disease in women of reproductive age that is diagnosed by the presence of serum intrinsic factor antibodies), and in those with malabsorption (e.g. Crohn's disease or ileal resection). *Folate deficiency* is less common today given the supplementation of foods with folate and universal folic acid supplementation in pregnancy. Recommended folate requirements are 400 mcg/day during pregnancy, with higher doses recommended in the presence of multiple gestations, hemolytic disorders such as sickle cell anemia or thalassemia, and in patients taking antiepileptic therapies or sulfa drugs (e.g. sulfasalazine). In addition to macrocytic anemia, folate deficiency may also cause thrombocytopenia. If a diagnosis of folate deficiency is made, or the woman had a prior pregnancy affected by a neural tube defect, the recommended dose of folic acid is 4 mg/day. Higher dosages are also recommended for women with multiple gestations, hemolytic disorders, and those taking antiepileptic therapies. Anemia due to folate or B_{12} deficiency should respond briskly, with an elevated reticulocyte count within 4 to 7 days of beginning treatment. In the case of macrocytic anemia with normal folate and

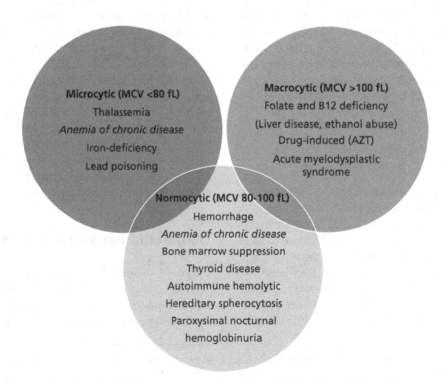

Microcytic (MCV <80 fL)
Thalassemia
Anemia of chronic disease
Iron-deficiency
Lead poisoning

Macrocytic (MCV >100 fL)
Folate and B12 deficiency
(Liver disease, ethanol abuse)
Drug-induced (AZT)
Acute myelodysplastic syndrome

Normocytic (MCV 80-100 fL)
Hemorrhage
Anemia of chronic disease
Bone marrow suppression
Thyroid disease
Autoimmune hemolytic
Hereditary spherocytosis
Paroxysimal nocturnal hemoglobinuria

Figure 12.1 Causes of maternal anemia, classified by mean corpuscular volume (MCV). AZT, azidothymidine.

vitamin B_{12} levels, a consultation with a hematologist is indicated for bone marrow biopsy.

Normocytic anemia

Evaluation of normocytic (MCV 80–100 fL) anemia should begin with evaluation of a reticulocyte count. A high reticulocyte count indicates either hemolysis or blood loss with resultant bone marrow activation. If a normocytic anemia with an elevated reticulocyte count is found, a careful history and evaluation of laboratory studies for hemolysis, such as Coombs test, peripheral smear, and lactate dehydrogenase level should be performed. A normal or low reticulocyte count in the setting of anemia raises concern for iron deficiency or bone marrow suppression/disorders. A ferritin level less than 10–15 µg/dL is diagnostic for iron-deficiency anemia, indicating depleted iron stores. Low reticulocyte count with normal or high serum ferritin levels can be seen in the presence of hypothyroidism or chronic disorders, such as inflammatory bowel disease, systemic lupus erythematosus, granulomatous infections, malignant neoplasms and rheumatoid arthritis. Hematology consultation for further assessment is indicated in these circumstances.

Mixed nutritional deficiencies (folate and iron) may lead to normocytic anemia in pregnancy, but routine supplementation makes the risk of such a scenario low. If concern for a mixed nutritional deficiency does arise, the red cell distribution width (RDW), a marker of increased variability in RBC size or anisocytosis, is a useful indicator as an RDW greater than 15% indicates the presence of nutritional deficiencies.

Microcytic anemia

As most cases of microcytic anemia in pregnancy are due to iron-deficiency anemia, evaluation of a ferritin level should be the first step in evaluation. Serum ferritin is the most sensitive and specific screening test for iron deficiency, with a level less than 10–15 µg/dL indicating depleted iron stores. If serum ferritin is normal or high, the next step is hemoglobin electrophoresis to evaluate for thalassemias (Table 12.2). Such situations usually warrant consultation with a hematologist for further evaluation.

Table 12.2 Electrophoresis results consistent with beta thalassemia or hemoglobin C traits

Condition	HbA	HbA2	HbF	HbS	HbC
Normal	95–98%	<3%	<2%	0	0
Beta-thalassemia trait	90–95%	>3.5%	1–3%	0	0
Hemoglobin C trait	50–60%	<3.5%	<2%	0%	40–50%

Because most cases of microcytic anemia (MCV <80 fL) in pregnancy are due to iron deficiency and because serum ferritin is an excellent indicator of body iron stores, the initial step should be assessment of serum ferritin levels. Low serum ferritin would diagnose iron deficiency. A high or normal serum ferritin level should indicate performance of a hemoglobin electrophoresis, which would allow identification of heterozygous thalassemia (characterized by high percentage levels of Hb A_2 and F). Normal hemoglobin A_2 and F should prompt DNA probes for alpha-thalassemia and a request for hematology consultation.

Iron supplementation in pregnancy

In a typical singleton gestation, maternal iron requirements (including blood volume expansion as well as fetal and placental requirements) average 1 g for the entire pregnancy, with this requirement further increased in the setting of multiple gestations. In a landmark study of healthy, nonanemic, menstruating young women who agreed to bone marrow biopsy, 66% had inadequate iron stores [19]. For these reasons, and because gastrointestinal side effects of oral iron supplementation (constipation, nausea, and diarrhea) are negligible with doses less than 45–60 mg, supplementation with elemental iron (30 mg/day) is recommended for all pregnant women in the United States, regardless of indices [20,21]. Supplementation should be continued until 3 months postpartum in areas with high prevalence of anemia. A review of randomized clinical trials (most performed in Western countries) shows that routine supplementation in nonanemic women results in higher maternal hemoglobin levels at term and 1 month postpartum. Additionally, women receiving routine supplementation have higher serum ferritin levels, lower rates of anemia at term (risk ratio [RR] 0.27, 95% confidence interval [CI] 0.17–0.42), and of iron deficiency anemia in particular (RR 0.33, 95% CI 0.16–0.69), and higher serum ferritin levels in the infants [22]. However no differences were noted in clinical outcomes such as preterm delivery, preeclampsia, or need for transfusion, birthweight, small for gestational age, perinatal mortality or need for neonatal intensive care unit admissions.

Treatment of iron deficiency anemia

Compared to routine supplementation in pregnancy, higher doses of iron, up to 200 mg/day, are required for the treatment of maternal anemia. *Oral iron* therapy is most often used, with a list of the most commonly available formulations provided in Table 12.3. Enteric-coated forms should be avoided because they are poorly absorbed; absorption is increased by intake of iron on an empty stomach and with vitamin C or orange juice.

Table 12.3 Oral preparations for therapy of iron deficiency anemia

Type of iron	Elemental iron (mg)	Brand
Ferrous fumarate	64–200	Femiron, Feostat, Ferrets, Fumasorb, Hemocyte, Ircon, Nephro-Fer, Vitron-C
Ferrous sulfate	40–65	Chem-Sol, Fe50, Feosol, Fergensol, Ferinsol, Ferogradumet, Ferosul, Ferratab, FerraTD, Ferrobob, Ferrospace, Ferrotime, Moliron, Slowfe, Yieronia
Ferrous gluconate	38	Fergon, Ferralet, Simron
Ferric	50–150	Ferrimin, Fe-Tinic, Hytinic, Niferex, Nu-iron

Adapted from ACOG Practice Bulletin No. 107: induction of labor. Obstet Gynecol. 2009 Aug;114(2 Pt 1):386–97.

Although several trials have been conducted to compare iron formulations, it is not possible to assess the efficacy of the treatments due to the use of different drugs, doses, and routes. Gut absorption decreases with increasing doses of iron; therefore, it is best to divide the total daily dose into 2–3 doses. A relationship is present between dose of oral iron and gastrointestinal side effects, with worsening of symptoms as dosages increase. Such side effects lead to discontinuation of therapy in up to 50% of women. To encourage compliance it is important to minimize side effects by increasing the dose gradually with larger doses in the evening, and consideration for the use of an iron sulfate elixir, which allows more gradual titration of dose. Stool softeners are often required to prevent constipation. Serum reticulocyte count should be elevated within 7–10 days of treatment initiation, with a more gradual improvement in hemoglobin levels – the hemoglobin deficit should be expected to halve in 1 month and normalize by 6–8 weeks after initiation of treatment. To replenish iron stores, oral therapy should be continued for 3 months after the anemia has been corrected.

Intravenous (IV) iron therapy is generally reserved for women that can or will not take oral iron preparations, or those whose anemia has not responded to oral supplementation. Hemoglobin indices are equivalent after 40 days of treatment in women receiving IV iron therapy as compared to those receiving oral therapy, but the rate of rise is more rapid in women receiving IV therapy. Multiple metanalysis of randomized controlled trials have found that pregnant women were more likely to achieve target hemoglobin levels with IV vs. oral iron supplementation (odds ratio [OR] 2.7, 95% CI 2.0–3.6), postpartum hemoglobin concentrations were higher, and adverse reactions or side effects were less common with IV vs. oral iron (OR 0.54, 95% CI

0.41–0.72) [23,24]. Randomized trials have not shown significant differences in need for maternal blood transfusion between the two forms of supplementation, and studies have demonstrated a preference for oral supplementation among most women [25]. Additionally, IV therapy is more costly and requires greater resources than oral supplementation. Therefore, at this time IV therapy is indicated only in patients with anemia with intolerance to oral therapy or malabsorption. Iron dextran is associated with a greater risk of anaphylaxis and is not recommended in the light of other available formulations with a lower risk of anaphylaxis: those tested in pregnancy or puerperium is shown in Table 12.4. The required dose of IV iron can be calculated according to the formula:

$$\text{Total IV iron dose (mg)} = \text{Hb deficit (g/dL)} \times \text{body weight (kg)} \times 2.145$$
$$(\textit{i.e.}, \text{Hb deficit is the desired Hb} - \text{observed Hb level})$$

Assumes blood volume is 65 mL/kg body weight and 3.3 mg of iron per g of Hb. Desired Hb is usually 12–14 g/dL and additional iron may be indicated to replete body stores (up to 500 mg iron)

Erythropoietin is not indicated in the treatment of iron deficiency anemia unless the anemia is caused by chronic renal failure or other serious chronic medical conditions and is expensive with many associated side effects – its use should be reserved for treatment by a hematologist. *Blood transfusion* is indicated only for anemia associated with hypovolemia from blood loss or in preparation for a cesarean delivery in the presence of severe anemia.

Table 12.4 Intravenous preparations for therapy of iron deficiency anemia

Type of intravenous iron	Commercial names	Dose
Iron dextran LMW	INFeD, Cosmofer	1000 mg/60 min (diluted in 250–1000 mL of normal saline)
Ferric gluconate	Ferlecit	125 mg IV infusion* over 30 min or slow IV push over 10 min
Iron sucrose	Venofer	Multiple formulations: 200 mg IV infusion* over 15 min or slow IV push over 2–5 min
Ferric carboxymaltose	Injectafer	750 mg IV infusion* over 15 min or slow IV push over 7.5 min

*diluted in 100 mL 0.9% sodium chloride. IV, intravenous.
Adapted from ACOG Practice Bulletin No. 107: induction of labor. Obstet Gynecol. 2009 Aug;114(2 Pt 1):386–97.

CASE PRESENTATION

A 28-year-old gravida 5 para 4 presented for prenatal care at 9 weeks gestation. Routine prenatal laboratory studies at that time revealed a hematocrit of 32.4%. The patient denied any personal or family history of blood disorders and had previously tested negative for sickle cell trait. She was diagnosed with mild anemia and instructed to take oral ferrous sulfate (45 mg elemental iron daily) in addition prenatal vitamins. She received routine prenatal care until a repeat complete blood count at 31 weeks gestation demonstrated a hematocrit of 22.5%, hemoglobin of 6.2 g/dL, and MCV of 72.2, consistent with a diagnosis of microcytic anemia. Further laboratory evaluation revealed iron deficiency as the cause of her anemia with low serum ferritin (6 ng/mL), low serum iron (27 mcg/dL), elevated total iron binding capacity (590 mcg/dL), and low percent saturation (5%). She was asymptomatic from her anemia.

Given the presence of severe iron deficiency despite oral iron supplementation, she was offered intravenous iron therapy, which she accepted. Her calculated iron deficit was 1088mg, given a body weight of 65 kg and a target hemoglobin of 14 g/dL. It was determined that nine doses of ferric gluconate or six doses of iron sucrose would be required, while only two doses of ferric carboxymaltose would be needed. Two doses of 750 mg ferric carboxymaltose were administered 1 week apart. By 36 weeks gestation, the patient's hematocrit had increased to 35.3% with a hemoglobin of 10.2 g/dL and MCV of 86.5. The patient continued oral iron and prenatal vitamins until she delivered by uncomplicated spontaneous vaginal delivery at term. The patient was discharged home with instructions to continue oral iron supplementation for 3 months postpartum.

References

1. Means RT. Iron deficiency and iron deficiency anemia: implications and impact in pregnancy, fetal development, and early childhood parameters. Nutrients. 2020;12(2):447.

2. Centers for Disease Control and Prevention. Recommendations to prevent and control iron deficiency in the United States. MMWR Recomm Rep. 1998 Apr 3;47(RR-3):1–29. PMID: 9563847.

3. Centers for Disease Control and Prevention. CDC criteria for anemia in children and childbearing-aged women. MMWR Morb Mortal Wkly Rep. 1989;38:400–4.

4. Adebisi OY, Strayhorn G. Anemia in pregnancy and race in the United States: blacks at risk. Fam Med. 2005;37:655–62.

5. Mei Z, Cogswell ME, Looker AC, Pfeiffer CM, Cusick SE, Lacher DA, et al. Assessment of iron status in US pregnant women from the National Health and Nutrition Examination Survey (NHANES), 1999-2006. Am J Clin Nutr. 2011;93: 1312–20.

6. Igbinosa I, Leonard SA, Noelette F, Mujahid M, Main EK, Lyell DJ. Health disparities in antepartum anemia: the intersection of race and social determinants of health. Am J Obstet Gynecol. Jan 2022;S529–30.

7. Zofkie AC, Garner WH, Schell RC, Ragsdale AS, McIntire DD, Roberts SW, et al. An evidence-based definition of anemia for singleton, uncomplicated pregnancies. PLoS One 2022 Jan 13;17(1):e0262436. doi: 10.1371/journal.pone.0262436. PMID: 35025925; PMCID: PMC8758102.

8. Hamm RF, Wang EY, Levine LD, Srinivas SK. Association between race and hemoglobin at delivery or need for transfusion when using race-based definitions for treatment of antepartum anemia. Obstet Gynecol. 2021 Jul 1;138(1):108–10. doi: 10.1097/AOG.0000000000004439. PMID: 34259472; PMCID: PMC8288460.

9. Kadyrov M, Kosanke G, Kingdom J, Kaufmann P. Increased fetoplacental angiogenesis during first trimester in anaemic women. Lancet 1998;352:1747.

10. Klebanoff MA, Shiono PH, Selby JV, Trachtenberg AI, Graubard BI. Anemia and spontaneous preterm birth. Am J Obstet Gynecol. 1991;164(1 Pt 1):59–63.

11. Lieberman E, Ryan KJ, Monson RR, Schoenbaum SC. Risk factors accounting for racial differences in the rate of premature birth. N Engl J Med. 1987;317:743–8.

12. Scanlon KS, Yip R, Schieve LA, Cogswell ME. High and low hemoglobin levels during pregnancy: differential risk for preterm birth and small for gestational age. Obstet Gynecol. 2000;96(5 Pt 1):741–8.

13. Smith C, Teng F, Branch E, Chu S, Joseph KS. Maternal and perinatal morbidity and mortality associated with anemia in pregnancy. Obstet Gynecol. 2019;134(6):1234–44. doi: 10.1097/AOG.0000000000003557

14. Scholz R, Young D, Scavone B, Hofer J, Siddiqui M. Anemia in pregnancy and risk of blood transfusion. Obstet Gynecol. 2018;131:33S. doi: 10.1097/01.AOG.0000532951.93536.70

15. Sutherland S, O'Sullivan D, Mullins J. An association between anemia and postpartum depression. Obstet Gynecol. 2018; 131:–39S. doi: 10.1097/01.AOG.0000532975.79181.b6

16. Alamri SH, Abdeen GN. Maternal nutritional status and pregnancy outcomes post-bariatric surgery. Obes Surg. 2022; 32:1325–40. https://doi.org/10.1007/s11695-021-05822-y

17. American College of Obstetricians and Gynecologists. Committee Opinion No. 691: carrier screening for genetic conditions. Obstet Gynecol. 2017;129:e41–55.

18. Zakama AK, Gaw SL. Malaria in pregnancy: what the obstetric provider in nonendemic areas needs to know. Obstet Gynecol Surv. 2019 Sep;74(9):546–56. doi:0.1097/OGX.0000000000000704. PMID: 31830300; PMCID: PMC7560991.

19. Scott DE, Pritchard JA. Iron deficiency in healthy young college women. JAMA. 1967;199(12):897–900.

20. Centers for Disease Control and Prevention. Recommendations to prevent and control iron deficiency in the United States. MMWR Recomm Rep 1998 Apr 3;47(RR-3):1–29. PMID: 9563847.

21. American College of Obstetricians and Gynecologists. ACOG Practice Bulletin No. 233: anemia in pregnancy. Obstet Gynecol 2021;138:e55–64.

22. Pena-Rosas JP, Viteri FE. Cochrane Pregnancy and Childbirth Group. Effects of routine oral iron supplementation with or

without folic acid for women during pregnancy. Cochrane Database Syst Rev. 2009;3:CD004736. doi: 10.1002/14651858. CD004736.pub2.

23. Sultan P, Bampoe S, Shah R, Guo N, Estes J, Stave C. Oral versus intravenous iron therapy for postpartum anemia: a systematic review and meta-analysis. Am J Obstet Gynecol. 2019; 221(1):19–29.e3. doi: 10.1016/j.ajog.2018. 12.016.

24. Govindappagari S, Burwick RM. Treatment of iron deficiency anemia in pregnancy with intravenous versus oral iron: a meta-analysis of RCTs. Obstet Gynecol. 2018;131:3S–4S. doi: 10.1097/01.AOG.0000533298.46904.df.

25. Nguyen V, Wuebbolt D, Thomas H, Murphy K, D'Souza R. Iron deficiency anemia in pregnancy and treatment options: a patient-preference study. Obstet Gynecol 2017;129(5):22S. doi: 10.1097/01.AOG.0000514632.23408.54.

Chapter 13
Thrombocytopenia

Ann M. Bruno and Robert M. Silver
Department of Obstetrics and Gynecology, University of Utah School of Medicine, Salt Lake City, UT, USA

Traditionally, thrombocytopenia in pregnancy has been defined as a platelet count less than 150 000/μL. Platelets nadir peridelivery but <10% of pregnant individuals have a platelet count less than 150 000/μL at term. Considering normative curves of platelets in pregnancy, further workup is often not indicated until platelets are below a threshold of 115 000–120 000/μL [1–3].

Maternal thrombocytopenia

Gestational thrombocytopenia

Gestational thrombocytopenia (GTP), also termed incidental thrombocytopenia of pregnancy, describes a mild (usually more than 70 000/μL platelet count), common (up to 5% of pregnant individuals), asymptomatic thrombocytopenia that occurs during pregnancy [4,5]. This accounts for more than 70% of thrombocytopenia in pregnant individuals [5,6]. The cause of thrombocytopenia is unclear but may be an acceleration of a physiologic pattern of increased platelet destruction [4]. Those with this diagnosis are healthy, not at risk for fetal thrombocytopenia or bleeding complications, and have no history of autoimmune thrombocytopenia. GTP is often incidentally identified through routine prenatal screening labs [4]. Platelet counts return to normal after delivery. It can be difficult to distinguish GTP from autoimmune thrombocytopenia. If thrombocytopenia is found late in pregnancy and counts are more than 70 000/μL, GTP is the most likely diagnosis. However, other causes of thrombocytopenia, including preeclampsia, should be excluded. Individuals with GTP do not require additional testing or specialized care.

Autoimmune thrombocytopenia

Autoimmune thrombocytopenia, also termed idiopathic thrombocytopenic purpura (ITP), is characterized by immunologically mediated thrombocytopenia. The disorder is caused primarily by autoantibodies to platelet membrane glycoproteins, leading to increased platelet destruction. Unlike GTP, platelet counts are usually less than 100 000/μL [7]. In adults, ITP is typically a chronic disorder. It can be difficult to distinguish from other causes of thrombocytopenia and is a diagnosis of exclusion. The most common signs and symptoms include petechiae, ecchymoses, easy bruising, epistaxis, gingival bleeding, and menorrhagia. Serious spontaneous bleeding complications are rare, even in severely thrombocytopenic individuals with platelet counts of less than 10 000/μL [8]. When thrombocytopenia is profound and detected early in pregnancy, suspicion is high that the diagnosis is ITP. It often coexists with pregnancy because the disease usually presents in the second to third decades of life and has a female preponderance of 3:1 in the mid-adult years (30–60 years) [9].

Few diagnostic tests are useful in the evaluation of ITP. A complete blood count (CBC) and peripheral blood smear are helpful to exclude other causes of thrombocytopenia (e.g. pancytopenia, leukemias). The peripheral smear may show an increased proportion of slightly enlarged platelets. Bone marrow biopsy is sometimes helpful, although rarely used given its invasive nature, to clarify the diagnosis as increased numbers of immature megakaryocytes may be seen and inadequate platelet production may be excluded [9]. Although antiplatelet antibodies are present in most individuals with ITP, they are very nonspecific and testing is not recommended for the routine evaluation of maternal thrombocytopenia [10].

The focus of maternal therapy is to avoid bleeding complications associated with severe thrombocytopenia. Because labor and delivery pose a substantial risk for bleeding, most authorities recommend more aggressive medical therapy for individuals in the late second or third trimesters. Current recommendations on maternal therapy for ITP are derived largely from expert opinion. Pregnant individuals who are asymptomatic and who have platelet counts of over 50 000/μL do not require treatment. In the first and second trimesters, asymptomatic individuals with platelet counts of

Queenan's Management of High-Risk Pregnancy: An Evidence-Based Approach, Seventh Edition. Edited by Catherine Y. Spong and Charles J. Lockwood.
© 2024 John Wiley & Sons Ltd. Published 2024 by John Wiley & Sons Ltd.

30 000–50 000/μL also do not require treatment. Treatment is considered appropriate [10,11]:

- for individuals with platelet counts of less than 20 000/μL at any gestational age
- for individuals with mucocutaneous bleeding and thrombocytopenia at any gestational age
- to produce an increase in platelet count to a level considered safe for procedures. This is controversial but is considered to be 50 000/μL for cesarean delivery and 75 000/μL for regional anesthesia [12]. Thus, more aggressive treatment is often considered during the third trimester in anticipation of delivery.

Glucocorticoids are standard first-line treatment in both pregnant and nonpregnant adults. Prednisone is initiated at a dosage of 1–2 mg/kg/day and is typically continued for 2–3 weeks. If platelet counts reach acceptable levels, the drug is tapered by 10–20% per week until the lowest dosage required to maintain the platelet count at an acceptable level is achieved. Some increase in platelet count occurs in approximately 70% of patients, and complete remission has been reported in up to 25% of cases [11]. A response to glucocorticoids is usually apparent in 3–7 days and will reach a maximum in 2–3 weeks [9–11]. Described adverse effects include hypertension, glucose intolerance, psychosis, and an association with preterm premature rupture of membranes. Long-term use is associated with adrenal insufficiency and osteoporosis [11]. The benefits of steroids appear to outweigh the risks in those requiring treatment for ITP but the lowest effective dose for the shortest time necessary are recommended. Dexamethasone is an alternative glucocorticoid for ITP treatment but is less preferred due to its known transplacental transfer to the fetus.

Intravenous immunoglobulin (IVIG) is an appropriate initial treatment for pregnant individuals with platelet counts of:

- less than 10 000/μL in the third trimester
- 10 000–30 000/μL who are bleeding.

Intravenous immunoglobulin is also used in cases refractory to treatment with glucocorticoids. IVIG is a pooled immunoglobulin concentrate produced from donor blood. The optimal dose for treatment is uncertain. IVIG 400 mg/kg/day given for 2–5 consecutive days is the most widely used regimen, although similar results have been obtained using higher doses for a shorter duration. This dose of IVIG will substantially increase the platelet count in 75% of patients and will restore normal platelet counts in 50% of patients [11,13]. Peak platelet account is usually achieved within 7 to 9 days. However, in 70% of cases, the platelet count will return to pretreatment levels within 1 month after treatment [11]. Mild side effects of IVIG are common (e.g. nausea, headache), but serious side effects are rare (e.g. liver dysfunction, neutropenia anaphylaxis reaction) [14]. The most substantial

drawback of IVIG therapy is expense. It should therefore be used in cases of severe thrombocytopenia, hemorrhage, or nonresponse to steroids.

Intravenous anti-D immunoglobulin has been used to treat ITP successfully and safely in rhesus (Rh)-positive individuals [15–17]. There is a theoretical risk of causing fetal anemia by administering high doses to pregnant individuals with Rh-positive fetuses. Acute hemolysis and disseminated intravascular coagulation (DIC) may be rare but potentially severe complications of anti-D administration [18]. In general, anti-D antibodies appear to be safe for both mother and fetus [15–17]. The use of anti-D is attractive because it is less expensive and has a shorter infusion time than IVIG.

Splenectomy was the first therapy recognized to be effective for ITP and induces complete remission in approximately 80% of patients. The post-splenectomy platelet counts increase rapidly and are often normal within 1–2 weeks. The procedure is usually avoided during pregnancy but can be safely accomplished, although preferably in the second trimester. Splenectomy during pregnancy is reserved for those with platelet counts of less than 10 000/μL who are bleeding and who fail to respond to steroids and IVIG [11]. The procedure is not recommended for asymptomatic individuals with platelet counts of more than 10 000/μL.

There are few data regarding the use of other medical therapies for ITP during pregnancy. One approach in refractory cases is to combine treatment with IVIG and steroids. Azathioprine, cyclosporine, and rituximab may be reasonable choices in extremely refractory cases [11,19]. Small observational studies have described successful use of thrombopoietin receptor antagonists (TPO-RAs) for refractory cases. TPO-RAs cross the placenta but adverse fetal/neonatal risks have not been identified [20–22]. Other drugs, such as cyclophosphamide, danazol, and alkaloids, that may be effective are avoided in pregnancy due to known adverse fetal effects [11].

Platelet transfusions should be used only as a temporary measure to prepare a patient for splenectomy or surgery or for life-threatening hemorrhage. However, the usual elevation in platelet counts of approximately 10 000/μL per unit of platelet concentrate transfused is not achieved in patients with ITP because antiplatelet antibodies also bind to donor platelets. Thus, 6–10 units of platelet concentrate should be transfused. The ITP practice guideline recommends platelet transfusions before delivery in individuals with platelet counts of less than 10 000/μL undergoing planned cesarean delivery or with mucous membrane bleeding and anticipated vaginal delivery [10,11]. Concurrent administration of IVIG and platelets may increase platelets more quickly than either alone if life-threatening bleeding is present [23].

Mothers with ITP require little specialized care beyond attention to platelet count. These patients should be instructed to avoid salicylates, nonsteroidal anti-inflammatory agents, and trauma. Regardless of route of delivery, platelets, fresh frozen plasma, and IVIG should be readily available.

HELLP

HELLP, or hemolysis, elevated liver enzymes, and low platelet count, is a severe form of preeclampsia. The diagnosis of HELLP includes the constellation of elevated aspartate aminotransferase (AST) and alanine aminotransferase (ALT) above twice the upper limits of normal for laboratory standards, platelets less than 100 000/μL, and evidence of hemolysis with lactate dehydrogenase (LDH) elevated over 600 IU/L [24,25]. The underlying pathophysiology of preeclampsia is incompletely understood but often attributed to inflammation and an imbalance in angiogenic factors [26,27]. The resultant thrombocytopenia is consumptive. HELLP is most commonly a condition of the third trimester but may also have onset earlier in pregnancy or postpartum. Findings of HELLP should prompt delivery with concomitant standard management for preeclampsia, including use of magnesium sulfate for maternal neuroprotection and hypertension control [28]. Management of thrombocytopenia secondary to HELLP in labor and delivery is supportive therapy. Platelet transfusion may be considered for procedural indications (e.g. cesarean or regional anesthesia) at similar thresholds to those outlined previously. After delivery, platelets return to normal range within 2–4 days on average [29].

Thrombotic thrombocytopenic purpura and atypical hemolytic uremic syndrome

Thrombotic thrombocytopenic purpura (TTP) and *atypical hemolytic uremic syndrome (HUS)* are thrombotic microangiopathies that manifest with thrombocytopenia [30]. Both can masquerade as preeclampsia/HELLP [31,32]. Unlike HELLP, which demonstrates laboratory improvements following delivery, TTP and HUS require additional therapy for resolution [30,31]. Therefore, high clinical suspicion most be maintained to differentiate these conditions from HELLP.

TTP results from a deficiency of a metalloproteinase enzyme, ADAMTS13, that is responsible for cleavage of von Willebrand factor multimers. In the setting of decreased enzyme activity, large multimers produce platelet aggregation and formation of microthrombi within the circulation [33]. The condition manifests with the classically described pentad: hemolytic anemia, renal dysfunction, thrombocytopenia, altered mental status, and fever. However, all features are not always present. ADAMTS13 deficiency can be acquired from autoantibodies or result from a congenital gene mutation [34–36]. The condition is rare with pregnancy-associated TTP described in less than 1 in 100,000 pregnancies [37,38].

If suspected, diagnosis is made by demonstration of low ADAMTS13 activity levels (<10% diagnostic) [30]. These enzyme studies, however, are not readily available or quick resulting in all institutions, which may delay care [39,40]. Additional studies include CBC demonstrating thrombocytopenia, and peripheral blood smear findings consistent with microangiopathic hemolytic anemia (e.g. presence of schistocytes). Other findings of hemolysis are often present including elevated bilirubin and LDH levels, reticulocytosis, and low haptoglobin. Treatment for TTP is plasmapheresis with a described survival rate of 80% [41,42]. Clinical suspicion and diagnosis are key to allow appropriate management. Immunosuppressive therapy may be necessary for refractory cases and *platelet transfusion should be avoided.*

HUS is rarer than TTP and manifests with the trio: hemolytic anemia, acute renal failure, and thrombocytopenia. HUS results from dysregulation of the complement pathway but similarly produces inflammation and platelet activation resulting in thrombotic microangiopathy [43,44]. Hemolytic uremic syndrome, as compared to TTP, usually manifests with milder thrombocytopenia but more severe renal manifestations including elevated creatinine and blood urea nitrogen [45]. The peripheral blood smear findings are similar. Unlike TTP, there is no specific study to confirm the diagnosis and therefore HUS is a diagnosis of exclusion [30]. Depending on the severity of renal dysfunction, dialysis may be required. Treatment standards are evolving with the best evidence of efficacy for anticomplement antibodies [46,47].

HUS and TTP are most commonly suspected in the postpartum setting in those presumed to have HELLP but with subsequent lack of laboratory improvements. However, both can manifest earlier in pregnancy and are associated with severe maternal morbidity and placental insufficiency. Antenatal diagnosis can be managed with outlined treatments (e.g. plasmapheresis for TTP, anticomplement antibodies for HUS) but depending on gestational age, delivery may be recommended weighing the risks of prematurity and theoretical but uncertain maternal benefit [48–50]. Recurrence of TTP/HUS in future pregnancies is a concern, and these patients should be seen in follow-up with experts in the area [51].

Other causes

Other causes of thrombocytopenia during pregnancy include systemic lupus erythematosus, antiphospholipid syndrome, human immunodeficiency virus (HIV) infection, hepatitis C virus (HCV) infection, DIC, drug-induced thrombocytopenia, and pseudothrombocytopenia as a result of laboratory artifact. These disorders can be excluded with an appropriate history, physical examination, assessment of blood pressure, HIV and HCV serology, and laboratory studies (e.g. liver function tests).

Fetal thrombocytopenia

Autoimmune thrombocytopenia

Fetal thrombocytopenia and, rarely, bleeding complications may occur with ITP because maternal immunoglobulin G (IgG) antiplatelet antibodies are actively transported across the placenta. Occasionally, minor clinical bleeding such as purpura, ecchymoses, hematuria, or melena is observed. Extremely rarely, fetal thrombocytopenia can lead to intracranial hemorrhage (ICH), which can result in severe neurologic impairment or even death. It is important to emphasize that the risk of serious fetal bleeding with maternal ITP is very low [6].

Strategies intended to minimize or avoid fetal bleeding complications include corticosteroids, IVIG, and splenectomy. Currently, no maternal treatment has been found to be consistently effective in the prevention of fetal/neonatal thrombocytopenia or to improve fetal outcome [52–55]. The risk of neonatal bleeding is inversely proportional to the fetal/neonatal platelet count and bleeding complications are rare with platelet counts over 50 000/μL [6,54]. Attempts have been made to determine which fetuses are severely thrombocytopenic and at higher risk for ICH. Unfortunately, no maternal factor has been identified that can predict fetal thrombocytopenia in all cases and current evidence does not support the routine use of fetal scalp sampling and cordocentesis in individuals with ITP [56,57].

Route of delivery was once considered critical to neonatal outcome in individuals with ITP. Passage through the birth canal was proposed as the reason for bleeding in thrombocytopenic fetuses and this together with anecdotal reports and case series led to recommendations for delivery by cesarean section [58]. However, vaginal delivery has never been proven to cause ICH and several studies have shown no association between route of delivery and neonatal bleeding complications [6,54,59]. Thus, it seems prudent to deliver by cesarean only for the usual obstetric indications without determination of the fetal platelet count.

In all cases of possible fetal thrombocytopenia, whether secondary to ITP or alloimmune thrombocytopenia, a neonatologist or other clinician familiar with the condition should be present to care for potential bleeding complications and the anticipated decrease in neonatal platelet count during the first several days after birth. The use of scalp electrodes, forceps, and vacuum extractors should be avoided in these patients. Although there is a theoretical risk of neonatal thrombocytopenia, individuals with ITP should not be discouraged from breastfeeding [60].

Alloimmune thrombocytopenia

Fetal and neonatal alloimmune thrombocytopenia (NAIT) is a serious and potentially life-threatening disorder that affects 1 in 1000–2000 liveborn infants [61–64]. Incidence varies by ethnicity with highest prevalence among the European White population [65]. The condition is analogous to Rh isoimmunization, except that maternal IgG alloantibodies are directed against fetal platelet antigens. Several polymorphic, diallelic platelet antigen systems are responsible for this condition. Uniform nomenclature has been adopted describing these antigen systems as human platelet antigens (e.g. HPA-1, HPA-2), with alleles designated as "a" or "b." The most frequent cause of severe NAIT in Europeans is the HPA-1a antigen. Although approximately 1 in 42 pregnancies is incompatible for HPA-1a, NAIT develops in only about 10% of these cases [66]. This may be because the disorder is subclinical in some cases, and it may also be because, in addition to antigen exposure, an immunologic susceptibility is necessary [67]. The human leukocyte antigen (HLA) DRB3*0101 has emerged as the immunologic antigen type resulting in clinically meaningful NAIT [68]. When done, HLA typing can be used to inform risk.

In contrast to Rh isoimmunization, NAIT can occur during a first pregnancy without prior exposure to the offending antigen. It is usually diagnosed after birth when an infant is found to have thrombocytopenia, petechiae, or ecchymoses. Affected infants are often severely thrombocytopenic, and 10–20% have ICH [69,70]. The rate of ICH is considerably lower in cases detected by routine screening rather than based on thrombocytopenic infants [66]. Fetal ICH can occur in utero and a significant number of cases can be diagnosed by antenatal ultrasound. The recurrence risk is substantial and has been estimated to be up to 100% in cases of HPA-1a incompatibility, depending upon paternal zygosity for HPA-1a [62,71]. Thrombocytopenia tends to worsen as pregnancy progresses in untreated fetuses.

The goal of the obstetric management of pregnancies at risk of NAIT is to prevent ICH and its associated complications. In contrast to ITP, the dramatically higher frequency of ICH associated with NAIT justifies more aggressive interventions. Also, therapy must be initiated antenatally because of the risk of in utero ICH. Possible NAIT should be suspected in cases of otherwise unexplained fetal or neonatal thrombocytopenia, ICH, or porencephaly. In most cases, the diagnosis of NAIT can be determined by testing the parents; testing fetal or neonatal blood is confirmatory and occasionally helpful. Appropriate assays include serologic confirmation of maternal antiplatelet antibodies that are specific for paternal or fetal/neonatal platelets. In addition, individuals should undergo platelet typing with paternal zygosity testing. This can be determined serologically or with DNA-based tests [72]. It is unnecessary to repeat testing in a family with a previously confirmed case of NAIT. Antibody titers are poorly predictive of risk to the current pregnancy and need not be obtained once the diagnosis is made. If the father is heterozygous for the offending antigen, fetal HPA typing can be accomplished with chorionic villi or amniocytes, or using free fetal DNA in maternal blood. Use of free fetal DNA offers an early (performed as soon as 10 weeks gestation), noninvasive option. Advances in next generation sequencing technologies have improved the accuracy and clinical utility of this testing in recent years [73]. Fetal genotyping avoids additional expensive and risky interventions in approximately 50% of such cases.

If the fetus is determined to be at risk, cordocentesis may be considered to determine the fetal platelet count. This strategy avoids treatment of fetuses that have normal platelet counts and provides feedback about treatment response in cases of thrombocytopenia. However, the risk of hemorrhagic complications with cordocentesis is increased in pregnancies affected by NAIT [74]. The overall perinatal loss rate for cordocentesis has been reported to be 2.7% [75] and is likely higher in the setting of severe fetal thrombocytopenia. Even with prophylactic transfusion of maternal platelets at the time of cordocentesis, the percentage of bleeding complications may be unchanged [76]. The risk of bleeding at the site of cordocentesis has prompted most clinicians to empirically treat pregnancies at risk for NAIT without determining the fetal platelet count. This strategy is usually reserved for cases of HPA-1a sensitization with a known antigen-positive fetus and is strongly recommended in cases with severely affected siblings [77].

Proposed therapies to increase fetal platelet counts and prevent ICH include maternal treatment with steroids and IVIG, fetal treatment with IVIG, and fetal platelet transfusions. No therapy is effective in all cases. Low dose maternal steroids do not appear to improve fetal platelet counts. The efficacy of high-dose steroids is uncertain. IVIG administered directly to the fetus has had inconsistent results. Fetal platelet transfusions are effective but the short half-life of transfused platelets requires weekly procedures [78]. The potential risks involved with multiple transfusions as well as the potential for increased sensitization limit the attractiveness of this treatment. Platelet transfusions are likely best reserved for severe cases refractory to other therapies. Administration of IVIG to the mother appears to be the most consistently effective antenatal therapy for NAIT. Weekly infusions of 1 g/kg maternal weight of IVIG will often stabilize or increase the fetal platelet count [70,79,80]. ICH is extremely rare in pregnancies treated with IVIG [70].

Berkowitz et al. and Bussel et al. further refined the optimal therapy for NAIT during pregnancy (HPA-1a sensitization and antigen-positive fetus) in several clinical trials [65,79,80–83]. According to available data, it seems appropriate to stratify treatment based on the level of risk for neonatal AIT. Pacheco and coworkers stratified the following management recommendations using such an approach [84]:

1. Stratum 1 includes families with an uncertain diagnosis (e.g. prior infant with thrombocytopenia, ICH, but no specific HPA antibodies or incompatibility). These patients should be screened for maternal anti-HPA antibodies.
2. Stratum 2 includes confirmed NAIT with a prior fetus having thrombocytopenia but not ICH. These pregnancies are treated with 1 g/kg/wk of IVIG and 0.5 mg/kg/d of prednisone or 2 g/kg/wk of IVIG starting at 20 weeks gestation. They all receive empiric salvage therapy with both 2 g/kg/wk of IVIG and 0.5 mg/kg/d of prednisone at 32 weeks gestation without assessment of fetal platelet count. They have an elective cesarean delivery at 37 to 38 weeks gestation, and cordocentesis is performed only if the patient desires a vaginal delivery.
3. Stratum 3 consists of women with confirmed NAIT and a prior infant with antenatal ICH at 28 weeks gestation or later or with peripartum ICH. These women start treatment with 1 g/kg/wk of IVIG at 12 weeks gestation. Their treatment at 20 and 28 weeks is the same as for stratum 2. They deliver by cesarean at 35 to 36 weeks gestation after documentation of lung maturity or undergo trial of labor after cordocentesis.
4. Stratum 4 includes women with a prior infant with antenatal intraventricular hemorrhage before 28 weeks gestation. These women are treated with 2 g/kg/wk of IVIG at 12 weeks gestation, and 0.5 mg/d of prednisone is added at 20 weeks gestation. Delivery is the same as for women in stratum 3.

Bussel and colleagues provide similar recommendations with slight modifications [85].

Most authorities recommend cesarean delivery for fetuses with platelet counts less than 50 000/μL. As discussed in the section on ITP, vaginal delivery has never been shown to cause ICH and cesarean delivery has never been shown to prevent it. Nonetheless, the substantial rate of ICH probably justifies cesarean delivery in pregnancies with severe NAIT. Cordocentesis at about 37 weeks gestation is used to document a safe platelet count for vaginal delivery. It is reasonable to consider a platelet count >100 000/μL at 32 weeks to be an adequate threshold for allowing a trial of labor. Currently, most clinicians perform cesarean delivery unless a fetal platelet count is documented to be greater than 50 000/uL [83–85].

There are no compelling data to support population-wide screening for HPA incompatibility. Population screening studies in Europe suggest cases identified by systematic screening are phenotypically different in severity as compared to clinically diagnosed cases (e.g. previously affected child, in utero concern for ICH) [86]. Studies are ongoing to address the efficacy and cost-effectiveness of such programs and the issue remains controversial [87,88]. Noninvasive free fetal DNA may afford the ability to routinely screen for HPA-1a susceptibility in the future but this is not routinely used in current clinical practice [85]. Screening relatives of affected individuals also remains of unproven benefit.

Ongoing research to elucidate alternative interventions for the prevention and treatment of NAIT is underway. Just as Rh-D immune globulin (Rhogam) is used to prevent sensitization in at-risk Rh-negative individuals, the concept of an immune globulin directed at HPA-1a is under study. Produced from human plasma of individuals with antibodies against HPA-1a, NAITgam is a concentrated immune globulin [85,89]. Biologic application has been demonstrated in animal models [89].

Concentration, dose, and timing data for administration of NAITgam in humans are still needed, as well as a population model for identification of those at-risk for receipt of prophylaxis [85].

Therapeutic inhibitors of the Fc receptor are another novel approach to NAIT prevention and therapy. Fc receptors have an integral role in the transendothelial transfer of IgG antibodies. Inhibition of Fc receptors has demonstrated efficacy in other autoimmune conditions. In pregnancy, use results in diminished IgG antibodies in mother and fetus. Ongoing trials are underway to evaluate the utility and safety of these medications for alloimmunization conditions (Clinical Trials: NCT03842189) [85].

CASE PRESENTATION 1

A healthy 34-year-old gravida 3, para 2002, at 36 weeks gestation, presents for evaluation of regular contractions. The cervix is 3 cm dilated and 50% effaced. Routine CBC is notable for a platelet count of 94000/μL. Her blood pressure is 116/72 mmHg. She denies headache, visual changes, abdominal pain, or bleeding of any type. Prenatal HIV serology is negative, and hematocrit, liver enzymes, and creatinine are normal. A platelet antibody test is positive. The clinician is concerned about possible ITP and wonders about the need for treatment.

When a clinician evaluates a mother with thrombocytopenia, a careful history should be obtained with emphasis on discovering a history of underlying bleeding diathesis, medication use, and medical conditions associated with thrombocytopenia. A physical examination should be performed to look for petechiae or ecchymoses. A peripheral smear should be considered to evaluate platelet morphology and to exclude platelet clumping. Although antiplatelet antibodies are present in most individuals with ITP, tests for these antibodies are nonspecific, poorly standardized, and subject to a large degree of interlaboratory variation. Antiplatelet antibody tests cannot distinguish between GTP and ITP and are not recommended for the routine evaluation of maternal thrombocytopenia.

In this case, there is no evidence of preeclampsia or other medical conditions associated with thrombocytopenia. Gestational thrombocytopenia is the most likely diagnosis and no additional testing or treatment is warranted.

CASE PRESENTATION 2

A 26-year-old gravida 2, para 1001 presents for prenatal care at 8 weeks gestation. Her prior pregnancy was uncomplicated, resulting in vaginal birth of a healthy infant at 39 weeks gestation. However, her infant had petechiae and neonatal platelet count was determined to be 22000/μL. There was no evidence of sepsis, preeclampsia, or other explanation for the thrombocytopenia. The platelet count increased after platelet transfusion and the child has had no medical problems or persistent thrombocytopenia. The couple asks whether the current fetus is at risk for thrombocytopenia and if anything can be done to prevent it.

The clinician should consider a diagnosis of NAIT in any case of current or prior unexplained fetal or neonatal thrombocytopenia. Both parents should be tested for platelet antigen type and zygosity, and the mother should be tested for specific antiplatelet antibodies against paternal platelet antigens. Testing is best accomplished in a specialized laboratory with expertise in NAIT; testing for generic antiplatelet antibodies in the mother is not clinically useful.

In this case, the mother is HPA-1b homozygous and the father is HPA-1a/HPA-1b heterozygous. The mother has specific antibodies against HPA-1a. The couple should be advised that there is a 50% chance that the fetus carries the HPA-1a gene and is at risk for NAIT. Testing for fetal platelet antigen genotyping should be offered. If the fetus is HPA-1b, no further evaluation is required. If the fetus is HPA-1a, the fetus should be treated as for stratum 2 as described previously. The couple should be referred for consultation with a maternal-fetal medicine specialist to discuss the risks and benefits of specific management options. Trial of labor should be allowed only in cases wherein fetal platelet count is documented to be more than 50000/μL and delivery should occur in a setting with neonatal expertise in NAIT.

References

1. Boehlen F, Hohlfeld P, Extermann P, Perneger TV, de Moerloose P. Platelet count at term pregnancy: a reappraisal of the threshold. Obstet Gynecol. 2000;95(1):29–33.

2. Reese JA, Peck JD, McIntosh JJ, Vesely SK, George JN. Platelet counts in women with normal pregnancies: a systematic review. Am J Hematol. 2017;92(11):1224–32.

3. Reese JA, Peck JD, Deschamps DR, McIntosh JJ, Knudtson EJ, Terrell DR, et al. Platelet counts during pregnancy. N Engl J Med. 2018;379(1):32–43.

4. Burrows RF, Kelton JG. Incidentally detected thrombocytopenia in healthy mothers and their infants. N Engl J Med. 1988;319:142–5.

5. Burrows RF, Kelton JG. Thrombocytopenia at delivery: a prospective survey of 6715 deliveries. Am J Obstet Gynecol. 1990;162:731–4.

6. Burrows RF, Kelton JG. Fetal thrombocytopenia and its relation to maternal thrombocytopenia. N Engl J Med, 1993;329:1463–6.

7. Rodeghiero F, Stasi R, Germersheimer T, Michel M, Provan D, Arnold DM, et al. Standardization of terminology, definitions and outcome criteria in immune thrombocytopenic purpura of adults and children: report from an international working group. Blood. 2009;113:2386–93.

8. Lacey JV, Penner JA. Management of idiopathic thrombocytopenic purpura in the adult. Semin Thromb Hemost. 1977;3:160–74.

9. George JN, El-Harake MA, Raskob GE. Chronic idiopathic thrombocytopenic purpura. N Engl J Med. 1994;331:1207–11.

10. Provan D, Stasi R, Newland AC, Blanchette VS, Bolton-Maggs P, Bussel JB, et al. International report on the investigation and management of primary immune thrombocytopenia. Blood. 2010:115:168–207.

11. Provan D, Arnold DM, Bussel JB, Chong BH, Cooper N, Gernsheimer T, et al. Updated international consensus report on the investigation and management of primary immune thrombocytopenia. Blood Adv 2019;3:3780–817.

12. Bauer ME, Arendt K, Beilin Y, Gernsheimer T, Perez Botero J, James AH, et al. The Society for Obstetric Anesthesia and Perinatology Interdisciplinary Consensus Statement on Neuraxial Procedures in Obstetric Patients with Thrombocytopenia. Anesth Analg. 2021;132(6):1531–44.

13. Bussel JB, Pham LC. Intravenous treatment with gamma globulin in adults with immune thrombocytopenia purpura: review of the literature. Vox Sang. 1987;52:206–11.

14. Ben-Chetrit E, Putterman C. Transient neutropenia induced by intravenous immune globulin. N Engl J Med. 1992;326:270–1.

15. Boughton BJ, Chakraverty R, Baglin TP, Simpson A, Galvin G, Rose P, et al. The treatment of chronic idiopathic thrombocytopenia with anti-D (Rho) immunoglobulin: its effectiveness, safety, and mechanism of action. Clin Lab Haematol. 1988;10:275–84.

16. Michel M, Novoa MV, Bussel JB. Intravenous anti-D as a treatment for immune thrombocytopenic purpura (ITP) during pregnancy. Br J Haematol. 2003;123:142–6.

17. Sieunarine K, Shapiro S, Al Obaidi MJ, Girling J. Intravenous anti-D immunoglobulin in the treatment of resistant immune thrombocytopenic purpura in pregnancy. Br J Obstet Gynaecol. 2007;114:505–7.

18. Gaines AR. Disseminated intravascular coagulation associated with acute hemoglobinemia or hemoglobinuria following Rh(0)(D) immune globulin intravenous administration for immune thrombocytopenic purpura. Blood. 2005;106:1532–7.

19. Chakravarty EF, Murray ER, Kelman A, Farmer P. Pregnancy outcomes after maternal exposure to rituximab. Blood. 2011;117(5):1499–506.

20. Michel M, Ruggeri M, Gonzalez-Lopez TJ, Alkindi S, Cheze S, Ghanima W, et al. Use of thrombopoietin receptor agonists for immune thrombocytopenia in pregnancy: results from a multicenter study. Blood. 2020;136(26):3056–61.

21. Decroocq J, Marcellin L, Le Ray C, Willems L. Rescue therapy with romiplostim for refractory primary immune thrombocytopenia during pregnancy. Obstet Gynecol. 2014;124(2 Pt 2 Suppl 1):481–3.

22. Patil AS, Dotters-Katz SK, Metjian AD, James AH, Swamy GK. Use of a thrombopoietin mimetic for chronic immune thrombocytopenic purpura in pregnancy. Obstet Gynecol. 2013;122(2 Pt 2):483–5.

23. Spahr JE, Rodgers GM. Treatment of immune-mediated thrombocytopenia purpura with concurrent intravenous immunoglobulin and platelet transfusion: a retrospective review of 40 patients. Am J Hematol. 2008;83(2):122–5.

24. Martin JN Jr, Blake PG, Perry KG Jr, McCaul JF, Hess LW, Martin RW. The natural history of HELLP syndrome: patterns of disease progression and regression. Am J Obstet Gynecol. 1991;164(6 Pt 1):1500–9.

25. Barton JR, Sibai BM. Diagnosis and management of hemolysis, elevated liver enzymes, and low platelets syndrome. Clin Perinatol. 2004;31(4):807–33, vii.

26. Sargent IL, Germain SJ, Sacks GP, Kumar S, Redman CW. Trophoblast deportation and the maternal inflammatory response in pre-eclampsia. J Reprod Immunol. 2003;59(2):153–60.

27. Walsh SW. Low-dose aspirin: treatment for the imbalance of increased thromboxane and decreased prostacyclin in preeclampsia. Am J Perinatol. 1989;6(2):124–32.

28. Fishel Bartal M, Sibai BM. Eclampsia in the 21st century. Am J Obstet Gynecol. 2020;S0002-9378(20)31128-5.

29. Neiger R, Contag SA, Coustan DR. The resolution of preeclampsia-related thrombocytopenia. Obstet Gynecol. 1991;77(5):692–5.

30. Scully M, Cataland S, Coppo P, de la Rubia J, Friedman KD, Kremer Hovinga J, et al.; International Working Group for Thrombotic Thrombocytopenic Purpura. Consensus on the standardization of terminology in thrombotic thrombocytopenic purpura and related thrombotic microangiopathies. J Thromb Haemost. 2017;15(2):312–22.

31. Sibai BM. Imitators of severe preeclampsia. Obstet Gynecol. 2007;109(4):956–66.

32. Rehberg JF, Briery CM, Hudson WT, Bofill JA, Martin JN Jr. Thrombotic thrombocytopenic purpura masquerading as hemolysis, elevated liver enzymes, low platelets (HELLP) syndrome in late pregnancy. Obstet Gynecol. 2006;108:817–20.

33. Furlan M, Robles R, Galbusera M, Remuzzi G, Kyrle PA, Brenner B, et al. Von Willebrand factor-cleaving protease in thrombotic thrombocytopenic purpura and the hemolytic uremic syndrome. N Engl J Med. 1998;339:1578–84.

34. Levy GG, Nichols WC, Lian EC, Foroud T, McClintick JN, McGee BM, et al. Mutations in a member of the ADAMTS gene

family cause thrombotic thrombocytopenic purpura. Nature. 2001;413:488–94.

35. Starke R, Machin S, Scully M, Purdy G, Mackie I. The clinical utility of ADAMTS13 activity, antigen and autoantibody assays in thrombotic thrombocytopenic purpura. Br J Haematol. 2007;136:649–55.

36. Sánchez-Luceros A, Farías CE, Amaral MM, Kempfer AC, Votta R, Marchese C, et al. Von Willebrand factor-cleaving protease (ADAMTS13) activity in normal non-pregnant women, pregnant and post-delivery women. Thromb Haemost. 2004;92(6):1320–6.

37. Scully M, Thomas M, Underwood M, Watson H, Langley K, Camilleri RS, et al.; collaborators of the UK TTP Registry. Thrombotic thrombocytopenic purpura and pregnancy: presentation, management, and subsequent pregnancy outcomes. Blood. 2014;124(2):211–9.

38. Delmas Y, Helou S, Chabanier P, Ryman A, Pelluard F, Carles D, et al. Incidence of obstetrical thrombotic thrombocytopenic purpura in a retrospective study within thrombocytopenic pregnant women. A difficult diagnosis and a treatable disease. BMC Pregnancy Childbirth. 2015;15:137.

39. Shah N, Rutherford C, Matevosyan K, Shen YM, Sarode R. Role of ADAMTS13 in the management of thrombotic microangiopathies including thrombotic thrombocytopenic purpura (TTP). Br J Haematol. 2013;163(4):514–9.

40. Kim CH, Simmons SC, Wattar SF, Azad A, Pham HP. Potential impact of a delayed ADAMTS13 result in the treatment of thrombotic microangiopathy: an economic analysis. Vox Sang. 2020;115(5):433–42.

41. Rock GA, Shumak KH, Buskard NA, Blanchette VS, Kelton JG, Nair RC, et al. Comparison of plasma exchange with plasma infusion in the treatment of thrombotic thrombocytopenic purpura. Canadian Apheresis Study Group. N Engl J Med. 1991;325(6):393–7.

42. Saha M, McDaniel JK, Zheng XL. Thrombotic thrombocytopenic purpura: pathogenesis, diagnosis and potential novel therapeutics. J Thromb Haemost. 2017;15(10):1889–900. doi: 10.1111/jth.13764.

43. George JN. ADAMTS13, thrombotic thrombocytopenic purpura, and hemolytic syndrome. Curr Hematol Rep. 2005;4:167–9.

44. Bruel A, Kavanagh D, Noris M, Delmas Y, Wong EKS, Bresin E, et al. hemolytic uremic syndrome in pregnancy and postpartum. Clin J Am Soc Nephrol. 2017;12(8):1237–47. doi: 10.2215/CJN.00280117.

45. Gupta M, Feinberg BB, Burwick RM. Thrombotic microangiopathies of pregnancy: Differential diagnosis. Pregnancy Hypertens. 2018;12:29–34.

46. Legendre CM, Licht C, Muus P, Greenbaum LA, Babu S, Bedrosian C, et al. Terminal complement inhibitor eculizumab in atypical hemolytic-uremic syndrome. N Engl J Med. 2013;368(23):2169–81.

47. Zuber J, Fakhouri F, Roumenina LT, Loirat C, Frémeaux-Bacchi V; French Study Group for aHUS/C3G. Use of eculizumab for atypical haemolytic uraemic syndrome and C3 glomerulopathies. Nat Rev Nephrol. 2012;8(11):643–57.

48. Fakhouri F, Scully M, Provôt F, Blasco M, Coppo P, Noris M, et al. Management of thrombotic microangiopathy in pregnancy and postpartum: report from an international working group. Blood. 2020;136(19):2103–17.

49. Martin JN, Bailey AP, Rehberg JF, Owens MT, Keiser SD, May WL. Thrombotic thrombocytopenic purpura in 166 pregnancies: 1955-2006. Am J Obstet Gynecol. 2008;199:98–104.

50. Esplin MS, Branch DW. Diagnosis and management of thrombotic microangiopathies during pregnancy. Clin Obstet Gynecol. 1999;42:360–7.

51. Raman R, Yang S, Wu HM, Cataland SR. ADAMTS13 activity and the risk of thrombotic thrombocytopenic purpura relapse in pregnancy. Br J Haematol. 2011;153:277–8.

52. Kaplan C, Daffos F, Forestier F, Tertian G, Catherine N Pons JC, et al. Fetal platelet counts in thrombocytopenic pregnancy. Lancet 1990;336:979–82.

53. Christiaens GCML, Nieuwenhuis HK, von dem Borne AE, Ouwehand WH, Helmerhorst FM, van Dalen CM, et al. Idiopathic thrombocytopenic purpura in pregnancy: a randomized trial on the effect of antenatal low dose corticosteroids on neonatal platelet count. Br J Obstet Gynaecol. 1990;97:893–8.

54. Cook RL, Miller RC, Katz VL, Cefalo RC. Immune thrombocytopenic purpura in pregnancy: a reappraisal of management. Obstet Gynecol. 1991;78:578–83.

55. Scott JR, Rote NS, Cruikshank DP. Antiplatelet antibodies and platelet counts in pregnancies complicated by autoimmune thrombocytopenic purpura. Am J Obstet Gynecol. 1983;145:932–9.

56. Silver RM. Management of idiopathic thrombocytopenic purpura in pregnancy. Am J Obstet Gynecol. 1998;41:436–48.

57. Silver RM, Branch DW, Scott JR. Maternal thrombocytopenia in pregnancy: time for a reassessment. Am J Obstet Gynecol. 1995;173:479–82.

58. Carlos HW, McMillan R, Crosby WH. Management of pregnancy in women with immune thrombocytopenic purpura. JAMA. 1980;224:2756–8.

59. Laros RK, Kagan R. Route of delivery for patients with immune thrombocytopenia. Am J Obstet Gynecol. 1984;148:901–8.

60. American Society of Hematology ITP Practice Guideline Panel. Diagnosis and treatment of idiopathic thrombocytopenic purpura: recommendation of the American Society of Hematology. Ann Intern Med. 1997;126:319–26.

61. Blanchette VS, Chen L, de Friedberg ZS, Hogan VA, Trudel E, Decary F. Alloimmunization to the PLA1 platelet antigen: results of a prospective study. Br J Haematol. 1990;74:209–15.

62. Bussel JB, Zabusky MR, Berkowitz RL, McFarland JG. Fetal alloimmune thrombocytopenia. N Engl J Med. 1997;337:22–26.

63. Dreyfus M, Kaplan C, Verdy E, Schlegel N, Durand-Zaleski I, Tchernia G. Frequency of immune thrombocytopenia in newborns: a prospective study: Immune Thrombocytopenia Working Group. Blood, 1997;89:4402–6.

64. Williamson LM, Hackett G, Rennie J, Palmer CR, Maciver C, Hadfield R, et al. The natural history of fetomaternal alloimmunization to the platelet-specific antigen HPA-1a (PLA1, Zwa) as determined by antenatal screening. Blood. 1998;92:2280–7.

65. Berkowitz RL, Bussel JB, McFarland JG. Alloimmune thrombocytopenia: state of the art 2006. Am J Obstet Gynecol. 2006;195:907–13.

66. Kjeldsen-Kragh J, Killie MK, Tomter G, Golebiowska E, Randen I, Hauge R, et al. A screening and intervention program aimed to reduce mortality and serious morbidity associated with

severe neonatal alloimmune thrombocytopenia. Blood. 2007;110:833–9.

67. L'abbe D, Tremblay L, Filion M, Busque L, Goldman M, Decary F, Chartrand P. Alloimmunization to platelet antigen HPA-1a (PLA1) is strongly associated with both HLA-DRB3*0101 and HLA-DQB1*0201. Hum Immunol. 1992;34:107–14.

68. Kjeldsen-Kragh J, Fergusson DA, Kjaer M, Lieberman L, Greinacher A, Murphy MF, et al. Fetal/neonatal alloimmune thrombocytopenia: a systematic review of impact of HLA-DRB3*01:01 on fetal/neonatal outcome. Blood Adv. 2020;4(14):3368–77.

69. Mueller-Eckhardt C, Kiefel V, Grubert A, Kroll H, Weisheit M, Schmidt S, et al. 348 cases of fetal alloimmune thrombocytopenia. Lancet. 1989;1:363–6.

70. Bussel JB, Skupski DW, McFarland JG. Fetal alloimmune thrombocytopenia: consensus and controversy. J Matern Fetal Med. 1996;5:281–92.

71. Kaplan C, Murphy MF, Kroll H, Waters AH. Feto-maternal alloimmune thrombocytopenia: antenatal therapy with IvIgG and steroids: more questions and answers. European Working Group on Feto-maternal Alloimmune Thrombocytopenia. Br J Haematol. 1998;100:62–5.

72. McFarland JG, Aster RH, Bussel JB, Gianopoulos JG, Derbes RS, Newman PJ. Prenatal diagnosis of neonatal alloimmune thrombocytopenia using allele-specific oligonucleotide probes. Blood. 1991;78:2276–82.

73. Nogués N. Recent advances in non-invasive fetal HPA-1a typing. Transfus Apher Sci. 2020;59(1):102708.

74. Paidas MJ, Berkowitz RL, Lynch L, Lockwood CJ, Lapinski R, McFarland JG, et al. Alloimmune thrombocytopenia: fetal and neonatal losses related to cordocentesis. Am J Obstet Gynecol. 1995;172:475–9.

75. Ghidini A, Sepulveda W, Lockwood CJ, Romero R. Complications of fetal blood sampling. Am J Obstet Gynecol. 1993;168:1339–44.

76. Silver RM, Porter TF, Branch DW, Esplin MS, Scott JR. Neonatal alloimmune thrombocytopenia: antenatal management. Am J Obstet Gynecol. 1999;182:1233–8.

77. Murphy MF, Bussel JB. Advances in the management of alloimmune thrombocytopenia. Br J Haematol. 2007;136:366–78.

78. Overton TG, Duncan KR, Jolly M, Letsky E, Fisk NM. Serial platelet transfusion for fetal alloimmune thrombocytopenia: platelet dynamics and perinatal outcome. Am J Obstet Gynecol. 2002;186:826–31.

79. Berkowitz RL, Lesser ML, McFarland JG, Wissert M, Primiani A, Hung C, et al. Antepartum treatment without early cordocentesis for standard risk alloimmune thrombocytopenia: a randomized controlled trial. Obstet Gynecol. 2007;110:249–55.

80. Bussel JB, Berkowitz RL, McFarland JG, Lynch L, Chitkara U. Antenatal treatment of neonatal alloimmune thrombocytopenia. N Engl J Med. 1988;319:1374–8.

81. Lynch L, Bussel JB, McFarland JG, Chitkara U, Berkowitz RL. Antenatal treatment of alloimmune thrombocytopenia. Obstet Gynecol. 1992;80:67–71.

82. Berkowitz RL, Kolb EA, McFarland JG, Wissert M, Primani A, Lesser M, et al. Parallel randomized trials of risk-based therapy for fetal alloimmune thrombocytopenia. Obstet Gynecol. 2006;107:91–6.

83. Bussel JB, Berkowitz RL, Hung C, Kolb EA, Wissert M, Primiani A, et al. Intracranial hemorrhage in alloimmune thrombocytopenia: stratified management to prevent recurrence in the subsequent affected fetus. Am J Obstet Gynecol. 2010;203:135.e1–14.

84. Pacheco LD, Berkowitz RL, Moise KJ Jr, Bussel JB, McFarland JG, Saade GR. Fetal and neonatal alloimmune thrombocytopenia: a management algorithm based on risk stratification. Obstet Gynecol. 2011;118(5):1157–63.

85. Bussel JB, Vander Haar EL, Berkowitz RL. New developments in fetal and neonatal alloimmune thrombocytopenia. Am J Obstet Gynecol. 2021;225(2):120–7.

86. Husebekk A, Killie MK, Kjeldsen-Kragh J, Skogen B. Is it time to implement HPA-1 screening in pregnancy? Curr Opin Hematol. 2009;16:497–502.

87. Tiller H, Killie MK, Skogen B, Øian P, Husebekk A. Neonatal alloimmune thrombocytopenia in Norway: poor detection rate with nonscreening versus a general screening programme. BJOG. 2009;116(4):594–8.

88. Kjeldsen-Kragh J, Bengtsson J. Fetal and neonatal alloimmune thrombocytopenia-new prospects for fetal risk assessment of HPA-1a-negative pregnant women. Transfus Med Rev. 2020;34(4):270–6.

89. Tiller H, Killie MK, Chen P, Eksteen M, Husebekk A, Skogen B, et al. Toward a prophylaxis against fetal and neonatal alloimmune thrombocytopenia: induction of antibody-mediated immune suppression and prevention of severe clinical complications in a murine model. Transfusion. 2012;52(7):1446–57.

Chapter 14
Inherited and Acquired Thrombophilias

Pouya Abhari[1] and Michael J. Paidas[2]

[1] Department of Obstetrics, Gynecology and Reproductive Sciences, University of Miami/Jackson Memorial Hospital, Miami, FL, USA
[2] Department of Obstetrics, Gynecology and Reproductive Sciences, Miller School of Medicine, University of Miami, Miami, FL, USA

Hormonal changes, specifically increases in estrogen and progesterone, coupled with anatomic changes, lead to a transient hypercoagulable state. This state was most likely evolutionarily developed to protect against fatal hemorrhage at birth or with miscarriage, given the invasive nature of the hemochorial placentation in humans [1]. Several coagulation factor levels increase during pregnancy and in parallel, there are changes in the anticoagulant and antifibrinolytic systems which also contribute to the overall prothrombotic tendency (Figure 14.1) [2]. Inherited and acquired thrombophilic conditions have varied clinical consequences, ranging from asymptomatic to severe life-threatening thrombotic conditions affecting maternal and fetal/neonatal outcome [3]. This chapter addresses both inherited and acquired thrombophilic conditions encountered in the context of pregnancy.

Overview of hemostasis changes during pregnancy

Factor levels that increase during pregnancy include factors I (fibrinogen), VII, VIII, X, von Willebrand factor (vWF), and plasminogen activator inhibitor (PAI-I and PAI-2), all of which return to normal beginning 2 to 3 weeks postpartum [4]. Concurrently, there is substantial decrease in anticoagulant free protein S levels because of increased levels of its C4b binding protein. In fact, protein S levels are as low as 30% in the second trimester and 26% in the third trimester of normal pregnancies [5]. Thus diagnosing a true hereditary protein S deficiency requires genetic testing and not measurement of protein S levels. An increase in activated protein C (APC) resistance in the absence of the factor V Leiden mutation (FVL), unexplained by the decrease in free protein S, also is observed in some pregnant patients, particularly in the third trimester. There also is a decrease in fibrinolytic tissue plasminogen activator activity. Besides these prothrombotic changes, there are several acquired prothrombotic risks that arise in pregnancy, including progressive venous obstruction from the enlarging uterus, relative immobility if it occurs as the pregnancy progresses (particularly if transient bed rest is prescribed); the presence of varicose veins; or the postoperative state (from cesarean delivery for example), further exacerbating the tendency toward clotting, resulting in overt thrombosis.

Thus, the hypercoagulable state of pregnancy is almost always a multifactorial process. The result of this transient hypercoagulable state is a 5- to 10-fold increased risk of venous thromboembolism (VTE). In absolute terms, the risk of VTE is approximately 1:1000 (0.66 to 2.22 of 1000 pregnancies) compared to 1:10000 in age-matched, nonpregnant females not on oral contraceptives [6]. VTE is also a leading cause of death worldwide [7–10]. There is an approximately 5- to 10-fold increased risk for VTE in the antepartum period and a 22- to 84-fold increased risk in the postpartum period. Although the risk in the postpartum period appears to be the highest, probably due to pronounced vascular congestion and continued changes in the hemostatic factors, substantial thrombotic risk is present as early as the first trimester, before anatomical changes ensue.

The majority of VTEs are deep venous thrombosis (DVT) and 20% are pulmonary emboli (PE). The risk for PE is far greater in the postpartum period; and although the risk for VTE is greatest for the first 6 weeks postpartum, it persists up to 12 weeks. The VTE risk is four- to fivefold greater after an emergency cesarean delivery when compared to a vaginal delivery. Pregnancy-associated DVT is more often proximal and massive compared to the nonpregnant setting and preferentially occurs in the left lower extremity. In contrast, distal DVT

Queenan's Management of High-Risk Pregnancy: An Evidence-Based Approach, Seventh Edition. Edited by Catherine Y. Spong and Charles J. Lockwood.

Intrinsic Pathway

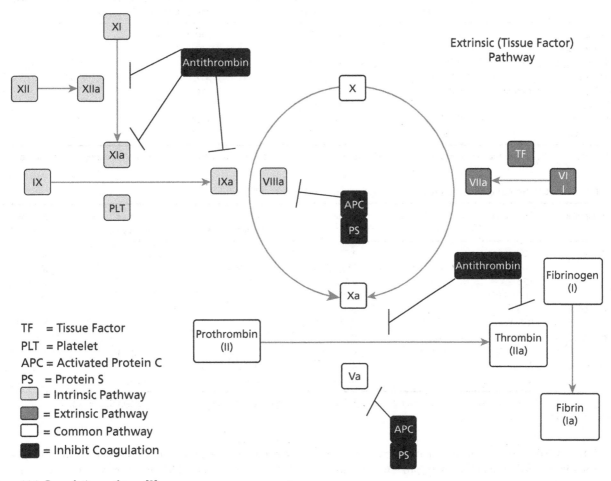

Figure 14.1 Coagulation pathway [2].

occurs with similar frequency in the left and right lower extremities. The left-sided and proximal over distal vein predominance of VTE may reflect compression by the gravid uterus of the left iliac vein as it crosses between the right iliac artery and lumbar vertebrae. Regarding superimposed genetic thrombophilia, between 20% and 50% of all thromboembolic events that occur in pregnant women are associated with a thrombophilic disorder. There is a concurrent three- to fourfold risk of arterial thromboembolism in pregnant women.

Given the differing absolute risks of thrombosis, thromboprophylaxis should be individualized based on the type of thrombophilia, presence of homozygous or heterozygous mutations, history of past VTE or pregnancy complications, and presence or absence of a family history of VTE, as well as the presence of additional prothrombotic conditions. The cumulative VTE risk then must be weighed against the bleeding risk with unfractionated or low molecular weight heparin, with the bleeding risk being at most approximately 3%.

Inherited thrombophilias

Inherited thrombophilias are a heterogeneous group of disorders associated with varying degrees of increased thrombotic risk. The occurrence of a thromboembolic event, even in pregnant women with an inherited thrombophilia, is highly dependent on other predisposing risk factors such as immobility, obesity, surgery, infection, etc. The most important risk modifier is a personal or family history of venous thrombosis (Table 14.1). Any woman who presents with VTE during pregnancy or the postpartum period should undergo an appropriate workup for inherited thrombophilias. Current guidance is to follow a tailored approach to thrombophilia screening. Consider screening for thrombophilic conditions in the following circumstances: when there is a personal history of VTE, with or without a recurrent risk factor, and no prior thrombophilia testing; and in the setting of a patient who has a first degree relative with a high-risk thrombophilia. A common approach is to perform genetic screening for FVL and the prothrombin G20210A

Table 14.1 Inherited thrombophilia, personal history of VTE and pregnancy VTE risk

Thrombophilia	Prevalence in general population (%)	VTE risk per pregnancy (no Hx) (%)	VTE risk per pregnancy (previous VTE) (%)	Percentage of all VTE
FVL heterozygous	1–15	0.5–1.2	10	40
FVL homozygous	<1	2.2–14.0	17	2
PGM heterozygous	2–5	0.4–2.6	>10	17
PGM homozygous	<1	2–4	>17	0.5
FVL/PGM double heterozygous	0.01	4–8.2	>20	1–3
AT deficiency	0.02	0.2–11.6	40	1
PC deficiency	0.2–0.4	0.1–1.7	4–17	14
PS deficiency	0.03–0.13	0.3–6.6	0–22	3

Adapted from [4]. AT, antithrombin; FVL, factor V Leiden; PC, protein C; PGM, prothrombin mutation; PS, protein S; VTE, venous thromboembolism.

Table 14.2 Inherited thrombophilia and pregnancy complications (odds ratio [95% confidence interval])

Thrombophilia	Preeclampsia	Fetal growth restriction	Abruption	Nonrecurrent pregnancy loss	Late nonrecurrent pregnancy loss	Recurrent pregnancy loss
FVL	1.23 (0.89–1.7)	1.0 (0.8–1.25)	1.85 (0.92–3.7)	1.52 (1.06–2.19)	2.06 (1.1–3.86)	3.04 (2.16–4.3)
PGM	1.25 (0.79–1.99)	1.25 (0.92–1.7)	2.02 (0.81–5.02)	1.13 (0.64–2.01)	2.66 (1.28–5.53)	2.05 (1.18–3.54)
PC deficiency	21.5 (1.1–414.4)	NA	5.93 (0.23–151.58)	1.4 (0.9–2.2)	NA	1.57 (0.23–10.54)
PS deficiency	2.83 (0.76–10.57)	10.2 (1.1–91)	0.3 (0–70.1)	1.3 (0.8–2.1)	7.39 (1.28–42.83)	14.72 (0.99–218.01)
AT deficiency	7.1 (0.4–117.4)	NA	4.1 (0.3–49.9)	2.1 (1.2–3.6)	5.2 (1.5–18.1)	NA

Adapted from [2,13–17]. AT, antithrombin; FVL, factor V Leiden; PC, protein C; PGM, prothrombin mutation; PS, protein S; VTE, venous thromboembolism.

mutation (PGM) and obtain functional screening for antithrombin activity, protein C activity, protein S free antigen and activity, and lupus anticoagulant. Functional screening should occur remote from a thrombotic event (>6 weeks), in nonpregnant individuals, among patients not on anticoagulation and not on hormonal therapy. Screening for antiphospholipid antibodies consist of anticardiolipin IgG and IgM, and β-2-glycoprotein 1 IgG and IgM antibodies. See the section on Antiphospholipid Antibody Syndrome for screening indications.

Factor V Leiden

FVL is a relatively common mutation, present in 5% of American Caucasians, 1% of African-Americans, and 5–9% of Europeans but is rare in Asian and African populations. The FVL mutation is associated with resistance to APC and is inherited primarily in an autosomal-dominant fashion. Heterozygosity is found in 20–40% of nonpregnant patients with thromboembolic disease, whereas homozygosity confers a >100-fold risk of thromboembolic disease. Well-conducted prospective studies suggest that lower-risk inherited thrombophilias, including FVL, have a weaker association with maternal thrombosis than that reported by prior retrospective studies [11,12]. In a study of 4885 low-risk

women screened in the first trimester for thrombophilias, 134 (2.7%) carried the FVL mutation but none experienced a thromboembolic event during pregnancy or the in puerperium (95% confidence interval [CI] 0–2.7%). Another two studies screening for FVL in early pregnancy also found no thrombotic episodes in women found to carry heterozygous mutations. FVL has been weakly associated with pregnancy loss [13]. See Table 14.2 for a summary of inherited thrombophilic conditions and pregnancy complications.

Prothrombin gene mutation (G2021A)

PGM has been found to increase circulating prothrombin levels and, hence, the risk of both thrombosis and pregnancy complications. In women with a history of VTE during pregnancy, PGM was found in 17% of patients compared with 1% of age-matched controls, and FVL was found in nearly 45% of patients. Homozygosity for PGM confers an equivalent risk of VTE to that of FVL homozygosity.

The pregnancy associated VTE risk in women without any prior history of VTE who have deficiencies of the natural anticoagulants, protein S, protein C and antithrombin are 0.3–6.6%, 0.1–1.7%, and 0.2–11.6%, respectively [18]. Antithrombin deficiency is the rarest and the most thrombogenic of the inherited thrombophilic conditions.

Protein C deficiency

Protein C is an anticoagulant responsible for the deactivation of factor Va and factor VIIIa. It is activated by thrombin to APC, which then degrades factors Va and VIIIa, inhibiting clot formation. Protein C synthesis or functional deficiency is found in 0.2–0.3% of individuals of European descent. Protein C deficiency is more common in those of Asian and African descent. The gene coding for protein C is located on chromosome 2. It is vitamin K dependent and is synthesized by the liver. Two major subtypes of protein C deficiencies have been delineated. The more common phenotype, type I, has both reduced immunoreactive protein C levels and reduced functional activity. Type II phenotypes have quantitatively normal immunoreactive levels of protein C but have compromised functional activity. Laboratory evaluation includes determination of both protein C antigen and activity levels. Laboratories typically use activity levels of <50–60% to define abnormalities. Testing is unreliable during an acute thrombosis or during anticoagulation therapy.

Regarding thrombotic event risk in pregnancy, protein C deficiency is moderately prothrombogenic. The risk is likely proportional to the deficiency of substrate and/or function. The relative risk (RR) of a first VTE in pregnancy is 3.0 (95% CI 1.4–6.5) when using a <73% of normal protein C activity cutoff and increases to 13.0 (95% CI 1.4–123) if using a <50% cutoff according to a case-control study of 173 women with VTE compared to 325 normal controls. A 2006 systemic review of available retrospective case-controlled studies showed a modest risk of VTE (OR 4.76, 95% CI 2.15–10.57) in patients with hereditary protein C deficiency. Because both DVT and protein C deficiency are uncommon, large prospective studies regarding their association are prohibitive.

Data regarding the association of protein C deficiency and poor obstetrical outcomes are sparse, and studies available are underpowered. The diverse genetic variants and phenotypes make it difficult to make any conclusion regarding management strategies. Many studies that do include protein C deficiency pool data with protein S and antithrombin deficiency. There is no clear association between recurrent early pregnancy loss and protein C deficiency. In systemic review of retrospective case-controlled studies, protein C deficiency was associated with preeclampsia (OR 21.5, 95% CI 1.1–414.4), however, all included studies were limited by small study size and large CIs.

Protein S deficiency

Protein S is a vitamin K-dependent anticoagulant cofactor in the clotting cascade. It accelerates APC's disruption of factor Va and factor VIIIa, ultimately suppressing thrombin formation. It is a less common thrombophilia with prevalence of 0.03–0.13% in the Caucasian European population. The coding gene, PROS1, is located on chromosome 3. There have been over 130 mutations found to cause protein S deficiency with variable expression. Deficiency of protein S has been divided into three major phenotypes. Type I disease has quantitatively low levels of protein S antigen, both free and total, and decreased function. Type II is characterized by normal free and total protein S levels but compromised functional activity. Type III disease has normal total antigen levels but low free protein S antigen and activity levels. Protein S activity is variable secondary to fluctuating levels of complement 4B-binding protein, a regulator in the compliment system. Free protein S levels fall throughout pregnancy due to increasing C4b-binding protein. Protein S levels are influenced by pregnancy, anticoagulation, and the presence of active thrombosis. During gestation, free protein S levels are substantially lower than nonpregnant values, with free levels of 38.9 ± 10.3% in the second trimester and 31.2 %± 7.4% in the third trimester [5]. When indicated, testing for hereditary protein S deficiency is generally deferred until at least 8–12 weeks postpartum to avoid confounding information. Free antigen levels below 60% are considered abnormal, but a diagnosis of hereditary protein S deficiency cannot be made based on protein S activity or free antigen levels when these levels are determined only in pregnancy. Protein S levels must be determined outside of pregnancy and the postpartum period, as well as in the absence of hormonal contraception to confirm the presence of a hereditary protein S deficiency.

Because of the relative infrequency of protein S deficiency, the number of studies regarding its risks during pregnancy is limited. A systematic review of available case-controlled studies in 2006 showed an odds ratio (OR) of 3.19 (95% CI 1.48–6.88) for VTE in pregnancy. An evaluation of 44 pregnancies in 17 patients with congenital protein S deficiency showed no thrombosis during pregnancies without anticoagulation but 5 thrombotic events in the postpartum period (17%, 95% CI 3–31). A systemic review found a relatively strong association with stillbirth defined as unexplained fetal loss after 20 weeks with no fetal abnormalities (OR 16.2, 95% CI 5–52.3). There are conflicting data in the literature regarding associations with other poor obstetrical outcomes.

Antithrombin deficiency

A less common but more thrombogenic hereditary dysfunction is caused by mutation in the serine protease inhibitor antithrombin (AT) gene. Sometimes referred to as antithrombin III, AT inhibits active thrombin's conversion of fibrinogen to fibrin. It is also a known inhibitor of factors Xa, IXa, XIa, and XIIa, as well as trypsin, plasmin, and kallikrein. Besides its role as anticoagulant, AT has also been found to have anti-inflammatory characteristics. Over 250 mutations have been identified at the AT gene loci that provide a wide spectrum of phenotypes. Type I disease infers a quantitative dysfunction. Type II is the qualitative class of dysfunction, which is further divided into subtypes. Type IIa is characterized by a defect in the reactive site of the protein and is generally more thrombogenic. Type IIb dysfunctions have a defect in the heparin-binding site and are less prone to thrombosis. Type IIc has defects in both binding sites. Type I makes up only 12% of the total of cases of AT deficiency, but it is much more thrombogenic, accounting for 80% of symptomatic cases. The prevalence of AT deficiency in Caucasian Europeans is estimated at 0.02–1.15%. It has been found to be even more common in some Asian populations, with a prevalence of up to 2–5%.

The laboratory assay of choice is plasma AT activity using heparin measures how well AT inhibits thrombin or factor Xa. Activity <80 % is considered abnormal, but most patients with hereditary AT deficiency have levels <60%. Testing can be abnormal secondary to anticoagulation and acute thrombosis and should be delayed until after completing treatment. The risk of VTE in pregnancy can be high with AT deficiency, though there is large variability among phenotypes. A systemic review reported an OR of 4.69 (95% CI 1.30–16.96) regarding VTE and pregnancy. A systemic review that included 112 pregnancies with AT deficiency without a personal history of VTE, found the incidence risk of VTE to be 11.6% in each pregnancy (OR 6.09, 95% CI 1.58–24.43). Retrospective studies have, however, estimated the risk for the more thrombogenic type I disease (OR 282, 95% CI 31–2532) compared to a much lower risk with type II disease (OR 28, 95% CI 5.5–142). It is estimated that the lifetime risk of VTE in those with type I disease is 50%. One case series of 63 untreated women with type I AT deficiency who went through pregnancy without anticoagulation found that 18% had a thrombotic complication during pregnancy and another 33% had a thrombotic complication postpartum.

Though AT deficiency is the first inherited thrombophilia identified, data regarding its association to poor obstetrical outcomes are less robust due to its rarity. Regarding early fetal loss, a retrospective cohort found a modest risk of a fetal loss < 28 weeks in patients with AT deficiency (OR 1.7, 95% CI 1–2.8). A meta-analysis did not find a significant increased risk of recurrent loss before 17 weeks (OR 0.88, 95% CI 0.17–4.48) or nonrecurrent loss at any gestational age (1.54, 95% CI 0.97–2.45). Other studies have failed in demonstrating an association with AT deficiency and early pregnancy loss. Studies investigating the relationship between stillbirth, fetal growth restriction and abruption, and AT deficiency are limited due the infrequency of both diagnoses [19].

Regarding AT levels in pregnancy, a gradual decline in AT activity during the late stage of pregnancy, namely, pregnancy-induced AT deficiency, has been reported in literature, in healthy parturients at term. Decreased AT activity levels have been inconsistently reported in patients complicated by preeclampsia. Initial studies reported lower mean AT activity levels in patients with preeclampsia compared to non-preeclamptic patients (60% ± 15 % vs. 85% ± 15 %) and falling AT levels with worsening preeclampsia. However, data from a recent pivotal randomized clinical trial found that the majority of patients of preterm preeclampsia (indicating a severe spectrum of preeclampsia) did not have low AT levels. It has been well known that AT concentrates (plasma-derived or recombinant forms) have potent anticoagulant, anti-inflammatory properties. Initial studies with plasma-derived AT administered to preeclamptic patients demonstrated success in prolonging pregnancy in early onset preeclampsia. However, a recent large, multicenter, double-blinded trial evaluating recombinant AT therapeutic benefits in patients with preterm preeclampsia between 23 and 30 weeks did not find a benefit in prolonging latency in preterm preeclampsia [20].

Acquired thrombophilia

Antiphospholipid antibody syndrome

Antiphospholipid antibody syndrome (APS) is defined by the combination of VTE, obstetric complications, and antiphospholipid antibodies (APA) [21]. Potential mechanism(s) by which APA induce arterial and venous thrombosis as well as adverse pregnancy outcomes include APA-mediated impairment of endothelial thrombomodulin and APC-mediated anticoagulation, induction of endothelial tissue factor expression, impairment of fibrinolysis and antithrombin activity, augmented platelet activation and/or adhesion, impairment of the anticoagulant effects of the anionic phospholipid binding proteins β2-glycoprotein-1 and annexin V. APA induction of complement activation has been suggested to play a role in fetal loss, with heparin preventing such aberrant activation.

Venous thrombotic events associated with APA include DVT with or without acute PE. The most common arterial events include cerebral vascular accidents and transient ischemic attacks. Anticardiolipin antibodies are associated with an OR of 2.17 (95% CI 1.51—3.11; 14 studies) for any thrombosis, 2.50 (95% CI 1.51–4.14) for DVT and PE, and 3.91 (95% CI 1.14–13.38) for recurrent VTE. Patients with systemic lupus erythematosus and lupus anticoagulants are at a sixfold greater risk of VTE compared with systemic lupus erythematosus patients without lupus anticoagulants, and systemic lupus erythematosus patients with anticardiolipin antibodies have a twofold greater risk of VTE compared with systemic lupus erythematosus patients without these antibodies. The lifetime prevalence of arterial or venous thrombosis in affected patients with APA is about 30%, with an event rate of 1% per year. These antibodies are present in up to 20% of individuals with VTE. A review of 25 prospective, cohort, and case-control studies involving more than 7000 patients observed an OR range for arterial and venous thromboses in patients with lupus anticoagulants of 8.65–10.84 and 4.09–16.2, respectively, and 1.0–18.0 and 1.0–2.51 for anticardiolipin antibodies [22].

There is a 5% risk of VTE during pregnancy and the puerperium among patients with APA despite treatment. Recurrence risks of up to 30% have been reported in APA-positive patients with a prior VTE; thus, long-term prophylaxis is required in patients with APS and a prior VTE. A severe form of APS is termed catastrophic APS, or CAPS, which is defined as a potentially life-threatening variant with multiple vessel thromboses leading to multiorgan failure.

APA-related thrombosis can occur in any tissue or organ except superficial veins, and accepted associated obstetric complications include at least one fetal death at or beyond the 10th week of gestation, or at least one premature birth at or before the 34th week, or at least three consecutive spontaneous abortions before the 10th week. All other causes of pregnancy morbidity must be excluded. APAs must be present on two or more occasions at least 12 weeks apart. A positive test occurs with detection of IgG and/or IgM of one of three APAs. Positive test results are as follows: anticardiolipin antibodies IgG or IgM greater than 40 GPL (1 GPL unit is 1 μg of IgG antibody) or 40 MPL (1 MPL unit is 1 μg of IgM antibody) or greater than the 99th percentile), anti–β-2 glycoprotein-I (IgG or IgM greater than the 99th percentile), or lupus anticoagulant. APAs are detected by screening for antibodies that: directly bind these protein epitopes (e.g. anti-β2-glycoprotein-1, prothrombin, annexin V, activated protein C, protein S, protein Z, Z protein Inhibitor, high- and low-molecular-weight kininogens, tissue plasminogen activator, factors VIIa and XII, the complement cascade constituents, C4 and CH, and oxidized low-density lipoprotein antibodies); or are bound to proteins present in an anionic phospholipid matrix (e.g. anticardiolipin and phosphatidylserine antibodies); or exert downstream effects on prothrombin activation in a phospholipid milieu (i.e. lupus anticoagulants).

Management considerations in patients with inherited or acquired thrombophilia

Inherited thrombophilia

As noted, among pregnant patients who have had a previous VTE, recurrence risks are highly dependent on the presence of a thrombophilia and the nature of the risk factors associated with the prior thrombus. See Table 14.3 for summary recommendations. Whereas VTE recurrences were not observed in women without detectable thrombophilias whose VTE was associated with a temporary risk factor, 5.9% of thrombophilic patients who did not receive thromboprophylaxis during pregnancy had

an antepartum recurrence of VTE. The Thrombophilia in Pregnancy Prophylaxis Study (TIPPS) trial results reported that antepartum prophylactic dalteparin did not reduce occurrence of VTE in high-risk settings or improve pregnancy outcomes.

The largest, prospective, randomized controlled trials have failed to demonstrate a benefit of anticoagulation therapy to improve pregnancy outcomes in the presence or absence of common inherited thrombophilia. Those patients with highly thrombogenic thrombophilias (e.g. antithrombin deficiency, homozygosity or joint heterozygosity for the FVL or PGM mutations) should receive both postpartum anticoagulation and therapeutic or subtherapeutic dosages of low molecular weight heparin (LMWH) throughout pregnancy. However, such therapy is not justified during the antepartum period in patients with less thrombogenic thrombophilias (e.g. heterozygosity for FVL or PGM, protein C deficiency, protein S deficiency) who are without a personal or strong family history of VTE.

Patients with new-onset VTE during pregnancy should receive therapeutic anticoagulation for a minimum of 3–6 months, depending on the clinical scenario, and including at least the first 6 weeks after delivery [23,24]. During pregnancy, either LMWH or unfractionated heparin (UFH) is a suitable anticoagulant, given their similar efficacy and safety profiles. Neither formulation crosses the placenta nor poses teratogenic risks. After delivery, oral anticoagulation with warfarin may be started and is considered safe in breastfeeding mothers. The primary risks of long-term heparin therapy in pregnancy are hemorrhage and osteoporosis. Although direct oral anticoagulants (DOACs) have largely replaced warfarin in the nonpregnant setting, DOACs are not recommended in pregnancy given limited data and concern for deleterious fetal effects.

Patients with AT deficiency represent the highest thrombogenic risk among inherited thrombophilias. Patients with hereditary AT deficiency and especially those with a prior thrombotic history or strong family of thrombosis are likely to benefit from receiving a plasma-derived or recombinant AT during periods of highest thromboembolic risk, namely delivery or surgery, when anticoagulation cannot be administered due to the risk of bleeding. The baseline AT level is expressed as the percentage of the normal level based on the functional AT III assay. The goal is to increase the AT levels to those found in normal human plasma (around 100%). These patients require a multidisciplinary approach to care, including participation from transfusion medicine, laboratory medicine, anesthesia, hematology, pediatric hematology, and maternal–fetal medicine [25].

Antiphospholipid antibody syndrome

Multiple randomized (not placebo controlled) studies have examined the effect of treatment of women with APSs with aspirin, heparin, or both. These studies,

Table 14.3 Anticoagulation considerations in pregnancy: indications, dosing, timing

Indication	Description	Antepartum	Postpartum
VTE in current pregnancy		Therapeutic LMWH/UFH from diagnosis until delivery	Therapeutic LMWH or UFH for at least 6 wk postpartum, depending on timing of VTE in pregnancy. Oral AC may be an option.
High-risk thrombophilia • FVL homozygous • PGM homozygous • FVL/PGM double heterozygous • Antithrombin deficiency	History of one prior VTE (not on long term AC)	Prophylactic or intermediate dose or therapeutic LMWH/UFH	Prophylactic AC or intermediate or therapeutic dose LMWH/UFH for 6 wk (therapy level should be equal to antepartum treatment)
	No history of VTE	Prophylactic or intermediate dose LMWH/UFH	Antenatal and 6-wk postpartum prophylactic AC or intermediate-dose LMWH/UFH
Low-risk thrombophilia • FVL heterozygous • PGM heterozygous • Protein C deficiency • Protein S deficiency	History of one prior VTE (not on long term AC)	Prophylactic or intermediate dose or therapeutic LMWH/UFH	Prophylactic or intermediate dose or therapeutic LMWH/UFH
	No history of VTE	Surveillance without AC	Surveillance without AC OR antenatal and 6-wk postpartum prophylactic AC if patient has additional risk factors
No thrombophilia	History of one prior VTE (pregnancy or estrogen related)	Prophylactic or intermediate dose or therapeutic LMWH/UFH	Therapeutic LMWH/UFH for at least 6 wk postpartum, longer duration may be indicated depending upon clinical scenario
	History of one prior VTE (specific event, nonestrogen related)	Surveillance without AC	Surveillance without AC or prophylactic LMWH if patient has additional risk factors
Two or more prior VTE episodes (thrombophilia or no thrombophilia)	On long-term AC	Therapeutic LMWH/UFH	Resumption of long-term AC. Oral AC may be considered depending upon the clinical scenario.
	Not on long-term AC	Intermediate dose or therapeutic dose LMWH/UFH	AC therapy with intermediate dose or therapeutic LMWH/UFH for 6 wk (therapy level should be equal to antepartum treatment)

Adapted from [4]. AC, anticoagulation; FVL, factor V Leiden; LMWH/UFH, low molecular weight heparin/unfractionated heparin; PGM, prothrombin mutation; PS, protein S; VTE, venous thromboembolism.

small and with heterogeneous criteria, generally have demonstrated an advantage of aspirin and heparin over either aspirin or heparin alone. However, one randomized trial found no benefit of LMWH and aspirin compared to aspirin alone; almost 80% of women in both arms had successful pregnancies. For women who fulfill laboratory and clinical criteria for APS, antepartum prophylactic-or intermediate-dose UFH or prophylactic LMWH combined with low-dose aspirin, 75 to 100 mg daily, is recommended but aspirin alone is an option until further data comparing LMWH plus aspirin vs. aspirin alone are available [26–28]. For patients with thrombotic events associated with APS, see Table 14.2 for anticoagulation management recommendations. Other potential treatment modalities that have been explored include hydroxychloroquine, as well as plasma exchange and pravastatin for difficult APS

cases, but more data are needed. A tumor necrosis factor blocking agent is also being evaluated as a treatment option for APS. In addition to routine obstetric management, inherited thrombophilias and APS require a tailored approach to maternal and fetal surveillance, the latter consisting of tests for fetal well-being and ultrasound assessment of fetal growth and optimizing time and mode of delivery.

Summary

Inherited and acquired thrombophilic conditions are a heterogenous group of disorders that require tailored approaches to screening, especially considering personal, familial, and obstetric history; prevention and treatment strategies; and obstetrical management.

CASE PRESENTATION

A 35-year-old gravida 2 para 1 (G2 P1001) patient presents at 7 weeks gestation for prenatal care. Her past medical history is significant for a pulmonary embolism at 19 years old in setting of initiating a combined oral contraceptive. She received 6 months of anticoagulation and then remained off anticoagulation. Two months following discontinuation of anticoagulation, and in the first half of her menstrual cycle, she underwent inherited and acquired thrombophilia evaluation, consisting of both genetic and functional screening. Factor V Leiden heterozygosity was identified. At 31 years old, she became pregnant and was given prophylactic anticoagulation antepartum with subcutaneous enoxaparin 40 mg daily. At 35 weeks gestation, she was converted to prophylactic subcutaneous unfractionated heparin 10 000 units twice daily until delivery. She also was diagnosed with chronic hypertension at her first prenatal visit, requiring labetalol 100 mg orally twice daily. She was induced at 39 weeks gestation and developed superimposed preeclampsia with severe features. She was delivered a healthy boy, birthweight 3200 g, Apgars 9 and 9, by primary low transverse Cesarean delivery due to arrest of dilation at 7 cm. Postpartum, she was started on subcutaneous enoxaparin 40 mg daily for 6 weeks. For contraception, a progestin-only intrauterine device was placed at her 6-week postpartum visit and was removed 2½ years later. The patient breastfed for 6 months. In her second pregnancy, in addition to her history of chronic hypertension requiring labetalol 100 mg twice daily, FVL, and previous cesarean delivery, she was diagnosed with an increased body mass index (36 kg/m2). The patient was again given prophylactic anticoagulation antepartum with subcutaneous enoxaparin 40 mg daily. At 12 weeks gestation, low dose aspirin for preeclampsia prevention was initiated. At 35 weeks gestation, she was converted to prophylactic subcutaneous unfractionated heparin 10 000 units twice daily until delivery. The patient declined a trial of labor and elected repeat cesarean delivery, which was performed uneventfully at 39 weeks gestation along with a bilateral tubal ligation for desired sterility. She delivered a healthy baby girl, 3500 g, Apgars 9 and 9. The patient had an uneventful postpartum course. She received subcutaneous enoxaparin 40 mg daily for 6 weeks postpartum and the anticoagulation was then discontinued. The patient breastfed for 8 months. The patient followed up with her internal medicine physician 2 months postpartum to manage her chronic hypertension long term, and her hematologist as needed.

References

1. American College of Obstetricians and Gynecologists' Committee on Practice Bulletins–Obstetrics. ACOG Practice Bulletin No. 197: inherited thrombophilias in pregnancy. Obstet Gynecol. 2018;132(1):e18–34.

2. American College of Obstetricians and Gynecologists' Committee on Practice Bulletins–Obstetrics. ACOG Practice Bulletin no. 196: thromboembolism in pregnancy. Obstet Gynecol. 2018;132:e1–e17.

3. Bourjeily G, Paidas MJ, Khalil H, Rosene-Montella K, Rodger M. Pulmonary embolism in pregnancy. Lancet. 2010 Feb 6;375(9713):500–12.

4. Kouides PA, Paidas M. Consultative hematology II: women's health issues. In: Cuker A, Altman JK, Gerds AT, Wun T, editors. American Society of Hematology self-assessment program. 7th ed. Washington, DC: American Society of Hematology; 2019. p.61–95.

5. Nelson-Piercy C, MacCallum P, Mackillop L. Reducing the risk of thrombosis and embolism during pregnancy and the puerperium (Green-top guideline no. 37a). London: Royal College of Obstetricians and Gynaecologists; 2015.

6. Ozimek JA, Kilpatrick SJ. Maternal mortality in the twenty first century. Obstet Gynecol Clin N Am. 2018;45:175–86.

7. van der Pol LM, Tromeur C, Bistervels IM, Ni Ainle F, van Bemmel T, Bertoletti L, Couturaud F, et al. Pregnancy-adapted YEARS algorithm for diagnosis of suspected pulmonary embolism. N Engl J Med. 2019 Mar 21;380(12):1139–49.

8. Virkus RA, Løkkegaard EC, Bergholt T, Mogensen U, Langhoff-Roos J, Lidegaard Ø. Venous thromboembolism in pregnant and puerperal women in Denmark 1995–2005. A national cohort study. Thromb Haemost. 2011 Aug;106(2):304–9.

9. Robertson L, Wu O, Langhorne P, Twaddle S, Clark P, Lowe G, et al. Thrombophilia in pregnancy: a systematic review. Br J Haematol. 2006;132(2):171–96.

10. Rodger MA, Betancourt MT, Clark P, Lindqvist PG, Dizon-Townson D, Said J, et al. The association of factor V Leiden and prothrombin gene mutation and placenta-mediated pregnancy complications: a systematic review and meta-analysis of prospective cohort studies. PLoS Med. 2010;7(6):728.

11. Petersen EE, Davis NL, Goodman D, Cox S, Mayes N, Johnston E, et al. Vital signs: pregnancy-related deaths, United States, 2011 2015, and strategies for prevention, 13 states, 2013–2017. MMWR Morb Mortal Wkly Rep. 2019 May 10;68(18):423–9.

12. Alfirevic Z, Roberts D, Martlew V. How strong is the association between maternal thrombophilia and adverse pregnancy outcome?: a systematic review. Eur J Obstet Gynecol Reprod Biol. 2002;101(1):6–14.

13. Preston FE, Rosendaal FR, Walker ID, Briet E, Berntorp E, Conard J, et al. Increased fetal loss in women with heritable thrombophilia. Lancet. 1996;348(9032):913–16.

14. Rey E, Kahn SR, David M, Shrier I. Thrombophilic disorders and fetal loss: a meta-analysis. Lancet. 2003;361(9361):901–8.

15. Roqué H, Paidas MJ, Funai EF, Kuczynski E, Lockwood CJ. Maternal thrombophilias are not associated with early pregnancy loss. Thromb Haemost. 2004;91(2):290–5.

16. Lykke J, Bare L, Olsen J, Lagier R, Arellano A, Tong C, et al. Thrombophilias and adverse pregnancy outcomes: results from the Danish National Birth Cohort. J Thromb Haemost. 2012;10(7):1320–5.

17. Silver RM, Zhao Y, Spong CY, Sibai B, Wendel G Jr, Wenstrom K et al. Prothrombin gene G20210A mutation and obstetric complications. Obstet Gynecol. 2010;115(1):14–20.

18. Paidas M, Ku DH, Lee MJ, Manish S, Thurston A, Lockwood C, Arkel Y. Protein Z, protein S levels are lower in patients with thrombophilia and subsequent pregnancy complications. J Thromb Haemost. 2005;3(3):497–501.

19. Conard J, Horellou M, Van Dreden P, Lecompte T, Samama M. Thrombosis and pregnancy in congenital deficiencies in AT III, protein C or protein S: study of 78 women. Thromb Haemost. 1990;63(2):319–20.

20. Ornaghi S, Mueller M, Barnea ER, Paidas MJ. Thrombosis during pregnancy: Risks, prevention, and treatment for mother and fetus–harvesting the power of omic technology, biomarkers and in vitro or in vivo models to facilitate the treatment of thrombosis. Birth Defects Res C Embryo Today Rev. 2015;105(3): 209–25.

21. Paidas MJ, Tita ATN, Macones GA, Saade GA, Ehrenkranz RA, Triche EW, et al. Prospective, randomized, double-blind, placebo-controlled evaluation of the pharmacokinetics, safety and efficacy of recombinant antithrombin versus placebo in preterm preeclampsia. Am J Obstet Gynecol. 2020 Nov;223(5): 739.e1–13.

22. Pritchard AM, Hendrix PW, Paidas MJ. Hereditary thrombophilia and recurrent pregnancy loss. Clin Obstet Gynecol. 2016 Sep;59(3):487–97.

23. James AH, Bates SM, Bauer KA, Branch W, Mann K, Paidas M, et al. Management of hereditary antithrombin deficiency in pregnancy. Thromb Res. 2017 Sep;157:41–5.

24. Miyakis S, Lockshin MD, Atsumi T, Branch DW, Brey RL, Cervera R, et al. International consensus statement on an update of the classification criteria for definite antiphospholipid syndrome (APS). J Thromb Haemost. 2006;4(2):295–306.

25. Galli M, Lucian D, Bertolini G, Barbui T. Anti-beta 2-glycoprotein I, antiprothrombin antibodies, and the risk of thrombosis in the antiphospholipid syndrome. Blood. 2003;102:2717–23.

26. Bates SM, Rajasekhar A, Middeldorp S, McLintock C, Rodger MA, James AH, et al. American Society of Hematology 2018 guidelines for management of venous thromboembolism: venous thromboembolism in the context of pregnancy. Blood Adv. 2018 Nov 27;2(22):3317–59.

27. Empson M, Lassere M, Craig J, Scott J. Prevention of recurrent miscarriage for women with antiphospholipid antibody or lupus anticoagulant. Cochrane Database Syst Rev. 2005 Apr 18;2005(2):CD002859. doi: 10.1002/14651858.CD002859.pub2.

28. Guerby P, Fillion A, O'Connor S, Bujold E. Heparin for preventing adverse obstetrical outcomes in pregnant women with antiphospholipid syndrome, a systematic review and meta-analysis. J Gynecol Obstet Hum Reprod. 2021 Feb;50(2):101974.

Chapter 15
Thromboembolic Disorders

Audrey A. Merriam and Christian M. Pettker

Department of Obstetrics, Gynecology and Reproductive Sciences, Yale University School of Medicine, New Haven, CT, USA

Complicating 1 in 1500 pregnancies, venous thromboembolism (VTE) is a leading cause of maternal morbidity and mortality [1–9]. Moreover, despite this seemingly low prevalence, pregnancy confers a nearly 6–10-fold increased risk of VTE in women of comparable childbearing age. In one large retrospective cohort study, 94 of 127 (74.8%) pregnant women with documented deep venous thrombosis (DVT) developed their clot during the antepartum period, with half detected before 15 weeks and fewer than 30% diagnosed after 20 weeks [10]. In contrast, most cases of pulmonary embolism (PE) developed during the postpartum period (23 of 38; 60.5%) and PE was strongly associated with cesarean delivery. However, the per diem risk of VTE is approximately threefold to eightfold higher in the puerperium than during an equivalent antepartum interval [9]. Pulmonary embolism is a leading cause of maternal mortality in the United States, contributing to 9.6% of such deaths [11]. An untreated DVT presents a 25% risk of PE, with a mortality rate of approximately 15% if undetected and untreated [12]. On the other hand, if a DVT is promptly diagnosed and treated, the risk of PE is less than 5% and the risk of maternal mortality is less than 1% [13].

The increased risk of pregnancy-associated VTE reflects local and systemic mechanisms that mitigate the risk of hemorrhage during placentation and the third stage of labor. Appreciation of the thrombotic risk of pregnancy demands knowledge of the sophisticated systems of coagulation and fibrinolysis and their inhibitors.

Physiology of hemostasis

Platelet plug formation

Vasoconstriction and platelet aggregation are the initial constraints on hemorrhage following vascular disruption, particularly in arteries. Vasoconstriction limits total blood flow to promote platelet plug formation. It also limits the size of the plug required to obstruct blood flow through the vascular defect. Platelet adhesion is initially mediated through von Willebrand factor (vWF), which is synthesized by megakaryocytes and endothelial cells. It is constitutively secreted but the most active forms are stored in endothelial Weibel-Palade bodies or platelet α-granules where the molecule is released upon activation [14]. Upon vascular wall disruption and after binding to subendothelial collagen, vWF undergoes a conformational change. This change permits it to also bind to the platelet glycoprotein (GP) Ib/IX/V receptor to establish a hemostatic bridge between collagen in the damaged vessel wall and the platelet. The resultant GPIb/IX/V-vWF-collagen interaction facilitates platelet adhesion in the high-flow (shear stress) state induced by vasoconstriction. A second platelet–collagen interaction is mediated by the binding of collagen I and IV to the platelet GPIa/IIa (integrin α2β1) receptor in the low-flow settings created by the expanding platelet plug.

Following collagen-mediated attachment, a second platelet receptor, GPIIb/IIIa (integrin α-IIb/β-3), is now positioned to serve as an alternative extracellular matrix adhering site on platelet cell membranes, permitting attachment to subendothelial laminin, thrombospondin, fibronectin, vitronectin, and possibly also vWF. Moreover, GPIIb/IIIa-mediated platelet adhesion then triggers calcium-dependent protein kinase C (PKC) activation that induces thromboxane A_2 (TXA$_2$) synthesis and platelet granule release. Beside vWF, platelet α-granules also contain various other clotting factors while densegranules contain adenosine diphosphate (ADP) and serotonin, which combine with TXA$_2$ to potentiate vasoconstriction and further promote platelet activation. Platelets can also be activated by thrombin, epinephrine, arachidonic acid, and platelet-activating factor. Platelet activation, in turn, releases more platelet surface GPIIb/IIIa receptors that promote aggregation by forming interplatelet fibrinogen, fibronectin, and vitronectin bridges [15]. Platelet aggregation in the setting of intact endothelium is prevented by active blood flow and prostacyclin, nitric oxide, and ADPase.

Queenan's Management of High-Risk Pregnancy: An Evidence-Based Approach, Seventh Edition. Edited by Catherine Y. Spong and Charles J. Lockwood.

During the platelet activation process, anionic (negatively charged) phospholipids are exteriorized on the cell membrane, creating an ideal clotting surface (discussed later). Platelet and endothelial cell activation also induces release of P-selectins from platelet α-granules and endothelial Weibel-Palade bodies that embed in the cell walls to further promote platelet and enhance monocyte adherence. P-selectin binding also induces expression of the potent procoagulant, tissue factor (TF), on monocytes to further enhance clotting (discussed later). These steps underscore the critical role played by platelets, monocytes, and endothelial cells in promoting the classic coagulation cascade.

The coagulation cascade

Platelet plug aggregation in the absence of fibrin generation is inadequate to control the hemorrhage following significant vascular injury. Thus, adequate hemostasis also requires fibrin plug formation which follows exposure of circulating factor VII to perivascular TF (Figure 15.1). The TF molecule is a cell membrane-bound glycoprotein, constitutively expressed by most nonendothelial extravascular cells and present in the blood in an encrypted (nonclotting) form [16]. This distribution reduces the likelihood of inappropriate activation of the clotting cascade in physiologic states, though obstetric sepsis can induce TF expression on monocytes and endothelial cells to generate thrombosis and disseminated intravascular coagulation (DIC) [16]. It is also highly induced by progesterone in perivascular decidualized endometrial stromal cells, first-trimester decidual cells, and term decidual cells where it is positioned to promote perinatal hemostasis [17].

The high levels of TF in the decidua also account for the intense thrombin generation and DIC accompanying decidual hemorrhage (i.e. abruption) [18]. It is also present in high levels in the amniotic fluid, perhaps accounting for the coagulopathy observed in amniotic fluid embolism [19]. Following vascular injury, perivascular TF binds circulating factor VII which attaches to negatively charged phospholipids via divalent calcium ions. Factor VII is autoactivated after binding to TF and can be externally activated by thrombin, factors IXa, Xa, or XIIa [20]. (The activated form of clotting factors is denoted by the letter "a" after the Roman numeral.) The TF/VIIa complex can directly activate factor X (see Figure 15.1) or indirectly activate Xa by activating factor IX (IXa), which then complexes with its co-factor, VIIIa, to activate factor X. In either case, factor Xa next complexes with its co-factor, Va, to convert prothrombin (factor II) to thrombin (factor IIa), which converts fibrinogen to fibrin and activates platelets. The co-factors V and VIII are activated by either thrombin or factor Xa. Thrombin, kallikrein-kininogen, and plasmin can each activate factor XII on the surface of platelets (see Figure 15.1). Factor XIIa can activate factor XI, providing another route of factor IX activation. All of these reactions occur on negatively charged phospholipids and require ionized calcium. Ultimately, thrombin cleaves fibrinogen to fibrin monomers which self-polymerize and are cross-linked via thrombin-activated factor XIIIa.

Endogenous anticoagulants

There is evidence that the clotting system "idles" (i.e. is active at a low level) to optimize the immediate response to vascular injury [20]. This chronic basal level of thrombin activation underscores the critical role of the endogenous anticoagulant system in preventing thrombosis (see Figure 15.1). The TF pathway inhibitor (TFPI) is the first agent in this system and acts on the factor Xa/TF/VIIa

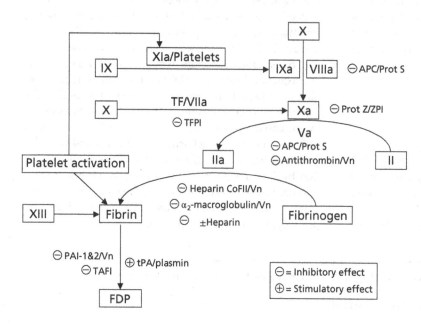

Figure 15.1 An outline of the mechanisms defining the careful balance of thrombosis and hemostasis vs. anticoagulation and fibrinolysis. APC, activated protein C; FDP, fibrin degradation products; PAI-1, plasminogen activator inhibitor 1; TAFI, thrombin activatable fibrinolysis inhibitor; TF, tissue factor; TFPI, tissue factor pathway inhibitor; tPA, tissue-type plasminogen activator; Vn, vitronectin; ZPI, protein Z-dependent protease inhibitor.

complex to inhibit TF-mediated clotting. The TFPI molecule is synthesized by endothelial cells and uses protein S as a co-factor [21]. Most TFPI (80%) is associated with the vessel wall, while the remainder circulates in plasma at a concentration of approximately 2.5 nM. However, factor XIa can bypass this TFPI-induced coagulation block and sustain clotting on the surface of activated platelets for some time. As a result, additional endogenous anticoagulant molecules are required to avoid thrombosis, including activated protein C, protein S, and protein Z.

Thrombin binds thrombomodulin on perturbed endothelial cell membranes, producing a conformational change that allows activation of protein C [22]. Activated protein C (APC) binds to anionic endothelial cell membrane phospholipids or to the endothelial cell protein C receptor (EPCR) to inactivate factors Va and VIIIa [23]. In addition to its potentiation role in the TFPI pathway, protein S also serves as a co-factor for both Va and VIIIa inactivation by APC. More than half of the total protein S exists in a high-affinity complex with C4b-binding protein, with the remainder circulating freely [24]. Protein Z-dependent protease inhibitor (ZPI) can also impede factor Xa activity. When bound to its co-factor, protein Z, the inhibitory activity of ZPI, is increased 1000-fold [25].

Serine protease inhibitors (SERPINs), which include heparin co-factor II, α2-macroglobulin and antithrombin, account for most of the thrombin inhibitory activity of plasma (see Figure 15.1). Antithrombin alone accounts for 80% of plasma antithrombin activity and also inactivates factors IXa, Xa, and XIa [26]. Heparins and circulating vitronectin bind to SERPINs and together augment anticoagulant activity 1000-fold [27,28].

Fibrinolysis

Fibrinolysis is initiated by tissue-type plasminogen activator (tPA), embedded in fibrin, which cleaves plasminogen to generate plasmin. Plasmin, in turn, cleaves fibrin into fibrin degradation products (FDPs), which are often used clinically as indirect measures of fibrinolysis. These FDPs can also inhibit thrombin action, a salutary result when limited but when generated in excess can contribute to DIC. Inhibitors of fibrinolysis include α2-plasmin inhibitor and type 1 and 2 plasminogen activator inhibitors (PAI-1 and PAI-2) which inactivate tPA. The endothelium and uterine decidua are primary sources of PAI-1 while the placenta produces PAI-2 [29,30]. The thrombin activatable fibrinolysis inhibitor (TAFI) modifies fibrin by cleaving carboxy-terminal lysine (Lys) residues from partially degraded fibrin. This in turn blocks tPa-mediated cleavage of plasminogen by preventing the formation of the tPA/plasminogen/fibrin complex. Thus, TAFI renders fibrin resistant to inactivation by plasmin [31]. Like activation of protein C, activation of TAFI by thrombin is greatly enhance by thrombin binding to thrombomodulin.

Pathophysiology of and risk factors for thrombosis in pregnancy

Risk factors for thrombosis not unique to pregnancy include age over 35 years, obesity (body mass index ≥30kg/m²), paralysis, infection, smoking, nephrotic syndrome, hyperviscosity syndromes, malignancies, trauma, surgery, orthopedic procedures, and a prior history of VTE [32]. There are also severe pregnancy-specific nonreversible and reversible risk factors that increase VTE risk. The nonreversible risk-factors include increased parity, multiple gestation, preeclampsia, postpartum endomyometritis, postpartum hemorrhage requiring transfusion, operative vaginal delivery and cesarean delivery [33,34]. Emergent cesarean delivery increases the risk of VTE even further than the fourfold increase in VTE risk associated with nonemergent cesarean deliveries [35]. Pregnancy-associated reversible risk factors include ovarian hyperstimulation syndrome, immobility, long distance travel (>4–6 hours), hyperemesis associated with dehydration, and hospital stay [34]. The risk for VTE persists for up to 28 days after a hospital stay during pregnancy [36].

All three components of Virchow's triad – vascular stasis, hypercoagulability, and vascular injury – are present in pregnancy. Stasis results from increases in deep vein capacitance secondary to increased circulating levels of estrogen and endothelial production of prostacyclin and nitric oxide, coupled with compression of the inferior vena cava and pelvic veins by the enlarging uterus [37–38]. Interestingly, over 85% of DVT cases in pregnancy are left-sided, likely due to compression of the left iliac vein by the right iliac artery and the gravid uterus [10,39].

Pregnancy-associated hypercoagulability results from changes in decidual and systemic hemostatic factors that likely meet the hemorrhagic challenges posed by vascular injury occurring in implantation, placentation, the third stage of labor, and particularly cesarean delivery. Decidual TF and PAI-1 expression is increased in response to progesterone, and levels of placental PAI-2, which are negligible prior to pregnancy, increase until term [17,29,30]. By term, circulating levels of fibrinogen double and levels of factors VII, VIII, IX, X, XII, and vWF increase 20–1000% [40,41]. Additionally, levels of free protein S antigen and activity decrease by approximately 40% due to hormonal induction of C4b-binding protein, conferring overall resistance to APC [42]. Further reductions in free protein S concentrations are seen after cesarean delivery and in the context of infection, both of which augment C4b-binding protein levels, helping to explain the ninefold higher incidence of VTE after cesarean compared with vaginal delivery and why 80% of fatal PE episodes in pregnancy follow cesarean delivery [43,44]. In general, normalization of these coagulation parameters occurs by 6 weeks postpartum. Although these mechanisms generally prevent puerperal hemorrhage, they predispose to thrombosis, a tendency aggravated by maternal thrombophilias.

Diagnosis of venous thromboembolism

Deep venous thrombosis

Clinical presentation

Typical clinical findings seen in the presence of a DVT are nonspecific and include erythema, warmth, pain, edema, localized tenderness and, occasionally, a palpable cord. Homan's sign–pain and tenderness with dorsiflexion of the foot or compression of the calf muscles with palpation. Chan and colleagues conducted a cross-sectional study over 7 years at five university-affiliated, tertiary care centers in Canada of 194 pregnant women with suspected DVT [45]. The prevalence of the disorder was 8.8% and the three most predictive clinical variables were left leg symptoms (adjusted odds ratio [aOR] 44.3, 95% confidence interval [CI] 3.2–609.7), calf circumference difference of 2 cm or more (adjusted OR 26.9, 95% CI 6.1–118.5), and onset of presentation in the first trimester (aOR 53.4, 95% CI 7.1–401). Among patients with a subsequently confirmed DVT, all had at least one variable, and 82.4% had two variables. Among patients without a confirmed DVT, half had no variables and only 5.7% had two or more variables. None of the pregnant patients with suspected DVT who failed to manifest any of the three variables had subsequent documentation of a DVT. When one or more variables were present, DVT was diagnosed in 16.4% and when two or three variables were present, DVT was diagnosed in 58.3% of cases (95% CI 35.8–75.5%). However, other studies have shown that in the presence of clinical symptoms DVT is only confirmed with objective testing in about 30% of patients [46,47].

Laboratory assays

D-dimer assays, which measures the product of the degradation of fibrin by plasmin, are useful in the nonpregnant population as a screening tool for DVT. The most accurate and reliable tests being two rapid enzyme-linked immunosorbent assays (ELISAs) (Instant-IA D-dimer, Stago, Asniéres, France and VIDAS DD, bioMérieux, Marcy-l'Etoile, France) and a rapid whole-blood assay (SimpliRED D-dimer, Agen Biomedical, Brisbane, Australia). The D-dimer assay is limited in pregnancy due to the physiologic increase in D-dimer seen in pregnancy. These levels are greater than the threshold for normal in 78% of women in the second trimester and 100% of women in the third trimester [48].

Chan and associates evaluated the sensitivity and specificity of D-dimer measurements using the SimpliRED assay for diagnosing DVT in 149 at-risk pregnant women [49]. They tested whole blood for D-dimer elevations at initial presentation, and the results were correlated with compression venous ultrasonography (VUS). The prevalence of DVT was 8.7% and the sensitivity of the D-dimer assay was 100% (95% CI 77–100%); however, the specificity was 60% (95% CI 52–68%). Of note, pregnancy itself is associated with progressive elevations in D-dimer generation. Chan et al. noted that the SimpliRED assay was "falsely" positive in 0% (95% CI 0–60%), 24% (95% CI 14–37%), and 51% (95% CI 40–61%) of women in the first, second, and third trimesters, respectively.

Given the lack of specificity of D-dimer assays for evaluating women with suspected DVT in pregnancy other laboratory studies have been evaluated including B-type naturietic peptide, C-reactive protein, plasmin-antiplasmin complexes and soluble tissue factor. Unfortunately, none of these other laboratory assays have been found to have clinically useful positive or negative predictive values when screening pregnant women for VTE [50].

Venous imaging

Intravenous contrast venography is the gold standard for DVT diagnosis but is no longer used for the diagnosis of DVT in pregnancy since it has no greater diagnostic efficacy than VUS and is associated with appreciable radiation exposure (Table 15.1). Compression venous ultrasonography with or without color Doppler has emerged as the preferred initial imaging modality. It requires sonographic imaging of the common femoral vein at the inguinal ligament, and then assessment of the other major venous systems of the leg, including the greater saphenous, the superficial femoral, and the popliteal veins to the deep veins of the calf. Pressure is applied to the transducer to determine the compressibility of the vein lumen under duplex and color flow Doppler imaging [51]. Noncompressibility of the venous lumen in a transverse plan with gentle pressure from the ultrasound probe using duplex and color flow Doppler imaging would be

Table 15.1 Fetal radiation exposure of various ionizing modalities

Radiological modality	Fetal radiation exposure (rad)
Chest X-ray	0.01
Venography	
Limited, shielded	0.05
Full (unilateral), unshielded	0.31
Pulmonary angiography	
Brachial vein	0.05
Femoral vein	0.22–0.37
V/Q scan	
Ventilation scan	0.001–0.019
Perfusion scan	0.006–0.012
CTPA	0.013

CTPA, computed tomography pulmonary angiography; V/Q, ventilation/perfusion.
Adapted from Toglia and Weg [6].

diagnostic for a venous thrombosis [47]. The overall sensitivity and specificity of VUS approach 100% for proximal vein thromboses [52] with slightly less efficacy for detecting isolated calf vein DVT (sensitivity 92.5%, specificity 98.7%, and accuracy 97.2%) [53].

A meta-analysis of 14 studies comparing the efficacy of magnetic resonance imaging (MRI) venography with a reference standard in nonpregnant patients with suspected DVT showed a pooled sensitivity of 91.5% and a pooled specificity of 94.8%, with a higher sensitivity for proximal than distal DVT [54]. Thus, MRI has equivalent sensitivity and specificity to VUS for the diagnosis of DVT. It may, however, be useful for detecting iliofemoral/pelvic vein thromboses which are poorly visualized by VUS and account for 11% of DVT in pregnancy, compared with just 1% in the nonpregnant state [55].

Diagnostic algorithm for suspected deep venous thrombosis

Based on the available data, we propose the diagnostic algorithm in Figure 15.2 that allows the diagnosis of DVT with highest sensitivity and specificity. We suggest the initial use of VUS. If the patient has a VUS, the presence of a clinically significant DVT is remote and therapy is withheld. If such a patient is considered at very high risk because of a prior VTE, thrombophilia, the presence of all three characteristic clinical findings, consideration should be given to either repeating the evaluation in 3 and 7 days or carrying out MRI interrogation of the leg and pelvic veins. If the VUS or MRI is positive, initiate therapeutic anticoagulation with low molecular weight heparin.

Pulmonary embolus

Clinical presentation
Gherman and colleagues analyzed the presenting signs and symptoms of pregnant women with confirmed PE and observed that 62% had shortness of breath, 55.3% had pleuritic chest pain, 23.7% cough, 18.4% diaphoresis, 7.9% hemoptysis, and 5.3% syncope [10]. In a retrospective cohort study of 304 pregnant and puerperal women consecutively evaluated for the clinical suspicion of PE, the most common signs and symptoms were dyspnea (60%), followed by tachycardia (54%) and desaturation to less than 95% (40%) [56]. However, none of these variables was significantly associated with subsequent documentation of a PE (i.e. all relative risks were nonsignificant). Factors significantly linked to a diagnosed PE included chest pain (relative risk [RR] 1.7, 95% CI 1.1–2.6) and a PaO_2 less than 65 mmHg (RR 2.8, 95% CI 1.4–5.8), but neither was sufficiently predictive of PE to be useful clinically (positive likelihood ratios of <3). Presyncope and syncope are rare, although these symptoms may indicate a massive and potentially fatal PE [57].

Nonspecific studies
Nonspecific studies sometimes employed in the evaluation of patients with suspected PE include electrocardiogram (ECG), blood gases, oxygen saturation levels, chest X-ray (CXR), and echocardiography. An abnormal ECG is present in 70–90% of nonpregnant patients with proven PE who do not have underlying cardiopulmonary disease, but these findings are generally nonspecific [58,59]. The classic ECG changes associated with PE are S1, Q3, and inverted T3, but other findings such as atrial fibrillation, nonspecific

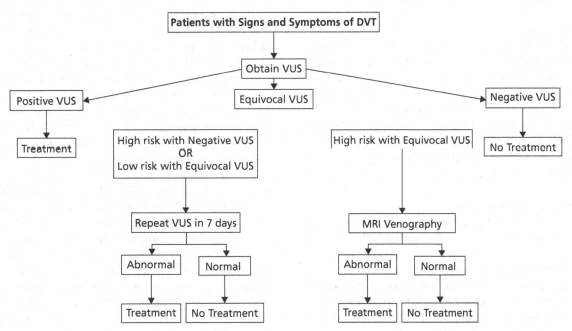

Figure 15.2 Diagnostic algorithm for the diagnosis of deep venous thrombosis in pregnant women. DVT, deep venous thrombosis; MRI, magnetic resonance imaging; VUS, venous ultrasonography.

ST changes, right bundle branch block, or right axis deviation may also be present. The latter two findings are usually associated with cor pulmonale and right heart strain or overload, reflective of more serious cardiopulmonary compromise. The Urokinase Pulmonary Embolism Trial found that 26–32% of patients with a massive PE had these ECG changes [58]. However, a lack of ECG changes should not reassure the physician when there is the clinical suspicion of PE. CXR findings commonly seen with PE include pleural effusion, pulmonary infiltrates, atelectasis and elevated hemidiaphragm. Traditional CXR findings of pulmonary infarction, such as a wedge-shaped infiltrate ("Hampton hump") or decreased vascularity ("Westermark sign"), are rare but up to 84% of patients can present with some degree of abnormal CXR findings [60,61]. The CXR may be valuable in ruling out other causes of hypoxemia, such as pulmonary edema or pneumonia. Thus, although a normal CXR in the setting of dyspnea, tachypnea, and hypoxemia in a patient without preexistent pulmonary or cardiovascular disease is suggestive of PE, a chest radiograph cannot confirm the diagnosis [60].

Large PE can create changes consistent with cor pulmonale and right heart strain, potentially identifiable on echocardiography. Abnormalities of right ventricular size or function on echocardiogram are seen in 30–80% of patients with PE although similar changes can be seen in exacerbations of chronic obstructive pulmonary disease [62–64]. Typical echocardiographic findings include a dilated and hypokinetic right ventricle or tricuspid regurgitation, in the absence of preexisting pulmonary arterial or left heart pathology. These findings indicate a large embolus and poor prognosis. Transesophageal echocardiography improves the sensitivity of diagnosing main or right pulmonary artery emboli [65].

D-dimer assays

Consistent with their limited utility in DVT assessment in pregnancy, D-dimer assays have limited utility in the evaluation of PE in pregnancy., There are reported false-negative D-dimer results in pregnant women with documented PE [66]. The sensitivity and specificity of D-dimer as a test for suspected PE in pregnancy were 73% and 15%, respectively [67]. Thus, D-dimer testing appears to be associated with an unacceptable false-negative rate in pregnancy and should not be used.

Pulmonary arteriography

Intravenous contrast pulmonary arteriography or angiography has been abandoned in the work-up of PE since it has a relative low sensitivity for smaller peripheral lesions [60,68,69], and is highly invasive, with a 0.5% mortality risk and a 3% complication rate, primarily as a result of the risks of contrast injection and catheter placement, including respiratory failure (0.4%), renal failure (0.3%), cardiac perforation (1%), and groin hematoma requiring transfusion (0.2%) [57,68,70].

Ventilation/perfusion scanning vs. spiral computed tomographic pulmonary angiography

Ventilation/perfusion scintigraphy (V/Q scan) involves comparative imaging of the pulmonary vascular bed and airspaces using intravenous and aerosolized radiolabeled markers [51]. The comparison of the resultant two images allows for differential diagnostic probabilities (high, intermediate, low, or normal). The Prospective Investigation of Pulmonary Embolism Diagnosis (PIO-PED) study evaluated the accuracy of V/Q scanning in nearly 1000 nonpregnant adults with suspected PE [58]. Overall, high-probability V/Q scans correlated with PE in 87.2% of cases; however, only 41% of patients with PE had high-probability scans, yielding a sensitivity of 41% and a specificity of 97%. However, in young healthy pregnant women, without severe asthma or chronic lung disease, the diagnostic accuracy of V/Q scanning is expected to be optimal.

Computed tomographic pulmonary angiography (CTPA) scanning uses intravenous contrast injection to visualize the pulmonary vasculature during scanning with highly sensitive multidetector-row CT technology [59]. Sensitivity of this testing is high for large vessel emboli, but more limited for small subsegmental vessels or vessels oriented horizontally (e.g. in the right middle lobe). Given its broad diagnostic capabilities, CT can be helpful in detecting nonembolic etiologies for the patient's signs and symptoms, such as pneumonia or pulmonary edema.

Comparisons of spiral CT with V/Q scanning for patients with suspected PE indicate that when the CXR is normal, V/Q scanning is more accurate. In a retrospective cohort study, Cahill and associates evaluated 304 consecutive women who were either pregnant or within 6 weeks postpartum, with a clinical suspicion of PE [55]. Of these, 108 (35.1%) underwent initial CTPA and 196 (64.9%) initial V/Q/ scanning. In the subgroup of women with a normal CXR, CTPA was five times more likely to produce a nondiagnostic result than V/Q scanning, even after adjusting for relevant confounding effects (30.0% compared with 5.6%; aOR 5.4, 95% CI 1.4–20.1). Even in patients with asthma with a normal chest radiograph V/Q scan and CTPA have similar nondiagnostic results [71]. In a smaller study, Ridge and associates compared the diagnostic accuracy of CTPA and V/Q scans in 28 and 25 pregnant patients with suspected PE, respectively [72]. They also found CTPA less reliable than V/Q scanning (inadequate diagnosis rate of 35.7% for CTPA vs. 4% for V/Q scans, P <0.001). The authors also compared the relative efficiency of CTPA in pregnant vs. nonpregnant women and noted that CTPA had a higher diagnostic inadequacy rate among pregnant compared with nonpregnant women (35.7% vs. 2.1%) (P <0.001). This was ascribed to more frequent interruption of contrast material by unopacified blood from the inferior vena cava in pregnancy, likely due to increased plasma volume.

Several other studies have also demonstrated that the quality of CTPA is lower in pregnancy. Andreou and colleagues compared contrast enhancement in 16 pregnant and 16 nonpregnant women and found significantly less pulmonary artery enhancement in the pregnancy group [73]. Similarly, U-King-Im and associates compared CTPA studies between 40 pregnant and 40 nonpregnant women and observed that pregnant women had more than triple the proportion of suboptimal studies (27.5% vs. 7.5%, $P = 0.015$) [74]. Similar findings were noted by Litmanovich and colleagues [75]. Taken together, these studies strongly indicate that VQ is the preferred test in pregnant women with suspected PE when the CXR is normal and that CTPA should be reserved for at-risk pregnant women with abnormal CXRs.

In addition to its higher diagnostic accuracy, V/Q scanning also results in substantially lower breast and lung irradiation. It has been estimated that CTPA exposes the mother's breasts to about 150 times more radiation than V/Q scans [44].

CTPA generates only slightly less fetal irradiation than V/Q scanning (see Table 15.1). Winer-Muram and associates calculated that the maximal fetal irradiation attributable to CTPA compared with V/Q scans was 131 μGy vs. 370 μGy [76]. To put this dose in perspective, in utero radiation exposures of up to 50 000 μGy result in negligible increased childhood cancer risk, and fetal doses resulting from both CTPA and V/Q scanning are substantially less than the fetus receives from background radiation (1150–2550 μGy) [77]. Given the diagnostic accuracy coupled with the radiation level concerns, V/Q scans are the modality of choice when evaluating pregnant patients with suspected PE and a normal CXR.

Magnetic resonance angiography

Magnetic resonance angiography (MRA) involves the use of IV contrast (gadolinium) during MRI. Meaney and colleagues assessed use of this modality in pregnancy and found a sensitivity of 100%, specificity of 95%, and positive and negative predictive values of 87% and 100%, respectively, when compared to use of pulmonary angiography [78]. A subsequent study involving 141 patients showed a lower overall sensitivity (77%), which was noted to be as low at 40% for diagnosis isolated subsegmental PE [79]. The lack of radiation may make MRA an appealing alternative to V/Q scans and CTPA; however, the need for IV contrast with gadolinium makes this modality an unideal choice for PE evaluation in pregnancy. A retrospective study using Canadian birth certificate data from approximately 1.4 million deliveries found an increase in stillbirth and neonatal demise and a range of rheumatologic, inflammatory, and infiltrative skin conditions in infants when they were exposed to gadolinium with MRI in utero compared to pregnancies where there was MRI exposure without gadolinium. Given these findings, gadolinium use in pregnancy should be used with caution, especially in the first trimester [80].

Lower extremity venous ultrasonography evaluation

Reports in nonpregnant patients indicate that the prevalence of DVT among those with a documented PE ranges from 58% to 82% [81–83]. Meta-analysis suggests that in nonpregnant adults, the prevalence of DVT in those with suspected PE is 18% [84]. Le Gal and associates observed that VUS had a sensitivity of 39% and a specificity of 99% in nonpregnant patients with confirmed PE [85]. Although it is uncertain whether comparable rates and diagnostic accuracy exist for pregnant women with coexisting DVT and PE, it seems reasonable to use this test first in stable patients with symptoms of both DVT and PE, as a positive VUS result would mandate the same treatment as a documented PE and would avoid breast and/or fetal irradiation. However, a negative VUS study is still associated with a 25% risk of PE, so a negative VUS in patients with symptoms concerning for a PE, additional imaging is imperative [86].

Workup of patients with suspected pulmonary embolism

Evaluation of patients with suspected PE should begin with assessment of their cardio-respiratory status. For stable patients with oxygen saturation levels above 92% and no hemodynamic instability, assessment should proceed in an ordered fashion, outlined in in Figure 15.3, an algorithm developed with expert guidance from the American Thoracic Society, the Society of Thoracic Radiology, and the American College of Obstetricians and Gynecologists. The work-up begins with assessment of possible signs and symptoms of lower extremity thrombosis. The presence of left leg symptoms should prompt VUS, and if positive, anticoagulation should commence. If the VUS is negative or the patient has no suggestive leg symptoms, proceed to a CXR. A negative CXR should prompt a V/Q scan as the initial imaging modality. If the CXR is positive, CTPA should be the definitive test. If either the V/Q scan or CTPA is positive for PE, treatment is begun. In the case of a nondiagnostic V/Q scan result–intermediate probability/equivocal in any patient and a low-probability result in a high-risk patient (history of prior VTE, known thrombophilia, family history of VTE in a first-degree relative <50 years old or other clinical risk factors–CTPA should be performed. For patients where the CTPA is nondiagnostic, consider further testing with MRA or serial lower extremity VUS studies.

In any critically ill patient with hemodynamic instability, therapeutic anticoagulation should be initiated while the testing algorithm in Figure 15.4 in initiated. Alternative causes of the hypoxia and/or hemodynamic instability must be excluded (e.g. sepsis with adult respiratory distress syndrome, pneumothorax, cardiomyopathy with pulmonary edema). Consideration should be given to

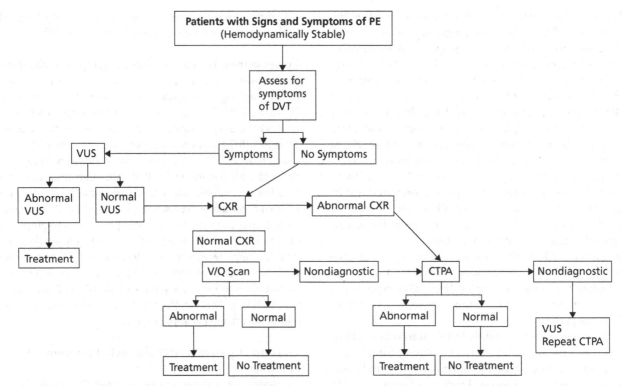

Figure 15.3 Diagnostic algorithm for the diagnosis of pulmonary embolism in hemodynamically stable pregnant women. CTPA, computed tomographic pulmonary angiography; CXR, chest X-ray; DVT, deep venous thrombosis; PE, pulmonary embolism; V/Q, ventilation/ perfusion; VUS, venous ultrasonography.

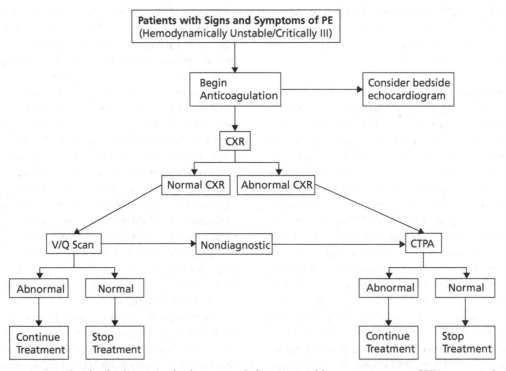

Figure 15.4 Diagnostic algorithm for the diagnosis of pulmonary embolism in unstable pregnant women. CTPA, computed tomographic pulmonary angiography; CXR, chest X-ray; PE, pulmonary embolism; V/Q, ventilation/perfusion.

performing a bedside echocardiogram (transthoracic or transesophageal, as appropriate) in very unstable patients as this is more likely to be diagnostic in this setting and avoids transporting a critically ill patient.

Conclusion

Avoidance of hemorrhage and thrombosis presents paradoxical challenges to the pregnant patient. Processes promoting hemostasis and endogenous anticoagulation are held in delicate equipoise, and the adaptations to and conditions of pregnancy predispose the gravid woman to increased risk of thromboembolic disease. Careful evaluation of risk of thromboembolic disease and elicitation of signs and symptoms are critical to making the diagnosis. The use of VUS is a simple and effective strategy for ruling out DVT. Lower extremity VUS and/or the combination of CXR with either V/Q scan or CTPA are the mainstays of diagnosing PE in pregnancy and the puerperium.

CASE PRESENTATION 1

A 42-year-old gravida 1, para 0 infertility patient has undergone in vitro fertilization with transfer of one embryo resulting in conception. Following several admissions for recurrent severe nausea and vomiting with weight loss, she has been resting at home for the past 4 days. She awakens late at night with left calf and thigh pain. She is seen in her physician's office the following morning. She denies dyspnea but notes mild calf and posterior thigh tenderness to palpation and has no other signs or symptoms of DVT. A VUS is ordered and she is found to have thrombosis involving the proximal thigh and calf veins. She is begun on therapeutic doses of low molecular weight heparin.

CASE PRESENTATION 2

A 27-year-old gravida 2, para 1 at 27 weeks gestation complains of left calf pain, which she believes began following the development of a painful muscle cramp after an intense exercise session, which awoke her the night before. She is seen in her physician's office and has an unremarkable exam except for bilateral trace lower extremity edema. She is quite healthy, exercises regularly, and has no personal or family history of thrombosis. A VUS is ordered, which returns negative. She is given instructions to call if the pain worsens or she develops unilateral lower extremity swelling, or dyspnea.

References

1. Ginsberg J, Brill-Edwards P, Burrows R, Bona R, Prandoni P, Büller HR, et al. Venous thrombosis during pregnancy: leg and trimester of presentation. Thromb Haemost. 1992;67:519–20.

2. Jacobsen A, Skjeldestad F, Sandset P. Incidence and risk patterns of venous thromboembolism in pregnancy and puerperium: a register-based case-control study. Am J Obstet Gynecol. 2008;198:e1–7.

3. Creanga AA, Syverson C, Seed K, Callaghan WM. Pregnancy-related mortality in the United States, 2011-2013. Obstet Gynecol. 2017;130:366–73.

4. Simpson E, Lawrenson R, Nightingale A, Farmer R. Venous thromboembolism in pregnancy and the puerperium: incidence and additional risk factors from a London perinatal database. Br J Obstet Gynaecol. 2001;108:56–60.

5. Stein P, Hull R, Jayali F, Olson RE, Alshab AK, Meyers FA, et al. Venous thromboembolism in pregnancy: 21-year trends. Am J Med. 2004;117:121–5.

6. Toglia M, Weg J. Venous thromboembolism during pregnancy. N Engl J Med. 1996;335:108–14.

7. O'Connor DJ, Scher LA, Gargiulo III NJ, Jang J, Suggs WD, Lipsitz EC. Incidence and characteristics of venous thromboembolic disease during pregnancy and the postnatal period: a contemporary series. Am Vasc Surg. 2011;25:9–14.

8. James K, Lohr J, Deshmukh R, Cranley J. Venous thrombotic complications of pregnancy. Cardiovasc Surg. 1996;4:777–82.

9. McColl M, Ramsay J, Tait R, Walker ID, McCall F, Conkie JA, et al. Risk factors for pregnancy associated venous thromboembolism. Thromb Haemost. 1997;78:1183–8.

10. Gherman RB, Goodwin TM, Leung B, Byrne JD, Hethumumi R, Montoro M. Incidence, clinical characteristics, and timing of objectively diagnosed venous thromboembolism during pregnancy. Obstet Gynecol. 1999;94:730–4.

11. Centers for Disease Control and Prevention. Pregnancy mortality surveillance system. [last reviewed 2023 Mar 23; cited 2022 Feb 18]. Available from: https://www.cdc.gov/reproductivehealth/maternal-mortality/pregnancy-mortality-surveillance-system.htm.

12. Wessler S. Medical management of venous thrombosis. Annu Rev Med. 1979;27:313–19.

13. Vallasanta U. Thromboembolic disease in pregnancy. Am J Obstet Gynecol. 1965;93:142–60.

14. Löwenberg EC, Meijers JC, Levi M. Platelet-vessel wall interaction in health and disease. Neth J Med. 2010; 68:242–51.

15. Pytela R, Pierschbacher M, Ginsberg M, Plow E, Ruoslahti E. Platelet membrane glycoprotein IIb/IIIa: member of a family of Arg-Gly-Asp-specific adhesion receptors. Science. 1986;231:1559–62.

16. Mackman N. Role of tissue factor in hemostasis and thrombosis. Blood Cells Mol Dis. 2006;36:104–7.

17. Lockwood CJ, Murk W, Kayisli UA, Buchwalder LF, Huang ST, Funai EF, et al. Progestin and thrombin regulate tissue factor expression in human term decidual cells. J Clin Endocrinol Metab. 2009;94:2164–70.

18. Lockwood CJ, Paidas M, Murk WK, Kayisli UA, Gopinath A, Huang SJ, et al. Involvement of human decidual cell-expressed tissue factor in uterine hemostasis and abruption. Thromb Res. 2009;124:516–20.

19. Lockwood C, Bach R, Guha A, Zhou X, Miller W, Nemerson Y. Amniotic fluid contains tissue factor, a potent initiator of coagulation. Am J Obstet Gynecol. 1991;165:1335–41.

20. Mackman N. The role of tissue factor and factor VIIa in hemostasis. Anesth Analg. 2009;108:1447–52.

21. Hackeng TM, Maurissen LF, Castoldi E, Rosing J. Regulation of TFPI function by protein S. J Thromb Haemost. 2009;7(Suppl 1):165–8.

22. Esmon C. The protein C pathway. Chest. 2003;124(3 Suppl):26S–32S.

23. Dahlback B. Progress in the understanding of the protein C anticoagulant pathway. Int J Hematol. 2004;79:109–16.

24. Dahlback B. The tale of protein S and C4b-binding protein, a story of affection. Thromb Haemost. 2007;98:90–6.

25. Broze G. Protein Z-dependent regulation of coagulation. Thromb Haemost. 2001;86:8–13.

26. Perry D. Antithrombin and its inherited deficiencies. Blood Rev. 1994;8:37–55.

27. Preissner K, Zwicker L, Muller-Berghaus G. Formation, characterization and detection of a ternary complex between protein S, thrombin and antithrombin III in serum. Biochem J. 1987;243:105–11.

28. Bouma B, Meijers J. New insights into factors affecting clot stability: a role for thrombin activatable fibrinolysis inhibitor. Semin Hematol. 2004;41:13–19.

29. Schatz F, Lockwood C. Progestin regulation of plasminogen activator inhibitor type-1 in primary cultures of endometrial stromal and decidual cells. J Clin Endocrin Metab. 1993; 77:621–5.

30. Lockwood C, Krikun G, Schatz F. The decidua regulates hemostasis in the human endometrium. Semin Reprod Endocrinol. 1999;17:45–51.

31. Bouma BN, Mosnier LO. Thrombin activatable fibrinolysis inhibitor (TAFI) – how does thrombin regulate fibrinolysis? Ann Med. 2006;38(6):378–88.

32. Girling J, de Swiet M. Inherited thrombophilia and pregnancy. Curr Opin Obstet Gynecol. 1998;10:135–44.

33. Thurn L, Wikman A, Lindqvist PG. Postpartum blood transfusion and hemorrhage as independent risk factors for venous thromboembolism. Thromb Res. 2018;165:54–60.

34. Nelson-Piercy C, MacCallum P, Mackillop L. Reducing the risk of thrombosis and embolism during pregnancy and the puerperium (Green-top guideline no. 37a). London: Royal College of Obstetricians and Gynaecologists; 2015.

35. Blondon M, Casini A, Hoppe KK, Boehlen F, Righini M, Smith NL. Risks of venous thromboembolism after cesarean sections: a meta-analysis. Chest. 2016; 150:572–96.

36. Abdul Sultan A, West J, Tata LJ, Fleming KM, Nelson-Piercy C, Grainge MJ. Risk of first venous thromboembolism in pregnant women in hospital: population based cohort study from England. BMJ. 2013;347:f6099.

37. Wright H, Osborn S, Edmunds D. Changes in the rate of flow of venous blood in the leg during pregnancy, measured with radioactive sodium. Surg Gynecol Obstet. 1950;90:481.

38. Goodrich S, Wood J. Peripheral venous distensibility and velocity of venous blood flow during pregnancy or during oral contraceptive therapy. Am J Obstet Gynecol. 1964;90:740–4.

39. Macklon N, Greer I, Bowman A. An ultrasound study of gestational and postural changes in the deep venous system of the leg in pregnancy. Br J Obstet Gynaecol. 1997;104:191–7.

40. Ray JG, Chan WS. Deep vein thrombosis during pregnancy and the puerperium: a meta analysis of the period of risk and the leg of presentation, Obstet Gynecol Surv. 1999;54:265–71.

41. Hellgren M, Blomback M. Studies on blood coagulation and fibrinolysis in pregnancy, during delivery and in the puerperium. Gynecol Obstet Invest. 1981;12:141–54.

42. Bremme K. Haemostatic changes in pregnancy. Baillière's Best Pract Res Clin Haematol. 2003;16:153–68.

43. Macklon N, Greer I. Venous thromboembolic disease in obstetrics and gynecology: the Scottish experience. Scott Med J. 1996;41:83–6.

44. Bourjeily G, Paidas M, Khalil H, Rosene-Montella K, Rodger M. Pulmonary embolism in pregnancy. Lancet. 2010; 375(9713):500–12.

45. Chan WS, Lee A, Spencer FA, Crowther M, Rodger M, Ramsay T, et al. Predicting deep venous thrombosis in pregnancy: out in "LEFt" field? Ann Intern Med. 2009;151:85–92.

46. Sandler D, Martin J, Duncan J, Blake GM, Ward P, Ramsay LE, et al. Diagnosis of deep-vein thrombosis: comparison of clinical evaluation, ultrasound, plethysmography, and venoscan with x-ray venogram. Lancet. 1984;8405:716–19.

47. Hirsh J, Hoak J. Management of deep vein thrombosis and pulmonary embolism: a statement for healthcare professionals from the Council on Thrombosis (in consultation with the Council on Cardiovascular Radiology), American Heart Association. Circulation. 1996;93:2212–45.

48. Kline JA, Williams GW, Hernandez-Nino J. D-dimer concentrations in normal pregnancy: new diagnostic thresholds are needed. Clin Chem. 2005;51(5):825–9.

49. Chan WS, Chunilal S, Lee A, Crowther M, Rodger M, Ginsberg JS. A red blood cell agglutination D-dimer test to exclude deep venous thrombosis in pregnancy. Ann Intern Med. 2007; 147:165–70.

50. Hunt BJ, Parmar K, Horspool K, et al. The DiPEP (Diagnosis of PE in pregnancy) biomarker study: an observational cohort study augmented with additional cases to determine the diagnostic utility of biomarkers for suspected venous thromboembolism during pregnancy and puerperium. Br J Haematol. 2018; 180:694–704.

51. Kassai B, Boissel J, Cucherat M, Sonie S, Shah N, Leizorovicz A systematic review of the accuracy of ultrasound in the diagnosis of deep venous thrombosis in asymptomatic patients. Thromb Haemost. 2004;91:655–66.

52. Gottlieb R, Widjaja J, Tian L, Rubens D, Voci S. Calf sonography for detecting deep venous thrombosis in symptomatic patients: experience and review of the literature. J Clin Ultrasound. 1999;27:415–20.

53. Sampson FC, Goodacre SW, Thomas SM, van Beek EJ. The accuracy of MRI in diagnosis of suspected deep vein thrombosis: systematic review and meta-analysis. Eur Radiol. 2007;17(1):175–81.

54. James AH, Tapson VF, Goldhaber SZ. Thrombosis during pregnancy and the postpartum period, Am J Obstet Gynecol. 2005;193:216–19.

55. Cahill AG, Stout MJ, Macones GA, Bhalla S. Diagnosing pulmonary embolism in pregnancy using computed-tomographic angiography or ventilation-perfusion. Obstet Gynecol. 2009; 114:124–9.

56. Fedullo P, Tapson V. The evaluation of suspected pulmonary embolism. N Engl J Med. 2003;349:1247–56.

57. Urokinase Pulmonary Embolism Trial: a national cooperative study. Circulation. 1973;47(Suppl II):1–108.

58. PIOPED Investigators. Value of the ventilation/perfusion scan in acute pulmonary embolism. Results of the prospective investigation of pulmonary embolism diagnosis (PIOPED). JAMA. 1990;263:2653–9.

59. Tapson V, Carroll B, Davidson B, Elliott CG, Fedullo PF, Hales CA, et al. The diagnostic approach to acute venous thromboembolism. Clinical practice guideline. American Thoracic Society. Am J Respir Clin Care Med. 1999;160:1043–66.

60. Come P. Echocardiographic evaluation of pulmonary embolism and its response to therapeutic interventions. Chest. 1992;101:151S–62S.

61. Stein P, Terrin M, Hales C, Palevsky HI, Saltzman HA, Thompson BT, et al. Clinical, laboratory, roentgenographic, and electrocardiographic findings in patients with acute pulmonary embolism and no pre-existing cardiac or pulmonary disease. Chest. 1991;100:598–603.

62. Kasper W, Meinertz T, Kersting F, Lollgen H, Limbourg P, Just H. Echocardiography in assessing acute pulmonary hypertension due to pulmonary embolism. Am J Cardiol. 1980;45:567–72.

63. Gibson N, Sohne M, Buller H. Prognostic value of echocardiography and spiral computed tomography in patients with pulmonary embolism. Curr Opin Pulm Med. 2005;11:380–4.

64. Pruszczyk P, Torbicki A, Pacho R, Chlebus M, Kuch-Wocial A, Pruszynski B, et al. Noninvasive diagnosis of suspected severe pulmonary embolism: transesophageal echocardiography vs spiral CT. Chest. 1997;112:722–8.

65. Stein P, Athanasoulis C, Alavi A, Greenspan RH, Hales CA, Saltzman HA, et al. Complications and validity of pulmonary angiography in acute pulmonary embolism. Circulation. 1992;85:462–8.

66. To MS, Hunt BJ, Nelson-Piercy C. A negative D-dimer does not exclude venous thromboembolism (VTE) in pregnancy. J Obstet Gynaecol. 2008;28:222–3.

67. Damodaram M, Kaladindi M, Luckit J, Yoong W. D-dimers as a screening test for venous thromboembolism in pregnancy: is it of any use? J Obstet Gynaecol. 2009;29:101–3.

68. Henry JW, Relyea B, Stein PD. Continuing risk of thromboemboli among patients with normal pulmonary angiograms. Chest. 1995;107(5):1375–8.

69. Mills S, Jackson D, Older R, Heaston D, Moore A. The incidence, etiologies, and avoidance of complications of pulmonary angiography in a large series. Radiology. 1980;136:295–9.

70. Dalen J, Brooks H, Johnson L, Meister S, Szucs MJ, Dexter L. Pulmonary angiography in acute pulmonary embolism: indications, techniques, and results in 367 patients. Am Heart J. 1971;81:175–85.

71. Sheen J-J, Haramati LB, Natenzon A, Ma H, Tropper P, Bader AS, et al. Performance of low-dose perfusion scintigraphy and CT pulmonary angiography for pulmonary embolism in pregnancy. Chest. 2018; 153:152–60.

72. Ridge CA, McDermott S, Freyne BJ, Brennan DJ, Collins CD, Skehan SJ. Pulmonary embolism in pregnancy: comparison of pulmonary CT angiography and lung scintigraphy. Am J Roentgenol. 2009;193(5):1223–7.

73. Andreou AK, Curtin JJ, Wilde S, Clark A. Does pregnancy affect vascular enhancement in patients undergoing CT pulmonary angiography? Eur Radiol. 2008;18(12):2716–22.

74. U-King-Im JM, Freeman SJ, Boylan T, Cheow HK. Quality of CT pulmonary angiography for suspected pulmonary embolus in pregnancy. Eur Radiol. 2008;18(12):2709–15.

75. Litmanovich D, Boiselle PM, Bankier AA, Kataoka ML, Pianykh O, Raptopoulos V. Dose reduction in computed tomographic angiography of pregnant patients with suspected acute pulmonary embolism. J Comput Assist Tomogr. 2009;33:961–6.

76. Winer-Muram HT, Boone JM, Brown HL, Jennings SG, Mabie WC, Lombardo GT. Pulmonary embolism in pregnant patients: fetal radiation dose with helical CT. Radiology. 2002;224(2):487–92.

77. Winer-Muram HT, Boone JM, and National Council on Radiation Protection. Exposure of the population in the United States and Canada to natural background radiation. Report No. 94. Bethesda, MD: National Council on Radiation Protection; 1987.

78. Meaney J, Weg J, Chenevert T, Stafford-Johnson D, Hamilton B, Prince M. Diagnosis of pulmonary embolism with magnetic resonance angiography. N Engl J Med. 1997;336:1422–7.

79. Oudkerk M, van Beek EJ, Wielopolski P, van Ooijen PM, Brouwers-Kuyper EM, Bongaerts AH, et al. Comparison of contrast-enhanced magnetic resonance angiography and conventional pulmonary angiography for the diagnosis of pulmonary embolism: a prospective study. Lancet. 2002;359(9318):1643–7.

80. Ray JG, Vermeulen MJ, Bharatha A, Montanera WJ, Park AL. Association between MRI exposure during pregnancy and fetal and childhood outcomes. JAMA. 2016; 316:952–61.

81. Yamaki T, Nozaki M, Sakurai H, Takeuchi M, Soejima K, Kono T. Presence of lower limb deep vein thrombosis and prognosis in patients with symptomatic pulmonary embolism: preliminary report. Eur J Vasc Endovasc Surg. 2009;37:225–31.

82. Girard P, Musset D, Parent F, Maitre S, Phlippoteau C, Simonneau G. High prevalence of detectable deep venous thrombosis in patients with acute pulmonary embolism. Chest. 1999;116:903–8.

83. Girard P, Sanchez O, Leroyer C, Musset D, Meyer G, Stern JB, et al. Deep venous thrombosis in patients with acute pulmonary embolism: prevalence, risk factors, and clinical significance. Chest. 2005;128:1593–600.

84. Van Rossum AB, van Houwelingen HC, Kieft G J, Pattynama PM. Prevalence of deep vein thrombosis in suspected and proven pulmonary embolism: a meta-analysis. Br J Radiol. 1998;71:1260–5.

85. Le Gal G, Righini M, Sanchez O, Roy PM, Baba-Ahmed M, Perrier A, et al. A positive compression ultrasonography of the lower limb veins is highly predictive of pulmonary embolism on computed tomography in suspected patients. Thromb Haemost. 2006;95:963–6.

86. Stein P, Hull R, Saltzman H, Pineo G. Strategy for diagnosis of patients with suspected pulmonary embolism. Chest. 1993;103:1553–9.

Chapter 16
Cardiac Disease in Pregnancy

Sarah Rae Easter

Division of Maternal-Fetal Medicine, Department of Obstetrics and Gynecology; Division of Critical Care Medicine, Department of Anesthesiology, Perioperative and Pain Medicine; Brigham and Women's Hospital, Harvard Medical School, Boston, MA, USA

Improvements in care for people with cardiovascular disease (CVD) coupled with evidence about the safety of pregnancy inform consensus guidelines. Pregnancy may not be contraindicated, but it is also not without risk. CVD has emerged to be the leading cause of pregnancy-related mortality emphasizing the need for close monitoring and early intervention [1]. Despite this, mortality reviews demonstrate failure to refer patients for risk-appropriate care as contributors to death in this population [2]).

These data alongside the clinical complexity for patients with CVD in pregnancy inform guidelines supporting the care for patients as a part of a cardio-obstetrics team. Disparities in timely access to risk-appropriate care as well as the possibility of new-onset CVD in pregnancy reinforce the need for all obstetric care providers to have a framework for the management of CVD in pregnancy. This protocol outlines an approach to the management of CVD to prioritize risk assessment, antenatal optimization, multidisciplinary delivery planning, and postpartum and interconception monitoring.

Risk assessment and risk-appropriate care

A key component of optimizing care for women with CVD is frequent risk assessment. Ideally patients with CVD will seek a preconception consultation. This centers on the risks of pregnancy through the lens of a patient's diagnosis and functional status and can provide opportunities to intervene medically or surgically to optimize a patient's cardiovascular status prior to pregnancy. With the prevalence of unplanned pregnancy as well as disparities in access to care the first interaction between a patient and the cardio-obstetrics team may be in the setting of pregnancy. Facilitating access to multidisciplinary risk assessment and counseling prior to

pregnancy is one assumed benefit of a coordinated cardio-obstetrics team [3].

Regardless of the timing of the initial encounter, risk assessment is the requisite first step in any clinical interaction for a person with CVD and plans for or ongoing pregnancy. Multiple risk-stratification tools and classification systems for patients with CVD have been derived and validated. The World Health Organization (WHO) classification system outlines four groups according to underlying diagnosis. These groups range from low-risk disease in which outcomes are similar to a patient without CVD (Group 1) to the highest risk group (Group 4) where risk of maternal morbidity or mortality is so high that pregnancy is contraindicated [4–6]. This disease-based classification system differs from tools such as ZAHARA and CARPREG, which incorporate clinical history with underlying diagnosis to assess risk of cardiac complication in pregnancy [7,8]. Both tools use a weighted point system to assign points for high-risk features and sum points to generate an overall score. Higher scores are associated with a higher risk of adverse cardiac events during pregnancy or delivery. Both CARPREG and ZAHARA highlight a history of arrhythmias, New York Heart Association functional status, cyanotic heart disease, left-ventricular obstruction, and the presence of a mechanical valve as high-risk features. Validation studies comparing CARPREG, ZAHARA, and the WHO classification scheme yield inconsistent findings, which may reflect differences in methodology or population in the derivation and validation cohorts. From the clinical perspective they are comparable with relative merits and limitations that may differ according to the time of intended use.

The WHO tool can be helpful in the preconception or early pregnancy setting to identify patients who have a contraindication to pregnancy or warrant a higher level of care. Decisions related to risk assessment and subsequent management for patients with the range of conditions captured in WHO class II and III may be clarified by

Queenan's Management of High-Risk Pregnancy: An Evidence-Based Approach, Seventh Edition. Edited by Catherine Y. Spong and Charles J. Lockwood.

Table 16.1 Framework for risk-appropriate care according to cardiovascular risk state

	Average risk	Increased risk	Highest risk
Clinical classification	Patients with similar risk to population without CVD allowing standard approach to management with increased surveillance.	Patients with low-risk disease but high-risk features or patients with compensated but high-risk disease.	Decompensated patients or those at high risk of decompensation with potential need for inotropes or mechanical circulatory support.
WHO class	I and II	II and III	III and IV
Example conditions	Repaired septal defects Regurgitant valvular lesions Mild pulmonary stenosis Supraventricular arrhythmias	Tetralogy of Fallot Mitral or aortic stenosis, asymptomatic Aortic coarctation Fontan circulation Systemic right ventricle Hypertrophic cardiomyopathy Unrepaired septal defects	Pulmonary hypertension Symptomatic left-sided obstructive lesions Decompensated heart failure Aortopathies associated with connective tissue disorders
Minimum level of care	Specialist obstetric care with cardiology and maternal-fetal medicine available for consultation	Care in cardio-obstetrics program with delivery at center with cardiology and MFM readily available to provide inpatient care	Management by cardio-obstetrics team with delivery at center with cardiac surgery and mechanical circulatory support
Anesthetic plan	Epidural	Slow epidural	Slow epidural with invasive hemodynamic monitoring
Intrapartum cardiac monitoring	None	Pulse oximetry	Telemetry Arterial line Pulmonary artery catheter[a]
Delivery location[2]	Labor and delivery	Labor and delivery with L&D OR available for space	L&D with critical care services available Surgical or cardiac ICU Cardiac OR[b]

[a]Reserved for patients with pulmonary artery hypertension or undifferentiated shock when invasive hemodynamic data may influence approach to treatment without other reasonable approach.
[b]Used for patients at high risk of mechanical circulatory support (e.g. severe left heart failure, right heart failure, pulmonary hypertension) or urgent cardiopulmonary bypass (e.g. aortic dissection).
CVD, cardiovascular disease; ICU, intensive care unit; L&D, labor and delivery; MFM, maternal–fetal medicine; OR, operating room.

incorporating clinical history. Regardless of the specific risk assessment tool or framework most patients with CVD can be easily situated into one of three categories: average risk, increased risk, and highest risk. Table 16.1 outlines a proposed framework for risk assessment in the setting of CVD that relies on the WHO categories but accounts for high-risk features identified by clinical scoring systems.

The choice of tool is less important than ensuring a system for universal assessment and frequent reassessment as all systems serve the same fundamental role – to standardize communication of level of risk to the patient and members of her multidisciplinary care team. Standardized assessment of risk then allows for informed discussion of the components of each patient's care plan including antenatal screening, intrapartum planning, and postpartum monitoring. This type of standardized and frequent risk assessment also has the potential to optimize risk-appropriate care.

National guidelines suggest patients with CVD seek delivery in level III or IV centers characterized by an obstetrician-gynecologist (OB-GYN) and anesthesiologist in house at all times with availability for inpatient support from cardiology and maternal–fetal medicine (MFM) when required [9]. Access to the full range of diagnostic services as well as an intensive care unit (ICU) are requisite in these centers with the availability of cardiac surgery as a distinguishing feature between level III and level IV centers. Patients with average risk disease without high-risk historical features or complicating diagnoses may consider care in level II centers in settings where access to subspecialty care is limited. In these cases antenatal consultation with a cardiologist and obstetric care provider with experience in CVD in pregnancy should be sought to outline delivery considerations and contingency plans as well as facilitate access to transfer should it be warranted.

In an ideal setting all patients with CVD would have access to the aforementioned resources and personnel facilitated by a dedicated cardio-obstetrics team consisting of a cardiologist, obstetrician, anesthesiologist, and nurse with familiarity and experience with CVD in pregnancy at a minimum. With an increasingly complex patient population additional contributors to the team should include specialists with subspecialty expertise in electrophysiology, heart failure, imaging, cardiac catheterization, and cardiac surgery. Establishing relationships with subspecialists across the medical and procedural disciplines of cardiology facilitates timely consultation from providers with experience with cardiac adaptations, diagnostic challenges, and therapeutic options in pregnancy.

This multidisciplinary team approach not only optimizes a holistic approach to patient care but has the potential to improve outcomes over time through concentrating experience and interdisciplinary education. Data from high-risk specialized diagnoses such as placenta accreta spectrum demonstrate not only improved outcomes when care is managed by a multidisciplinary team but show that outcomes improved for patients managed by the team over time. Extrapolating from this literature and comparison of outcomes between the CARPREG-I and CARPREG-II studies also showing lower adverse cardiovascular events over time suggests that coordinated multidisciplinary care could improve outcomes for patients with CVD in pregnancy. In some settings such as congenital heart disease (CHD) or valvular disorders cardiologists from the multidisciplinary team provide a key role in longitudinal preconception and postpartum follow-up for high-risk patients.

Antenatal care and optimization

Regardless of the care setting providers caring for patients with CVD in pregnancy should adopt a standard approach to antenatal care that can be individualized based on underlying diagnosis and risk state viewed through the lens of pregnancy physiology. The hallmark physiologic change of pregnancy is an increase in cardiac output (CO) that comes from a gradual longitudinal increase in both heart rate (HR) and stroke volume (SV). Stroke volume is first increased by a decrease in afterload due to a decrease in systemic vascular resistance (SVR) that characterizes the first and second trimesters. Physiologic changes in the kidney coupled with a reset osmostat then support the increase in SV leading to a slow increase in plasma volume that reaches its peak around 32 weeks of pregnancy. This evolving physiology underscores the role for frequent risk assessment in prenatal care with the use of diagnostic studies and preventive therapy as appropriate. Figure 16.1 proposes one standardized approach to care according to trimester of pregnancy and underlying cardiovascular diagnosis [10].

First trimester
The preconception or initial prenatal visit provides an opportunity to review clinical history and diagnostic studies. An increased heart rate alongside the compensated respiratory alkalosis of pregnancy are the primary physiologic changes in early pregnancy making this time period well tolerated from a cardiopulmonary standpoint. Obtaining a baseline brain-natriuretic peptide (BNP) and electrocardiogram (ECG) can be helpful for all patients for comparison over time.

For most patients a transthoracic echocardiogram (TTE) performed within the past 12 months will be adequate to confirm disease stability. A first-trimester TTE should be considered for patients with connective tissue disease or highest risk disease to monitor the size of the aortic root and biventricular function, respectively. For patients with more than average risk disease or those with a history of arrhythmias ambulatory Holter monitoring can be helpful to identify subclinical ectopy warranting further monitoring or therapy.

Cardiopulmonary exercise testing (CPET) can be helpful to objectively assess functional capacity and unmask any exercise-associated hemodynamic changes or arrhythmias. Patients in the highest risk category or those of increased risk with features raising concern for the patient's ability to tolerate pregnancy. Guidelines encourage the use of semirecumbent cycle ergometry reaching 80% of the predicted maximal heart rate [4]. Obtaining a CPET during the first or early second trimester may optimize timing for an appropriate clinical response. For patients with valvular heart disease or coronary artery disease CPET can unmask changes warranting cardiac intervention that is best timed in the second trimester. For patients with highest-risk disease objective findings from CPET may motivate the care team to counsel the patients toward pregnancy termination further underscoring the importance of this test early in pregnancy when indicated.

Counseling patients about maternal risk in the setting of CVD is of paramount importance but noting fetal risks associated with the underlying cardiac state or other obstetric conditions is also warranted. Patients with congenital heart disease have an increased risk of CHD in their fetus suggesting a role for nuchal translucency screening—even in the setting of low-risk laboratory screening or diagnostic testing. Patients with a history of dilated cardiomyopathy, aortopathy, or CVD as a part of an underlying genetic syndrome will benefit from the input of genetic counseling to assess risk of transmission to the fetus and review options for diagnostic testing. The biologic and epidemiologic associations between preeclampsia and cardiac disease suggest low-dose aspirin therapy prior to 14 weeks should be initiated in the setting of CVD. Ensuring patients understand the rationale for this therapy as well as the importance of continuing medications for CVD is a critical component of prenatal care.

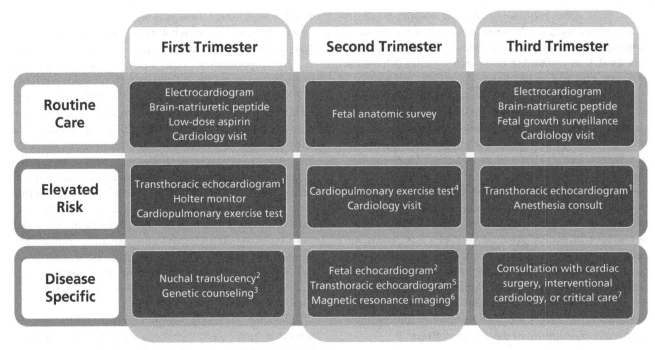

	First Trimester	**Second Trimester**	**Third Trimester**
Routine Care	Electrocardiogram Brain-natriuretic peptide Low-dose aspirin Cardiology visit	Fetal anatomic survey	Electrocardiogram Brain-natriuretic peptide Fetal growth surveillance Cardiology visit
Elevated Risk	Transthoracic echocardiogram[1] Holter monitor Cardiopulmonary exercise test	Cardiopulmonary exercise test[4] Cardiology visit	Transthoracic echocardiogram[1] Anesthesia consult
Disease Specific	Nuchal translucency[2] Genetic counseling[3]	Fetal echocardiogram[2] Transthoracic echocardiogram[5] Magnetic resonance imaging[6]	Consultation with cardiac surgery, interventional cardiology, or critical care[7]

Figure 16.1 Risk-based approach to antenatal care for cardiac disease in pregnancy.
Monitoring considerations for the antenatal care of patients with cardiac disease by trimester in addition to routine prenatal care. Patients with high-risk disease warrant additional testing as outlined whereas those with increased-risk disease may warrant these studies in response to clinical risk assessment.
[1]Consider either first or third trimester transthoracic echocardiogram (TTE) for patients with low-risk disease if not done within past year.
[2]Patients with congenital heart disease.
[3]Patients with dilated cardiomyopathy, aortopathy, or underlying genetic cause of CVD.
[4]Patients with dilated cardiomyopathy, aortopathy, or underlying genetic cause of CVD.
[5]Patients with aortopathy or concern for evolving left ventricular dysfunction for longitudinal assessment of echocardiographic parameters.
[6]Cardiac magnetic resonance imaging (MRI) without gadolinium should be performed for patients with aortic disease without an assessment of thoracic and abdominal aorta. Cardiac MRI may also be considered in patients in whom TTE was insufficient for diagnosis.
[7]Consultation between patient and provider or between providers for patients with potential need for critical care services or mechanical circulatory support including extracorporeal membrane oxygenation at delivery.

Second trimester

The notable hemodynamic event of the second trimester is the physiologic nadir in SVR that can be accompanied by postural hypotension and tachycardia. This normal physiology can present symptomatically as palpitations and presyncope, which may be impossible to distinguish between new-onset arrhythmias or cardiac decompensation in the setting of underlying CVD. With this in mind a low threshold for repeat testing with a Holter monitor, TTE, or CPET (if not performed in the second trimester) is warranted in the setting of new cardiopulmonary complaints. A repeat TTE may be considered for patients with highest risk disease including heart failure with reduced ejection fraction, valvular or structural disease leading to left ventricular outflow tract obstruction, and aortopathy. The value of TTE in this setting is to monitor for concerning trends that may prompt intervention or termination of pregnancy prior to the third trimester of pregnancy.

The fetal anatomic survey is a critical screening test for all pregnant patients but is of particular importance in the setting of CVD. The aforementioned increased risk of CHD in patients with CHD underscores the recommendation for fetal echocardiography in patients with CHD. Pursuing an early anatomic survey around 17 to 19 weeks followed by dedicated fetal echocardiography at 20 to 22 weeks gestation may balance early detection of CHD in the fetus with optimization of views obtained on fetal echo. The diagnosis of CHD in the fetus should prompt a referral for genetic counseling for consideration of diagnostic testing if this was not discussed in the first trimester.

Third trimester

Monitoring for cardiac or obstetric complications and planning for delivery characterize the third trimester of pregnancy. The known association between CVD and fetal growth restriction (FGR) suggests routine fetal growth surveillance with ultrasound is warranted for patients with CVD independent of the presence of medications such as beta blockers that may increase the risk of

FGR. A baseline assessment of fetal weight at 28 to 32 weeks and again at 36 weeks should be considered to help monitor for fetal complications and develop a timeline for delivery planning in the event earlier delivery is warranted for fetal indications.

A dedicated visit with the cardiologist including repeat BNP and ECG as well as a consultation with an anesthesiologist are key additions to routine prenatal care in the setting of CVD. For patients with increased or high-risk disease repeating TTE to ensure patients tolerate the volume load of pregnancy is of critical importance. The peak increase in plasma volume is reached at 32 weeks, suggesting TTE should be timed at this time point in pregnancy in the absence of other indications. This third-trimester assessment of cardiac function is a key data point for delivery planning and may be planned earlier in pregnancy to facilitate this process–particularly for patients with an increased risk of preterm birth or with the potential need for additional subspecialty involvement (such as cardiac surgery or interventional cardiology for mechanical circulatory support) at the time of delivery.

Multidisciplinary delivery planning

The aforementioned increase in HR and plasma volume happen gradually across pregnancy but encounter acute stress at the time of labor and delivery (L&D). Labor is accompanied by an increase in catecholamines leading to a physiologic increase in HR with the potential for significant hemodynamic impact. The gradual increase in plasma volume occurring over the first 32 weeks of pregnancy must be managed at the time of delivery leading to an acute increase in preload for the maternal circulation. This physiologic stress coupled with the possibility of competing events such as intrapartum cesarean delivery (CD) or infection is a hemodynamic challenge for all birthing persons, but one that may have greater physiologic impact in the setting of underlying CVD. In addition to assessment of cardiopulmonary status delivery planning must account for interactions between the patients CVD and other medical and obstetric comorbidities as well as the patient's goals of care. Integrating cardiovascular risk with other obstetric and anesthetic risk factors is critical to creating a comprehensive birth plan for this patient.

Mode of delivery

Table 16.1 includes an approach to delivery planning based on cardiovascular risk state. Evidence-based guidelines and expert opinion encourage an attempted vaginal delivery for the vast majority of patients with CVD and emphasize reserving CD for routine obstetric indications [4,11]. Obstetric care providers are familiar with the short- and long-term benefits of attempted vaginal delivery and serve a key role educating patients and nonobstetric providers

about available literature. Highlighting the psychological benefit of experiencing what most consider to be a "normal" process and part of life is key–particularly when caring for a population with more exposure to medical interventions in childhood and early adulthood.

Although intrapartum changes in HR and volume state are a primary concern, the second stage of labor has been considered a hemodynamically vulnerable time with the need for recurrent Valsalva to affect delivery. Valsalva is characterized hemodynamically by an increase in intrathoracic pressure with a subsequent decrease in preload and increase in afterload in the thoracic aorta. Historically, patients with preload dependent lesions or aortic disease may have been counseled towards an assisted second stage with an operative vaginal delivery using vacuum or forceps. The rationale for this approach is to shorten the time of the second stage and decrease the impact of Valsalva on maternal hemodynamics.

There may be a physiologic argument to shorten the second stage for the sake of hemodynamics, but there is a lack of evidence supporting this approach. The unproven benefit coupled with the known increase in maternal and neonatal complications associated with operative vaginal delivery support an unassisted second stage for patients with CVD. Planning for an unassisted second stage should be focused on a multidisciplinary understanding of the patient's CVD and hemodynamic vulnerabilities. For patients with complex CHD diagrams can be helpful to develop a common mental model of hemodynamic vulnerabilities while all patients will benefit from the documentation of changes in vital signs such as narrowing of the pulse pressure or rebound tachycardia that may signal impending decompensation.

Analgesia and anesthesia

Neuraxial analgesia is encouraged for all patients with CVD to minimize the pain-mediated increase in HR and facilitate rapid access to surgical analgesia should the need for intrapartum CD or postpartum procedures arise [12]. Though epidural analgesia offers benefits beyond pain control in terms of hemodynamics, its administration is associated with a decrease in SVR leading to decreased afterload and preload most often manifest as hypotension. For patients with preload dependent lesions and left-ventricular outflow tract obstruction, this change in physiology can predispose them to hemodynamic instability or even collapse. In these settings the routine approach to administration of neuraxial can be replaced with a slow infusion of medication over time either during epidural placement or in anticipation of CD. For patients with increased or highest risk disease predelivery consultation with an anesthesiologist with expertise in obstetrics should be pursued to allow the anesthesia care team to integrate available data with a functional assessment and outline an anesthetic plan including contingency planning for intrapartum and postpartum emergencies.

Monitoring and emergency preparedness

Despite the need for advanced planning, the majority of patients with CVD can be safely managed without additional intrapartum cardiac monitoring. Any monitoring plan should take into account the patient's underlying hemodynamic vulnerabilities and outline changes warranting intervention with an emphasis on maintaining cardiac output. CO optimization will vary according to underlying pathophysiology with available frameworks emphasizing control of HR and preload and afterload optimization.

All patients warrant meticulous documentation of intake and output with the use of an indwelling urinary catheter for most patients once neuraxial analgesia is in place. Patients with preload dependent lesions or those whose CO depends on passive filling in the case of Fontan circulation may warrant more fluids during labor, the routine use of maintenance intravenous fluids without frequent reassessment of hemodynamics should be avoided. Point-of-care ultrasound has been adopted with enthusiasm across specialties for dynamic assessment of volume status and can be a useful tool on L&D to optimize hemodynamics in vulnerable patients.

For many patients with increased or high-risk CVD continuous pulse oximetry may provide sufficient cardiopulmonary monitoring mitigating the need for routine telemetry or invasive hemodynamic monitoring. Patients with decreasing oxygenation or concern for arrhythmia on pulse oximetry can be transitioned to telemetry intrapartum should concerns about pathologic arrhythmia arise. Patients who have a history of pathologic ventricular arrhythmias, are vulnerable to the impacts of tachycardia on hemodynamics, or are at an increased risk of hemodynamically significant arrhythmias due to cardiac structure or function may require telemetry to facilitate early identification and intervention.

Maintaining normal sinus rhythm for high-risk patients is of paramount importance. Not only does tachycardia decrease the diastolic filling time essential to maintaining CO but it also reduces the time for filling of the coronary arteries and therefore coronary perfusion pressure. For patients with mitral stenosis the chronic stress on the left atrium may predispose them to atrial arrhythmias that further reduce end-diastolic volume by effectively removing the increased filling that occurs with atrial contraction. Direct cardioversion should be considered in the face of new-onset atrial arrhythmias to restore sinus rhythm and optimize hemodynamics in patients whose cardiac output depends on atrial contraction.

Early identification of hypotension or respiratory variation in pulse pressure informs the rationale supporting invasive hemodynamic monitoring with an arterial line in highest risk patients. Arterial line placement also facilitates frequent laboratory draws and may be useful in patients with mechanical valves requiring intrapartum heparin administration or those requiring frequent electrolyte monitoring and repletion. Medical therapy including vasopressors may be required in response to hypotension in patients with high-risk disease states. Patients with Eisenmenger physiology, right heart failure, and pulmonary hypertension may benefit from prophylactic use of vasopressors or inotropes to optimize biventricular function. An arterial line facilitates safe administration of continuous vasopressors in these settings. Further invasive hemodynamic monitoring with pulmonary artery catheters can typically be avoided with rare exception.

Regardless of vasopressor or disease state, ensuring euvolemia to maximize preload and therefore contractility via the Frank–Starling mechanism is imperative. For all patients who may be particularly vulnerable to even slight hemodynamic changes, a vasopressor strategy to address hypotension associated with neuraxial analgesia or hemorrhage should be discussed and documented as a part of multidisciplinary team planning with key clinical considerations.

Some L&D units can provide these services in the presence of trained nurses supported by obstetric anesthesiologists, maternal-fetal medicine specialists, and intensivists. Ease of access to the operating room for emergencies, the availability of medications and tools that are unique to the obstetric environment, and normalization of the birth process for the patient and multidisciplinary care team motivate this approach. In some settings, however, the resources and personnel to facilitate safe delivery for patients with highest risk CVD may be limited to the ICU or cardiac operating room. In these settings planning with the cardio-obstetrics team should include physician and nurse members of both the critical care, L&D, and neonatal ICU with input from pharmacy and respiratory therapy to ensure timely access to medications and equipment not routinely found outside of L&D.

Postpartum and interconception care

Though L&D represents a particularly vulnerable time for patients with CVD the recovery from intrapartum events and reversal of pregnancy physiology that characterizes the postpartum period is not without risk. Contemporary guidelines encourage an early postpartum visit 7 to 14 days after delivery to monitor for and educate patients about signs and symptoms that may signal cardiovascular decompensation [5]. New complaints or evolving symptoms should prompt timely diagnostic testing and engagement of the cardio-obstetrics team for close clinical monitoring. Routine anticipatory guidance including introductory conversations about postpartum contraception are key components of this visit.

This early postpartum visit can happen with any member of the cardio-obstetrics team but most centers emphasize the importance of a dedicated cardiology visit as a part of routine postpartum care. Scheduling this visit at or beyond 6 weeks affords the opportunity to pursue a TTE for increased or high-risk patients to monitor for postpartum cardiovascular function and dictate ongoing care. An added benefit of this cardiology visit is the potential to facilitate transition back to primary care—particularly for patients whose cardiovascular care was transitioned to a member of the cardio-obstetrics team for pregnancy. Additional considerations include transition of medications back to the prepregnancy regimen and incorporating the events of pregnancy into a longitudinal care plan using the lens of pregnancy as a window to future health.

The routine 6-week postpartum visit should ensure the receipt of reliable contraception with an emphasis on user-independent methods such as intrauterine devices due to their reliability and lower potential to interact with underlying CVD. The postpartum visit should allow for adequate time to debrief the patient's birthing experience through the lens of trauma-informed care, which may warrant a longer session to ensure adequate time to address these needs. Ensuring adequate time to address psychosocial concerns has the potential to improve postpartum mental health, ensure unmet social needs are identified and addressed, and solidify trust with the patient and her care team. Emphasizing the importance of planning for the next pregnancy is a key part of counseling as the postpartum visit for the current pregnancy may serve as a preconception consultation for the next.

Conclusion

The hemodynamic and psychosocial complexities of pregnancy for people with CVD demand early and frequent risk assessment with a goal of optimizing risk-appropriate care. The involvement of a cardio-obstetrics team with a standard approach to antenatal, intrapartum, and interconception care has the potential to optimize outcomes and is requisite for patients with increased and high-risk disease. Integrating input from obstetric care providers, cardiologists, anesthesiologists, and nurses is a critical component of holistic multidisciplinary care for all patients and must include contingency plans to address unanticipated events of labor delivery. Ensuring adequate person-centered postpartum follow-up may reduce the risk of morbidity and mortality through early recognition and response and has the potential to optimize outcomes for subsequent pregnancies. The rising prevalence of persons with CVD seeking pregnancy and growing contribution of CVD to pregnancy-related mortality underscore the importance of equitable and timely access to risk-appropriate care for patients with CVD.

CASE PRESENTATION

A 32-year-old gravida 1 para 0 presents to clinic at 12 weeks gestation with past medical history notable for mitral stenosis (MS) as a consequence of rheumatic heart disease as a child. She moved to town a couple of years ago to be closer to family and has yet to establish care with a cardiologist. She denies any complications of her cardiac disease since childhood but is concerned about worsening dyspnea challenging her ability to work as a server at a busy local restaurant. She is well appearing on exam with a heart rate of 90 beats per minute, blood pressure of 90/50 mmHg, breathing 14 times per minute with an oxygen saturation of 100% on room air. A transthoracic echocardiogram (TTE) is ordered urgently along with ambulatory Holter monitor while awaiting expedited intake to see one of the cardiology members of the cardio-obstetrics team. Her TTE demonstrates moderate MS with a valve area of 1.4 cm^2, a mean pressure gradient of 11 mmHg, left atrial enlargement, and ejection fraction of 60% without regional wall motion abnormalities. An ambulatory Holter monitor was unrevealing and a cardiopulmonary exercise test demonstrated rare premature ventricular complexes without associated symptoms.

She has a routine antepartum course but presents for follow-up at 32 weeks with TTE noting severe MS based on mean pressure gradient of 15 mmHg with stable valve area of 1.4 cm^2. She is started on metoprolol to lower heart rate to enhance ventricular filling time. The cardio-obstetrics team recommends early epidural with telemetry in labor to reduce the risk of catecholamine-associated atrial arrhythmias and aid in early identification. Her intrapartum plan also includes targeting even to slightly positive fluid balance, twice daily electrolytes, a preference for phenylephrine to address any epidural-associated hypotension, and intravenous (IV) metoprolol readily available in the event of arrhythmia. She undergoes induction of labor at 39 weeks that results in spontaneous vaginal birth. She receives 20 mg IV furosemide on postpartum day 2 in response to oxygen saturation of 96% with mild pulmonary edema on chest X-ray. She is stable and asymptomatic at a 1-week postpartum check-in and recovering well at her 6-week postpartum visit. She elects for an intrauterine device for contraception but notes her interest in pursuing another pregnancy within the next 2 years. She is scheduled for an interconception consultation with the cardio-obstetrics team to optimize medications and discuss the role of valve replacement prior to another pregnancy.

References

1. Creanga AA, Syverson C, Seed K, Callaghan WM. Pregnancy-related mortality in the United States, 2011-2013. Obstet Gynecol. 2017 Aug;130(2):366–73.

2. Briller J, Koch AR, Geller SE. Maternal cardiovascular mortality in Illinois, 2002-2011. Obstet Gynecol. 2017 May;129(5):819–26.

3. Easter SR, Valente AM, Economy KE. Creating a multidisciplinary pregnancy heart team. Curr Treat Options Cardiovasc Med. 2020 Jan 27;22(1):3.

4. Regizt-Zagrosek V, Roos-Hesselink JW, Bauersachs J, Blomstrom-Lundgvist C, Cifkova R, De Bonis M, et al. 2018 ESC guidelines for the management of cardiovascular diseases during pregnancy. Eur Heart J. 2018 Sep 7;39(34):3165–3241.

5. American College of Obstetricians and Gynecologists' Presidential Task Force on Pregnancy and Heart Disease and Committee on Practice Bulletins—Obstetrics. ACOG Practice Bulletin No. 212: pregnancy and heart disease. Obstet Gynecol. 2019 May;133(5):e320–65.

6. Mehta LS, Warnes CA, Bradley E, Burton T, Economy K, Mehran R, et al. Cardiovascular considerations in caring for pregnant patients: A scientific statement from the American Heart Association. Circulation. 2020;141:e884–903.

7. Silversides CK, Grewal J, Mason J, Sermer M, Kiess M, Rychel V, et al. Pregnancy outcomes in women with heart disease: The CARPREG II Study. J Am Coll Cardiol. 2018 May 29;71(21):2419–30.

8. Balci A, Sollie-Szarynska KM, van der Bijl AG, Ruys TP, Mulder BJ, Roos-Hesselink JW, et al. Prospective validation and assessment of cardiovascular and offspring risk models for pregnant women with congenital heart disease. Heart. 2014 Sep;100(17):1373–81.

9. American Association of Birth Centers; Association of Women's Health, Obstetric, and Neonatal Nurses; American College of Obstetricians and Gynecologists and Society for Maternal-Fetal Medicine, Kilpatrick SJ, Menard MK, Zahn CM; Centers for Disease Control and Prevention, Callaghan WM. Obstetric Care Consensus No. 9: levels of maternal care. Am J Obstet Gynecol. 2019 Dec;221(6):B19–B30.

10. Valente AM, Landzberg MJ Gauvreau K, Egidy-Assenza G, Barker N, Partington S, et al. Standardized outcomes in reproductive cardiovascular care: The STORCC initiative. Am Heart J. 2019 Aug 9;217:112–20.

11. Ruys TP, Roos-Hesselink JW, Pijuan-Domenech A, Vasario E, Gaisin IR, Iung B, et al. Is a planned caesarean section in women with cardiac disease beneficial? Heart. 2015 Apr;101(7):530–6.

12. Meng ML, Arendt KW. Obstetric anesthesia and heart disease: practical clinical considerations. Anesthesiology. 2021 Jul 1;135(1):164–83.

Chapter 17
Renal Disease

Shivani Patel

Division of Maternal-Fetal Medicine, Department of Obstetrics and Gynecology, University of Texas Southwestern Medical School, Dallas, TX, USA

Physiological changes in renal function during pregnancy

Renal function, water metabolism, and sodium homeostasis are among the systems undergoing physiologic changes during pregnancy, and these normal changes are critical to identify pathologic changes. The volume expansion of pregnancy is characterized by an increase in extracellular fluid and peripheral vasodilation that begins in the first trimester and continues until delivery. Of the 6–8 L of body water accumulated during pregnancy, the majority is held in the extracellular compartment with about 1200 mL accounted for in the plasma volume and the rest distributed to the interstitial space. Plasma osmolality drops as the osmostat is reset from 280 mOsm/kg H_2O to about 270 mOsm/ kg H_2O [1].

Glomerular filtration rate (GFR) begins to increase early in pregnancy and rises by 50% at the early second trimester that is sustained for the remainder of pregnancy [2]. Renal plasma flow also rises and peaks in the second trimester at about 60–80% above baseline prepregnancy levels. It falls back to about 50–60% above baseline in the third trimester [3,4]. This increase in GFR and renal plasma flow may be mediated by the hormone relaxin. This hormone increases renal nitric oxide production, which causes renal vasodilation and decreased renal afferent and efferent arteriolar resistance. Thus, there is a reliable fall in the serum creatinine from an average of 0.67 ± 0.2 mg/dL in the nonpregnant state to about 0.5 ± 0.1 mg/dL during pregnancy. This fall is reliable such that a level above 0.9 mg/dL raises suspicion for renal disease [5]. Prepregnancy levels are returned within 3 months after delivery.

Other changes are also noted in renal tubular function with regard to electrolytes and nonelectrolyte solutes. These alterations result in an increase in the fractional excretion of glucose, amino acids, and small peptides [6]. Glucosuria may be found in the setting of diabetes mellitus and glucose tolerance testing may be indicated. Protein excretion can be double nongravid levels. Indeed, the mean 24-hour urinary protein in pregnancy is 117 mg, and the upper 95% confidence limit is 259 mg, approaching the level of 300 mg/24 hours that defines proteinuria [7]. Although these findings suggest that there is a generalized reduction in the reabsorption of nonelectrolyte solutes during pregnancy, as was noted for sodium, there is a net retention of 350 mEq of potassium due to increased proximal tubular reabsorption [8]. Understanding these physiologic changes promotes recognition of renal disease and insufficiency.

Anatomic changes in the urinary tract during pregnancy

The kidney increases in size during pregnancy by about 1–1.5 cm in length and about 30% in volume [9,10]. The urinary collecting system dilates, with the right side more affected than the left [11,12]. The enlarging, dextrorotated uterus, enlarged right ovarian vein plexuses, and hormonal influences, primarily from progesterone, play a role in creating the physiologic hydronephrosis and ureteric dilation of pregnancy. These anatomic changes must be borne in mind when interpreting imaging studies in pregnant patients. As a result, there is a higher incidence of pyelonephritis complicating asymptomatic bacteriuria, especially on the right side.

Renal disease in pregnancy

Renal disease can be broadly characterized into primary and secondary, based on whether the disorder is inherent to the kidney or caused by other systemic diseases. When considering secondary etiologies in pregnancy, pregnancy-associated conditions such as preeclampsia should be

Queenan's Management of High-Risk Pregnancy: An Evidence-Based Approach, Seventh Edition. Edited by Catherine Y. Spong and Charles J. Lockwood.

considered. However, when renal disease is diagnosed before 20 weeks gestation, it is very rarely related to a pregnancy associated condition. The main markers for diagnosis of renal disease during pregnancy are the same markers identified outside of pregnancy: proteinuria and an elevated serum creatinine. Assessment of serum creatinine levels and urinalysis for proteinuria in the first trimester may identify preexisting renal disease or serve as baselines for later comparison later in pregnancy.

Proteinuria

Abnormal proteinuria in pregnancy is defined as urinary protein excretion greater than 300 mg/24 hours. Proteinuria is usually indicative of renal disease and can be characterized based on the site of the injury – glomerular or tubulointerstitial. Although this distinction is not always critical to management of the disease, it can be. When the excretion is >2.0 g/24 hours, the injury is usually glomerular. Symptoms increase as the amount of proteinuria rises. Although excretion <3.0 g/24 hours is usually asymptomatic, above that level, there may be edema due to the retention of sodium and water. Nephrotic syndrome is defined as proteinuria >3.0 g/24 hours with a serum albumin level <3.0 g/dL. Edema can develop only in the presence of hypoalbuminemia, and when this is present, edema will form when the sodium intake exceeds the maximum capacity for sodium excretion. Edema formation with nephrotic syndrome can be profound, affecting the legs, arms, and vulva. Vulvar edema can make the patient extremely uncomfortable and may increase the likelihood of vaginal lacerations at the time of delivery.

Although some women may enter pregnancy with proteinuria in nephrotic syndrome range secondary to known renal disease, it may also be caused by intrinsic renal disease that is unmasked by the pregnancy. Proteinuria may also result from renal disease that is secondary to a chronic systemic disease such as diabetes, hypertension, and lupus. The most common cause for the new onset of proteinuria in pregnancy is preeclampsia, a condition defined by new-onset hypertension (blood pressure >140/90 on two occasions at least 4 hours apart) and a 24-hour urine protein collection >300 mg.

If nephrotic syndrome is diagnosed, management is focused on limiting edema formation. Dietary sodium restriction should be limited to 1.5 g sodium daily. Prophylactic anticoagulation in nephrotic pregnant women has been recommended by some specialists, but there are few, if any, data to prove the efficacy of such treatment. In general, diuretics are avoided as these women already have reduced plasma volume and further intravascular volume depletion may impair uteroplacental perfusion. Furthermore, because blood pressure normally declines during pregnancy, saluretic therapy could precipitate circulatory collapse or thromboembolic episodes. However, in cases of severe edema, low doses of

loop diuretics may be used to reduce edema while minimizing the risk of excessive reduction of plasma volume. Note that the reduced circulating plasma volume that characterizes preeclampsia generally precludes using diuretics in the setting of edema secondary to proteinuria in severe preeclampsia.

Chronic kidney disease

Chronic kidney disease is classified based on GFR (Table 17.1). The severity of renal insufficiency during pregnancy is classified based on the creatinine at initial presentation or a serum creatinine within 6 months of conception if the patient presents for care late in her pregnancy. Using serum creatinine levels, mild insufficiency is defined as serum creatinine >0.8 to ≤1.4 mg/dL, moderate as >1.4 to ≤2.5 mg/dL, and severe as >2.5 mg/dL.

Adverse maternal and pregnancy-related outcomes are generally related to the degree of renal impairment and the presence or absence of hypertension [13]. Severity of chronic kidney disease is classified by the National Kidney Foundation based on GFR. Usually, women with mild renal dysfunction have successful obstetric outcomes and pregnancy does not appear to adversely affect their underlying renal condition. About 20% of women with mild renal impairment experience worsening proteinuria and 8% have a shift in the stage of kidney disease (Table 17.2). Of women with moderate to severe kidney dysfunction, 16–20% have a change in stage and 70–86% have worsening proteinuria. Based on serum creatinine, the greatest risk for accelerated progression to end-stage renal disease is seen in women with a serum creatinine above 2.0 mg/dL (177 µMol/L) in early pregnancy. Within 6 months postpartum, 23% of these women progress to end-stage renal disease.

Perinatal outcomes for women with mild renal disease are minimally affected compared to other stages (Table 17.3) [14]. Women with moderate to severe kidney

Table 17.1 Classification of chronic kidney disease

Stage	Glomerular filtration rate (mL/min/1.73m²)	Description
1	≥90	Normal
2	60–89	Mildly decreased
3	30–59	Moderately decreased
4	29–15	Severely decreased
5	<15	Kidney failure

Table 17.2 Classification of chronic kidney disease

	Stage 1	Stage 2	Stage 3	Stage 4–5
New-onset hypertension	8%	18%	47%	50%
Worsening proteinuria	21%	38%	87%	70%
Change in stage or initiation of renal replacement therapy	8%	13%	16%	20%

Table 17.3 Pregnancy-related outcomes by chronic kidney disease stage

	Stage 1	Stage 2	Stage 3	Stages 4–5
Cesarean delivery	48–57%	40–70%	78–82%	70–75%
Preterm birth	24–33%	40–50%	78–91%	90–100%
Fetal growth restriction	13%	7–18%	19–27%	50–75%
Admission to the neonatal intensive care unit	10–18%	20–28%	44–55%	70–100%

disease are at increased risk for adverse pregnancy outcomes. The presence of chronic hypertension further increases the risk for adverse pregnancy outcomes. Whether that is because of the inherent risks of hypertension-preeclampsia, fetal growth restriction, and preterm birth or because the presence of hypertension signifies a worst disease state is unknown.

Mild renal insufficiency

Women with mild renal insufficiency can be expected to have relatively uncomplicated pregnancies. In a large series examining pregnancy complicated by mild renal insufficiency, it was shown that new-onset hypertension or exacerbation of hypertension was seen in about 25%. In 63% of the women, new-onset proteinuria occurred during pregnancy. Decrease in renal function was seen in 16% but was small and generally reversible [15]. Several other authors documented similar findings [16–18]. Indeed, there is no evidence that pregnancy alters the long-term natural course of renal disease in these cases.

Moderate and severe renal insufficiency

Early reports of pregnancies in women with moderate and severe renal disease suggested that pregnancy accelerated progression of renal disease in about 50% of cases [19,20]. However, with improvements in management of hypertension, recent reports have been more encouraging. Two series suggest that about one third of women with moderate renal insufficiency would experience a permanent deterioration in their renal function [21,22]. Only 21% of women with a decline in renal function during pregnancy recovered to prepregnancy levels. Most women with stable renal function through the 6-week postpartum visit remained stable at 6 months postpartum.

Among pregnant women with moderate and severe renal insufficiency, <10% of the pregnancies showed a decline to end-stage disease within 12 months of delivery [23]. Significantly, the risk appeared to be low for women with baseline creatinine <2.0 mg/dL, with only 2% of these women showing an accelerated decline in renal function. The risk of a rapid decline to end-stage disease was significantly higher for women with baseline creatinine levels between 2.0 and 2.5 mg/dL. Among women with only moderate renal insufficiency, the most common maternal complications were worsening hypertension and worsening proteinuria (Table 17.2).

Fetal complications include preterm birth, fetal-growth restriction, and admission to the neonatal intensive care unit. In the subset of women with severe disease, 33% had an accelerated decline in renal function and obstetric complications were more frequent.

In summary, although neonatal outcomes are generally good for women with moderate and severe renal insufficiency, these pregnancies carry significant risks of obstetric and maternal complications, including a risk of accelerated loss of renal function, particularly for women with baseline creatinine levels >2.0 mg/dL.

Hypertensive disorders with renal insufficiency

Pregnant women with preexisting renal disease or essential hypertension are more susceptible to superimposed preeclampsia, which frequently occurs in midpregnancy or early in the third trimester. Superimposed preeclampsia, however, may be difficult to differentiate from aggravation of the underlying renal disorder. This is especially true in women with a glomerular disease that is prone to hypertension and proteinuria. In these situations, the patient should be hospitalized and managed as if she has superimposed preeclampsia. Detection of fetal growth restriction or fetal compromise, or both, is important and, will influence the timing of delivery.

Although obstetricians have traditionally preferred to use α-methyldopa as their antihypertensive of choice due to its long track record of safety for the fetus, other medications have been gaining in popularity, particularly labetalol and calcium channel blockers. Diltiazem has been proposed as an appropriate antihypertensive medication to use in pregnant women with renal disease, as it decreases proteinuria and preserves renal structure and function [24]. A small series suggested trends towards improved pregnancy outcomes in women treated with diltiazem compared to no therapy, but there were no statistically significant findings. Angiotensin-converting enzyme inhibitors and angiotensin receptor blockers are contraindicated in pregnancy due to their fetotoxic effects. Poorly controlled blood pressure has been implicated in the progressive decline in renal function in women with chronic renal disease [25].

Renal dialysis

In the setting of end-stage renal disease requiring dialysis, although less common, pregnancies can occur and be managed with both peritoneal dialysis and hemodialysis. In the largest series of pregnancies from a single center, 52 pregnancies were followed with hemodialysis [26]. Forty-seven of 54 fetuses survived, and four stillbirths and three neonatal deaths occurred for a perinatal mortality rate of 13%. The preterm delivery rate was 85% with a mean gestational age at delivery of 32 weeks. The authors found that preeclampsia was diagnosed in 19% of pregnancies, but these pregnancies accounted for a disproportionate share of the other obstetric complications, such as preterm birth and perinatal loss. Another small series suggested that increasing time on dialysis improves pregnancy outcomes [27]. The authors followed seven pregnancies in five women who were treated with an average dialysis time of 36 hours/week prior to conception and 48 hours/week during pregnancy. One pregnancy was terminated due to suspicion of a molar pregnancy; however, all six of the others survived with a mean gestational age at delivery of 36 weeks. Women requiring dialysis often have anemia, and erythropoietin is required.

During pregnancy, the frequency of peritoneal dialysis should be increased, and the exchange volumes decreased. The frequency of hemodialysis also should be increased to five to seven sessions per week to optimize control of uremia. Additionally, it should consist of slow-rate ultrafiltration, bicarbonate buffer, and minimal heparinization to avoid dialysis-induced hypotension and volume contraction.

Renal transplantation

Pregnancy following transplantation yields a live birth in 70–90% of cases [28,29]. The common adverse pregnancy outcomes are preterm birth, low birthweight, fetal growth restriction, and preeclampsia. Hypertension is seen in about 70% and preeclampsia in 30% [30]. Over 50% of these pregnancies are delivered preterm with a mean gestational age of about 36 weeks.

Graft rejection affects 2–4% of pregnancies in women with renal transplants [31]. It does not appear that pregnancy decreases long-term graft survival. As might be expected, pregnancy outcomes are improved in transplant recipients with serum creatinine levels ≤1.4 mg/dL, but fetal survival is about 75%, even with moderate renal insufficiency. Women should be counseled to wait 1 year before attempting pregnancy after a living related donor transplantation and 2 years after unrelated deceased donor transplantation to avoid problems with immunotherapy and rejection. Pregnancy has little, if any, effect on kidney function in women with renal allograft.

Management of pregnancies complicated by renal disease

As stated previously, a multidisciplinary approach is best under the coordinated care of an obstetrician, maternal–fetal medicine subspecialist, and a nephrologist. The initial laboratory tests should include those that help in the early detection of renal impairment, as well as provide a baseline for comparison later when superimposed

preeclampsia may need to be assessed. Thus, besides the usual prenatal screening tests, the following baseline parameters should be determined:
• Serum creatinine, blood urea nitrogen, albumin, and electrolytes.
• 24-hour urine collection for volume, protein, and creatinine clearance. Quantification of urine protein can also be done by a random protein-to-creatinine ratio.
• Urinalysis and urine culture (to detect and treat asymptomatic bacteriuria).
• Uric acid level, aspartate and alanine aminotransferases, complete blood count, and platelet count.
• Lactic dehydrogenase, prothrombin time, and partial thromboplastin time may also be considered in the baseline assessment.

Generally, women can be followed every 2 weeks until 30 to 32 weeks gestation and weekly thereafter. The number and frequency of prenatal visits should be based on the severity of renal disease and the presence of other complications, such as hypertension and fetal growth restriction. Maternal renal parameters should be assessed every 4 weeks throughout pregnancy unless more frequent evaluations become necessary. Low-dose aspirin is recommended for prevention of preeclampsia [32].

Fetal surveillance such as biophysical profile testing is best started at approximately 32 weeks gestation, especially in nephrotic patients with hypoalbuminemia. Ultrasonographic examinations for pregnancy dating, fetal anatomy and monitoring fetal growth are also an integral part of surveillance. Early delivery is not undertaken solely for renal impairment, but rather may be indicated for obstetric indications or acutely worsening renal disease [33].

Anemia is a common clinical issue in pregnant women requiring dialysis. Treatment of anemia includes blood transfusions as indicated and administration of erythropoietin to maintain hemoglobin of at least 10 or 11 g/dL. Vitamin supplementation is also part of the dialysis regimen.

Renal biopsy during pregnancy is important in the setting of rapid unexplained renal function deterioration or profound symptomatic nephrotic syndrome prior to 32 weeks gestation. In experienced clinicians, a renal biopsy, if indicated, can be safely done in pregnant women with controlled blood pressures and normal coagulation studies.

Conclusion

In summary, although many women with renal disease have successful pregnancy outcomes, significant risks remain for both fetus and mother, especially when maternal serum creatinine levels are >2.0 mg/dL. Women with severe renal insufficiency should be counseled about the risks, and preferably undergo preconception counseling to optimize disease prior to pregnancy.

CASE PRESENTATION

A 32-year-old woman with history of renal transplant at the age of 26 due to lupus nephritis presented for care during her first pregnancy. Her medical history was also complicated by chronic hypertension for which she takes nifedipine XL 30 mg daily. She has a baseline serum creatinine of 0.6 mg/dL and no proteinuria. During pregnancy, her creatinine increased to 1.0 mg/dL. She was maintained on tacrolimus, which required increased dosing during pregnancy due to the normal pregnancy-associated plasma volume expansion. Her fetus was followed with serial growth ultrasounds and weekly biophysical profiles beginning at 34 weeks gestation. She underwent induction of labor at 39 weeks gestation. She had a normal vaginal delivery without complications.

This case illustrates a successful pregnancy outcome in the setting of a kidney transplant, normal renal function, and chronic hypertension. It illustrates that despite the comorbidity of hypertension and an increase in serum creatinine, most patients with normal renal function 1–2 years following renal transplant will have a successful pregnancy outcome.

References

1. Lindheimer MD, Davison JM, Katz AI. The kidney and hypertension in pregnancy: twenty exciting years. Semin Nephrol. 2001 Mar;21(2):173–89.

2. Lopes van Balen VA, van Gansewinkel TAG, de Haas S, Spaan JJ, Ghossein-Doha C, van Kuijk SMJ, et al. Maternal kidney function during pregnancy: a systematic review and meta-analysis. Ultrasound Obstet Gynecol. 2019 Sep;54(3):297–307.

3. Pregnancy and renal disease. Lancet. 1975;2:801–2.

4. Conrad KP, Gaber LW, Lindheimer MD. The kidney in normal pregnancy and preeclampsia. In: Taylor RN, Roberts JM, Cunningham FG, editors. Chesley's hypertensive disorders in pregnancy. 4th ed. Amsterdam: Academic Press; 2015. p.335–77.

5. Wiles K, Bramham K, Seed PT, Nelson-Piercy C, Lightstone L, Chappell LC. Serum creatinine in pregnancy: a systematic review. Kidney Int Rep. 2018 Oct 29;4(3):408–19.

6. Davison JM, Hytten FE. The effect of pregnancy on the renal handling of glucose. Br J Obstet Gynaecol. 1975;82:374–81.

7. Higby K, Suiter CR, Phelps JY, Siler-Khodr T, Langer O. Normal values of urinary albumin and total protein excretion during pregnancy. Am J Obstet Gynecol. 1994;171:984–9.

8. Lindheimer MD, Richardson DA, Ehrlich EN, Katz AI. Potassium homeostasis in pregnancy. J Reprod Med. 1987;32:517–22.

9. Bailey RR, Rolleston GL. Kidney length and ureteric dilatation in the puerperium. J Obstet Gynaecol Br Commonw. 1971;78:55–61.

10. Christensen T, Klebe JG, Bertelsen V, Hansen HE. Changes in renal volume during normal pregnancy. Acta Obstet Gynecol Scand. 1989;68:541–3.

11. Fried AM, Woodring JH, Thompson DJ. Hydronephrosis of pregnancy: a prospective sequential study of the course of dilatation. J Ultrasound Med. 1983;2:255–9.

12. Schulman A, Herlinger H. Urinary tract dilatation in pregnancy. Br J Radiol. 1975;48:638–45.

13. Fischer MJ, Lehnerz SD, Hebert JR, Parikh CR. Kidney disease is an independent risk factor for adverse fetal and maternal outcomes in pregnancy. Am J Kidney Dis. 2004;43(3):415–23.

14. Hladunewich MA, Melamed N, Bramham K. Pregnancy across the spectrum of chronic kidney disease. Kidney Int. 2016;89(5):995–1007.

15. Katz AI, Davison JM, Hayslett JP, Singson E, Lindheimer MD. Pregnancy in women with kidney disease. Kidney Int. 1980;18:192–206.

16. Jungers P, Forget D, Henry-Amar M, Albouze G, Fournier P, Vischer U, et al. Chronic kidney disease and pregnancy. Adv Nephrol Necker Hosp. 1986;15:103–41.

17. Abe S, Amagasaki Y, Konishi K, Kato E, Sakaguchi H, Iyori S. The influence of antecedent renal disease on pregnancy. Am J Obstet Gynecol. 1985;153:508–14.

18. Barceló P, López-Lillo J, Cabero L, del Río G. Successful pregnancy in primary glomerular disease. Kidney Int. 1986;30:914–19.

19. Bear RA. Pregnancy in patients with renal disease. A study of 44 cases. Obstet Gynecol. 1976;48:13–18.

20. Kincaid-Smith P, Fairley KF, Bullen M. Kidney disease and pregnancy. Med J Aust. 1967;2:1155–9.

21. Hou SH, Grossman SD, Madias NE. Pregnancy in women with renal disease and moderate renal insufficiency. Am J Med. 1985;78:185–94.

22. Imbasciati E, Pardi G, Capetta P, Ambroso G, Bozzetti P, Pagliari B, et al. Pregnancy in women with chronic renal failure. Am J Nephrol. 1986;6:193–8.

23. Jones DC, Hayslett JP. Outcome of pregnancy in women with moderate or severe renal insufficiency. N Engl J Med. 1996;335:226–32.

24. Khandelwal M, Kumanova M, Gaughan JP, Reece EA. Role of diltiazem in pregnant women with chronic renal disease. J Matern Fetal Neonat Med. 2002;12:408–12.

25. Zucchelli P, Zuccalà A, Borghi M, Fusaroli M, Sasdelli M, Stallone C, et al. Long-term comparison between captopril and nifedipine in the progression of renal insufficiency. Kidney Int. 1992;42:452–8.

26. Luders C, Castro MC, Titan SM, De Castro I, Elias RM, Abensur H, et al. Obstetric outcome in pregnant women on long-term dialysis: a case series. Am J Kidney Dis. 2010;56:77–85.

27. Barua M, Hladunewich M, Keunen J, Pierratos A, McFarlane P, Sood M, et al. Successful pregnancies on nocturnal home hemodialysis. Clin J Am Soc Nephrol. 2008;3:392–6.

28. Deshpande NA, James NT, Kucirka LM, Boyarsky BJ, Garonzik-Wang JM, Montgomery RA, et al. Pregnancy outcomes in kidney transplant recipients: a systematic review and meta-analysis. Am J Transplant. 2011 Nov; 11(11):2388–404.

29. Bramham K, Nelson-Piercy C, Gao H, Pierce M, Bush N, Spark P, et al. Pregnancy in renal transplant recipients: a UK national cohort study. Clin J Am Soc Nephrol. 2013 Feb;8(2):290–8.

30. Fuchs KM, Wu D, Ebcioglu Z. Pregnancy in renal transplant recipients. Semin Perinatol. 2007;31:339–47.

31. Mastrobattista JM, Gomez-Lobo V. Pregnancy after solid organ transplantation. Obstet Gynecol. 2008;112:919–32.

32. ACOG Committee Opinion No. 743: low-dose aspirin use during pregnancy. Obstet Gynecol. 2018 Jul;132(1):e44–e52.

33. ACOG Committee Opinion No. 764: medically indicated late-preterm and early-term deliveries. Obstet Gynecol. 2019 Feb;133(2):e151–5.

Chapter 18
Pregnancy in Transplant Patients

Lisa A. Coscia[1], Serban Constantinescu[1,2], and Michael J. Moritz[1,3,4]

[1]Transplant Pregnancy Registry International, Philadelphia, PA, USA
[2]Department of Medicine, Section of Nephrology, Hypertension and Kidney Transplantation, Lewis Katz School of Medicine at Temple University, Philadelphia, PA, USA
[3]Deparment of Surgery, Section of Transplantation, Lehigh Valley Health Network, Allentown, PA, USA
[4]Morsani College of Medicine, University of South Florida, Tampa, FL, USA

Transplantation has evolved as a treatment of choice for many people with end-stage organ disease. In the United States in 2021, 15604 females received a solid organ transplant [1]. With the advancement of transplant technique and immunosuppression and increased quality of life post transplant, having a family is an option for transplant recipients. This chapter reviews maternal and newborn outcomes and prepregnancy, antepartum, and postpartum care.

It has been over 60 years since the first child was born to a kidney transplant recipient, and women with virtually all types of organ transplants have now had successful pregnancies. Recently, patients with Mayer-Rokitansky-Kuster-Hauser syndrome have received uterus transplants [2]. Nevertheless, these are high-risk pregnancies that require expert obstetric care in coordination with other specialists [3].

Prepregnancy assessment and counseling

Contraceptive and preconception counseling is important for transplant recipients of childbearing age before the transplant, continuing post transplant, and before a pregnancy is attempted [3,4]. Transplant recipients contemplating pregnancy should be in good health with no evidence of graft rejection (Box 18.1). Other comorbid conditions such as diabetes mellitus, hypertension, and cardiovascular or pulmonary disease should be under good control prior to pregnancy. The ideal time for pregnancy has not been established; however, based on data from the Transplant Pregnancy Registry International (TPRI) and meta-analyses, it is advisable to wait for transplant function to be stable, immunosuppression to have tapered to maintenance doses, and for the transplant to be

rejection free for at least 1 year before conceiving. Practically, this means waiting at least 1–2 years after transplant [5,6] An assessment of the recipient's family and partner support as well as a tactful but honest discussion of her life expectancy and potential pregnancy complications is important. Long-term organ allograft survival rates have improved, but the transplant recipient and family should be aware that she may not live to raise her child into adulthood.

Most posttransplant pregnancy information comes from the TPRI. TPRI is a voluntary pregnancy registry that has been collecting information from all types of solid organ transplant recipients since 1991 [7].

Antepartum care

The greatest experience is with pregnancy after kidney transplantation, which is applicable to the other organs though there are obviously differences. Early diagnosis of pregnancy is important, and an early, first-trimester ultrasound examination will establish an accurate due date. Antenatal management includes frequent prenatal visits with serial assessment of maternal allograft function and immunosuppressive drug levels plus prompt diagnosis and treatment of infections, anemia, hypertension, and preeclampsia. Nausea and vomiting or hyperemesis gravidarum can lead to decreased absorption of and inadequate immunosuppression. In the second and third trimesters, altered gut motility, increasing volume of distribution, and increasing fetal liver metabolism can negatively impact immunosuppressive medication exposure [8]. Close fetal surveillance for preterm labor is necessary, and the risk of fetal growth restriction is monitored by serial ultrasound examinations. Theoretically, women can become Rh sensitized from the allograft or transfusions which will be detected on the routine first-trimester screen.

The incidence of intraepithelial and invasive cancer of the genital tract in patients taking immunosuppressive drugs is increased, and regular cervical cytology and screening for malignancies are vital components of clinical care [9]. Condyloma and human papillomavirus (HPV) are common in transplant patients, but if the patient is negative for HPV, she should receive the HPV vaccine. Vaccine responsiveness is less in the immunosuppressed, so pretransplant vaccination is best. All immunosuppressive regimens are associated with increased risk of neoplasia, particularly lymphoma and skin cancer (squamous cell). Age-appropriate cancer screening is strongly recommended.

Urinary tract infections are particularly common in kidney transplant patients with up to a twofold increase in the incidence of pyelonephritis. Asymptomatic bacteriuria should be treated for at least 7 days with follow-up urine cultures, and suppressive doses of antibiotics may be needed. Most infections during pregnancy are manageable and are not life threatening. Other bacterial and fungal infections associated with immunosuppression include endometritis, wound infections, skin abscesses, and pneumonia, often with unusual organisms.

Transplant recipients are susceptible to reactivation of viral infections such as cytomegalovirus (CMV), herpes genitalis (herpes simplex, HSV), and HPV. The transplanted organ is a source of CMV, and recipients typically receive prophylaxis against CMV for 3–7 months post transplant when the risk of infection is highest. The greatest risk of congenital infection in the fetus is with primary CMV infection during pregnancy, but reactivation CMV infection in immunosuppressed women has caused congenital CMV in the infant [10].

Hepatitis B (HBV) and C (HCV) pose a risk for both the mother and her fetus. Effective curative antihepatitis C treatment is available and should be completed before pregnancy as the antivirals have potential toxicity. Vertical transmission of hepatitis C occurs in 5–15% of live births, and about half of the infants will acquire chronic infection. Hepatitis B's vertical transmission rate exceeds 90%, but >95% of transmissions can be stopped with administration of hepatitis B immunoglobulin and HBV vaccine to the newborn with completion of the vaccination series. Acyclovir as prophylaxis or treatment of HSV can be used safely during pregnancy.

Review of common agents for maintenance immunosuppression

Obstetricians should understand the impact of immunosuppressive therapies on pregnancy and potential side effects. Maintenance immunosuppression begins at transplant and absent the development of a new problem, does not change. The most common regimen of immunosuppression is tacrolimus, a mycophenolic acid (MPA, mycophenolate mofetil or mycophenolic acid) product with or without prednisone [11]. Steroid sparing regimens have become more common since 2000. Multidrug regimens are standard. New agents occasionally become available. This review does not include immunosuppression used peri transplant or to treat acute rejection episodes [12] (Table 18.1).

Prednisone or prednisolone is the usual maintenance corticosteroid and intravenous corticosteroids are used to treat acute rejection episodes. As prednisone is largely metabolized by placental 11-hydroxygenase to the relatively inactive 11-keto form, the fetus is exposed to only

Table 18.1 Common transplant maintenance immunosuppressive medications

	Branded name in the United States	Old FDA category[a]
Relatively safe at contemporary clinical dosing:		
Prednisone, prednisolone		B
Azathioprine	Imuran®	C
Cyclosporine	Sandimmune®, Neoral®, Gengraf®	C
Tacrolimus	Prograf®	C
Tacrolimus once daily	Astagraf XL®, Envarsus XR®	C
Contraindicated during pregnancy		
Mycophenolate mofetil	CellCept®	D
Mycophenolic acid	Myfortic®	D
Insufficient data to affirm safety		
Sirolimus	Rapamune®	C
Everolimus	Zortress®	C
Belatacept	Nulojix®	C

[a]Category A, controlled studies, no risk; Category B, no evidence of risk in humans; Category C, risk cannot be ruled out; Category D, positive evidence of risk; Category X, contraindicated in pregnancy. FDA, Food and Drug Administration.

10% of the maternal dose of the active drug. Most patients are maintained on moderate doses of prednisone (5–10 mg/day), which are relatively safe with few fetal effects [13].

Azathioprine and its more toxic metabolite 6-mercaptopurine are purine analogs whose principal action is to decrease lymphocyte proliferation by inhibiting DNA replication; hence they are classified as antimetabolites. The primary maternal hazards of azathioprine administration are increased risks of infection and neoplasia. Between 64% and 90% of azathioprine crosses the placenta in human pregnancies, but the majority is the inactive form thiouric acid. Assessment of teratogenicity is based largely on two early series that reported an incidence of congenital anomalies of 9% and 6.4% [14]. Larger data sets have not seen a specific pattern of defects emerge, and azathioprine is not associated with more congenital malformations than seen in the general population [15–17]. This agent is not commonly initiated since the advent of the more effective MPA products, except for pregnancy where azathioprine is used to replace MPA products prepregnancy (or during pregnancy when an unplanned pregnancy is discovered) as its safety profile is much better than MPA's.

Cyclosporine is a cyclic polypeptide whose major inhibitory effect is on T-cell-mediated responses by inhibiting production of interleukin (IL)-2 via the calcineurin-dependent pathway and is classified as a calcineurin inhibitor. It became a standard component of immunosuppressive regimens in the 1980s. The drug has a propensity for nephrotoxicity and hypertension. Other side effects include hirsutism, tremor, and gingival hyperplasia. Cyclosporine readily crosses the placenta, but there is no evidence of teratogenicity in humans [16,18–20].

Tacrolimus, also a calcineurin inhibitor, is a macrolide widely used in solid organ transplantation, replacing cyclosporine [11]. Side effects include an increase in glucose intolerance and new-onset diabetes mellitus, nephrotoxicity, and neurotoxicity (headache, tremor, peripheral neuropathy) [21]. Cord blood concentrations are approximately 50% of maternal levels. Neonatal hyperkalemia has been reported [22]. Tacrolimus has not been associated with congenital malformations [12,19,23].

MPA, an antimetabolite, is a reversible inhibitor of inosine monophosphate dehydrogenase which blocks *de novo* purine synthesis via a pathway that lymphocytes are much more dependent on than other cell types. Side effects include bone marrow suppression specifically leukopenia, abdominal pain, and diarrhea. MPA is destroyed by gastric acidity and so is available in two forms, an enteric coated tablet released downstream and mycophenolate mofetil, where the mofetil moiety lends acid-degradation resistance. MPA is a teratogen and exposure results in a very high incidence of first-trimester miscarriage (up to 52%) and in liveborn babies a pattern of malformations that form the distinctive mycophenolate embryopathy [24,25]. The specific structural anomalies in these newborns are microtia, auditory canal atresia, cleft lip and palate, micrognathia, hypertelorism, ocular coloboma, short fingers, and hypoplastic nails and are seen in up to 14% of first-trimester MPA exposed liveborn babies. In 2008, the Food and Drug Administration (FDA) issued a black box warning for increased risk of miscarriage and increase and pattern of congenital malformations with MPA exposure in utero and changed the FDA pregnancy category to D. Patients taking this agent should use effective contraception beginning 4 weeks before starting MPA and continued for 6 weeks after the last dose. Most transplant recipients can be switched to azathioprine preconception for a planned pregnancy.

For new classes of immunosuppressant agents, less is known about their teratogenic potential or safety during pregnancy. Sirolimus and everolimus are lymphocyte inhibitors downstream from IL-2 generation. The major adverse effects are edema, hypercholesterolemia, hypertriglyceridemia, and thrombocytopenia. Based on limited experience, they have not been associated with specific fetal malformations [26]. Belatacept is a selective T cell costimulation blocker that is parenteral only, given via monthly infusion, and is used in place of calcineurin inhibitors. Belatacept is used with MPA and steroids [27] There are only a few reports of pregnancy exposure with no reports of congenital malformations [7,28, 29].

Before discussing specific types of organ recipients, a comment on interpreting outcome results. As may be evident from the preceding discussion, the factor that most heavily affects outcomes, particularly live birth rate, miscarriage rate, and birth defect rate, is the proportion of pregnancies with first-trimester exposure to MPA. This is more influential than type of transplanted organ, original disease causing organ failure, additional immunosuppressants, or other factors. MPA use varies widely across time (approved for clinical use in the United States in 1995, European Union in 1996) and with recognition of teratogenicity in 2006 [30], and across geography due to its high cost relative to azathioprine. Single-center or single-country reports can vary widely in reported outcomes and MPA use can be difficult to assess, depending on the level of detail of immunosuppressants provided in the report. TPRI data are summarized in Table 18.2.

Kidney transplant

End-stage renal disease requiring dialysis affects about 800 000 people in the United States, where 42% are female, and 15% are <44 years of age [31]. Kidney transplantation is associated with longer survival than dialysis and can

Table 18.2 Transplant Pregnancy Registry International: Newborn outcomes across solid organ transplant recipients

	Kidney	Liver	Kidney-pancreas	Heart	Lung
Live births	**1735**	**528**	**94**	**131**	**35**
Mean gestational age (wk)	35.8	36.7	34.1	36.2	34.0
Late preterm (32–<37 wk)	37%	26%	51%	32%	34%
Very preterm (28–<32 wk)	6%	5%	12%	5%	20%
Mean birthweight (g)	2555	2772	2142	2595	2192
Low (<2500 g)	42%	28%	62%	37%	66%
Very low (<1500 g)	10%	7%	21%	10%	23%
Birth defects	4.6%	5.5%	2.1%	8.4%	8.6%
Child follow-up (yr)	14.0	9.1	9.9	7.9	8.3

restore a better quality of life than dialysis. It is also more cost effective for the health care system. With steady growth, more than 24 000 kidney transplants were performed in 2019 [32].

A meta-analysis examined 4174 kidney recipients with 6712 pregnancies [6]. Overall, the rate of live birth was 72.9%. Preeclampsia occurred in 21.5%. The rate of cesarean delivery was 62.6% and 43.1% were premature (<37 weeks) with neonatal mortality of 3.8%. The rate of acute rejection during pregnancy was 9.4%.

If preconception graft function is adequate, as evidenced by a serum creatinine of less than 1.5 mg/dL and no or minimal proteinuria, a pregnancy can be expected to progress normally. Glomerular filtration rate may decrease during the third trimester but returns to prepregnancy function postpartum. Chronic hypertension and preeclampsia are the most common complications in pregnant female kidney recipients and contribute to the increase in preterm births, and perinatal mortality [6,7]. Hypertension is present in at least half of these pregnancies, and over 20% develop preeclampsia.

Pregnancy is more complicated in patients with prepregnancy elevated creatinine, proteinuria, or chronic rejection [6,7]. Acute rejection is usually asymptomatic, diagnosed only by evaluation of a rise in creatinine or worsening proteinuria, and worked up by ultrasound and biopsy. Clinically, the diagnosis is difficult because of overlap with other disorders including pyelonephritis, preeclampsia, and nephrotoxicity from immunosuppressant drugs. It is crucial to establish the diagnosis of rejection before initiating antirejection therapy. A recent study of TPRI recipients compared those with rejection to those with preeclampsia. Those with acute rejection had relatively higher serum creatinine levels whereas preeclampsia was associated with relatively increased proteinuria. It is imperative to differentiate the two diagnoses as acute rejection in pregnancies confers higher

risk of prematurity and eventual transplant loss for the mother in contrast to those diagnosed with preeclampsia [33,34]. Treatment of acute rejection during pregnancy is complex, balancing the need to restore and preserve the integrity and function of the transplant organ with potential fetotoxicity, and is not discussed here in further detail.

Other organ transplant patients

Kidney-pancreas

Pancreas transplantation, usually in conjunction with a kidney transplant, is a treatment option for patients with type 1 insulin-dependent diabetes mellitus with advanced diabetic nephropathy. One-year graft survival rate for female recipients is approximately 95%, with a 5-year graft survival rate of 79% [1]. Most pancreas transplants are performed simultaneously with the kidney transplant, but a minority are performed in patients who previously received a kidney transplant, often from a living donor.

Antepartum and intrapartum management is similar to that for kidney transplant patients. However, the diabetogenic effects of pregnancy, corticosteroids, and other immunosuppressive drugs can all lead to or aggravate hyperglycemia, macrosomia, and other diabetic sequelae. Euglycemia should be present preconception, and glucose tolerance testing (GTT) is warranted prior to 20 weeks. If hyperglycemia is present, diet and insulin therapy should be instituted at that time. If the GTT screen is normal, it should be repeated at 24–28 weeks as with any pregnant patient. Most pancreas transplant patients have maintained euglycemia throughout pregnancy and labor. Kidney-pancreas recipients tend to have more preeclampsia, 34% compared to their kidney-alone counterparts at 29%. The infants tend to be born at an earlier gestational age (GA) 34.1 weeks compared to kidney alone recipients with a mean GA of 35.8 weeks, and have lower birthweight newborns 2142 g compared to kidney recipients, 2555 g [7].

Liver

In the United States 9000 liver transplants are performed annually, 5% from living donors [1,32]. Of the solid organs transplanted, the liver is the least likely to develop rejection, and consequently liver recipients take less immunosuppression than other transplant recipients. Liver recipients have a liveborn rate of 71–100% with a rejection rate of 4.8% [7,35,36]. The rate of preeclampsia is lower than for kidney recipients, 12.8%. Akin to kidney, episodes of liver rejection are not symptomatic, presenting with elevated liver tests (transaminases, bilirubin, biliary enzymes), which can overlap with cholestasis of pregnancy. Cholestasis of pregnancy is much more common in liver recipients, 17%, compared to 1–5% in the general population. Suspected graft rejection needs biopsy confirmation.

Heart

Since 1988, 22 341 US women have undergone heart transplants. About 20% of recipients are <34 years of age. One-year graft survival in women is 91% and 5-year survival is 76% [1]. The denervated heart will not respond reliably to vagally mediated medications (specifically little or no response to atropine) but does respond to direct acting medications (e.g. isoproterenol as a chronotrope). The transplanted heart may be more sensitive to β-adrenergic agonists because of an increase in β-receptors [37].

The transplanted heart must adapt to the physiologic changes of pregnancy. One third of patients have tricuspid regurgitation 1 year post transplant, which may worsen with the increased blood volume associated with pregnancy. Almost one third of cardiac transplant patients have coronary artery disease by 3 years after the transplant and up to 50% have coronary atherosclerosis at 5 years [38]. Myocardial ischemia does not cause chest pain with no afferent innervation, and paroxysmal dyspnea may be the only presenting symptom. Maternal graft rejection episodes occur in approximately 7.1–11.8% of pregnancies [38,39], but most are not clinically evident and are diagnosed by routine surveillance biopsy. Cardiac biopsies are obtained from the right ventricle guided by fluoroscopy or echocardiography. The increased rates of hypertension, preeclampsia, prematurity, and low birthweight are similar to those of other transplant patients [7,38,39]. It is vital to involve an anesthesiologist to formulate a well-organized plan for labor and delivery because these patients are very sensitive to volume shifts and to catecholamines.

Lung

Of the 2759 lung transplants in the United States in 2019, 282 or 10% were performed in recipients less than 34 years of age [32]. One-year survival rate is 89%, which decreases to 56% at 5 years [1,7,40–42]. The lung is relatively immunogenic and more prone to rejection, and lung recipients take more immunosuppression and have higher rejection risks and rates. The higher attrition after the first post-transplant year is attributable to chronic rejection, its presence, severity, and progression. Before any consideration of pregnancy, assessment of the lungs to characterize the presence of chronic rejection is vital. Noninvasively, lungs are assessed via serial measurements of forced expiratory volume 1, but again rejection is a biopsy diagnosis. Lung functions, gas exchange, lymphatic drainage, etc. are not typically normal post transplant, and susceptibility to pulmonary edema from fluid overload is a definite possibility. Lung recipients tend to deliver earlier,

mean GA 34.0 weeks and long-term survival continues to be a concern for these recipients post partum [40].

Other transplant groups

In addition to the major organ groups, other smaller cohorts exist including small bowel, pancreas alone, dual transplants (heart-kidney, liver-kidney), multivisceral, and the newly emerging uterus transplant [7]. Overall, these recipients have greater risks than other solid-organ recipients. Caution is warranted as there are often multiple disease processes responsible, transplant function in multiple organs must be assessed and managed, and rejection risks are higher. Obstetric outcomes have been reported in small numbers for these groups.

Uterus

Although considered an experimental therapy for uterine factor infertility in the United States, reports are growing of live births after living and deceased donor uterus transplant [2,43]. There are obvious differences compared to "vital" organ transplants. The cervix is surgically closed at transplant and the first posttransplant year immunosuppression is tacrolimus-MPA product based while the uterus is assessed for rejection by biopsy. After the first year, if the patient is rejection free, MPA is switched to azathioprine and in vitro fertilization can proceed. Cesarean delivery is mandatory. After one, or at most two successful pregnancies, the transplant uterus is removed, and the immunosuppression stopped. Thus, the period of immunosuppression is limited, avoiding its chronic consequences. Uterine transplant recipients will be an emerging recipient cohort in the future.

Intrapartum management

The timing of delivery is often dependent on events such as premature labor, premature ruptured membranes, or severe preeclampsia. The extraperitoneal location of the transplanted kidney in the iliac fossa usually does not interfere with vaginal delivery. There are no particular contraindications to induction, labor, or vaginal delivery in organ transplant recipients. Based on data from 1865 pregnancies with a trial of labor vs. scheduled cesarean section, a trial of labor was associated with improved neonatal and maternal outcomes among kidney and liver transplant recipients [44]. Because of an increased susceptibility to infection, vaginal examinations should be kept to a minimum and artificial rupture of membranes and internal monitoring performed only when specifically indicated.

Cesarean delivery should be based on accepted obstetric indications. Operative deliveries in these patients are managed with prophylactic antibiotics and corticosteroids when indicated and require strict asepsis and careful attention to hemostasis. A lower midline vertical incision provides the greatest exposure and avoids the region of the transplanted kidney and the transplant ureter. A low transverse uterine incision is possible, but the obstetrician should be aware of the anatomic alterations associated with the transplanted kidney and to avoid inadvertent damage to the blood supply, urinary drainage, or bladder in kidney recipients. A subset of pancreas transplants have a duodenal-bladder diagnosis (bladder-drained pancreas) and this is in danger at Cesarean—a transplant surgeon should be present at the time of Cesarean surgery.

Obstetric emergencies

Acute emergencies may arise in pregnant transplant patients with severe consequences that require aggressive management and intensive care. These are best managed in a tertiary setting where the transplant surgeon, high-risk obstetrician, medicine subspecialists, intensivists, and neonatologists can work together. Most difficult is severe and chronic rejection or allograft vasculopathy with loss of graft function threatening the life of the mother and fetus. That is why establishment of adequate prepregnancy transplant organ function is critical when planning a pregnancy. Kidney transplant recipients with deteriorating function may require dialysis, and other organ recipients may require a variety of supportive measures or retransplantation. Sepsis and overwhelming infections are a constant threat in these women, and patients have died of meningitis, pneumonia, gastroenteritis, HCV, HBV, and HIV [1, 2, 23, 24]. With the high incidence of hypertension and preeclampsia, it is not surprising that HELLP (hemolysis, elevated liver enzymes, low platelets) syndrome, stroke, and eclampsia have occurred [1,2,23,24]. Other causes of morbidity that have required emergency procedures or surgery include obstruction of the transplant ureter, antepartum bleeding, uterine rupture, small bowel injury at cesarean delivery (including injury to the transplant duodenum as part of a pancreatic transplant), postpartum hemorrhage, abdominal wound dehiscence, and pelvic abscess.

The baby

All immunosuppressive drugs cross the placental barrier and diffuse into the fetal circulation. As there is no convincing evidence that prednisone, azathioprine, cyclosporine, or tacrolimus produces congenital abnormalities in the human fetus, they are the immunosuppressants of choice for pregnancy. Other than preterm birth, most offspring born to these mothers have had relatively uncomplicated neonatal courses. Mothers have historically been advised against breastfeeding, but the dosage of immunosuppressive drugs detected in breastmilk and delivered to the infant is quite small and breastfeeding should no longer be viewed as absolutely contraindicated [45,46]. Comparison of mean gestational ages and birthweights among TPRI recipients is shown in Table 18.2.

Most infants have progressed normally through childhood [7,47–50]. Theoretical concerns have been raised about the potential for delayed adverse effects in adulthood such as late development of fertility problems, autoimmune disorders, or neoplasia [49,50]. This is difficult to study lacking suitable controls and the reluctance to expose ostensibly healthy infants to any invasive procedures including phlebotomy, but observational studies although imperfect have thus far not detected any worrisome signals. It remains important that all offspring exposed to these agents in utero have appropriate follow-up and participation in a registry such as the TPRI, constantly watching for evidence of health risks to the offspring.

CASE PRESENTATION

A 26-year-old primigravida underwent heart transplantation for idiopathic dilated cardiomyopathy and intractable congestive heart failure. When she conceived 4 years after the transplant, she was receiving conventional doses of cyclosporine, azathioprine, and prednisone.

The patient was followed from 7 weeks gestation with frequent antepartum visits and serial sonograms for fetal growth. Right heart catheterizations and cardiac biopsies showed stable cardiac function throughout pregnancy. The pregnancy progressed normally until 33 weeks. At that time, she developed pruritus, slight icterus, and a blood pressure of 130/90 mmHg. Admission laboratory tests were normal except for a hematocrit of 28.5%, platelet count 99 000/μL, alkaline phosphatase 12 IU/L, lactic dehydrogenase 345 IU/L, and total bilirubin 2.8 mg/dL. Despite bed rest, her blood pressure gradually rose to 150/100 mmHg, and she developed proteinuria. A diagnosis of preeclampsia was made, and labor was induced at 34 weeks gestation. The patient delivered a healthy 2500 g female infant.

Over the first 4 postpartum days, the mother had three intermittent episodes of sudden vaginal bleeding, which were treated with uterine massage, intravenous oxytocin, intramuscular prostaglandin $F_2\alpha$, uterine curettage, and blood transfusions. Persistent uterine bleeding on the fifth

Continued

postpartum day prompted an abdominal hysterectomy. The uterus contained an unusual arteriovenous malformation likely unrelated to her heart transplant. She had an uneventful postoperative course and her infant did well.

The patient developed coronary artery arteriosclerosis and gradual compromise of cardiac function over the next decade. She was otherwise in relatively good health except for chronic vulvar condylomata unresponsive to multiple therapeutic regimens. At age 35, 14 years after her transplant and 9 years after her delivery, a vulvar biopsy revealed invasive vulvar carcinoma which was

treated with a radical vulvectomy and bilateral inguinal lymphadenectomy. One year later, her allograft vasculopathy was progressing and she was hospitalized and treated for an acute myocardial infarction and a pulmonary embolism. She was admitted to the intensive care unit 3 weeks later with herpes encephalitis where she developed acute tachycardia, severe hypoxia despite intubation, rapidly deteriorated, and died. She is survived by her husband and her daughter, who is now 14 years old.

This case illustrates short- and long-term problems that can occur in transplant patients of reproductive age.

References

1. Organ Procurement and Transplant Network. National data. [cited 2022 Feb 16]. Available from: https://optn.transplant.hrsa.gov/data/view-data-reports/national-data/#.

2. Jones BP, Kasaven L, Vali S, Saso S, Jalmbrant M, Bracewell-Milnes T, et al. Uterine transplantation: review of livebirths and reproductive implications. Transplantation. 2021;105(8):1695–707.

3. Klein CL, Josephson MA. Post-transplant pregnancy and contraception. Clin J Am Soc Nephrol. 2021 Mar 17:CJN.14100820. doi: 10.2215/CJN.14100820.

4. Sarkar M, Bramham K, Moritz MJ, Coscia L. Reproductive health in women following abdominal organ transplant. Am J Transplant. 2018;18(5):1068–76. doi: 10.1111/ajt.14697.

5. McKay DB, Josephson MA, Armenti VT, August P, Coscia LA, Davis CL, et al. Reproduction and transplantation: report on the AST Consensus Conference on Reproductive Issues and Transplantation. Am J Transplant. 2005;5(7):1592–9. doi: 10.1111/j.1600-6143.2005.00969.x.

6. Shah S, Venkatesan RL, Gupta A. Pregnancy outcomes in women with kidney transplant: Meta analysis and systematic review. BMC Nephrol. 2019;20(1):24.

7. Moritz M, Constantinescu S, Coscia L. 2020 annual report, Transplant Pregnancy Registry International (TPRI). Philadelphia, PA: TPRI; 2020.

8. Zheng S, Easterling TR, Umans JG, Miodovnik M, Calamia JC, Thummel KE, et al. Pharmacokinetics of tacrolimus during pregnancy. Ther Drug Monit. 2012;34:660–70.

9. Dantal J, Soulillou J-P. Immunosuppressive drugs and the risk of cancer after organ transplantation. N Engl J Med 2005;352:1271–3.

10. American College of Obstetricians and Gynecologists. ACOG Practice Bulletin No. 20: perinatal viral and parasitic infections. Int J Gynaecol Obstet 2002;76(1):95–107.

11. OPTN/SRTR 2019 annual data report: preface. Am J Transplant. 2021;21(S2):1–10. doi: 10.1111/ajt.15670.

12. Coscia LA, Constantinescu S, Davison JM, Moritz MJ, Armenti VT. Immunosuppressive drugs and fetal outcome. Best Pract Res Clin Obstet Gynaecol. 2014;28(8):1174–87. doi: 10.1016/j.bpobgyn.2014.07.020.

13. Kemp MW, Newnham JP, Challis JG, Jobe AH, Stock SJ. The clinical use of corticosteroids in pregnancy. Hum Reprod Update. 2016;22(2):240–59. doi: 10.1093/humupd/dmv047.

14. Registration Committee of the European Dialysis and Transplant Association. Successful pregnancies in women treated by dialysis and kidney transplantation. Br J Obstet Gynaecol 1980;87:839–45.

15. Cleary BJ, Kallen B. Early pregnancy azathioprine use and pregnancy outcomes. Birth Defects Res A Clin Mol Teratol. 2009;85:647–54.

16. Armenti VT, Ahlswede KM, Ahlswede BA, Jarrell BE, Moritz MJ, Burke JF. National Transplantation Pregnancy Registry – outcomes of 154 pregnancies in cyclosporine-treated female kidney transplant recipients. Transplantation. 1994;57(4):502–6.

17. Langagergaard V, Pedersen L, Gislum M, Nørgard B, Sørensen HT. Birth outcome in women treated with azathioprine or mercaptopurine during pregnancy: A Danish nationwide cohort study. Aliment Pharmacol Ther. 2007;25(1):73–81. doi: 10.1111/j.1365-2036.2006.03162.x.

18. Paziana K, Del Monaco M, Cardonick E, Moritz M, Keller M, Smith B, et al. Ciclosporin use during pregnancy. Drug Saf. 2013 May;36(5):279–94. doi:10.1007/s40264-013-0034-x.

19. Gong X, Li J, Yan J, Dai R, Liu L, Chen P, Chen X. Pregnancy outcomes in female patients exposed to cyclosporin-based versus tacrolimus-based immunosuppressive regimens after liver/kidney transplantation: A systematic review and meta-analysis. J Clin Pharm Ther. 2021;46(3):744–53. doi: 10.1111/jcpt.13340.

20. Bar Oz B, Hackman R, Einarson T, Koren G. Pregnancy outcome after cyclosporine therapy during pregnancy: a meta-analysis. Transplantation. 2001;71(8):1051–5. doi: 10.1097/00007890-200104270-00006.

21. Barbarino JM, Staatz CE, Venkataramanan R, Klein TE, Altman RB. PharmGKB summary: cyclosporine and tacrolimus pathways. Pharmacogenet Genomics. 2013 Oct;23(10):563–85. doi: 10.1097/FPC.0b013e328364db84.

22. Vyas S, Kumar A, Piecuch S, Hidalgo G, Singh A, Anderson V, Markell MS, Baqi N. Outcome of twin pregnancy in a renal transplant recipient treated with tacrolimus. Transplantation. 1999 Feb 15;67(3):490–2. doi: 10.1097/00007890-199902150-00028.

23. Kainz A, Harabacz I, Cowlrick IS, Gadgil D, Hagiwara D. Review of the course and outcome of 100 pregnancies in 84 women treated with tacrolimus. Transplantation. 2000;70:1718–21.

24. Coscia LA, Armenti DP, King RW, Sifontis NM, Constantinescu S, Moritz MJ. Update on the teratogenicity of maternal mycophenolate mofetil. J Pediatr Genet. 2015;4(2):42–55. doi: 10.1055/s-0035-1556743.

25. Perez-Aytes A, Ledo A, Boso V, Sáenz P, Roma E, Poveda JL, et al. In utero exposure to mycophenolate mofetil: a characteristic phenotype? Am J Med Genet. 2008;146A:1–7.

26. Framarino dei Malatesta M, Corona LE, De Luca L, Rocca B, Manzia TM, Orlando G, et al. Successful pregnancy in a living-related kidney transplant recipient who received sirolimus throughout the whole gestation. Transplantation. 2011;91(9):e69–71. doi: 10.1097/TP.0b013e3182154267.

27. Nulojix (belatacept) [package insert]. Princeton, NJ: Bristol-Myers Squibb Co.; 2014.

28. Combs J, Kagan A, Boelkins M, Coscia L, Moritz M, Hofmann RM. Belatacept during pregnancy in renal transplant recipients: Two case reports. Am J Transplant. 08 2018;18(8):2079–82. doi: 10.1111/ajt.14911.

29. Klintmalm GB, Gunby RT. Successful pregnancy in a liver transplant recipient on belatacept. Liver Transpl. 09 2020;26(9):1193–4. doi: 10.1002/lt.25785.

30. Sifontis N, Coscia LA, Constantinescu S, Lavelanet AF, Moritz MJ, Armenti VT. Pregnancy outcomes in solid organ transplant recipients with exposure to mycophenolate mofetil and sirolimus. Transplantation. 82:1698–702; 2006.

31. National Institute of Diabetes and Digestive and Kidney Disease. United States Renal Data System. [cited 2022 Feb 28]. Available from: https://www.usrds.org/esrd-quarterly-update/.

32. Health Resources and Services Administration. OPTN/SRTR 2019 annual data report. [cited 2023 May 25]. Available from: https://srtr.transplant.hrsa.gov/annual_reports/2019_ADR_Preview.aspx.

33. van Buren MC, Schellekens A, Groenhof TKJ, van Reekum F, van de Wetering J, Paauw ND, et al. Long-term graft survival and graft function following pregnancy in kidney transplant recipients: a systematic review and meta-analysis. Transplantation. 08 2020;104(8):1675–85. doi: 10.1097/TP.0000000000003026.

34. Yin O, Kallapur A, Coscia L, Constantinescu S, Moritz M, Afshar Y. Differentiating acute rejection from preeclampsia after kidney transplantation. Obstet Gynecol. 2021 Jun 1;137(6):1023–31. doi: 10.1097/AOG.0000000000004389.

35. Lim TY, Gonsalkorala E, Cannon MD, Gabeta S, Gabeta S, Penna L, Heaton ND, et al. Successful pregnancy outcomes following liver transplantation is predicted by renal function. Liver Transpl. 2018;24(5):606–15.

36. Marson EJ, Kamarajah SK, Dyson JK, White SA. Pregnancy outcomes in women with liver transplants: systematic review and meta-analysis. HPB (Oxford). 2020;22(8):1102–11. doi: 10.1016/j.hpb.2020.05.001.

37. Camann WR, Goldman GA, Johnson MD, Moore J, Greene M. Cesarean delivery in a patient with a transplanted heart. Anesthesiology 1989;71:618–20.

38. Punnoose LR, Coscia LA, Armenti DP, Constantinescu S, Moritz MJ. Pregnancy outcomes in heart transplant recipients. J Heart Lung Transplant. 2020;39(5):473–80. doi: 10.1016/j.healun.2020.02.005.

39. Souza R, Soete E, Silversides CK, Zaffar N, Van Mieghem T, Van Cleemput J, et al. Pregnancy outcomes following cardiac transplantation. J Obstet Gynaecol Can. 2018;40(5):566–71. doi: 10.1016/j.jogc.2017.08.030.

40. Shaner J, Coscia LA, Constantinescu S, McGrory CH, Doria C, Moritz MJ, et al. Pregnancy after lung transplant. Prog Transplant. 2012;22(2):134–40. doi: 10.7182/pit2012285.

41. Bry C, Hubert D, Reynaud-Gaubert M, Dromer C, Mal H, Roux A, et al. Pregnancy after lung and heart-lung transplantation: a French multicentre retrospective study of 39 pregnancies. ERJ Open Res. 2019;5(4):00254.

42. Thakrar MV, Morley K, Lordan JL, Meachery G, Fisher AJ, Parry G, et al. Pregnancy after lung and heart-lung transplantation. J Heart Lung Transplant. 2014;33(6):593–8. doi: 10.1016/j.healun.2014.02.008.

43. Daolio J, Palomba S, Paganelli S, Falbo A, Aguzzoli L. Uterine transplantation and IVF for congenital or acquired uterine factor infertility: a systematic review of safety and efficacy outcomes in the first 52 recipients. PLoS One. 2020;15(4):e0232323. doi: 10.1371/journal.pone.0232323.

44. Yin O, Kallapur A, Coscia L, Kwan L, Tandel M, Constantinescu SA, et al. Mode of obstetric delivery in kidney and liver transplant recipients and associated maternal, neonatal, and graft morbidity during 5 decades of clinical practice. JAMA Netw Open. 2021;4(10):e2127378.

45. Constantinescu S, Pai A, Coscia LA, Davison JM, Moritz MJ, Armenti VT. Breast-feeding after transplantation. Best Pract Res Clin Obstet Gynaecol. 2014;28(8):1163–73. doi: 10.1016/j.bpobgyn.2014.09.001.

46. Bramham K, Chusney G, Lee J, Lightstone L, Nelson-Piercy C. Breastfeeding and tacrolimus: serial monitoring in breast-fed and bottle-fed infants. Clin J Am Soc Nephrol. 2013;8(4):d–7. doi: 10.2215/CJN.06400612.

47. Dinelli MIS, Ono E, Viana PO, Dos Santos AMN, de Moraes-Pinto MI. Growth of children born to renal transplanted women. Eur J Pediatr. 2017 Sep;176(9):1201–7. doi: 10.1007/s00431-017-2965-1.

48. Nulman I, Sgro M, Barrera M, Chitayat D, Cairney J, Koren G. Long-term neurodevelopment of children exposed in utero to ciclosporin after maternal renal transplant. Paediatr Drugs. 2010;12(2):113–22. doi: 10.2165/11316280-000000000-00000. PMID: 20095652.

49. Boulay H, Mazaud-Guittot S, Supervielle J, Chemouny JM, Dardier V, Lacroix A. Maternal, foetal and child consequences of immunosuppressive drugs during pregnancy in women with organ transplant: a review. Clin Kidney J. 2021;14(8):1871–8. doi: 10.1093/ckj/sfab049.

50. Scott JR. Development of children born to mothers with connective tissue diseases. Lupus 2002;11:655–60.

Chapter 19
Gestational Diabetes Mellitus

Angela R. Boyd and Deborah L. Conway
Department of Obstetrics and Gynecology, Joe R. and Teresa Lozano Long School of Medicine, San Antonio, TX, USA

Normal pregnancy is a state of insulin resistance. To spare glucose for the developing fetus, the placenta produces hormones that antagonize maternal insulin, shifting the principal energy source from glucose to ketones and free fatty acids. Most pregnant women maintain normal blood glucose levels despite the increased insulin resistance through enhanced insulin production and release by the pancreas, both in the basal state, and in response to meals.

Gestational diabetes mellitus (GDM) is a state of carbohydrate intolerance that develops or is first recognized during pregnancy. In some women, β-cell production of insulin cannot keep pace with the resistance to insulin produced by the diabetogenic hormones from the placenta. The prevalence of GDM in the United States is estimated to be 5–7% and continues to increase with the increasing prevalence of type 2 diabetes mellitus (T2DM) in the population under examination [1,2]. It is the most common medical complication of pregnancy and is clearly linked to several maternal and fetal complications including fetal macrosomia, operative delivery, birth trauma, preeclampsia and hypertensive disorders, and metabolic complications in the neonate including hypoglycemia, hypocalcemia, hyperbilirubinemia, prematurity, and perinatal mortality.

Risk factors for gestational diabetes

Rigorous identification and effective treatment of diabetes minimizes the occurrence of pregnancy complications that can result from maternal hyperglycemia [3,4]. In 2014, the US Preventive Services Task Force recommended universal screening of all pregnant women at or beyond 24 weeks gestation to identify GDM [5]. They concluded that the evidence was insufficient to recommend screening prior to 24 weeks gestation. However, the American College of Obstetricians and Gynecologists (ACOG) and the American Diabetes Association (ADA) suggest early screening for the presence of pregestational diabetes or early-onset GDM in those with risk factors [6,7]. Women at high risk include those with a history of GDM, macrosomia, stillbirth, or congenital anomaly in a prior pregnancy; a first-degree relative with T2DM; polycystic ovarian syndrome; or a history of glucose intolerance or "prediabetes" (see Box 19.1 for a detailed list of risk factors).

There are two accepted methods to identify GDM: the two-step screening approach (1-hour screening test, followed by diagnostic testing) or the one-step, 2-hour 75-g oral glucose tolerance test (OGTT). The two-step screening approach involves a 1-hour 50-g OGTT screening test, followed by a diagnostic 2-hour or 3-hour OGTT. The most commonly employed cutoff value for the 1-hour 50-g screening test is 140 mg/dL, which results in an approximately 15% test positive rate. By reducing the cutoff to 130 mg/dL, the sensitivity of the test (i.e. the proportion of women with GDM who have a "positive" screen) improves to nearly 100%, at the expense of specificity [10]. In a low-risk population (i.e. one with a low burden of type 2 diabetes), the actual number of extra cases identified with this increase in sensitivity is greatly outweighed by the number of false-positive screens between 130 and 140 mg/dL. Conversely, in a high-risk population in which T2DM is common, the number missed by using the higher cutoff may be unacceptable. Therefore, the population characteristics should be taken into consideration when selecting the appropriate cut-off for gestational diabetes screening.

After a positive screening test result is obtained, a diagnostic test is performed. The 3-hour OGTT is a 100-g oral glucose load after a fasting plasma glucose. Plasma glucose levels are then obtained at 1, 2, and 3 hours. According to the recommendations by the ADA's Fourth International Workshop Conference on Gestational Diabetes, the Carpenter and Coustan modification of O'Sullivan and Mahan's original values should be used [8] (Table 19.1).

Queenan's Management of High-Risk Pregnancy: An Evidence-Based Approach, Seventh Edition. Edited by Catherine Y. Spong and Charles J. Lockwood.

Therapeutic modalities in gestational diabetes

Medical management of GDM aims to optimize glycemic control to prevent or minimize complications while avoiding ketosis and poor nutrition. The cornerstone of care is diet. Medical nutrition therapy for GDM is aimed at optimizing metabolic outcomes and improving health by encouraging healthy food choices, while addressing personal and cultural preferences and providing adequate energy and nutrients for optimal pregnancy outcomes [13]. Elements of dietary therapy include total calorie allocation, calorie distribution, and nutritional component management. Total daily calorie intake is based on ideal bodyweight. For example, overweight and obese women can be given approximately 25 kcal/kg, up to a total of 2800–3000 kcal/day. Women with normal prepregnancy body mass index (BMI) receive approximately 30 kcal/kg, with a minimum intake of 1800 kcal/day. These calories are typically distributed between three meals and two to four snacks during the day. Smaller, more frequent meals lead to better satiety, improved compliance with the diet, and reduced magnitude of postprandial peak glucose levels.

Postprandial glucose measurements are directly influenced by the amount of carbohydrate consumed. A traditional diet typically contains 55–60% carbohydrate. Major et al. [14], described their success with a diet containing 40–42% carbohydrate. Mild carbohydrate restriction resulted in improved glycemic control, less need for insulin, and fewer large-for-gestational-age (LGA) infants.

Exercise is another key component. Cardiovascular exercise reduces insulin resistance and reduces the frequency of GDM [15,16]. Fasting and postprandial glucose levels are lower in women with GDM who exercise, possibly avoiding the need for insulin treatment in some women [17]. The physiologic and anatomic changes of pregnancy should be taken into consideration when counseling pregnant women about exercise.

There is no established standard on frequency of glucose monitoring in GDM. The goal is to identify if glycemic targets are met. Commonly used targets include fasting values below 95 mg/dL and 2-hour postprandial values below 120 mg/dL. Alternatively, 1-hour postprandial values may be used, with a target below 140 mg/dL. Many recommend daily monitoring. One trial suggested that monitoring postprandial glucose was more effective than preprandial values in managing GDM [18]. The women randomized to postprandial readings had significantly less fetal overgrowth, fewer cesarean deliveries for cephalopelvic disproportion, and less neonatal hypoglycemia, compared with women who checked their glucose levels before meals.

Ultimately, some with GDM will not be able to meet glycemic targets with diet therapy alone and will require

Box 19.1 Criteria for early screening for pregestational diabetes or early-onset gestational diabetes

• Consider in overweight and obese (body mass index ≥25 kg/m² or ≥23 kg/m² in Asian Americans) women with one or more of the following:
  – First-degree relative with diabetes mellitus
  – High-risk race/ethnicity (African American, Hispanic, Native American, Asian American, or Pacific Islander)
  – History of gestational diabetes
  – History of cardiovascular disease
  – Prior birth of an infant weighing more than 4000 g
  – Chronic hypertension (140/90 mmHg or on therapy for hypertension)
  – Women with polycystic ovarian syndrome
  – Physical inactivity
  – A1c greater than or equal to 5.7%, impaired glucose tolerance, or impaired fasting glucose on prior testing
  – Other clinical conditions associated with insulin resistance (e.g. body mass index >40 kg/m², acanthosis nigricans)

Adapted from [6,7].

Table 19.1 Diagnostic thresholds for gestational diabetes

Time	ADA/Carpenter and Coustan thresholds[a] [8](mg/dL)	IADPSG thresholds[b] [9] (mg/dL)
Fasting	95	92
1-h	180	180
2-h	155	152
3-h	140	n/a

[a]If two or more values *meet or exceed* these thresholds, the diagnosis of gestational diabetes is made.
[b]If one or more values *meet or exceed* these thresholds, the diagnosis of gestational diabetes is made.
ADA, American Diabetes Association; IADPSG, International Association of Diabetes and Pregnancy Study Groups.

Alternatively, the 2-hour 75 g OGTT may be used after a positive screening test or as a one-step screening approach. The diagnostic thresholds (Table 19.1) are values above which there is an increased risk of neonatal adiposity and elevated cord blood insulin levels [11]. Use of the one-step screening approach may improve patient compliance with completion of diagnostic testing; however, using the 2-hour approach will increase the number of women diagnosed with GDM given the lower thresholds and diagnosis with only one abnormal value. A randomized trial comparing women diagnosed with GDM with the one- vs. the two-step approach resulted in more women diagnosed and treated for GDM with the one-step approach with no difference in maternal or neonatal outcomes [12]. Institutions and practices should take into account available resources when adopting a one-step or two-step screening approach.

medical intervention. This can be determined once dietary therapy has been in place for 2 weeks [19]. Insulin does not cross the placenta and remains the first-line agent for management of GDM [20]. Insulin dosage is calculated according to body weight, starting in the range of 0.7–1.0 units/kg of current body weight, usually given in the form of long-acting or intermediate-acting insulin with short-acting insulin analogues in divided doses. The pregnant woman with diabetes demonstrates both insulin resistance and relative insulin deficiency; thus, it is typical to require large doses of insulin to achieve adequate glycemic control [21]. It is important to remember that with advancing gestational age, the patient will become more insulin resistant and therefore insulin requirements will increase. The insulin dose can be adjusted as frequently as every 3–4 days and can be increased 10–20% depending on the corresponding values obtained from patient self-monitoring.

Women who have mild hyperglycemia despite dietary changes and decline insulin therapy may be offered oral antidiabetic treatment with metformin. In a randomized trial comparing metformin to insulin, women taking metformin gained less weight and had lower rates of cesarean delivery with no difference in mean birthweight and rates of macrosomia (birthweight over 4000 g) [22]. Metformin readily crosses the placenta, and the long-term effects of this exposure are unknown [23]. A prospective follow-up study of children with in utero exposure to either metformin or insulin at 2 years of age found no difference in neurodevelopmental outcomes [24]. However, a meta-analysis that examined growth of children exposed to metformin vs. insulin found that metformin-exposed children had significantly higher body weight percentile at 18–24 months and higher BMIs at 5–9 years of age [25].

Another treatment option for women whose diabetes is not controlled on diet alone is the sulfonylurea drug glyburide. Glyburide also crosses the placenta [26]. In a randomized trial comparing insulin with glyburide in women with GDM, no differences were found between groups in terms of mean maternal blood glucose, LGA infants, macrosomia (greater than 4000 g), lung complications, hypoglycemia, or cord blood insulin levels [27]. Thus, both metformin and glyburide have been found to achieve adequate glycemic control with less risk for maternal hypoglycemia compared to insulin-treated women [22,27]. It should be noted when counseling patients that if they are unable to reach recommended glycemic targets with metformin or glyburide, insulin should be started to minimize adverse maternal and neonatal outcomes associated with maternal hyperglycemia [20,28].

Antenatal testing

Antenatal testing is recommended with pregestational diabetes, GDM treated with medication or with poor glycemic control, and GDM with another pregnancy complication such as hypertension or abnormal fetal growth [29]. The method of testing (e.g. nonstress testing, biophysical profile) is left to the discretion of the provider, guided by local practice. In addition, all women with GDM should be instructed to perform fetal kick counts daily, beginning in the third trimester, and to notify their care provider promptly if fetal movements are diminished.

Delivery: when and how to deliver

Few prospective trials have been undertaken to optimize delivery outcomes in women with diabetes. What has been consistently shown is that the cesarean delivery rate is higher in women with diabetes [30], even when careful antenatal care has achieved near normal rates of fetal overgrowth [31].

Women with well-controlled GDM should not undergo delivery prior to 39 weeks gestation [32]. Women with well-controlled GDM on diet, should be allowed to enter spontaneous labor up to 40 6/7 weeks gestation. Comparison of this approach to planned labor induction at 38 weeks gestation in a randomized trial of women with class A2 and B diabetes showed that expectant management prolonged gestation by 1 week, resulted in a doubling in the rate of macrosomic infants but with similar rates of cesarean delivery [33]. In women with GDM well controlled with medication, delivery is recommended at 39 0/7 to 39 6/7 weeks gestation. Indications for delivery prior to 39 weeks gestation include inability to achieve adequate glucose control; poor compliance with visits or prescribed treatment, prior stillbirth or abnormal antenatal testing, and the presence of chronic hypertension. Delivery prior to 37 weeks should be reserved for women with abnormal antenatal testing or those with additional indications for preterm delivery.

Macrosomia and shoulder dystocia occur more frequently in pregnancies complicated by diabetes than in the general obstetric population. Shoulder dystocia remains most often an unpredictable and unpreventable obstetric emergency. Based on the observation that most cases of shoulder dystocia in diabetic women occur when birthweight is > 4000 g [32], our practice has been to recommend cesarean delivery without a trial of labor to women with an estimated fetal weight above 4250 g who have diabetes. By implementing this practice, our shoulder dystocia rate in women with diabetes has been reduced by 80%, and shoulder dystocia rates among macrosomic infants fell from 19% to 7% after implementing this practice. There was a small but significant increase in the cesarean delivery rate [34]. ACOG recommends that planned cesarean delivery to prevent shoulder dystocia may be considered for suspected fetal macrosomia with estimated fetal weight exceeding 4500 g in women with diabetes [35].

Postpartum considerations

Gestational diabetes may be the first signal of inherent insulin resistance. Women with GDM need to have glucose tolerance reassessed in the postpartum period. Use of the 2-hour OGTT permits identification of both impaired glucose tolerance and overt diabetes. When tested early in the postpartum period, 20–30% of women with GDM will have abnormal values [36]. A comparative study found that performing the 2-hour OGTT on postpartum day 2 was able to identify women with impaired glucose tolerance or diabetes at 1 year after delivery with similar diagnostic value to routine testing at 4–12 weeks

postpartum [37]. It is estimated that <50% of women complete the recommended OGTT at 4–12 weeks postpartum, and thus testing prior to hospital discharge may improve compliance with postpartum assessment for impaired glucose tolerance and T2DM without sacrificing accuracy.

The importance of postpartum testing cannot be overstated. Within 5–6 years after a pregnancy complicated with GDM, up to 50% of women will have type 2 diabetes [20]. Early identification of impaired glucose tolerance affords the opportunity to institute therapeutic measures such as exercise, diet, and weight control, perhaps preventing progression to diabetes. Identification and treatment of overt diabetes early in the course of the disease offer the best opportunity to delay or avoid the micro and macrovascular complications associated with the disease.

CASE PRESENTATION

A 27-year-old woman, gravida 2, para 1001, at 12 weeks gestation presents for initial prenatal care. She denies a history of GDM. Her first child, born by uncomplicated spontaneous vaginal delivery, weighed 4100 g at 38 weeks gestation. Her records indicate that the 3-hour GTT performed at 25 weeks in her first pregnancy had the following values: fasting 96 mg/dL, 1-hour 191 mg/dL, 2-hour 152 mg/dL, 3-hour 122 mg/dL. Her mother and her older sister have type 2 diabetes mellitus.

A 50 g GCT is performed with her initial prenatal laboratory tests, and it is abnormal. A 3-hour GTT performed at 13 weeks gestation is normal (96/177/148/125). However, repeat testing at 25 weeks reveals she has GDM (99/202/168/141). In initiating treatment, she is prescribed medical nutrition therapy comprised of 40–45% carbohydrates, 30–35% protein, and 25% fat. Total energy supplied is calculated to be 2500 kcal/day, based on her prepregnancy weight of 100 kg (BMI 35 obese, 25 kcal/kg).

She is instructed to perform self-monitored blood glucose readings. After 1 week of therapy, her fasting glucose levels are consistently above 95 mg/dL, and more than 50% of her postprandial glucose values are also above target range. Insulin is initiated, but despite increasing doses over the subsequent weeks, she remains poorly controlled as term approaches. Her fundal height at 38 weeks measures 41 cm, and an ultrasound reveals a fetal weight estimate of 4600 g. Given these findings, in the setting of poorly controlled GDM, the patient is counseled about and accepts a cesarean delivery. The infant's birthweight is 4450 g, and the neonatal course is complicated by hypoglycemia that requires intravenous glucose infusion.

At the time of the postpartum visit, a 2-hour GTT is obtained and indicates impaired glucose tolerance (fasting 97 mg/dL, 2-hour 178 mg/dL). Lifestyle modifications are recommended to prevent progression to type 2 DM, and annual screening for diabetes is suggested.

References

1. Correa A, Bardenheier B, Elixhauser A, Geiss LS, Gregg E. Trends in prevalence of diabetes among delivery hospitalizations, United States, 1993-2009. Matern Child Health J. 2015;19(3):635–42.
2. Hunt KJ, Schuller KL. The increasing prevalence of diabetes in pregnancy. Obstet Gynecol Clin North Am. 2007;34(2):173–99, vii.
3. Crowther CA, Hiller JE, Moss JR, McPhee AJ, Jeffries WS, Robinson JS, et al. Effect of treatment of gestational diabetes mellitus on pregnancy outcomes. N Engl J Med. 2005;352(24):2477–86.
4. Landon MB, Spong CY, Thom E, Carpenter MW, Ramin SM, Casey B, et al. A multicenter, randomized trial of treatment for mild gestational diabetes. N Engl J Med. 2009;361(14):1339–48.
5. Moyer VA, U.S. Preventive Services Task Force. Screening for gestational diabetes mellitus: U.S. Preventive Services Task Force recommendation statement. Ann Intern Med. 2014;160(6):414–20.
6. ACOG Practice Bulletin No. 190: gestational diabetes mellitus. Obstet Gynecol. 2018;131(2):e49–e64.
7. American Diabetes Association. 2. Classification and diagnosis of diabetes. Diabetes Care. 2017;40(Suppl 1):S11–S24.
8. Carpenter MW, Coustan DR. Criteria for screening tests for gestational diabetes. Am J Obstet Gynecol. 1982;144(7):768–73.
9. International Association of Diabetes and Pregnancy Study Groups Consensus Panel; Metzger BE, Gabbe SG, Persson B, Buchanan TA, et al. International Association of Diabetes and Pregnancy study groups recommendations on the diagnosis

and classification of hyperglycemia in pregnancy. Diabetes Care. 2010;33(3):676–82.

10. Coustan DR, Widness JA, Carpenter MW, Rotondo L, Pratt DC, Oh W. Should the fifty-gram, one-hour plasma glucose screening test for gestational diabetes be administered in the fasting or fed state? Am J Obstet Gynecol. 1986;154(5):1031–5.

11. Group HSCR, Metzger BE, Lowe LP, Dyer AR, Trimble ER, Chaovarindr U, et al. Hyperglycemia and adverse pregnancy outcomes. N Engl J Med. 2008;358(19):1991–2002.

12. Hillier TA, Pedula KL, Ogasawara KK, Vesco KK, Oshiro CES, Lubarsky SL, et al. A pragmatic, randomized clinical trial of gestational diabetes screening. N Engl J Med. 2021; 384(10):895–904.

13. Franz MJ, Bantle JP, Beebe CA, Brunzell JD, Chiasson JL, Garg A, et al. Nutrition principles and recommendations in diabetes. Diabetes Care. 2004;27 Suppl 1:S36–46.

14. Major CA, Henry MJ, De Veciana M, Morgan MA. The effects of carbohydrate restriction in patients with diet-controlled gestational diabetes. Obstet Gynecol. 1998;91(4):600–4.

15. Wang C, Wei Y, Zhang X, Zhang Y, Xu Q, Sun Y, et al. A randomized clinical trial of exercise during pregnancy to prevent gestational diabetes mellitus and improve pregnancy outcome in overweight and obese pregnant women. Am J Obstet Gynecol. 2017;216(4):340–51.

16. Ehrlich SF, Ferrara A, Hedderson MM, Feng J, Neugebauer R. Exercise during the first trimester of pregnancy and the risks of abnormal screening and gestational diabetes mellitus. Diabetes Care. 2021;44(2):425–32.

17. Jovanovic-Peterson L, Durak EP, Peterson CM. Randomized trial of diet versus diet plus cardiovascular conditioning on glucose levels in gestational diabetes. Am J Obstet Gynecol. 1989;161(2):415–9.

18. de Veciana M, Major CA, Morgan MA, Asrat T, Toohey JS, Lien JM, et al. Postprandial versus preprandial blood glucose monitoring in women with gestational diabetes mellitus requiring insulin therapy. N Engl J Med. 1995;333(19):1237–41.

19. McFarland MB, Langer O, Conway DL, Berkus MD. Dietary therapy for gestational diabetes: how long is long enough? Obstet Gynecol. 1999;93(6):978–82.

20. American Diabetes Association. 14. Management of diabetes in pregnancy: standards of medical care in diabetes–2020. Diabetes Care. 2020;43(Suppl 1):S183–92.

21. Langer O, Anyaegbunam A, Brustman L, Guidetti D, Mazze R. Gestational diabetes: insulin requirements in pregnancy. Am J Obstet Gynecol. 1987;157(3):669–75.

22. Picon-Cesar MJ, Molina-Vega M, Suarez-Arana M, Gonzalez-Mesa E, Sola-Moyano AP, Roldan-Lopez R, et al. Metformin for gestational diabetes study: metformin vs insulin in gestational diabetes: glycemic control and obstetrical and perinatal outcomes: randomized prospective trial. Am J Obstet Gynecol. 2021;225(5):517.e1–e17.

23. Elliott BD, Langer O, Schuessling F. Human placental glucose uptake and transport are not altered by the oral antihyperglycemic agent metformin. Am J Obstet Gynecol. 1997;176(3):527–30.

24. Wouldes TA, Battin M, Coat S, Rush EC, Hague WM, Rowan JA. Neurodevelopmental outcome at 2 years in offspring of women randomised to metformin or insulin treatment for gestational diabetes. Arch Dis Child Fetal Neonatal Ed. 2016;101(6):F488–93.

25. Tarry-Adkins JL, Aiken CE, Ozanne SE. Neonatal, infant, and childhood growth following metformin versus insulin treatment for gestational diabetes: a systematic review and meta-analysis. PLoS Med. 2019;16(8):e1002848.

26. Hebert MF, Ma X, Naraharisetti SB, Krudys KM, Umans JG, Hankins GD, et al. Are we optimizing gestational diabetes treatment with glyburide? The pharmacologic basis for better clinical practice. Clin Pharmacol Ther. 2009;85(6):607–14.

27. Langer O, Conway DL, Berkus MD, Xenakis EM, Gonzales O. A comparison of glyburide and insulin in women with gestational diabetes mellitus. N Engl J Med. 2000;343(16):1134–8.

28. Rowan JA, Hague WM, Gao W, Battin MR, Moore MP, Mi GTI. Metformin versus insulin for the treatment of gestational diabetes. N Engl J Med. 2008;358(19):2003–15.

29. American College of Obstetricians and Gynecologists' Committee on Practice Bulletins—Obstetrics. ACOG Practice Bulletin No. 229: antepartum fetal surveillance. Obstet Gynecol. 2021;137(6):1134–6.

30. Jacobson JD, Cousins L. A population-based study of maternal and perinatal outcome in patients with gestational diabetes. Am J Obstet Gynecol. 1989;161(4):981–6.

31. Naylor CD, Sermer M, Chen E, Sykora K.; Toronto Trihospital Gestational Diabetes Investigators. Cesarean delivery in relation to birth weight and gestational glucose tolerance: pathophysiology or practice style? JAMA. 1996;275(15):1165–70.

32. Spong CY, Mercer BM, D'Alton M, Kilpatrick S, Blackwell S, Saade G. Timing of indicated late-preterm and early-term birth. Obstet Gynecol. 2011;118(2 Pt 1):323–33.

33. Kjos SL, Henry OA, Montoro M, Buchanan TA, Mestman JH. Insulin-requiring diabetes in pregnancy: a randomized trial of active induction of labor and expectant management. Am J Obstet Gynecol. 1993;169(3):611–5.

34. Conway DL, Langer O. Elective delivery of infants with macrosomia in diabetic women: reduced shoulder dystocia versus increased cesarean deliveries. Am J Obstet Gynecol. 1998;178(5):922–5.

35. Practice Bulletin No 178: shoulder dystocia. Obstet Gynecol. 2017;129(5):e123–33.

36. Conway DL, Langer O. Effects of new criteria for type 2 diabetes on the rate of postpartum glucose intolerance in women with gestational diabetes. Am J Obstet Gynecol. 1999;181(3):610–4.

37. Society for Maternal-Fetal Medicine, Werner EF, Has P, Rouse D, Clark MA. Two-day postpartum compared with 4- to 12-week postpartum glucose tolerance testing for women with gestational diabetes. Am J Obstet Gynecol. 2020;223(3):439 e1–e7.

Chapter 20
Diabetes Mellitus

George R. Saade

Department of Obstetrics and Gynecology, Eastern Virginia Medical School, Norfolk, VA, USA

As more women with diabetes are contemplating pregnancy and more women are delaying pregnancy, health care providers should expect to see more pregnant patients with pregestational as well as gestational diabetes. The goal of management is to decrease the risk for congenital anomalies secondary to preconception hyperglycemia, as well as to reach term without maternal complications such as preeclampsia or fetal complications such as uteroplacental insufficiency, fetal death, macrosomia, birth injury, and postnatal hypoglycemia. This includes frequent glucose monitoring, dietary and pharmacologic interventions, diligent fetal surveillance, appropriate timing of delivery, and judicious choice of delivery route. In most cases, patients with diabetes can reach term, and perinatal mortality from stillbirth, prematurity, and birth injury can be markedly reduced. It is important that the obstetrician who infrequently manages patients with diabetes is familiar with the uses and limitations of established treatments. This chapter concentrates on the pregestational patient with diabetes. For discussion of gestational diabetes, see Chapter 19.

The leading cause of perinatal mortality in pregnancies complicated by insulin-dependent diabetes mellitus is congenital malformation. The risk of major malformations in such pregnancies is increased three- to fourfold over the 2–3% incidence noted in the general population. There is good evidence that these anomalies are a result of marked alterations in maternal glycemic control during the critical period of fetal embryogenesis, at 5–8 weeks gestation. Patients whose diabetes is poorly regulated are also at greater risk for a spontaneous abortion.

There is a direct correlation between maternal glycosylated hemoglobin (hemoglobin [Hb] A$_{1c}$) levels and the risk for fetal anomalies [1] (Table 20.1). Women with pregestational diabetes had an 8% major anomaly rate; an HbA1c of 10% was associated with a 10% anomaly rate and an HbA1c of 13% with a 20% anomaly rate. The risks of spontaneous abortion and major malformations are reported as 12.4% and 3.0%, respectively, with first-trimester HbA1c ≤9.3%, versus risks of 37.5% and 40%, respectively, with HbA1c >14.4% [2]. Preconception care in diabetic women is associated with fewer maternal hospitalizations, less use of neonatal intensive care, and a reduction in major congenital anomalies and perinatal deaths [3]. The aim should be to maintain HbA1c as close to normal as possible without significant hypoglycemia, but certainly less than 7%. For this reason, treatment of the woman with insulin-dependent diabetes who is considering a pregnancy should be initiated before conception [4]. In addition, the preconception patient should be placed on 4 mg/day folic acid supplementation in order to reduce the risk for neural tube defect. Thorough evaluation should be undertaken to detect evidence of maternal retinopathy, nephropathy, or coronary artery disease. For the most recent classification, diagnostic criteria, and practice guidelines for pregestational diabetes, refer to the Standards of care in Diabetes from the American Diabetes Association [5] and the American College of Obstetricians and Gynecologists technical bulletin addressing pregestational diabetes [6].

Initial evaluation

For women with previously diagnosed diabetes, it is important to take a careful history and perform a physical examination as soon as pregnancy is diagnosed, paying special attention to the following:
- Careful dating of the pregnancy by history, ultrasound, and physical signs.
- Evaluation for presence of other comorbid conditions.
- Progress and outcome of any previous pregnancies.
- Careful fundoscopic examination for the presence of retinopathy.
- Findings of urinalysis and culture, as well as 24-hour urine collection for creatinine clearance and protein.
- Baseline blood pressure measurement, electrocardiogram (ECG), and thyroid function tests.

Queenan's Management of High-Risk Pregnancy: An Evidence-Based Approach, Seventh Edition. Edited by Catherine Y. Spong and Charles J. Lockwood.

Table 20.1 Risk of major malformation in fetuses of women with insulin-dependent diabetes according to HbA1c levels in a contemporary cohort of 1573 pregestational diabetics with singleton gestation

	<6% (n=113)	6–6.9% (n=168)	7–7.9% (n=155)	8–8.9% (n=147)	10–10.9% (n=126)	11–11.9% (n=84)	>12% (n=79)	*P* value
Major malformations	1 (1%)	6 (4%)	8 (5%)	6 (4%)	15 (10%)	12 (14%)	12 (15%)	<0.001

HbA1c, glycosylated hemoglobin.
Adapted from Martin et al. [1].

- Baseline glycosylated hemoglobin measurement.
- Review of insulin dosage, nutrition, physical activity, and logs of home glucose monitoring.

Regulating maternal glycemia

Careful control of maternal glucose levels significantly improves perinatal outcome. Except during brief periods after meals, glucose should normally remain below 100 mg/dL. Maternal hyperglycemia and rapid fluctuations in blood glucose produce similar changes in the fetal compartment. Fetal hyperglycemia leads to β-cell hyperplasia and hyperinsulinemia. Also, there is a significant correlation between maternal glucose levels and subsequent adiposity in the infant. Ketoacidosis at any time during pregnancy may lead to death in utero. Management of diabetic ketoacidosis includes aggressive fluid and electrolyte replacement, in addition to insulin administration.

Maintenance of euglycemia depends not only on diligent regulation of diet and insulin but also on strict attention to physical activity and stress. Patients should eat three meals and three snacks each day, adding up to 30–35 cal/kg of ideal bodyweight.

The most successful regimen of insulin administration usually includes combinations of short-acting insulin (regular insulin; onset of action 30–60 minutes) or rapid-acting insulin analogues (e.g. insulin lispro, insulin aspart; onset of action 1–15 minutes) plus longer-acting insulins (e.g. neutral protamine Hagedorn [NPH], insulin detemir, insulin glargine) given in two or more injections daily. The rapid-acting insulin analogues are preferred over regular insulin as they can be given right before the meal rather than needing to anticipate a meal when giving regular insulin. The limited data on the longer-acting insulins do not point to a benefit of one over the others. The amount of NPH insulin given in the morning generally exceeds that of regular insulin by a 2:1 ratio. In the evening, equal amounts of NPH and regular insulin are given. If several fasting or postprandial glucose levels are not acceptable (usually more than one third of values), insulin doses are increased by 20%. Several days are then allowed to pass before further changes are made. The use of other insulin administration routes (e.g. insulin pump), as well as oral hypoglycemic agents, should be individualized

and reserved for special circumstances [7]. Limited evidence suggests that women with pregestational diabetes who continue oral hypoglycemics when they become pregnant are at higher risk for complications [8]. Generally pregestational women with diabetes are best switched to and managed with insulin during pregnancy [9]. During labor, a continuous insulin infusion is best to stabilize maternal glucose levels and reduce neonatal hypoglycemia. The goal is to maintain hourly glucose levels at less than 110 mg/dL.

Glycemic control cannot be accurately assessed by random blood glucose determinations or by testing urine specimens for glucose. The patient should be taught to assess her capillary glucose levels by using reagent strips and a blood glucose reflectance meter. Determinations should be made in the fasting state and 2 hours after meals. The goal of therapy is to maintain capillary whole-blood glucose levels as close to normal as possible, including a fasting glucose level of 95 mg/dL or less, and 2-hour postprandial values of 120 mg/dL or less. When using a meter, it is imperative to determine whether it tests whole blood, serum, or plasma, as results may vary (plasma levels approximately 10 mg/dL higher than whole blood). A blood glucose sample drawn 80 minutes after breakfast correlates well with the mean amplitude of glycemic excursions throughout the day. Measurements made before lunch, dinner, and bedtime may also be helpful; these premeal values should be 100 mg/dL or less. Some prefer to monitor 1-hour postpartum glucose levels, which should be at 140 mg/dL or less.

A useful parameter for assessing control over a prolonged period (4–8 weeks) is HbA1c, a minor variant of HbA, produced by the addition of a single glucose moiety to the terminal valine of the β-chain. This glycosylated hemoglobin is synthesized throughout the red blood cell's life cycle in amounts that reflect the degree of chronic hyperglycemia present. Levels correlate significantly with mean fasting glucose, mean daily glucose, and highest daily glucose values. In normal pregnancy, glycosylated hemoglobin declines during the first and second trimesters, returning to baseline levels at term. To convert the HbA1c level to the mean glucose level, one can use the "rule of 8s." An HbA1c level of 8% reflects a mean glucose level of 180 mg/dL in most laboratories. Each change of 1% in the HbA1c value indicates a change of 30 mg/dL in mean glucose. There is a direct correlation between maternal third-trimester HbA1c levels and increased birthweight [10]. HbA1c should be checked every trimester.

The insulin requirement postpartum decreases dramatically (usually by 50%) and thus must be carefully monitored. Patients with type 1 diabetes are at increased risk for postpartum thyroiditis, so a high index of suspicion should be maintained.

Management during pregnancy

Major fetal malformations occur in around 5–8% of women with type 1 diabetes. Diabetes is not associated with an increase in the risk of fetal chromosomal abnormalities. During the second trimester, a careful evaluation for fetal malformations includes obtaining a maternal serum α-fetoprotein level at 16 weeks (helpful in detecting neural tube defects), a targeted ultrasound at 18–20 weeks, and fetal echocardiography at 20 weeks [11]. In addition, the rate of fetal growth, development of early signs of preeclampsia, and incidence of infection of the urinary tract or other sites are closely monitored. By accurately assessing fetal health and maturity, clinicians can prevent intrauterine deaths while safely prolonging pregnancy to avoid the hazards of iatrogenic prematurity.

Low-dose aspirin to prevent preeclampsia is recommended, starting before 28 weeks (optimally between 12 and 16 weeks). At 28 weeks, daily maternal assessment of fetal activity is started. Twice-weekly nonstress tests (NSTs) are started at 32 weeks, or earlier if there are other maternal or fetal complications (e.g. hypertension, growth restriction) [12]. A nonreactive NST must be followed by a biophysical profile or contraction stress test. Antepartum heart rate testing using the twice-weekly NSTs has proved to be a reliable index of fetal well-being in a metabolically stable patient [13]. Timing of delivery should be individualized and depends on glycemic control, presence of associated maternal complications, and fetal status [14]. Ideally, the pregnant patients with diabetes should not go beyond 40 weeks gestation. In general, presence of comorbidity (hypertension), complications of diabetes (vasculopathy, nephropathy), poor glycemic control, or fetal growth abnormalities would favor earlier delivery

(36 0/7 to 38 6/7 weeks), whereas absence of any of these factors would favor expectant management until 39 0/7 weeks. Presence of more than one of these factors would tip the balance further toward earlier delivery.

Finally, in order to avoid birth injury from fetal macrosomia, a liberal attitude toward cesarean delivery (CD) should be employed in such cases. Sonographic assessment of estimated fetal weight and growth of the abdominal circumference is of value in detecting fetal macrosomia. If the estimated fetal weight exceeds 4500 g, delivery by elective CD should be considered. A macrosomic fetus, particularly in the presence of polyhydramnios, is usually an indication of poor glycemic control. Although macrosomia by itself is not an indication for delivery before 39 0/7 weeks, its presence in a diabetic patient is usually an indication of poor glycemic control, particularly if associated with polyhydramnios or increased abdominal circumference, and delivery may be considered if the patient is at 36 0/7 weeks or later [15].

Management of insulin during labor

When delivery is scheduled, the usual dose of insulin should be given at bedtime and the morning dose should be withheld [6]. The patient should be admitted early in the morning and a saline infusion started. Glucose levels should be checked hourly, and the infusion changed to 5% dextrose if the glucose level drops below 70 mg/dl. The rate of glucose infusion should be adjusted to keep the glucose level at about 100 mg/dl. If the glucose level is above 100 mg/dl on saline infusion, then infusion of regular insulin is needed. Regular short-acting insulin can be started at 1 U/h and titrated to keep the glucose level below 100 mg/dL. When the delivery is unscheduled, then the patient's usual intermittent insulin doses should be withheld and she should be managed similar to the scheduled patient. If the patient is on subcutaneous insulin pump, she may continue her basal rate.

Insulin requirements decrease rapidly after delivery. The patient can be restarted on half of her predelivery insulin dose as soon as she is eating regular food. For postoperative patients, sliding scale insulin regimen may be instituted until the patient is tolerating regular food.

CASE PRESENTATION

A 30-year-old gravida 4, para 3 was first seen at 18 weeks gestation. Her past obstetric history included the vaginal delivery of a 4100 g baby boy, who suffered a fractured humerus during delivery. The patient's mother had diabetes mellitus. Plasma glucose was obtained 1 h after a 50 g oral glucose load and was found to be 175 mg/dL. A 3-hour oral glucose tolerance test (OGTT) was then ordered. The results were as follows: fasting, 110 mg/dL; 1 hour, 243 mg/dL; 2 hour, 176 mg/dL; and 3 hour, 154 mg/dL. Pregestational diabetes was suspected.

Continued

The patient was started on a 2200-calorie diet with strict avoidance of concentrated sweets. Fasting and postprandial capillary glucose determinations were obtained daily. The fasting values ranged from 100 to 110 mg/dL, so she was started on split-dose insulin. Fetal growth was normal, and the patient remained normotensive.

Antepartum fetal evaluation was initiated with twice-weekly nonstress testing initiated at 32 weeks. Her glucose levels remained within the acceptable range. At 40 weeks, the estimated fetal weight was 4600 g. A cesarean delivery was performed. A 2-hour OGTT performed at 6 weeks postpartum confirmed type 2 diabetes.

References

1. Martin RB, Duryea E, Amnia A, Ragsdale A, McIntire D, Wells CE, et al. Congenital malformation risk according to hemoglobin A1c values in a contemporary cohort with pregestational diabetes. Am J Perinatol. 2021;38:1217–22.
2. Greene MF, Hare JW, Cloherty JP, Benacerraf BR, Soeldner JS. First-trimester hemoglobin A1 and risk for major malformation and spontaneous abortion in diabetic pregnancy. Teratology. 2002;65:97–101.
3. Korenbrot CC, Steinberg A, Bender C, Newberry S. Preconception care: a systematic review. Matern Child Health J. 2002;6:75–88.
4. American Diabetes Association. Preconception care of women with diabetes. Diabetes Care. 2004;27(Suppl 1):S76–8.
5. Standards of care in diabetes–2023. Diabetes Care. 2023;46(Suppl 1):S1–291.
6. American College of Obstetricians and Gynecologists. ACOG Practice Bulletin No. 201: pregestational diabetes mellitus. Obstet Gynecol. 2018;132:e228–47.
7. Siebenhofer A, Plank J, Berghold A, Horvath K, Semlitsch T, Berghold A, et al.; Cochrane Metabolic and Endocrine Disorders Group. Short acting insulin analogues versus regular human insulin in patients with diabetes mellitus. Cochrane Database Syst Rev. 2006;2:CD003287. doi: 10.1002/14651858.CD012161.
8. Hughes RC, Rowen JA. Pregnancy in women with type 2 diabetes: who takes metformin and what is the outcome? Diabet Med. 2006;23:318–22.
9. Ekpebegh CO, Coetzee EJ, van der Merwe L, Levitt NS. A 10-year retrospective analysis of pregnancy outcome in pregestational type 2 diabetes: comparison of insulin and oral glucose-lowering agents. Diabet Med. 2007;24(3):253–8.
10. Widness JA, Schwartz HC, Thompson D, King KC, Kahn CB, Oh W, et al. Glycohemoglobin (HbA1c): a predictor of birth weight in infants of diabetic mothers. J Pediatr. 1978;92:8–12.
11. Albert TJ, Landon MB, Wheller JJ, Samuels P, Cheng RF, Gabbe S. Prenatal detection of fetal anomalies in pregnancies complicated by insulindependent diabetes mellitus. Am J Obstet Gynecol. 1996; 174:1424–8.
12. Landon MB, Langer O, Gabbe SG, Schick C, Brustman L. Fetal surveillance in pregnancies complicated by insulin-dependent diabetes mellitus. Am J Obstet Gynecol. 1992;167:617–21.
13. Gabbe SG, Graves CR. Management of diabetes mellitus complicating pregnancy. Obstet Gynecol. 2003;102:857–68.
14. Boulvain M, Stan C, Irion O.; Cochrane Pregnancy and Childbirth Group. Elective delivery in diabetic pregnant women. Cochrane Database Syst Rev. 2006;2:CD000451. doi: 10.1002/14651858.CD001997.
15. American College of Obstetricians and Gynecologists. ACOG Practice Bulletin No. 216: macrosomia. Obstet Gynecol. 2020; 135:e18–e35.

Chapter 21
Thyroid Disorders

Elizabeth O. Buschur[1] and Stephen F. Thung[2]

[1]Department of Internal Medicine, Division of Endocrinology, Metabolism, and Diabetes, The Ohio State University College of Medicine, Columbus, OH, USA

[2]Department of Obstetrics, Gynecology and Reproductive Sciences, Yale School of Medicine, New Haven, CT, USA

Thyroid disease in pregnancy is second only to diabetes amongst endocrine disorders. The overlap between common pregnancy complaints and physiological changes and the signs and symptoms of both hyperthyroidism and hypothyroidism can make recognition challenging.

Maintenance of maternal euthyroid status is critical for maternal and fetal health and development. The fetal thyroid becomes active as early as 12 weeks of gestation [1,2] and until this time the fetus is dependent upon transplacental transport of maternal thyroid hormone.

Pregnancy induces thyroid-related physiological changes. Estrogens stimulate rapid production of both thyroid-binding globulins as well as total thyroid hormones (T3 and T4) to levels significantly greater than in the nonpregnant state. Despite this rapid increase, active free thyroid hormone levels (free T3 and free T4) do not change significantly from nonpregnant levels. Thyroid-stimulating hormone (TSH) changes modestly during pregnancy, particularly in the first trimester when levels are commonly reduced below nonpregnant norms as a result of the thyrotropic effects of human chorionic gonadotropin (hCG), which is structurally similar to TSH [3].

Diagnosis

TSH and free T4 assessments are required to make the diagnosis for thyroid disorders (Table 21.1) [3,4].

Additional studies

• *T3 levels*: when there is a strong clinical suspicion for hyperthyroidism with a low or suppressed TSH and normal free T4, testing a T3 may be useful to determine etiology. Isolated T3 thyrotoxicosis can be found in Graves' disease. During pregnancy, the reference range for total T3 is typically 1.5 times higher than outside pregnancy.

• *TSH-receptor antibodies (TRAb)* include thyroid-stimulating immunoglobulin and thyroid inhibitory antibodies that stimulate or inhibit, respectively, the TSH receptor resulting in Graves' disease. TRAb are the pathological antibodies found in Graves' disease-related hyperthyroidism that mediate the signs and symptoms of the disorder and can confirm the diagnosis. Moreover, TRAb cross the placenta (IgG) and on rare occasions stimulate the fetal thyroid leading to fetal or neonatal Graves' disease regardless of maternal thyroid state. Testing for TRAb is recommended in women who have active or treated Graves' disease including those who have had either radioactive iodine ablation or surgery (thyroidectomy) in the past. Pregnant women with high TRAb (>3 times the upper limit of normal) should have close fetal and neonatal follow-up, similar to mothers with active hyperthyroidism, as the fetus and neonate remain at risk.

• *Antithyroid peroxidase antibodies (TPO) or antithyroglobulin (TG) antibodies* are antibodies commonly associated with Hashimoto's thyroiditis and hypothyroidism and can be positive in 2–18% of unselected pregnant women. TPO antibodies in euthyroid women have been associated with future thyroiditis risks (especially postpartum thyroiditis) as well as pregnancy loss. TPO testing may be indicated in women with recurrent pregnancy loss, as some studies demonstrate that low-dose thyroid hormone supplementation may reduce the risk of recurrent loss or prematurity in euthyroid women. Women with positive TPO or TG antibodies should have a TSH checked at pregnancy confirmation and monthly in the first half of pregnancy.

Hypothyroidism

Unrecognized overt hypothyroidism is uncommon during pregnancy due to a high prevalence of infertility. However, pregnant women with medically managed pre-existing hypothyroidism is common. In the United States, Hashimoto's thyroiditis is the most common etiology due

---

Queenan's Management of High-Risk Pregnancy: An Evidence-Based Approach, Seventh Edition. Edited by Catherine Y. Spong and Charles J. Lockwood.

Table 21.1 Diagnosis of thyroid disorders

Condition	TSH	Free T4
Overt hypothyroidism	High	Low
Subclinical hypothyroidism	High	Normal range
Overt hyperthyroidism	Low (commonly undetectable)	High
Subclinical hyperthyroidism	Low	Normal range
Hypothyroxinemia	Normal range	Low

TSH, thyroid-stimulating hormone.

to autoimmune–mediated inflammation and destruction of thyroid gland [3]. Surgical thyroidectomy or radioactive iodine ablation are other causes.

Worldwide, iodine deficiency is the most common etiology for maternal hypothyroidism and is the leading cause of offspring intellectual deficits (cretinism). Even in the United States, moderate iodine deficiency is a growing concern as Americans consume less salt due to cardiovascular concern, and salt-containing foods consumed daily lack significant iodine supplementation such as processed foods and popular salt products (sea salt and kosher salts).

Implications for pregnancy

Overt hypothyroidism is clearly associated with adverse pregnancy outcomes. When managed judiciously, outcomes can be similar to uncomplicated low-risk gestations. Adverse pregnancy outcomes due to hypothyroidism can include:
• spontaneous abortion and fetal demise
• placental abruption
• gestational hypertension and preeclampsia
• idiopathic preterm birth
• low birthweight
• offspring developmental delay

Subclinical hypothyroidism is commonly defined by an elevated TSH above 95% or 97.5% for pregnancy and a normal free T4. Large randomized controlled trials of pregnant women with subclinical hypothyroidism and hypothyroxinemia found that treatment did not improve maternal or fetal outcome, including IQ at age 5 [5,6]. Many women with subclinical hypothyroidism are TPO antibody positive, which may be associated with poor outcomes in the absence of any thyroid hormone derangements.

TPO antibody-positive women may be a special population. Routine screening for this condition is not recommended and there is no consensus guideline on treatment if identified. In our opinion, among women with a history of recurrent pregnancy loss, levothyroxine supplementation for TPO antibody-positive women with normal free T4 levels may be considered, especially for women with TSH levels above the pregnancy reference range. Typically, a low dose of levothyroxine such as 50 µg daily should not pose maternal risks [3].

Hypothyroxinemia has not been clearly associated with adverse pregnancy outcomes and thyroid hormone supplementation is not recommended [5,6]. Attention to diet and adequate iodine intake is prudent in these cases.

Thyroid cancer is rare during pregnancy. In general, most thyroid neoplasms are slow growing, and surgery may be deferred until after delivery. That being said, data suggest no differences in pregnancy outcome if thyroidectomy is performed in the second trimester [7]. Lifelong thyroid hormone replacement is essential after thyroidectomy.

Treatment

Therapy for overt hypothyroidism is straightforward in most cases.
• Oral levothyroxine (T4) is recommended. Combined T4/T3 products are not recommended for management of hypothyroidism [3].
• Levothyroxine dosing for overt hypothyroidism is typically 100–125 µg daily but may be significantly higher in women who have had a thyroidectomy/ablation. For mild to moderate cases 1 µg/kg/day is appropriate as an initial dose, and severe cases may require 1.5 µg/kg/day.
• Dosing typically increases in the first trimester, approximately 20–30%. Some experts empirically increase dosing once pregnancy is determined while others determine dosing changes based upon TSH and free T4 levels at a first prenatal visit. Both approaches are acceptable [3].
• For women with hypothyroidism, TSH should be checked at pregnancy confirmation and every 4 weeks until halfway through pregnancy then once per trimester.
• Be aware that iron and/or calcium supplementation can interfere with thyroid hormone absorption and dosing should be staggered, 4–6 hours before or after levothyroxine.
• TSH goals for levothyroxine titration are not agreed upon. If the lab provides a trimester-specific reference range in your region, the dose of levothyroxine should be adjusted to achieve a TSH in the lower half of the pregnancy reference range, or if not provided TSH <2.5 mIU/L.
• In the postpartum period, levothyroxine dosing should be returned to prepregnancy dose. TSH should be tested at the routine postpartum visit (~6 weeks) in those on levothyroxine and to rule out postpartum thyroiditis in those with positive TPO or TG antibodies not on thyroid hormone replacement. There are no concerns with breastfeeding and levothyroxine therapy.

Hyperthyroidism

Hyperthyroidism affects approximately 0.2% of pregnancies. The overwhelming majority have Graves' disease. Other etiologies include active thyroid adenomas and toxic nodular goiter, thyroiditis, and transient gestational thyrotoxicosis (hCG induced).

Graves' disease is an autoimmune disorder that may involve several organ systems, including the thyroid and the eyes. TRAb mediate the disease state including triggering overactivity of the thyroid gland. These IgG autoantibodies cross the placenta to stimulate fetal disease in rare cases (1–5%) [6]. Even when the maternal thyroid gland is removed (thyroidectomy) or destroyed (radioactive iodine ablation), circulating TRAb may mediate fetal disease in a euthyroid mother.

Implications for pregnancy

This is related to severity of the disease state. Mild disease can be tolerated while moderate and severe disease generally requires pharmacotherapy or thyroidectomy in recalcitrant cases. Women not optimally managed face risks of preeclampsia/gestational hypertension and tachycardia. In severe cases, particularly in thyroid storm, women are at significant risk for cardiac heart failure and death.

Thyroid storm is an acute medical emergency characterized by a hypermetabolic state that when unmanaged results in heart failure and death. Recognition and aggressive management in an intensive care setting are essential.

Fetal consequences include growth restriction, fetal/neonatal tachycardia, and demise. Neonatal hyperthyroidism is found in 1–5% of Graves' disease pregnancies, mediated by TRAb that cross the placenta. Findings include fetal tachycardia, fetal goiter, cardiac heart failure/hydrops, accelerated bone maturity, and craniosynostosis. On ultrasound, a fetal goiter may be seen as a homogenous echogenic vascular anterior neck mass measuring more than 95th percentile.

Transient gestational thyrotoxicosis is generally a self-limited consequence of the common alpha subunits of hCG and TSH. As such, hCG is a weak stimulator of thyroid hormone release and as hCG levels rise in the first trimester, so does the potential for subclinical hyperthyroidism or mild overt hyperthyroidism. As hCG levels taper in the second trimester, so does the associated thyrotoxicosis. Typically, therapy is not required beyond reassurance. HCG-mediated thyrotoxicosis is more common in pregnant women with hyperemesis or multiple fetuses.

Management

Subclinical hyperthyroidism does not require treatment, but follow-up for development to overt hyperthyroidism may be prudent, particularly in the postpartum period.

Pharmacotherapy management of overt maternal hyperthyroidism alleviates maternal and fetal risks, but may result in unintentional fetal hypothyroidism due to placental transfer of the antithyroid medication. As such, using minimal dosing of pharmacological agents is necessary. Titrating therapy to achieve a euthyroid state bordering upon subclinical hyperthyroidism is ideal.

Antithyroid therapy. Two therapeutic options are available. Propylthiouracil (PTU) has been used due to concerns of small but increased risks of teratogenicity with methimazole (MMI). PTU has been associated with fulminant hepatitis for all users (1/10000) that may result in death or liver transplantation. As such, MMI is now the first-line hyperthyroidism therapy for nonpregnant users due to its safer side effect profile and once-daily dosing. This is the case for pregnancy, except in the first trimester.

Current recommendations are to use PTU preconception and first trimester followed by MMI for the remainder of pregnancy to minimize both fetal and maternal risks. For mild hyperthyroidism or early Graves' disease, it is reasonable to postpone treatment until organogenesis is complete.

• *MMI* use has concerns including maternal hepatitis and *possible* concerns for fetal abnormalities such as aplasia cutis, choanal atresia, and tracheoesophageal fistulas [8]. Absolute risks are low and if a woman enters prenatal care past the period of organogenesis, MMI therapy should be maintained, rather than changed to alternative agents. Initial dosing commonly ranges from 5 to 10 mg daily with upward titration to 10–30 mg daily.

• *PTU* side effects include rash, and rare hepatitis and liver failure (1/10000) resulting in death or liver transplant, as well as agranulocytosis (first 3 months typically less than 1% risk) [9]. Typical starting dose should be determined by severity of disease, but we commonly start with 50 mg three times daily and increase monthly to a typical 100–150 mg every 8 hours. Serial liver function tests are not useful due to rapid progression of hepatitis when it occurs. For both PTU and MMI, a baseline complete blood count and hepatic panel prior to starting the medication is recommended. There is no evidence that monitoring serial liver enzymes will prevent liver failure from PTU and therefore this is not recommended by the Food and Drug Administration or American Thyroid Association [3]. Some clinicians choose to repeat liver enzymes monthly with thyroid lab draws. Agranulocytosis with antithyroid medications has typically occurred within the first 2–3 months of treatment so monitoring at dose initiation or reinitiation is best.

• *Changing between PTU and MMI.* MMI is 20–30-fold more potent per milligram than PTU [3]. As such, a patient requiring 300 mg (total daily dose) of PTU could be expected to require 10 to 15 mg of MMI daily. For both therapies, monthly thyroid function follow-up is needed to actively titrate dosing. In more severe cases, free T4 can be measured more frequently to guide increasing dosage. The goal of treatment is to maintain the free T4 level at high normal or even slightly elevated to minimize fetal thyroid suppression. The goal is not to normalize the TSH. Requirements typically fall in the third trimester due to reduced disease activity, and some women are able to discontinue medication in later pregnancy. Both therapies are acceptable for breastfeeding [3], but the infant's pediatrician should be advised that the mother uses the medication. With higher doses of PTU or MMI or with infant growth restriction, the infant's thyroid hormone level should be checked.

For *severe cases with symptoms*, propranolol 20 mg every 6–8 hours can be used.

Fetal surveillance. Given the fetal risks, a detailed anatomical survey is indicated with serial ultrasound for growth, commonly monthly. For women with a history of Graves' disease, fetal hyperthyroidism is a concern through TRAb-mediated pathogenesis. In these cases, TRAb can be measured to determine if there is fetal risk (higher risk with TRAb levels more than three times the upper reference for the assay), but attention to the presence of fetal tachycardia and subsequent sonographic evaluation of the fetal neck for goiter (homogenous echogenic enlargement on the anterior neck more than 95%) is typically sufficient [3]. Women with a history of Graves' disease or hyperthyroidism treated with radioactive iodine ablation, thyroidectomy, or antithyroid medications should have TRAb measured with the first prenatal labs and, if elevated, again at 18–22 weeks and 24–28 weeks gestation. A TRAb value above three times the upper limit of normal is associated with neonatal Graves' disease [3].

In rare cases of treated hyperthyroidism when a fetal goiter is identified, determining whether the fetus is hyperthyroid or hypothyroid can be difficult. In these cases, using cordocentesis to sample fetal blood and thyroid levels for therapy guidance has been described. However, our own experience suggests that identifying persistent fetal tachycardia with heart rate variability is sufficient to exclude fetal hypothyroidism and confirm a diagnosis of fetal hyperthyroidism. In these cases, additional dosing of antithyroid medication (+/− maternal levothyroxine supplementation) may be required with a goal of normalizing the fetal heart rate. These cases should be referred to a tertiary center that has experience with this management.

In *recalcitrant cases* that do not respond to pharmacotherapy, thyroidectomy may be considered. Surgical removal can be done safely, especially in the second trimester. Radioactive iodine is contraindicated as it is concentrated in the fetal thyroid.

Thyroid storm management [3,4,10]

- This is a medical emergency that requires immediate admission to a medical intensive care unit.
- Common symptoms include fever, agitation, delirium, tachycardia, and congestive heart failure.
- Therapy is no different than the nonpregnant state.
- Immediate intravenous (IV) access and hydration.
- PTU 600–800 mg PO/crushed in a nasogastric tube, followed by 150–200 mg every 4–6 hours.
- Iodide product to suppress T3 and T4 release from thyroid gland; options include:
  - sodium iodide 500–1000 mg IV (1 hour after PTU administration) every 8 hours (or)
  - potassium iodide (SSKI) 5 drops every 8 hours (or)
  - lugol solution 8 drops PO every 6 hours (or)
  - lithium carbonate 300 mg every 6 hours (if allergic to the above)
  - dexamethasone 2 mg IV every 6 hours for 4 doses (blocks peripheral conversion of T4 to T3).
- Beta blockers if the patient is not hypotensive or in heart failure. Options include:
  - propranolol 1 mg IV (slow) every 5 minutes for a total of 6 mg followed by 1–10 mg IV every 4 hours (or)
  - propranolol 20–80 mg PO or nasogastric tube every 4–6 hours (or)
  - esmolol drip, 250–500 µg/kg with continuous drip of 50–100 µg/kg/min.

CASE PRESENTATION

A healthy 36-year-old G1P0 woman at 7 weeks gestation presents with fatigue and constipation at her first prenatal visit. She also complains of dry hair and brittle nails. TSH is found to be 11 (0.45–4.5 mIU/L) and free T4 is normal. Anti-TPO antibody is positive. What is the next best step?

(A) Start levothyroxine 25 mcg daily
(B) No follow-up is needed
(C) Repeat TSH in 6–8 weeks
(D) Start armour thyroid 90 mg daily
(E) Start levothyroxine 100 mcg daily

The correct answer is (E). This pregnant patient has symptoms of hypothyroidism and elevated TSH in setting of Hashimoto's thyroiditis. It is recommended to start thyroid hormone replacement with levothyroxine weight-based 1.6 mcg/kg (~100 mcg/kg). Follow-up is needed as TSH is recommended to be less than 2.5 mIU/L in women with Hashimoto's thyroiditis during pregnancy for optimal outcomes. Treatment should begin immediately. Mixed thyroid hormone preparations such as armour thyroid (containing T4 and T3) are not recommended in pregnancy due to T3 not readily crossing the placenta, and these preparations are not recommended by the American Thyroid Association for treatment of hypothyroidism in nonpregnant or pregnant patients.

References

1. Calvo RM, Jauniaux E, Gulbis B, Asuncion M, Gervy C, Contempre B, et al. Fetal tissues are exposed to biologically relevant free thyroxine concentrations during early phases of development. J Clin Endocrinol Metab. 2002;87(4):1768–77.
2. Gorman CA. Radioiodine and pregnancy. Thyroid. 1999;9(7):721–6.
3. Alexander EK, Pearce E, Brent G, Brown RS, Chen H, Dosiou C, et al. 2017 Guidelines of the American Thyroid Association for the diagnosis and management of thyroid disease during pregnancy and the postpartum. Thyroid. 2017;27(3):315–89.
4. American College of Obstetricians and Gynecologists. ACOG Practice Bulletin No. 223: thyroid disease in pregnancy. Obstet Gynecol. 2020;135(6):e261–74.
5. Casey BM, Thom EA, Peaceman AM, Varner MW, Sorokin Y, Hirtz DG, et al. Treatment of subclinical hypothyroidism or hypothyroxinemia in pregnancy. N Engl J Med. 2017;376:815–25.
6. Cooper DS, Laurberg P. Hyperthyroidism in pregnancy. Lancet Diabetes Endocrinol. 2013;1(3):238–49.
7. Gharib H, Papini E, Garber JR, Duick DS, Harrell RM, Hegedüus L, AACE/ACE/AME Task Force on Thyroid Nodules. American Association of Clinical Endocrinologists, American College of Endocrinology, and Associazione Medici Endocrinologi medical guidelines for clinical practice for the diagnosis and management of thyroid nodules–2016 update. Endocr Pract. 2016;22(5):622–39.
8. Andersen SL, Olsen J, Laurberg P. Antithyroid drug side effects in the population and in pregnancy. J Clin Endocrinol Metab. 2016;101(4):1606–14.
9. Chalasani NP, Hayashi PH, Bonkovsky HL, Navarro VJ, Lee WM, Fontana RJ, Practice Parameters Committee of the American College of Gastroenterology. ACG Clinical Guideline: the diagnosis and management of idiosyncratic drug-induced liver injury. Am J Gastroenterol. 2014;109(7):950–66; quiz 967.
10. Hamidi OP, Barbour LA. Endocrine emergencies during pregnancy: diabetic ketoacidosis and thyroid storm. Obstet Gynecol Clin North Am. 2022;49(3):473–89.

Chapter 22
Asthma

Jennifer Namazy[1] and Michael Schatz[2]
[1]Department of Allergy and Immunology, Scripps Clinic, San Diego, CA, USA
[2]Department of Allergy, Kaiser Permanente Medical Center, San Diego, CA, USA

Asthma affects 4–8% of pregnant women [1] and thus is a common medical problem in pregnancy. Moreover, the prevalence of asthma during pregnancy is increasing. Prevalence was 5.5% in 2001, which increased to 7.8% in 2007 [1,2]. Maternal asthma increases the risk of perinatal mortality, preeclampsia, preterm birth, and low-birth-weight infants. More severe asthma is associated with increased risks [3]. This chapter reviews the definition and diagnosis of asthma and the interrelationships between asthma and pregnancy as a prelude to discussing the management of asthma in pregnant women.

Definition of asthma

Asthma is an inflammatory disease of the airways that is associated with reversible airway obstruction and airway hyperreactivity. A number of clinical triggering factors exist, including viral infections, allergens, exercise, sinusitis, reflux, weather changes, and stress.

Airway obstruction can be produced by varying degrees of mucosal edema, bronchoconstriction, mucus plugging, and airway remodeling. In acute asthma, these changes can lead to ventilation/perfusion imbalance and hypoxia. Although early acute asthma is typically associated with hyperventilation and hypocapnea, progressive acute asthma can cause respiratory failure with associated carbon dioxide retention and acidosis.

Effect of pregnancy on the course of asthma

Clinical observations

A metaanalysis of 14 studies found that asthma severity improves in one-third of women, worsens in one-third, and remains unchanged in one third [4]. However, a critical review of the literature found only three studies of 54 women that were prospective, enrolled women before the third trimester, and assessed their patients with objective measures of asthma severity or validated severity scales [5]. In a recent large prospective study of 1739 pregnant asthmatic women, severity classification (based on symptoms, pulmonary function, and medication use) worsened in 30% and improved in 23% of patients during pregnancy [6]. Asthma is more likely to be more severe or to worsen during pregnancy in women who have more severe asthma before becoming pregnant.

The course of asthma may vary by stage of pregnancy. The first trimester is generally well tolerated, with infrequent acute episodes [7]. Increased symptoms and more frequent exacerbations occur between weeks 17 and 36 of gestation [7]. In contrast, asthmatic women tend to experience fewer symptoms and less frequent exacerbations during weeks 37–40 of pregnancy [7]. These studies suggest that the first trimester and the last month of pregnancy are relatively free of asthma exacerbations and that the second and earlier third trimester have more potential for increased asthma symptoms.

The variable effect of pregnancy on the course of asthma appears to be more than just random fluctuation in the natural history of the disease because pregnancy-associated changes usually revert toward the prepregnancy state by 3 months postpartum. It is also of interest that asthma is often consistent in an individual woman during successive pregnancies [8].

Mechanisms

The mechanisms responsible for the altered clinical course of asthma during pregnancy are unknown and represent a fertile area for additional research. There are multiple biochemical and physiologic changes during pregnancy that could potentially ameliorate or exacerbate gestational asthma [9]. However, it is not clear which, if any, of these factors are important in determining the course of asthma during pregnancy.

Effect of asthma on pregnancy

Clinical observations
A meta-analysis from Murphy et al. found that pregnant women with asthma are at a significantly increased risk of a range of adverse perinatal outcomes including low birthweight and preterm birth [10].

This is supported by a study from Sweden, which reported an increased risk of preeclampsia, emergency cesarean section, and small for gestational age, even when controlled for familial confounding factors [11]. Data from two US health claims databases found increased risks of prematurity, small for gestational age, and neonatal intensive care unit (ICU) admissions among women with asthma. Women with uncontrolled asthma demonstrated increased risks of preterm birth and neonatal ICU admission. Those with more severe asthma had an increased risk of small for gestational age infants [12].

Mechanisms
Definition of the mechanism(s) of maternal asthma's adverse effect on pregnancy outcomes reported should allow institution of optimal intervention strategy. Mechanisms postulated to explain these increased perinatal risks have included:
• hypoxia and other physiologic consequences of poorly controlled asthma
• medications used to treat asthma
• demographic or pathogenic factors *associated with* asthma but not actually caused by the disease or its treatment

The latter would imply that asthma and adverse perinatal outcomes may share the same underlying pathogenetic mechanism (such as a predisposition to inflammation) or demographic associations (such as smoking), but that inadequately controlled asthma or asthma treatment is not causally related to the adverse perinatal outcome.

Available information, however, suggests that adequate asthma control during pregnancy is important in improving maternal and fetal outcomes. Oral corticosteroids have also been associated with increased risks of preeclampsia [13] and prematurity [14] in pregnant asthmatic women. However, whether this represents a drug effect, an effect of inadequately controlled asthma, or a marker for common pathogenesis factors associated with more severe asthma is not clear from the data.

Maternal use of bronchodilators has been associated with an increased risk of infant cardiac defects [15] and gastroschisis [16]. However, because women experiencing asthma exacerbations during the first trimester of pregnancy have been reported to have an increased risk of congenital malformations in their infants compared to infants of asthmatic women not experiencing exacerbations [17], the reported relationships between congenital malformations and bronchodilators may be confounded by severe asthma episodes.

Diagnosis of asthma during pregnancy

Many patients with asthma during pregnancy have a diagnosis of asthma. A new diagnosis is usually suspected on typical symptoms – wheezing, chest tightness, cough, and associated shortness of breath – which tend to be episodic fluctuating in intensity and are typically worse at night. Identification of the characteristic triggers further supports the diagnosis. Wheezing may be present on auscultation of the lungs, but the absence of wheezing on auscultation does not exclude the diagnosis. The diagnosis is confirmed by spirometry that shows a reduced forced expiratory volume in 1 second (FEV_1; <80% predicted) with an increase in FEV_1 of 12% or more after an inhaled short-acting bronchodilator.

It is sometimes difficult to demonstrate reversible airway obstruction in patients with mild or intermittent asthma. Although methacholine challenge testing may be considered in nonpregnant patients with normal pulmonary function to confirm asthma, such testing is not recommended during pregnancy. Exhaled nitric oxide (eNO) is elevated in pregnant patients with asthma [18]. If available, an elevated eNO (>25 ppb) would support a diagnosis of asthma during pregnancy. If eNO is not available therapeutic trials of asthma therapy should generally be used. Improvement with asthma therapy supports the diagnosis, which can then be confirmed postpartum with additional testing if necessary.

The most common differential diagnosis is dyspnea of pregnancy, which may occur in early pregnancy in approximately 70% of women. This dyspnea is differentiated from asthma by its lack of association with cough, wheezing, or airway obstruction.

Management

Asthma guidelines include four categories.
• Assessment and monitoring
• Control of factors contributing to severity
• Patient education
• Pharmacologic therapy

The Global Initiative for Asthma Strategy report of 2021 [19] had key changes for the treatment of asthma. These include that asthma in adults and adolescents should not be treated with short acting beta-agonists (SABA) alone but rather with an inhaled corticosteroid (ICS) to reduce overuse and exacerbation risk. The preferred method is to use low-dose ICS–formoterol–as the reliever option. This, however, has not been studied in pregnant asthmatic women.

Assessment and monitoring

Once the diagnosis of asthma is confirmed, the severity (in patients not already on controller medications) or assessment of control (in patients already on controller medications) is assessed. Severity is based on the frequency of daytime and nighttime symptoms and pulmonary function (ideally spirometry, minimally peak flow rate) (Table 22.1). Based on this, controller therapy is initiated (if indicated).

In treated patients (either initially or with follow-up), it is important to determine whether their asthma is controlled (Table 22.2). Like severity, assessment of control depends on frequency of symptoms, nighttime awakening, interference with normal activity, exacerbations, and

Table 22.1 Stepwise approach for managing asthma during pregnancy in patients not on controllers

Clinical features before treatment	Symptoms/day Daily medications	PEFR or FEV$_1$	Medications required to maintain long-term control

Severe persistent	Symptoms/night Continual Frequent	≤60%	• Preferred treatment:
			  – High-dose inhaled corticosteroid *and*
			  – Long-acting inhaled β2-agonist and, if needed,
			  – Corticosteroid tablets or syrup long term (starting at 1 mg/kg/day, reducing systemic corticosteroid to lowest effective dose)
			• Alternative treatment:
			  – High-dose inhaled corticosteroid *and*
			  – Sustained release theophylline to serum concentration of 5–12 µg/mL

Moderate persistent	Daily >1 night/wk	>60–<80%	• Preferred treatment:
			either
			  – Low-dose inhaled corticosteroid and long-acting β2-agonist *or*
			  – Medium-dose inhaled corticosteroid
			If needed (particularly in patients with recurring severe exacerbations):
			  – Medium-dose inhaled corticosteroid and long-acting inhaled β2-agonist
			• Alternative treatment:
			  – Low-dose inhaled corticosteroid and either theophylline or leukotriene receptor antagonist.
			If needed:
			  – Medium-dose inhaled corticosteroid and either theophylline or leukotriene receptor antagonist

Mild persistent	>2 d/wk but <daily >2 nights/m	>80%	• Preferred treatment: – Low-dose inhaled corticosteroid • Alternative treatment: leukotriene receptor antagonist *or* sustained-release theophylline to serum concentration of 5–12 µg/mL
Mild intermittent	≤2 d/wk ≤2 nights/m	≥80%	• No daily medication needed • Severe exacerbations may occur, separated by long periods of normal lung function and no symptoms

FEV$_1$, forced expiratory volume in 1 sec; PEFR, peak expiratory flow rate.

Table 22.2 Assessment of asthma control in pregnant women

Components of control	Classification of control[a]		
	Well controlled	Not well controlled	Very poorly controlled
Symptoms	≤2 d/wk	>2 d/wk	Throughout the day
Nighttime awakening	≤2 times/m	1–3 times/wk	≥4 times/wk
Interference with normal activity	None	Some limitation	Extremely limited
Short-acting β2-agonist use for symptom control FEV$_1$ or peak flow	≤2 d/wk >80%[b]	>2 d/wk 60–80%[b]	Several times per day <60%[b]
Exacerbations requiring systemic corticosteroids	0–1 in past 12 m	≥2 in past 12 m	

[a]The level of control is based on the most severe category. Assess symptom frequency and impact by patient's recall of previous 2–4 weeks.
[b]Predicted or personal best.
FEV$_1$, forced expiratory volume in 1 second. Adapted from [23].

pulmonary function. Therapy is adjusted based on this assessment of control. Validated questionnaires are used to assess asthma control, the pregnancy Asthma Control Test (p-ACT) has been shown to be valid and reliable to monitor asthma control during pregnancy. CARAT or "control of Allergic Rhinitis and Asthma Test" is a brief self-administered questionnaire to quantify the degree of control of allergic rhinitis and asthma. It was preliminarily validated in 42 pregnant asthmatic patients [20,21]. Patients with persistent asthma should be monitored monthly for asthma control. This is due to asthma changes in approximately two thirds of women during pregnancy. Home peak flow monitoring should be considered for patients with moderate-to-severe asthma, especially for those who have difficulty perceiving signs of worsening asthma.

FeNO may also be useful in the management of asthma during pregnancy. A double-blind, parallel-group tested the value of measurement of fraction of exhaled nitric oxide (F(E)NO) to guide management of pregnant asthmatic women finding that the exacerbation rate was lower in the group using F(E)NO to adjust asthma therapies [22].

Because asthma is associated with intrauterine growth restriction and preterm birth, pregnancy dating should be established accurately. All should be instructed to be attentive to fetal activity. The intensity of antenatal testing of fetal well-being should be considered on the basis of the severity and control of the asthma. Evaluation of fetal activity and growth by serial ultrasounds should be considered for women:

• who have suboptimally controlled asthma
• with moderate-to-severe asthma (starting at 32 weeks)
• who are recovering from a severe asthma exacerbation

Control of factors contributing to severity

The control of maternal asthma is essential to reduce the risk of perinatal complications. There are several factors that remain barriers to asthma control in this group of patients. They include adherence, physician undertreatment, obesity, smoking, and infections.

Genetic factors may influence asthma during pregnancy and act as confounders when interpreting outcomes studies. Rejno et al. [11] performed an analysis of perinatal outcomes in full cousin and sister pairs. They found that outcomes including preeclampsia, low birthweight, cesarean section, and gestational age were more common in women with asthma, suggesting that these associations are not confounded by genes but rather a true effect of asthma on pregnancy.

Medication nonadherence during pregnancy is a significant clinical problem. A cohort study of 115 169 pregnant asthmatics in South Korea reported that women tended to rapidly reduce their asthma medication use during the beginning of their pregnancy. This led to a greater number of exacerbations in a small proportion of the study population [24]. Kim et al. found that use of ICS-long-acting beta agonists, systemic steroids, and SABA was less in likely in pregnant women [25]. Another study found that about one third of pregnant asthmatics discontinued asthma medications during pregnancy, often without consulting their physicians [26]. Lim et al. [27] examined nonadherence in pregnant asthmatic women. Concerns about medication use, specifically steroid use, overshadowed concerns about the potential risks of uncontrolled asthma. Many were content to rely on their reliever therapy and decreased preventive therapy without consulting their doctors. Interestingly, the majority complained about the lack of information available regarding asthma during pregnancy. Lack of support was also common. Many felt that the information they were receiving was contradictory, leading them to make their own choices about medication management. As a result, many decreased or discontinued their asthma medications or withheld doses during pregnancy. According to the study, women felt it would have been helpful if asthma had been discussed further by their health care professionals, providing opportunities for pursuing more reliable information. Robijn et al. found that persistent nonadherence to ICS was associated with lower maternal age, higher parity, and no prescribed ICS at baseline [28].

Unfortunately, over a quarter of family physicians would instruct their patients to decrease or discontinue asthma medication during pregnancy when asthma was well controlled by current therapy [29]. Furthermore, almost 30% of physicians would not perform spirometry in pregnant asthmatic patients, and only 64% reported that they followed the asthma guidelines in the management of pregnant asthmatic patients [30].

Physician reluctance may also affect the course of asthma during pregnancy. One study identified 51 pregnant women and 500 nonpregnant women presenting to the emergency department with acute asthma. Although asthma severity appeared to be similar, pregnant women were significantly less likely to be discharged on oral corticosteroids (38% vs. 64%). Presumably related to this undertreatment, pregnant women were three times more likely than nonpregnant women to report an ongoing exacerbation 2 weeks later. [31,32]

Obesity has been shown to be an inflammatory state that may play an important role in asthma initiation and control. Obesity is associated with adverse perinatal outcomes including gestational diabetes, preeclampsia, thromboembolic disorders, postpartum hemorrhage, large for gestational age, fetal death, and congenital anomalies. The mechanisms are thought to be due to a heightened inflammatory response. Airway macrophages from obese adults have impaired function in clearing apoptotic inflammatory cells [11]. This was associated with inflammation measured by increased oxidant levels and decreased corticosteroid responsiveness. Higher body mass index has been associated with an increased risk for asthma exacerbations in both nonpregnant and pregnant women. In one study of pregnant asthmatic women, 30.7% of participants were obese (body mass index ≥30 kg/m2), and obesity was associated with an increase in asthma exacerbations (odds ratio [OR] 1.3, 95% confidence interval [CI] 1.1–1.7) compared to nonobese pregnant asthmatic women [12]. Another study reported that women with asthma exacerbations had a larger gestational weight gain in the first trimester of pregnancy and increased total gestational weight gain compared with women without exacerbation. In fact, more than 5 kg first-trimester weight gain was associated with a large increased risk of asthma exacerbation (OR 9.35, 95% CI 6.39–13.68, $P<0.01$) [33].

Population-based studies have shown a relationship between smoking and airway hyperresponsiveness [34]. Tobacco smoke is also a common airway irritant. Although asthma and smoking during pregnancy have been separately linked to adverse perinatal outcomes such as low birthweight and preterm birth, the combination increases the risk [35]. Even passive smoke exposure has been associated with an increased risk of uncontrolled asthma during pregnancy [36,37].

An increased risk of preterm birth has been linked to exposure to traffic-related air pollutants [38]. Infections during pregnancy can affect the course of gestational asthma and be a barrier to asthma control. Some degree of decrease in cell-mediated immunity may make the pregnant patient more susceptible to viral infection, and upper respiratory tract infections have been reported to be the most common precipitants of asthma exacerbations during pregnancy [7]. Sinusitis, a known asthma trigger, has been reported to be six times more common in pregnant compared to nonpregnant women [39]. In addition, pneumonia has been reported to be greater than five times more common in asthmatic than nonasthmatic women during pregnancy [40].

Pregnant women are at an increased risk for respiratory viral infections including influenza A (H1N1) [41] and rhinovirus [42]. These infections may be complicated by bronchitis, bacterial pneumonia, and bacterial sinusitis, all of which may have adverse effects on both mother and baby. Therefore, vaccination for influenza for the pregnant asthmatic is an important part of management. More research is needed on the prevention of viral-induced asthma exacerbations during pregnancy.

Patient education

Controlling asthma during pregnancy is important for the well-being of the fetus as well as for the mother's well-being, and the pregnant woman must understand that it is safer to be treated than to have uncontrolled symptoms.

Uninformed decisions by pregnant asthmatic patients or those managing their asthma may lead to exacerbations during pregnancy and adverse perinatal outcomes. Therefore, asthma education is a critical component in the management =. One successful approach was recently reported in the multidisciplinary approach to management of maternal asthma study or MAMMA. Subjects were randomized to either receive a pharmacist-led intervention (consisting of self-management strategies, such as proper inhaler technique, adherence support, monthly Asthma Control Questionnaire (ACQ) assessments, FEV1, and action plans) or usual care. There was communication between the pharmacist, family physician, midwife, and the patient. At the end of 6 months there was a significant reduction in ACQ (improved asthma control) compared to the group that received usual care [43]. A recent prospective cohort study of over 800 pregnant women with asthma found a high prevalence of nonadherence and poor self-management skills. After three educational sessions on medication knowledge, maximal improvements in adherence were seen [44].

The pregnant woman should be instructed regarding optimal inhaler technique. She must be able to recognize symptoms of worsening asthma and know what to do about them. She should be given an individualized action plan that defines:

* maintenance medication
* symptoms (and possibly peak flow levels) that indicate exacerbations
* rescue therapy and increases in maintenance medications in response to her level of exacerbation
* how and when to contact her asthma clinician for uncontrolled symptoms.

Pharmacologic therapy

Asthma medicines include relievers and long-term controllers. Relievers provide quick relief of bronchospasm and include short-acting β-agonists (albuterol is preferred during pregnancy, two to four puffs every 3–4 hours when required) and the anticholinergic bronchodilator ipratropium (generally used as second-line therapy for acute asthma–discussed later). Long-term control medications are described in Table 22.3. Inhaled corticosteroids (Table 22.4) are the most effective controller asthma medications.

Chronic asthma

Patients with intermittent asthma do not need controller therapy. In patients with persistent asthma not already on controller therapy, it should be initiated as shown in

Table 22.3 Safety of commonly used medications for the treatment of asthma during pregnancy

Medication	Major birth defects	Other birth outcomes
Systemic corticosteroids	Meta-analysis of cohort studies showed no overall increased risk of major birth defects in pooled 535 exposed pregnancies; meta-analysis of four case-control studies showed an increased risk of ~threefold for oral clefts [46]. However, most recent and largest case control study from US National Birth Defects Prevention Study showed no increased risk for oral clefts with first-trimester systemic steroid use for any indication in 2372 cases and 5922 controls [47].	Preterm delivery, low birthweight or reduced birthweight, preeclampsia, and gestational diabetes have all been reported to occur more frequently in women treated with systemic steroids in pregnancy; however, studies that attempted to control for underlying maternal disease and disease activity typically find the associated risks for these outcomes reduced or eliminated [48].
Any inhaled corticosteroids (ICS) including beclomethasone, budesonide, flunisolide, fluticasone, triamcinolone	No increased risk for major birth defects in 396 exposed compared with the general population [49]. A meta-analysis of studies of inhaled steroids did not find increased risk of major birth defects overall [50].	No increased risks for preterm delivery, low birthweight or pregnancy-induced hypertension in 396 exposed or in meta-analysis [49].
Budesonide	No increased risk for major birth defects overall or oral clefts among 2014 exposed in population-based Scandinavian register [51].	No increased risks for preterm birth, reduced birthweight or length, or stillbirths in 2968 exposed in population-based Scandinavian register [52].
Fluticasone	No increased risk of major congenital malformations overall in a cohort study of 1602 mother—infant pairs exposed to fluticasone compared to 3678 exposed to other ICS, stratified by severity [53].	No increased risk of low birthweight, preterm birth, or small for gestational age in retrospective database study of infants of 3190 mothers exposed to fluticasone compared to 608 mothers exposed to budesonide [54].
Cromolyn Nedocromil	No increase in major birth defects overall in 296 pregnancies exposed throughout pregnancy [55]. No increase in major birth defects overall in 151 exposed pregnancies [56]. No overall increase in major birth defects in case control study of 5124 malformed compared to 30053 controls; nine cases exposed to cromones; some suggestion of an increased risk for musculoskeletal malformations among the nine cases but no specific pattern noted [57].	No increased risk for premature delivery or spontaneous abortion/stillbirth in 296 pregnancies exposed throughout pregnancy [55]. No increased risk for premature delivery, preeclampsia, or low birthweight in 243 women exposed anytime in pregnancy [56].
Montelukast	No increased risk of major birth defects overall in 74 and 180 exposed pregnancies [58,59]. No increased risk in major birth defects overall or specific birth defects in 1164 exposed pregnancies in claims study [60]. No increased risk in major birth defects in 1827 exposed pregnancies in Danish register study [61].	No increased risk for reduced birthweight or shortened gestational age in 180 exposed when compared to other asthmatics [58]. No increased risk for preterm delivery, low birthweight, or preeclampsia in 1827 exposed compared to other treated asthmatics [61].
Omalizumab	No increased risk compared to general population for major birth defects overall in 169 exposed pregnancies (156 live births) enrolled in a registry [62].	
Short-acting beta agonists (primarily albuterol)	No increase in major birth defects over expected among 1090 albuterol-exposed pregnancies in a claims database [63]. No increase in major birth defects in 1753 albuterol-exposed pregnancies compared to other asthmatic pregnancies [64]. Modest increased risk in isolated cleft lip or cleft palate (odds ratios 1.65–1.79) in albuterol-exposed pregnancies in case control study of 2711 cases of oral clefts and 6482 controls [65]. Several additional studies have suggested modest increased risks (odds ratios <3) for specific birth defects such as any cardiac or gastroschisis, esophageal atresia, omphalocele [15,66,67].	No increase in preterm delivery, low birthweight, or small for gestational age infants in 1828 pregnancies exposed to short-acting beta agonists compared to other asthmatic pregnancies [64].

(Continued)

Table 22.3 (*Continued*)

Medication	Major birth defects	Other birth outcomes
Short-acting beta agonists (others)	Ephedrine: No increased risk in major birth defects in 373 exposed [68]. Epinephrine: Increased risk for major and minor birth defects overall and specifically for inguinal hernia in 189 exposed [68]. Metaproterenol: No excess in major birth defects noted in 361 exposed pregnancies from a database [63]. Terbutaline: No increased risk for major birth defects in 149 exposed [63].	
Long-acting beta agonists	No evidence of increased risk in major birth defects in 65 salmeterol exposed pregnancies [69]. In one analysis of a database, increased risks for major cardiac and major "other" birth defects were seen with first-trimester exposure in 165 pregnancies [70]. However, in a later study from the same database, 841 pregnancies exposed to long-acting beta agonists with low or medium dose inhaled corticosteroids showed no increased risk of major birth defects overall compared to pregnancies exposed to medium to high dose inhaled corticosteroids alone [71].	No difference in low birthweight, preterm birth, or small for gestational age was noted in infants of mothers exposed to salmeterol vs. formoterol in a retrospective database study [54].
Theophylline	No increase in major birth defects overall in 212, 292, and 273 pregnancies [56,64,72]. Three case reports of severe cardiac defects in exposed [73].	

Adapted from [74].

Table 22.4 Clinically comparable doses of inhaled corticosteroids

Drug	Low daily dose (µg)	Medium daily dose (µg)	High daily dose (µg)
Beclomethasone HFA MDI	80–240	>240–480	>480
Budesonide DPI	200–600	>600–1200	>1200
Ciclesonide HFA MDI	160–320	>320–640	>640
Flunisolide	500–1000	>1000–2000	>2000
CFC MDI	320	>320–640	>640
HFA MDI			
Fluticasone	88–264	>264–440	>440
HFA MDI	100–300	>300–500	>500
DPI	220	440	>440
Momethasone DPI	300–750	>750–1500	>1500
Triamcinolone acetonide CFC MDI			

CFC MDI, chlorofluorocarbon-propelled metered dose inhaler; DPI, dry powder inhaler; HFA MDI, hydrofluoroalkaline-propelled metered dose inhaler.
Adapted from [75].

Table 22.1. Controller therapy should be progressed in steps (Table 22.5) until adequate control is achieved, as defined previously. Therapy should be increased one step for patients whose asthma is not well controlled despite attention to the nonpharmacologic strategies described previously. A two-step increase, a course of oral corticosteroids, or both should be recommended for women whose asthma is very poorly controlled.

Once control is achieved and sustained for several months, a stepdown to less intensive therapy is encouraged for nonpregnant patients to identify the minimum therapy necessary to maintain control. Although a similar stepdown approach can be considered for pregnant patients, it should be undertaken cautiously and gradually to avoid compromising the patient's asthma control [45]. For some patients it may be prudent to postpone attempts to reduce therapy that is effectively controlling the woman's asthma until after the infant's birth.

Inhaled corticosteroids are the mainstay of controller therapy during pregnancy. Because it has the most published

Table 22.5 Steps of asthma therapy during pregnancy[a]

Step	Preferred controller medication	Alternative controller medication
1	None	–
2	Low-dose ICS	LTRA, theophylline ICS+albuterol PRN[b] ICS/formoterol PRN[b]
3	Medium-dose ICS	Low-dose ICS + either LABA, LTRA or theophylline ICS/Formoterol PRN[b]
4	Medium-dose ICS + LABA	Medium-dose ICS + LTRA or theophylline
5	High-dose ICS + LABA	Omalizumab-
6	High-dose ICS + LABA + oral prednisone	Omalizumab

[a]Data modified from Schatz M, Dombrowski M. Clinical practice. Asthma in pregnancy. N Engl J Med. 2009;360:1862–9 [23].
[b]Updated recommendations on asthma therapy from the 2020 Global Initiative for Asthma report; however, these recommendations have not been studied specifically during pregnancy.
ICS, inhaled corticosteroids; LABA, long-acting beta agonists; LTRA, leukotriene-receptor antagonists; PRN, pro re nata.

reassuring human gestational safety data, budesonide is considered the preferred inhaled corticosteroid for asthma during pregnancy. It is important to note that no data indicate that the other inhaled corticosteroid preparations are unsafe. Therefore, inhaled corticosteroids other than budesonide may be continued in patients who were well controlled by these agents prior to pregnancy, especially if it is thought that changing formulations may jeopardize asthma control. Based on longer duration of availability in the United States, salmeterol is considered the long-acting β-agonist of choice during pregnancy. As described in Table 22.3, theophylline (primarily because of increased side-effects compared with alternatives) and leukotriene receptor antagonists (because of the limited published human gestational data for these drugs) are considered by the National Asthma Education and Prevention Program to be alternative, but not preferred, treatments for persistent asthma during pregnancy. Although oral corticosteroids have been associated with possible increased risks during pregnancy, such as oral clefts, preeclampsia, and prematurity as described, if needed during pregnancy, they should be used because these risks are less than the potential risks of severe uncontrolled asthma, which include maternal mortality, fetal mortality, or both.

Acute asthma

A major goal of chronic asthma management is the prevention of acute asthmatic episodes. When increased asthma does not respond to home therapy, expeditious acute management is necessary for the health of both the mother and fetus.

As a result of progesterone-induced hyperventilation, normal blood gases during pregnancy reveal a higher PO_2 (100–106 mmHg) and a lower PCO_2 (28–30 mmHg) than in the nonpregnant state. The changes in blood gases that occur secondary to acute asthma during pregnancy will be superimposed on the "normal" hyperventilation of pregnancy. Thus, a $PCO_2 > 35$ or a $PO_2 < 70$ associated with acute asthma will represent more severe compromise during pregnancy than will similar blood gases in the nongravid state.

The recommended pharmacologic therapy of acute asthma during pregnancy is summarized in Box 22.1 [45]. Intensive fetal monitoring as well as maternal monitoring is essential. In addition to pharmacologic

Box 22.1 National Asthma Education and Prevention Program (NAEPP) recommendations for the pharmacologic management of acute asthma during pregnancy

1 Initial therapy

A FEV$_1$ or PEFR ≥50% predicted or personal best
  1 Short-acting inhaled β2-agonist by metered dose inhaler or nebulizer, up to three doses in first hour
  2 Oral systemic corticosteroid if not immediate response or if patient recently took oral systemic corticosteroid
B FEV$_1$ or PEFR <50% predicted or personal best (severe exacerbation)
  1 High-dose short-acting inhaled β2-agonist by nebulization every 20 min or continuously for 1 h plus inhaled ipratropium bromide
  2 Oral systemic corticosteroid

2 Repeat assessment

A Moderate exacerbation (FEV$_1$ or PEFR 50–80% predicted or personal best, moderate symptoms)
  1 Short-acting inhaled β2-agonist every 60 min
  2 Oral systemic corticosteroid (if not already given)
  3 Continue treatment 1–3 h, provided there is improvement
B Severe (FEV$_1$ or PEFR <50% predicted or personal best, severe symptoms at rest)
  1 Short-acting inhaled β2-agonist hourly or continuously plus inhaled ipratropium bromide
  2 Systemic corticosteroid (if not already given)

3 Response and disposition

A Good (FEV$_1$ or PEFR ≥70% predicted or personal best, no distress, response sustained 60 min after last treatment). Discharge home
B Incomplete (FEV$_1$ or PEFR ≥50% predicted or personal best but <70%, mild or moderate symptoms). Individualize decision regarding discharge home vs. admit to hospital ward
C Poor (FEV$_1$ or PEFR <50% predicted or personal best, $PCO_2 > 42$ mmHg, severe symptoms, drowsiness, confusion). Admit to hospital intensive care

FEV$_1$, forced expiratory volume in 1 second; PEFR, peak expiratory flow rate.
Adapted from [45].

therapy, supplemental oxygen (initially 3–4 L/min by nasal cannula) should be administered, adjusting fraction of inspired oxygen (FiO_2) to maintain at $PO_2 \geq 70$ and/or O_2 saturation by pulse oximetry >95%. Intravenous fluids (containing glucose if the patient is not hyperglycemic) should also be administered, initially at a rate of at least 100 mL/h

Systemic corticosteroids (approximately 1 mg/kg) are recommended for patients who do not respond well (FEV_1 or peak expiratory flow rate [PEFR] $\geq 70\%$ predicted) to the first β-agonist treatment as well as for patients who have recently taken systemic steroids and for those who present with severe exacerbations (FEV_1 or PEFR $\leq 50\%$ predicted). Patients with good responses to emergency therapy (FEV_1 or PEFR $\geq 70\%$ predicted) can be discharged home, generally on a course of oral corticosteroids. Inhaled corticosteroids should also be continued or initiated upon discharge until review at medical follow-up. Hospitalization should be considered for patients with an incomplete response (FEV_1 or PEFR $\geq 50\%$ but <70% predicted). Admission to an intensive care unit should be considered for patients with persistent FEV_1 or PEFR <50% predicted, $PCO_2 > 42$, or sensorium changes.

Management during labor and delivery

Asthma medications should be continued during labor and delivery. If systemic corticosteroids have been used in the previous 4 weeks, then stress-dose steroids (e.g. 100 mg hydrocortisone every 8 hours IV) should be administered during labor and for the 24-hour period after delivery to prevent maternal adrenal crisis [45].

Prostaglandin (PG) E_2 or E_1 can be used for cervical ripening, the management of spontaneous or induced abortions, or postpartum hemorrhage. However, 15-methyl-PGF_2-α and methylergonovine can cause bronchospasm. There is no contraindication to the use of oxytocin for postpartum hemorrhage. Magnesium sulfate and β-adrenergic agents, which are bronchodilators, can be used to treat preterm labor. Indomethacin can induce bronchospasm in the aspirin-sensitive patient and thus must be avoided in such patients [45].

Epidural anesthesia has the additional benefit of reducing oxygen consumption and minute ventilation during labor. If a general anesthetic is necessary, preanesthetic use of atropine and glycopyrrolate may provide bronchodilation. Ketamine is the agent of choice for induction of anesthesia because it decreases airway resistance and can prevent bronchospasm. Low concentrations of halogenated anesthetics are recommended as inhalation anesthetic agents in pregnant asthmatic patients because they also cause bronchodilation [45].

Conclusion

Asthma is a common medical problem during pregnancy. Optimal diagnosis and management of asthma during pregnancy should maximize maternal and fetal health.

CASE PRESENTATION

The patient is a 23-year-old gravida 2, para 1 woman who is seen during her first trimester for asthma. Her asthma was first diagnosed at age 15. She has not been hospitalized for asthma but did require an emergency department visit for asthma 6 months previously. She was worse during her prior pregnancy 2 years ago. She is currently having daily asthma symptoms, nocturnal symptoms twice a week, and using her albuterol inhaler 3–4 times per day. She was given a steroid inhaler but was afraid to use it while she was pregnant. She has noticed that cleaning the house triggers her asthma. She has had a cat at home for 1 year, has been worse over this period, but does not think the cat affects her asthma. She has had some daily sneezing and nasal congestion since childhood, which she considers mild. She does not smoke cigarettes, has not been previously evaluated for allergies, and denies any other significant medical history.

Auscultation of the lungs was normal, and examination of the nose revealed mild mucosal edema. Spirometry showed an FEV_1 of 70% predicted. The diagnostic impression was moderate persistent asthma with a probable mite and dander allergy component and mild allergic rhinitis. The initial plan included education regarding asthma and pregnancy, an allergy evaluation (in vitro tests), environmental control instructions based on the testing, initiation of medium-dose inhaled budesonide with instructions on inhaler technique, provision of a symptom-based home action plan, and scheduled follow-up in 1 month.

References

1. Kwon HL, Triche E, Belanger K, Bracken M. The epidemiology of asthma during pregnancy: prevalence, diagnosis, and symptoms. Immunol Allergy Clin North Am. 2006;26(1):29–62.

2. Hansen C, Joski P, Freiman H, Andrade S, Toh S, Dublin S, et al. Medication exposure in pregnancy risk evaluation program: the prevalence of asthma medication use during pregnancy. Matern Child Health J. 2013;17(9):1611–21.

3. Perlow JH, Montgomery D, Morgan MA, Towers CV, Porto M. Severity of asthma and perinatal outcome. Am J Obstet Gynecol. 1992;167(4 Pt 1): 963–7.

4. Juniper E, Daniel E, Roberts R, Kline P, Hargreave F, Newhouse M. Improvement in airway hyperresponsiveness and asthma severity during pregnancy. a prospective study. Am Rev Resp Dis. 1989;140:924–31.

5. Kwon HL, Belanger K, Bracken MB. Asthma prevalence among pregnant and childbearing-aged women in the United States: estimates from national health surveys. Ann Epidemiol. 2003;13(5):317–24.

6. Schatz M, Dombrowski M, Wise R. Asthma morbidity during pregnancy can be predicted by severity classification. J Allergy Clin Immunol. 2003;112:283–8.

7. Murphy VE, Gibson P, Talbot PI, Clifton VL. Severe asthma exacerbations during pregnancy. Obstet Gynecol. 2005;106 (5 Pt 1):1046–54.

8. Gluck J, Gluck P. The effect of pregnancy on the course of asthma. Immunol Allergy Clin N Am. 2000;20:729–43.

9. Murphy VE, Gibson PG, Smith R, Clifton VL. Asthma during pregnancy: mechanisms and treatment implications. Eur Respir J. 2005;25(4):731–50.

10. Murphy V, Namazy J, Powell H, Schatz M, Chambers C, Attia J, et al. A meta-analysis of adverse perinatal outcomes in women with asthma. BJOG. 2011;118(11):1314–23.

11. Rejno G, lundholm C, Larsson K, Larsson H, Lichtenstein P, D'Onofrio BM, et al. Adverse pregnancy outcomes in asthmatic women: a population-based family design study. J Allergy Clin Immunol Pract. 2017;6(3):916–22.

12. Yland J, Bateman B, Huybrecht K, Schatz M, Wurst K, Hernandez-Diaz S. Perinatal outcomes associated with maternal asthma and its severity and control during pregnancy. J Allergy Clin Immunol Pract. 2020 Jun;8(6):1928–1937.e3.

13. Martel MJ, Rey E, Beauchesne MF, Perreault S, Lefebvre G, Forget A, et al. Use of inhaled corticosteroids during pregnancy and risk of pregnancy induced hypertension: nested case-control study. BMJ. 2005;330(7485):230.

14. Bakhireva LN, Schatz M, Jones KL, Chambers CD. Asthma control during pregnancy and the risk of preterm delivery or impaired fetal growth. Ann Allergy Asthma Immunol. 2008;101(2):137–43.

15. Lin S, Herdt-Losavio M, Gensburg L, Marshall E, Druschel C. Maternal asthma medication use and the risk of congenital heart defects. Birth Defects Res A Clin Mol Teratol. 2009;85:161–8.

16. Lin S, Munsie J, Herdt-Losavio M, Bell E, Druschel C, Romitti PA, et al. Maternal asthma medication use and the risk of gastroschisis. Am J Epidemiol. 2008;168:73–9.

17. Blais L, Kettani FZ, Forget A, Beauchesne MF, Lemiere C. Asthma exacerbations during the first trimester of pregnancy and congenital malformations:revisisting the association in a large representative cohort. Thorax. 2015;70:647–52.

18. Tamasi L, Bohacs A, Bikov A, Andorka C, Rigó J Jr, Losonczy G, et al. Exhaled nitric oxide in pregnant healthy and asthmatic women. J Asthma. 2009;46(8):786–91.

19. Global Initiative for Asthma. Global strategy for asthma management and prevention. Fontana, WI: GINA; 2021 [cited 2023 Jun 22]. Available from: https://ginasthma.org/wp-content/uploads/2023/04/GINA-Main-Report-2021-V2-WMSA.pdf.

20. Amaral L, Martins C.,Coimbra A. Use of the control of allergic rhinitis and asthma test and pulmonary function tests to assess asthma control in pregnancy. Aust N Z J Obstet Gynaecol. 2017;58:1–5.

21. Palmsten K, Schatz M, Chan PH, Johnson DL, Chambers CD. Validation of the Pregnancy Asthma Control Test. J Allergy Clin Immunol. 2016 Mar-Apr;4(2):310-5.e1.

22. Powell H, Murphy VE, Taylor DR, Hensley MJ, McCaffery K, Giles W, et al. Management of asthma in pregnancy guided by measurement of fraction of exhaled nitric oxide: a double-blind, randomised controlled trial. Lancet. 2011;378(9795): 983–90.

23. Schatz M, Dombrowski MP. Clinical practice. Asthma in pregnancy. N Engl J Med. 2009 Apr 30;360(18):1862–9.

24. Koo SM, Kim Y, Park C, Park GW, Lee M, Won S, et al. Effect of pregnancy on quantitative medication use and relation to exacerbations in asthma. Biomed Res Int. 2017;8276190. doi: 10.1155/2017/8276190. Epub 2017 Jul 20.

25. Kim S, Kim J, Park SY, Um HY, Kim K, Kim Y, et al. Effect of pregnancy in asthma on health care use and perinatal outcomes. J Allergy Clin Immunol. 2015;136(5):1215–23.

26. Sawicki E, Stewart K, Wong S, Paul E, Leung L, J G. Management of asthma by pregnant women attending an Australian maternity hospital. Aust N Z J Obstet Gynaecol. 2012;52(2):183–8.

27. Lim AS, Stewart K, Abramson MJ, Ryan K, George J. Asthma during pregnancy: the experiences, concerns and views of pregnant women with asthma. J Asthma. 2012;49(5):474–9.

28. Robijn AL, Barker D, Gibson P, Giles WB, Clifton VL, Mattes J, et al. Factors associated with nonadherence to inhaled corticosteroids for asthma during pregnancy. J Allergy Clin Immunol Pract. 2020;9(3):1242–52.

29. Lim A, Stewart K, Abramson M, George J. Management of pregnant women with asthma by Australian general practitioners. BMC Fam Pract. 2011;12:121.

30. Cimbollek S, Plaza V, Quirce S, Costa R, Urrutia I, Ojeda P, et al. Knowledge, attitude and adherence of Spanish healthcare professionals to asthma management recommendations during pregnancy. Allergol Immunopathol (Madr). 2013 Mar-Apr; 41(2):114–20.

31. Cydulka R, Emerman C, Schreiber D, Molander K, Woodruff P, Camargo C. Acute asthma among pregnant women presenting to the emergency department. Am J Respir Crit Care Med. 1999;160:887–92.

32. McCallister J, Benninger C, Frey H, Phillips G, Mastronarde J. Pregnancy related treatement disparities of acute asthma exacerbations in the emergency department. Respir Med. 2011 Oct;105(10):1434–40.

33. Ali Z, Ulrik CS. Incidence and risk factors for exacerbations of asthma during pregnancy. J Asthma Allergy. 2013;6:53–60.

34. Bokem MP, Robijn AL, Jensen ME, Barker D, Callaway L, Clifton V, et al. Factors associated with asthma exacerbations during pregnancy. J Allergy Clin Immunol Pract. 2021; 9(12):4343–52.

35. Hodyl NA, Stark MJ, Schell W, Grzeskowiak LE, Clifton VL. Perinatal outcomes following maternal asthma and cigarette smokin during pregnancy. Eur Respir J. 2014;43(3):704–16.

36. Murphy VE, Clifton, V.L, Gibson, P.G. The effect of cigarette smoking on asthma control during exacerbations in pregnant women. Thorax. 2010;65(8):739–44.

37. Grarup PA, Janner JH, Ulrik CS. Passive smoking is associated with poor asthma control during pregnancy: a prospective study of 500 pregnancies. PLoS One. 2014;9(11):e112435.

38. Mendola P, Wallace M, Hwang BS. Preterm birth and air pollution: critical windows of exposure for women with asthma. J Allergy Clin Immunol. 2016;138(2):432–40.

39. Sorri M, Hartikainen A, Karja I. Rhinitis during pregnancy. Rhinology. 1980;18(2):83–6.

40. Munn M, Groome L, Atterbury J. Pneumonia as a complication of pregnancy. J Matern Fetal Med. 1999;8:151–54.

41. Cox S, Posner SF, McPheeters M, Jamieson DJ, Kourtis AP, Meikle S. Hospitalizations with respiratory illness among pregnant women during influenza season. Obstet Gynecol. 2006;107:1315–22.

42. Forbes RL, Wark PAB, Murphy VE, Gibson P. Pregnant women have attenuated innate interferon responses to 2009 pandemic influenza A virus subtype H1N1. J Infect Dis. 2012; 206:646–53.

43. Lim AS, Stewart K, Abramson MJ, Walker S, Smith CL, George J. Multidisciplinary Approach to Management of MAternal ASthma (MAMMA): a randomized controlled trial. Chest. 2014;145(5):1046–54.

44. Robijn AL, Jensen, M.E.,Gibson, P.G.,et al. Trends in asthma self-management skills and inhaled corticosteroid use during pregnancy and postpartum from 2004-2017. J Asthma. 2018;56(6):594–602.

45. Busse WW. NAEPP expert panel report. Managing asthma during pregnancy: recommendations for pharmacologic treatment-2004 update. J Allergy Clin Immunol. 2005; 115(1):34–46.

46. Park-Wyllie L MP, Pastuszak A, et al. Birth defects after maternal exposure to corticosteroids: Prospective cohort study and meta-analysis of epidemiologic studies. Teratology, 62, 385–392 (2000).

47. Skuladottir H, Wilcox AJ, Ma C, Lammer EJ, Rasmussen SA, Werler MM, et al. Corticosteroid use and risk of orofacial clefts. Birth Defects Res A Clin Mol Teratol. 2014;100(6):499–506.

48. Palmsten K, Bandoli G, Watkins J, Vazquez-Benitez G, Gilmer TP, Chambers C. Oral corticosteroids and risk of preterm borth in the California Medicaid program. J Allergy Clin Immunol Pract. 2021;9:375–84.

49. Namazy J, Schatz M, Long L et al. Use of inhaled steroids by pregnant asthmatic women does not reduce intrauterine growth. J Allergy Clin Immunol. 2004;113(3):427–32.

50. Rahimi R, Nikfar S, Abdollahi M. Meta-analysis finds use of inhaled corticosteroids during pregnancy safe: a systematic meta-analysis review. Hum Exp Toxicol. 2006;25(8):447–52.

51. Kallen B, Rydhstroem H, Aberg A. Congenital malformations after the use of inhaled budesonide in early pregnancy. Obstet Gynecol. 1999;93(3):392–95.

52. Norjavaara E, de Verdier MG. Normal pregnancy outcomes in a population-based study including 2968 pregnant women exposed to budesonide. J Allergy Clin Immunol. 2003; 111(4):736–42.

53. Charlton RA, Hutchison A, Davis KJ, de Vries CS. Asthma management in pregnancy. PLoS One. 2013;8(4):e60247.

54. Cossette B, Beauchesne MF, Forget A, Lemière C, Larivée P, Rey E, et al. Relative perinatal safety of salmeterol vs formoterol and fluticasone vs budesonide use during pregnancy. Ann Allergy Asthma Immunol. 2014;112(5):459–64.

55. Wilson J. Use of sodium cromoglycate during pregnancy: results on 296 asthmatic women. Acta Therap. 1982; 8(Suppl):45–51.

56. Schatz M, Zeiger RS, Harden K, Hoffman CC, Chilingar L, Petitti D. The safety of asthma and allergy medications during pregnancy. J Allergy Clin Immunol. 1997;100(3):301–6.

57. Tata LJ, Lewis SA, McKeever TM, Smith CJ, Doyle P, Smeeth L, et al. A comprehensive analysis of adverse obstetric and pediatric complications in women with asthma. Am J Respir Crit Care Med. 2007;175(10):991–7.

58. Sarkar M, Koren G, Kalra S, Ying A, Smorlesi C, De Santis M, et al. Montelukast use during pregnancy; a multicentre, prospective, comparative study of infant outcomes. Eur J Clin Pharmacol. 2009;65(12):1259–64.

59. Bakhireva LN, Jones KL, Schatz M, Klonoff-Cohen HS, Johnson D, et al. Safety of leukotriene receptor antagonists in pregnancy. J Allergy Clin Immunol. 2007;119(3):618–25.

60. Nelsen LM, Shields KE, Cunningham ML, Stoler JM, Bamshad MJ, Eng PM, et al. Congenital malformationsamong infants born to women receiving montelukast, inhlaed corticosteroids, and other asthma medications. J Allergy Clin Immunol. 2012;129(1):251–4.e256.

61. Cavero-Carbonell C, Vinketl-Hansen A, Rabanque-Hernandez MJ, Martso C, Garne E. Fetal exposure to montelukast and congenital anomalies: a population based study in Denmark. Birth Defects Res. 2017;109:452–9.

62. Namazy J, Cabana M, Scheuerle A, Thorp JM Jr, Chen H, Miller MK, et al. The Xolair Pregnancy Registry (EXPECT): an observational study of omalizumab during pregnancy in women with asthma. Am J Respiratory Crit Care Med. 2012;(185):A4221.

63. Briggs GG, Freeman RK, Towers CV, Forinash AB. Drugs in pregnancy and lactation : a reference guide to fetal and neonatal risk. Philadelphia, PA: Wolters Kluwer; 2017.

64. Schatz M, Dombrowski MP, Wise R, Momirova V, Landon M, Mabie W, et al. The relationship of asthma medication use to perinatal outcomes. J Allergy Clin Immunol. 2004;113(6): 1040–5.

65. Munsie JP, S. L, Browne ML, Caton AR, Bell EM, Rasmussen SA, et al. Maternal bronchodilator use and the risk of orofacial clefts. Hum Reprod. 2011;26:3147–54.

66. Garne E, Hansen AV, Morris J, Zaupper L, Addor MC, Barisic I, et al. Use of asthma medication during pregnancy and risk of specific congenital anomalies: a European case-malformed control study. J Allergy Clin Immunol. 2015;136:1496–502.

67. Lin S, Munsie JPW, Herdt-Losavio ML et al. Maternal asthma medication use and the risk of selected birth defects. Pediatrics, 129, e317–e324 (2012).

68. Heinonen OP, Slone D, Shapiro S. Birth defects and drugs in pregnancy. Littleton, MA: Publishing Sciences Group; 1977.

69. Wilton LV, Pearce GL, Martin RM, Mackay FJ, Mann RD. The outcomes of pregnancy in women exposed to newly marketed drugs in general practice in England. BJOG. 1998;105(8):882–9.

70. Eltonsy S, Forget A, Blais L. Beta2-agonists use during pregnancy and the risk of congenital malformations. Birth Defects Res A Clin Mol Teratol. 2011;91(11):937–47.

71. Eltonsy S, Forget A, Beauchesne MF, Blais L. Risk of congenital malformations for asthmatic pregnant women using long-acting beta-agonist and inhaled corticosteroid combination versus higher-dose inhlaed corticosteroid monotherapy. J Allergy Clin Immunol. 2015;135(1):123–30.

72. Stenius-Aarniala B, Riikonen S, Teramo K. Slow-release theophylline in pregnant asthmatics. Chest. 1995;107(3):642–7.

73. Park JM, Schmer V, Myers TL. Cardiovascular anomalies associated with prenatal exposure to theophylline. South Med J. 1990;83:487–8.

74. Namazy, J, Schatz, M, editors. Asthma, allergic and immunologic diseases during pregnancy: a guide to management. Springer; 2019.

75. Kelly HW. Comparison of inhaled corticosteroids: an update. Ann Pharmacother. 2009;43(3):519–27.

Chapter 23
Epilepsy

Regan J. Lemley[1] and P. Emanuela Voinescu[2]

[1] Department of Neurology – Division of Epilepsy, Brigham and Women's Hospital and Harvard Medical School, Boston, MA, USA

[2] Division of Women's Medicine, Brigham and Women's Hospital and Harvard Medical School, Boston, MA, USA

Epilepsy is a brain disease characterized by recurrent unprovoked seizures, though individuals with a single unprovoked seizure but high probably of further seizures can also be diagnosed with epilepsy [1]. A seizure clinically manifests as a stereotyped, episodic alteration in behavior or perception and is the result of excessive synchronous neuronal activity. Depending upon the location and extent of neural involvement, seizures may or may not involve loss of awareness and involuntary movements. The majority of people with epilepsy have seizures that can be well controlled by antiseizure medications (ASMs). Epilepsy can begin at any age of life and has a bimodal distribution of incidence with peaks in young children and the elderly [2]. Active epilepsy affects approximately 1.2% of individuals in the United States [3] and although the prevalence of epilepsy is reported to be slightly higher in men, there are over 1.5 million women with epilepsy (WWE) of childbearing age in the United States [4].

Although uncontrolled seizures and some medications may increase maternal and fetal risks compared to the general population [5], most women with epilepsy will have a normal pregnancy with favorable outcomes. Thoughtful management of epilepsy in a woman of reproductive age to minimize these risks should start in the preconception years. The initial visit between the physician and a woman with epilepsy of childbearing age should include a discussion about family planning. Topics should include effective birth control, the importance of planned pregnancies with ASM optimization and folate supplementation prior to conception, teratogenicity of ASMs vs. the risks of seizures during pregnancy, and obstetric complications. The primary goal is effective control of maternal seizures with the least risk to the fetus.

Contraception

Contraceptive counseling is an important component to epilepsy care for women, as there can be significant interactions between antiseizure medications and hormonal contraceptives. Unfortunately, only 37% women are counseled on contraception by their neurologists in the first few clinic visits [6]. In a survey of women with epilepsy in the United States and internationally, 46.6% use hormone containing birth control including hormonal oral contraceptives, hormonal patch, vaginal ring, progestin implant, or depomedroxyprogesterone [7].

Exogenous hormones are metabolized by the cytochrome P450 enzyme system, and there are also several ASMs that are P450 enzyme inducers. When taken concurrently, enzyme inducing ASMs can therefore promote the conversion of exogenous hormones to their inactive compounds and effectively decrease hormonal birth control effectiveness. Women on enzyme-inducing ASMs have several options, listed in order of effectiveness: intrauterine device (copper or progestin-based), depot medroxyprogesterone, progestin implant, (combined) cervical ring, (combined) patch, or pill with high progestin dose along with an additional contraceptive method such a barrier method [8,9]. Contraceptive adjustments are not needed for most non-enzyme-inducing ASMs. However, lamotrigine is an exception because estrogen containing birth control acts on glucuronidation pathways and increases the metabolism of lamotrigine, therefore decreasing lamotrigine levels. When a woman stops taking the active combined birth control pills and starts on placebo pills for menstruation, lamotrigine levels will rise and may cause toxic medication side effects in some individuals [10]. Lamotrigine dosing may therefore need to change during the placebo pill phase, or the placebo pills may need to be skipped altogether.

Queenan's Management of High-Risk Pregnancy: An Evidence-Based Approach, Seventh Edition. Edited by Catherine Y. Spong and Charles J. Lockwood.

Table 23.1 Interactions between antiseizure medication (ASM) and exogenous sex hormones (hormonal contraceptives)

	Lowers hormone levels	ASM reduced by hormones
Carbamazepine	✓	
Clobazam	n.a.	
Eslicarbazepine	✓	
Felbamate	✓	
Gabapentin	x	
Lacosamide	x	
Lamotrigine	✓ (progestin only)	✓
Levetiracetam	x	
Oxcarbazepine	✓	✓
Perampanel	✓ (progestin only)	
Phenobarbital	✓	
Phenytoin	✓	
Pregabalin	n.a.	
Primidone	✓	
Rufinamide	✓	✓
Topiramate	✓ (ethinyl estradiol only)	
Valproate	x	✓
Zonisamide	x	

Table 23.1 lists the interactions of individual ASMs and oral hormonal contraceptives [9,10].

Fertility

There have been previous concerns that WWE may have a higher rate of infertility. These beliefs may be due to findings of lower birth rates in WWE when compared to reference cohorts [11]. However, there are many socioeconomic reasons why these rates may differ. Recent studies have largely alleviated concerns about differing fertility. A retrospective web-based survey of WWE revealed an infertility rate of 9.2%, which is comparable to national rates, though there was a trend toward higher infertility as the number of ASMs increased [12]. A prospective observational study that enrolled WWE and controls seeking pregnancy and excluded those with known infertility showed that WWE have the same pregnancy rate, time to pregnancy, ovulatory rates, and live birth rates when compared to controls [13]. Additionally, WWE are just as likely to conceive via assisted reproductive technology as women without epilepsy, and ASMs do not seem to affect success rates [14].

Preconception counseling

Women with epilepsy are concerned about how their epilepsy and ASMs may affect a future child and how pregnancy affects seizures, and these concerns should be addressed through high-quality comprehensive preconception counseling [15]. Approximately 50% of pregnancies in WWE are unplanned, so information should

ideally be shared to all individuals of childbearing potential [16].

Folic acid

Daily folic acid is recommended to all women planning for pregnancy as supplementation in the preconception and early stages of pregnancy has been shown to reduce major congenital malformations and to offer neurodevelopmental benefits. Unfortunately, only 47.6% of women with epilepsy at risk of becoming pregnant are taking folic acid, though the percentage does increase to 61.7% as women are purposely trying for pregnancy [17,18]. The current dose recommended to all women is 0.4 mg, and a higher dose of 4 mg is suggested for women who have had previous pregnancies complicated by major congenital malformations. The ideal dose for women with epilepsy is not entirely clear, as higher folic acid doses may not necessarily counteract the neurodevelopmental side effects of higher risk ASMs such as valproic acid [19]. An observational study in children of women with epilepsy showed that there is a five to nine times lower risk of autism in children whose mothers took >0.4 mg of folic acid compared to those who did not [20]. The Neurodevelopmental Effects of Antiepileptic Drugs (NEAD) study showed that at age 6, children whose mothers took folic acid had, on average, a seven-point higher IQ than children whose mothers did not take folic acid [21], but an independent analysis including many of the children in the NEAD study showed no significant difference in IQs [22]. More recently, there have been some concerns that oversupplementation of folic acid may cause neurodevelopmental complications in offspring [23]. Guidelines vary on the recommended dose of folic acid for pregnant women, but a daily dose of 0.4–1 mg is recommended for most women with epilepsy and 4 mg for those on ASMs that may interfere with folate metabolism, such as valproate [24].

Seizures during pregnancy

Generalized convulsive seizures carry the highest health risk to the mother and fetus, as the mother may suffer injury during the seizure that could harm both herself and her baby, and depression of fetal heart rate occurs both during and several minutes after the seizure [25]. One retrospective study showed that more than one generalized convulsive seizure during pregnancy was found to be associated with smaller gestational age and higher risk of prematurity [26]. Focal seizures with intact awareness experienced during pregnancy have been reported to have no immediate measurable effect on the fetus [27], whereas focal seizures with impaired awareness may be associated with fetal bradycardia [28]. In regard to longer term outcomes, five or more generalized tonic–clonic seizures during a pregnancy have been associated with lower IQ and other neurodevelopmental deficits [29,30].

Pregnancy itself may not necessarily contribute to seizure worsening. A prospective multicenter cohort study found that with active drug monitoring, the percentage of women who experienced seizure worsening during pregnancy (23%) was the same as those who were not pregnant (25%) [31]. When women are not treated for their epilepsy during pregnancy, they do have higher rates of seizures overall compared to those who are treated (56.1% vs. 46.9%) [32]. One of the best predictors for seizure frequency during pregnancy is the seizure rate in the year prior to pregnancy, so a woman who has achieved seizure freedom in the year prior to pregnancy is most likely to have a seizure-free pregnancy [33,34].

Certain epilepsy subtypes are associated with a higher risk of seizure worsening during pregnancy. In a prospective study from 2013 to 2018, more women with focal epilepsy had seizure worsening during pregnancy compared to women with generalized epilepsy (21.1% to 5.3%, respectively), and of women with focal epilepsies, seizures occurred most often in women with frontal lobe epilepsy [35,36]. Generalized epilepsy seems to confer a greater degree of seizure freedom during pregnancy compared to focal epilepsy, regardless of the prepregnancy seizure rate [37].

Some studies have indicated that certain ASMs, particularly lamotrigine, may be associated with relatively higher risk of seizure worsening during pregnancy [38]. However, we now know that medications such as lamotrigine undergo significant clearance changes during pregnancy and must be actively monitored with dose adjustments, and more recent studies have not shown seizure worsening when lamotrigine doses are adequately increased.

ASM risks: Structural and neurodevelopmental teratogenicity

Epilepsy alone does not increase the risk of major congenital malformations (MCMs). Metanalyses have shown that there is not a significant difference in MCM rates of children whose mothers had nontreated epilepsy compared to the general population, however the children whose mothers were treated with ASMs during pregnancy had an increased risk of MCMs (odds ratio [OR] of 3.26) compared to controls [39]. Multiple prospective, observational pregnancy registries have been established around the world to understand the structural and neurodevelopment effects of ASMs on exposed children. These registries include the North American Antiepileptic Drug Pregnancy Registry (NAAPR), the European Registry of Antiepileptic Drugs and Pregnancy (EURAP), Australian Pregnancy Registrar (APR), the UK and Ireland Epilepsy Pregnancy Register, and Kerala Registry of Epilepsy and Pregnancy. Every woman with epilepsy on medical therapy who becomes pregnant should be encouraged to enroll in their respective registry. Overall, these registries have shown that there is a broad spectrum of risk across currently prescribed ASMs, with medications such as valproate at the highest end of risk and levetiracetam and lamotrigine at the lowest end. The ASM monotherapy risk spectrum is shown in Figure 23.1. Furthermore, ASM monotherapy typically poses a lower risk than ASM polytherapy, particularly when polytherapy includes higher risk medications such as valproate and topiramate [40]. Rates of MCMs have been reported as high as 16.78% on ASM polytherapy [41].

The highest risk ASM is valproate. The MCM rate of newborns exposed to valproate is 10.3% (95% confidence interval [CI] 8.8–12.0,) according the latest data from EURAP, and the risk increases as the daily dose is increased above 650 mg [42]. The malformations associated with valproate exposure are neural tube defects such as spina bifida, cardiovascular malformations, cleft palate, anorectal atresia, and hypospadias [43]. In regard to neurodevelopmental side effects, valproate-exposed children have lower IQs (7–10 points) when assessed at ages 3 and 6 years and have lower verbal, nonverbal, and spatial scores with higher likelihood of educational intervention – especially at doses >800 mg [22]. The risk of autism spectrum disorder is also higher, with a hazard ratio of 1.7 [44]. It is recommended that women with childbearing capacity not be prescribed valproate.

Intermediate risk ASMs include phenobarbital with an MCM rate of 6.5% (95% CI 4.2–9.9), phenytoin of 6.4% (2.8–12.2), carbamazepine of 5.5% (3.1–9.6), and topiramate of 3.9% (1.5–8.4) [24]. Phenobarbital is specifically associated with an increased risk of ventricular septal defects as well as other cardiac defects, and topiramate with increased risk of cleft lip and cleft palate [43]. In utero exposure to carbamazepine may be associated with reduced verbal ability, though there is no difference in overall IQ [21,22].

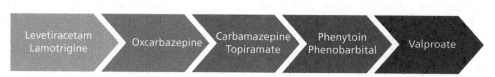

Figure 23.1 Degree of structural teratogenicity, from the lowest (on the left) to the highest (on the right).

NEAD reveals overall normal IQs for phenytoin-exposed children as well [21]. Neurodevelopmental outcome data on phenobarbital and topiramate monotherapy exposure is more limited.

Oxcarbazepine has an MCM prevalence of 1.6% (0.6–4.0) according to the most recent NAAPR data, and studies assessing neurodevelopmental outcomes of oxcarbazepine-exposed children have found no major differences compared to controls [45]. The number of oxcarbazepine monotherapy pregnancies is significantly lower than the number of lamotrigine or levetiracetam pregnancies, but oxcarbazepine may also be considered lower risk.

The lowest risk ASMs are lamotrigine and levetiracetam, and recent systemic metanalysis has shown that they are not associated with an increased risk of MCMs compared to controls [46]. Studies of neurodevelopment in children exposed to lamotrigine have overall shown no increased risk of neurodevelopmental disorders or difference in IQs compared to controls; however, there may be a dose-dependent association of reduced motor and sensory functions [47]. Children exposed to levetiracetam have had no reported developmental outcomes that differ from controls from ages 2 to 8 [48,49].

There are limited outcome data on ASMs such as perampanel, clobazam, cenobamate, lacosamide, and zonisamide, so conclusions cannot yet be definitively drawn. According to the latest data from the NAAPR, there have been 0% (95% CI 0–7.1%) of MCMs in 64 lacosamide-exposed pregnancies and 1.5% (95% CI 0.4–4.6%) in 205 zonisamide-exposed pregnancies [50].

Importantly, there are dose-dependent trends in rates of MCMs even in drugs that are less risky, such as lamotrigine. At doses of >325 mg/day of lamotrigine, the prevalence of MCMs begin to be similar to that of lower dose (<700 mg/day) of carbamazepine at 4.3–4.5% or so. As carbamazepine, valproate, and phenobarbital increase, there are definite increases in MCM prevalence [51].

In the preconception phase, a woman with epilepsy should ideally be transitioned to a low-risk ASM and be maintained on the lowest dose to control her seizures. As prescription trends have changed to safer ASM therapies, the overall prevalence of MCMs in offspring of mothers treated for epilepsy has significantly decreased without increasing the risk of generalized seizures in epileptic mothers [52]. Medication transitions prior to pregnancy may of course be limited by aggressive or refractory epilepsies.

Management during pregnancy

Prenatal screening

Women on ASMs during pregnancy should undergo prenatal screening to detect fetal MCMs, especially if their ASM regimen is considered higher risk. In addition to routine screening measures, this includes ultrasonographic measurements of nuchal translucency in combination with levels of placenta-associated pregnancy protein A, α-fetoprotein, and human chorionic gonadotropin to detect congenital malformations. A detailed anatomic ultrasound at 18–22 weeks can further evaluate for malformations, and if there are any cardiac concerns, fetal echocardiography should also be done. Amniocentesis (with measurements of amniotic fluid α-fetoprotein and acetylcholinesterase) is not performed routinely but should be offered if any screening tests are equivocal, increasing the sensitivity for detection of neural tube defects to greater than 99%.

ASM levels

There are several physiological factors unique to pregnancy that alter ASM metabolism and lead to a decrease in serum concentration of most ASMs, with the most drastic changes in the first more than second trimester. These factors include hormonal variations, change in drug absorption and distribution, and altered ASM pharmacokinetics and clearance [53]. In a prospective, observational study in women taking ASM monotherapy, serum drug levels and ASM doses were recorded four times during pregnancy and three times postpartum. It was found that for lamotrigine, dose-normalized concentrations decreased by 56.1% and for levetiracetam, 36.8% [54]. Reported ASM clearance changes are shown in Table 23.2 [24]. The greatest change in clearance for each medication can occur at different time points throughout pregnancy; for example, the greatest change occurs for levetiracetam in the first trimester, oxcarbazepine and topiramate in the second trimester, and for lamotrigine there are significant changes in all trimesters [55,56]. Carbamazepine levels appear to remain relatively stable throughout pregnancy [57]. Robust published pharmacokinetic data for newer ASMs such as brivaracetam and perampanel are lacking. Decreased drug levels are associated with seizure worsening, particularly when drug levels decrease <60–65% from the prepregnancy level [55].

Ideally, a prepregnancy ASM serum level should be acquired when seizures are under good control, and a goal serum concentration range should be established so that proactive dose adjustments to stay in that range can

Table 23.2 Total antiseizure medication (ASM) serum decreases during pregnancy

ASM	% decrease
Phenytoin	60–70
Lamotrigine	17–69
Oxcarbazepine	36–62
Levetiracetam	40–60
Phenobarbital	to 55
Zonisamide	to 35
Topiramate	to 30
Valproate	to 23
Carbamazepine	0–12

be made throughout the pregnancy [58]. Serum levels should be taken at the beginning of every trimester and again 4 weeks prior to delivery. There can be substantial variation in drug metabolism in each patient, so monthly levels may also be appropriate [24].

Peripartum care

Labor and delivery

Most women with epilepsy will not have a delivery complicated by seizures. Prior studies have found that 1–3.5% of women had seizures near the time of delivery [59]. One study found that women with generalized epilepsy had more seizures than women with focal epilepsy (12.5% in 32 women vs. none in 57 women) at delivery, though what was most striking was that these seizures occurred in the setting of subtherapeutic ASM levels [60]. Should a convulsive or repeated seizure occur, standard treatment with a benzodiazepine such as 2–4 mg of intravenous lorazepam is appropriate. Benzodiazepines can cause neonatal respiratory depression, decreased heart rate, and maternal apnea if given in large doses, and these potential side effects need to be monitored closely. If convulsive seizures occur, oxygen should be administered to the patient and she should be placed on her left side to increase uterine blood flow and decrease the risk of maternal aspiration. Prompt cesarean delivery should be performed when repeated generalized tonic–clonic seizures cannot be controlled during labor or when the mother is unable to cooperate during labor because of impaired awareness during repetitive absence or complex partial seizures.

Though epilepsy itself is not an indication for a cesarean delivery, the rate of cesarean delivery tends to be higher in women with epilepsy [61,62]. Uncontrolled seizures during pregnancy may influence the decision on delivery method (OR 3.39 comparing women who had seizures during pregnancy to women with epilepsy who did not) [63].

Maternal outcomes

There are several adverse outcomes increased in women with epilepsy. A meta-analysis that included 38 studies and close to 3 million pregnancies showed that women with epilepsy had an increased odds of induction of labor (OR 1.67), spontaneous miscarriage (OR 1.54), antepartum hemorrhage (OR 1.49), hypertensive disorders (OR 1.37), postpartum hemorrhage (OR 1.29), and preterm birth (OR 1.16) when compared to women without epilepsy [64]. In a retrospective cohort study, women with epilepsy had an elevated risk of severe maternal morbidity compared to women without epilepsy (4.3% vs. 1.4%, adjusted OR 2.91) [65]. Severe maternal morbidity includes medical complications such as myocardial infarction, eclampsia, and need for transfusion [66]. When ASM exposure was examined, women who were ASM

exposed had higher odds of postpartum hemorrhage (OR 1.33) and induction of labor (OR 1.40) compared to women who did not take ASMs [64]. In a register-based cohort study in Norway, lamotrigine monotherapy increased the odds of preeclampsia (OR 7.5) and hemorrhage (OR 6.2) in women with epilepsy compared to women on other ASMs [67]. There is, however, an overall paucity of data regarding individual ASM risk on pregnancy complications, so clinical conclusions cannot yet be made.

Mortality is higher during and just after pregnancy in women with epilepsy. A retrospective cohort study using hospital records from the Nationwide Inpatient Sample found that there were 80 deaths per 100 000 delivery hospitalizations in women with epilepsy compared to 6 deaths per 100 000 in women without epilepsy, giving an odds ratio of 11.46 (95% CI 8.64–15.19) [68]. The risk of sudden unexpected death in epilepsy (SUDEP) also appears to be higher in WWE and is a major contributor to overall increased mortality in this population. In a UK study examining deaths during or shortly after pregnancy in women with epilepsy, 11 of 14 deaths were attributable to SUDEP and the authors estimated the SUDEP rate to be 1:1000 [69].

The majority of studies that examine maternal morbidity and mortality must include large numbers to the infrequency of events, and details such as access to specialized epilepsy care, high-risk obstetrical care, or proactive ASM drug monitoring are often not included. There is hope that specialty care of women with epilepsy during pregnancy may result in reduced pregnancy complication risks, as we know that better control of generalized seizures does decrease the risk of events such as SUDEP [70].

Postpartum care

ASM management and seizure risk

In the postpartum weeks, ASM clearance rates that have been affected by pregnancy will rapidly change and return to the prepregnancy baseline. A postpartum ASM taper plan should be made prior to delivery to avoid supratherapeutic drug levels and associated toxicity, and lamotrigine in particular needs to be tapered within the first few days of delivery [56]. Due to the major life changes that come after having a child including decreased and interrupted sleep, providers may continue a ASM at a slightly higher than preconception dose due the increased seizure risk from sleep deprivation [71]. Women should be encouraged to make arrangements so that they can get at least 4 uninterrupted hours of sleep and obtain 6 hours in a 24 hour period. Other practical advice is to not bathe the baby alone, not co-sleep, and change the baby on the floor so that the baby is not harmed should a maternal seizure occur [72].

Women with epilepsy tend to have higher 30- and 90-day readmissions after the delivery hospitalization compared to women without epilepsy (OR 1.86 and 2.04, respectively), though admission rates are still relatively low (2.4% and 3.7%, respectively) [73]. Readmissions are due to obstetrical complications rather than breakthrough seizures; seizures were the fourth most common reason for admission at day 30 and second most common reason at day 90 [73].

Breastfeeding

A woman with epilepsy on ASM therapy should not be discouraged from breastfeeding. Data from the Maternal Outcomes and Neurodevelopmental Effects of Antiepileptic Drugs (MONEAD) study showed that infants breastfed by mothers on antiseizure medication therapy had ASM levels 0.3% to 44.2% of maternal levels, and almost half of the ASMs studied had infant levels that were under the lower limits of quantification [74]. Reported percentages are listed in Table 23.3. When these children were followed up at 6 years of age and underwent cognitive testing, no adverse effects were seen and children who were breastfed exhibited higher IQs [75]. Unfortunately, women with

Table 23.3 Median percentage of infant-to-mother antiseizure medication (ASM) concentration

ASM	% medication concentration
Oxcarbazepine	0.3
Levetiracetam	5.3
Carbamazepine	5.4
Topiramate	17.2
Valproate	21.4
Lamotrigine	28.9
Zonisamide	44.2

epilepsy have lower rates of breastfeeding compared to women without epilepsy after delivery (50.9% vs. 87.6%), which may be influenced by concerns of infant ASM exposure and inappropriate discouragement [76]. Breastfeeding rates can be improved with education and lactation consultation.

Postpartum depression

Depression during pregnancy and in the postpartum period is more common in women with epilepsy. A prospective cohort study of 55 pregnant women with and without epilepsy in Italy found that postpartum depression was present in 39% of women with epilepsy as opposed to 12% of controls [77]. Choice of ASM did not affect depression rates. Uncontrolled seizures are a predictive factor for postpartum depression, so effective seizure control as well as appropriate psychiatric screening and care are vital for prevention and treatment [78].

Summary

Women with epilepsy can have excellent maternal and fetal outcomes, and the majority will have uneventful pregnancies. Providers should be mindful of ASM interactions with contraception, the teratogenic risks of medications such as valproate, and the medications that undergo major clearance changes during pregnancy such as lamotrigine. Due to a high percentage of unplanned pregnancies, the topic of pregnancy and epilepsy-specific management concerns should be brought up early to women with epilepsy of childbearing potential.

CASE PRESENTATION

A 29-year-old female with well-controlled epilepsy presented after a miscarriage. She reported a history of febrile seizures in childhood, recurrence at age 16 (thought to be provoked) and again at age 24, leading to a burn injury and initiation of antiseizure medications. Her seizures were described as generalized tonic–clonic convulsions. She was initially prescribed levetiracetam, but she was not consistently compliant because of significant irritability. She became pregnant and stopped her medication for fear that she would harm her child. She had a breakthrough seizure at 13 weeks of gestation leading to a miscarriage.

She presented to our clinic determined to improve her compliance with medication for a future successful planned pregnancy. She was transitioned to lamotrigine, started on folic acid 1 mg daily and prenatal vitamins. She was worried because she read that pregnant women on

lamotrigine are at a higher risk of seizures and of dying during pregnancy yet encouraged to hear that monitoring during pregnancy reduces the risk of seizure breakthrough. She has breakthrough seizures on lower doses and concentrations of lamotrigine, so her individualized target concentration is established at 6–8 mcg/mL during her preconception year. She was concerned because she read that lamotrigine has a dose-dependent risk of malformations but reassured to hear that the largest neurodevelopmental study to date showed no dose-dependent effects on cognition. During her second pregnancy, she was referred to a maternal–fetal medicine specialist and followed closely both in the epilepsy and obstetric clinics. Shortly after conception, monthly serum lamotrigine levels were obtained for therapeutic drug monitoring to maintain her individualized target concentration, through dosage adjustments. She remained seizure free throughout

Continued

pregnancy and, in agreement with her obstetric providers, opted for a vaginal delivery. She refused an epidural, despite recommendations, and after a prolong labor delivered a healthy 8 lb 10 oz baby boy. Shortly after delivery, she had a staring spell that resolved with lorazepam 1 mg. Because of this breakthrough absence seizure, she delayed starting her postpartum taper, but at 5 days postpartum she reached out to report double vision and significant balance problems and followed recommendations for gradually reducing her lamotrigine dose every

2–3 days to a dose slightly higher to her preconception dose. She breastfed her son until he was 1 year old.

She returned to clinic the next year, planning for another pregnancy, and she delivered a full-term healthy 7 lb 13 oz baby girl following another uneventful seizure-free pregnancy with therapeutic drug monitoring of lamotrigine. She had an epidural and no seizures during her delivery admission. She followed her postpartum taper as instructed with no side effects or breakthrough seizures postpartum.

References

1. Fisher RS, Acevedo C, Arzimanoglou A, Bogacz A, Cross JH, Elger CE, et al. ILAE Official Report: A practical clinical definition of epilepsy. Epilepsia. 2014;55(4):475–82. doi: 10.1111/epi.12550.
2. Beghi E. The epidemiology of epilepsy. Neuroepidemiology. 2020;54(2):185–91. doi: 10.1159/000503831.
3. Zack MM, Kobau R. National and state estimates of the numbers of adults and children with active epilepsy – United States, 2015. Morb Mortal Wkly Rep. 2017;66(31):821–5. doi: 10.15585/mmwr.mm6631a1.
4. Hessler A, Dolbec K. Seizures: clinical updates in women's health care primary and preventive care review. Obstet Gynecol. 2021;137(1):207. doi: 10.1097/AOG.0000000000004211.
5. Harden CL, Hopp J, Ting TY, Pennell PB, French JA, Hauser WA, et al. Practice parameter update: management issues for women with epilepsy – focus on pregnancy (an evidence-based review): obstetrical complications and change in seizure frequency. Neurology. 2009;73(2):126–32. doi: 10.1212/WNL.0b013e3181a6b2f8.
6. Espinera AR, Gavvala J, Bellinski I, Kennedy J, Macken MP, Narechania A, et al. Counseling by epileptologists affects contraceptive choices of women with epilepsy. Epilepsy Behav. 2016;65:1–6. doi: 10.1016/j.yebeh.2016.08.021.
7. Herzog AG, Mandle HB, Cahill KE, Fowler KM, Hauser WA, Davis AR. Contraceptive practices of women with epilepsy: findings of the epilepsy birth control registry. Epilepsia. 2016;57(4):630–7. doi: 10.1111/epi.13320.
8. Harden CL, Leppik I. Optimizing therapy of seizures in women who use oral contraceptives. Neurology. 2006;67(12 Suppl 4):S56–8. doi: 10.1212/wnl.67.12_suppl_4.s56.
9. Reimers A. Contraception for women with epilepsy: counseling, choices, and concerns. Open Access J Contracept. 2016;7:69–76. doi: 10.2147/OAJC.S85541.
10. Sidhu J, Job S, Singh S, Philipson R. The pharmacokinetic and pharmacodynamic consequences of the co-administration of lamotrigine and a combined oral contraceptive in healthy female subjects. Br J Clin Pharmacol. 2006;61(2):191–9. doi: 10.1111/j.1365-2125.2005.02539.x.
11. Artama M, Isojärvi JIT, Auvinen A. Antiepileptic drug use and birth rate in patients with epilepsy—a population-based cohort study in Finland. Hum Reprod. 2006;21(9):2290–5. doi: 10.1093/humrep/del194.
12. MacEachern DB, Mandle HB, Herzog AG. Infertility, impaired fecundity, and live birth/pregnancy ratio in women with epilepsy in the USA: Findings of the Epilepsy Birth Control Registry. Epilepsia. 2019;60(9):1993–8. doi: 10.1111/epi.16312.
13. French J, Harden C, Pennell P, Bagiella E, Andreopoulos E, Lau C, et al. A Prospective Study of Pregnancy in Women with Epilepsy Seeking Conception (The WEPOD Study) (I5.001). Neurology. 2016;86(16 Suppl) [cited 2022 Apr 27]. Available from: https://n.neurology.org/content/86/16_Supplement/I5.001.
14. Larsen MD, Jølving LR, Fedder J, Nørgård BM. The efficacy of assisted reproductive treatment in women with epilepsy. Reprod Biomed Online. 2020;41(6):1015–22. doi: 10.1016/j.rbmo.2020.07.019.
15. Crawford P, Hudson S. Understanding the information needs of women with epilepsy at different lifestages: results of the "Ideal World" survey. Seizure–Eur J Epilepsy. 2003;12(7):502–7. doi: 10.1016/S1059-1311(03)00085-2.
16. Johnson EL, Burke AE, Wang A, Pennell PB. Unintended pregnancy, prenatal care, newborn outcomes, and breastfeeding in women with epilepsy. Neurology. 2018;91(11):e1031–9. doi: 10.1212/WNL.0000000000006173.
17. Herzog AG, MacEachern DB, Mandle HB, Cahill KE, Fowler KM, Davis AR, et al. Folic acid use by women with epilepsy: findings of the Epilepsy Birth Control Registry. Epilepsy Behav. 2017;72:156–60. doi: 10.1016/j.yebeh.2017.05.007.
18. Ban L, Fleming KM, Doyle P, Smeeth L, Hubbard RB, Fiaschi L, et al. Congenital anomalies in children of mothers taking antiepileptic drugs with and without periconceptional high dose folic acid use: a population-based cohort study. PloS One. 2015;10(7):e0131130. doi: 10.1371/journal.pone.0131130.
19. Vajda FJE, O'Brien TJ, Graham JE, Hitchcock AA, Perucca P, Lander CM, et al. Folic acid dose, valproate, and fetal malformations. Epilepsy Behav. 2021;114(Pt A):107569. doi: 10.1016/j.yebeh.2020.107569.
20. Bjørk M, Riedel B, Spigset O, Veiby G, Kolstad E, Daltveit AK, et al. Association of folic acid supplementation during pregnancy with the risk of autistic traits in children exposed to antiepileptic drugs in utero. JAMA Neurol. 2018;75(2):160–8. doi: 10.1001/jamaneurol.2017.3897.
21. Meador KJ, Baker GA, Browning N, Cohen MJ, Bromley RL, Clayton-Smith J, et al. Fetal antiepileptic drug exposure and cognitive outcomes at age 6 years (NEAD study): a prospective observational study. Lancet Neurol. 2013;12(3):244–52. doi: 10.1016/S1474-4422(12)70323-X.
22. Baker GA, Bromley RL, Briggs M, Cheyne CP, Cohen MJ, García-Fiñana M, et al. IQ at 6 years after in utero exposure to antiepileptic drugs. Neurology. 2015;84(4):382–90. doi: 10.1212/WNL.0000000000001182.

23. Murray LK, Smith MJ, Jadavji NM. Maternal oversupplementation with folic acid and its impact on neurodevelopment of offspring. Nutr Rev. 2018;76(9):708–21. doi: 10.1093/nutrit/nuy025.

24. Tomson T, Battino D, Bromley R, Kochen S, Meador K, Pennell P, et al. Management of epilepsy in pregnancy: a report from the International League Against Epilepsy Task Force on Women and Pregnancy. Epileptic Disord. 2019;21(6):497–517. doi: 10.1684/epd.2019.1105.

25. Teramo K, Hiilesmaa V, Bardy A, Saarikoski S. Fetal heart rate during a maternal grand mal epileptic seizure. J Perinat Med. 1979;7(1):3–6. doi: 10.1515/jpme.1979.7.1.3.

26. Rauchenzauner M, Ehrensberger M, Prieschl M, Kapelari K, Bergmann M, Walser G, et al. Generalized tonic–clonic seizures and antiepileptic drugs during pregnancy – a matter of importance for the baby? J Neurol. 2013;260(2):484–4. doi: 10.1007/s00415-012-6662-8.

27. Christiana A, Della Torre M, Serafini A. Two cases of focal status epilepticus in pregnancy. Epilepsy Behav Rep. 2021; 16:100483. doi: 10.1016/j.ebr.2021.100483.

28. Sahoo S, Klein P. Maternal complex partial seizure associated with fetal distress. Arch Neurol. 2005;62(8):1304–5. doi: 10.1001/archneur.62.8.1304.

29. Cummings C, Stewart M, Stevenson M, Morrow J, Nelson J. Neurodevelopment of children exposed in utero to lamotrigine, sodium valproate and carbamazepine. Arch Dis Child. 2011;96:643–7. doi: 10.1136/adc.2009.176990.

30. Adab N. The longer term outcome of children born to mothers with epilepsy. J Neurol Neurosurg Psychiatry. 2004;75(11): 1575–83. doi: 10.1136/jnnp.2003.029132.

31. Pennell PB, French JA, May RC, Gerard E, Kalayjian L, Penovich P, et al. Changes in seizure frequency and antiepileptic therapy during pregnancy. N Engl J Med. 2020;383(26): 2547–56. doi: 10.1056/NEJMoa2008663.

32. Vajda FJE, O'Brien TJ, Graham J, Lander CM, Eadie MJ. The outcomes of pregnancy in women with untreated epilepsy. Seizure. 2015;24:77–81. doi: 10.1016/j.seizure.2014.08.008.

33. Vajda FJE, Hitchcock A, Graham J, O'Brien T, Lander C, Eadie M. Seizure control in antiepileptic drug-treated pregnancy. Epilepsia. 2008;49(1):172–6. doi: 10.1111/j.1528-1167.2007.01412.x.

34. Thomas SV, Syam U, Devi JS. Predictors of seizures during pregnancy in women with epilepsy. Epilepsia. 2012;53(5): e85–8. doi: 10.1111/j.1528-1167.2012.03439.x.

35. Voinescu PE, Ehlert AN, Bay CP, Allien S, Pennell PB. Variations in seizure frequency during pregnancy and postpartum by epilepsy type. Neurology. 2022;98(8):e802–7. doi: 10.1212/WNL.0000000000013056.

36. Mostacci B, Troisi S, Bisulli F, Zenesini C, Licchetta L, Provini F, et al. Seizure worsening in pregnancy in women with sleep-related hypermotor epilepsy (SHE): a historical cohort study. Seizure. 2021;91:258–62. doi: 10.1016/j.seizure.2021.06.034.

37. Vajda FJE, Brien TJO, Graham JE, Hitchcock AA, Perucca P, Lander CM, et al. The control of treated generalized and focal epilepsies during pregnancy. Epilepsy Behav. 2021;125. doi: 10.1016/j.yebeh.2021.108406.

38. Battino D, Tomson T, Bonizzoni E, Craig J, Lindhout D, Sabers A, et al. Seizure control and treatment changes in pregnancy: observations from the EURAP epilepsy pregnancy registry. Epilepsia. 2013;54(9):1621–27. doi: 10.1111/epi.12302.

39. Fried S, Kozer E, Nulman I, Einarson TR, Koren G. Malformation rates in children of women with untreated epilepsy. Drug Saf. 2004;27(3):197–202. doi: 10.2165/00002018-200427030-00004.

40. Keni RR, Jose M, Sarma PS, Thomas SV, Kerala Registry of Epilepsy and Pregnancy Study Group. Teratogenicity of antiepileptic dual therapy: dose-dependent, drug-specific, or both? Neurology. 2018;90(9):e790–6. doi: 10.1212/WNL.0000000000005031.

41. Meador K, Reynolds MW, Crean S, Fahrbach K, Probst C. Pregnancy outcomes in women with epilepsy: a systematic review and meta-analysis of published pregnancy registries and cohorts. Epilepsy Res. 2008;81(1):1–13. doi: 10.1016/j.eplepsyres.2008.04.022.

42. Hernandez-Díaz S. Comparative safety of antiepileptic drugs during pregnancy. Neurology. 2012 May 22;78(21):1692–9.

43. Blotière PO, Raguideau F, Weill A, Elefant E, Perthus I, Goulet V, et al. Risks of 23 specific malformations associated with prenatal exposure to 10 antiepileptic drugs. Neurology. 2019;93(2):e167–80. doi: 10.1212/WNL.0000000000007696.

44. Christensen J, Grønborg TK, Sørensen MJ, Schendel D, Parner ET, Pedersen LH, et al. Prenatal valproate exposure and risk of autism spectrum disorders and childhood autism. JAMA. 2013;309(16):1696–703. doi: 10.1001/jama.2013.2270.

45. Knight R, Wittkowski A, Bromley RL. Neurodevelopmental outcomes in children exposed to newer antiseizure medications: a systematic review. Epilepsia. 2021;62(8):1765–79. doi: 10.1111/epi.16953.

46. Veroniki AA, Cogo E, Rios P, Straus SE, Finkelstein Y, Kealey R, et al. Comparative safety of anti-epileptic drugs during pregnancy: a systematic review and network meta-analysis of congenital malformations and prenatal outcomes. BMC Med. 2017;15:95. doi: 10.1186/s12916-017-0845-1.

47. Rihtman T, Parush S, Ornoy A. Developmental outcomes at preschool age after fetal exposure to valproic acid and lamotrigine: cognitive, motor, sensory and behavioral function. Reprod Toxicol. 2013;41:115–25. doi: 10.1016/j.reprotox.2013.06.001.

48. Shallcross R, Bromley RL, Irwin B, Bonnett LJ, Morrow J, Baker GA; Liverpool Manchester Neurodevelopment Group; UK Epilepsy and Pregnancy Register. Child development following in utero exposure: levetiracetam vs sodium valproate. Neurology. 2011;76(4):383–9. doi: 10.1212/WNL.0b013e3182088297.

49. Cognition in school-age children exposed to levetiracetam, topiramate, or sodium valproate Neurology. 2016;87(18): 1943–53 [cited 2022 Apr 29]. Available from: https://n.neurology.org/content/87/18/1943.short.

50. North American Antiepileptic Drug Pregnancy Registry. Annual update for 2022–AED. [cited 2022 May 2]. Available from:https://www.aedpregnancyregistry.org/annual-update-for-2022/.

51. Tomson T, Battino D, Bonizzoni E, Craig J, Lindhout D, Perucca E, et al. Comparative risk of major congenital malformations with eight different antiepileptic drugs: a prospective cohort study of the EURAP registry. Lancet Neurol. 2018;17(6):530–8. doi: 10.1016/S1474-4422(18)30107-8.

52. Tomson T, Battino D, Bonizzoni E, Craig J, Lindhout D, Perucca E, et al. Declining malformation rates with changed antiepileptic drug prescribing: an observational study. Neurology. 2019;93(9):e831–40. doi: 10.1212/WNL.0000000000008001.

53. Voinescu PE, Pennell PB. Management of epilepsy during pregnancy. Expert Rev Neurother. 2015;15(10):1171–87. doi: 10.1586/14737175.2015.1083422.

54. Pennell PB, Karanam A, Meador KJ, Gerard E, Kalayjian L, Penovich P, et al. Antiseizure medication concentrations during pregnancy: results from the Maternal Outcomes and Neurodevelopmental Effects of Antiepileptic Drugs (MONEAD) study. JAMA Neurol. 2022;79(4):370–9. doi: 10.1001/jamaneurol.2021.5487.

55. Voinescu PE, Park S, Chen LQ, Stowe ZN, Newport DJ, Ritchie JC, et al. Antiepileptic drug clearances during pregnancy and clinical implications for women with epilepsy. Neurology. 2018;91(13):e1228–36. doi: 10.1212/WNL.0000000000006240.

56. Pennell PB, Peng L, Newport DJ, Ritchie JC, Koganti A, Holley DK, et al. Lamotrigine in pregnancy: clearance, therapeutic drug monitoring, and seizure frequency. Neurology. 2008;70(22 Pt 2):2130–6. doi: 10.1212/01.wnl.0000289511.20864.2a.

57. Johnson EL, Stowe ZN, Ritchie JC, Newport DJ, Newman ML, Knight B, et al. Carbamazepine clearance and seizure stability during pregnancy. Epilepsy Behav. 2014;33:49–53. doi: 10.1016/j.yebeh.2014.02.011.

58. Arfman IJ, Wammes-van der Heijden EA, ter Horst PGJ, Lambrechts DA, Wegner I, Touw DJ. Therapeutic drug monitoring of antiepileptic drugs in women with epilepsy before, during, and after pregnancy. Clin Pharmacokinet. 2020;59(4):427–45. doi: 10.1007/s40262-019-00845-2.

59. EURAP Study Group. Seizure control and treatment in pregnancy: observations from the EURAP epilepsy pregnancy registry. Neurology. 2006;66(3):354–60. doi: 10.1212/01.wnl.0000195888.51845.80.

60. Katz JM, Devinsky O. Primary generalized epilepsy: a risk factor for seizures in labor and delivery? Seizure. 2003;12(4):217–19. doi: 10.1016/S1059-1311(02)00288-1

61. Huang C-Y, Dai Y-M, Feng L-M, Gao W-L. Clinical characteristics and outcomes in pregnant women with epilepsy. Epilepsy Behav. 2020;112:107433. doi: 10.1016/j.yebeh.2020.107433.

62. Mari L, Placidi F, Romigi A, Tombini M, Del Bianco C, Ulivi M, et al. Levetiracetam, lamotrigine and carbamazepine: which monotherapy during pregnancy? Neurol Sci. 2022;43(3):1993–2001. doi: 10.1007/s10072-021-05542-2.

63. Melikova S, Bagirova H, Magalov S. The impact of maternal epilepsy on delivery and neonatal outcomes. Childs Nerv Syst. 2020;36(4):775–82. doi: 10.1007/s00381-019-04435-2.

64. Viale L, Allotey J, Cheong-See F, Arroyo-Manzano D, Mccorry D, Bagary M, et al. Epilepsy in pregnancy and reproductive outcomes: a systematic review and meta-analysis. Lancet. 2015;386(10006):1845–52. doi: 10.1016/S0140-6736(15)00045-8.

65. Panelli DM, Leonard SA, Kan P, Meador KJ, McElrath TF, Darmawan KF, et al. Association of epilepsy and severe maternal morbidity. Obstet Gynecol. 2021;138(5):747–54. doi: 10.1097/AOG.0000000000004562.

66. Centers for Disease Control and Prevention. How does CDC Identify severe maternal morbidity? 2021 Feb 8 [cited 2022 May 2]. Available from: https://www.cdc.gov/reproductive health/maternalinfanthealth/smm/severe-morbidity-ICD. htm.

67. Borthen I, Eide MG, Veiby G, Daltveit AK, Gilhus NE. Complications during pregnancy in women with epilepsy: population-based cohort study. BJOG. 2009;116(13):1736–42. doi: 10.1111/j.1471-0528.2009.02354.x.

68. MacDonald SC, Bateman BT, McElrath TF, Hernández-Díaz S. Mortality and morbidity during delivery hospitalization among pregnant women with epilepsy in the United States. JAMA Neurol. 2015;72(9):981–8. doi: 10.1001/jamaneurol.2015.1017.

69. Edey S, Moran N, Nashef L. SUDEP and epilepsy-related mortality in pregnancy. Epilepsia. 2014;55(7):e72–4. doi: 10.1111/epi.12621.

70. Devinsky O, Hesdorffer DC, Thurman DJ, Lhatoo S, Richerson G. Sudden unexpected death in epilepsy: epidemiology, mechanisms, and prevention. Lancet Neurol. 2016;15(10):1075–88. doi: 10.1016/S1474-4422(16)30158-2.

71. Dell KL, Payne DE, Kremen V, Maturana MI, Gerla V, Nejedly P, et al. Seizure likelihood varies with day-to-day variations in sleep duration in patients with refractory focal epilepsy: a longitudinal electroencephalography investigation. eClinicalMedicine. 2021;37. doi: 10.1016/j.eclinm.2021.100934.

72. Crawford P. Best practice guidelines for the management of women with epilepsy. Epilepsia. 2005;46(Suppl 9):117–24. doi: 10.1111/j.1528-1167.2005.00323.x.

73. Decker BM, Thibault D, Davis KA, Willis AW. A nationwide analysis of maternal morbidity and acute postpartum readmissions in women with epilepsy. Epilepsy Behav. 2021;117:107874. doi: 10.1016/j.yebeh.2021.107874.

74. Birnbaum AK, Meador KJ, Karanam A, Brown C, May RC, Gerard EE, et al. Antiepileptic drug exposure in infants of breastfeeding mothers with epilepsy. JAMA Neurol. 2020;77(4):441–50. doi: 10.1001/jamaneurol.2019.4443.

75. Meador KJ, Baker GA, Browning N, Cohen MJ, Bromley RL, Clayton-Smith J, et al. Breastfeeding in children of women taking antiepileptic drugs. JAMA Pediatr. 2014;168(8):729–36. doi: 10.1001/jamapediatrics.2014.118.

76. Al-Faraj AO, Pandey S, Herlihy MM, Pang TD. Factors affecting breastfeeding in women with epilepsy. Epilepsia. 2021;62(9):2171–9. doi: 10.1111/epi.17003.

77. Turner K, Piazzini A, Franza A, Marconi AM, Canger R, Canevini MP. Epilepsy and postpartum depression. Epilepsia. 2009;50(s1):24–7. doi: 10.1111/j.1528-1167.2008.01965.x.

78. Bjørk MH, Veiby G, A. Engelsen B, Gilhus NE. Depression and anxiety during pregnancy and the postpartum period in women with epilepsy: a review of frequency, risks and recommendations for treatment. Seizure. 2015;28:39–45. doi: 10.1016/j.seizure.2015.02.016.

Chapter 24
Chronic Hypertension

Christina L. Herrera

Department of Obstetrics and Gynecology, Division of Maternal-Fetal Medicine, University of Texas Southwestern Medical Center, Dallas, TX, USA

Chronic hypertension is one of the most serious pregnancy complications with resultant maternal and perinatal mortality. Its cited incidence ranges from 2% to 6% [1,2]. Recent contemporaneous increases in obesity and advancing maternal age have contributed to an increase in the number of individuals beginning pregnancy with chronic hypertension [3]. Therefore, familiarity with diagnosis, management, and sequelae of chronic hypertension during pregnancy remains paramount for all obstetric providers.

Definition

Chronic hypertension in pregnancy is defined as hypertension diagnosed or present before 20 weeks of gestation [4]. Classically, 140/90 mmHg has been used as the upper limit of normal for blood pressure in pregnancy despite known racial and ethnic variation [5]. Recent recommendations from the American College of Cardiology and the American Heart Association have suggested lower criteria for diagnosis outside of pregnancy in order to enhance modification of long-term cardiovascular risk [6]. These recommendations include a lower threshold of 130/80 mmHg for stage 1 hypertension and 140/90 mmHg for stage 2 hypertension (Table 24.1). At present there are not clear data on what should be done in a pregnant people without a prior diagnosis of chronic hypertension who has stage 1 hypertension prior to 20 weeks [7]. It is reasonable in such individuals to take a conservative approach with a higher degree of observation, particularly if she is multiparous or has a history of hypertensive disorders of pregnancy or family history of chronic hypertension. The diagnosis may be missed during the first half of pregnancy because of the physiologic decrease in vascular resistance that nadirs at 16–18 weeks. As a result, chronic hypertension may be diagnosed as gestational hypertension or preeclampsia in late pregnancy.

Diagnosis

Chronic hypertension is diagnosed ≥140/90 mmHg and classified as severe (≥160/110 mmHg) based on measurements on two occasions at least 4 hours apart [7]. The blood pressures meeting these criteria should be documented only after the patients has been in the sitting position for at least 10 minutes with legs uncrossed and back supported. To reduce inaccurate readings, an appropriate size cuff should be used – length 1.5 times upper arm circumference or a cuff with a bladder that encircles 80% or more of the upper arm. Obesity can make measurement of the blood pressure more challenging due to arm/cuff mismatch. Documentation should note if a larger- or smaller-than-normal cuff size is used [6]. The patient should not use tobacco or caffeine for 30 minutes preceding the measurement [8]. Uterine size and compression of the inferior vena cava and aorta are factors (especially in the supine position) that alter blood pressure readings as the uterus enlarges.

Preconceptional counseling

Preconceptional counseling is important for pregnant people with chronic hypertension. Ideally the duration of hypertension, degree of control, medications taken, and presence of end-organ damage are established. Those with poor control, requiring multiple medications, or with significant end-organ damage (e.g. severe renal or cardiac dysfunction) should be advised of the greater risk of adverse outcomes. Pregnant individuals with chronic hypertension should be taught self-blood pressure monitoring, and home measurement devices checked for accuracy. Medication should be adjusted to those acceptable during pregnancy. Angiotensin-converting enzyme (ACE) inhibitors and angiotensin receptor blockers (ARB) are contraindicated in the periconceptual period and the first trimester due to associations with cardiac and central

Queenan's Management of High-Risk Pregnancy: An Evidence-Based Approach, Seventh Edition. Edited by Catherine Y. Spong and Charles J. Lockwood.
© 2024 John Wiley & Sons Ltd. Published 2024 by John Wiley & Sons Ltd.

Table 24.1 Criteria for diagnosis of hypertension

Blood pressure (mmHg)		Nonpregnant ACC/AHA	Pregnant ACOG
SBP	DBP		
<120	<180	Normal	Normal
120–129	<80	Elevated	Normal
130–139	80–89	Stage 1 HTN	Normal
140–159	≥90	Stage 2 HTN	HTN
≥160	≥110	Stage 2 HTN	Severe HTN

ACC, American College of Cardiology; AHA, American Heart Association; ACOG, American College of Obstetricians and Gynecologists; DBP, diastolic blood pressure; HTN, hypertension; SBP, systolic blood pressure.

nervous system anomalies [9]. Past the first trimester, they are associated with fetal hypocalvaria, lung hypoplasia renal anomalies, and renal failure that may not be reversible [10–12]. Mineralocorticoid receptor antagonists are likewise not recommended due to concern for under-virilization of male fetuses and theoretical concern for placental perfusion late in pregnancy [13].

Morbidity and mortality

Chronic hypertension in pregnancy is associated with a number of adverse pregnancy outcomes (Table 24.2). Complications are more likely with severe baseline hypertension and in the presence of concomitant end-organ damage [14,15]. Maternal complications include preeclampsia, placental abruption, stroke, hypertensive cardiomyopathy, pulmonary edema, myocardial infarction, and a five-fold increased risk of death [16,17]. Fetal complications include growth restriction (FGR), stillbirth, preterm birth, and a four-fold increase in perinatal mortality [1]. Up to 30% of pregnant individuals with chronic hypertension are delivered preterm from complications of super-imposed preeclampsia or FGR [18]. The risk of preeclampsia is directly related to the severity of baseline hypertension [19]. Pregnant individuals with chronic

Table 24.2 Adverse outcomes associated with chronic hypertension

Maternal	Fetal
Superimposed preeclampsia	Stillbirth
HELLP syndrome	Growth restriction
Placental abruption	Preterm birth
Stroke	Neonatal morbidity
Acute kidney injury	Neonatal death
Heart failure	
Hypertensive cardiomyopathy	
Myocardial infarction	
Death	

HELLP, hemolysis, elevated liver enzymes, and low platelet count.

hypertension develop preeclampsia and FGR at rates of 20–50% and 25–40% respectively [18,20]. Despite this increased risk, there are currently no useful tests for predicting superimposed preeclampsia; because of this, heightened vigilance is necessary.

Diagnosis and evaluation in pregnancy

When hypertension is present or suspected, additional testing should be carried out based on clinical considerations. If a practitioner has not had extensive experience with hypertension during pregnancy, consultative advice should be sought from a maternal-fetal medicine specialist. As the kidneys are often the first organ affected by chronic hypertension, assessment of renal function commonly includes serum creatinine and spot urine protein-to-creatinine ratio. If the latter is greater than 0.15, a 24-hour urinary protein excretion is measured. Baseline assessments of complete blood count with platelet count and liver function testing (aspartate aminotransferase, alanine aminotransferase), should also be performed. Serum electrolytes (specifically potassium) should be assessed in individuals taking diuretics. If the hypertension has been present for at least 5 years, additional consideration should be given to obtaining an electrocardiogram and echocardiogram.

Although uncommon, secondary causes of hypertension should be evaluated based on clinical presentation. Consideration should be given to underlying renal disease, connective tissue disease, primary aldosteronism, Cushing syndrome, pheochromocytoma, or other causes. In particular, a young patients with severe hypertension (especially with no family history) may need Doppler flow studies to evaluate for renal artery stenosis. Generally, the presence of diabetes mellitus is known, but in patients with proteinuria this should remain a consideration. A toxicology screen should be considered in all patients with severe and/or accelerated hypertension to examine for illicit substance abuse, such as cocaine or methamphetamine. Obstructive sleep apnea should be suspected and appropriate referral for evaluation should be undertaken in obese individuals with hypertension who snore loudly while asleep, awake with headache, and fall asleep inappropriately during the day.

Treatment during pregnancy

Home blood pressure monitoring may be a useful adjunct, especially in the second half of pregnancy. Procedures for the use of home blood pressure monitoring emphasize patient training, use of an appropriately calibrated device, and clear instructions [6]. Home measurement should be compared with office measurements to verify calibration and assist with adjusting medication when there is uncertainty [21]. Home monitoring will augment tele-health visits.

The precise blood pressure levels that require antihypertensive therapy in pregnancy remains debatable. A previous Cochrane review concluded that treatment of mild chronic hypertension reduced the incidence of severe hypertension but did not reduce the frequency of preeclampsia, preterm birth, or other adverse pregnancy outcomes [22]. Moreover, overtreatment was a concern as other meta-analyses had demonstrated a twofold increased risk of small for gestational age (SGA) infants [23,24]. The Chronic Hypertension and Pregnancy (CHAP), a large, pragmatic, randomized control trial, recently found that treatment of mild hypertension reduced the risk of maternal and perinatal morbidity without an increase in the risk of SGA infants. Specifically, they found a number need to treat of 14.7 to reduce the primary composite outcome of preeclampsia with severe features, medically indicated preterm birth <35 weeks, placental abruption, and fetal or neonatal death <28 days. Due to the study findings, both the American College of Obstetricians and Gynecologists and the Society for Maternal-Fetal Medicine released statements revising recommendations of a treatment threshold from 160/110 to 140/90 mm Hg [25,26]. However, as others have favored using a goal of 150/100 in all pregnant individuals, the benefit of this lower threshold remains unclear [4,27]. For those with associated comorbid conditions, even lower blood pressure goals may be desired, and consultation with subspecialties should be pursued to optimize care.

Although the most extensively studied antihypertensive agent is methyldopa, it is currently rarely used in pregnant people. Labetalol and extended-release nifedipine, though introduced as second-line agents, are commonly used as first-line agents for control of hypertension in pregnancy. Nifedipine is an ideal first-line antihypertensive agent in pregnancy due to its low maternal side effect profile and steady blood pressure control with extended-release dosing. The effect of calcium channel blockade is vasodilation, and it may have a salutary effect on the uterine blood flow similar to its effect on renal blood flow. Labetalol is an alternative medication that has α-adrenergic and central β-blocking effects. Other β-blocking medications do not have this dual effect, which may explain why they are associated with fetal growth restriction [28]. Thiazides may curtail the expected volume expansion in pregnancy. Despite similar perinatal outcomes in individuals on this medication, this concern has led to the withholding of thiazides as a first line therapy, particularly after 20 weeks [4]. A table of the commonly used oral antihypertensive medications is included for reference (Table 24.3).

All of the aforementioned drugs probably cross the placenta and enter the fetal circulation but have not been known to cause birth defects. As mentioned above, antihypertensive medications that work through the renin–angiotensin system including ARBs and ACE inhibitors are contraindicated. These drugs are associated with various congenital anomalies and subsequent renal defects, oligohydramnios, and skeletal deformities. Mineralocorticoid receptors antagonists are also avoided. Using two antihypertensive medications of the same class whenever a patient needs more than one agent to control the hypertension should be avoided. This is most likely to occur for agents acting on the adrenergic system (e.g. avoid combining methyldopa with labetalol).

Antihypertensive treatment is given for acute onset severe hypertension that is sustained: ≥160/110 mmHg for 15 minutes or more. Agents should be administered within 30–60 minutes [7]. This lower threshold for treatment has been established to prevent cerebrovascular accidents of hypertensive encephalopathy [29]. Randomized controlled trials for the acute treatment of severe-range blood pressure during pregnancy are limited and have not established a favored therapy [30,31]. Drug selection should be individualized based on side effect profile and patient co-morbidities. Agents for the treatment of acute blood pressure management are highlighted in Table 24.4.

Because pregnant individuals with chronic hypertension are at high risk for the development of preeclampsia, the US Preventive Service Task Force, the American College

Table 24.3 Commonly used oral antihypertensive medications for chronic hypertension in pregnancy

Medication	Daily dose	Side effects	Comment
Labetalol	100 mg BID to 800 mg TID	Tremulousness, flushing, headache; agents may lead to decreased placental perfusion	β-blocker with α-blocking activity
Nifedipine (extended-release)	30 mg to 120 mg; 60 mg BID recommended for 120 mg dosing	Headache, tachycardia, orthostatic hypotension; avoid use in the setting of coronary artery disease	Calcium channel blocker
Methyldopa	250 mg BID to 1000 mg TID	Lethargy, fever, hepatitis, hemolytic anemia, positive Coombs test	Centrally acting α-agonist
Thiazide diuretics	12.5 to 25 mg	May be harmful in volume-contracted states such as preeclampsia; initial effect is to decrease plasma volume	Second- or third-line agent unless patient enters pregnancy with medication

Table 24.4 Antihypertensive agents for acute blood pressure control in pregnancy

Medication	Dose	Side effects	Onset
Hydralazine	5–10 mg IV or IM, then 10 mg every 20 minutes as needed	Maternal hypotension, headaches, and tracing abnormalities with high and frequent dosing	10–20 min
Labetalol	20 mg IV, then 40 then 80 mg every 20 minutes as needed; max 300 mg	Tachycardia less common. Avoid with asthma and preexisting cardiac disease.	1–2 min
Nifedipine (immediate release)	10 mg orally, then 20 mg then 20 mg every 20 minutes as needed	Reflex tachycardia, headaches	5–10 min

IM, intramuscular; IV, intravenous.

of Obstetricians and Gynecologists, and the Society for Maternal-Fetal Medicine recommend low-dose aspirin (81 mg/day) for prevention of preeclampsia [32,33]. Low-dose aspirin is given beginning between 12 and 28 weeks of gestation and optimally before 16 weeks and continued daily until delivery. The impact of this recommendation is debatable, as use has not led to a change in rates of superimposed preeclampsia or fetal growth restriction in pregnant people with chronic hypertension [34].

Antepartum fetal assessment

Antepartum fetal evaluation should include sonography for the establishment of optimal dating criteria [35]. Careful dating of gestation is important so that fetal growth may be assessed accurately, and appropriate timing of delivery planning may be undertaken. Third-trimester sonography for assessment of fetal growth with subsequent follow-up as indicated is appropriate. Fetal growth restriction is usually not clinically apparent until after 30–32 weeks gestation in most pregnant people with mild to moderate hypertension not requiring pharmacotherapy. Those individuals on multiple agents, poorly controlled hypertension, or associated medical co-morbidities may require earlier serial assessment.

Even uncomplicated pregnant patients with chronic hypertension or gestational hypertension carry an increased risk of perinatal mortality. Therefore, many recommend antenatal fetal surveillance beginning at 32 weeks gestational age [36]. Those on multiple agents, with poorly controlled hypertension, or associated medical co-morbidities may require a more individualized approach. In the presence of fetal growth restriction or

superimposed preeclampsia, antenatal fetal surveillance is recommended at diagnosis or at a gestational age when delivery would be of benefit. Twice weekly testing is recommended for those without severe features. Daily testing is recommended for those when severe features are present [37].

Delivery

For pregnant people with chronic hypertension without additional complications, delivery is recommended beginning at 38 0/7 weeks of gestation for those not taking antihypertensive therapy, and at 37 0/7 weeks of gestation in those requiring antihypertensive therapy [7]. Expectant management beyond 39 0/7 weeks of gestation is not recommended due to the increased incidence of superimposed preeclampsia [38]. Pregnant individuals with severe acute hypertension or superimposed preeclampsia with severe features should be delivered when the diagnosis is made after 34 0/7 weeks of gestation. Those who develop preeclampsia without severe features can be expectantly managed until 37 0/7 weeks of gestation. Prior to 34 0/7 weeks of gestation, expectant management of superimposed preeclampsia with severe features may be considered with inpatient management. In the setting of fetal growth restriction, the decision to deliver is often made by clinical judgement based on maternal and fetal risks.

Postpartum care

Pregnant people with chronic hypertension are at increased risk for metabolic syndrome, renal dysfunction, and lifetime cardiovascular morbidity, including myocardial infarction and cerebrovascular disease. These risks are further increased when associated comorbid conditions are present. Thus, optimized blood pressure control should be continued into the postpartum period and beyond remains critically important. Mobilization of extravascular fluid may result in postpartum elevations of blood pressure that can result in additional morbidity if unaddressed. Early visits in the first 1–2 weeks after delivery and home monitoring are recommended to enable optimal blood pressure control.

Contraception should also be reviewed. Individuals who have completed their childbearing can be offered a permanent form of contraception. Combined hormonal contraceptives even in well-controlled hypertension are linked to greater risks than non-users for stroke, acute myocardial infraction, and peripheral arterial disease, and are considered US Medical Eligibility Criteria for Contraceptive Use category 3, which concludes that risks usually outweigh the advantages [39]. Progestin-based oral contraception is considered safe. Depot-medroxyprogesterone acetate (DMPA) may be considered in those with well-controlled hypertension, but has been found to have a higher risk of stroke in those with severe hypertension [40]. Other contraceptive options that may be considered include the intrauterine device (levonorgestrel or copper), contraceptive vaginal ring, etonogestrel contraceptive implant, or a barrier method.

Long-term follow-up includes referral to an appropriate primary care physician who can facilitate routine monitoring of blood pressure, appropriate laboratory studies, and lifestyle interventions to maximize cardiovascular health and decrease hypertension-related morbidity and mortality.

CASE PRESENTATION

A 40-year-old gravida 3, para 2 presented to her obstetrician at 18 weeks age of gestation with systolic blood pressures of 145/90 and 148/96 mmHg. Urine dipstick for protein was 2+. A 24-hour urine collection disclosed a total protein excretion of 420 mg. The remaining laboratory findings were in the accepted normal range of reference for pregnancy. Because she had evidence of end-organ damage, antihypertensive medications were started. Echocardiography showed normal ventricular indices with an ejection fraction of 60%. The electrocardiogram was also normal. Blood pressures at subsequent visits were within normal limits. She underwent a rate of growth sonogram at 32 weeks and thereafter weekly biophysical profiles that were normal. She subsequently presented at 36 weeks with an increase in her blood pressure to 150/100 and 152/96 mmHg despite antihypertensive medication and repeat 24-hour urine collection resulted in 930 mg of protein. Superimposed preeclampsia without severe features was diagnosed and labor was induced at 37 weeks of gestation. She stopped her medication during the postpartum period and 12 weeks after delivery still had blood pressures greater than 140/90 mmHg. She was referred for follow-up by a primary care physician for long-term management of hypertension and to address her cardiovascular health and lifestyle modifications.

References

1. Bateman BT, Huybrechts KF, Fischer MA, Seely EW, Ecker JL, Oberg AS, et al. Chronic hypertension in pregnancy and the risk of congenital malformations: a cohort study. Am J Obstet Gynecol. 2015;212(3):337e1–14.

2. Fryar CD, Ostchega Y, Hales CM, Zhang G, Kruszon-Moran D. Hypertension prevalence and control among adults: United States, 2015-2016. NCHS Data Brief. 2017;(289):1–8.

3. Martin JA, Hamilton BE, Osterman MJK, Driscoll AK. Births: final data for 2019. Natl Vital Stat Rep. 2021;70(2):1–51.

4. Report of the National High Blood Pressure Education Program Working Group on High Blood Pressure in Pregnancy. Am J Obstet Gynecol. 2000;183(1):S1–s22.

5. Kotchen TA. Hypertensive vascular disease. In: Jameson JL, Fauci AS, Kasper DL, Hauser SL, Longo DL, Loscalzo J, editors. Harrison's principles of internal medicine. 20th ed. New York, NY: McGraw-Hill Education; 2018.

6. Whelton PK, Carey RM, Aronow WS, Casey DE Jr., Collins KJ, Dennison Himmelfarb C, et al. 2017 ACC/AHA/AAPA/ABC/ACPM/AGS/APhA/ASH/ASPC/NMA/PCNA Guideline for the prevention, detection, evaluation, and management of high blood pressure in adults: A Report of the American College of Cardiology/American Heart Association Task Force on Clinical Practice Guidelines. Hypertension. 2018;71(6):e13–e115.

7. American College of Obstetricians and Gynecologists' Committee on Practice Bulletins—Obstetrics. ACOG Practice Bulletin No. 203: chronic hypertension in pregnancy. Obstet Gynecol. 2019;133(1):e26–e50.

8. The sixth report of the Joint National Committee on prevention, detection, evaluation, and treatment of high blood pressure. Arch Intern Med. 1997;157(21):2413–46.

9. Cooper WO, Hernandez-Diaz S, Arbogast PG, Dudley JA, Dyer S, Gideon PS, et al. Major congenital malformations after first-trimester exposure to ACE inhibitors. N Engl J Med. 2006;354(23):2443–51.

10. Piper JM, Ray WA, Rosa FW. Pregnancy outcome following exposure to angiotensin-converting enzyme inhibitors. Obstet Gynecol. 1992;80(3 Pt 1):429–32.

11. Martinovic J, Benachi A, Laurent N, Daikha-Dahmane F, Gubler MC. Fetal toxic effects and angiotensin-II-receptor antagonists. Lancet. 2001;358(9277):241–2.

12. Bullo M, Tschumi S, Bucher BS, Bianchetti MG, Simonetti GD. Pregnancy outcome following exposure to angiotensin-converting enzyme inhibitors or angiotensin receptor antagonists: a systematic review. Hypertension. 2012;60(2):444–50.

13. Riester A, Reincke M. Progress in primary aldosteronism: mineralocorticoid receptor antagonists and management of primary aldosteronism in pregnancy. Eur J Endocrinol. 2015;172(1):R23–30.

14. Czeizel AE, Bánhidy F. Chronic hypertension in pregnancy. Curr Opin Obstet Gynecol. 2011;23(2):76–81.

15. Morgan JL, Nelson DB, Roberts SW, Wells CE, McIntire DD, Cunningham FG. Association of baseline proteinuria and adverse outcomes in pregnant women with treated chronic hypertension. Obstet Gynecol. 2016;128(2):270–6.

16. Gilbert JS, Ryan MJ, LaMarca BB, Sedeek M, Murphy SR, Granger JP. Pathophysiology of hypertension during preeclampsia: linking placental ischemia with endothelial dysfunction. Am J Physiol Heart Circ Physiol. 2008;294(2):H541–50.

17. Creanga AA, Bateman BT, Butwick AJ, Raleigh L, Maeda A, Kuklina E, et al. Morbidity associated with cesarean delivery in the United States: is placenta accreta an increasingly important contributor? Am J Obstet Gynecol. 2015;213(3):384 e1–11.

18. Seely EW, Ecker J. Chronic hypertension in pregnancy. Circulation. 2014;129(11):1254–61.

19. Morgan JL, Nelson DB, Roberts SW, Wells CE, McIntire DD, Cunningham FG. Blood pressure profiles across pregnancy in women with chronic hypertension. Am J Perinatol. 2016;33(12):1128–32.

20. Sibai BM, Lindheimer M, Hauth J, Caritis S, VanDorsten P, Klebanoff M, et al. Risk factors for preeclampsia, abruptio placentae, and adverse neonatal outcomes among women with chronic hypertension. National Institute of Child Health and Human Development Network of Maternal-Fetal Medicine Units. N Engl J Med. 1998;339(10):667–71.

21. Staessen JA, Den Hond E, Celis H, Fagard R, Keary L, Vandenhoven G, et al. Antihypertensive treatment based on blood pressure measurement at home or in the physician's office: a randomized controlled trial. JAMA. 2004;291(8):955–64.

22. Abalos E, Duley L, Steyn DW, Gialdini C. Antihypertensive drug therapy for mild to moderate hypertension during pregnancy. Cochrane Database Syst Rev. 2018;10(10):Cd002252. doi: 10.1002/14651858.CD002252.pub4.

23. Magee LA, Elran E, Bull SB, Logan A, Koren G. Risks and benefits of beta-receptor blockers for pregnancy hypertension: overview of the randomized trials. Eur J Obstet Gynecol Reprod Biol. 2000;88(1):15–26.

24. von Dadelszen P, Ornstein MP, Bull SB, Logan AG, Koren G, Magee LA. Fall in mean arterial pressure and fetal growth restriction in pregnancy hypertension: a meta-analysis. Lancet. 2000;355(9198):87–92.

25. Society for Maternal-Fetal Medicine. SMFM statement: antihypertensive therapy for mild hypertension in pregnancy: The CHAP Trial. Washington, DC: SMFM; 2022.

26. Kaimal AJ, Gandhi M, Pettker CM, Simhan H. ACOG practice advisory: clinical guidance for the integration of the findings of the Chronic Hypertension and Pregnancy (CHAP) Study. Washington, DC: ACOG; 2022.

27. Cunningham GC, Nelson DB. Chronic hypertension. In: Cunningham F, Leveno KJ, Bloom SL, Dashe JS, Hoffman BL, Casey BM, Spong CY, editors. Williams obstetrics. 25th ed. New York: McGraw-Hill Education; 2018. P. 755–802.

28. Bayliss H, Churchill D, Beevers M, Beevers DG. Antihypertensive drugs in pregnancy and fetal growth: evidence for "pharmacological programming" in the first trimester? Hypertens Pregnancy. 2002;21(2):161–74.

29. Varon J, Marik PE. The diagnosis and management of hypertensive crises. Chest. 2000;118(1):214–27.

30. Zulfeen M, Tatapudi R, Sowjanya R. IV labetalol and oral nifedipine in acute control of severe hypertension in pregnancy: a randomized controlled trial. Eur J Obstet Gynecol Reprod Biol. 2019;236:46–52.

31. Raheem IA, Saaid R, Omar SZ, Tan PC. Oral nifedipine versus intravenous labetalol for acute blood pressure control in hypertensive emergencies of pregnancy: a randomised trial. BJOG. 2012;119(1):78–85.

32. LeFevre ML. Low-dose aspirin use for the prevention of morbidity and mortality from preeclampsia: U.S. Preventive Services Task Force recommendation statement. Ann Intern Med. 2014;161(11):819–26.

33. ACOG Committee Opinion No. 743: low-dose aspirin use during pregnancy. Obstet Gynecol. 2018;132(1):e44–52.

34. Banala C, Moreno S, Cruz Y, Boelig RC, Saccone G, Berghella V, et al. Impact of the ACOG guideline regarding low-dose aspirin for prevention of superimposed preeclampsia in women with chronic hypertension. Am J Obstet Gynecol. 2020;223(3):419.e1–16.

35. Committee Opinion No 700: methods for estimating the due date. Obstet Gynecol. 2017;129(5):e150–4.

36. American College of Obstetricians and Gynecologists' Committee on Obstetric Practice, Society for Maternal-Fetal Medicine. ACOG Committee Opinion No. 828: indications for outpatient antenatal fetal surveillance. Obstet Gynecol. 2021;137(6):e177–97.

37. ACOG Practice Bulletin No. 202: gestational hypertension and preeclampsia. Obstet Gynecol. 2019;133(1):1–25.

38. Harper LM, Biggio JR, Anderson S, Tita ATN. Gestational age of delivery in pregnancies complicated by chronic hypertension. Obstet Gynecol. 2016;127(6):1101–9.

39. Curtis KM, Tepper NK, Jatlaoui TC, Berry-Bibee E, Horton LG, Zapata LB, et al. U.S. medical eligibility criteria for contraceptive use, 2016. MMWR Recomm Rep. 2016;65(3):1–103.

40. Cardiovascular disease and use of oral and injectable progestogen-only contraceptives and combined injectable contraceptives. Results of an international, multicenter, case-control study. World Health Organization Collaborative Study of Cardiovascular Disease and Steroid Hormone Contraception. Contraception. 1998;57(5):315–24.

Chapter 25
Systemic Lupus Erythematosus

Michael Richley and Christina S. Han
Department of Obstetrics and Gynecology, University of California at Los Angeles, Los Angeles, CA, USA

Systemic lupus erythematosus (SLE) is a chronic autoimmune disorder characterized by disease flares and remissions. It is a heterogeneous disorder with a variety of clinical and laboratory manifestations. Affected patients can have a relatively benign course, affecting only the skin and musculoskeletal system, or be affected by aggressive, life-threatening visceral involvement.

Systemic manifestations include arthralgias, rashes, renal abnormalities, neurologic complications, thromboemboli, myocarditis, and serositis [1]. Box 25.1 outlines the revised diagnostic criteria by the American College of Rheumatology [2,3]. Patients must fulfil at least 4 of the 11 criteria. These criteria have been found to be 96% sensitive and 96% specific for the diagnosis of SLE [2].

Epidemiology

The prevalence of SLE varies is generally 5–125 per 100 000 and affects approximately 1% of pregnancies [4]. The lifetime risk 1 in 700, with a peak incidence at age 30 [5]. The prevalence is affected by sex, race, and geography. Lupus affects women 3–10 times as often as men, and disproportionately affects African-Americans, Afro-Caribbeans, Asians, and Hispanics [1,5].

Etiology

The etiology of SLE is multifactorial and studies have suggested a combination of genetic, epigenetic, and environmental factors. Major advances have identified several independently replicated SLE linkage regions, contributing to specific clinical or immunologic SLE features. Key candidate genes with strong evidence for a role in pathogenesis of SLE include *MHC, ITGAM, IRF5, BLK, STAT4, PTPN22*, and *FCGR2A* [7]. Specific genes are associated with clinical subsets of SLE, such as nephritis (*2q34*), hemolytic anemia (*11q14*), or development of specific autoantibodies, such as anti-double-stranded DNA (*19p13.2*). Although these genetic factors influence risk of SLE, additional factors are necessary to trigger onset of the disease [8].

Hormonal and environmental factors contribute to the disease process. Early menarche, estrogen-containing contraceptive use, and hormone replacement therapy are associated with increased risk of SLE [9]. Viral infections, ultraviolet light, and medications have also all been implicated in the disease process [10,11].

Pathogenesis

Pathogenesis of SLE begins with recognition of autoantigens and activation of the innate immune system. Dysregulated response to initial cytokine signals from both the innate and adaptive immune systems results in an overactive, proinflammatory response to the autoantigens [7].

Autoantibodies in SLE include antinuclear antibodies (ANA), anti-double-stranded DNA (anti-dsDNA), anti-Smith (anti-Sm), anti-ribonucleoprotein (anti-RNP), anti-Ro/SSA, and anti-La/SSB antibodies. These autoantibodies carry diagnostic and prognostic implications, and contribute to the wide spectrum of clinical manifestations. ANA is the most common antibody for screening for autoimmune syndromes. However, 10% of asymptomatic pregnant women without autoimmune disease have ANA antibodies compared to 2% of nonpregnant controls [12]. Because of the high prevalence in the general population, ANA is used mainly as a screening test for lupus.

Anti-dsDNA and anti-Sm are highly specific for lupus. Anti-dsDNA has been correlated with disease activity, particularly lupus nephritis. Renal damage is secondary

Queenan's Management of High-Risk Pregnancy: An Evidence-Based Approach, Seventh Edition. Edited by Catherine Y. Spong and Charles J. Lockwood.

Box 25.1 Criteria for diagnosis of SLE

1 Malar rash
Fixed erythema, flat or raised, over the malar eminences, tending to spare the nasolabial folds

2 Discoid rash
Erythematous raised patches with adherent keratotic scaling and follicular plugging; atrophic scarring may occur in older lesions

3 Photosensitivity
Skin rash as a result of unusual reaction to sunlight, by patient history or physician observation

4 Oral ulcers
Oral or nasopharyngeal ulceration, usually painless, observed by a physician

5 Arthritis
Nonerosive arthritis involving two or more peripheral joints, characterized by tenderness, swelling, or effusion

6 Serositis
  (a) Pleuritis: convincing history of pleuritic pain or rub heard by a physician or evidence of pleural effusion
  or
  (b) Pericarditis: documented by ECG or rub or evidence of pericardial effusion

7 Renal disorder
Persistent proteinuria greater than 0.5 g/d or greater than 3+ proteinuria if quantitation is not performed
or
Cellular casts: may be red cell, hemoglobin, granular, tubular, or mixed

8 Neurologic disorder
Seizures, in the absence of offending drugs or known metabolic derangements (e.g. uremia, ketoacidosis, or electrolyte imbalance)
or
Psychosis, in the absence of offending drugs or known metabolic derangements (e.g. uremia, ketoacidosis, or electrolyte imbalance)

9 Hematologic disorder
Hemolytic anemia, with reticulocytosis
or
Leukopenia: less than 4000/mm³ on two or more occasions
or
Lymphopenia: less than 1500/mm³ on two or more occasions
or
Thrombocytopenia: less than 100 000/mm³ in the absence of offending drugs

10 Immunologic disorder Anti-ds DNA antibody or anti-Sm antibody
or
Positive findings of antiphospholipid antibodies based on:
  (a) Abnormal serum level of IgG or IgM anticardiolipin antibodies
  or
  (b) Positive test result for lupus anticoagulant
  or
  (c) False-positive serologic test for syphilis known to be positive for at least 6 months and confirmed by *Treponema pallidum* immobilization or fluorescent treponemal antibody absorption test

11 Antinuclear antibody
An abnormal titer of antinuclear antibody by immunofluorescence or an equivalent assay at any point in time and in the absence of drugs known to be associated with "drug-induced lupus" syndrome

A person is classified as having SLE if any 4 of the 11 criteria are present (serially or simultaneously) during any interval of the evaluation.
Adapted from Tan et al. [2] and Hochberg [13].

---

to immune complex deposition, complement activation, and inflammation and subsequent fibrosis [1].

Anti-RNP can be found in SLE, mixed connective tissue disease, and scleroderma and is associated with myositis, Raynaud phenomenon, and less severe lupus. Anti-Ro/SSA and anti-La/SSB are more often associated with Sjögren syndrome but are also found in 20–40% of women with SLE. Anti-Ro/SSA and anti-La/SSB are of particular significance in pregnancy due to the association with neonatal lupus syndrome[14,15]. Lastly, antiribosomal P protein is associated with lupus cerebritis and neuropsychiatric manifestations [16].

Lupus flares are difficult to characterize, as they represent worsening of a heterogeneous disease process. Scoring systems have been developed to measure SLE disease status and aid the diagnosis of a flare. In one retrospective study, flares occurred in 68% of SLE pregnancies, the majority of which were mild to moderate [17]. Symptoms of flares include fatigue, fever, arthralgias, myalgias, weight loss,

rash, renal deterioration, serositis, lymphadenopathy, and central nervous system symptoms. The titer of autoantibodies to Sm, RNP, Ro/ SSA, or La/SSB may or may not fluctuate in parallel with disease flares. However, rising titers of anti-dsDNA (particularly in the setting of falling complement levels) may suggest an impending flare of disease and thus should trigger closer surveillance of the patient [18].

Patients with SLE may also form antibodies to cell membrane phospholipids. Approximately 30% of women with SLE have antiphospholipid antibodies (APA), which increase the risk for thrombosis and adverse pregnancy outcomes [19]. Placentas from women with SLE demonstrate characteristic changes: reduction in size, placental infarctions, intraplacental hemorrhage, deposition of immunoglobulin and complement, and thickening of the trophoblast basement membrane [20,21]. These changes appear to be responsible for many of the effects of SLE (e.g. increased rates of preeclampsia, fetal growth restriction [FGR], preterm delivery).

Differential diagnosis

The main differential diagnosis for SLE is rheumatologic and connective tissue disorders. Many of these share common diagnostic criteria and it may take time for diagnosis.

Differentiation of SLE can be challenging, given the frequency of vague musculoskeletal complaints or symptoms of fatigue. In addition, differentiation of SLE flare from preeclampsia can be even more challenging. The difficult diagnosis results from a high rate of chronic hypertension and disproportionately high rate of preeclampsia in SLE pregnancies. Chronic hypertension was reported in 28% of SLE patients, with preeclampsia in 32% of the hypertensive pregnancies [22].

Lupus flares often feature inflammatory arthritis, significant leukopenia or thrombocytopenia, inflammatory rashes, pleuritis, and fevers. Many of the manifestations of SLE flare can be similar to preeclampsia (hypertension, proteinuria, activation of the coagulation cascade) although the treatment is different. The treatment for severe preeclampsia often involves delivery, while lupus flares can be treated conservatively. A rising anti-dsDNA titer, active urinary sediment, and low complement levels (C3, C4, and CH50) suggest a lupus flare [18,23,24]. In general, complement levels rise in pregnancy and are unaffected by uncomplicated preeclampsia.

Conversely, rising uric acid levels or a greater coagulopathy suggest severe preeclampsia and HELLP (hemolysis, elevated liver enzymes, and low platelet count) syndrome. As the pregnancy approaches term, efforts at discriminating between the two are not likely to be worthwhile: delivery will cure preeclampsia and if the symptoms do not improve, treatment of lupus flare can be initiated.

Morbidity

General morbidity and mortality

Women with SLE are more prone to cardiovascular disease, thromboembolic phenomena, infection, and renal disease [4]. Survival rates are improved with 5-, 10-, 15-, and 20-year survival rates of 93%, 85%, 79%, and 68%, respectively [25]. Risk factors for mortality include renal damage, thrombocytopenia, lung involvement, high disease activity at diagnosis, and age ≥50 at diagnosis [25]. A summary of the effects of SLE on pregnancy and pregnancy on SLE can be found in Table 25.1.

Effects of pregnancy on systemic lupus erythematosus

The effect of pregnancy on SLE is widely debated. A shift in cytokines from a type 1 helper T response (Th1) to a type 2 helper T response (Th2) pattern is seen, with predominance of the anti-inflammatory and pro-B-cell

Table 25.1 Systemic lupus erythematosus and pregnancy

Effect of SLE on pregnancy	Effect of pregnancy on SLE
Increased stillbirth rate (25 times baseline)	Worsening of renal status if nephropathy present
Increased preeclampsia rate (20–30%)	Increased flare rates (higher if active at start of pregnancy)
Increased growth restriction rate (12–32%)	
Increased preterm delivery rate (50–60%)	
Increased PPROM rate	
Neonatal lupus (1–2% if anti-SSA/SSB present)	

PPROM, preterm premature rupture of membranes; SLE, systemic lupus erythematosus.

cytokines interleukin (IL)-4 and IL-10 [5]. Because the autoimmunity in SLE is largely humorally mediated, one might expect that this cytokine shift may worsen the disease process or increase the rate of lupus flares [5].

The reported incidence of lupus flares in pregnancy, however, ranges from 13% to 74% [26–29]. The discrepancies in can be attributed to variations in criteria for diagnosing lupus flares and the inherent heterogeneity of patients [5].

Ruiz-Irastorza et al. [30] found that flare rates were higher in pregnant women than in nonpregnant controls. When the pregnant women were followed for the year postpartum, it was found that they flared more frequently during pregnancy compared to the year following their deliveries. However, the flares during pregnancy were no more severe than nonpregnant controls or postpartum. Other authors have found equivalent rates of flares in pregnancy compared with nonpregnant controls [31,32].

It is generally believed that the risk for flare in pregnancy is increased if women are not in remission prior to becoming pregnant [5,31]. Approximately 35% of flares occur in the second trimester with 35% postpartum [27,30]. The majority are minor and do not require immunosuppressive therapy; however, serious manifestations can occur.

Lupus nephropathy is the result of autoimmune-mediated inflammation and renal damage. Pregnancy causes a worsening in renal function in approximately 20% of women with nephropathy but is reversible 95% of the time [25]. The risk of renal deterioration is directly correlated with prepregnancy renal status.

The impact of pregnancy on postpartum damage accrual in SLE was reported in 2006 by Andrade et al. [33]. The Systemic Lupus International Collaborating Clinics Damage Index (SDI) score was strongly associated with longer pregnancy duration ($P = 0.006$), disease activity ($P = 0.001$), damage prior to pregnancy ($P <0.001$), and total disease duration ($P = 0.039$) by multivariable analyses [33].

Effects of systemic lupus erythematosus on pregnancy

Systemic lupus erythematosus in pregnancy can affect both the mother and offspring. Maternal and obstetric sequelae include hypertension, preeclampsia, worsening renal disease, and thrombosis. Fetal effects include stillbirth, FGR, abnormal fetal testing, neonatal lupus erythematosus (NLE), and preterm birth (both iatrogenic and spontaneous).

Adverse pregnancy outcomes are seen more frequently in women with SLE than in controls or in women who later develop SLE [34]. Preeclampsia occurs in 20–30% of women with SLE, with higher rates seen in women with underlying hypertension, renal disease, or antiphospholipid syndrome (APS) [21,35,36]. Intrauterine growth restriction has been reported in 12–32% of lupus pregnancies, which was higher than in control populations [28,36,37]. Preterm birth is increased in SLE pregnancies, with rates as high as 50–60% resulting from preeclampsia, FGR, abnormal fetal testing, and preterm premature rupture of membranes (PPROM) [28,37–39]. Rupture of membranes in women with SLE is more common in preterm and term pregnancies when compared with controls and appears to be unrelated to disease status, treatment, or serology [38]. Factors that were associated with premature delivery included prednisone use at conception (relative risk [RR] 1.8), the use of antihypertensive medications (RR 1.8), and a severe flare during pregnancy (RR 2.0) [16]. A recent study by Kim et al. demonstrated that if patients have increased baseline complement activation, this is associated with an increased risk of adverse pregnancy outcomes with an OR of 2.01 [40].

Pregnancy outcome and risk of stillbirth are related to the baseline disease status prior to pregnancy and do not appear to be affected by the presence or absence of flares in pregnancy [41]. Fewer pregnancies among women with high-activity lupus ended with live births compared to those with low-activity lupus (77% vs. 88%, P = 0.063) [42]. Stillbirth rates in women with SLE have been found to be 150 per 1000 births, 25 times the national average [36]. Much of the effect of SLE on fetal loss rates has been attributed to concomitant APS [41,43]. If initial diagnosis of SLE is made during pregnancy, complication rates and fetal loss rates are further increased.

Risk factors for pregnancy loss identified in the first trimester include secondary APS (adjusted odds ratio [aOR] 3.4, 95% confidence interval [CI] 1.1–10.5), thrombocytopenia (aOR 4.4, 95% CI 1.4–13.4), and hypertension (aOR 3.0, 95% CI 1.1–8.5) [44]. In women with active renal disease, stillbirth rates are as high as 30%, and for women with more advanced renal disease, fetal loss rates approach 60%. Active renal disease also prognosticates risks of hypertensive disorders of pregnancy, FGR, and premature birth. However, women with stable lupus nephritis, plasma creatinine values less than 1.5 mg/dL, proteinuria less than 2 g/24 hours, and no hypertension have lower risks of adverse pregnancy outcome [35].

NLE occurs in 1–2% of women with anti-Ro/SSA or anti-La/SSB antibodies regardless of whether they also have SLE [14]. The pathophysiology is thought to be transplacental passage of autoantibodies that target the developing fetus with resulting inflammation. The syndrome is most commonly characterized by fetal and neonatal congenital heart block (CHB), dermatologic findings, and occasionally thrombocytopenia, anemia, and hepatitis [14].

Approximately 50% of women whose fetuses or infants have CHB are asymptomatic, but more than 85% are anti-Ro/SSA or anti-La/SSB positive [14,45]. Approximately half of these women will eventually develop symptoms of a rheumatic disease, most commonly Sjögren syndrome. These women should be reassured that they do not have SLE in the absence of other clinical features and have <50% likelihood of developing SLE in the future.

Although other manifestations are transient humorally mediated effects with resolution in the first few months of life, CHB is a permanent condition. The anti-Ro/SSA and anti-La/SSB maternal antibodies cross the placenta and can damage the fetal atrioventricular conducting system, which results in varying degrees of heart block and, less often, fetal myocarditis. Fetal CHB is most commonly diagnosed between 18 and 24 weeks gestation [46]. These autoantibodies may act via apoptosis [47] or by direct interference with cardiac conduction through calcium channels [48]. There was a study by Cuneo et al. that demonstrated that home monitoring for fetal heart rate changes showed that there was a rapid progression from normal to CHB [49]. They additionally showed that early intervention can improve outcomes if intervention is done within 12 hours of intervention with steroids [49]. The PRIDE Study showed that there was rapid progression from normal to CHB but that CHB was not always proceeded by first- and second-degree heart blocks [50].

The risk of CHB in women with anti-Ro/SSA antibodies and no prior affected infants is 1–2% [13,14] but increases to 19% with a prior affected child [45]. Although third-degree or "complete" CHB is permanent, there are some observational data that first- or second-degree disease can be reversed with antenatal fluorinated steroid therapy, and that progression to more severe forms of heart block may be prevented [51]. Additionally, steroid therapy has shown some reversal of hydropic features in fetuses with CHB and evidence of cardiac failure [51]. At present, there is no evidence supporting the routine use of prophylactic steroid therapy in women with anti-Ro/SSA or anti-La/SSB antibodies to prevent the onset of CHB [47]. A 2016 study showed that early intervention can improve outcomes and reduce the risk of progression to complete heart block however intervention would need to be done within 24 hours of initial atrioventricular

(AV) block meaning that in order to reduce risk of AV block, daily fetal monitoring would be needed [52]. Cost-effectiveness analysis showed that using risk stratification based on antibody levels to determine testing frequency supported using at least weekly testing for high-risk patients and routine screening for low-risk patients [53–56]. Recent studies have found that the risk of fetal heart block and the degree of tissue damage is related to the level on anti-Ro/SSA antibodies seen in maternal serum [57]. A critical titer was found to be 100 U/ml [57].

Management during pregnancy

Prior to conception, maternal disease status should be assessed and risks of pregnancy discussed. Evaluation for preexisting renal disease is performed with a 24-hour urine collection and serum creatinine. Remission for 6 months prior to pregnancy reduces adverse outcomes.

Early pregnancy assessment should include assessment of maternal disease status including 24-hour urine collection, plasma creatinine, complete blood count, anti-Ro/SSA antibody, anti-La/SSB antibody, anti-dsDNA antibody, C3, and C4 levels. Baseline presence of lupus anticoagulant (LAC), anticardiolipin antibody (ACA), and anti-β_2-glycoprotein-I (anti-β_2GPI) antibody should also be evaluated.

Early ultrasound and establishment of reliable dating are particularly important given the risks of premature delivery and fetal growth restriction. In patients with severe disease, early assessment may expedite the diagnosis of nonviable pregnancy.

Repeat anti-dsDNA, 24-hour urine collection, plasma creatinine, C3, and C4 levels to monitor disease status may be considered each trimester. LAC, ACA, and anti-β_2GPI antibody can also be repeated in the second trimester to screen for development of APS.

Medication regimens should be adjusted prior to conception to achieve optimal disease status with minimal teratogenicity. Medication classes include nonsteroidal glucocorticoids drugs (pregnancy class B), antimalarials (pregnancy class C), glucocorticoids (pregnancy class C), and immunosuppressive agents (pregnancy categories D and X). If APS is also present, anticoagulation can reduce the associated complications [4].

Prepregnancy drug regimens, if safe in pregnancy, should be continued to maintain remission. Nonsteroidal glucocorticoids are contraindicated after 28 weeks due to the risk of closure of the fetal ductus arteriosus. Hydroxychloroquine, an antimalarial medication, is often maintained to decrease rates of prematurity, decrease required dose of glucocorticoids and decrease risk of neonatal lupus. [58–60] In addition, hydroxychloroquine decreases postpartum lupus flares if continued for 3 months postpartum [61]. Hydroxycholorquine (400 mg daily) reduces the risk of congenital heart block in patients with anti-Ro/SSA or anti-La/SSB antibodies [62]. Glucocorticoids require stress-dose at delivery for patients requiring chronic use. Azathioprine (pregnancy class D) is an immunosuppressive agent that is metabolized to 6-mercaptopurine and is a cytotoxic purine analog. Most have found azathioprine to be acceptable in pregnancy although there is a risk of growth restriction and fetal immunosuppression. Other cytotoxic agents such as cyclophosphamide (pregnancy class D) and methotrexate (pregnancy class X) are contraindicated. A summary of medications used in the management of SLE is given in Table 25.2.

Fetal growth assessment is performed at 4-week intervals. Doppler evaluation is reserved for assessment of fetal well-being if estimated fetal weight is less than the 10th percentile. Weekly nonstress testing with assessment of amniotic fluid can begin at 30–32 weeks. Additional

Table 25.2 Systemic lupus erythematosus therapeutic agents

Drug	Safety in pregnancy	Comments
Hydroxychloroquine	Generally considered safe pregnancy class C	Antimalarial. Reduces disease flares. Reduces risk of congenital heart block in patients with anti-Ro/SSA or anti-La/SSB
NSAIDs	Pregnancy class B	Association with oligohydramnios and ductus arteriosus closure. Avoid after 28 wk
Glucocorticoids	Safe pregnancy class C	Association with growth restriction at high dose, need stress-dose steroids at delivery or for medical illnesses if chronic use through pregnancy. Increased risk of PPROM and preterm delivery
Azathioprine	Pregnancy class D	Risk of fetal growth restriction and immunosuppression. Use as second-line agent
Cyclophosphamide	Unsafe pregnancy class D	Alkylating agent. Skeletal and palate defects, also defects in eyes and limbs
Methotrexate	Unsafe pregnancy class X	Folic acid antagonist. Abortifacient and teratogen

NSAIDs, nonsteroidal anti-inflammatory drugs; PPROM, preterm premature rupture of membranes.

surveillance with mechanical P-R intervals should be initiated at regular intervals if maternal anti-Ro/SSA or anti-La/SSB is present beginning at 16–20 weeks.

Lupus flares can be managed conservatively with adjustment of medication regimen or addition of analgesics such as acetaminophen. Glucocorticoid therapy can be initiated.

When women are followed in an intensive multidisciplinary clinic with pregnancies initiated during disease quiescence and treatment of underlying disease, fetal outcomes appear to be improved. Diagnosis and treatment of APS further decrease fetal loss rates.

Antiphospholipid antibodies

Antiphospholipid antibodies can be present alone or in conjunction with APS. APS has specific diagnostic criteria, which were revised by an international consensus conference in 2006 [63]. The clinical and laboratory criteria are listed in Box 25.2.

Clinical complications of APS include thrombosis, adverse pregnancy outcome (including FGR and third trimester fetal death), and recurrent pregnancy loss [63]. Prospective studies of women with APS without treatment have shown fetal loss rates as high as 50–90% [64]. APA and LAC are found in 1–5% of asymptomatic pregnant women but are higher in SLE patients (12–30% and 15–34%, respectively) [19].

The laboratory component for diagnosis of APS tests for ACA, LAC, and anti-β_2GPI antibody. ACA and LAC bind to β_2GPI, other phospholipid-associated proteins, or the phospholipids themselves. β GPI and annexin V are associated with phospholipids in the cell membrane and inhibit platelet and clotting cascade activation. Both molecules are found endogenously in high concentrations on the endothelium and syncytiotrophoblast and are thought to provide a protective layer. ACA, LAC, and anti-β_2GPI antibodies disrupt this protective layer, activating the clotting cascade and allowing complement-mediated injury to the placental vasculature to occur [65].

LAC is detected by the prolongation of various clotting assays with failure to normalize with the addition of control plasma (to exclude factor deficiencies). One common test is the dilute Russell viper venom test (dRVVT), and is reported as present or absent. ACA are detected by direct β_2GPI-dependent immunoassays and are reported by antibody class and low or high titer. Medium or high titers of IgG or IgM (i.e. >40 GPL or MPL, respectively, or >99th percentile) are clinically relevant [66]. Although LAC and ACA are frequently concordant and sometimes share epitope specificity, they are distinct entities. The presence of LAC is more specific for APS than ACA. Anti-β_2GPI antibodies are considered positive if they are >99th percentile.

Box 25.2 Criteria for the classification of antiphospholipid antibody syndrome. Presence of at least one clinical criterion and one laboratory criterion necessary for the diagnosis of APAS

Clinical criteria

1 Nonobstetric morbidity: thrombosis in any tissue, diagnosed via objective validated criteria, such as diagnostic imaging or histopathologic diagnosis.
  (a) Arterial thrombosis, including cerebrovascular accidents, transient ischemic attacks, myocardial infarction, amaurosis fugax
  (b) Venous thromboembolism, including deep venous thrombosis, pulmonary emboli, or small vessel thrombosis
2 Obstetric morbidity
  (a) Unexplained IUFD at ≥10 wk in a morphologically and karyotypically normal fetus
  (b) Three or more unexplained spontaneous abortions at ≤10 wk
  (c) History of preterm delivery <34 weeks, as a sequela of preeclampsia or uteroplacental insufficiency, including the following:
    (i) Nonreassuring fetal testing indicative of fetal hypoxemia (e.g. abnormal Doppler flow velocimetry waveform)
    (ii) Oligohydramnios
    (iii) FGR <10th percentile
    (iv) Placental abruption

Laboratory criteria

Positive testing for APA is required on two occasions, at least 12 wk apart, and no more than 5 y prior to clinical manifestations.
1 Anticardiolipin antibody (ACA): IgG or IgM isotype, present in moderate or high titers (i.e. >40 GPL or MPL, or >99th percentile)
2 Anti-β_2-glycoprotein-I (anti-β_2GPI): IgG or IgM isotype (>99th percentile)
3 Presence of lupus anticoagulant (LAC)

APA, antiphospholipid antibody; FGR, fetal growth restriction; GPL, IgG phospholipid units; Ig, immunoglobulin; IUFD, intrauterine fetal death; MPL, IgM phospholipid units.
Adapted from [63].

Treatment goals for APS include improvement of fetal outcomes and reduction in risk for maternal thrombosis. Current accepted therapies include heparin anticoagulation and low-dose aspirin (LDA). Heparin has been shown to prevent both thromboembolic events and pregnancy loss. Either unfractionated heparin (UFH, pregnancy class C) and low molecular weight heparin (LMWH, pregnancy class B) can be used. Multiple mechanisms of action for heparin in treatment of APS have been proposed. UFH potentiates the effects of antithrombin, increases levels of factor Xa inhibitor, and inhibits platelet aggregation. Heparins may also render APA inactive via binding [67]. LMWH in vitro has been shown to counteract APA-induced trophoblast inflammation. However, in the absence of APA, LMWH in vitro induces potentially detrimental proinflammatory and antiangiogenic profile in the trophoblast. Therefore, anticoagulation should only be used when truly indicated [68].

A meta-analysis showed that the live birth rate was improved by 54% with heparin and aspirin therapy [69]. One cautionary note is that despite anticoagulation, 20–30% of women with APS have fetal losses, which may be explained by the in vitro effects of the medications on trophoblast function [68]. Intravenous immunoglobulin (IVIG) has been shown to be effective, although the cost and side effects currently limit it to women with severe APS or those who have been refractory to heparin therapy.

Aspirin therapy can be initiated at the first positive pregnancy test and heparin therapy can be initiated at 5–7 weeks gestation. As there is no maternal blood flow through the placenta prior to 5–7 weeks, heparin is not necessary before this point and may exacerbate implantation bleeding. Heparin therapy can either be therapeutic (i.e. 1 mg/kg enoxaparin every 12 hours with maintenance of anti-Xa levels between 0.5 and 1.0) or prophylactic (i.e. 40 mg/day enoxaparin). It is not our practice to follow anti-Xa levels in those women receiving prophylactic heparin treatment. Although heparin-induced thrombocytopenia is a rare occurrence with LMWH, a platelet count should be obtained within 2 weeks of initiation of therapy. Because of the 1–2% risk of osteoporosis and fracture with UFH anticoagulation in pregnancy [70,71], we recommend daily calcium, vitamin D supplementation, and daily weight-bearing exercise as tolerated. Data suggest that LMWH anticoagulation during pregnancy does not significantly affect bone mineral density [13]. At 36 weeks, aspirin can be discontinued and LMWH switched to UFH to facilitate anticoagulation management at delivery. Postpartum anticoagulation (if indicated) can be with either warfarin or LMWH.

Treatment of APS during pregnancy with active fetal surveillance has shown improved outcomes. Nonetheless, antepartum complications remain common with elevated rates of preeclampsia, growth restriction, and premature birth [5].

CASE PRESENTATION

A 32-year-old gravida 5, para 1 at 7 weeks gestation has a history of a term vaginal delivery 7 years ago of an infant with second-degree heart block. She had three subsequent miscarriages at approximately 10 weeks gestation. An evaluation revealed the presence of anti-Ro/SSA antibodies, positive ANA, positive dRVVT, as well as high-titer ACA IgG. She also complains of periodic arthralgias and has had persistent proteinuria. What is her diagnosis and what therapy recommendations and prognosis can be given for her current pregnancy?

The patient can be diagnosed with APS because of her high-titer ACA and recurrent first-trimester miscarriages. Additionally, she meets the criteria for SLE (ANA, ACA, arthralgias, renal disease). She has a 19% chance of another child with CHB and a substantial risk of miscarriage given her prior losses. Additionally, she has increased risk for preeclampsia, FGR, PPROM, and preterm delivery. She can be offered aspirin and LMWH therapy for her APS and close fetal surveillance to monitor for the development of heart block or FGR. In recent years, hydroxychloroquine has been shown to reduce the incidence of recurrent of congenital heart block secondary to anti-Ro/SSA or anti-La/SSB antibodies [66]. A recommendation to start hydroxychloroquine before 10 weeks (400 mg daily) should be made. Therapy for SLE should be reviewed and optimized for her pregnancy. Her baseline renal status should be assessed and a baseline cardiac evaluation including electrocardiography would not be unreasonable.

References

1. Mills JA. Systemic lupus erythematosus. N Engl J Med. 1994;330:1871–9.
2. Tan EM, Cohen AS, Fries JF, Masi AT, McShane DJ, Rothfield NF, et al. The 1982 revised criteria for the classification of systemic lupus erythematosus. Arthritis Rheum. 1982;25:1271–7.
3. Hochberg MC. Updating the American College of Rheumatology revised criteria for the classification of systemic lupus erythematosus. Arthritis Rheum. 1997;40:1725.
4. Ruiz-Irastorza G, Khamashta MA, Castellino G, Hughes GR. Systemic lupus erythematosus. Lancet. 2001;357:1027–32.
5. Buyon JP. The effects of pregnancy on autoimmune diseases. J Leukoc Biol. 1998;63:281–7.
6. Chakravarty EF, Bush TM, Manzi S, Clarke AE, Ward MM. Prevalence of adult systemic lupus erythematosus in California and Pennsylvania in 2000: estimates obtained using hospitalization data. Arthritis Rheum. 2007;56:2092.
7. Rhodes B, Vyse TJ. The genetics of SLE: an update in the light of genome-wide association studies. Rheumatology. 2008;47(11):1603-11.
8. Sestak AL, Nath SK, Sawalha AH, Harley JB. Current status of lupus genetics. Arthritis Res Ther. 2007;9(3):210.
9. Costenbader KH, Feskanich D, Stampfer MJ, Karlson EW. Reproductive and menopausal factors and risk of systemic lupus erythematosus in women. Arthritis Rheum. 2007;56(4):1251–62.
10. Cooper GS, Dooley MA, Treadwell EL, St Clair EW, Gilkeson GS. Risk factors for the development of systemic lupus erythematosus: allergies, infections, and family history. J Clin Epidemiol. 2002; 55(10):982–9
11. Lehmann P, Holzle E, Kind P, Goerz G, Plewig G. Experimental reproduction of skin lesions in lupus erythematosus by UVA

and UVB radiation. J Am Acad Dermatol. 1990; 22(2 Pt 1):181–7.

12. Farnam J, Lavastida MT, Grant JA, Reddi RC, Daniels JC. Antinuclear antibodies in the serum of normal pregnant women: a prospective study. J Allergy Clin Immunol. 1984;73: 596–9.

13. Dahlman TC. Osteoporotic fractures and the recurrence of thromboembolism during pregnancy and the puerperium in 184 women undergoing thromboprophylaxis with heparin. Am J Obstet Gynecol. 1993;168(4):1265–70.

14. Gladman G, Silverman ED, Yuk L, Luy L, Boutin C, Laskin C, et al. Fetal echocardiographic screening of pregnancies of mothers with anti-Ro and/or anti-La antibodies. Am J Perinatol. 2002;19:73–80.

15. Lee LA. Neonatal lupus erythematosus. J Invest Dermatol. 1993;100:9S–13S.

16. Schneebaum AB, Singleton JD, West SG, Blodgett JK, Allen LG, Cheronis JC, et al. Association of psychiatric manifestations with antibodies to ribosomal P proteins in systemic lupus erythematosus. Am J Med, 1991;90(1):54–62.

17. Chakravarty EF, Colón I, Langen ES, Nix DA, El-Sayed YY, Genovese MC, et al. Factors that predict prematurity and preeclampsia in pregnancies that are complicated by systemic lupus erythematosus. Am J Obstet Gynecol. 2005;192(6):1897–904.

18. Repke JT. Hypertensive disorders of pregnancy: differentiating preeclampsia from active systemic lupus erythematosus. J Reprod Med. 1998;43:350–4.

19. Levine JS, Branch DW, Rauch J. The antiphospholipid syndrome. N Engl J Med. 2002;346:752–63.

20. Hanly JG, Gladman DD, Rose TH, Laskin CA, Urowitz MB. Lupus pregnancy: a prospective study of placental changes. Arthritis Rheum 1988;31:358–66.

21. Lockshin MD, Sammaritano LR. Lupus pregnancy. Autoimmunity. 2003;36:33–40.

22. Egerman RS, Ramsey RD, Kao LW, Bringman JJ, Bush AJ, Wan JY. Hypertensive disease in pregnancies complicated by systemic lupus erythematosus. Am J Obstet Gynecol. 2005;193: 1676–9.

23. Buyon JP, Tamerius J, Ordorica S, Young B, Abramson SB. Activation of the alternative complement pathway accompanies disease flares in systemic lupus erythematosus during pregnancy. Arthritis Rheum. 1992;35:55–61.

24. Abramson SB, Buyon JP. Activation of the complement pathway: comparison of normal pregnancy, preeclampsia, and systemic lupus erythematosus during pregnancy. Am J Reprod Immunol. 1992;28:183–7.

25. Abu-Shakra M, Urowitz MB, Gladman DD, Gough J. Mortality studies in systemic lupus erythematosus. Results from a single center. II. Predictor variables for mortality. J Rheumatol. 1995;22:1265–70.

26. Lockshin MD. Pregnancy does not cause systemic lupus erythematosus to worsen. Arthritis Rheum. 1989;32:665–70.

27. Carmona F, Font J, Cervera R, Munoz F, Cararach V, Balasch J. Obstetrical outcome of pregnancy in patients with systemic lupus erythematosus: a study of 60 cases. Eur J Obstet Gynecol Reprod Biol. 1999;83:137–42.

28. Mintz G, Niz J, Gutierrez G, Garcia-Alonso A, Karchmer S. Prospective study of pregnancy in systemic lupus erythematosus: results of a multidisciplinary approach. J Rheumatol. 1986;13:732–39.

29. Nossent HC, Swaak TJ. Systemic lupus erythematosus. VI. Analysis of the interrelationship with pregnancy. J Rheumatol. 1990;17:771–6.

30. Ruiz-Irastorza G, Lima F, Alves J, Khamashta MA, Simpson J, Hughes GR, et al. Increased rate of lupus flare during pregnancy and the puerperium: a prospective study of 78 pregnancies. Br J Rheumatol. 1996;35:133–8.

31. Urowitz MB, Gladman DD, Farewell VT, Stewart J, McDonald J. Lupus and pregnancy studies. Arthritis Rheum. 1993;36: 1392–7.

32. Lockshin MD, Reinitz E, Druzin ML, Murrman M, Estes D. Lupus pregnancy: case-control prospective study demonstrating absence of lupus exacerbation during or after pregnancy. Am J Med. 1984;77:893–8.

33. Andrade RM, McGwin G Jr, Alarcón GS, Sanchez ML, Bertoli AM, Fernández M, et al. Predictors of post-partum damage accrual in systemic lupus erythematosus: data from LUMINA, a multiethnic US cohort (XXXVIII). Rheumatology (Oxford). 2006;45:1380.

34. Kiss E, Bhattoa HP, Bettembuk P, Balogh A, Szegedi G. Pregnancy in women with systemic lupus erythematosus. Eur J Obstet Gynecol Reprod Biol. 2002;101:129–34.

35. Hayslett JP, Lynn RI. Effect of pregnancy in patients with lupus nephropathy. Kidney Int. 1980;18:207–20.

36. Simpson LL. Maternal medical disease: risk of antepartum fetal death. Semin Perinatol. 2002;26:42–50.

37. Lima F, Buchanan NM, Khamashta MA, Kerslake S, Hughes GR. Obstetric outcome in systemic lupus erythematosus. Semin Arthritis Rheum. 1995;25:184–92.

38. Johnson MJ, Petri M, Witter FR, Repke JT. Evaluation of preterm delivery in a systemic lupus erythematosus pregnancy clinic. Obstet Gynecol. 1995;86:396–9.

39. Hochberg MC. Updating the American College of Rheumatology revised criteria for the classification of systemic lupus erythematosus (letter). Arthritis Rheum. 1997;40(9):1725.

40. Kim AHJ, Strand V, Sen DP, Fu Q, Mathis NL, Schmidt MJ, et al. Association of blood concentrations of complement split product iC3b and serum C3 with systemic lupus erythematosus disease activity. Arthritis Rheumatol. 2019 Mar;71(3):420–30. doi: 10.1002/art.40747. Epub 2019 Jan 24. PMID: 30294950; PMCID: PMC6393208.

41. Faussett MB, Branch DW. Autoimmunity and pregnancy loss. Semin Reprod Med. 2000;18:379–92.

42. Clowse ME, Magder LS, Witter F, Petri M. The impact of increased lupus activity on obstetric outcomes. Arthritis Rheum. 2005;52:514–21.

43. Ginsberg JS, Brill-Edwards P, Johnston M, Denburg JA, Andrew M, Burrows RF, et al. Relationship of antiphospholipid antibodies to pregnancy loss in patients with systemic lupus erythematosus: a cross-sectional study. Blood. 1992;80:975–80.

44. Clowse ME, Magder LS, Witter F, Petri M. Early risk factors for pregnancy loss in lupus. Obstet Gynecol. 2006;107:293–9.

45. Buyon JP, Rupel A, Clancy RM. Neonatal lupus syndromes. Lupus. 2004;13:705–12.

46. Buyon JP, Waltuck J, Kleinman C, Copel J. In utero identification and therapy of congenital heart block. Lupus. 1995;4:116–21.

47. Buyon JP, Clancy RM. Maternal autoantibodies and congenital heart block: mediators, markers, and therapeutic approach. Semin Arthritis Rheum. 2003;33:140–54.

48. Izmirly P, Kim M, Friedman DM, Costedoat-Chalumeau N, Clancy R, Copel JA, et al. Hydroxychloroquine to prevent recurrent congenital heart block in fetuses of anti-SSA/Ro-positive mothers. J Am Coll Cardiol. 2020 Jul 21;76(3):292–302. doi: 10.1016/j.jacc.2020.05.045. PMID: 32674792; PMCID: PMC7394202.

49. Cuneo BF, Sonesson SE, Levasseur S, Moon-Grady AK, Krishanan A, Donofrio MT, et al. Home monitoring for fetal heart rhythm during anti-Ro pregnancies. J Am Coll Cardiol. 2018 Oct 16;72(16):1940–51. doi: 10.1016/j.jacc.2018.07.076. Erratum in: J Am Coll Cardiol. 2019 Jan 8;73(1):120. PMID: 30309472.

50. Boutjdir M. Molecular and ionic basis of congenital complete heart block. Trends Cardiovasc Med. 2000;10:114–22.

51. Friedman DM, Kim MY, Copel JA, Davis C, Phoon CKL, Glickstein JS, et al. Utility of Cardiac monitoring for fetuses at risk for congenial heart block: the PR Interval and Dexamethasone Evaluation (PRIDE) prospective study. Circulation. 2008 Jan 29;117(4):485–93. doi: 10.1161/CIRCULATIONAHA.107.707661. Epub 2008 Jan 14. PMID: 118195175.

52. Cuneo BF, Ambrose SE, Tworezky W. Detection and successful treatment of emergent anti-SSA-mediated fetal atrioventricular block. Am J Obstet Gynecol. 2016 Oct;215(4):527–8. doi:10.1016/j.ajog.2016.07.002.Epub 2016 Jul 12. PMID: 227418449.

53. Evers PD, Alsaied T, Anderson JB, Cnota JF, Divanovic AA. Prenatal heart block screening in mothers with SSA/SSB autoantibodies: targeted screening protocol is a cost-effective strategy. Congenit Heart Dis. 2019 Mar;14(2):221–9. doi: 10.1111/chd.12713.Epub 2018 Nov 16. PMID: 30444309.

54. Kim MY, Guerra MM, Kaplowitz E, Laskin CA, Petri M, Branch DW, et al. Complement activation predicts adverse pregnancy outcome in patients with systemic lupus erythematosus and/or antiphospholipid antibodies. Ann Rheum Dis. 2018 Apr;77(4):549–55.

55. Kan N, Silverman ED, Kingdom J, Dutil N, Laskin C, Jaeggi E. Serial echocardiography for immune-mediated heart disease in the fetus: results of a risk-based prospective surveillance strategy. Prenat Diagn. 2017 Apr;37(4):375–82. doi: 10.1002/pd.5021. Epub 2017 Feb 27. PMID: 28177533.

56. Jaeggi E, Laskin C, Hamilton R, Kingdom J, Silverman E. The importance of the level of maternal anti-Ro/SSA antibodies as prognostic marker of the development of cardiac neonatal lupus erythematosus: a prospective study of 186 antibody-exposed fetuses and infants. J Am Coll Cardiol. 2010;55(24):2778–84. PMID: 20538173.

57. Vanoni F, Lava SAG, Fossali EF, Cavalli R, Simonetti GD, Bianchetti MG, et al. Neonatal systemic lupus erythematosus syndrome: a comprehensive review. Clinic Rev Allerg Immunol. 2017;53:469–76.

58. Sciascia S, Hunt BJ, Talavera-Garcia E, et al. The impact of hydroxychloroquine treatment on pregnancy outcome in women with antiphospholipid antibodies. Am J Obstet Gyneco.l 2016;214:273.e1–8.

59. Leroux M, Desveaux C, Parcevaux M, Julliac B, Gouyon JB, Dallay D, et al. Impact of hydroxychloroquine on preterm delivery and intrauterine growth restriction in pregnant women with systemic lupus erythematosus: a descriptive cohort study. Lupus 2015;24:1384–91.

60. Levy RA, Vilela VS, Cataldo MJ, Ramos RC, Duarte JL, Tura BR, et al. Hydroxychloroquine (HCQ) in lupus pregnancy: double-blind and placebo-controlled study. Lupus. 2001;10:401–4.

61. Eudy AM, Siega-Riz AM, Engel SM, Franceschini N, Howard AG, Clowse MEB, et al. Effect of pregnancy on disease flares in patients with systemic lupus erythematosus. Ann Rheum Dis. 2018;77:855–60.

62. Saleeb S, Copel J, Friedman D, Buyon JP. Comparison of treatment with fluorinated glucocorticoids to the natural history of autoantibody-associated congenital heart block: retrospective review of the research registry for neonatal lupus. Arthritis Rheum. 1999;42:2335–45.

63. Miyakis S, Lockshin MD, Atsumi T, Branch DW, Brey RL, Cervera R, et al. International consensus statement on an update of the classification criteria for definite antiphospholipid syndrome (APS). J Thromb Haemost. 2006;4:295–306.

64. Warren JB, Silver RM. Autoimmune disease in pregnancy: systemic lupus erythematosus and antiphospholipid syndrome. Obstet Gynecol Clin North Am. 2004;31:345-72, vi–vii.

65. Salmon JE, Girardi G, Holers VM. Activation of complement mediates antiphospholipid antibody-induced pregnancy loss. Lupus. 2003;12:535–8.

66. Silver RM, Porter TF, van Leeuween I, Jeng G, Scott JR, Branch DW. Anticardiolipin antibodies: clinical consequences of "low titers." Obstet Gynecol. 1996;87:494–500.

67. Franklin RD, Kutteh WH. Effects of unfractionated and low molecular weight heparin on antiphospholipid antibody binding in vitro. Obstet Gynecol. 2003;101(3):455–62.

68. Han CS, Mulla MJ, Brosens JJ, Chamley LW, Paidas MJ, Lockwood CJ, et al. Aspirin and heparin effect on basal and antiphospholipid antibody modulation of trophoblast function. Obstet Gynecol. 2011 Nov;118(5):1021–8.

69. Empson M, Lassere M, Craig JC, Scott JR. Recurrent pregnancy loss with antiphospholipid antibody: a systematic review of therapeutic trials. Obstet Gynecol. 2002;99:135–44.

70. Dahlman TC. Osteoporotic fractures and the recurrence of thromboembolism during pregnancy and the puerperium in 184 women undergoing thromboprophylaxis with heparin. Am J Obstet Gynecol. 1993;168:1265–70.

71. Pettila V, Leinonen P, Markkola A, Hiilesmaa V, Kaaja R. Postpartum bone mineral density in women treated for thromboprophylaxis with unfractionated heparin or LMW heparin. Thromb Haemost. 2002;87:182–6.

Chapter 26
Perinatal Infections

Michelle E. Whittum and Stephanie T. Ros
Department of Obstetrics and Gynecology, University of South Florida, Tampa, FL, USA

Infections can be transmitted from the pregnant person to the fetus at any time, including in utero or during the birthing process. Infection can also be transmitted to the newborn during breastfeeding. In some cases, the infections would be of little clinical consequence to the adult, sometimes even escaping clinical notice. However, these same infections can lead to long-lasting effects for the fetus and newborn. Perinatal infections are a major contributor to morbidity and mortality both in the United States and worldwide. In this chapter, we review some of the most common infections, their mode of transmission and clinical manifestations, methods for diagnosis, and any available strategies for treatment and prevention of infection.

Parvovirus B$_{19}$

The parvoviruses are single-stranded DNA viruses. Parvovirus B$_{19}$ is the only one known to cause human infection and causes primarily childhood illness (erythema infectiosum/EI or fifth disease); by adulthood approximately 60% have evidence of prior exposure. It primarily targets rapidly proliferating cells, the most concerning of which for the fetus are the erythroid progenitor cells, which can result in a severe anemia. This virus is predominantly transmitted via respiratory droplets but can also be transmitted via transfusion or vertical transmission, which happens in approximately one third of infected pregnancies [1,2].

The incubation period for this virus ranges between 4 to 20 days, although in fetuses it can be much longer, up to 8 weeks. If symptoms present, they are contagious for 1–2 days after the onset of the rash and are also contagious before the skin findings. Unlike the herpesviruses, there is no documentation of reactivation with parvovirus.

Clinical manifestations

Adults are often asymptomatic (20–30% of cases). When symptoms present, they include:
- Erythema infectiosum or fifth disease: mild flulike symptoms including fever and headache, followed by rash. In children, the classic appearance is the "slapped cheek" distribution of facial erythema. This is often not the case with adults. In both children and adults, there can be a lacy reticular rash on the body.
- Polyarthralgias/arthritis may be noted in adults particularly.
- Parvovirus B$_{19}$ targets erythrocyte progenitors. Adults with immunodeficiency or chronic hemolytic anemia are at risk for transient aplastic crisis.
- Fetuses are at risk of aplastic anemia, leading to high output cardiac failure and fetal hydrops. The virus can also directly damage myocardial cells, further contributing to heart failure. Fetuses are also at risk of thrombocytopenia [3].

In fetuses, the illness has the potential to be much more severe. Fetal infection has been associated with pregnancy loss [2–6] with an increased risk of death with earlier infection (<20 weeks gestation) [7]. Infected fetuses are at risk of hydrops. It can resolve in 4–6 weeks in the absence of intervention. The risk of hydrops is higher the earlier the infection occurs: prior to 12 weeks gestation, the risk is 5–10%, but after 20 weeks gestation the risk is <1% [7,8].

Diagnosis

Serologic testing is the most effective way to determine infection. In order to distinguish between prior infection/immunity, recent infection, and past infection one must compare the serum IgG and IgM. Anti-parvovirus IgM is detectable within days of infection and will remain detectable for 2–3 months; IgG is present about 1 week after infection. Therefore, the presence of IgM alone indicates a new infection, both IgM and IgG positive indicates infection in the recent past, and presence of IgG alone indicates prior immunity. The absence of any antibodies indicates either very early infection or susceptible individuals [9,10] (Figure 26.1).

In cases of hydrops, evaluation for parvovirus infection should be considered. Besides maternal serum testing, detection of parvovirus DNA within the amniotic fluid and from fetal blood samples are preferred due to sensitivity and specificity over serology.

Management of parvovirus B$_{19}$ in pregnancy

Given that hydrops in the setting of parvovirus infection has onset within 10 weeks after infection, fetuses should be

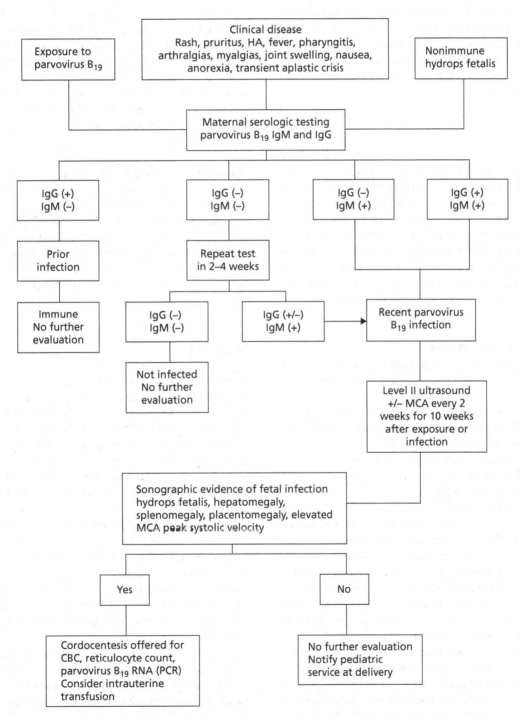

Figure 26.1 Algorithm for evaluation and management of parvovirus B19 infection in pregnancy. CBC, complete blood count; HA, headache; MCA, middle cerebral artery Doppler measurements; PCR, polymerase chain reaction.

evaluated for anemia throughout this period. Figure 26.1 details the evaluation and management of human parvovirus B_{19} infection in pregnancy. Once hydrops is present, the fetal hematocrit can be estimated at <20%. Screening for fetal anemia using middle cerebral artery Doppler assessing peak systolic velocity allows the opportunity for intervention with fetal blood transfusion [11,12]. In cases where transfusion is indicated, only one is typically necessary given the relatively quick resolution of fetal anemia from parvovirus. The overall mortality rate is <10%, and in those who undergo transfusion 94% of survivors fully recover within 6 weeks [13,14]. There are conflicting reports on neurodevelopmental consequences for fetuses with a history of parvovirus infection and resulting anemia and transfusion [15,16].

Rubella

Rubella, also referred to as German measles, is an RNA togavirus. It is transmitted via respiratory droplets and is highly virulent, with almost 80% of susceptible individuals infected after exposure. Viremia takes place 5–7 days after exposure, and the virus disseminates widely, including the placenta and fetus. The introduction of a live virus vaccine in 1969 led to a marked decrease in the incidence of rubella and the congenital rubella syndrome. In the United States there are fewer than 200 cases documented per year.

Clinical manifestations

Many infections are asymptomatic in adults and in children. However, when symptoms are present, they include:

• Flulike illness – fever, malaise, headache, arthralgia
• The key finding is a maculopapular rash which begins in the face but spreads throughout the body
• Pharyngitis and conjunctivitis may be present
• Lymphadenopathy is common (posterior cervical, postauricular, and occipital)

One particularly concerning consequence of rubella infection is congenital rubella syndrome. In the first trimester the likelihood of fetal infection is highest – 85% to 90% of pregnancies infected with rubella in the first trimester will result in a neonate with congenital infection. Very few are affected with infections occurring on or after 18 weeks gestation. Complications of fetal infection with rubella include fetal death. Those who live are at risk of severe morbidity including sensorineural deafness (60–75%), eye disease such as cataracts or retinopathy, microcephaly, developmental delay, cardiac defects, and more. Those who are asymptomatic at birth can still develop sequelae as adolescents or teens; these include type 1 diabetes and thyroid disease. An infant with congenital infection can shed virus for 6–12 months [17].

Diagnosis

The diagnosis of rubella can be made using maternal serology. The IgM from a primary infection is detectable at 5–7 days and can persist for 2 months; it should be noted that small amounts of IgM will be found in the circulation when there is reexposure. In the case of a positive result for both IgM and IgG, in order to distinguish between a past infection and current immunity vs. a recent infection (2 weeks to 2 months prior), the next best step is IgG avidity testing [18]. Detection of rubella DNA in amniotic fluid by polymerase chain reaction (PCR) is also possible. It should be noted that detection of viral DNA in the fetal compartment is not indicative of the degree of future morbidity, and many of the sequelae of congenital rubella are not detectable on ultrasound. Additionally, false-positive and -negative results have been reported in the literature [19].

Management and prevention

Rubella has no treatment. Supportive therapy is appropriate. Prevention is the key to reducing congenital rubella syndrome. The MMR vaccine (confers immunity to measles, mumps, and rubella) should not be administered during pregnancy because it is a live-attenuated vaccine. Women who are rubella nonimmune during pregnancy should be offered the MMR vaccine in the postpartum period [20].

Syphilis

Syphilis is caused by a spirochete, *Treponema pallidum*. According to the Centers for Disease Control and Prevention (CDC), rates of syphilis have increased since 2001. During 2018–2019 the rate increased by 11.2%, and in 2019, 129813 cases were reported in the United States. Correspondingly, the rate of congenital syphilis has increased every year since 2013, and in 2019 there were 1870 cases of congenital syphilis – a 291.1% increase relative to 2015.

Syphilis is acquired primarily through sexual contact. The incubation period is approximately 3 weeks but can vary (3–90 days) [21]. Syphilis has defined stages of disease (primary, secondary, early latent, late latent, and tertiary). Exposure to an infected individual during the earliest stages is most likely to result in transmission, although this is not the case for perinatally acquired infection [22,23].

Fetal infection most commonly occurs via transplacental passage; however, it can also occur via direct contact with lesions at delivery. *T. pallidum* spirochetes have been isolated from placenta, umbilical cord, and amniotic fluid [24–28]. Risk factors associated with maternal syphilis include young age, Black and Hispanic ethnicity, single, low socioeconomic status, less education, inadequate prenatal care and screening, prostitution, and substance abuse [29–32].

Clinical manifestations

Syphilis in the adult manifests in distinct stages:
- Primary syphilis: the predominant finding is a syphilitic chancre–characteristically painless and ulcerated, with a raised border. This appears at the site of entry, which is often at the cervix or vagina for women and can go unrecognized. Even without treatment, this lesion resolves spontaneously in 3–6 weeks.
- Secondary syphilis: defined by bacteremia and manifestations involving all organ systems including skin, with a macular rash on the trunk, extremities, and commonly includes plantar and palmar lesions. These lesions are highly infectious. Mucosal lesions are highly infectious, as well as genital lesions called condyloma lata, which are raised plaques. Generalized lymphadenopathy is common. At this stage many will experience a flulike illness (70%) with low-grade fever, malaise, arthralgias, myalgias, anorexia, and headache. All of these will resolve without treatment.
- Latent stage: this is a period of asymptomatic quiescence, termed "early latent" in the first 12 months and "late latent" beginning 12 months after symptom onset. Without treatment, 20–30% will progress to tertiary syphilis.
- Tertiary: this stage is rarely seen due to the responsiveness of this organism to treatment. In tertiary syphilis, there is major damage to the organ systems including cardiovascular and neurologic.

Fetal risks include stillbirth, nonimmune hydrops, neonatal demise, preterm birth, and congenital infection. Congenital infection is more likely when the exposure is later in the pregnancy; adverse outcomes for the fetus are more severe when the pregnant patient has primary or secondary syphilis. In the neonate, there is a distinction between early congenital syphilis which can manifest with central nervous system (CNS) involvement, rash, osteochondritis, hepatosplenomegaly, and chorioretinitis and late congenital syphilis which presents after the second year of life (sometimes into adolescence) and involves such findings as Hutchinson teeth, Cranial Nerve VIII deafness, developmental delay, saddle nose deformity, and saber shins. Neonates who become infected as a result of contact with lesions during birth may present with the chancre of primary syphilis.

Diagnosis

The diagnosis is through serology, and in pregnancy the recommendations are for screening at initial visit, at 28–32 weeks if at high risk, and again at delivery; per CDC guidelines, all children delivered should have maternal syphilis serostatus determined prior to leaving the hospital. The method for screening is via one of two algorithms.

In the traditional algorithm, the initial test is a nontreponemal test such as the rapid plasma reagin or the Venereal Disease Research Laboratory, then positive results are confirmed using a treponemal test such as fluorescent treponemal antibody absorption test, the microhemagglutination assay for antibodies to *T. pallidum*, and the *T. pallidum* passive particle agglutination test. The reverse algorithm begins with the treponemal test and confirms positive results with a nontreponemal test. Neither algorithm has been conclusively determined to be superior [33].

Congenital syphilis can be challenging to diagnose. If there are no characteristic ultrasound findings, PCR testing of amniotic fluid may be done. Performing serologic tests either on the umbilical cord blood or a neonatal blood sample is not easy to interpret because of the transplacental passage of maternal antibodies.

Treatment

Penicillin is the drug of choice for treatment of syphilis in pregnancy:
- Primary, secondary, and early latent: Benzathine penicillin G, 2.4 million units IM x 1
- Late latent or latent of unknown duration and tertiary: Benzathine penicillin G, 7.2 million units administered as 2.4 million units IM weekly for 3 weeks

No other antimicrobial agent is recommended in pregnancy. If a woman reports a penicillin allergy, a skin test for major or minor determinant antigens of penicillin should be performed if possible. If reactive, penicillin desensitization should be performed orally (Table 26.1) or intravenously [34]. Up to 50% of women treated for early-stage syphilis will have a systemic

Table 26.1 Oral desensitization protocol for penicillin-allergic patients

Dose[a]	Phenoxymethyl penicillin (units/mL)[b]	Dose (units)	Cumulative dose (units)
1	1000	100	100
2	1000	200	300
3	1000	400	700
4	1000	800	1500
5	1000	1600	3100
6	1000	3200	6300
7	1000	6400	12700
8	10000	12000	24700
9	10000	24000	48700
10	10000	48000	96700
11	80000	80000	176000
12	80000	160000	336700
13	80000	320000	636700
14	80000	640000	1296700

Observe for 30 min prior to parenteral benzathine penicillin G.
[a]15-min intervals.
[b]250 mg/5 mL equals 80000 units/mL.
Reproduced from [34]/with permission from Massachusetts Medical Society.

reaction called the Jarisch–Herxheimer reaction. Though transient with only mild constitutional symptoms, preterm labor and fetal distress may complicate treatment. Treatment after 20 weeks gestation should be preceded by an ultrasound to assess possible fetal infection. If abnormal, antepartum fetal heart rate monitoring should accompany treatment. In fetuses at or near term, delivery with treatment of the mother and infant postpartum may be warranted.

Careful follow-up after treatment should be performed to determine treatment failure (rare) or reinfection. Nontreponemal tests should be performed every month during pregnancy because the consequence of a treatment failure or reinfection in these high-risk women is a congenitally infected infant.

Toxoplasmosis

Toxoplasmosis is a protozoal disease caused by infection with *Toxoplasma gondii*. This organism can be found in undercooked raw meat and cat feces. The protozoan can cross the placenta and cause fetal infection with approximately 400–4000 cases per year in the United States [35,36]. The protozoal life cycle includes an oocyst, which is produced in the intestine of feral or domestic cats and then excreted in their feces. Other mammals ingest the oocyte, which is then disrupted and results in the release of the trophozoite. This disseminates and forms cysts within the brain and muscle tissue. If a human ingests infected meat or is in contact with cat feces (particularly from nonindoor cats who might themselves eat infected meat), they are at risk of infection. Congenital infection is more likely with advancing gestation. In the first trimester, the likelihood of transmission is between 10–25%; in the third trimester that increases to 60%. However, the sequelae for the infant are more severe with earlier infection than with later infection.

Clinical manifestations
Although often asymptomatic, fetal infection can cause severe morbidity including developmental delay, epilepsy, and visual impairment. Symptomatic maternal infection consists of a flulike illness, with fever, malaise, fatigue, and lymphadenopathy. There can also be a maculopapular rash. In patients who are immunocompromised this is as expected more severe; in fact, in people with HIV, toxoplasmosis of the brain is considered to be an AIDS-defining illness.

For the fetus, the risks include fetal death and growth restriction. Even for those who are asymptomatic at birth, up to 80% will develop learning and visual disturbances. On ultrasound, findings consistent with infection include hyperechoic bowel, ascites, growth restriction, liver calcifications, intracranial calcifications, ventriculomegaly,

and placental thickening. Those who are symptomatic at birth experience a disseminated rash, hepatosplenomegaly, chorioretinitis, CNS changes including ventriculomegaly and periventricular calcifications, seizures, and developmental delay [37,38].

Diagnosis
The diagnosis of toxoplasmosis is quite challenging. There is a specific laboratory, the Toxoplasma Serology Laboratory in Palo Alto, California, that can be consulted. The utility of IgG and IgM is not comparable to other infections, and in some cases IgA and IgE antibodies are more useful for the diagnosis of an acute infection. The Toxoplasma Serology Laboratory uses a Toxoplasma Serologic Profile that can be employed to assist with the diagnosis [39].

When evaluating for congenital toxoplasmosis, PCR for toxoplasmosis DNA can be performed on a sample obtained from the amniotic fluid [40]. It is also possible to test maternal serum for anti-toxoplasma IgM and IgA, but the sensitivity is low.

Management and prevention
Treatment is recommended for acute infection in pregnancy. Although spiramycin is not readily available in the United States, it can be obtained through the compassionate use pathway provided by the Food and Drug Administration. Confirmed fetal infection requires multiagent therapy, with a combination of pyrimethamine, folinic acid, and sulfadiazine.

Patient education on the prevention of maternal toxoplasmosis infection is paramount. Pregnant patients should be counseled to avoid raw meat and close contact with cat feces. Any fruits and vegetables should be washed prior to consumption and hand washing after contact with soil or raw meat is also important.

Herpes simplex infection

Herpes simplex virus (HSV) is caused by two different herpesviruses, HSV-1 and HSV-2. The virus causes infection of the oral cavity, lower genital tract, and skin; contrary to previously held beliefs, both viruses can cause lesions in all areas. It is a highly prevalent sexually transmitted illness in the United States, with over 1.6 million new infections per year. Approximately 25% of women in the United States are seropositive for HSV-2, with rates even higher in high-risk populations [41–43]. HSV is spread by sexual contact. After intimate contact, the incubation period is 3–6 days long. Following the initial infection, the virus travels along sensory nerves and remains latent; it can reactivate and cause recurrent mucocutaneous lesions. The frequency of reactivation is variable.

Fetuses can rarely be infected in utero due to transplacental passage or ascending infection from the genital tract. However, it should be noted that the majority of neonatal herpes (85%) occurs as a result of direct contact during the birth process. This is not necessarily limited to visible lesions; it could be due to asymptomatic shedding [44].

Clinical manifestations

Genital HSV infection can manifest in the following ways:
• First episode primary herpes: this is diagnosed when a patient has a first-time lesion that contains HSV-1 or -2 without any serum antibodies. This phase may be symptomatic or asymptomatic. There may be a flulike illness with fever, malaise, inguinal lymphadenopathy, dysuria, and vulvar pruritus. Vesicles are the classic lesion in HSV; they may present as abrasions if the surface of the vesicle has been removed. Unlike the lesions in syphilis, the lesions of HSV are very painful. They last 3–6 weeks.
• First episode nonprimary herpes: this refers to the first time a patient experiences lesions and has antibodies to the other HSV serotype. Given the natural cross-reactivity between the antibodies, patients with first episode nonprimary herpes have a clinical presentation similar to a recurrent infection.
• Recurrent herpes: this refers to an outbreak that is milder than initial outbreaks, typically with fewer lesions that don't remain present as long. The risk of transmission to the fetus in cases of recurrent herpes is low.
• Asymptomatic shedding: this refers to detectable HSV on the skin and mucosal surfaces without signs or symptoms of an outbreak. The majority of HSV transmission occurs during this phase.

Neonatal HSV is at high risk of acquisition during delivery when the fetus directly contacts virus in the lower genital tract. If the birth takes place during a first episode, this confers the highest risk of neonatal infection. Infants can demonstrate infection in the skin, eyes, mucous membranes, encephalitis, or disseminated disease including the liver which is associated with a high mortality rate [47,48].

Diagnosis

In most cases, clinical diagnosis is sufficient when a patient presents with an outbreak of the typical appearing group of vesicular or ulcerated lesions. The lesions can be probed and fluid sent for viral culture, but PCR is more sensitive. One can also perform serologic testing, which can distinguish between HSV-1 and HSV-2 antibodies; however, this testing is somewhat controversial given the seroprevalence of anti-HSV antibodies [33,49,50].

Management and prevention

The treatment for symptomatic outbreaks is to use an antiviral such as acyclovir, valacyclovir, or famcyclovir.

The goal is to reduce symptoms and duration of outbreak. Acyclovir or valacyclovir can be used beginning at approximately 36 weeks gestation to decrease the likelihood of an HSV outbreak at term and also decrease the quantity of asymptomatic shedding.

At the time of delivery, women with known HSV should be evaluated for symptoms and examined for any lesions. If there is a lesion in the genital tract or symptoms consistent with prodromal HSV, the patient should be offered cesarean delivery, although delivery by cesarean does not fully prevent the transmission to the neonate. Nongenital HSV is not an indication for cesarean. Breastfeeding is not contraindicated unless there is an HSV lesion on the breast.

Patients with a history of HSV seropositivity should be counseled regarding these risks, suggested safe sexual practices, and offered prophylaxis in the third trimester. If a patient does not have HSV but her partner does, they should avoid intercourse during pregnancy, particularly in the third trimester when risk of transmission is highest.

Cytomegalovirus

Cytomegalovirus, also known as CMV, is a herpesvirus. It is the most common cause of perinatal infection in the United States, with rates as high as 2% [52,53]. CMV is typically found in children. The virus is spread through close contact with infected saliva, nasopharyngeal secretions, urine, blood or through sexual contact. Neonates can acquire the virus through transplacental passage or during birth via direct contact. Seropositivity is common in pregnant women, however the presence of antibodies does not protect against reinfection and resulting vertical transmission. However, it should be noted that the highest rate of vertical transmission is in those women who are infected with primary CMV during pregnancy (Figure 26.2).

Women with primary CMV infections during pregnancy will transmit the virus to the fetus 40% of the time. In contrast, of women with recurrent infection, only 0.15–1% will transmit the virus to the fetus. The risk of clinically apparent disease or sequelae in the neonate is higher in those infants infected during a primary maternal infection. As with many other congenital infections, perinatal transmission is more likely in the third trimester, but outcomes are more severe the earlier in gestation transmission occurs. Recent evidence has shown that reinfection with a different strain of CMV can also lead to intrauterine transmission [56,57].

Clinical manifestations

Most adults with CMV are asymptomatic. In those with symptoms, CMV infection may include a flulike illness

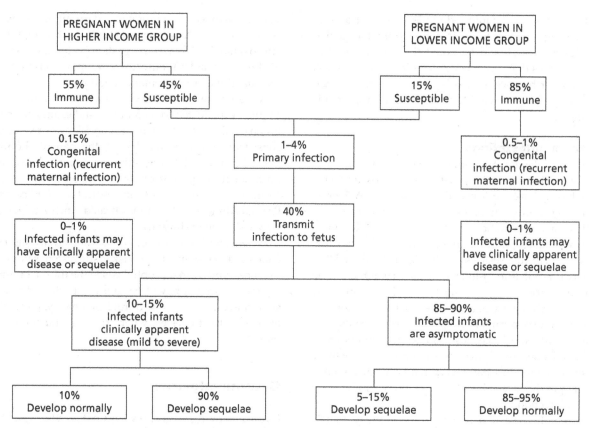

Figure 26.2 Characteristics of CMV infection in pregnancy. Reproduced from Stagno and Whitley (1985)/with permission from the Massachusetts Medical Society. CMV, cytomegalovirus.

including fever, malaise, headache, arthritis, pharyngitis, and lymphadenopathy. It should be noted that immunocompromised patients can develop much more morbid complications involving almost every organ system. Reactivation of CMV is usually asymptomatic but is associated with viral shedding.

Congenital CMV infection may present with hepatosplenomegaly, thrombocytopenia, jaundice, and petechiae ("blueberry muffin"). Low birthweight, microcephaly, intracranial calcifications, chorioretinitis, hearing deficits, pneumonitis, microphthalmia, and seizures are also not uncommon. Though the majority of infected infants are asymptomatic at birth, some will develop late onset sequelae. These commonly include psychomotor retardation, hearing loss, neurologic deficits, chorioretinitis, and learning disabilities. CMV is the leading cause of sensorineural hearing loss in children that is attributed to infection.

Diagnosis

Primary symptomatic maternal CMV infection presents similarly to Epstein–Barr virus. However, heterophile antibody testing will be negative. CMV IgM is detected within a few days of infection but is only found in 75–90% of women with acute infection [55]. CMV IgM

may remain positive for 4–8 months and reemerge with recurrent infection, making it problematic for diagnosis of acute disease. CMV IgG testing is more reliable – a fourfold rise in paired acute and convalescent sera indicates acute infection. CMV viral culture remains the gold standard for diagnosis though a minimum of 21 days is required for a culture to be reported as negative. Avidity testing is now available to determine disease acuity [33].

Perinatal infection may be suspected on ultrasound. Though nonspecific, fetal hydrops, intrauterine growth restriction, microcephaly, ventriculomegaly, hepatomegaly, cerebral calcifications, hyperechoic bowel, and amniotic fluid abnormalities have all been described. If suspected, amniotic fluid for DNA amplification testing has become the gold standard, though a negative result does not exclude fetal infection [58]. Finally, amniotic fluid for CMV culture may be useful but requires a long incubation period.

Management and prevention

There is no known pharmacologic therapy that can prevent congenital CMV. Studies have evaluated acyclovir and have not demonstrated benefit. A large randomized trial recently demonstrated that administration of hyperimmune globulin does not improve rates of congenital CMV [59]. If recent primary infection is diagnosed, invasive testing can be offered to identify infected fetuses. Counseling then is performed regarding the stage of infection and gestational age, understanding that the majority of fetuses develop normally. Pregnancy termination may be an option in rare cases.

Routine serologic screening for CMV is not recommended. Preventive measures including handwashing and minimizing exposure to CMV from high-risk areas such as day care centers and nurseries are the mainstays of preventing primary CMV infection. A CMV vaccine is not available currently for use in pregnancy.

Varicella zoster virus

Varicella zoster virus (VZV) is a DNA virus from the herpesvirus family. It is the most contagious viral infection complicating pregnancy. It is unusual to occur during pregnancy (0.1–0.4 cases per 1000 pregnant patients each year in the United States), with most of the US population showing evidence of immunity due to childhood illness. However, if a pregnant patient does become infected, the morbidity is greater than with childhood infection.

Similar to the other herpesviruses, VZV presents with an initial infection (varicella or chicken pox) then remains latent in the neurons and can reactivate, in this case as herpes zoster, also known as shingles. Transmission occurs through direct contact with lesions but can also occur via respiratory droplets. The incubation period is 1–2 weeks long; individuals become contagious one day before manifestation of the rash until the lesions have crusted over. There is a possibility of transplacental passage leading to congenital varicella; this is more likely if it occurs prior to 20 weeks gestation. Neonatal infection is also possible if there is exposure 5 days prior to delivery up to 2 days postpartum.

Clinical manifestations
Individuals infected with VZV can demonstrate the following signs and symptoms:
• A 1–2 day prodrome of a flulike illness, with fever, malaise, myalgias, and headache
• The classic lesions then appear, and undergo a typical cycle—initially papular, then a clear vesicle surrounded by an erythematous halo, then the vesicle is unroofed and crusts over. These are extremely pruritic and appear in irregular crops. The typical presentation begins with the head and trunk then progresses through the rest of the body.
• Varicella pneumonia is a potentially serious complication of varicella that is more common in adults than

children, and more common in pregnant patients (5.2%) [60]. The likelihood of varicella pneumonia is further increased in smokers and in those with >100 skin lesions. Mortality was once as high as 40%, but with advances in care and aggressive antivirals the rate of mortality has decreased to <2%. Because initial symptoms may be mild, a chest X-ray should be considered in all pregnant women presenting with varicella.
• Herpes zoster or shingles is the reactivation of VZV. This occurs along a dermatomal pattern. Pain precedes the appearance of papules, which become vesicles. Those can coalesce or rupture, then ultimately crust over.

Congenital varicella can result in multiple morbidities for the neonate. These include limb abnormalities (cutaneous scarring, hypoplasia, muscle atrophy) and also CNS effects (chorioretinitis, microcephaly, microphthalmia, seizures, cortical atrophy, and developmental delay). In contrast neonatal varicella, which occurs if there is exposure proximal to delivery, has a mortality rate of approximately 25%. These infants present with disseminated mucocutaneous lesions but also visceral infection and pneumonia.

Diagnosis
The diagnosis of varicella is usually made clinically. The characteristic rash in susceptible individuals allows for accurate diagnosis in the majority of cases. If the diagnosis is not readily apparent, VZV can be isolated by scraping the base of the vesicles during the acute phase of the infection. Tzanck smear, tissue culture, and direct fluorescent antibody testing are all available to test the vesicle specimen. DNA amplification techniques of body fluid or tissue are very sensitive and are rapidly becoming the gold standard. Seroconversion can be documented by antibody assay using acute and convalescent sera. VZV IgM develops rapidly and will remain positive for 4–5 weeks and may be useful in the acute setting. Fetal varicella can be diagnosed using DNA amplification techniques on amniotic fluid specimens, though it often does not correlate with clinical disease [61].

Management and prevention
The pregnant woman with primary VZV infection should be isolated and evaluated for pneumonia. Chest X-ray is useful. Hospitalization and antiviral therapy are reserved for those complicated by pneumonia or with systemic symptoms requiring intravenous fluids and symptomatic relief. If antiviral therapy is required, acyclovir (500 mg/m^2 or $10–15 \text{ mg/kg}$ every 8 hours) should be started as soon as possible. Oral administration is indicated for those with active lesions, but if pneumonia or encephalitis are diagnosed, or if immunocompromised, then intravenous acyclovir should be administered.

Prevention is the mainstay of population-based VZV management. The infected individual should be isolated. An exposed pregnant woman should be evaluated as to past disease – if no history of varicella infection, an IgG titer can be rapidly performed. At least 70% of individuals without reported history of VZV actually have VZV IgG. An exposed pregnant woman who is deemed susceptible may be given passive immunity using varicella zoster immune globulin (VariZIG). This is a human globulin fraction produced in Canada and available under an expanded access protocol. Contact information is at www.cdc.gov [62]. VariZIG should be given within 96 h of exposure to maximize the effect. As VariZIG is limited in quantity and is expensive, IgG testing is essential to limit the number of women requiring its administration.

The varicella vaccine currently available is a live attenuated vaccine (Varivax). It is not recommended in pregnancy and pregnancy should be avoided within 1 month of administration, but pregnant patients who are found to be seronegative should be counseled to receive the vaccine after delivery. To date, there have been no adverse outcomes in women inadvertently receiving the vaccine immediately before or during pregnancy.

Group B *Streptococcus*

Group B Streptococcus, also referred to as Group B Strep or GBS, is a gram-positive coccus. This bacterium can be found colonizing the gastrointestinal tract and vagina in 10–30% of women, and approximately 50% of pregnant patients who are colonized transmit the bacterium to their infant during labor or after rupture of membranes in a nonlaboring patient. GBS is associated with perinatal sepsis. According to the CDC, in the United States each year 930 infants are diagnosed with GBS early-onset disease (EOD) (<7 days of life) and 1050 are diagnosed with late-onset GBS disease (7–90 days); of those infants, 4–6% do not survive. Development of GBS EOD is more likely in pregnancies with previous GBS bacteriuria, preterm delivery, very low birthweight, intra amniotic infection, and prolonged rupture of membranes (>18 hours), and in those with a previous infant with GBS disease. There is also evidence of disparities in maternal health care, with Black race being associated with greater likelihood of GBS EOD [63]. GBS EOD is most often acquired as the neonate traverses the birth canal, but that is not the case for late-onset disease, which is thought to be acquired through nosocomial infection.

Clinical manifestations

GBS can be an asymptomatic colonizer of the urogenital tract. However, it can also cause cystitis, intraamniotic infection, endometritis, wound infection preterm labor, and has been associated with stillbirth. For the newborn, GBS EOD manifests as sepsis, pneumonia, and meningitis; infants who develop respiratory distress can die quickly. Late-onset disease manifests as bacteremia, meningitis, and can involve organ and soft tissue infection. Mortality is lower with late-onset disease, but there is a risk of long-term neurological sequelae including cerebral palsy [64].

Diagnosis

The diagnosis of Group B Strep, is preferred by culture. An accurate culture includes a swab of the distal half of the vagina, the perineum, and the outer portion of the anus. Some centers may offer a nucleic acid amplification test but the sensitivity and specificity are not as high as with culture unless the sample is first incubated in broth. American College of Obstetricians and Gynecologists guidelines recommend a GBS culture at 36–37+6 weeks gestation. If a patient presents with preterm labor, a GBS test should be done at presentation. If negative, and delivery has not taken place within 5 weeks, the test should be repeated with recurrent preterm labor or at 36-37+6 weeks. If positive at any point in pregnancy, whether from a rectovaginal swab or detected on a urine culture, the patient should have treatment during labor [65].

Management and prevention

Treatment with antibiotics is indicated during labor in order to prevent perinatal transmission. Antibiotic prophylaxis is necessary during labor in the following circumstances:

• A positive rectovaginal GBS swab, unless a cesarean is performed prior to membrane rupture
• Prior neonate with invasive GBS disease
• GBS bacteriuria during pregnancy
• Unknown GBS status and preterm labor, rupture of membranes >18 hours, fever, or known GBS positive in a prior pregnancy

Penicillin is the antibiotic of choice for GBS prophylaxis. In patients with a penicillin allergy, the choice of antibiotic is more complex. In patients with a high risk of severe penicillin allergy (for example anaphylaxis, hypotension, or a pruritic urticarial rash), the next most appropriate step is to obtain clindamycin susceptibility testing on the sample submitted for culture. If susceptible, clindamycin is an appropriate choice. If resistant, the recommended antibiotic is vancomycin. In patients with a low risk of severe allergic reaction (report gastrointestinal discomfort, pruritus without rash, family history but no personal history of allergy), cefazolin is the antibiotic of choice. If the risk is unclear, consider penicillin allergy testing or administration of any of the aforementioned alternatives. Erythromycin is no longer recommended.

The goal is to administer the antibiotic for 4 hours or more before birth, but even 2 hours has been shown to decrease neonatal sepsis [66–68].

CASE PRESENTATION

A 28-year-old female presents to your office for ultrasound at 20 weeks gestation. The fetus is noted to have growth restriction and echogenic bowel. She reports that approximately 2 weeks prior to the office visit, she had a low-grade fever, myalgias and arthralgias. She agrees to an amniocentesis, and serologies. Serum testing reveals positive IgM and low avidity IgG for CMV; CMV DNA is detected in the amniotic fluid by PCR. You review with her that there is no known treatment for presumed congenital CMV and describe some of the potential sequelae including sensorineural hearing loss. She goes on to deliver at a tertiary care center and the newborn is transferred to the neonatal intensive care unit for further care and evaluation.

References

1. Public Health Laboratory Service Working Party on Fifth Disease. Prospective study of human parvovirus (B19) infection in pregnancy. BMJ. 1990;300:1166–70.

2. De Jong EP, de Haan TR, Kroes AC, Beersma MF, Oepkes D, Walther FJ. Parvovirus B19 infection in pregnancy. J Clin Virol. 2006;36:1–7.

3. Melamed, W Whittle, EN Kelly, Windrim R, Seaward PG, Keunen J, et al. Fetal thrombocytopenia in pregnancies with fetal human parvovirus-B19 infection. Am J Obstet Gynecol. 2015;212:793.e1–8.

4. Harger JH, Adler SP, Koch WC, Harger GF. Prospective evaluation of 618 pregnant women exposed to parvovirus B19: risks and symptoms. Obstet Gynecol. 1998;91:413–20.

5. Rodis JF, Quinn DL, Garry GW, Anderson LJ, Rosengren S, Cartter ML, et al. Management and outcomes of pregnancies complicated by human B19 parvovirus infection: a prospective study. Am J Obstet Gynecol. 1990;163:1168–71.

6. Brown T, Anand A, Ritchie LD. Intrauterine parvovirus infection associated with hydrops fetalis. Lancet. 1984;2: 1033–4.

7. Crane J; Society of Obstetricians and Gynaecologists of Canada. Parvovirus B19 infection in pregnancy. J Obstet Gynaecol Can. 2002;24:727–43.

8. Enders M, Weidner A, Zoellner I, Searle K, Enders G. Fetal morbidity and mortality after acute human parvovirus B19 infection in pregnancy: prospective evaluation of 1018 cases. Prenat Diagn. 2004;24:513–18.

9. Enders M, Schalasta G, Baisch C, Weidner A, Pukkila L, Kaikkonen L, et al. Human parvovirus B19 infection during pregnancy value of modern molecular and serological diagnosis. J Clin Virol. 2006;35:400–6.

10. Butchko AR, Jordan JA. Comparison of three commercially available serologic assays used to detect human parvovirus B19-specific immunoglobulin M (IgM) and IgG antibodies in sera of pregnant women. J Clin Microbiol. 2004;42:3191–5.

11. Delle Chiaie L, Buck G, Grab D, Terinde R. Prediction of fetal anemia with doppler measurement of the middle cerebral artery peak systolic velocity in pregnancies complicated by maternal blood group alloimmunization or parvovirus B19 infection. Ultrasound Obstet Gynecol. 2001;18:232–6.

12. Cosmi E, Mari G, delle Chiaie L, Detti L, Akiyama M, Murphy J, et al. Noninvasive diagnosis by doppler ultrasonography of fetal anemia resulting from parvovirus infection. Am J Obstet Gynecol. 2002;187: 1290–3.

13. Schild RL, Bald R, Plath H, Eis-Hübinger AM, Enders G, Hansmann M. Intrauterine management of fetal parvovirus B19 infection. Ultrasound Obstet Gynecol. 1999;13:161–6.

14. Von Kaisenberg CS, Jonat W. Fetal parvovirus B19 infection. Ultrasound Obstet Gynecol. 2001;18:280–8.

15. Dembinski J, Haverkamp F, Maara H, Hansmann M, Eis-Hübinger AM, Bartmann P. Neurodevelopmental outcome after intrauterine red cell transfusion for parvovirus B19-induced fetal hydrops. Br J Obstet Gynaecol. 2002;109:1232–4.

16. Nagel HT, de Haan TR, Vandenbussche FP, Oepkes D, Walther FJ. Long-term outcome after fetal transfusion for hydrops associated with parvovirus B19 infection. Obstet Gynecol. 2007;109(1):42–7.

17. Webster WS. Teratogen update: congenital rubella. Teratology. 1998;58:13–23.

18. Mubareka S, Richards H, Gray M, Tipples GA. Evaluation of commercial rubella immunoglobulin G avidity assays. J Clin Microbiol. 2007;45:231–3.

19. Tang JW, Aarons E, Hesketh LM, Strobel S, Schalasta G, Jauniaux E, et al. Prenatal diagnosis of congenital rubella infection in the second trimester of pregnancy. Prenat Diagn. 2003;6:509–12.

20. Haas DM, Flowers CA, Congdon CL. Rubella, rubeola, and mumps in pregnant women. Obstet Gynecol. 2005;106:295–300.

21. Larsen SA, Hunter EF, McGrew BE. Syphilis. In: Wentworth BB, Judson FN, editors. Laboratory methods for the diagnosis of sexually transmitted diseases. Washington, DC: American Public Health Association; 1984. p.1–42.

22. Sanchez PJ, Wendel GD. Syphilis in pregnancy. Clin Perinatol. 1997;24:71–90.

23. Maruti S, Hwany LY, Ross M, Leonard L, Raffel J, Hollins L. The epidemiology of early syphilis in Houston, TX, 1994-1995. Sex Transm Dis. 1997;24: 475–80.

24. Wendel GE, Sanchez PJ, Peters MT, Harstad TW, Potter LL, Norgard MV. Identification of *Treponema pallidum* in amniotic fluid and fetal blood from pregnancies complicated by congenital syphilis. Obstet Gynecol. 1991;78:890–5.

25. Qureshi F, Jacques SM, Reyes MP. Placental histopathology in syphilis. Human Pathol. 1993;24:779–84.

26. Genest DR, Choi-Hong SR, Tate JE, Qureshi F, Jacques SM, Crum C. Diagnosis of congenital syphilis from placental examination. Human Pathol. 1996;27:366–72.

27. Grimprel E, Sanchez PJ, Wendel GD, Burstain JM, McCracken GH Jr, Radolf JD. Use of polymerase chain reaction and rabbit infectivity testing to detect *Treponema pallidum* in amniotic fluids, fetal and neonatal sera, and cerebrospinal fluid. J Clin Microbiol. 1991;29:1711–18.

28. Wendel GD, Maberry MC, Christmas JT, Goldberg MS, Norgard MV. Examination of amniotic fluid in diagnosing congenital syphilis with fetal death. Obstet Gynecol. 1989;74:967–70.

29. Johnson HL, Erbelding EJ, Zenilman JM, Ghanem KG. Sexually transmitted diseases and risk behaviors among pregnant women attending inner city public sexually transmitted diseases clinics in Baltimore, MD, 1996-2002. Sex Transm Dis. 2007;34:991–4.

30. Trepka MJ, Bloom SA, Zhang G, Kim S, Nobles RE. Inadequate syphilis screening among women with prenatal care in a community with a high syphilis incidence. Sex Transm Dis. 2006;33:670–4.

31. Taylor MM, Mickey T, Browne K, Kenney K, England B, Blasini-Alcivar L. Opportunities for the prevention of congenital syphilis in Maricopa County, Arizona. Sex Transm Dis. 2008;35:341–3.

32. Wilson EK, Gavin NI, Adams EK et al. Patterns in prenatal syphilis screening among Florida Medicaid enrollees. Sex Transm Dis. 2007;34:378.

33. Ortiz DA, Shukla MR, Loeffelholz MJ. The traditional or reverse algorithm for diagnosis of syphilis: pros and cons. Clin Infect Dis. 2020;71(Suppl 1):S43–S51.

34. Wendel GD, Stark BJ, Jamison RB, Molina RD, Sullivan TJ. Penicillin allergy and desensitization in serious infections during pregnancy. N Engl J Med. 1985;312:1229–32.

35. Centers for Disease Control and Prevention. CDC recommendations regarding selected conditions affecting women's health. MMWR Morb Mortal Wkly Rep. 2000;49(RR-2):59–75.

36. Jones JL, Kruszon-Moran D, Wilson M. *Toxoplasma gondii* infection in the United States, 1999-2000. Emerg Infect Dis. 2003 Nov;9(11):1371–4 [cited 2023 May 26]. Available from: https://wwwnc.cdc.gov/eid/article/9/11/03-0098_article.

37. Carter AO, Frank JW. Congenital toxoplasmosis: epidemiologic features and control. Can Med Assoc J. 1986;135:618–23.

38. Wilson CB, Remington JS, Stagno S, Reynolds DW. Development of adverse sequelae in children born with subclinical congenital *toxoplasma* infection. Pediatrics. 1980;66:767–74.

39. Montoya JG. Laboratory diagnosis of *Toxoplasma gondii* infection and toxoplasmosis. J Infect Dis. 2002;185(Suppl 1):573–82.

40. Thalib L, Gras L, Roman S, Prusa A, Bessieres MH, Petersen E, et al. Prediction of congenital toxoplasmosis by polymerase chain reaction analysis of amniotic fluid. Br J Obstet Gynaecol. 2005;11:567–74.

41. Fleming D, McQuillan G, Johnson R, Nahmias AJ, Aral SO, Lee FK, et al. Herpes simplex virus type 2 in the United States, 1976 to 1994. N Engl J Med. 1997;337:1105–11.

42. Xu F, Markowitz LE, Gottlieb SL, Berman SM. Seroprevalence of herpes simplex virus types 1 and 2 in pregnant women in the United States. Am J Obstet Gynecol. 2007;196:43.e1–6.

43. Xu F, Sternberg MR, Kottiri BJ, McQuillan GM, Lee FK, Nahmias AJ, et al. Trends in herpes simplex virus type 1 and type 2 seroprevalence in the United States. JAMA. 2006;30:964–73.

44. Brown ZA, Wald A, Morrow RA, Selke S, Zeh J, Corey L. Effect of serologic status and cesarean delivery on transmission rates of herpes simplex virus from mother to infant. JAMA. 2003;289:203–9.

45. Mahnert N, Roberts SW, Laibl VR, Sheffield JS. The incidence of neonatal herpes infection. Am J Obstet Gynecol. 2007;196:e55–6.

46. Whitley R, Davis EA, Suppapanya N. Incidence of neonatal herpes simplex virus infections in a managed-care population. Sex Transm Dis. 2007;34:704–8.

47. Kimberlin DW, Rouse DJ. Genital herpes. N Engl J Med. 2004;350:1970–7.

48. Kimberlin DW. Neonatal herpes simplex infection. Clin Microbiol Rev. 2004;17:1–13.

49. Anzivino E, Fioriti D, Mischitelli M, Bellizzi A, Barucca V, Chiarini F, et al. Herpes simplex virus infection in pregnancy and in neonate: status of art of epidemiology, diagnosis, therapy and prevention. Virol J. 2009;6:40.

50. Laderman EI, Whitworth E, Dumaual E, Jones M, Hudak A, Hogrefe W, et al. Rapid, sensitive, and specific lateral-flow immunochromatographic point-of-care device for detection of herpes simplex virus type 2-specific immunoglobulin G antibodies in serum and whole blood. Clin Vaccine Immunol. 2008;15:159.

51. American College of Obstetricians and Gynecologists. Practice Bulletin No. 82: management of herpes in pregnancy. Obstet Gynecol. 2007;109:1489–98.

52. Stagno S, Pass RF, Dworsky ME, Henderson RE, Moore EG, Walton PD, et al. Congenital cytomegalovirus infection. The relative importance of primary and recurrent maternal infection. N Engl J Med. 1982;306:945–9.

53. Stagno S, Cloud G, Pass RF, Britt WJ, Henderson RE, Walton PD, et al. Primary cytomegalovirus infections in pregnancy: incidence, transmission to the fetus and clinical outcome. JAMA. 1986;256:1904–8.

54. Hughes BL, Gyamfi-Bannerman C, Society for Maternal-Fetal Medicine (SMFM). Diagnosis and antenatal management of congenital cytomegalovirus infection. Am J Obstet Gynecol. 2016;214(6):B5–B11.

55. Stagno S, Tinker MK, Irod C, Fuccillo DA, Cloud G, O'Beirne AJ. Immunoglobulin M antibodies detected by enzyme-linked immunosorbent assay and radioimmunoassay in the diagnosis of cytomegalovirus infections in pregnant women and newborn infants. J Clin Microbiol. 1985;21:930–5.

56. Yamamoto AY, Mussi-Pinhata MM, Boppana SB, Novak Z, Wagatsuma VM, Oliveira Pde F, et al. Human cytomegalovirus reinfection is associated with intrauterine transmission in a highly CMV immune maternal population. Am J Obstet Gynecol. 2010;202(3):297.e1–8.

57. Ross SA, Arora N, Novak Z, Fowler KB, Britt WJ, Boppana SB. Cytomegalovirus reinfections in healthy seroimmune women. J Infect Dis. 2010;201:386–9.

58. Revello MG, Genna G. Pathogenesis and prenatal diagnosis of human cytomegalovirus infection. J Clin Virol. 2004;29:71–83.

59. Hughes BL, Clifton RG, Rouse DJ, Saade GR, Dinsmoor MJ, Reddy UM, et al. A trial of hyperimmune globulin to prevent congenital cytomegalovirus infection. N Engl J Med. 2021;385(5):436–44.

60. Harger JH, Ernest JM, Thurnau GR, Moawad A, Momirova V, Landon MB, et al. Risk factors and outcome of varicella-zoster virus pneumonia in pregnancy women. J Infect Dis. 2002;185:422–7.

61. Mendelson E, Aboundy Y, Smetana Z, Tepperberg M, Grossman Z. Laboratory assessment and diagnosis of congenital viral infections: rubella, cytomegalovirus (CMV), varicella-zoster virus (VZV), herpes simplex virus (HSV), parvovirus B19 and human immunodeficiency virus (HIV). Reprod Toxicol. 2006;21:350–82.

62. Centers for Disease Control and Prevention. A new product (VariZIG) for postexposure prophylaxis of varicella available under an investigational new drug application expanded access protocol. MMWR Morb Mortal Wkly Rep. 2006;55:209–10.

63. ACOG Committee on Obstetric Practice. Committee Opinion 797: prevention of Group B Streptococcal early-onset disease in newborns., Obstet Gynecol. 2020 Feb;135(2):e51–e72.

64. Nanduri SA, Petit S, Smelser C, Apostol M, Alden NB, Harrison LH, et al. Epidemiology of invasive early-onset and late-onset group B streptococcal disease in the United States, 2006 to 2015: multistate laboratory and population-based surveillance. JAMA Pediatr. 2019 Mar 1;173(3):224–33. doi: 10.1001/jamapediatrics.2018.4826.

65. Jamie WE, Edwards RK, Duff P. Vaginal-perianal compared with vaginal-rectal cultures for identification of group B streptococci. Obstet Gynecol. 2004 Nov;104(5 Pt 1):1058–61.

66. De Cueto M, Sanchez JM, Sampedro A, Miranda JA, Herruzo AJ, Rosa-Fraile M. Timing of intrapartum ampicillin and prevention of vertical transmission of group B streptococcus. Obstet Gynecol. 1998;91:112–14.

67. McNanley A, Glantz C, Hardy DJ, Vicino D. The effect of intrapartum penicillin on vaginal group B streptococcus colony counts. Am J Obstet Gynecol. 2007;197:583.e1–4.

68. Barber EL, Zhao G, Buhimschi IA, Illuzzi JL. Duration of intrapartum prophylaxis and concentration of penicillin G in fetal serum at delivery. Obstet Gynecol. 2008 Aug;112(2 Pt 1):265–70.

Chapter 27
Malaria

Richard M.K. Adanu

University of Ghana School of Public Health and Ghana College of Physicians and Surgeons, Accra, Ghana

Malaria is caused by the protozoon *Plasmodium*, which is transmitted through the bite of the female *Anopheles* mosquito. The four species of *Plasmodium* responsible for malaria are *P. falciparum*, *P. vivax*, *P. ovale*, and *P. malariae*. *Plasmodium falciparum* is responsible for most of the cases. There are about 400 million cases of malaria annually with 1–3 million deaths [1,2]. Malaria in pregnancy is responsible for 75 000–200 000 infant deaths per year [1]. Over 90% of malaria cases occur in sub-Saharan Africa [2].

Clinical features

Malaria usually begins with a nonspecific flulike reaction. The patient usually complains of fever, headaches, and general malaise; some complain of abdominal pains and vomiting.

Malaria is characterized by febrile paroxysms that last for 6–10 hours and are characterized by three stages. The patient first experiences a cold stage in which there is intense shivering. The next stage is the occurrence of a high-grade fever that later breaks and brings on the sweating stage of the febrile paroxysm. After the resolution of these stages, symptoms subside for a time and then the cycle is repeated within 36–48 hours.

Clinical examination usually reveals a woman who is febrile with a temperature of 38°C or higher. Depending on whether the disease has been going on for some time and on the hemoglobin level, pallor of the mucous membranes may be present. The degree of pallor is worst in women who suffer from hemoglobinopathies such as sickle cell disease. Other signs that could be present in malaria are jaundice and splenomegaly. Jaundice and splenomegaly are usually found in people who live outside holoendemic areas and thus who have no immunity to malaria and in patients with preexisting hemoglobinopathies. Women living in holoendemic areas usually only have fever as the sign that is noted on clinical examination.

Diagnosis

To successfully diagnose malaria the clinician needs to have a high index of suspicion. A history of travel to a malaria endemic area should lead to malaria being considered when a fever occurs. In holoendemic areas, however, there is a risk of clinicians over diagnosing malaria from clinical signs and symptoms. Because malaria is a common condition in such places, a thorough workup on the cause of a fever is often overlooked.

To diagnose malaria correctly, laboratory investigation using a thick or thin peripheral blood film for microscopic examination is essential. The thick blood film is used for low parasitemias and the thin blood film for high parasitemias [2,3]. The level of parasitemia as well as the species of *Plasmodium* responsible is revealed by microscopic examination. Microscopy is the gold standard for routine laboratory diagnosis of malaria and is a very reliable way of diagnosing the condition [3].

In areas where malaria cases are not commonly seen, polymerase chain reaction procedures are more accurate In areas where there is no laboratory support for the clinician, rapid diagnostic tests to determine the presence of plasmodial antigens can be used [4].

Treatment

The medications that can be used in the treatment of malaria in pregnancy depend on the stage of pregnancy at which the disease is diagnosed and the condition of the patient.

A combination of quinine and clindamycin is recommended when malaria is diagnosed in the first trimester. Quinine can be used alone if clindamycin is unavailable or unaffordable [5]. In the second and third trimesters, artemisinin-based combination therapy (ACT) is used for treatment. The recommended forms of ACT are artemether-lumefantrine, artesunate plus amodiaquine, artesunate plus mefloquine, and artesunate plus sulfadoxine-pyrimethamine [5].

There are limited data on the safety of ACT in the first trimester even though it is recommended that ACT be used in the first trimester if it is the only available treatment [5].

Antiemetics and analgesics are used to manage severe vomiting, headaches, and myalgia associated with malaria in pregnancy. In severe cases of vomiting, patients are unable to take oral medication and are also unable to eat. These patients are managed with fluid and electrolyte replacement therapy, parenteral quinine and parenteral antiemetic agents. Oral medication is begun once the vomiting stops.

Complications

Malaria affects both the mother and the fetus. Malaria has been reported to cause severe anemia leading to cardiac failure. It can lead to acute renal failure as a result of infected red blood cells causing endothelial damage and resultant reduced blood flow to the kidneys. It also causes hypoglycemia leading to central nervous complications of cerebral malaria characterized by seizures and loss of consciousness. Malaria causes maternal mortality through these complications.

Malaria causes miscarriages when it occurs in the first trimester. Intrauterine growth restriction and intrauterine fetal death from malaria are caused by the reduction in oxygen and nutrient delivery due to placental malaria. Malaria causes low birthweight because of the associated maternal anemia and the intrauterine growth restriction. Intrauterine infection of the fetus with malaria–congenital malaria–results from placental malaria. The febrile paroxysms due to malaria could precipitate preterm labor and prematurity.

Prevention

In holoendemic areas, malaria and its complications in pregnancy are prevented by the following measures:
- Intermittent preventive treatment [6,7]
- Use of insecticide-treated nets [8]
- Effective case management of malaria and anemia

Intermittent preventive treatment is the use of antimalarial medications at specific intervals during the pregnancy in the absence of clinical malaria. The World Health Organization recommends that all pregnant women in holoendemic areas should receive three or more doses of sulfadoxine-pyrimethamine at monthly intervals after quickening. The first dose should not be administered earlier than 16 weeks gestation and the last dose should not be after 36 weeks gestation [5,6].

Pregnant women in holoendemic areas are advised to sleep under insecticide-treated bed-nets in order to reduce the frequency of mosquito bites.

Effective diagnosis and treatment of malaria will prevent the occurrence of maternal and fetal complications.

CASE PRESENTATION

A 26-year-old primigravida at 33 weeks gestation presented to the clinic with complaints of recurrent lower abdominal pain radiating to her back and thighs. She also complained of a mild fever and chills but no dysuria.

On examination, the patient appeared to be in moderate pain but did not appear acutely ill. She was warm to touch with a temperature of 38° C. She was neither pale nor jaundiced. Examination of her abdomen showed a uterus that was appropriate for dates. She had a singleton pregnancy in cephalic presentation with a normal fetal heart rate. She was having two contractions in 10 minutes with each contraction lasting about 20 seconds. Speculum examination showed that her cervix was about 3 cm long and not dilated.

Laboratory tests ordered were urine microscopy, biochemistry and culture, complete blood count, blood film for malaria parasites, and an ultrasound scan.

The urine tests were normal; hemoglobin level was 9.5 g/dL; thick film smear for malaria parasites showed 2 + parasitemia. The ultrasound examination did not show any abnormalities.

A diagnosis of malaria complicated by preterm contractions was made. She was put on a course of artemether lumefantrine and the dosage of her regular hematinic was doubled. She was admitted for observation because of the preterm contractions.

By the second day of admission, she was feeling better and the contractions had stopped. She was discharged home to complete the antimalarial treatment. On her return visit a week later, she was in a very good state of health with no complaints.

References

1. Lagerberg RE. Malaria in pregnancy: a literature review. J Midwifery Womens Health. 2008;53(3):209–15.

2. World Health Organization. World malaria report 2008. Geneva: World Health Organization; 2008.

3. World Health Organization. Role of laboratory diagnosis to support malaria disease management. Report of a WHO consultation. Geneva: World Health Organization; 2006.

4. World Health Organization. The use of malaria rapid diagnostic tests. 2nd ed. Geneva: World Health Organization; 2006.

5. World Health Organization. Guidelines for the treatment of malaria. Geneva: World Health Organization, 2006.

6. WHO Global Malaria Programme. WHO policy brief for the implementation of intermittent preventive treatment of malaria in pregnancy using sulfadoxine pyrimethame (IPTp-SP). Geneva: World Health Organization; 2014.

7. Kayentao K, Kodio M, Newman RD, Maiga H, Doumtabe D, Ongoiba A, et al. Comparison of intermittent preventive treatment with chemoprophylaxis for the prevention of malaria during pregnancy in Mali. J Infect Dis. 2005; 191(1):109–16.

8. Kabanywanyi AM, Macarthur JR, Stolk WA, Habbema JD, Mshinda H, Bloland PB, et al. Malaria in pregnant women in an area with sustained high coverage of insecticide-treated bed nets. Malar J. 2008;7:133.

Chapter 28
Hepatitis in Pregnancy

Asa Oxner[1], Andrew Myers[1], and Sarah G. Običan[2]

[1]University of South Florida Health Morsani College of Medicine, Department of Internal Medicine, Tampa, FL, USA
[2]Department of Obstetrics and Gynecology, University of South Florida, Tampa, FL, USA

Hepatitis is a common and often serious inflammation of the liver caused by a viral infection with specific RNA and DNA viruses. The manifestations of hepatitis can range from no or minimal symptoms to severe fulminant liver failure, encephalopathy, and hepatocellular carcinoma. The purpose of this chapter is to review six different types of viral hepatitis: A, B, C, D, E, and G; describe the diagnostic tests for each of these infections; and define the perinatal complications and management associated with each form of viral hepatitis. The chapter is written in order of viral mode of transmission rather than alphabetically (Table 28.1).

Hepatitis A

Hepatitis A infection is caused by an RNA virus transmitted via fecal-oral contact that results in the second most common form of viral hepatitis in the United States. The disease is most prevalent in areas of poor sanitation and overcrowded housing [1]. The typical clinical manifestations of hepatitis A infection include low grade fever, malaise, anorexia, right upper quadrant pain and tenderness, jaundice, and acholic stools. Infections in children are usually asymptomatic; infections in adults are usually symptomatic. The diagnosis is most easily confirmed by detection of serum immunoglobin M (IgM) antibody specific for the hepatitis A virus (HAV).

Hepatitis A does not cause a chronic carrier state. Perinatal transmission virtually never occurs, and, therefore, the infection does not pose a major risk to either the mother or baby unless the mother develops fulminant hepatitis and liver failure, which is extremely rare [1].

Hepatitis A can be prevented by administration of an inactivated vaccine. There are limited data on vaccination use in pregnancy; however, the vaccine is composed of inactivated HAV and the risk to the developing fetus is expected to be low to none. As with most vaccines and medications, the risk of the vaccine should be weighed with the risk of acquiring HAV. Two monovalent formulations of the vaccine are available: Vaqta and Havrix. Both vaccines require an initial intramuscular injection, followed by a second dose 6–12 months later. The vaccine should be offered to the following individuals:

- International travelers
- Children in endemic areas
- Intravenous drug users
- Individuals who have occupational exposure
- Residents and staff of chronic care institutions
- Individuals with liver disease
- Homosexual men
- Individuals with clotting factor disorders

The vaccine can also be given in a bivalent form in combination with hepatitis B vaccine. Hepatitis A vaccination is now the agent of choice for postexposure prophylaxis as well. It is normally readily available and provides both short- and long-term protection against hepatitis A. Standard immunoglobulin provides reasonably effective passive immunization for hepatitis A if it is given within 2 weeks of exposure for patients younger than 12 months, those with chronic liver disease, or who are immunocompromised. The standard intramuscular dose of immunoglobulin is 0.1 ml/kg [2].

Hepatitis E

Hepatitis E is caused by an RNA virus also transmitted via fecal-oral route and thus most common among populations living in poor sanitation housing. Symptoms are very similar to hepatitis A infection except that maternal infection with hepatitis E has an alarmingly high mortality, in the range of 10–20%. This high mortality is thought to result from underlying poor nutrition, poor general health, and lack of access to medical care [1]. Hepatitis E does not cause a chronic carrier state and there

Table 28.1 Viral hepatitis in pregnancy: summary of key facts

Infection	Mechanism of transmission	Best diagnostic test	Carrier state	Perinatal trans-mission	Vaccine	Points of interest
A	Fecal–oral	Antibody detection	No	No	Yes	Pre- or postexposure prophylaxis–either standard immunoglobulin or hepatitis A vaccine
E	Fecal–oral	Antibody detection	No	Rare	No	High maternal mortality in developing countries. No immunoprophylaxis available
B	Parenteral/sexual contact/placental transfer	Antibody detection	Yes	Yes	Yes	Postexposure prophylaxis–hepatitis B immunoglobulin (HBIG) and booster dose of hepatitis B vaccine
D	Parenteral/sexual contact	Antibody detection	Yes	Yes	Prevented by hepatitis B vaccine	Virus cannot replicate in absence of hepatitis B infection
C	Blood-borne during delivery/parenteral/sexual contact	Antibody detection	Yes	Yes	No	No immunoprophylaxis is available. High risk of coinfection with hepatitis B and HIV
G	Parenteral/sexual contact	Antibody detection	Yes	Yes	No	Infection has no clinical significance

are no vaccines or immunoprophylaxis against it. Diagnosis is confirmed via IgM serology. Perinatal transmission can occur but is extremely rare [3].

Hepatitis B

Hepatitis B (HBV) is a DNA virus infecting up to 8% of pregnant women in endemic countries and populations, making it the most common hepatitis virus worldwide. HBV is known to be highly transmissible via mother to child route with a likelihood of transmission as high as 90%, however, this vertical transmission is largely preventable with maternal screening and treatment and newborn postexposure prophylaxis. Acute HBV infection during pregnancy is associated with low birth weight and maternal chronic HBV infection is associated with increased risk of gestational diabetes, antepartum hemorrhage, and preterm delivery. Because hepatitis B is so common and actionable by maternal and child health care workers, we review in detail recommendations and data supporting screening, prevention, and treatment of pregnant women and management of prophylaxis in newborns for HBV.

Interaction of HBV with physiology of the pregnant immune system

Worldwide, 296 million individuals are infected with chronic HBV according to World Health Organization (WHO) 2019 data; an estimated half of these infections were acquired perinatally or during early childhood. The largest burden of HBV infection is in China, followed by the rest of the WHO Western Pacific Region and African Region [4].

HBV DNA is found in the umbilical cord blood and placental cells of mothers with detectable viral load and hepatitis B e antigen (HBeAg) can pass through placenta from mother to fetus where it induces fetal T cell tolerance in utero. Because of this in utero tolerance, up to 90% of infants exposed to HBV perinatally or in early childhood develop chronic HBV infection with progression to cirrhosis and hepatocellular carcinoma in 15–40% of chronic cases [5,6]. In 2019, 820,000 deaths resulted from hepatitis B, mostly due to cirrhosis and hepatocellular carcinoma [4]. Conversely, adults who become infected with HBV have <5% chance of developing chronic HBV. Thus, reducing mother-to-child transmission of HBV and early childhood bloodborne horizontal transmission is essential in controlling the global burden of infection and morbidity.

Additionally, HBV increases potential postpartum complications in mothers. Pregnancy is an immunosuppressed state with increased Th2 regulatory T cells allowing increased HBV viral multiplication during gestation. After delivery, when the mother's immune system restores balance between Th2 and Th1 cells, there is a 45–65% chance of HBV flare due to immune reconstitution [5].

Maternal screening

Maternal screening for hepatitis B surface antigen (HBsAg) is universally recommended in the first trimester of pregnancy in all countries by the WHO. Point-of-care capillary tests for HBsAg are available with a sensitivity of 99%, specificity of 95–99% depending on manufacturer, and a cost of US$0.63–1.20 per test [7]. As noted, the risk of transmission from mother to child without prophylaxis is as high as 90% in mothers with HBeAg-positivity, and even in HbeAg-negative/anti-Hbe-antibody-positive mothers without prophylaxis the rate of antenatal infection of the newborn is 12% [8].

Diagnosis of HBV infection in newborns is defined as HBsAg positivity at 6 months of age or greater [7]. Antibodies against HBeAg antigen and core antigen both cross the placenta and persist in newborns up to 24 months of age; thus they cannot be used to diagnose HBV infection in children [7].

Prevention of HBV infection

The HBV vaccine is safe and effective, offering 95–100% protection against hepatitis B infection when given to young individuals who have not yet been exposed to the virus [6,8]. The vaccine is made from recombinant HBsAg and induces anti-HBsAg antibody seropositivity. The HBV vaccine is also safe to administer to pregnant women whose screening is negative for chronic infection. Vaccination schedule for adults (including pregnant women) is 1 mL intramuscular injection initially, then 1 month and 6 months after the first dose. Protective immunity from the vaccine series lasts at least 20 years and is lifelong in many individuals.

Newborns born of HBsAg-positive mothers should receive both passive and active immunoprophylaxis within 12 hours of birth to reduce their risk of acquiring HBV infection [6,8]. Passive immunoprophylaxis is the administration of hepatitis B immune globulin (HBIG) and active immunoprophylaxis is administration of HBV vaccine. The infant should receive two additional doses of HBV vaccine

over the next 6 months. Even with correct administration of HBIG and HBV vaccine, however, 3–13% of children will have chronic HBV infection (most commonly those born to HBeAg-positive mothers) [8]. Newborns of HBV-negative mothers should also receive the HBV vaccine initial dose within 24 hours of birth, before being discharged from the hospital or birthing center.

Treatment of mothers with HBV

Overall, the American Association for the Study of Liver Diseases (AASLD) recommends tenofovir or entecavir as the preferred antiviral therapy for pregnant women with chronic HBV because of the drugs' higher threshold to develop resistance and, in the case of tenofovir, more extensive safety data in pregnancy [9]. The dose and frequency of each recommended nucleoside analog (NA) regimen for treatment of chronic HBV infected adults and mothers is summarized in Table 28.2. Tenofovir and lamivudine have widespread evidence of fetal safety during gestational treatment for HIV, with no increased rate of birth defects. Telbivudine, entecavir, and adefovir have less extensive data.

Pegylated interferon (Peg-IFN) has not been studied in pregnant women and should be avoided during pregnancy [9]. Peg-IFN is still a recommended therapy for some patients with chronic HBV but has limited tolerability, higher cost, and several contraindications including autoimmune disease, uncontrolled psychiatric disease, cytopenia, severe cardiac disease, seizures, and decompensated cirrhosis. All medications are proven safe and

Table 28.2 Nucleos(t)ide analogs recommended for treatment of chronic hepatitis B viral infection in adults including pregnant women

Tenofovir disoproxil fumarate (TDF)*	300 mg PO daily	Higher barrier to resistance than lamivudine, first-line recommended antiviral
		Needs renal dose adjustment with creatinine clearance (CrCl) <50 ml/min
		Should monitor bone density every 2 y in patients taking TDF chronically with other risk factors for osteoporosis
Lamivudine	100 mg PO daily (HBV mono-infection)	Resistance is common, should be considered for HBV treatment only when an alternative antiviral is not available or appropriate
	Or	Needs renal dose adjustment with CrCl <50 ml/min
	150 mg PO daily (HIV/ HBV coinfection)	
Telbivudine	600 mg PO daily	Cross-resistance with lamivudine is expected, use only for treatment naïve HBV and monitor HBV viral load
		Needs renal dose adjustment with CrCl <50 ml/min
Entecavir	0.5 mg PO daily	High barrier of resistance, equally efficacious as TDF
		Needs renal dose adjustment with CrCl <50 ml/min
Adefovir	10 mg PO daily	Needs renal dose adjustment with CrCl <50 ml/min

effective regardless of the degree of cirrhosis or decompensation except Peg-IFN.

There are three important treatment precautions in all adults who start antiviral therapy for HBV [9]:

1. Patients who are coinfected with HIV must have triple-agent highly active antiretroviral therapy, which can include tenofovir or lamivudine to treat both HIV and HBV. Single-agent antiviral therapy for HBV will cause resistance of HIV virus because it is also active against HIV.
2. Lactic acidosis and fatal hepatomegaly have been reported with the use of all nucleoside analog antivirals alone or in combination with antiretrovirals. Monitoring of liver function tests (LFTs) at 4 weeks after initiation of antivirals is recommended.
3. Severe acute exacerbations of hepatitis B, including fatal cases, have been reported in patients who discontinue antihepatitis B therapy. Patients who discontinue should have office visits and LFT monitoring every 3 months for at least 6 months and resumption of antiviral therapy if LFTs exceed the upper limit of normal.

The biggest treatment decision for mothers infected with HBV is the timing of initiation of anti-HBV antivirals. For pregnant women already in treatment with antivirals or those with confirmed fibrosis/cirrhosis on liver imaging, therapy should be continued or initiated immediately to reduce the risk of decompensation of liver disease during delivery and the postpartum immune reconstitution period. For women who are newly diagnosed during antenatal screening and who have no laboratory or imaging findings of advanced liver disease (normal alanine transaminase [ALT]), the decision to start antiviral medications should be based on the HBV DNA viral load or HBeAg status when viral load testing is not available. HBeAg-positive mothers should begin antiviral therapy in the third trimester; HBeAg-negative mothers could delay antiviral therapy until after the delivery [6,9]. In settings where HBV viral load quantification is available, initiation of antiviral therapy should be triggered when HBV DNA levels are above 1,000,000 copies (200,000 IU/mL), regardless of HBeAg status [6,9].

Discontinuation of HBV therapy is a debated topic but can be considered in noncirrhotic patients with HBeAg positivity once they experience seroconversion to anti-HBe. For these patients, it is recommended to continue therapy for 12 months of persistently normal ALT and undetectable HBV DNA levels, then discontinue therapy with monitoring of ALT every 3 months for 1 year after discontinuation [9]. Patients who were HBeAg-negative when beginning therapy are less likely to fully clear their chronic infection, thus although discontinuation of therapy can be considered if they have loss of HBsAg-positivity and normalization of ALT, the AASLD recommends indefinite therapy. All individuals with cirrhosis from HBV should continue their antiviral therapy indefinitely regardless of antibody seroconversion.

Additionally, all women who are HBsAg-positive should receive liver ultrasonography to screen for cirrhosis. If pregnant women are cirrhotic from any cause, they should undergo upper endoscopy to screen for esophageal varices in the second trimester of pregnancy with endoscopic treatments (banding, laser therapy) and beta-blocker prescription if varices are found [6]. Esophageal rupture occurs in 20–25% of cirrhotic pregnancies [6]. Ascites and hepatic encephalopathy would be managed the same as in nonpregnant individuals [6].

Elective cesarean section vs. vaginal delivery

There is no strong evidence that elective cesarean delivery protects against mother-to-child transmission of HBV compared to vaginal delivery. Elective cesarean for reduction in maternal transmission of HBV is not recommended by the American College of Obstetricians and Gynecologists (ACOG) or the Centers for Disease Control and Prevention (CDC).

Breastfeeding

Breastfeeding is not contraindicated for newborns who receive their active and passive immunoprophylaxis against HBV. If the mother is taking antiviral therapy with tenofovir disoproxil fumarate or lamivudine, data from HIV cohorts indicate there is no risk to the newborn and breastfeeding is recommended by the WHO and AASLD. Breastfeeding while taking any of the other antiviral therapies is not recommended. If tenofovir is available, it would be preferable to switch mothers taking telbivudine, entecavir, or adefovir to tenofovir after delivery to allow for safe breastfeeding. If tenofovir is not available, mothers taking any of these antivirals during pregnancy and delivery should discontinue the therapies, then monitor mother's LFTs every 3 months and encourage breastfeeding with appropriate active and passive immunoprophylaxis of the infant.

Hepatitis D

Hepatitis D (HDV) is an incomplete, single stranded circular RNA virus that depends upon coinfection with hepatitis B for transmission and replication. Specifically, HDV requires hepatitis B surface antigen (HBsAg) to be infectious. Overall, 5% of chronic HBV carriers have coinfection with HDV, but in some high prevalence areas coinfection could reach closer to 15% [10].

The main mode of transmission is infected bodily fluid or blood and vertical transmission during pregnancy is rare though it is more likely with high levels of HBV DNA [11]. The diagnosis of hepatitis D can be established by detection of IgM and/ or IgG antibody in serum. Development of fulminant hepatis in pregnancy is rare [12]. However, hepatitis D can cause a chronic carrier state in conjunction with hepatitis B infection. Coinfection of HDV in chronic HBV carriers significantly increases the risk of earlier development of cirrhosis and hepatocellular carcinoma [1,10]. Immunoprophylaxis against HBV is also highly effective in preventing transmission of hepatitis D [1,6]. Breastfeeding is not contraindicated in women with HDV.

Hepatitis C

Hepatitis C virus (HCV) is a small, enveloped, single-stranded, positive sense RNA virus. It infects approximately 3% of the world's population [13]. In comparison to HBV infection, hepatitis C infection is less prevalent, mothers are less likely to transmit HCV to children during delivery and early childhood, and infected mothers are curable before or after pregnancy with newer medications [13]. There is no effective vaccine against HCV. The overall risk of mother to child transmission of HCV is about 5%, which is much lower than the rate of hepatitis B maternal transmission [13]. Infants born of mothers with HCV infection have a higher rate of low birthweight; but are unlikely to experience lasting health effects if they avoid HCV transmission during delivery. We discuss the epidemiology, screening, and treatment of hepatitis C in pregnant and breastfeeding women.

Epidemiology

In the United States, where an estimated 2.4 million people are living with HCV, this virus was responsible for more deaths than HIV, tuberculosis, and other reportable diseases combined [13]. Globally, HCV kills almost 400,000 people yearly. The major causes of mortality among individuals infected with HCV are the complications of cirrhosis and hepatocellular carcinoma. Once infected, ~ 80% of people develop chronic infection, 10–20% develop cirrhosis after 20 or more years of HCV infection, and 1–5% of cirrhotic patients develop hepatocellular carcinoma per year [13]. HCV infection prevalence has increased by about 3.5-fold from 2010 to 2016, especially in the 20- to 29-year-old age group [13]. The increased incidence in this young population is mostly due to intravenous drug use or snorting cocaine and thus overlaps with the demographics and geography of the opioid and HIV epidemics.

Screening

A recent metanalysis by Andres et al. found that up to 27% of all HCV positive women have no identifiable risk factor for infection [14]. In addition, using risk-based screening, two thirds of pregnant patients with a known risk factor were not appropriately screened. With increasing maternal infections there is an increase in perinatally acquired HCV infections. According to the Society for Maternal and Fetal Medicine (SMFM), 5.8% of all infants born to an HCV-positive individual will become infected [15]. Given the many factors including the rise of new cases among reproductive age adults, the subsequent expected increase in perinatal hepatitis C, the availability of treatment and the severe consequence of untreated HCV, there has been a significant shift in screening recommendations for HCV. ACOG, the CDC, and the US Preventive Services Task Force now recommend abolishing risk-based screening strategies in favor of universal screening of all pregnant adults in each pregnancy [13,16].

Diagnostic algorithm

The diagnosis of HCV infection is a two-step process [13]. First an anti-HCV antibody is checked. If it is negative, then the patient is presumed to never have been exposed to HCV (keeping in mind the 4-month window period). If the anti-HCV antibody screen is positive, then an HCV RNA test is performed. If HCV RNA is negative, then the patient does not have a current infection meaning the patient was infected with HCV previously but cleared the infection. If the HCV RNA study is positive, the patient has an active infection and nonpregnant females should be treated. This approach is summarized in Figure 28.1.

Children born of mothers with HCV should not be tested before 18 months of age because maternal anti-HCV antibodies persist until that age. At 18 months and

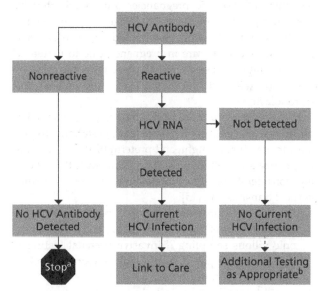

Figure 28.1 CDC-recommended diagnostic algorithm for identifying current HCV infection. CDC, Centers for Disease Control and Prevention; HCV, hepatitis C virus.

[a] If the antibody screen is negative but the exposure is recent, or the patient is immunocompromised then consider repeating antibody screen or use RNA study.

[b] In the case of a positive antibody but negative RNA study – this could be a cleared prior infection or false positive antibody result, thus, if this scenario fits with the clinical picture, no further studies are needed, if not, repeat the antibody test with another brand assay or repeat the RNA to confirm that is still negative.

older, testing with the normal algorithm of anti-HCV with HCV RNA confirmation is appropriate. If testing is needed prior to age 18 months, it would require HCV RNA testing only.

Additional monitoring and management considerations during pregnancy

Once a pregnant woman is confirmed to be HCV infected based on anti-HCV and HCV RNA testing, she should be referred to either an infectious disease, gastroenterology, or general internal medicine practice with experience in managing chronic HCV infection. Treatment must be delayed until after delivery (see next section), but additional laboratory studies should be ordered including HIV Ag/Ab test, HBsAg, HBsAb, complete blood count, LFTs, international normalized ratio, HCV genotype, alpha-fetoprotein tumor marker, liver ultrasound (to identify lesions of hepatocellular carcinoma), and fibroscan (to identify presence and stage of fibrosis) [16]. The current direct acting antiviral treatments (DAAs) are usually effective across all HCV genotypes. The choice of medication regimen may depend on the HCV genotype, HIV status, and presence or absence of cirrhosis.

As discussed in the HBV section, if a mother is found to have cirrhosis, aggressive management of esophageal varices should occur during pregnancy because about one third of cirrhotic pregnancies are complicated by variceal rupture. Management of hepatic encephalopathy would include standard care including lactulose and rifaximin. Ascites is rare in pregnancy due to increased intraperitoneal pressure but if present would also be managed with standard care of furosemide and spironolactone.

HCV carriers are more likely to have pregnancy complications such as gestational diabetes, gestational hypertension, low birth weight, and preterm birth [17]. During pregnancy and delivery, SMFM recommends the following considerations for HCV-positive women to reduce vertical transmission [15]:

1. Limited literature shows vertical transmission through amniocentesis is low and may be preferred over chorionic villous sampling if invasive prenatal testing is requested or required. Noninvasive screening modalities should be considered.
2. Avoid internal fetal monitoring and episiotomy during labor.
3. Avoid prolonged rupture of membranes.
4. Cesarean delivery should be reserved for obstetric indications.

Treatment

Fortunately, with advances in DAAs over the past 20 years, HCV infection is now curable for more than 90% of people with an 8- to 12-week course of medication [16]. Selection of DAA regimen (and single vs. dual antiviral agents) depends upon stage of fibrosis, coinfection with HIV, and HCV genotype of the patient. Although animal studies of most DAAs have shown a reasonable pregnancy safety profile, there is a paucity of human studies and thus DAAs remain contraindicated during pregnancy or breastfeeding. One small phase 1 study is ongoing for ledipasvir/sofosbuvir administration during pregnancy and animal studies suggest that ledipasvir, sofosbuvir, and dasabuvir are the DAAs that are not embryotoxic [18]. Whenever possible, expectant mothers should complete a course of DAA before becoming pregnant or after breastfeeding. If found to have HCV infection, children can be treated starting at age 12 in consultation with infectious disease or gastroenterology physicians [16]. In all cases of patients with HCV or any other liver disease, alcohol must be avoided.

Breastfeeding

There is limited evidence regarding the risk of transmission of HCV through breastfeeding. The CDC and AASLD both recommend that mothers who are infected with HCV should breastfeed their infants. Temporary formula feeding and pump-discard precautions could be taken in mothers with cracked or bleeding nipples. Pharmacologic studies show that all DAAs tested do pass into breastmilk; however, some compounds may be bound to human plasma proteins with limited access to milk. Some animal studies in rats have not shown adverse effects on the offspring development [19]. However, the effects of this on human infants have not been studied.

Hepatitis G

Hepatitis G is caused by an RNA virus that is related to HCV. Hepatitis G is more prevalent but less virulent than hepatitis C. Many patients who have hepatitis G are coinfected with hepatitis A, B, C, and HIV. Interestingly, coinfection with hepatitis G does not adversely affect the prognosis of these other infections. Most patients with hepatitis G are asymptomatic. The diagnosis is best established by detection of virus by polymerase chain reaction and by detection of antibody.

Hepatitis G may cause a chronic carrier state, and perinatal transmission has been documented. However, the clinical effect of infection in the mother and baby appears to be minimal. Accordingly, patients should not routinely be screened for this infection. There is no antiviral agent, vaccine, or immunoprophylaxis for hepatitis G, and no special treatment is indicated even if infection is confirmed [20–22].

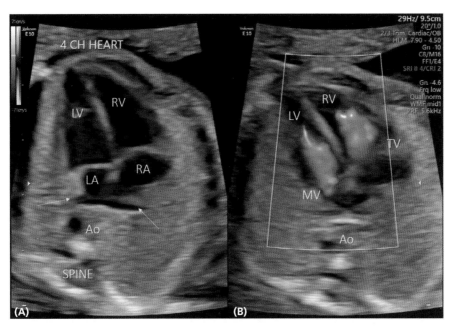

Plate 6.1 (A) A transverse view through the fetal chest demonstrating an apical four-chamber view. The most anterior chamber is the trabeculated right ventricle (RV) and the most posterior chamber adjacent to the spine is the left atrium (LA) into which are draining the left and right inferior pulmonary veins (arrows). The patent foramen ovale can be seen between the two atria. The atrioventricular valves are closed in systole. (B) Color flow Doppler demonstrating antegrade flow across the open tricuspid (TV) and mitral valves (MV) in diastole. The crux and interventricular septum appear intact. Ao, descending thoracic aorta; LV, left ventricle; RA, right atrium.

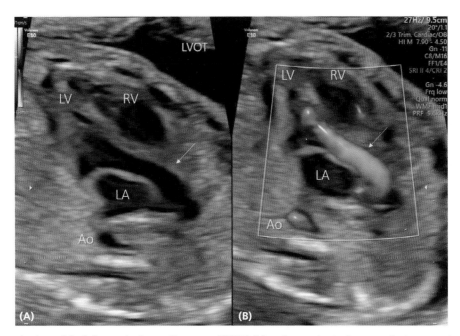

Plate 6.2 (A) Long-axis view of the left ventricular outflow tract (LVOT). Note the continuity between the interventricular septum and the anterior wall of the ascending aorta (arrow). (B) Color flow Doppler demonstrating normal laminar antegrade flow across the aortic valve in systole (arrow). Ao, descending thoracic aorta; LA, left atrium; LV, left ventricle; RV, right ventricle.

Queenan's Management of High-Risk Pregnancy: An Evidence-Based Approach, Seventh Edition. Edited by Catherine Y. Spong and Charles J. Lockwood.
© 2024 John Wiley & Sons Ltd. Published 2024 by John Wiley & Sons Ltd.

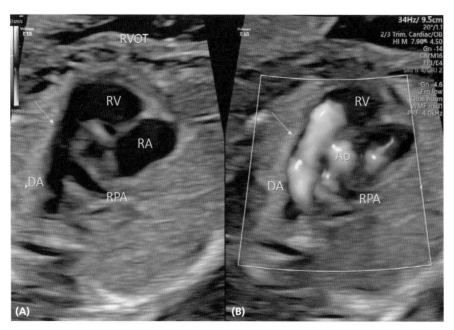

Plate 6.3 (A) Short-axis view of the right ventricular outflow tract (RVOT) wrapping around the aorta as it exits the right ventricle (RV) before dividing into the branch pulmonary arteries and ductus arteriosus (DA). (B) Color flow Doppler demonstrating normal laminar antegrade flow across the pulmonary valve. The main pulmonary artery (*arrow*) is similar in size to the aorta (Ao). RA, right atrium; RPA, right branch pulmonary artery.

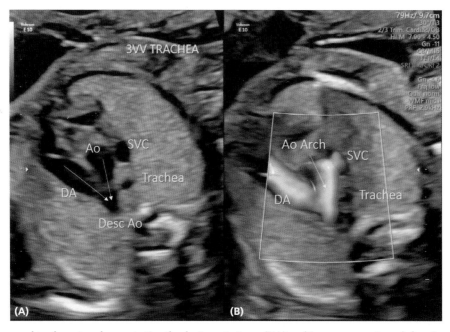

Plate 6.4 (A) Three-vessel trachea view demonstrating the ductus arteriosus (DA) and transverse aortic arch forming a "V" as they reach the descending thoracic aorta (Ao) toward the left of the fetal spine. The superior vena cava (SVC) and trachea are to the right of the great arteries. (B) Color flow Doppler demonstrating anterior-to-posterior flow in the DA and transverse aortic arch (*arrow*) to the descending thoracic aorta.

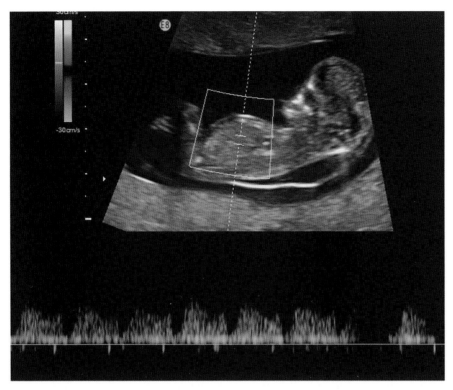

Plate 7.1 Septated cystic hygroma at 11 weeks' gestation: midsagittal view demonstrating increased NT space extending along the entire length of the fetus. The ductus venosus shows positive a-wave. Chorionic villus sampling revealed normal male karyotype. The pregnancy proceeded to full term with the delivery of a healthy infant. NT, nuchal translucency.

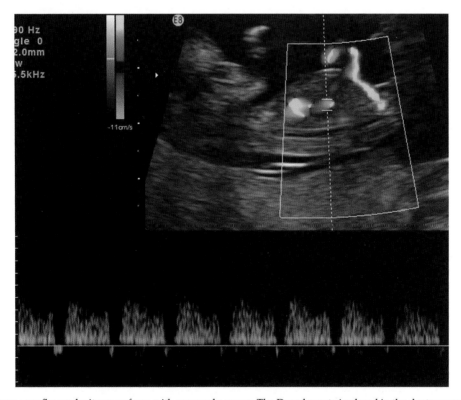

Plate 7.2 Ductus venosus flow velocity waveform with reversed a-wave. The Doppler gate is placed in the ductus venosus between the umbilical venous sinus and the inferior vena cava. Subsequent CVS confirmed a fetus affected by trisomy 21. CVS, chorionic villus sampling.

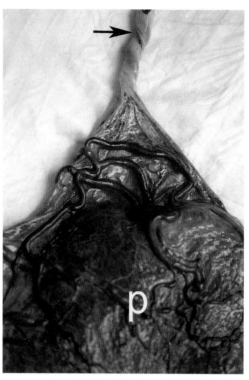

Plate 43.1 Vasa previa shown after cesarean delivery. In this case, the diagnosis had been made prenatally. The umbilical cord (arrow) inserts into the membranes through which prominent velamentous vessels travel to insert into the placenta (p).

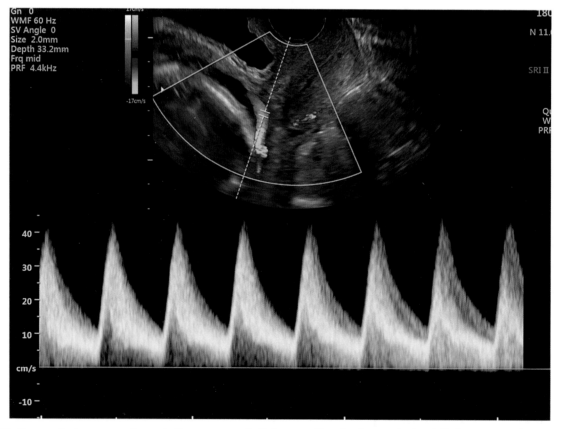

Plate 43.2 Transvaginal sonogram demonstrating a vasa previa. Pulse wave Doppler shows a fetal umbilical artery waveform.

CASE PRESENTATION 1

A 28-year-old woman, gravida 2, para 1001, at 8 weeks gestation is found to be seropositive for hepatitis B surface antigen and HIV. Additional testing shows that she is negative for hepatitis C, D, gonorrhea, chlamydia, and syphilis.

- What additional testing and counseling is indicated in this patient?
  - o Answer: Patients coinfected with hepatitis B and HIV are highly likely to develop chronic liver disease (including liver failure) and hepatocellular carcinoma. For HIV, she should begin highly active antiretroviral therapy immediately (HAART) with selection of antivirals to include anti-HBV activity; such as regimens containing lamivudine, emtricitabine, and tenofovir disoproxil fumarate or tenofovir alafenamide. In HBV mono-infection, patients would begin treatment if their viral load is >1000 copies/mL with oral lamivudine from 28 weeks gestation. Patients should be counseled that both HIV and HBV are unlikely to transmit to the fetus during pregnancy, delivery, or postpartum if they are taking their antiviral medications with high adherence.

- What interventions are appropriate for her sexual partner?
  - o Answer: The patient's sexual partner should be tested for hepatitis B, C, and HIV. If he is seronegative for hepatitis B, he should receive hepatitis B immunoglobulin and begin the hepatitis B vaccine series. This immunoprophylaxis will also protect against hepatitis D infection. If he is negative for HIV, he should be offered daily anti-HIV antiviral preexposure prophylaxis (PREP). If he is positive for HIV and/or HBV then he would start the same regimen as the mother.
- What type of immunoprophylaxis is indicated for this patient's neonate?
  - o Answer: The infant should receive hepatitis B immunoglobulin within 12 h of birth. Prior to discharge from hospital, the infant should receive the first dose of hepatitis B vaccine. A second and third dose should be administered at 1 month of age and 6 months of age.
- Is it safe for the baby to breastfeed?
  - o Answer: Yes, breastfeeding is safe in HIV and HBV infection when mothers are adherent to treatment.

CASE PRESENTATION 2

A 35-year-old woman, gravida 3, para 1111, at 20 weeks gestation is found to be seropositive for hepatitis C. Reflex viral load is >1 million but serologies are negative for hepatitis B, D, HIV, gonorrhea, chlamydia, or syphilis.

- What additional testing is indicated in this patient?
  - o Answer: None immediately, but patients with hepatitis C diagnosed during pregnancy should be referred to a maternal fetal medicine obstetrician to manage the pregnancy and also a hepatologist to get them set up for treatment immediately after delivery.
- What interventions are appropriate for her sexual partner?

  - o Answer: Her partner should be tested for HCV, HBV, and HIV and if he is found to be positive, he could begin direct anti-HCV therapy.
- What type of immunoprophylaxis is indicated for this patient's neonate?
  - o Answer: Unfortunately, there is no immunoprophylaxis for hepatitis C.
- Is it safe for the baby to breastfeed?
  - o Answer: Yes. Fortunately, even without immunoprophylaxis, breastfeeding does not appear to increase the risk of hepatitis C in the neonate.

References

1. Duff P. Hepatitis in pregnancy. Semin Perinatol. 1998;22:277–83.
2. Update: Recommendations of the Advisory Committee on Immunization Practices for use of hepatitis A vaccine for postexposure prophylaxis and for preexposure prophylaxis for international travel. MMWR Morb Mortal Wkly Rep. 2018 Nov 2;67(43):1216–20.
3. Khuroo MS, Kamili S, Jameel S. Vertical transmission of hepatitis E virus. Lancet. 1995 Apr 22;345(8956):1025–6.
4. World Health Organization. Hepatitis B. [last updated 2022 Jun 24; cited 2023 May 27]. Available from: https://www.who.int/news-room/fact-sheets/detail/hepatitis-b.
5. Borgia G, Carleo MA, Gaeta GB, Gentile I. Hepatitis B in pregnancy. World J Gastroenterol. 2012 Sep 14;18(34):4677–83.
6. American College of Obstetricians and Gynecologists. Practice Advisory: hepatitis B prevention. [last updated 2020 May 22; reaffirmed 2021 Oct; cited 2023 May 27]. Available from: https://www.acog.org/Clinical-Guidance-and-Publications/Practice-Advisories/Practice-Advisory-Hepatitis-B-Prevention.

7. World Health Organization. Hepatitis B surface antigen assays: operational characteristics. 2004 [cited 2023 Jun 6]. Available from: https://apps.who.int/iris/bitstream/handle/10665/43031/9241592206.pdf?sequence=1&isAllowed=y.

8. Schillie S, Vellozzi C, Reingold A, Harris A, Haber P, Ward JW, et al. Prevention of hepatitis B virus infection in the United States: Recommendations of the Advisory Committee on Immunization Practices. Centers for Disease Control and Prevention. MMWR Recomm Rep. 2018 Jan 12;67(1):1–31.

9. Terrault NA, Bzowej NH, Chang KM, Hwang JP, Jonas MM, Murad MH; American Association for the Study of Liver Diseases. AASLD guidelines for treatment of chronic hepatitis B. Hepatology. 2016 Jan;63(1):261–83.

10. Miao Z, Zhang S, Ou X, Li S, Ma Z, Wang W, et al. Estimating the global prevalence, disease progression, and clinical outcome of hepatitis delta virus infection. J Infect Dis. 2020 Apr 27;221(10):1677–87.

11. Cheung KW, Seto MTY, Kan ASY, Wong D, Kou KO, So PL, et al. Immunoprophylaxis failure of infants born to hepatitis B carrier mothers following routine vaccination. Clin Gastroenterol Hepatol. 2018 Jan;16(1):144–5.

12. Jaiswal SP, Jain AK, Naik G, Soni N, Chitnis DS. Viral hepatitis during pregnancy. Int J Gynaecol Obstet. 2001;72(2): 103–8.

13. Centers for Disease Control and Prevention. Hepatitis C questions and answers for health professionals. [last updated 2020 Aug 7; cited 2022 Feb 20]. Available from: https://www.cdc.gov/hepatitis/hcv/hcvfaq.htm.

14. Andes A, Ellenberg K, Vakos A, Collins J, Fryer K. Hepatitis C virus in pregnancy: a systematic review of the literature. Am J Perinatology. 2021 Aug;38(S 01):e1–13.

15. Society for Maternal-Fetal Medicine (SMFM). Hughes BL, Page CM, Kuller JA. Hepatitis C in pregnancy: screening, treatment, and management. Am J Obstet Gynecol. 2017 Nov;217(5):B2–12.

16. American Association for the Study of Liver Diseases (AASLD) and Infectious Diseases Society of America (IDSA). HCV testing and linkage to care. [last updated 2022 Oct 24; cited 2022Feb24].https://www.hcvguidelines.org/evaluate/testing-and-linkage.

17. Connell LE, Salihu HM, Salemi JL, August EM, Weldeselasse H, Mbah AK. Maternal hepatitis B and Hepatitis C carrier status and perinatal outcomes. Liver Int. 2011 Sep;31(8): 1163–70.

18. Chappell CA, Krans EE, Bunge K, Macio I, Bogen D, Scarsi KK, et al. A Phase 1 study of ledipasvir/sofosbuvir in pregnant women with hepatitis C virus. Conference on Retroviruses and Opportunistic Infections, Seattle, WA, 2019 Mar 7.

19. Merck and Co., Inc. Zepatier prescribing information. 2017 [revised 2018 Jun; cited 2023 May 27]. Available from: https://www.accessdata.fda.gov/drugsatfda_docs/label/2018/208261s005lbl.pdf.

20. Kew MC, Kassianides C. HGV: hepatitis G virus or harmless G virus? Lancet. 1996 Dec 21-28;348 Suppl 2:sII10.

21. Alter MJ, Gallagher M, Morris TT, Moyer LA, Meeks EL, Krawczynski K, et al. Acute non-A-E hepatitis in the United States and the role of hepatitis G infection. New Engl J Med. 1997;336:741–6.

22. Miyakawa Y, Mayuma M. Hepatitis G virus–a true hepatitis virus or an accidental tourist? New Engl J Med. 1997; 336:795–6.

Chapter 29
HIV Infection

Emily H. Adhikari

Department of Obstetrics and Gynecology, University of Texas Southwestern Medical Center, Dallas, TX, USA

Forty years after the human immunodeficiency virus (HIV) was first recognized in the United States, there is still work to be done to end the epidemic. An estimated 1.5 million individuals acquired HIV around the world in 2020 [1]. In the United States, Black or African American women make up 13% of the female population but account for 55% of new HIV infections – a statistic that has remained fairly consistent over decades [2]. In 2019, the US Department of Health and Human Services launched the Ending the HIV Epidemic Initiative, which aims to reduce new HIV infections in the United States by 90% by 2030 by targeting six key indicators: incident infections, knowledge of status, diagnosed infections, linkage to HIV care, viral suppression, and preexposure prophylaxis (PrEP) coverage (https://ahead.hiv.gov/). Obstetricians continue to play a pivotal role in prevention of both perinatal HIV transmission and horizontal transmission to women who are seronegative but at risk for HIV acquisition. Indeed, there is increased risk for acquisition of HIV during pregnancy that carries into the postpartum period [3]. This chapter is designed to provide guidance to physicians who can identify and treat pregnant women with HIV infection, as well as for those who have the opportunity to counsel and prevent HIV acquisition among those at high risk of infection.

Identifying infected patients

Approximately 13% of HIV-infected persons in the United States are unaware of their status [4]. To reduce this statistic, recommended practice is to use an "opt-out" approach, by which HIV testing is made a routine part of antenatal screening for every pregnant woman. This includes women without prenatal care, who present in labor or at delivery and whose HIV status is unknown [5].

The recommended laboratory-based HIV screening test now available at most clinical sites is a fourth-generation rapid immunoassay which detects both HIV-1 p24 *antigen* as well as *antibodies* to HIV-1 and 2 [6]. If negative, the patient is considered to be HIV negative. If recent HIV exposure is suspected, a quantitative viral load is also performed. If the HIV-1/2 antigen/antibody immunoassay is positive or reactive, a reflex HIV-1/HIV-2 *antibody differentiation assay* is necessary to determine which antibodies are present. This second test may be negative or nonreactive in early HIV infection. If antigen/antibody screening immunoassay is reactive but differentiation assay is nonreactive, a nucleic acid test (quantitative viral load or qualitative test) is recommended to evaluate for possible early or acute HIV infection. A thorough sexual history and risk factor assessment will also help the clinician to determine whether the patient with discordant laboratory test results is likely to have an early infection. Clinical history is particularly important for management of patients who present in labor or at delivery with little or no prenatal care, and especially if laboratory testing is delayed. Consultation with specialists experienced in interpreting HIV laboratory tests is imperative to identify early HIV infection, as well as to avoid misinterpretation and potential harm. The Perinatal HIV Consultation and Referral Services Hotline is available 24 hours/7 days per week for questions about diagnosis and management (888-448-8765) [7].

Posttest counseling of pregnant patients with HIV

When an individual's serostatus is determined to represent an incident infection, there is an acute need to provide appropriate posttest counseling, preferably in person. This counseling must address medical as well as

---

psychosocial aspects of the diagnosis, such as the need to dispel fears that may disrupt relationships with family, a partner, or other children. From a patient education standpoint, it is important to draw a clear distinction between HIV infection and acquired immunodeficiency syndrome (AIDS). The natural history of HIV disease, including the risks of AIDS and viral resistance with inconsistent use of antiretroviral therapy (ART) and benefits of long-term retention in HIV care should be outlined. Treatment with antiretrovirals should be presented as a path to a normal lifespan as well as a prevention strategy, given the understanding that maintaining a suppressed viral load following consistent use of a combined ART regimen prevents horizontal sexual transmission of HIV to partners [8]. Early on, a plan is established for postpartum engagement in HIV care with a primary infectious disease specialist, to minimize the risk of postpartum disengagement or loss to follow-up. Additionally, perinatal counseling focuses on the normalization of ART use during pregnancy, and the benefits of sustained viral suppression and ART for the patient, partner(s), and fetus. The discussion focuses on the risks of HIV to the pregnancy, rather than the risks of pregnancy on HIV control, which are thought to be minimal with access to highly efficacious ART. The expectation should be early rapid ART initiation and sustained viral suppression during pregnancy and thereafter, with viral suppression maintained between pregnancies for any patient who is of childbearing age.

Laboratory assessment of the pregnant patient with HIV

Although a focus of attention during pregnancy will be on the prevention of mother-to-child transmission of HIV, care begins with a focus on the health of the mother. For pregnant patients with known HIV, an assessment of prior ART regimens, side effects and adherence challenges, and prior genotype (viral resistance) testing should be obtained. For all patients, a baseline CD4 count and quantitative viral load provide a reliable picture of the patient's current viral and immune status, the likelihood of progression to clinical illness, and the need for instituting prophylaxis against opportunistic infection in addition to antiviral therapy. For patients with a new HIV diagnosis, presence of anti-toxoplasma immunoglobulin G (IgG) antibodies is assessed to determine latent infection and risk for reactivation. HIV genotype or resistance testing is usually performed at the initial visit for those who are ART naïve, or if virologic failure is suspected in a patient adherent to ART with a viral load (VL) >500 copies/mL. Baseline complete blood cell count and liver and renal function tests are obtained as well as routine sexually transmitted

infection screening for syphilis, chlamydial, or gonorrheal infection and trichomoniasis. Screening for hepatitis A virus (HAV), hepatitis C virus (HCV), and tuberculosis are recommended in addition to routine screening for hepatitis B virus (HBV). Finally, if the use of abacavir is anticipated or considered, HLA-B*5701 testing is indicated [9].

If the initial HIV viral load is suppressed and the patient is adherent to a recommended three-drug ART regimen, quantitative VL is repeated at least every 3 months or more frequently if ART adherence is questioned. For patients with detectable viremia, monthly VL is performed to establish a trend and determine whether the ART regimen should be altered (whether for virologic failure or poor adherence). The HIV VL is also assessed at around 34 to 36 weeks for delivery planning. A CD4 count is established at the initial visit and then every 3 months if ART use is less than 2 years or for those with CD4 counts <300 cells/mm^3 [9].

Recommended immunizations for pregnant patients with HIV

Pregnancy is an opportunity to optimize immunizations for patients living with HIV, who are at high risk of increased disease severity from secondary infectious diseases. For patients without evidence of HAV or HBV immunity (negative HAV IgG and HBV surface antibody titer <10 mIU/mL) who have not yet completed recommended vaccinations, and following negative HBV surface antigen screening, maternal vaccination is recommended [10]. Currently, a multidose immunization series is necessary for hepatitis B. Two hepatitis B vaccines are available for adults, include two recombinant HBsAg vaccines (Engerix-B and Recombivax-HB) and a newer, recombinant HBsAg vaccine conjugated to a cytosine phosphoguanine oligonucleotide (CpG 1018) adjuvant, which is a toll-like receptor 9 agonist (Heplisav-B). The Engerix-B and Recombivax-HB vaccines are currently recommended in pregnancy based on available safety data but require a prolonged dosing schedule (either 0, 1, and 6 or 0, 1, 2, and 6 months) for completion of the series. The newer Heplisav-B vaccine is a two-dose series (0 and 1 months) that has been shown to be more immunogenic in persons living with HIV, including those who have not responded to previous Engerix-B or Recombivax-HB series [11]. Although animal data are reassuring, data are currently limited for use of Heplisav-B in pregnancy [12]. For hepatitis A, either of two inactivated vaccines may be used on a two-dose schedule (Havrix and Vaqta at 0 and 6–12 or 6–18 months, respectively) [13]. If the CD4 count is <200 cells/mm^3 and risk assessment suggests risk of exposure to be low, waiting for CD4 >200 cells/mm^3 following ART initiation may be considered before beginning the HAV series, although delay is not recommended for hepatitis B immunization.

Additionally, vaccination against influenza, pneumococcus, Tdap (tetanus, diphtheria, and pertussis), and SARS-CoV-2 is recommended during pregnancy and for patients living with HIV [14]. These and other recommended immunizations may be distributed throughout pregnancy according to prevailing risk of exposure, gestational age, influenza season, SARS-CoV-2 prevalence, and patient preference. Vaccination against SARS-CoV-2 (COVID-19) is recommended regardless of CD4 count because the potential benefits outweigh potential risks, and because of the risk for severe or critical COVID-19 illness in pregnancy. For immunocompromised individuals, mRNA vaccines are preferred. An additional updated bivalent mRNA vaccine (including Omicron variant BA.4 and BA.5 as well as original strain) following a complete two-dose primary mRNA series is recommended for all individuals. Patients with moderate to severe immunocompromise, which includes those with advanced or untreated HIV infection or history of AIDS-defining illness without immune reconstitution, have the option to receive one additional dose of the bivalent mRNA vaccine at least 2 months following the last bivalent mRNA vaccine dose. Updated COVID vaccine guidelines may be found at https://www.cdc.gov/coronavirus/2019-ncov/vaccines/stay-up-to-date.html.

Antiretroviral treatment in pregnancy

At the initial prenatal visit, plans for initiation, continuation, or modification of an existing ART regimen should be established without regard to HIV RNA level (VL) or CD4 count [9]. For patients already adherent to a fully suppressive ART regimen, continuation is recommended in almost all cases.

For patients not initiated on, or adherent to, a three-drug regimen that is acceptable for use in pregnancy, initial laboratory assessment is previously described, and initiation of ART is not delayed for laboratory studies to result. The use of a three-drug regimen aimed at minimizing pill burden, side effects, and medication interactions is recommended and may be chosen in consultation with maternal–fetal medicine or infectious disease specialists with experience managing HIV in pregnancy. If necessary, a regimen may be modified based on laboratory and viral resistance studies. The typical regimen now initiated in pregnancy includes a dual-nucleoside reverse transcriptase inhibitor (NRTI) backbone plus either an integrase strand transfer inhibitor (INSTI) or a protease inhibitor (PI) (Table 29.1). Use of nonnucleoside reverse transcriptase inhibitors (NNRTIs) such as efavirenz or rilpivirine are no longer preferred as first line for initiation in ART-naïve pregnant patients. Considerations include timing of the dose (for example, INSTI dose should be taken at least 2 hours apart from iron or calcium

Table 29.1 Preferred antiretroviral regimens for initiation in ART-naïve pregnant people with HIV

Antiretroviral drug class	Pharmacokinetics in pregnancy	Dosing in pregnancy	Recommendations for use in pregnancy
Nucleoside reverse transcriptase inhibitor (NRTI) backbone	A dual-NRTI backbone is recommended for use as part of a combination regimen, usually either an INSTI or PI. There are no data on the use of two-drug oral regimens during pregnancy.		
Tenofovir alafenamide fumarate (TAF) with emtricitabine (FTC) or lamivudine (3TC)	No significant plasma pharmacokinetic changes in pregnancy No dose adjustments recommended during pregnancy	TAF/FTC available as fixed dose combination (Descovy): TAF 25 mg/FTC 200 mg tablet; one tablet daily without regard to food or TAF 25 mg (one tablet daily) plus 3TC 300 mg (one tablet daily) without regard to food	No evidence of teratogenicity in animals Alternative dosing/medication required for CrCl <30 mL/min
Tenofovir disoproxil fumarate (TDF) with emtricitabine (FTC) or lamivudine (3TC)	AUC lower in third trimester but trough levels are adequate No dose adjustments recommended during pregnancy	TDF/FTC available as fixed dose combination (Truvada): TDF 300 mg/FTC 200 mg tablet; one tablet daily without regard to food or TDF 300 mg (one tablet daily) plus 3TC 300 mg (one tablet daily) without regard to food	No evidence of human teratogenicity Alternative dosing/medication required for CrCl <50 mL/min

(Continued)

Table 29.1 (Continued)

Antiretroviral drug class	Pharmacokinetics in pregnancy	Dosing in pregnancy	Recommendations for use in pregnancy
Abacavir (ABC) with lamivudine (3TC)	No significant plasma pharmacokinetic changes in pregnancy No dose adjustments recommended during pregnancy	ABC/3TC available as fixed dose combination (Epzicom): ABC 600 mg / 3TC 300 mg tablet; one tablet daily without regard to food	No evidence of human teratogenicity Not for use in patients who test positive for HLA-B*5701 because of the risk of hypersensitivity reaction Not recommended for use with ATV/r if the pretreatment viral load is >100 000 copies/mL
Integrase strand transfer inhibitor (INSTI) regimens	Recommended for use in combination with dual-NRTI backbone		
Dolutegravir (DTG) *plus a preferred dual-NRTI backbone*	AUC may be decreased in third trimester but levels are adequate for inhibiting viral replication No dose adjustments recommended during pregnancy Associated with lower rates of INSTI resistance than RAL	DTG/ABC/3TC available as fixed drug combination (Triumeq): DTG 50 mg/ABC 600 mg/3TC 300 mg tablet; one tablet daily without regard to food DTG 50 mg tablet INSTI naïve: one tablet daily without regard to food INSTI experienced: one tablet twice daily without regard to food	No evidence of teratogenicity in animals Use of DTG/ABC/3TC requires HLA-B*5701 testing because of the risk of hypersensitivity reaction (see ABC) DTG should not be administered within 2 hours of minerals such as iron or calcium including prenatal vitamins DTG is preferred for acute HIV infection
Raltegravir (RAL) *plus a preferred dual-NRTI backbone*	Decreased concentration in third trimester but no dosing change recommended Must be dosed twice daily in pregnancy	400 mg tablet (one tablet twice daily) without regard to food RAL 100 mg chewable tablets are available	No evidence of human teratogenicity Rare cases of hypersensitivity reactions reported in nonpregnant adults RAL chewable tablets contain phenylalanine RAL should not be administered within 2 hours of minerals such as iron or calcium including prenatal vitamins
Protease inhibitor (PI) regimens	Recommended for use in combination with dual-NRTI backbone		
Atazanavir/ritonavir (ATV/r) *plus a preferred dual-NRTI backbone*	Decreased plasma ATV in second and third trimester with standard dosing, with further reduction if ATV is given concomitantly with TDF or H2-receptor antagonist Use of ATV is not recommended for ART-experienced pregnant patients who are taking *TDF and an H2-receptor antagonist. Not recommended for use with proton pump inhibitors (PPIs).* For pregnant patients receiving *either TDF or an H2-receptor antagonist*, a dose of ATV/r 400 mg/100 mg is recommended. Some experts recommend ATV/r 400 mg/100 mg dose in all women during second and third trimesters	ART naïve: ATV/r 300 mg/100 mg once daily with food ART experienced or taking either TDF or an H2-receptor antagonist: ATV/r 400 mg/100 mg once daily with food	No evidence of human teratogenicity ATV must be given with ritonavir boosting in pregnancy Oral powder (but *not* capsules) contains phenylalanine, which can be harmful to patients with phenylketonuria Avoid coadministration with H2-receptor antagonist: administer ATV/r 2 hours before or 10 hours after dose Use of ATV with cobicistat not recommended in pregnancy

Table 29.1 (Continued)

Antiretroviral drug class	Pharmacokinetics in pregnancy	Dosing in pregnancy	Recommendations for use in pregnancy
Darunavir/ritonavir (DRV/r) *plus a preferred dual-NRTI backbone*	Decreased exposure in pregnancy with use of DRV/r. Twice daily dosing is recommended for all pregnant patients	DRV/r 600 mg/100 mg twice daily with food	No evidence of human teratogenicity Use of DRV with cobicistat not recommended in pregnancy

ART, antiretroviral; AUC, area under the curve; CrCl, creatinine clearance; INSTI, integrase strand transfer inhibitor; NRTI, nucleoside reverse transcriptase inhibitor; PI, protease inhibitor. Adapted from [9].

supplements), pill burden and size, and drug interactions (azatanavir concentration is lower if the patient is concomitantly taking H2-receptor antagonists and tenofovir-containing regimens). If a regimen must be stopped during pregnancy for any reason, the entire ART regimen should be stopped and close follow up established until a complete regimen can be safely restarted. For third-trimester patients unable to tolerate a complete ART regimen, consideration is given to admission for directly observed therapy until a stable regimen is established, or until delivery if adherence to outpatient ART is unlikely.

Primary prophylaxis for prevention of *pneumocystis* pneumonia is indicated if CD4 T-cell count is <200 cells/mm³. The first-line regimen is trimethoprim-sulfamethoxazole, one double-strength tablet daily until the CD4 count is >200 cells/mm³ for at least 3 months. This regimen is also active for prevention of toxoplasma reactivation in those with CD4 <100 cells/mm³. Primary prophylaxis against *Mycobacterium avium* complex is no longer recommended for patients with CD4 <50 cells/mm³ who immediately initiate a complete ART regimen.

Labor and delivery care for pregnant patients living with HIV

Women living with HIV who are receiving oral ART should continue oral therapy during labor and delivery or on the day of cesarean delivery. During labor, intravenous administration of zidovudine (ZDV), which has high transplacental transfer, is recommended for patients with HIV RNA VL >1000 copies/mL or unknown HIV RNA near the time of delivery. Intrapartum prophylaxis is also recommended for patients with lower VLs who have questionable adherence, inconsistent virologic suppression, or limited prenatal care. Although there is less evidence for added benefit for use of intravenous ZDV for patients who have achieved and maintained virologic suppression <50 copies/mL with oral ART in the 4 weeks prior to delivery, clinical judgment and institutional practices may dictate its use. In one study, 6% of patients with suppressed VL during pregnancy had rebound detected

at delivery [15]. Intravenous ZDV is a 1-hour initial loading dose of 2 mg/kg, followed by a continuous infusion of 1 mg/kg/h for 2 hours, for a minimum of 3 hours before cesarean or until vaginal delivery. In select situations, urgent delivery following the loading dose may be necessary.

Cesarean delivery is recommended at 38 weeks, before the onset of labor and before rupture of membranes, among patients with either unknown VL or VL >1000 copies/mL near the time of delivery. Evaluating quantitative viral load at around 36 weeks for delivery planning purposes is common. Recommendations for mode and timing of delivery among women taking oral ART with VL <1000 copies/mL before delivery generally follow routine obstetric guidance [16]. This includes avoiding scheduled cesarean at less than 39 weeks in patients without another indication for early delivery. Similarly, there is no evidence for induction of labor before 39 weeks for the prevention of perinatal HIV transmission.

Use of invasive fetal scalp electrodes, intrauterine pressure catheter, and other invasive monitoring devices is avoided if possible, for patients with evidence of unsuppressed (>50 copies/mL) VL near delivery. Similarly, operative vaginal delivery with the use of vacuum extractor or obstetric is generally avoided if possible, for patients with unsuppressed VL. Management of intrapartum complications such as hemorrhage due to uterine atony requires consideration of the antiretroviral regimen due to the risk for medication interactions. The use of protease inhibitors or cobicistat, which are cytochrome P450 3A4 enzyme inhibitors, potentially increase the risk for an exaggerated vasoconstrictive response when combined with methergine [17]. In the case of uterine atony in a patient taking either of these agents, alternative treatments for uterine atony should be prioritized, or use of the lowest possible dose of methergine, if no alternative is available and the benefits outweigh the risks. Additionally, use of some NNRTIs such as nevirapine, efavirenz, and etravirine are CYP34A inducers and thus may decrease the level of methergine, so alternative agents for treatment of uterine atony should be considered.

Postpartum care for pregnant patients living with HIV

For all postpartum patients, ART should be continued after delivery, and any necessary changes in dosing or regimen anticipated and communicated before discharge. A contraceptive plan is determined ideally well before delivery, with discussion of future reproductive plans discussed in the context of the expectation of continued viral suppression for maternal, partner, and infant health. Importantly, a clear plan for follow-up with an infectious disease specialist as well as an obstetrician-gynecologist is critical to avoid a lapse in care or virologic rebound in the postpartum period, as well as to perform screening for postpartum depression. Additionally, the importance of infant follow-up and neonatal antiretroviral prophylaxis should be emphasized by the obstetrician. The neonatal antiretroviral regimen is determined by pediatric infectious disease specialists based on maternal oral ART adherence and VL near delivery, receipt of intravenous ZDV prophylaxis intrapartum, and other risk factors [18]. Single or dual antiretroviral agent prophylaxis is used for infants at low risk of perinatal HIV acquisition and includes zidovudine for 4 weeks with or without additional agents. For infants at highest risk of HIV acquisition, including those born to patients not adherent to oral ART regimen or who have an unsuppressed viral load near delivery, a three-drug regimen known as "presumptive HIV therapy" may be initiated.

Counseling regarding infant feeding practices remains consistent in the United States, and breastfeeding is not recommended regardless of maternal VL at delivery. The evidence for vertical transmission of 10–20% with breastfeeding over 2 years is from trials conducted before maternal ART was routine [19]. However, the PROMISE trial conducted between 2011 and 2014 demonstrated that among 2431 mother–infant pairs randomized to either maternal ART or infant prophylaxis until 18 months or breastfeeding cessation, the risk for vertical HIV transmission was 0.6% at 12 months [20]. Vertical transmission is higher if adherence to maternal ART or neonatal prophylaxis is inconsistent [21]. Additionally, although suppression of maternal cell-free viral RNA can be achieved with ART, evidence suggests that cell-associated virus in T lymphocytes may provide a latent reservoir of HIV-1 proviral DNA that is capable of establishing infection in the neonate [22]. Understanding and conveying the most current evidence is key to maintaining a physician–patient relationship. Ultimately, the choice for infant feeding is influenced by cultural, psychosocial, and economic factors, and the clinician should approach counseling in a nonjudgmental way. If after counseling, the patient elects to breastfeed, risk-reduction strategies are employed [23]. Although studies prior to widespread use of maternal ART have shown that limited (6 months) exclusive breastfeeding is associated with lower vertical HIV transmission compared with mixed breast and formula feeding, evidence from contemporaneous cohorts is lacking [24]. Risk-reduction measures include supporting maternal ART adherence and consistent virologic suppression throughout breastfeeding, with viral load monitoring every 2 months or if nonadherence is suspected. Gradual (over rapid) weaning while introducing complementary foods after 6 months is encouraged. A plan for infant prophylaxis and serial HIV screening is established in consultation with pediatric infectious disease expert. Monitoring for and treating maternal mastitis or infant thrush, both associated with increased HIV transmission, is recommended.

Ethical and legal considerations

The opportunity for HIV diagnosis should not be missed in pregnant patients. However, once diagnosed, ethical and legal obligations may differ according to jurisdiction. Obstetricians should be aware of the locally relevant statutes regarding HIV reporting and delivering of positive HIV results, and act as patient advocate while recognizing the need for public health intervention success. Importantly, a capable clinician should arrange prompt posttest counseling (preferably in-person in a private setting) to ensure the patient understands the result and is promptly linked to medical and social support services, whether pregnant or postpartum. Respect for the patient's confidentiality is paramount, and the clinician should encourage patient-initiated disclosure of serostatus to sexual partners only if safety is assured. Engagement of local or state health department disease intervention specialists for assistance with confidential partner services is encouraged.

Conclusion

In the twenty-first century, HIV has become a treatable infection whose transmission from mother to child can be eliminated. With advances in therapeutics that make ART tolerable and safe in pregnancy, as well as increasing access to new therapies in both developing countries and hard-to-reach populations in developed countries, the end of the HIV epidemic is achievable. With a renewed focus on increasing early diagnosis and maternal knowledge of HIV status, expediting linkage to HIV care and viral suppression during pregnancy, and optimizing management of labor and delivery and postpartum continuity to care, obstetricians can meaningfully contribute to the elimination of perinatal HIV infection.

CASE PRESENTATION

The patient is a 30-year-old gravida 1 para 0 at 12 weeks gestation who presented following routine HIV testing at her first prenatal visit. The fourth-generation combination p24 and HIV-1 and HIV-2 immunoassay was reactive, and the differentiation assay identified HIV-1 antibodies. Additionally, urine molecular testing for gonorrhea was positive. When the patient was informed of the results, she denied any history of intravenous drug use and reported a new sexual partner with unknown HIV status in the past 12 months and three lifetime sexual partners. She was unable to recall any symptoms suggestive of acute HIV infection. The initial evaluation included a CD4 count that was 380 cells/mm³ and a viral load of 12 000 copies/mL. HIV genotype, liver function tests, complete blood count, hepatitis serologies, and sexually transmitted infection screening was performed along with routine prenatal blood studies. Appropriate vaccinations were given. Treatment for gonorrhea was given, and she provided partner information that was conveyed to the local health department for partner services for both HIV and gonorrhea. She was informed about the importance of prompt treatment for maternal health, and for prevention of horizontal and vertical HIV transmission. After review of her other medications, an antiretroviral therapy regimen with dual-NRTI backbone (Descovy; tenofovir alafenamide fumarate [TAF] 25 mg with emtricitabine [FTC] 200 mg) once daily and INSTI (dolutegravir 50 mg) once daily was initiated. She was scheduled to return for repeat viral load testing in a month. Within 1 month, her viral load had decreased substantially, and by 2 months her viral load was undetectable. Her CD4 count rose to 440 cells/mm³ after 3 months. Repeat screening for gonorrhea was negative. At 36 weeks gestation, her viral load remained undetectable and vaginal delivery was planned. She arrived in early labor at 39 weeks, and an intravenous infusion of ZDV was begun. Oral ART was continued during labor. She had an uncomplicated spontaneous vaginal delivery, and elected formula feeding. A plan for contraceptive, infant prophylaxis and maternal and infant follow up with infectious disease specialists was established, and she continued the current ART regimen at discharge. At postpartum follow-up, the patient remained well and a long-acting reversible contraceptive was initiated. Her child remained uninfected and the patient had a negative screen for postpartum depression, with adequate social and mental health support in the postpartum period.

References

1. HIV global statistics. [updated 2022 Aug 3; cited 2022 Feb 20]. Available from: https://www.hiv.gov/hiv-basics/overview/data-and-trends/global-statistics.

2. Centers for Disease Control and Prevention. Diagnosis of HIV infection in the United States and dependent areas 2019: special focus profiles. [last reviewed 2021 Oct 15; cited 2022 Feb 20]. Available from: https://www.cdc.gov/hiv/library/reports/hiv-surveillance/vol-32/content/special-focus-profiles.html#Women.

3. Thomson KA, Hughes J, Baeten JM, John-Stewart G, Celum C, Cohen CR, et al. Increased risk of HIV acquisition among women throughout pregnancy and during the postpartum period: a prospective per-coital-act analysis among women with HIV-infected partners. J Infect Dis. 2018;218(1):16–25.

4. America's HIV epidemic analysis dashboard. 2021 [cited 2022 Feb 20]. Available from: https://ahead.hiv.gov/.

5. US Preventive Services Task Force. Human immunodeficiency screening. 2019 Jun 11 [cited 2022 Feb 20]. Available from: https://www.uspreventiveservicestaskforce.org/uspstf/recommendation/human-immunodeficiency-virus-hiv-infection-screening.

6. Centers for Disease Control and Prevention. FDA approved HIV tests. [last reviewed 2023 May 1; cited 2022 Feb 20]. Available from: https://www.cdc.gov/hiv/testing/laboratorytests.html.

7. AIDS Education and Training Center Program. [cited 2022 Feb 20]. Available from: https://aidsetc.org/.

8. Cohen MS, Chen YQ, McCauley M, Gamble T, Hosseinipour MC, Kumarasamy N, et al.; HPTN 052 Study Team. Antiretroviral therapy for the prevention of HIV-1 transmission. N Engl J Med. 2016 Sep 1;375(9):830–9.

9. Recommendations for the use of antiretroviral drugs during pregnancy and interventions to reduce perinatal HIV transmission in the United States. [updated 2023 Jan 31; cited 2022 Feb 20]. Available from: https://clinicalinfo.hiv.gov/en/guidelines/perinatal.

10. Celzo F, Buyse H, Welby S, Ibrahimi A. Safety evaluation of adverse events following vaccination with Havrix, Engerix-B or Twinrix during pregnancy. Vaccine. 2020 Sep 11; 38(40):6215–23.

11. Khaimova R, Fischetti B, Cope R, Berkowitz L, Bakshi A. Serological response with Heplisav-B® in prior Hepatitis B vaccine non-responders living with HIV. Vaccine. 2021 Oct 22;39(44):6529–34.

12. Centers for Disease Control and Prevention. Heplisav-B® (HepB-CpG) vaccine. [last updated 2018 Apr 24; cited 2022 Feb 20]. Available from: https://www.cdc.gov/vaccines/schedules/vacc-updates/heplisav-b.pdf.

13. Nelson NP, Weng MK, Hofmeister MG, Moore KL, Doshani M, Kamili S, et al. Prevention of hepatitis A virus infection in the United States: recommendations of the Advisory Committee on Immunization Practices, 2020. MMWR Recomm Rep. 2020;69(No. RR-5):1–38.

14. Guidelines for the prevention and treatment of opportunistic infections in adults and adolescents with HIV. [updated 2023

Apr 13; cited 2022 Feb 20]. Available from: https://clinicalinfo. hiv.gov/en/guidelines/adult-and-adolescent-opportunistic-infection/recommended-immunization-schedule.

15. Boucoiran I, Albert AYK, Tulloch K, Wagner EC, Pick N, van Schalkwyk J, et al. Human immunodeficiency virus viral load rebound near delivery in previously suppressed, combination antiretroviral therapy-treated pregnant women. Obstet Gynecol. 2017;130(3):497–501.

16. American College of Obstetricians and Gynecologists. Committee Opinion No. 751: labor and delivery management of women with human immunodeficiency virus infection. Obstet Gynecol. 2018 Sep;132(3):e131–7.

17. Navarro J, Curran A, Burgos J, Torrella A, Ocaña I, Falcó V, et al. Acute leg ischaemia in an HIV-infected patient receiving antiretroviral treatment. Antivir Ther. 2017;22(1):89–90. doi: 10.3851/IMP3075. Epub 2016 Aug 22.

18. Guidelines for the use of antiretroviral agents in pediatric HIV infection. [updated 2023 Apr 11; cited 2022 Feb 20]. Available from: https://clinicalinfo.hiv.gov/en/guidelines/pediatric-arv.

19. Nduati R, John G, Mbori-Ngacha D, Richardson B, Overbaugh J, Mwatha A, et al. Effect of breastfeeding and formula feeding on transmission of HIV-1: a randomized clinical trial. JAMA. 2000;283(9):1167–74.

20. Flynn PM, Taha TE, Cababasay M, Fowler MG, Mofenson LM, Owor M, et al. Prevention of HIV-1 transmission through breastfeeding: efficacy and safety of maternal antiretroviral therapy versus Infant nevirapine prophylaxis for duration of breastfeeding in HIV-1-infected women with high CD4 cell count (IMPAACT PROMISE): a randomized, open label, clinical trial. J Acquir Immune Defic Syndr. 2017;77(4):383–92.

21. Flynn PM, Taha TE, Cababasay M, Butler K, Fowler MG, Mofenson LM, et al. Association of maternal viral load and CD4 count with perinatal HIV-1 transmission risk during breastfeeding in the PROMISE Postpartum component. J Acquir Immune Defic Syndr. 2021;88(2):206–13.

22. Ndirangu J, Viljoen J, Bland RM, Danaviah S, Thorne C, Van de Perre P, et al. Cell-free (RNA) and cell-associated (DNA) HIV-1 and postnatal transmission through breastfeeding. PLoS One. 2012;7:e51493.

23. Levison J, Weber S, Cohan D. Breastfeeding and HIV-infected women in the United States: harm reduction counseling strategies. Clin Infect Dis. 2014;59(2):304–9.

24. Coovadia HM, Rollins NC, Bland RM, Little K, Coutsoudis A, Bennish ML, et al. Mother-to-child transmission of HIV-1 infection during exclusive breastfeeding in the first 6 months of life: an intervention cohort study. Lancet. 2007;369(9567):1107–16.

Chapter 30
Pregnancy in Women with Disabilities

Caroline Signore

Eunice Kennedy Shriver National Institute of Child Health and Human Development, Bethesda, MD, USA

Disability is defined in multiple ways, with common features including the existence of a bodily or mental impairment that, along with barriers in the built and attitudinal environment, makes certain activities more difficult and limits one's ability to participate in social, recreational, and/or community life. US data from 2016 (See Table 30.1) indicate that nearly 18% of women of reproductive age report at least one disability related to hearing, vision, cognition, mobility, self-care, or independent living [1]. Physical disabilities such as cerebral palsy, spinal cord injury, and multiple sclerosis are associated with limitations of mobility, flexibility, and/or dexterity; sensory disabilities include vision and hearing impairments; and cognitive or intellectual and developmental disabilities (IDD) are neurodevelopmental disorders characterized by limitations in cognitive, communication, and social domains [2,3].

Most women with disabilities (WWD) do not have impaired fertility, and many want to be mothers. The number of women of reproductive age with disabilities is increasing and rates of pregnancy among WWD are increasing. Statewide delivery data from California indicate that the proportion of all births among women with physical, sensory, or IDD more than doubled between 2000 and 2010 [4]. Multiple studies have shown that the prevalence of pregnancy is similar among women with and without disabilities, refuting pervasive stereotypes about reproductive choices among WWD [5–7]. Iezzoni and colleagues [5] found that, after adjusting for sociodemographic characteristics related to pregnancy, pregnancy rates among women with physical disabilities are similar to nondisabled women (adjusted odds ratio [aOR] of current pregnancy 0.83 (95% confidence interval [CI] 0.65–1.05, *P* = 0.12). In another study Iezzoni et al. [6] reported an annual pregnancy rate of 2% among women with spinal cord injury (SCI). Houtchens et al. used US administrative claims data to show that the proportion of women with pregnancy and multiple sclerosis (MS)

increased from 7.91% in 2006 to 9.47% in 2014 [8]. Pregnancy rates decrease with the severity of the limiting condition [5,7].

This chapter summarizes emerging evidence on pregnancy risks and outcomes among WWD, including those with physical, cognitive or intellectual and developmental, and sensory disabilities.

General considerations

Demographic disadvantages

It is well documented that WWDs experience persistent disparities in healthcare access and outcomes compared with nondisabled women [9]. Social determinants of health and risk factors for poor pregnancy outcomes are more prevalent in the disability community [2], with lower educational attainment and employment, higher poverty rates, higher rates of housing and food insecurity, and higher rates of social isolation [10–11].

Pregnant WWD share these disadvantages and are more likely than women without disabilities to be unemployed or unable to work, unmarried, publicly insured, or uninsured, live in poverty, and have lower educational attainment [12–16].

Prepregnancy health and wellness

Compared to women of reproductive age without disabilities, WWD are more likely to enter pregnancy in poorer health. Mitra et al. used 2010 Behavioral Risk Factor Surveillance System data to examine preconception health risk factors among women of reproductive age. Compared to women without disabilities, WWD who intended to conceive in the next 5 years (N = 1728) had a significantly higher adjusted prevalence ratio of self-reported fair or poor health [17]. Studies have shown that WWD have higher prevalence of many preconception risk factors, including obesity, diabetes, hypertension,

---

Queenan's Management of High-Risk Pregnancy: An Evidence-Based Approach, Seventh Edition. Edited by Catherine Y. Spong and Charles J. Lockwood.
© 2024 John Wiley & Sons Ltd. Published 2024 by John Wiley & Sons Ltd.

237

Table 30.1 Weighted unadjusted prevalence estimates of disability among US women aged 18–44 years, by type of disability – Behavioral Risk Factor Surveillance System, 2016

Type of disability[a]	%
Hearing	1.6
Vision	3.0
Cognition	11.7
Mobility	5.6
Self-care	1.7
Independent living	5.5
Any	17.9

[a]Each disability type might not be independent; a respondent might have two or more disability types. Adapted from Okoro, 2018 [1].

asthma, sexually transmitted infections, depressive symptoms, smoking, binge drinking, and drug use and rehabilitation [17–19].

These disadvantages are also prevalent during pregnancy among WWD, who also are more likely to rate their health as poor. An analysis of National Health Interview Survey data from 2006–2011 showed that among pregnant women with mobility difficulties, 29% reported fair or poor health compared to 3.2% of gravidas without impaired mobility [20]. Multiple studies have demonstrated a higher prevalence of coexisting health conditions across disability subtypes among pregnant WWD. Up to 75% of pregnant WWD have one or more preexisting health problems [20], including overweight and obesity [20]), hypertension [14,16,20–25], heart disease or stroke [8,16,20,25], pregestational diabetes [3,14,16,20,22,24], asthma [16,20,25], renal disease [16], HIV [16], and/or thyroid disease [16,25]. These conditions may be more likely to be poorly controlled among people with disabilities [26] and compounded among women at the intersection of disability and race or ethnicity [15] and other social determinants of health. Thus, it is recommended that WWD who desire pregnancy receive preconception care to optimize health status before pregnancy [15,20,26–29].

Medication use

Many women with disabilities use medication regularly for treatment of the underlying disorder or prevention and management of secondary conditions. Ideally, medication use should be evaluated preconceptionally and regimens modified or discontinued as appropriate. The effects of many drugs on fetal development may not be well understood. Women who must continue medications during pregnancy should be counseled about potential risks and fetal effects of treatment and the possible risks of nontreatment to the extent possible. The use of disease-modifying therapies during pregnancy and postpartum in MS and treatments for other conditions should be tailored according to a patient's age, disease activity, disability, risks of discontinuing treatment vs. maintaining therapy, and patient preference [30].

Psychosocial risk factors

All women are at risk for psychosocial concerns during pregnancy; however, a higher background prevalence of some psychosocial problems among WWD suggests careful screening is warranted.

Abuse

Multiple studies have demonstrated that people with disabilities experience higher rates of abuse than nondisabled peers. Beyond the threat of bodily harm (e.g. kicking, slapping) and sexual assault, abuse may take the form of refusal to provide needed assistance, withholding of medication or adaptive equipment, or neglect. Frequently, abuse against people with disabilities is perpetrated by personal attendants and health care providers [31]. Women with mobility impairments may find it difficult or impossible to extract themselves from abusive situations and thus are at risk for prolonged exposure to abuse as compared to able-bodied women [31]. A simple tool for screening for abuse among WWD is available [32]. Approximately two thirds of women with physical disabilities have experienced some form of physical violence or abuse [31]. A recent meta-analysis showed that people with disabilities are at higher risk of being sexually abused (aOR 1.49, 95% CI 1.27–1.76) [33]. WWD are significantly more likely to experience physical abuse during pregnancy as well [34,35]. An analysis of Massachusetts Pregnancy Risk Assessment Monitoring System (PRAMS) data demonstrated that physical abuse was significantly more common among WWD both before (13.6%) and during (8.1%) pregnancy, compared to women without disabilities (2.8% and 2.3%, respectively) [34].

Mental health

Compared to nondisabled women, women with disabilities report higher levels of perceived stress [36] and feelings of sadness, unhappiness, or depression [37]. Recent data show that symptomatology and diagnosed mental health conditions are more common among pregnant WWD as well. An analysis of National Health Interview Survey data from 2006 to 2011 showed that pregnant women with chronic physical disabilities are three to six times more likely to report having symptoms of a mental health problem (such as sadness, nervousness, hopelessness) than nondisabled pregnant women (67% vs. 30%, $P<0.0001$) [38]. Multiple investigators have found that pregnant WWD have a significantly higher prevalence of mental health diagnoses [22,24,26,39], including depression [8,16], anxiety [8,16], psychotic conditions [3], and substance use disorders [3]. An analysis of Rhode Island PRAMS data from 2009–2011 found that 25% of mothers with disabilities were diagnosed with depression during pregnancy compared to 7.6% of other mothers [13].

Perceived stress is common in pregnancy, and especially so for WWD. Mitra and colleagues [13] used PRAMS data to show that WWD had significantly increased rates of maternal stressors during pregnancy (86% vs. 71%, P< 0.001) [13]. Booth et al. [35] analyzed Massachusetts PRAMS data and found that, compared to women without disabilities, WWD were more likely to report stressful life events in the 12 months before birth (87% vs. 67%, P< 0.00001). Among those experiencing six or more stressors, WWD were nearly four times more likely than women without disabilities to report postpartum depressive symptoms. WWD describe struggling with feeling unsupported and isolated after delivery [40] and are more likely to report often or always feeling down, depressed, or sad postpartum (28.9% vs. 10%) [13]. In analyses adjusted for other factors associated with mental health outcomes, WWD were more likely than nondisabled women to report symptoms of postpartum depression (adjusted risk ratio [aRR] 1.6, 95% CI 1.1–2.2) [13]. In a population-based comparison of pregnancy outcomes among people with (n = 529) and without (n = 5282) congenital or acquired spinal cord lesions, women with spinal conditions had a greater than eightfold increased risk of rehospitalization for postpartum depression (RR 8.15, 95% CI 4.29–15.48) [41].

Tobacco, alcohol, and substance use and misuse

Smoking is more common among people with disabilities than the public generally, including during pregnancy [16,38]. In one study of Massachusetts PRAMS data, compared to nondisabled pregnant women, WWD were significantly more likely to smoke a pack or more of cigarettes per day and to smoke continuously before, during, and after pregnancy (aRR 1.8, 95% CI 1.2–2.8) [42]. Beyond the well-known adverse pregnancy effects of smoking, for women with physical disabilities and mobility impairment, tobacco use increases the risk of pressure ulcer formation and impairs wound healing.

Most reports indicate that nonpregnant WWD consume alcohol at rates and amounts similar to those of women in general [43]. Multiple studies [8,13,16] have found that pregnant WWD drink alcohol at rates similar to pregnant women without disabilities. In contrast, illicit drug use is more common among WWD than in the general population, with risk factors including chronic pain, use of prescription drugs, social adjustment difficulties, and being a victim of substance-abuse-related violence [19,44], but little is known about substance use during pregnancy among WWD. In one Canadian study, birthing people with IDD or multiple disabilities had a higher prevalence of substance use disorder than those without disabilities [26].

Weight gain, mobility, and skin integrity

For women with impaired mobility, weight gain and alterations in body mechanics associated with advancing pregnancy can pose special problems. Increased weight may make it difficult for women to propel a manual wheelchair, prevent them from accomplishing transfers (for example from wheelchair to bed) independently, or increase risk for falls. Additionally, extra weight increases the risk for pressure ulceration, a preventable condition that can cause substantial morbidity. Frequent skin inspection, weight-shifting maneuvers, and adjustments in wheelchair seating and cushioning may be needed to prevent this complication. Care must also be taken to shift positions frequently during labor and postpartum to prevent skin injury [28]. Women who are ambulatory may experience increased fatigue carrying pregnancy weight or may find that their altered center of gravity makes ambulation more difficult and increases risk for injury from falls.

Urinary tract function and infections

Bladder dysfunction and urinary tract infections (UTIs) are common among women with physical disabilities; these problems may be exacerbated by pregnancy. Spinal cord injury, MS, and spina bifida are frequently associated with neurogenic bladder. Pregnant women with SCI, for example, rely on permanent indwelling catheters (urethral or suprapubic 35%) or intermittent catheterization (25%) for urinary management [45], often reflecting a change from prepregnancy management [46]. New-onset incontinence may develop in nearly 50% of pregnant women with SCI [46]. Andretta et al. reported a retrospective cohort study of 52 primigravidas with spinal cord lesions and found frequent changes to bladder management, recurrent UTI, new or worsening urinary incontinence, and bowel dysfunction during pregnancy [46].

Among individuals with spinal injuries, rates of asymptomatic bacteriuria are 50% in those who void via intermittent catheterization and 100% in those with chronic indwelling catheters [47]. It is important to distinguish urinary tract colonization and bacteriuria from true UTI in the setting of a neurogenic bladder. Women with SCI may have unique symptoms of a UTI, including increased spasticity and autonomic dysreflexia (discussed later).

UTIs in patients with SCI [45] and MS [48] are common in pregnancy. According to a 2011 systematic review of 163 women with 226 pregnancies, among women with SCI, UTI occurred at least once during pregnancy in 64% and in 100% of those with indwelling catheters [45]. Several studies [41,45,49] suggest that the risk of pyelonephritis in pregnancy is higher among gravidas with disabilities. In one study, acute pyelonephritis (defined as UTI with fever >38° C) developed in 36% of pregnant women with cervical SCI, but just 7% of those with thoracic lesions in a single center retrospective study of 65 pregnancies [46].

Experts disagree about the use of antibiotics for UTI prophylaxis in pregnant WWD. In one small study, a weekly oral cyclic antibiotic regimen significantly decreased the incidence of UTI in pregnancy as compared to prepregnancy incidence in women with SCI [50]. Though antibiotic prophylaxis is prescribed for gravidas with SCI and other physical disabilities in some centers [45,49,51], there is no consensus in the literature about the optimal management of bacteriuria or UTI prevention in pregnant women with physical disabilities [47]. The American College of Obstetricians and Gynecologists (ACOG) concluded that evidence was insufficient to recommend frequent screening or treatment for asymptomatic bacteriuria in women with SCI, but recommended that clinicians consider extended course (14 days) antibiotics for treatment of symptomatic UTI in patients with SCI [52].

Respiratory complications

Conditions such as MS, SCI, spinal muscular atrophy, and spina bifida may weaken muscles of respiration and/or cause kyphoscoliosis [8,53–55], predisposing pregnant patients to respiratory compromise that may be worsened as the gravid uterus displaces the diaphragm upward. Some experts recommend baseline and serial pulmonary function tests in WWD to monitor vital capacity [53–55]. WWD may also have impaired coughing and be prone to atelectasis, which may increase the incidence and/or severity of perinatal pneumonia.

Venous thromboembolic disease

Limited mobility, obesity, and higher prevalence of smoking may increase the risk of venous thromboembolism (VTE) among pregnant people with disabilities. In a survey of 24 women with SCI who had completed 37 pregnancies, a thrombotic event occurred in 3 (8%) of pregnancies [56]. More recently, Crane et al. reported a greater than ninefold increased risk of VTE/pulmonary embolism during pregnancy among women with paralytic spinal cord disorders compared with controls (RR 9.16, 95% CI 2.17–38.60) [41]. Another recent study [16] reported a significantly greater than fivefold increase in VTE among women with physical disabilities and a significant 10-fold increase in women with hearing or vision impairments (aRR 10.65, 95% CI 4.73–24.04). Women with IDDs also may be at higher risk. In a population-based Canadian study [3], VTE occurred more often in women with IDDs than in control pregnancies (aRR = 1.60, 95% CI 1.17–2.19), but another study found no increased risk [16].

The use of routine thromboprophylaxis during pregnancy in women with paralysis or other mobility disorders has not been tested in clinical trials and the risk-benefit ratio of anticoagulation is unclear. Nevertheless, this therapy is instituted with some regularity; in a survey study of postpartum women with SCI, 19% received thromboprophylaxis during pregnancy [56],

and some experts recommend thromboprophylaxis from 28 weeks to 6 weeks postpartum [57]. A small survey of Canadian physicians revealed substantial variation in clinicians' use of VTE prophylaxis among women with physical disabilities in the antepartum and postpartum periods, with maternal–fetal medicine specialists more likely to prescribe antepartum thromboprophylaxis for a pregnant young woman using a wheelchair (73%) than internal medicine physicians (8%) [58]. ACOG suggests considering mechanical or pharmacologic VTE prophylaxis based on patient history, individual risk factors, and local practice [52].

Antepartum consultation

Depending upon the nature and severity of a woman's disability and condition, antepartum care could require coordination of care and consultation with several appropriate specialists. Obstetrician-gynecologists in general practice may seek consultation with maternal–fetal medicine specialists to plan obstetric management and monitor maternal and fetal well-being. All maternity care providers should seek and maintain contact with women's primary care providers and specialists (physiatrists, neurologists, rheumatologists, etc.) to collaboratively monitor the status of the disabling condition, development or progression of secondary conditions, recommend any medication use or changes, and to plan strategies for prevention and management of complications. Antepartum consultation with an obstetric anesthesiologist is highly recommended. For women who have had abdominal surgeries such as augmentation cystoplasty or ventriculoperitoneal shunting, prenatal consultation with the urologist or neurosurgeon is advisable; if cesarean delivery is required, these colleagues should be invited to assist at the time of surgery. Some recommend an upper uterine incision in these patients [55], but a low-transverse cesarean is possible in some cases [59].

Barriers to care

The Americans with Disabilities Act of 1990 (ADA) ushered in an era of improved access and participation in society for people with disabilities. Nevertheless, barriers remain, taking diverse forms, such as limitations in access to transportation, lack of health insurance or underinsurance, difficulty with physical access within health care facilities, fragmented care delivered by multiple providers, and stubbornly pervasive negative attitudes about disability [9].

In the office, WWD may have difficulty completing lengthy medical history forms, or require assistance to collect a urine specimen. Very few offices have a platform scale designed to weigh women seated in wheelchairs, thus making impossible one of the most fundamental assessments in prenatal care. Many women who use wheelchairs could transfer to an exam table independently but are prevented from doing so if the table cannot be lowered to wheelchair height (17–20 inches). Joint contractures or neuromuscular spasticity may make achieving and maintaining position for a pelvic exam difficult or impossible without adaptations. Individuals who are deaf or hard of hearing (DHH) are at higher risk of poorer health literacy than their hearing peers, and women who are DHH often report communication difficulties in prenatal care (and during labor and delivery), even though the ADA requires health providers to provide qualified interpreters [60]. Women who are blind or have low vision describe dissatisfaction with perinatal care that is not adapted for their needs, such as being asked to fill lengthy written forms, childbirth education materials that are not accessible (also required by the ADA) or providers neglecting to orient them to the physical layout of offices, exam rooms, or labor rooms [61]. Communication difficulties are also a major barrier for women with IDD, who may struggle to understand providers' instructions and recommendations [62].

WWD report being troubled by perceived negative attitudes from health care providers and others. When presenting for prenatal care, some women feel that their practitioners do not consider them capable or qualified to parent and that they are thought to be irresponsible for becoming pregnant with a disability [63,64]. It is not unusual for WWD to be afraid and have anxiety over the possibility that these biases may lead to referrals to child protective services and loss of custody before an adequate evaluation and provision of supports [62,65]. Another attitudinal barrier may arise in discussions of prenatal screening and genetic counseling. Some WWD may view these measures as devaluing and consider them an offensive attempt by society to eliminate people with bodily or mental differences.

Patients with disabilities and health care providers themselves recognize a substantial gap in training when it comes to provision of patient-centered disability-competent perinatal care [15,61,66,67]. Clinician education needs to include health aspects of maternal care for WWD and training to recognize and counter implicit biases toward disability, sexuality, pregnancy, and parenting by WWD [15,68].

Pregnancy outcomes

Across disability types

Most WWD can expect largely uneventful pregnancies and normal birth outcomes [14]. Nevertheless, a growing body of evidence suggests that risks for pregnancy complications are higher among WWD compared to their nondisabled counterparts. The reasons for these increased risks are not well understood but may involve interactions between the pregnant state and the condition causing the disability. In addition, it is plausible that poor outcomes are related to poor preconception health status among WWD generally [19], barriers to care, and/or

pervasive disparities in social determinants of health that disproportionally affect WWD. Unplanned pregnancy is common among WWD [69] and may reflect inadequate sexual and contraceptive counseling. Lack of practitioner training, poor communication, and other barriers to care unique to WWD may play a part. One research group [16] suggests that their findings of increased risk of adverse maternal outcomes in pregnant WWD may be related to underrecognition of the higher risks faced by WWD and lack of knowledge or discomfort providers experience while managing their pregnancies.

In an analysis of Medical Expenditure Panel Survey (MEPS) data from 1996–2007, Horner-Johnson et al. found few differences in the odds of live birth, miscarriage, and abortion among US women with and without disabilities [14]. An analysis of National Survey of Family Growth data showed that women with physical, cognitive, and independent living disabilities had significantly increased odds of experiencing at least one miscarriage in the last 5 years (aOR 1.65–1.99) [70]; however, reasons for these losses were not clear.

Multiple studies point to increased risk of adverse pregnancy outcomes across disability types. For example, Gleason and colleagues [16] analyzed data from the Consortium on Safe Labor, a cohort of deliveries from 19 US hospitals that included 2074 WWD and 221, 311 without. They found that WWD as a group had significantly higher risk of almost all adverse maternal outcomes examined, including hypertensive disorders, gestational diabetes, placenta previa, premature rupture of the fetal membranes (PROM), and preterm PROM (PPROM; see Figure 30.1). A recent systematic review and metanalysis of 23 studies representing >8.5 million women found that women with any disability had significantly increased risk of hypertensive disorders of pregnancy (OR 1.45, 95% CI 1.16–1.82) and cesarean delivery (OR 1.31, 95% CI 1.02–1.68) [29]. Biel and colleagues analyzed California statewide data comprising more than 2.4 million births and reported that, across every type of disability (physical, hearing, vision, IDD), WWD had significantly higher risk of gestational diabetes (except DHH women), gestational hypertension/preeclampsia, and preterm birth [24]. A population-based study from Canada showed that compared to women without disabilities, WWD (n >201K) have increased risk of a composite severe maternal morbidity and mortality outcome, with commonest indicators being postpartum hemorrhage, maternal intensive care unit (ICU) admission, puerperal sepsis, and severe preeclampsia and hemolysis, elevated liver enzymes, and low platelet count (HELLP) syndrome [26]. Barring any specific contraindication or expected drug interaction with low dose aspirin, in consultation with the provider managing the disabling condition, providers can initiate therapy in WWD at risk for preeclampsia as recommended for the wider obstetric population at risk.

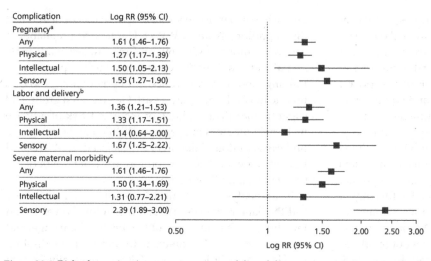

Complication	Log RR (95% CI)
Pregnancy[a]	
Any	1.61 (1.46–1.76)
Physical	1.27 (1.17–1.39)
Intellectual	1.50 (1.05–2.13)
Sensory	1.55 (1.27–1.90)
Labor and delivery[b]	
Any	1.36 (1.21–1.53)
Physical	1.33 (1.17–1.51)
Intellectual	1.14 (0.64–2.00)
Sensory	1.67 (1.25–2.22)
Severe maternal morbidity[c]	
Any	1.61 (1.46–1.76)
Physical	1.50 (1.34–1.69)
Intellectual	1.31 (0.77–2.21)
Sensory	2.39 (1.89–3.00)

Log RR (95% CI)

[a] Maternal pregnancy composite includes pregnancy-related hypertensive diseases, gestational diabetes, placental abruption, placenta previa, premature rupture of membranes, and preterm premature rupture of membranes.

[b] Labor and delivery composite includes chorioamnionitis, hemorrhage, blood transfusion, thromboembolism, postpartum fever, infection, cardiovascular events, cardiomyopathy, and maternal death.

[c] Severe maternal morbidity composite includes severe preeclampsia/eclampsia, hemorrhage, thromboembolism, fever, endometritis, major puerperal infection, wound infection/separation, sepsis, cardiomyopathy, and cardiovascular event.

Figure 30.1 Risk of experiencing any pregnancy or labor, delivery, or postpartum complication by disability status. CI, confidence interval; RR, risk ratio. Gleason JL et al. 2021/American Medical Association/Public Domain CC-BY License Permissions. This is an open access article distributed under the terms of the CC-BY license, which permits unrestricted use, distribution, and reproduction in any medium. You are not required to obtain permission to reuse this article content, provided that you credit the author and journal.

Cesarean delivery

Cesarean delivery rates are increased among WWD. People with sensory, physical, and IDD disabilities are more likely to have primary cesarean deliveries, although risk decreased over time, ranging from aOR 2.60 in 2000 to aOR 1.66 in 2010 in California data [4]. In this study, the highest rates of cesarean deliveries were among women with vision disabilities (38–54%) and women with IDD (29–45%). Multiple studies have shown that pregnant people with physical disabilities as a group are at significantly increased risk for cesarean delivery, with aRR/aOR ranging from 1.09–6.83 [16,22,29,41].

Disability, per se, is not an indication for cesarean delivery, but there may be disability-related conditions that warrant cesarean delivery, for example, respiratory compromise, pelvic deformity, or previous abdominal or pelvic surgery [27]. The question remains whether cesarean deliveries among WWD are fully clinically indicated. Gleason et al. used Consortium for Safe Labor data to examine indications for cesarean deliveries among WWD and found that persons with any disability were significantly less likely to have solely clinical obstetric indications for operative delivery, concluding that practitioners may prefer and overuse cesarean delivery in this population [16]. Biel and colleagues [24] analyzed California hospital discharge data and linked vital records of all nulliparous births (n >2.4 million, including >14000 WWD) and found that, overall, WWD were less likely to experience labor (77% vs. 91%, *P*<0.001; aOR 0.45, 95% CI 0.41–0.49), with rates of labor lowest among women with vision disabilities, and highest among women with hearing disabilities. Although the majority of WWD delivered vaginally, among laboring patients, WWD were significantly more likely to deliver by

cesarean. Among prelabor scheduled cesarean deliveries, WWD had a significantly lower proportion with medical indication (aOR 0.45, 95% CI 0.41–0.50). The authors concluded that their findings suggest a pattern of prelabor cesarean deliveries that are not medically indicated, even though the majority of women did labor and of those, the majority did deliver vaginally. In another study, analysis of population-based data in Canada showed that cesarean delivery rates were slightly increased among patients with IDD, but in mediation analyses found that the majority the elevated occurrence of cesarean was not explained by preexisting conditions or pregnancy complications [39]. Risks associated with cesarean deliveries are well-known, but WWD may have an especially difficult time recovering from even an uncomplicated cesarean [40].

Considerations for specific disability types and associated conditions

Physical disabilities

Physical disability in women may be related to arthritic and rheumatic conditions, back injury, multiple sclerosis, spinal cord injury, amputation, neural tube defect, or cerebral palsy, among other conditions. Studies have shown that, when considered as a group, pregnant people with physical disabilities have higher risk of complications and adverse outcomes than able-bodied counterparts. A recent systematic review [71] including 16 studies of pregnancy outcomes in women with physical disabilities reported higher number of prenatal care visits, emergency department visits, and observational inpatient visits (aRRs 1.30–2.90) among WWD. Hypertensive disorders and gestational diabetes were more common among women with diagnosed–but not self-reported–physical disabilities. Most studies included in this review found increased risk of preterm labor, preterm birth, cesarean delivery, and longer postdelivery hospitalization. Infants were generally more likely to be low birth weight (aRR 2.27–4.0) and small for gestational age infant (SGA) (aRR 1.1–1.65). Risk for these outcomes varied by the underlying disabling condition and was higher in people with more severe physical limitations [71].

In the Gleason et al. study of severe maternal morbidity and mortality (SMMM) among WWD [16], the risk of a composite outcome of pregnancy complications among women with physical disabilities was elevated 27% (aRR 1.27; 95% CI 1.16–1.38). A similar population-based Canadian study [26] included women with physical disabilities (n = 144,972) and without (n = 1,601,363) and examined risks for SMMM. Risk of a composite outcome including obstetric hemorrhage, cardiac conditions, severe preeclampsia/eclampsia/HELLP, sepsis, and ICU admission was significantly higher among women with physical disabilities during pregnancy (aRR 1.40), at birth to 42 days postpartum (aRR 1.24), and at 43 to 365 days postpartum (aRR 1.53) [26].

Spinal cord injury

Acute traumatic injury of the spinal cord occurs in approximately 3500 women per year in the United States and 22% of SCI occur in women of reproductive age [73]. The most common cause of injury is motor vehicle accident (39%), followed by falls (30%) and violence (14%) [74]. Approximately 60% of all injuries are to the cervical spinal cord, resulting in varying degrees of tetraplegia (weakness in all four limbs); the remainder are to the thoracic, lumbar, or sacral regions of the cord resulting in paraplegia (weakness of the lower limbs) [74]. Acute SCI during pregnancy is rare [53]; data on birth outcomes among women who sustain a SCI during pregnancy are limited to case reports.

Those caring for pregnant people with SCI must be aware of autonomic dysreflexia (ADR), one of the most feared complications of pregnancy and SCI. Characterized by acute increase of blood pressure as high as 300/200 mmHg, this syndrome is caused by unchecked sympathetic outflow in response to a stimulus below the level of the spinal cord lesion. ADR largely affects individuals with injuries at T6 and above but does occur rarely with lower-level lesions [75]. Common precipitants include dilation of a hollow viscus (e.g. bladder distension, fecal impaction), skin injury, bladder infection, or other stimuli. Labor is a potent inciting event. The literature is mixed on the incidence of ADR during pregnancy and delivery, with rates of 12–85% reported [10, 82–85]. Signs and symptoms of ADR include systolic hypertension of at least 20–40 mmHg over baseline, reflex bradycardia, tachycardia, or other cardiac rhythm disturbances,

severe headache, sweating, flushing, nasal congestion, piloerection, prickling sensation in the scalp, spasticity, and anxiety. Left untreated, ADR can result in fetal distress, maternal intracranial hemorrhage, coma, seizures, and death.

Care must be taken to distinguish ADR from preeclampsia. One key difference is that in ADR, blood pressure rises and falls with contractions, whereas in preeclampsia blood pressure is unrelated to contractions. General steps in the treatment of ADR include repositioning, elevation of the head, and eliminating the offending stimulus (e.g. full bladder, digital cervical exam). Obstetric clinicians should be aware of both ADR prevention and acute management in pregnancy.

To avoid ADR during labor and delivery, women with SCI should have epidural anesthesia instituted early in labor to block labor pain. Vital signs must be monitored frequently throughout labor, with pharmacologic control of refractory hypertension with rapid-acting agents with short duration such as oral and sublingual nifedipine, prazosin and other α-blockers, nitrates, hydralazine, and labetalol [30]. Some experts recommend offering a scheduled induction of labor to facilitate neuraxial analgesia for patients at risk for ADR in labor [27]. Postpartum, in susceptible patients, contractions of uterine involution and fundal massage may incite ADR. Continuing epidural analgesia for 48 hours postpartum may mitigate this risk [28].

Preterm birth (<37 weeks) occurs in 18–33% of women with SCI, and data from one study indicates the majority (77%) are spontaneous preterm deliveries [10,51,56,80–82]. Women with injuries at T10 or above may be unable to perceive contractions. In one study, 80% of women who delivered preterm could not feel contractions. Women can be taught to palpate uterine contractions and monitor for other unique symptoms of labor onset such as ADR, increased spasticity, or bladder spasms [10]. Sensation during the second stage of labor originates in S2–S4, so patients with SCI or other sensory impairments are at risk for unattended birth, which could be especially dangerous preterm [28]. Some suggest routine cervical examination after 28 weeks [83], or serial ultrasonographic assessment of cervical length [56], but neither practice has been tested in women with SCI.

Women with SCI are capable of vaginal delivery, which is achieved by 33–78%, and in most cases is spontaneous [10,80–82]. Cesarean delivery rates as high as 67% have been reported [10,80–82], though, as noted previously, it is not clear whether this reflects a true elevation in obstetrical indications for operative delivery.

Multiple sclerosis

This autoimmune demyelinating disorder most commonly affects women of childbearing age, with features including muscular weakness and spasticity, disrupted coordination and balance, disturbances of sensation, visual changes, and bowel and bladder dysfunction. The pregnancy course of MS resembles that of other autoimmune diseases. A large European prospective cohort study showed that MS flare rates tend to decrease during pregnancy but rise during the first 3 months postpartum, occurring in approximately 30% [84]. More recently, the use of disease-modifying therapies (DMTs) has led to improved disease control before pregnancy and a 14% risk of postpartum relapse [85]. Breastfeeding or early resumption of DMTs may reduce postpartum relapses [85,86].

In general, perinatal outcomes among women with MS are favorable [85,87], but several studies have suggested increased risk of adverse pregnancy outcomes in women with MS. Fong and colleagues [25] analyzed data from California births 2001–2009, including 1185 patients with MS and >4.4 million without. They found significant increases in UTI (aOR 1.8), induction of labor (aOR 1.4), and cesarean delivery (aOR 1.4), but not other complications, including gestational diabetes, preeclampsia, preterm birth, operative vaginal delivery, stillbirth, fetal growth restriction, endometritis, or VTE. A matched analysis of US claims data (>95% privately insured) found that, among women with and without MS and a live birth, women with MS had significantly higher rates of preterm labor and infection during pregnancy, but not gestational diabetes, hypertensive disorders of pregnancy, operative vaginal delivery, or cesarean delivery [8].

In a study of administrative data on more than 10,000 women with MS, Kelly and colleagues reported significantly higher rates of fetal growth restriction (OR 1.7, 95% CI 1.2–2.4), antenatal hospitalization (OR 1.3, 95% CI 1.2–1.5), and cesarean delivery (OR 1.3, 95% CI 1.1–1.4), but not hypertensive disorders or PROM [88]. Analysis of a population-based Danish national registry from 1997–2016 found no difference in gestational diabetes, preeclampsia, or intrapartum cesarean delivery among women with MS (n = 2930) but significantly increased risk of preterm birth (aOR 1.15), elective cesarean (aOR 1.89), and SGA (aOR 1.29) compared to controls (n = 56,958) [89]. A study of US administrative data sets found a 19–30% increase in preterm birth and suggested a 16% increased risk of cesarean delivery [48]. Risks of impaired fetal growth, preeclampsia, chorioamnionitis, postpartum hemorrhage, stillbirth, and congenital anomalies were not elevated in women with MS. A limitation of many of these studies is that, given the nature of the data sets used, they cannot account for disease activity and treatment prior to and throughout pregnancy and postpartum.

Rheumatoid arthritis

As with other autoimmune conditions, rheumatoid arthritis (RA) disease activity has traditionally been thought to decrease substantially during pregnancy and then flare in the postpartum period. However, more recent data suggest that in the third trimester, fewer than 25% of women are in remission and 10–20% have high disease activity [90,91]. A 2019 systematic review and meta-analysis found that 60% of patients with RA improve during pregnancy and 47% relapse postpartum [92].

An analysis of administrative data on 1425 delivery hospitalizations in US women with RA demonstrated increased risk of fetal growth restriction (OR 2.2, 95% CI 1.2–4.1]) and cesarean delivery (OR 1.5, 95% CI 1.2–1.9) compared to controls [93]. A similar, more recent study of US data including more than 31 000 women with RA found similar increases in risk for fetal growth restriction and cesarean delivery. In addition, women with RA had significantly increased risk of hypertensive disorders (aOR 1.16), antepartum hemorrhage (aOR 1.23), and preterm birth (aOR 1.46) [94].

Preterm birth rates of 6.4–26% have been reported and are positively associated with disease activity and systemic steroid use [95–97]. A Scandinavian matched cohort study including 1739 RA-pregnancies and 17 390 control pregnancies showed increased risks of spontaneous preterm birth (aOR 1.79, 95% CI 1.41–2.28), induced preterm birth (aOR 2.10, 95% CI 1.45–3.05), SGA infants (aOR 1.93, 95% CI 1.45–2.57), and elective cesarean delivery (aOR 1.41, 95% CI 1.20–1.67) but not large for gestational age infants (LGA) or stillbirth [98]. As previously, risk for preterm birth was associated with higher disease activity during pregnancy. Analyses of preterm birth risk by antirheumatic treatment during pregnancy stratified by disease activity found no significant increased risk. However, use of combination antirheumatic therapies before pregnancy was associated with increased risk of preterm birth and SGA infants.

Congenital neuromuscular disorders

A matched case-control study of those with congenital neuromuscular disabilities including spina bifida, cerebral palsy, muscular dystrophy, contractures, arthrogryposis, and other skeletal or connective tissue conditions (n = 125) and those without (n = 505) found a significant nearly fourfold increase in preterm birth [69]. In 315 gestations among 178 patients with hereditary neuromuscular disorders, including myotonic dystrophies and proximal spinal muscular atrophy, Awater et al. found significantly increased rates of polyhydramnios, placenta previa, UTI, preterm delivery, cesarean delivery, and nonvertex presentation [54].

Cerebral palsy

Women with cerebral palsy (CP) experience varying degrees of movement and posture disorders, spasticity, and joint contractures that may be associated with cognitive and communication difficulties. Data on pregnancy outcomes for women with CP are inconclusive. In one small descriptive study, pregnancies among women with CP were complicated by preeclampsia (17.9%), cesarean delivery (33%, most often for cephalopelvic disproportion and abnormal fetal position), and preterm birth (7.8%) [99]. Another study found a similar rate of cesarean delivery, but preeclampsia occurred in only 5% [100]. Difficulties in labor and delivery due to spasticity or joint contractures did not occur, but a small proportion of women reported increased physical disability postpartum [99]. A larger, more recent survey-based study (n=76 women with CP reporting 149 pregnancies) found that 71% experienced decreased mobility during pregnancy, but few were referred for physical or occupational therapy evaluation and assistance. There were not major differences in miscarriage, stillbirth, or preterm birth compared to population norms, but 50% of deliveries were by cesarean [101].

Spina bifida

Conditions associated with spina bifida include deformity of the spine or pelvis, spasticity, bowel and bladder dysfunction, ileal conduits and ventriculoperitoneal shunting for management of hydrocephalus. The enlarging uterus can cause shunt malfunction; thus, women should be monitored for headache, nausea/vomiting, and signs of increased pressure [55]. Allergy to latex is common, occurring in about 23% [102]. Offspring of mothers with spina bifida have a 4–7% rate of neural tube defects [103]. Women with spina bifida considering pregnancy should begin folic acid supplementation, 4 mg daily, before conception [104].

There are scant data on the course and outcomes of pregnancy in women with spina bifida. A survey of 17 women who had had 23 pregnancies revealed frequent antepartum admissions, recurrent UTIs, worsening pressure sores and stomal problems [105]. Hypertensive disorders occurred in 26%, preterm birth in 35%, cesarean delivery in 50%, and SGA infants in 47% of pregnancies. Regional anesthesia use was rare, and 92% of cesareans were performed under general anesthesia. Sterling et al. [51] conducted a single-center retrospective chart review of the course and outcomes of 37 pregnancies among 32 women with spinal cord lesions, 69% of whom had neural tube defects. Antenatal hospitalization occurred in 46%, most often for threatened preterm labor, 68% had at least one UTI, and 11% were hospitalized with pyelonephritis. Overall, 33% delivered vaginally; preterm birth occurred in 24%. Fifty-seven percent of cesarean deliveries occurred under general anesthesia, with the most frequent indications being elective repeat, failure to progress, and pelvic instability/contracture. Planned vaginal birth should consider the presence and extent of pelvic skeletal deformity and consideration of operative vaginal delivery to shorten the second stage to decrease elevation of maternal intracranial pressure [55].

A recent study [106] examined pregnancy and infant outcomes in a large, population-based Canadian cohort of 397 women with spina bifida who had 720 infants and compared them to >1 million women without spina bifida who had ~1.9 million infants. During the study period, from 1989 to 2013, births to women with spina bifida increased 14-fold. In adjusted analyses, women with spina bifida had increased prevalence of nearly every adverse outcome examined, with maternal death or near-miss mortality (adjusted prevalence ratio [aPR] 2.83), ICU admission (aPR 3.41), postpartum length of stay ≥14 days (aPR 4.01), cesarean delivery (aPR 1.98), and respiratory morbidity (aPR 9.46) reaching statistical significance. Among infants born to women with spina bifida, statistically significant increases in preterm birth, birth hypoxia, intracranial hemorrhage, intubation, delivery hospitalization >14 days, and oral clefts and abdominal wall/diaphragm defects (but not neural tube defects) were reported.

Intellectual and developmental disabilities

Conditions associated with IDD include fetal alcohol spectrum disorders, autism spectrum disorders, chromosomal abnormalities such as Down syndrome, and neurologic injuries. A growing body of evidence indicates that people with IDD are at increased risk for pregnancy complications and adverse outcomes. Gleason et al. [16] found that the risk of any pregnancy complication among women with IDD (n=91) was elevated 49% (aRR 1.49, 95% CI 1.06–2.10) compared to women without IDD (n=221311). A population-based Canadian study of data from 2003–2018, which included women with (n=2227) and without (n=1,601,363) IDD, investigated rates of SMMM up to 1 year postpartum. A SMMM composite outcome was significantly increased during pregnancy (aRR 1.63), birth to 42 days (aRR 1.56), and 43–365 days (aRR 2.18) among people with IDD [26].

Multiple studies [62] have reported significantly increased risk of cesarean delivery (aRR/aOR 1.09–2.43) [12,16,22,29,39,107]; hypertensive disorders of pregnancy (aRR/aOR 1.47–2.55) [3,16,29,107]; preterm birth (aOR/aRR 2.40–4.53) [3,21,72,107]; stillbirth [3,21,108]; and perinatal/neonatal death (aRR/aOR 2.66–4.25) in women with IDD [3,108]. Some studies have also found increased risk of PROM [16], PPROM [16], operative vaginal delivery [16], maternal sepsis [16], peripartum hemorrhage [3], VTE [3], placental abruption [3], low birth weight [21], and SGA infants [3,108].

The literature on the course and outcomes of pregnancy among people with specific conditions associated with IDD is sparse and largely limited to case reports or case series. An analysis of national Swiss hospitalization data from 1998–2009 included 97 pregnancies in women with Down syndrome, 82 in women with other forms of IDD, and 172 in women without IDD [109]. Women with Down syndrome had a significantly increased risk of abortion (63%) compared to women with other IDDs (22%) and women without IDD (15%, *P*<0.001). It is not clear what proportion of these were induced, medically indicated, or spontaneous losses. Among pregnancies resulting in a birth (n = 246), significant group differences were seen for hypertensive disorders of pregnancy and "other complications," which included cardiovascular, metabolic, and respiratory diagnoses, and were more common among women with IDD and women with Down syndrome compared to women without IDD.

A Swedish population-based analysis of birth registry data from 2006–2014 compared pregnancy outcomes among women with autism (n = 2198) and those without (n = 877,742). Women with autism had higher odds of moderately preterm birth at 32 to <37 weeks (aOR 1.32, 95% CI 1.10–1.58), medically indicated preterm birth (aOR 1.41, 95% CI 1.08–1.82), elective cesarean delivery (aOR 1.44, 95% CI 1.25–1.66), labor induction (aOR 1.52, 95% CI 1.37–1.70), and preeclampsia (aOR 1.34, 95% CI 1.08–1.66), but not SGA, stillbirth, or gestational diabetes [110].

Sensory disabilities

Visual impairment in adults of reproductive age is often caused by retinopathy from preterm birth, genetic conditions, refractive errors, amblyopia, accidental eye injury, diabetic retinopathy, and glaucoma [111]. Bilateral speech-frequency hearing impairment affects 1 to 3.4% of US women ages 20 to 49 years and increases with age [112]. Recent large studies have found that women with either vision or hearing loss have a significantly increased risk of pregnancy complications and severe maternal morbidity and mortality. The Gleason et al. secondary analysis of Consortium for Safe Labor data revealed the risk of a composite outcome of pregnancy complications among women with sensory disabilities was elevated 53% (aRR 1.53, 95% CI 1.26–1.86) [16]. The Canadian study by Brown et al. [3] that included more than 45000 women with sensory disabilities found that a composite outcome of SMMM was significantly increased during pregnancy (aRR 1.25), from birth–42 days postpartum (aRR 1.08), and from 43–365 days postpartum (aRR 1.30).

A 2020 systematic review and meta-analysis of 23 studies including more than 8.5 million women found in crude analyses that women with sensory disabilities had higher odds of gestational diabetes (crude OR 2.85, 95% CI 0.79–10.31), hypertensive disorders of pregnancy (crude OR 2.84, 95% CI 0.82–9.83), and cesarean delivery (crude OR 1.28, 95% CI 0.84–1.93), but these associations did not reach statistical significance [29]. In a combined group of

pregnant people with vision and/or hearing impairments, Gleason et al. [16] found no significant increased risk of gestational diabetes but a more than fourfold increased risk of severe preeclampsia/eclampsia (aRR 4.29, 95% CI 3.13–5.89) and cesarean delivery (aRR 1.39, 95% CI 1.17–1.67). In this study, risks of operative vaginal delivery, hemorrhage, blood transfusion, maternal VTE, major puerperal infection, and cardiovascular events during labor and delivery were also significantly increased.

In one study examining outcomes specifically among those with vision disability, Schiff and colleagues [113] conducted a population-based retrospective cohort study using 1987–2014 linked hospital discharge records and vital statistics data in Washington state. Compared to a random selection of women without visual impairment (n = 2362) women with low vision (n = 232) had a significant 3.8-fold increased risk of severe preeclampsia, and 1.6-fold increase in preterm birth but no significant difference in gestational diabetes, cesarean delivery, or SGA infants. The authors speculate that inaccessible education about warning signs and symptoms of preeclampsia may lead to late presentation for care for preeclampsia with severe features already manifest.

Mitra et al. [60] used nationally-representative administrative data including deliveries to 5258 DHH women and >8 million hearing women between 2007–2016 and found that DHH women had statistically significant increased risk for preeclampsia and eclampsia (aRR 1.20), placenta previa (aRR 1.39), chorioamnionitis (aRR 1.15), PROM (aRR 1.26), preterm birth (aRR 1.13), and prolonged hospitalization after vaginal or cesarean delivery (aRR 1.30) but not labor induction, operative vaginal delivery, cesarean delivery, antepartum/postpartum hemorrhage, stillbirth, SGA, or LGA infants.

Breastfeeding

Studies have shown lower rates of breastfeeding among WWD [49,114,115]. A recent systematic review found that women with physical disabilities were significantly less likely to breastfeed (OR 0.3, 95% CI 0.1–0.8) [71]. Patients with disabilities can be encouraged to breastfeed, but difficulties have been reported and supportive care and services are important. Some patients with SCI have reported ADR in response to infant suckling [28]. Breastfeeding difficulties in women with SCI, especially injuries above T6, can result from ADR and/or inhibition of the milk ejection reflex, which may shorten breastfeeding duration [52,116]. Women with SCI at any level report that their most difficult problem breastfeeding is positioning for feeds, perhaps related to arm and trunk paresis and instability [116].

Mothers with disabilities relate that facilitators to breastfeeding include adaptations to techniques, pillows and other supports and equipment, pumping and bottle-feeding, receiving physical assistance, and peer support [117]. They describe barriers such as lack of knowledge, experience, and cultural competence among lactation consultants or others, disability-related health concerns (medication use, bone loss), scant evidence-based practice, and difficulties with positioning and latching.

A qualitative study of lived experience of breastfeeding among WWD revealed that communication difficulties, intense pressure to breastfeed, difficulty with milk supply and infant latching could leave WWD feeling judged—by themselves and others—as inadequate, so much that some feared their baby would be taken from them on the presumption they were not fit to parent [118]. Accessible communication [119], cultural competence, and creativity from lactation consultants and health practitioners are needed to overcome breastfeeding barriers for WWD.

Conclusion

Most women with disabilities can expect an uneventful pregnancy and delivery of a healthy baby. Maternal care providers should be aware of problems that may arise more frequently in WWD as compared to their peers without disabilities. These include UTIs, VTE, respiratory compromise, decline in mobility, substance misuse, stress and depression, and limitations in access to care. Pregnancy course and outcomes depend on the nature and severity of the disabling condition. Though the mechanisms are unclear, a growing body of evidence suggests that women across the spectrum of disability are at increased risk of multiple adverse pregnancy outcomes. Management of these pregnancies should be by a multidisciplinary team, with vigilance for common complications and marshalling of needed supports for the transition to motherhood.

CASE PRESENTATION

The patient is a 29-year-old primigravida who sustained a complete thoracic (T4) spinal cord injury at age 19 years and presented for antenatal care at 10 weeks gestation. She was using a manual wheelchair for mobility, and aside from occasional episodes of autonomic dysreflexia (ADR) related to bladder distension and frequent UTIs (3 to 5 per year) she had no health complaints or complications from her injury. Bladder management was by clean intermittent catheterization, which she was able to perform independently. Her last known weight was 3 years ago, was 131 lb, corresponding to a body mass index of 23.3 kg/m². She was married, worked part time at a nonprofit organization, and did not smoke or use drugs or alcohol. Current medications were oxybutinin for bladder relaxation and oral baclofen for management of mild spasticity. Examination was unremarkable except for bilateral 2+ pitting edema in the lower extremities. Compression stockings were recommended.

Routine prenatal labs were normal except for mild anemia (Hct 36.3); the patient refused oral iron supplementation for fear of constipation. Her pregnancy progressed uneventfully through the second trimester except for a UTI treated with a 14-day course of nitrofurantoin. At 28 weeks, the patient was seen by an obstetric anesthesiologist to develop a plan for early induction of epidural anesthesia upon presentation for labor. Additionally, referrals to physical and occupational therapy were made to assist with current mobility and begin planning for adaptations for baby care after delivery. She was instructed on abdominal/uterine palpation to detect contractions.

At 30 weeks gestation, she experienced an episode of ADR because she found she was unable to self-catheterize; the ADR resolved when the bladder spontaneously emptied. After discussion, a Foley catheter was inserted, to remain until after delivery. By 32 weeks, she required assistance with transfers and propelling her wheelchair.

One evening at 35 weeks, she noted a substantial increase in spasticity, headache, skin tingling, and profuse sweating above the level of her injury. Upon presentation at labor and delivery, her blood pressure was 230/120 mmHg, with heart rate of 55 bpm. Urine dipstick for protein was negative. She was placed in a seated upright position with a wedge under her right hip and examined for the source of the presumed ADR. Her catheter was draining normally, there was no evidence of skin injury, and tocodynamometer revealed contractions occurring every 4 minutes. Fetal heart rate (FHT) was 120–130 bpm, with decreased variability and occasional late decelerations. Cervical exam was 3 cm dilated, 70% effaced and -3 station. She was admitted for labor and urgent epidural placement. Under epidural anesthesia to the T10 level, her blood pressure, heart rate, and FHT normalized and remained stable throughout labor. She underwent a spontaneous vaginal delivery of a 2515 g infant with Apgars of 7 and 9. A second-degree laceration was repaired. The infant was monitored for 2 days in the NICU. The patient's postpartum course was unremarkable, and she was discharged on postpartum day two with instructions to continue Foley catheterization, avoid ice or heat to the perineum, and continue working with her lactation consultant.

References

1. Okoro CA, Hollis ND, Cyrus AC, Griffin-Blake S. Prevalence of disabilities and health care access by disability status and type among adults–United States, 2016. MMWR Morb Mortal Wkly Rep. 2018 Aug 17;67(32):882–7. doi: 10.15585/mmwr.mm6732a3. PMID: 30114005; PMCID: PMC6095650.

2. Signore C, Davis M, Tingen CM, Cernich AN. The intersection of disability and pregnancy: risks for maternal morbidity and mortality. J Womens Health (Larchmt). 2021 Feb;30(2):147–53. doi: 10.1089/jwh.2020.8864. Epub 2020 Nov 19. PMID: 33216671; PMCID: PMC8020507.

3. Brown HK, Cobigo V, Lunsky Y, Vigod SN. Maternal and offspring outcomes in women with intellectual and developmental disabilities: a population-based cohort study. BJOG. 2017 Apr;124(5):757–65. doi: 10.1111/1471-0528.14120. Epub 2016 May 24. PMID: 27222439.

4. Horner-Johnson W, Biel FM, Darney BG, Caughey AB. Time trends in births and cesarean deliveries among women with disabilities. Disabil Health J. 2017 Jul;10(3):376–81. doi: 10.1016/j.dhjo.2017.02.009. Epub 2017 Apr 6. PMID: 28431988; PMCID: PMC5544013.

5. Iezzoni LI, Yu J, Wint AJ, Smeltzer SC, Ecker JL. Prevalence of current pregnancy among US women with and without chronic physical disabilities. Med Care. 2013 Jun;51(6):555–62. doi: 10.1097/MLR.0b013e318290218d. PMID: 23604018; PMCID: PMC3733491.

6. Iezzoni LI, Chen Y, McLain AB. Current pregnancy among women with spinal cord injury: findings from the US national spinal cord injury database. Spinal Cord. 2015;53(11):821–6. doi: 10.1038/sc.2015.88.

7. Horner-Johnson W, Darney BG, Kulkarni-Rajasekhara S, Quigley B, Caughey AB. Pregnancy among US women: differences by presence, type, and complexity of disability. Am J Obstet Gynecol. 2016 Apr;214(4):529.e1–9. doi: 10.1016/j.ajog.2015.10.929. Epub 2015 Nov 4. PMID: 26546851; PMCID: PMC4821180.

8. Houtchens MK, Edwards NC, Schneider G, Stern K, Phillips AL. Pregnancy rates and outcomes in women with and without MS in the United States. Neurology. 2018 Oct 23;91(17):e1559–69. doi: 10.1212/WNL.0000000000006384. Epub 2018 Sep 28. PMID: 30266889; PMCID: PMC6205683.

9. Wisdom JP, McGee MG, Horner-Johnson W, Michael YL, Adams E, Berlin M. Health disparities between women with and without disabilities: a review of the research. Soc Work Public Health. 2010 May;25(3):368–86. doi: 10.1080/19371910903240969. PMID: 20446182; PMCID: PMC3546827.

10. Jackson AB, Wadley V. A multicenter study of women's self-reported reproductive health after spinal cord injury. Arch Phys Med Rehabil. 1999 Nov;80(11):1420–8.

11. Barclay L. Are pregnant women with disabilities at higher risk for adverse maternal outcomes? Medscape. 2022 Jan 28 [cited 2023 Jun 11]. Available from: https://www.medscape.org/viewarticle/967089.

12. Höglund B, Lindgren P, Larsson M. Pregnancy and birth outcomes of women with intellectual disability in Sweden: a national register study. Acta Obstet Gynecol Scand. 2012 Dec;91(12):1381–7. doi: 10.1111/j.1600-0412.2012.01509.x. Epub 2012 Sep 18. PMID: 22881406; PMCID: PMC3549474.

13. Mitra M, Iezzoni LI, Zhang J, Long-Bellil LM, Smeltzer SC, Barton BA. Prevalence and risk factors for postpartum depression symptoms among women with disabilities. Matern Child Health J. 2015 Feb;19(2):362–72. doi: 10.1007/s10995-014-1518-8. PMID: 24889114; PMCID: PMC4254905.

14. Horner-Johnson W, Kulkarni-Rajasekhara S, Darney BG, Dissanayake M, Caughey AB. Live birth, miscarriage, and abortion among U.S. women with and without disabilities. Disabil Health J. 2017 Jul;10(3):382–6. doi: 10.1016/j.dhjo.2017.02.006. Epub 2017 Apr 6. PMID: 28431989; PMCID: PMC5544009.

15. Horner-Johnson W, Akobirshoev I, Amutah-Onukagha NN, Slaughter-Acey JC, Mitra M. Preconception health risks among U.S. women: disparities at the intersection of disability and race or ethnicity. Womens Health Issues. 2021 Jan-Feb;31(1):65–74. doi: 10.1016/j.whi.2020.10.001. Epub 2020 Nov 21. PMID: 33234388; PMCID: PMC7775679.

16. Gleason JL, Grewal J, Chen Z, Cernich AN, Grantz KL. Risk of adverse maternal outcomes in pregnant women with disabilities. JAMA Netw Open. 2021 Dec 1;4(12):e2138414. doi: 10.1001/jamanetworkopen.2021.38414. PMID: 34910153; PMCID: PMC8674748.

17. Mitra M, Clements KM, Zhang J, Smith LD. Disparities in adverse preconception risk factors between women with and without disabilities. Matern Child Health J. 2016 Mar;20(3):507–15. doi: 10.1007/s10995-015-1848-1. PMID: 26518009; PMCID: PMC4754136.

18. Nosek MA, Robinson-Whelen S, Hughes RB, Petersen NJ, Taylor HB, Byrne MM, Morgan R. Overweight and obesity in women with physical disabilities: associations with demographic and disability characteristics and secondary conditions. Disabil Health J. 2008 Apr;1(2):89–98. doi: 10.1016/j.dhjo.2008.01.003. PMID: 21122716.

19. Deierlein AL, Litvak J, Stein CR. Preconception health and disability status among women of reproductive age participating in the National Health and Nutrition Examination Surveys, 2013–2018. J Womens Health (Larchmt). 2022 Sep;31(9):1320–33. doi: 10.1089/jwh.2021.0420. Epub 2022 Jan 17. PMID: 35041530.

20. Iezzoni LI, Yu J, Wint AJ, Smeltzer SC, Ecker JL. General health, health conditions, and current pregnancy among U.S. women with and without chronic physical disabilities. Disabil Health J. 2014 Apr;7(2):181–8. doi: 10.1016/j.dhjo.2013.12.002. Epub 2014 Jan 2. PMID: 24680047; PMCID: PMC3971389.

21. Akobirshoev I, Parish SL, Mitra M, Rosenthal E. Birth outcomes among US women with intellectual and developmental disabilities. Disabil Health J. 2017 Jul;10(3):406–12. doi: 10.1016/j.dhjo.2017.02.010. Epub 2017 Apr 6. PMID: 28404230; PMCID: PMC5477666.

22. Darney BG, Biel FM, Quigley BP, Caughey AB, Horner-Johnson W. Primary cesarean delivery patterns among women with physical, sensory, or intellectual disabilities. Womens Health Issues. 2017 May-Jun;27(3):336–44. doi: 10.1016/j.whi.2016.12.007. Epub 2017 Jan 18. PMID: 28109562; PMCID: PMC5435518.

23. Mitra M, Akobirshoev I, McKee MM, Iezzoni LI. Birth outcomes among U.S. women with hearing loss. Am J Prev Med. 2016 Dec;51(6):865–73. doi: 10.1016/j.amepre.2016.08.001. Epub 2016 Sep 26. PMID: 27687529.

24. Biel F, Darney B, Caughey A, Horner-Johnson W. Medical indications for primary cesarean delivery in women with and without disabilities. J Matern Fetal Neonatal Med. 2020 Oct;33(20):3391–8. doi: 10.1080/14767058.2019.1572740. Epub 2019 Mar 18. PMID: 30879367; PMCID: PMC7780300.

25. Fong A, Chau CT, Quant C, Duffy J, Pan D, Ogunyemi DA. Multiple sclerosis in pregnancy: prevalence, sociodemographic features, and obstetrical outcomes. J Matern Fetal Neonatal Med. 2018 Feb;31(3):382–7. doi:10.1080/14767058.2017.1286314. Epub 2017 Apr 10. PMID: 28139946.

26. Brown HK, Ray JG, Chen S, Guttmann A, Havercamp SM, Parish S, Vigod SN, Tarasoff LA, Lunsky Y. Association of preexisting disability with severe maternal morbidity or mortality in Ontario, Canada. JAMA Netw Open. 2021 Feb 1;4(2):e2034993. doi: 10.1001/jamanetworkopen.2020.34993. PMID: 33555330; PMCID: PMC7871190.

27. Berndl A, Ladhani N, Wilson RD, Basso M, Jung E, Tarasoff LA, Angle P, Soliman N. Guideline No. 416: labour, delivery, and postpartum care for people with physical disabilities. J Obstet Gynaecol Can. 2021 Jun;43(6):769–80.e1. doi: 10.1016/j.jogc.2021.02.111. Epub 2021 Feb 22. PMID: 33631321.

28. Wendel MP, Whittington JR, Pagan ME, Whitcombe DD, Pates JA, McCarthy RE, Magann EF. Preconception, antepartum, and peripartum care for the woman with a spinal cord injury: a review of the literature. Obstet Gynecol Surv. 2021 Mar;76(3):159–65. doi: 10.1097/OGX.0000000000000868. PMID: 33783544.

29. Tarasoff LA, Ravindran S, Malik H, Salaeva D, Brown HK. Maternal disability and risk for pregnancy, delivery, and postpartum complications: a systematic review and meta-analysis. Am J Obstet Gynecol. 2020 Jan;222(1):27.e1–32. doi: 10.1016/j.ajog.2019.07.015. Epub 2019 Jul 12. PMID: 31306650; PMCID: PMC6937395.

30. Canibaño B, Deleu D, Mesraoua B, Melikyan G, Ibrahim F, Hanssens Y. Pregnancy-related issues in women with multiple sclerosis: an evidence-based review with practical recommendations. J Drug Assess. 2020;9(1):20–36. doi: 10.1080/21556660.2020.1721507.

31. Young ME, Nosek MA, Howland C, Chanpong G, Rintala DH. Prevalence of abuse of women with physical disabilities. Arch Phys Med Rehabil. 1997 Dec;78(12 Suppl 5):S34–S38.

32. McFarlane J, Hughes RB, Nosek MA, Groff JY, Swedlend N, Dolan MP. Abuse assessment screen-disability (AAS-D): measuring frequency, type, and perpetrator of abuse toward women with physical disabilities. J Womens Health Gend Based Med. 2001 Nov;10(9):861–6.

33. Amborski AM, Bussières EL, Vaillancourt-Morel MP, Joyal CC. Sexual violence against persons with disabilities: a meta-analysis. Trauma Violence Abuse. 2022 Oct;23(4):1330–43. doi: 10.1177/1524838021995975. Epub 2021 Mar 4. PMID: 33657931; PMCID: PMC9425723.

34. Mitra M, Manning SE, Lu E. Physical abuse around the time of pregnancy among women with disabilities. Matern Child Health J. 2012 May;16(4):802–6. doi: 10.1007/s10995-011-0784-y. PMID: 21556697.

35. Booth EJ, Kitsantas P, Min H, Pollack AZ. Stressful life events and postpartum depressive symptoms among women with disabilities. Womens Health (Lond). 2021 Jan-Dec;17:17455065211066186. doi: 10.1177/17455065211066186. PMID: 34904463; PMCID: PMC8679014.

36. Hughes RB, Taylor HB, Robinson-Whelen S, Nosek MA. Stress and women with physical disabilities: identifying correlates. Womens Health Issues. 2005 Jan;15(1):14–20.

37. Hughes RB, Robinson-Whelen S, Taylor HB, Petersen NJ, Nosek MA. Characteristics of depressed and nondepressed women with physical disabilities. Arch Phys Med Rehabil. 2005 Mar;86(3):473–9.

38. Iezzoni LI, Yu J, Wint AJ, Smeltzer SC, Ecker JL. Health risk factors and mental health among US women with and without chronic physical disabilities by whether women are currently pregnant. Matern Child Health J. 2015 Jun;19(6):1364–75. doi: 10.1007/s10995-014-1641-6. PMID: 25421328; PMCID: PMC4442759.

39. Brown HK, Kirkham YA, Cobigo V, Lunsky Y, Vigod SN. Labour and delivery interventions in women with intellectual and developmental disabilities: a population-based cohort study. J Epidemiol Community Health. 2016 Mar;70(3):238–44. doi: 10.1136/jech-2015-206426. Epub 2015 Oct 8. PMID: 26449738.

40. Becker H, Andrews E, Walker LO, Phillips CS. Health and well-being among women with physical disabilities after childbirth: an exploratory study. Womens Health Issues. 2021 Mar-Apr;31(2):140–7. doi: 10.1016/j.whi.2020.10.007. Epub 2020 Dec 1. PMID: 33272777.

41. Crane DA, Doody DR, Schiff MA, Mueller BA. Pregnancy outcomes in women with spinal cord injuries: a population-based study. PM R. 2019 Aug;11(8):795–806. doi: 10.1002/pmrj.12122. Epub 2019 Apr 26. PMID: 30729746; PMCID: PMC6675642.

42. Mitra M, Lu E, Diop H. Smoking among pregnant women with disabilities. Womens Health Issues. 2012 Mar;22(2):e233–9. doi: 10.1016/j.whi.2011.11.003. Epub 2012 Jan 21. PMID: 22265182.

43. Ford JA, Glenn MK, Li L, Moore DC. Substance abuse and women with disabilities. In: Welner SL, Haseltine F, editors. Welner's guide to the care of women with disabilities. Philadelphia, PA: Lippincott Williams & Wilkins; 2004.

44. Li L, Ford JA. Illicit drug use by women with disabilities. Am J Drug Alcohol Abuse. 1998 Aug;24(3):405–18.

45. Pannek J, Bertschy S. Mission impossible? Urological management of patients with spinal cord injury during pregnancy: a systematic review. Spinal Cord. 2011 Oct;49(10):1028–32. doi: 10.1038/sc.2011.66. Epub 2011 Jun 14. PMID: 21670736.

46. Andretta E, Landi LM, Cianfrocca M, Manassero A, Risi O, Artuso G. Bladder management during pregnancy in women with spinal-cord injury: an observational, multicenter study. Int Urogynecol J. 2019 Feb;30(2):293–300. doi: 10.1007/s00192-018-3620-8. Epub 2018 Mar 29. PMID: 29600402.

47. Nicolle LE. Urinary tract infections in patients with spinal injuries. Curr Infect Dis Rep. 2014 Jan;16(1):390. doi: 10.1007/s11908-013-0390-9. PMID: 24445675.

48. MacDonald SC, McElrath TF, Hernández-Díaz S. Pregnancy outcomes in women with multiple sclerosis. Am J Epidemiol. 2019;188(1):57–66. doi: 10.1093/aje/kwy197.

49. Morton C, Le JT, Shahbandar L, Hammond C, Murphy EA, Kirschner KL. Pregnancy outcomes of women with physical disabilities: a matched cohort study. PM R. 2013 Feb;5(2):90–8. doi: 10.1016/j.pmrj.2012.10.011. Epub 2012 Nov 27. PMID: 23200116.

50. Salomon J, Schnitzler A, Ville Y, Laffont I, Perronne C, Denys P, et al. Prevention of urinary tract infection in six spinal

cord-injured pregnant women who gave birth to seven children under a weekly oral cyclic antibiotic program. Int J Infect Dis. 2009 May;13(3):399–402.

51. Sterling L, Keunen J, Wigdor E, Sermer M, Maxwell C. Pregnancy outcomes in women with spinal cord lesions. J Obstet Gynaecol Can. 2013 Jan;35(1):39–43. doi: 10.1016/s1701-2163(15)31046-x. PMID: 23343795.

52. American College of Obstetricians and Gynecologists. ACOG committee opinion no. 808: obstetric management of patients with spinal cord injuries. Obstet Gynecol. 2020; 135(5):e230–6.

53. Pereira L. Spinal cord injury. Maternal-fetal evidence based guidelines. 2nd ed. Boca Raton, FL: CRC Press LLC; 2011.

54. Awater C, Zerres K, Rudnik-Schöneborn S. Pregnancy course and outcome in women with hereditary neuromuscular disorders: comparison of obstetric risks in 178 patients. Eur J Obstet Gynecol Reprod Biol. 2012 Jun;162(2):153–9. doi: 10.1016/j.ejogrb.2012.02.020. Epub 2012 Mar 28. PMID: 22459654.

55. Berndl A, Nosek M, Waddington A. Women's health guidelines for the care of people with spina bifida. J Pediatr Rehabil Med. 2020;13(4):655–62. doi: 10.3233/PRM-200757. PMID: 33325413; PMCID: PMC7838966.

56. Ghidini A, Healey A, Andreani M, Simonson MR. Pregnancy and women with spinal cord injuries. Acta Obstet Gynecol Scand. 2008;87(10):1006-10.

57. Bertschy S, Schmidt M, Fiebag K, Lange U, Kues S, Kurze I. Guideline for the management of pre-, intra-, and postpartum care of women with a spinal cord injury. Spinal Cord. 2020 Apr;58(4):449–58. doi: 10.1038/s41393-019-0389-7. Epub 2019 Dec 6. PMID: 31811245.

58. Kazi S, McLeod A, Berndl A. VTE prophylaxis in pregnant people with chronic physical disability: Data from a physicians survey and the need for guidance. Obstet Med. 2023 Mar;16(1):35–9. Epub 2022 Jan 27. doi: 10.1177/1753495X221074616

59. Kapoor D, Chipde SS, Agrawal S, Chipde S, Kapoor R. Delivery after augmentation cystoplasty: Implications and precautions. J Nat Sci Biol Med. 2014 Jan;5(1):206–9. doi: 10.4103/0976-9668.127334. PMID: 24678231; PMCID: PMC3961938.

60. Mitra M, McKee MM, Akobirshoev I, Ritter GA, Valentine AM. Pregnancy and neonatal outcomes among deaf and hard of hearing women: results from nationally representative data. Womens Health Issues. 2021 Sep-Oct;31(5):470–7. doi: 10.1016/j.whi.2021.03.005. Epub 2021 Apr 20. PMID: 33888398; PMCID: PMC8448895.

61. Mazurkiewicz B, Stefaniak M, Dmoch-Gajzlerska E. Perinatal care needs and expectations of women with low vision or total blindness in Warsaw, Poland. Disabil Health J. 2018 Oct;11(4):618–23. doi: 10.1016/j.dhjo.2018.05.005. Epub 2018 Jun 12. PMID: 29907533.

62. Potvin LA, Brown HK, Cobigo V. Social support received by women with intellectual and developmental disabilities during pregnancy and childbirth: An exploratory qualitative study. Midwifery. 2016 Jun;37:57–64. doi: 10.1016/j.midw.2016.04.005. Epub 2016 Apr 25. PMID: 27217238.

63. Tarasoff LA. "We don't know. We've never had anybody like you before": Barriers to perinatal care for women with physical disabilities. Disabil Health J. 2017 Jul;10(3):426–33. doi: 10.1016/j.dhjo.2017.03.017. Epub 2017 Apr 5. PMID: 28404229.

64. Iezzoni LI, Wint AJ, Smeltzer SC, Ecker JL. "How did that happen?" Public responses to women with mobility disability during pregnancy. Disabil Health J. 2015 Jul;8(3):380–7. doi: 10.1016/j.dhjo.2015.02.002. Epub 2015 Mar 10. PMID: 25944504; PMCID: PMC4795154.

65. Xie E, Gemmill M. Exploring the prenatal experience of women with intellectual and developmental disabilities: In a southeastern Ontario family health team. Can Fam Physician. 2018 Apr;64(Suppl 2):S70–5. PMID: 29650748; PMCID: PMC5906775.

66. Mitra M, Long-Bellil LM, Iezzoni LI, Smeltzer SC, Smith LD. Pregnancy among women with physical disabilities: unmet needs and recommendations on navigating pregnancy. Disabil Health J. 2016 Jul;9(3):457–63. doi: 10.1016/j.dhjo.2015.12.007. Epub 2016 Jan 2. PMID: 26847669; PMCID: PMC4903955.

67. Smeltzer SC, Mitra M, Long-Bellil L, Iezzoni LI, Smith LD. Obstetric clinicians' experiences and educational preparation for caring for pregnant women with physical disabilities: a qualitative study. Disabil Health J. 2018 Jan;11(1):8–13. doi: 10.1016/j.dhjo.2017.07.004. Epub 2017 Aug 1. PMID: 28784583; PMCID: PMC5723564.

68. Diamanti A, Sarantaki A, Gourounti K, Lykeridou A. Perinatal care in women with vision disorders: a systematic review. Maedica (Bucur). 2021 Jun;16(2):261–7. doi: 10.26574/maedica.2020.16.2.261. PMID: 34621349; PMCID: PMC8450664.

69. García MH, Parker SE, Petersen JM, Rubenstein E, Werler MM. Birth outcomes among women with congenital neuromuscular disabilities. Disabil Health J. 2022 Apr;15(2):101259. doi: 10.1016/j.dhjo.2021.101259. Epub 2021 Dec 1. PMID: 34980574.

70. Dissanayake MV, Darney BG, Caughey AB, Horner-Johnson W. miscarriage occurrence and prevention efforts by disability status and type in the United States. J Womens Health (Larchmt). 2020 Mar;29(3):345–52. doi: 10.1089/jwh.2019.7880. Epub 2019 Nov 21. PMID: 31750752; PMCID: PMC7097696.u

71. Deierlein AL, Antoniak K, Chan M, Sassano C, Stein CR. Pregnancy-related outcomes among women with physical disabilities: A systematic review. Paediatr Perinat Epidemiol. 2021 Nov;35(6):758–78. doi: 10.1111/ppe.12781. Epub 2021 Aug 24. PMID: 34431112.

72. Tarasoff LA, Murtaza F, Carty A, Salaeva D, Hamilton AD, Brown HK. Health of newborns and infants born to women with disabilities: a meta-analysis. Pediatrics. 2020 Dec;146(6):e20201635. doi: 10.1542/peds.2020-1635. Epub 2020 Nov 17. PMID: 33203648; PMCID: PMC7786829.

73. National Spinal Cord Injury Statistical Center. Spinal cord injury facts and figures at a glance. Birmingham, AL: University of Alabama; 2019 [cited 2022 Feb 13]. Available from: https://www.nscisc.uab.edu/Public/Facts%20and%20Figures%202020.pdf.

74. National Spinal Cord Injury Statistical Center. Recent trends in causes of spinal cord injury. Birmingham, AL: University of Alabama at Birmingham; 2015 [cited 2022 Mar 27]. Available from: https://www.nscisc.uab.edu/PublicDocuments/fact_sheets/Recent%20trends%20in%20causes%20of%20SCI.pdf.

75. Krassioukov A, Stillman M, Beck LA. A primary care provider's guide to autonomic dysfunction following spinal cord injury. Top Spinal Cord Inj Rehabil. 2020 Spring;26(2):123–7. doi: 10.46292/sci2602-123. PMID: 32760191; PMCID: PMC7384539.

76. Cross LL, Meythaler JM, Tuel SM, Cross AL. Pregnancy, labor and delivery post spinal cord injury. Paraplegia. 1992 Dec;30(12):890–902.

77. McGregor JA, Meeuwsen J. Autonomic hyperreflexia: a mortal danger for spinal cord-damaged women in labor. Am J Obstet Gynecol. 1985 Feb 1;151(3):330–3.

78. Wanner MB, Rageth CJ, Zach GA. Pregnancy and autonomic hyperreflexia in patients with spinal cord lesions. Paraplegia. 1987 Dec;25(6):482–90.

79. Hughes SJ, Short DJ, Usherwood MM, Tebbutt H. Management of the pregnant woman with spinal cord injuries. Br J Obstet Gynaecol. 1991 Jun;98(6):513–8. doi: 10.1111/j.1471-0528.1991.tb10361.x. PMID: 1873238.

80. Westgren N, Hultling C, Levi R, Westgren M. Pregnancy and delivery in women with a traumatic spinal cord injury in Sweden, 1980-1991. Obstet Gynecol. 1993 Jun;81(6):926–30.

81. Ghidini A, Simonson M. Pregnancy after spinal cord injury: a review of the literature. Top Spinal Cord Inj Rehabil. 2011;16:93–103.

82. Robertson K, Dawood R, Ashworth F. Vaginal delivery is safely achieved in pregnancies complicated by spinal cord injury: a retrospective 25-year observational study of pregnancy outcomes in a national spinal injuries centre. BMC Pregnancy Childbirth. 2020 Jan 29;20(1):56. doi: 10.1186/s12884-020-2752-2. PMID: 31996150; PMCID: PMC6988250.

83. Pereira L. Obstetric management of the patient with spinal cord injury. Obstet Gynecol Surv. 2003 Oct;58(10):678–87.

84. Vukusic S, Hutchinson M, Hours M, Moreau T, Cortinovis-Tourniaire P, Adeleine P, et al. Pregnancy and multiple sclerosis (the PRIMS study): clinical predictors of post-partum relapse. Brain. 2004 Jun;127(Pt 6):1353–60.

85. Andersen JB, Magyari M. Pharmacotherapeutic considerations in women with multiple sclerosis. Expert Opin Pharmacother. 2020 Sep;21(13):1591–602. doi: 10.1080/14656566.2020.1774554. Epub 2020 Jun 10. PMID: 32521172.

86. Krysko KM, Rutatangwa A, Graves J, Lazar A, Waubant E. Association between breastfeeding and postpartum multiple sclerosis relapses: a systematic review and meta-analysis. JAMA Neurol. 2020 Mar 1;77(3):327–38. doi: 10.1001/jamaneurol.2019.4173. PMID: 31816024; PMCID: PMC6902174.

87. Modrego PJ, Urrea MA, de Cerio LD. The effects of pregnancy on relapse rates, disability and peripartum outcomes in women with multiple sclerosis: a systematic review and meta-analysis. J Comp Eff Res. 2021 Feb;10(3):175–86. doi: 10.2217/cer-2020-0211. Epub 2021 Feb 10. PMID: 33565886.

88. Kelly VM, Nelson LM, Chakravarty EF. Obstetric outcomes in women with multiple sclerosis and epilepsy. Neurology. 2009 Dec 1;73(22):1831–6.

89. Andersen JB, Kopp TI, Sellebjerg F, Magyari M. Pregnancy-related and perinatal outcomes in women with multiple sclerosis: a nationwide Danish cross-sectional study. Neurol Clin Pract. 2021 Aug;11(4):280–90. doi: 10.1212/CPJ.0000000000001035. Epub 2021 Feb 3. PMID: 34484927; PMCID: PMC8382416.

90. de Man YA, Hazes JM, van de Geijn FE, Krommenhoek C, Dolhain RJ. Measuring disease activity and functionality during pregnancy in patients with rheumatoid arthritis. Arthritis Rheum. 2007 Jun 15;57(5):716–22.

91. de Man YA, Dolhain RJ, van de Geijn FE, Willemsen SP, Hazes JM. Disease activity of rheumatoid arthritis during pregnancy: results from a nationwide prospective study. Arthritis Rheum. 2008 Sep 15;59(9):1241–8.

92. Jethwa H, Lam S, Smith C, Giles I. Does rheumatoid arthritis really improve during pregnancy? a systematic review and metaanalysis. J Rheumatol. 2019 Mar;46(3):245–50. doi: 10.3899/jrheum.180226. Epub 2018 Nov 1. PMID: 30385703.

93. Chakravarty EF, Nelson L, Krishnan E. Obstetric hospitalizations in the United States for women with systemic lupus erythematosus and rheumatoid arthritis. Arthritis Rheum. 2006 Mar;54(3):899–907.

94. Kishore S, Mittal V, Majithia V. Obstetric outcomes in women with rheumatoid arthritis: Results from Nationwide Inpatient Sample Database 2003-2011. Semin Arthritis Rheum. 2019 Oct;49(2):236–40. doi: 10.1016/j.semarthrit.2019.03.011. Epub 2019 Mar 23. PMID: 30992155.

95. Chambers CD, Johnson DL, Jones KL. Pregnancy outcome in women exposed to anti-TNF-alpha medications: The OTIS Rheumatoid Arthritis in Pregnancy Study [abstract]. Arthritis Rheum. 2004;50:S479–80.

96. de Man YA, Hazes JM, van der Heide H, Willemsen SP, de Groot CJ, Steegers EA, et al. Association of higher rheumatoid arthritis disease activity during pregnancy with lower birth weight: results of a national prospective study. Arthritis Rheum. 2009 Nov;60(11):3196–206.

97. Skomsvoll JF, Ostensen M, Irgens LM, Baste V. Obstetrical and neonatal outcome in pregnant patients with rheumatic disease. Scand J Rheumatol. 1998;107 Suppl:109–12.

98. Hellgren K, Secher AE, Glintborg B, Rom AL, Gudbjornsson B, Michelsen B, Granath F, Hetland ML. Pregnancy outcomes in relation to disease activity and anti-rheumatic treatment strategies in women with rheumatoid arthritis. Rheumatology (Oxford). 2022 Aug 30;61(9):3711–22. doi: 10.1093/rheumatology/keab894. PMID: 34864891.

99. Winch R, Bengtson L, McLaughlin J, Fitzsimmons J, Budden S. Women with cerebral palsy: obstetric experience and neonatal outcome. Dev Med Child Neurol. 1993 Nov;35(11):974–82.

100. Foley J. The offspring of people with cerebral palsy. Dev Med Child Neurol. 1992 Nov;34(11):972–8.

101. Hayward K, Chen AY, Forbes E, Byrne R, Greenberg MB, Fowler EG. Reproductive healthcare experiences of women with cerebral palsy. Disabil Health J. 2017 Jul;10(3):413–18. doi: 10.1016/j.dhjo.2017.03.015. Epub 2017 Apr 5. PMID: 28428111.

102. Jackson AB, Mott PK. Reproductive health care for women with spina bifida. ScientificWorldJournal. 2007;7:1875–83.

103. Jackson AB, Sipski ML. Reproductive issues for women with spina bifida. J Spinal Cord Med. 2005;28(2):81–91.

104. American College of Obstetricians and Gynecologists. Practice Bulletin No. 187: neural tube defects. Obstet Gynecol. 2017;130:e279–90.

105. Arata M, Grover S, Dunne K, Bryan D. Pregnancy outcome and complications in women with spina bifida. J Reprod Med. 2000 Sep;45(9):743–8.

106. Auger N, Arbour L, Schnitzer ME, Healy-Profitós J, Nadeau G, Fraser WD. Pregnancy outcomes of women with spina bifida. Disabil Rehabil. 2019 Jun;41(12):1403–1409. doi: 10.1080/09638288.2018.1425920. Epub 2018 Jan 12. PMID: 29327608.

107. Parish SL, Mitra M, Son E, Bonardi A, Swoboda PT, Igdalsky L. Pregnancy outcomes among U.S. women with intellectual and developmental disabilities. Am J Intellect Dev Disabil. 2015 Sep;120(5):433–43. doi: 10.1352/1944-7558-120.5.433. PMID: 26322390.

108. Höglund B, Lindgren P, Larsson M. Newborns of mothers with intellectual disability have a higher risk of perinatal death and being small for gestational age. Acta Obstet Gynecol Scand. 2012 Dec;91(12):1409–14. doi: 10.1111/j.1600-0412.2012.01537.x. Epub 2012 Nov 1. PMID: 22924821; PMCID: PMC3549565.

109. Bless DO, Hoffman V. Pregnancies and births in women with Down syndrome–An analysis based on the Medical Statistics of Swiss Hospitals. J Intellect Dev Disabil. 2020;45(4):377–85. doi: 10.3109/13668250.2020.1767767.

110. Sundelin HE, Stephansson O, Hultman CM, Ludvigsson JF. Pregnancy outcomes in women with autism: a nationwide population-based cohort study. Clin Epidemiol. 2018 Nov 30;10:1817–26. doi: 10.2147/CLEP.S176910. PMID: 30555264; PMCID: PMC6280895.

111. Centers for Disease Control and Prevention. Vision loss and age. [last reviewed 2020 Jun 12; cited 2022 Mar 27]. Available from: https://www.cdc.gov/visionhealth/risk/age.htm.

112. Hoffman HJ, Dobie RA, Losonczy KG, Themann CL, Flamme GA. Declining prevalence of hearing loss in US adults aged 20 to 69 Years. JAMA Otolaryngol Head Neck Surg. 2017;143(3):274–85. doi: 10.1001/jamaoto.2016.3527

113. Schiff MA, Doody DR, Crane DA, Mueller BA. Pregnancy outcomes among visually impaired women in Washington State, 1987-2014. Disabil Health J. 2021 Jul;14(3):101057. doi: 10.1016/j.dhjo.2020.101057. Epub 2020 Dec 24. PMID: 33384279; PMCID: PMC8222420.

114. Mitra M, Parish SL, Clements KM, Cui X, Diop H. Pregnancy outcomes among women with intellectual and developmental disabilities. Am J Prev Med. 2015 Mar;48(3):300–8. doi: 10.1016/j.amepre.2014.09.032. Epub 2014 Dec 26. PMID: 25547927.

115. Mitra M, Clements KM, Zhang J, Iezzoni LI, Smeltzer SC, Long-Bellil LM. Maternal characteristics, pregnancy complications, and adverse birth outcomes among women with disabilities. Med Care. 2015 Dec;53(12):1027–32. doi: 10.1097/MLR.0000000000000427. PMID: 26492209; PMCID: PMC4648667.

116. Holmgren T, Lee AHX, Hocaloski S, Hamilton LJ, Hellsing I, Elliott S, Hultling C, Krassioukov AV. The influence of spinal cord injury on breastfeeding ability and behavior. J Hum Lact. 2018 Aug;34(3):556–65. doi: 10.1177/0890334418774014. Epub 2018 May 22. PMID: 29787691.

117. Powell RM, Mitra M, Smeltzer SC, Long-Bellil LM, Smith LD, Rosenthal E, Iezzoni LI. Breastfeeding among women with physical disabilities in the United States. J Hum Lact. 2018 May;34(2):253–61. doi: 10.1177/0890334417739836. Epub 2017 Nov 22. PMID: 29166569.

118. Andrews EE, Powell RM, Ayers KB. Experiences of breastfeeding among disabled women. Womens Health Issues. 2021 Jan-Feb;31(1):82–89. doi: 10.1016/j.whi.2020.09.001. Epub 2020 Oct 10. PMID: 33051056.

119. Hall J, Hundley V, Collins B, Ireland J. Dignity and respect during pregnancy and childbirth: a survey of the experience of disabled women. BMC Pregnancy Childbirth. 2018 Aug 13;18(1):328. doi: 10.1186/s12884-018-1950-7. PMID: 30103731; PMCID: PMC6088410.

Chapter 31
COVID-19 in Pregnancy

Carolynn M. Dude[1], Martina L. Badell[1], and Denise J. Jamieson[2]

[1]Department of Gynecology and Obstetrics, Emory University School of Medicine, Atlanta, GA, USA
[2]Vice President for Medical Affairs and Dean of the Roy J. and Lucille A. Carver College of Medicine, University of Iowa, Iowa City, IA, USA

In late December 2019, the first four cases of pneumonia of unknown etiology were identified in Wuhan, China [1]. Shortly after, coronavirus disease 2019 (COVID-19), the respiratory disease caused by the severe acute respiratory syndrome coronavirus 2 (SARS-CoV-2), spread rapidly across the world; on March 11, 2020, the WHO declared the SARS-CoV-2 outbreak a worldwide pandemic [2]. Early on, COVID-19 was noted to cause more severe disease in pregnant people when compared to their non-pregnant peers [3], and researchers and clinicians initially struggled to define appropriate treatment algorithms. Additionally, pregnant persons were often purposefully excluded from trials for many of the COVID-19 therapeutics, including the initial vaccine trials, and so there was a substantial lack of safety and efficacy data to help guide clinicians. Although the knowledge of COVID-19 in pregnancy is still evolving, much more is now known about the epidemiology, prevention, and treatment of COVID-19 in the pregnant patient.

Pathophysiology of COVID in pregnancy

The physiologic alterations of pregnancy mean that infectious diseases such as COVID-19 may affect pregnant persons differently than their nonpregnant peers. Prior to the COVID-19 pandemic, other respiratory viruses such as the H1N1 strain of influenza had been shown to disproportionately affect pregnant persons, with pregnant people being at higher risk for hospitalization, intensive care unit [ICU] admission, and death [4]. Additionally, pregnant persons were also at higher risk for severe disease and complications from other coronavirus infections including SARS and Middle Eastern Respiratory Syndrome (MERS) [5].

The reasons pregnant persons are at higher risk are multifactorial, but the changes in the physiology of the immune, respiratory, and hematologic systems during pregnancy likely play a role. Research done after the 2009 H1N1 influenza A pandemic showed that viral pathogens such as influenza can provoke an exaggerated inflammatory response in pregnant persons, with higher levels of proinflammatory cytokines correlating with disease severity [6,7]. While investigations into the pregnant immune response to SARS-CoV-2 infection are ongoing, much of the morbidity of COVID-19 infection comes from an unregulated inflammatory response, and so this may explain some of the clinical outcomes seen thus far.

In addition to changes in the immune system, significant changes to the respiratory system occur during pregnancy. As the gravid uterus displaces the diaphragm, the reduced chest volume results in a decrease of both the expiratory reserve volume and residual volume, which in turn results in a moderate decrease to the functional residual capacity. This decrease in reserve means that pregnant persons may not be able to tolerate prolonged periods of tachypnea and may require intubation earlier in their clinical course.

Finally, all pregnant persons are at an increased risk for venous thromboembolism, due to compression of the vena cava by the gravid uterus, increased vasodilation from increased progesterone, increased levels of clotting factors such as fibrinogen and thrombin, reduced levels of anti-clotting factors, resistance to activated protein C and elevated levels of antifibrinolytic proteins. COVID-19 disease has also been associated with high rates of thromboembolic events due to excessive inflammation, platelet activation, endothelial dysfunction and stasis [8], and, although data are still accumulating, the unique physiology of pregnancy means that pregnant persons with COVID-19 may be at even higher risk for thrombotic complications than the general population.

Epidemiology

There have been nearly 400 million confirmed cases of COVID-19 globally and more than 76 million cases in the United States by the beginning of 2022 [9]. As more than 20% of the global population is women of reproductive age, and approximately 5% of women of reproductive age are pregnant at any point in time [10], there have likely been several million cases of COVID-19 among pregnant persons. Although it is difficult to definitively determine, there do not seem to be large disparities in susceptibility to SARS-CoV-2 between pregnant and nonpregnant persons [11]. However, among pregnant persons, COVID-19 infection is more prevalent among those living in socially and economically disadvantaged settings, as is the case among nonpregnant persons [12,13]. Pregnant persons with symptomatic COVID-19 infection appear to be at increased risk for severe disease with increased rates of hospitalization, intensive care unit admission, intubation, and death [3,14]. Many of the same risk factors for severe disease found in the general population have also been found among pregnant persons including older age, obesity, and chronic medical conditions [15,16]. Furthermore, certain variants may cause more severe illness than others during pregnancy, as pregnant persons infected with SARS-CoV-2 when the Delta variant was the predominant stain were more severely affected when compared to pregnant persons infected prior to the wide circulation of the Delta variant [17].

Screening and Prevention

The primary mode of transmission of SARS-CoV-2 is via airborne droplets, and general prevention measures advocated by the Centers for Disease Control and Prevention (CDC) and other public healthcare organizations are aimed at decreasing transmission by reducing droplet spread [18]. These measures include universal masking in public, avoiding crowds and poorly ventilated spaces, staying at least six feet apart when in public and frequent hand washing during epidemics. Additionally, the CDC recommends frequent testing of those who were symptomatic and/or exposed, and mandatory isolation of anyone who tested positive. These general measures have been recommended from the beginning of the pandemic; later, as the COVID-19 vaccines were available, vaccination formed a cornerstone of prevention and/or mitigation guidelines.

In addition to these general principles, specific guidelines were quickly adapted for both the inpatient and outpatient obstetric settings. On the inpatient side, many obstetric governing bodies including the American College of Obstetricians and Gynecologists (ACOG) and the Society for Maternal-Fetal Medicine (SMFM) recommend testing all individuals with suspected COVID-19, all symptomatic patients, and universal screening on labor and delivery in areas of high community spread and/or in areas with low vaccination rates [19]. Additionally, most guidelines discuss appropriate personal protective equipment for all health care workers and call for universal masking and symptom screening for all visitors to labor and delivery [19]. In the outpatient setting, screening patients ahead of time for symptoms and/or COVID-19 exposure may help facilitate rescheduling and/or implementing telehealth appointments for those likely to be infectious; however, all guidelines do not recommend delaying time-sensitive care based on COVID status alone [20]. Visitor restrictions, physical distancing in the waiting rooms and universal masking may also help decrease transmission in the outpatient setting.

Vaccination

Vaccines typically require years of development and testing before they are adopted for widespread use; however, the coronavirus vaccines were developed and adopted for widespread use with rapid speed. There are currently three COVID-19 vaccines authorized for use in the United States, all of which may be used during any trimester of pregnancy. None of the available vaccines contain live virus. Two of the vaccines (Pfizer-BioNTEch BNT 162b2 and Moderna mRNA 1273) are two-dose messenger RNA (mRNA) vaccines of the SARS-CoV-2 spike S protein. These vaccines work by releasing the mRNA that codes for the SARS-CoV-2 spike protein; after the mRNA is taken up by cells and the protein is made, the mRNA is destroyed while the protein remains. The latter then facilitates an immune response without any sort of permanent host genetic modification. Everyone 18 years or older should receive a booster dose 6 months after completing the primary series. The other available vaccine (Janssen/Johnson & Johnson J&J Ad26.COV2.S) is a one-dose adenovirus vaccine, which uses the adenovirus vector to transfer the SARS-CoV-2 spike protein DNA into the cell, where the DNA is translated into mRNA, which then generates an immune response. The CDC recommends that persons 18 years and older receiving the Janssen/Johnson & Johnson vaccine receive a booster dose of either mRNA vaccine at least 2 months later.

The CDC and professional organizations such as ACOG and SMFM strongly recommend that all persons, including those who are pregnant, receive a primary COVID-19 vaccine series and booster vaccination [21,22]. For safety and efficacy reasons, an mRNA vaccine is preferred over the Janssen/Johnson & Johnson adenoviral vaccine for all adults including pregnant persons. A pregnancy test is not recommended prior to vaccination and there is no need to delay attempting pregnancy after vaccination.

Currently, there are no data to guide ideal timing of vaccination during pregnancy; therefore, like the influenza vaccine, which is given with the primary goal of preventing maternal infection, the COVID-19 vaccine is recommended regardless of trimester.

The initial reported efficacy of the Pfizer and Moderna vaccines was 95.0% and 94.1%, respectively, 2 weeks after the two-dose series [23,24]. The Janssen/Johnson & Johnson vaccine efficacy was 72% overall and 85% effective in preventing severe disease [25]. With the addition of booster doses and with new mutations of the SARS-CoV-2 virus, these efficacy rates may vary. Although pregnant persons were excluded from all the initial vaccine trials, observational data support a similar humoral and functional immune response to the vaccines in pregnant persons as compared to nonpregnant persons [26–29]. A few studies on the effectiveness of vaccination in pregnancy found that vaccinated pregnant persons were less likely (2/140; 1.4%) than unvaccinated pregnant persons (210/1862; 11.3%) to have COVID-19 illness [30] and a large study with over 10,000 pregnant people found COVID-19 vaccines as effective for pregnant persons as the general population [31]. Although the currently available COVID-19 vaccines have been shown to be less effective at preventing infection with the newer Omicron variant, they have been shown to have high vaccine effectiveness against severe disease and hospitalization in the general population [32,33]. Finally, vaccination during pregnancy may also provide protection for the newborn. Studies have documented binding and neutralizing antibodies in the cord blood of vaccinated mothers [28,34–38]. In addition, a case-control study demonstrated that maternal COVID-19 vaccination reduced the risk of COVID-19 hospitalization in infants <6 months of age [39]. The duration of clinical protection for newborns is currently unclear. A few studies have evaluated perinatal outcomes after maternal vaccination including spontaneous abortion, stillbirth, preterm birth, and fetal growth restriction and did not find increased risks for any of these outcomes [30,40–42]. The vaccine side effect profile also appears to be similar to that of nonpregnant people with pain at the injection site, fatigue, headache, and myalgias being the most frequent symptoms [41,43].

However, despite the known increased risks of COVID-19 disease in pregnancy, and the demonstrated safety of these vaccines, vaccine hesitancy remains high among some pregnant persons. As of early 2022, approximately 64% of the US population was fully vaccinated against COVID, and only 42% of pregnant people were vaccinated, with higher rates of vaccine hesitancy seen in people of non-Hispanic Black race, younger age, lower education, public health insurance, low parity, and substance use [44]. The lack of uptake in the pregnant population is worrisome, and the inclusion of pregnant people in vaccine research is paramount in helping to increase knowledge about and boosting confidence in these life-saving technologies.

Clinical course

As the pandemic has evolved, several large cohort studies have found that COVID-19 infection during pregnancy is associated with an increased risk of adverse maternal and obstetric outcomes [45–47]. Several small studies have suggested that COVID-19 infection in early pregnancy is not associated with an increased risk of spontaneous abortion or decreased fertility in women [48,49], although this will need to be validated with data from larger sample sizes. In contrast, the virus may have a negative impact on the male reproductive tract, as early studies done on men infected with COVID-19 suggest that infection with SARS-CoV-2 negatively affects sperm concentration and motility [50]. However, the relationship between these changes in sperm parameters and overall fertility rates remains unknown.

COVID-19 infection during pregnancy has been associated with several adverse maternal outcomes including an increased risk of venous thromboembolism, acute respiratory distress syndrome, acute renal failure, sepsis, shock, mechanical ventilation, ICU admission, and death [46,47,51]. These risks all increase with worsening disease severity, as well as with underlying medical comorbidities, especially increased body mass index [45]. Most [52,53] but not all [54] studies have found an increased risk of preterm birth, preeclampsia, and stillbirth associated with maternal COVID-19 infection, particularly among those with severe disease. Vaccination against COVID-19 appears to mitigate some of these risks, as at least one large cohort study from Scotland demonstrated that the severe complications resulting from COVID-19 such as ICU admission and perinatal mortality were significantly higher in unvaccinated women compared to their partially or fully vaccinated peers [47].

Vertical transmission

Based on what is known about SARS-CoV-2, as well as the transmission of other viral pathogens, several systems for classifying intrauterine transmission have been proposed. In general, required components for classifying a case of intrauterine transmission include documentation of maternal infection, identification of SARS-CoV-2 within the first 24 hours of neonatal life, and persistence of infection in the neonate [55–57]. Although several cases of intrauterine transmission have been carefully documented [58], the risk for vertical transmission appears low. The low risk for transmission may be the result of several factors including the low levels of maternal SARS-CoV-2 viremia, as well as the comparatively low

Clinical management

A pregnant person with a SARS-CoV-2 infection may be asymptomatic or have a wide range of clinical symptoms resulting in mild to severe disease. When diagnosed with COVID-19 in pregnancy, the patient should be evaluated for severity of infection, symptoms and underlying medical conditions to help determine acuity and need for in-person care (Figure 31.1). If a pregnant patient requires supplemental oxygen and/or has SpO2 ≤ 94% on room air, then hospitalization is indicated, and this should ideally occur at a facility that can provide maternal and fetal monitoring when appropriate. A multidisciplinary team approach is ideal and may include obstetrics, maternal fetal medicine, infectious diseases, pulmonary critical care, and neonatology.

Maternal COVID-19 is not an indication for delivery. For critically ill patients, the decision to proceed with delivery should be based on the understanding that delivery may improve maternal status or fetal status. If a patient is infected at or near term, the decision to deliver should be individualized. Considerations include risk of maternal deterioration, access to health services, separation from family, and exposure to health care workers. The mode of delivery does not appear to affect risk of perinatal infection and thus cesarean delivery is not indicated to prevent perinatal transmission.

After a COVID-19 infection in pregnancy, patients still need follow-up antenatal care. During the recommended quarantine time frame, if a patient is considered otherwise low risk, the next prenatal appointment may be delayed or occur via telehealth. However, in high-risk patients, antenatal surveillance may need to occur even during the quarantine period when indicated. Given lack of long-term follow-up data following COVID-19 infection in pregnancy, the ideal recommendation for future antenatal surveillance is unknown. A detailed mid-trimester anatomy ultrasound may be considered following periconception or first trimester maternal infection, and follow-up growth ultrasounds may be considered based on the timing of infection, disease severity, and other maternal risk factors. At this time, data on increased risk for stillbirth are inconclusive and therefore antenatal testing should be reserved for routine obstetric indications [62].

Treatment

Overall, management of pregnant patients with COVID-19 should be the same as nonpregnant patients. The COVID-19 Treatment Guidelines Panel recommends *against* withholding treatment for COVID-19 from pregnant people because of theoretical safety concerns [63]. Shared

decision-making discussions are recommended to review the use of investigational drugs for treatment of COVID-19 and particular considerations for safety in pregnancy. Figure 31.2 outlines current therapeutic management of COVID-19 in pregnancy. To date, pregnant women have been excluded from most clinical trials on drug treatments for COVID-19, which makes evidence-based recommendations challenging in this population. Anti-SARS-CoV-2 monoclonal antibodies should be offered when indicated given other immunoglobulin G (IgG) products have been safely used in pregnancy. Currently, several medications may be given in the outpatient setting to help prevent progression of severe disease, including various formulations of monoclonal antibodies and the antiviral medications remdesivir and nirmatrelvir/ritonavir (Figure 31.2). The specific monoclonal antibody recommended has changed over time; currently, due to the rise of variant, the National Institutes of Health (NIH) recommend using a single infusion of the monoclonal antibody sotrovimab 500 mg intravenous (IV) and recommends against using bamlanivimab/etesevimab or casirivimab/imdevimab, although this may change in the future [63]. In addition to remdesivir, which is given as an infusion over three days, an additional oral antiviral medication, nirmatrelvir/ritonavir (Paxlovid), maybe given as an outpatient therapy for high-risk patients. Another antiviral medication recently approved for outpatient therapy, molnupiravir, is not recommended in pregnancy due to concerns for fetal toxicity based on animal studies. Pregnancy is generally considered a risk factor for poor outcomes and thus pregnant patients should be a prioritized group for therapeutic management.

If hospitalized with COVID-19 disease, additional therapeutics are available (Figure 31.2). Remdesivir, an antiviral medication, is recommended for treatment of COVID-19 in hospitalized patients with SpO2 ≤ 94% on room air or those who require supplemental oxygen [64]. Dexamethasone 6 mg PO or IV daily for up to 10 days is recommended in patients with COVID-19 who are ventilated or require supplemental oxygen. SMFM recommends that remdesivir and dexamethasone should both be offered to pregnant patients requiring supplemental oxygen; if glucocorticoids are indicated for fetal lung maturity, dexamethasone can be given 6 mg IM every 12 hours for four doses followed by 6 mg PO or IV daily for up to a total of 10 days [62]. The COVID-19 Treatment Guidelines from the NIH are regularly updated to include new therapeutics, are easily accessible online and contain a specific section on "Special Considerations in Pregnancy" [63].

Postpartum care and newborns

The period of increased risk for severe disease from SARS-CoV-2 likely persists in the postpartum period [52,65]. Although this is extrapolated from what

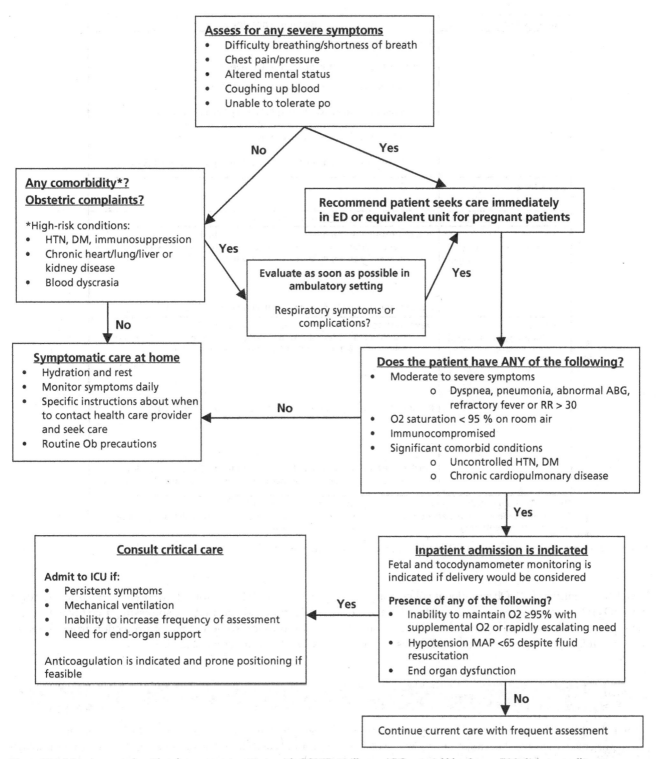

Figure 31.1 Management algorithm for pregnant patients with COVID-19 illness. ABG, arterial blood gass; DM, diabetes mellitus; HTN, hypertension; MAP, mean arterial pressure; RR, respiratory rate.

has been observed in cohorts of COVID-19 infected pregnant persons who are followed postpartum, it is not possible to carefully delineate when this period of increased risk ends.

SARS-CoV-2 IgG antibodies are found in the cord blood of infants born to mothers after natural infection [66] or vaccination [26,27]. Although this suggests maternal transfer of protective immunity, the degree of protection that these antibodies provide early in neonatal life is unknown.

No replication-competent virus has been identified in breastmilk, although nonreplicating viral fragments

Patient status	Recommendation
Outpatient	Symptomatic treatment
	Treatment to prevent progression to severe disease[a] - Administered as soon as possible and within 5 d of symptoms - Nirmatrelvir/Ritonavir (Paxlovid): 300 mg/100 mg BID x 5 d - Sotrovimab: 500 mg single IV infusion - Remdesivir: 200 mg IV on Day 1 then 100 mg IV daily on Days 2 and 3
Inpatient	
Normal O2 saturation	Dexamethasone is NOT recommended
Requires supplemental oxygen	[b]**Dexamethasone**: 6 mg po or IV daily for up to 10 d - If also indicated for fetal lung maturity: 6 mg IM q 12 hr x 4 doses followed by 6 mg po or IV daily for up to total of 10 d **+** **Remdesivir**: 200 mg IV once, then 100 mg IV daily for up to 4 d
Requires mechanical ventilation or Extracorporeal membrane oxygenation (ECMO)	**Dexamethasone**: 6 mg poor IV daily for up to 10 d - If also indicated for fetal lung maturity: 6 mg IM q 12 hr x 4 doses followed by 6 mg po or IV daily for up to total of 10 d **+** **Remdesivir**: 200 mg IV once, then 100 mg IV daily for up to 4 d **+** **Tocilizumab IV**: 8 mg/kg actual body weight (up to 800 mg) x 1 IV dose - If not available can use another Immunomodulatory drug (ex: sarilumab)

[a]Treatment listed in order of preference based on efficacy and convenience.
[b]For all medications: Ensure patient meets emergency use authorization criteria, when applicable give drug fact sheet to patient/caregiver and obtain verbal consent for treatment.

Figure 31.2 Therapeutic management of COVID-19 in pregnancy. IM, intramuscular; IV, intravenous.

have been identified [67]. Observational cohorts suggest that COVID-19 infected persons can safely breastfeed their infants with masking and careful hand and breast hygiene [68,69]. High titers of antibodies against SARS-COV-2 are found in breastmilk after natural infection and vaccination, suggesting that breastfeeding may provide some degree of protection from neonatal COVID-19 infection [26,27].

CASE PRESENTATION

The patient is a 28-year-old para 0 at 31 weeks gestation who presented to an outpatient appointment with a cough, myalgias, fevers, and shortness of breath for two days. On presentation, she was tachycardic to low 100s, and her O_2 saturation was 90% on room air. She was sent to OB triage for further workup, where she had a nasopharyngeal polymerase chain reaction test for SARS-CoV-2 that was positive; the remainder of her labs were within normal limits. Her chest X-ray showed patchy increased opacities concerning for pneumonia. On admission to the antepartum service, the patient was placed on 2 L of oxygen by nasal cannula and started on dexamethasone and IV remdesivir. On hospital day 2, she desaturated to the low 70s and a stat arterial blood gas showed decreasing O_2 levels (PaO_2 77 mmHg, normal 105 mmHg) and increased CO_2 (32 mmHg, normal 30 mmHg). A rapid response was called, and the patient was placed on high-flow oxygen (45 L/100% FiO_2). She was transferred to the stepdown unit for continued high-flow oxygen therapy and received monoclonal antibody treatment (tocilizumab) as well as heparin venous thromboembolism prophylaxis. Twice daily fetal monitoring was reassuring. She clinically improved over the next 4 days and was ultimately weaned off oxygen therapy prior to discharge. The remainder of her prenatal course was uncomplicated, and she delivered via spontaneous vaginal delivery at 38 weeks after presenting in active labor. She was eligible for and received the COVID-19 vaccination at her 6-week postpartum visit, as it had been 90 days since she received monoclonal antibody therapy.

References

1. Li Q, Guan X, Wu P, Wang X, Zhou L, Tong Y, et al. Early transmission dynamics in Wuhan, China, of novel coronavirus-infected pneumonia. N Engl J Med. 2020 Mar 26;382(13):1199–207.

2. Cucinotta D, Vanelli M. WHO declares COVID-19 a pandemic. Acta Biomed. 2020 Mar 19;91(1):157–60.

3. Zambrano LD, Ellington S, Strid P, Galang RR, Oduyebo T, Tong VT, et al. Update: characteristics of symptomatic women of reproductive age with laboratory-confirmed SARS-CoV-2 infection by pregnancy status–United States, January 22–October 3, 2020. MMWR Morb Mortal Wkly Rep. 2020 Nov 6;69(44):1641–7.

4. Mosby LG, Rasmussen SA, Jamieson DJ. 2009 pandemic influenza A (H1N1) in pregnancy: a systematic review of the literature. Am J Obstet Gynecol. 2011 Jul;205(1):10–8.

5. Di Mascio D, Khalil A, Saccone G, Rizzo G, Buca D, Liberati M, et al. Outcome of coronavirus spectrum infections (SARS, MERS, COVID-19) during pregnancy: a systematic review and meta-analysis. Am J Obstet Gynecol MFM. 2020 May;2(2):100107.

6. Le Gars M, Kay AW, Bayless NL, Aziz N, Dekker CL, Swan GE, et al. Increased proinflammatory responses of monocytes and plasmacytoid dendritic cells to influenza a virus infection during pregnancy. J Infect Dis. 2016 Dec 1;214(11):1666–71.

7. Periolo N, Avaro M, Czech A, Russo M, Benedetti E, Pontoriero A, et al. Pregnant women infected with pandemic influenza A(H1N1)pdm09 virus showed differential immune response correlated with disease severity. J Clin Virol. 2015 Mar;64:52–8.

8. Bikdeli B, Madhavan MV, Jimenez D, Chuich T, Dreyfus I, Driggin E, et al. COVID-19 and thrombotic or thromboembolic disease: implications for prevention, antithrombotic therapy, and follow-up: JACC state-of-the-art review. J Am Coll Cardiol. 2020 Jun 16;75(23):2950–73.

9. COVID 19 dashboard by the Center for Systems Science and Engineering (CSSE) at Johns Hopkins University (JHU). 2023 [cited 2023 Jun 7]. Available from: https://coronavirus.jhu. edu/map.html.

10. Curtin S, Abma J. 2010 pregnancy rates among U.S. women. Centers for Disease Control and Prevention. National Center for Health Statistics. [last reviewed 2015 Nov 6; cited 2023 Jun 7]. Available from: https://www.cdc.gov/nchs/data/hestat/ pregnancy/2010_pregnancy_rates.html.

11. Jamieson DJ, Rasmussen SA. An update on COVID-19 and pregnancy. Am J Obstet Gynecol. 2022 Feb;226(2):177–86.

12. Joseph NT, Stanhope KK, Badell ML, Horton JP, Boulet SL, Jamieson DJ. Sociodemographic predictors of SARS-CoV-2 infection in obstetric patients, Georgia, USA. Emerg Infect Dis. 2020 Nov;26(11):2787–9.

13. Emeruwa UN, Ona S, Shaman JL, Turitz A, Wright JD, Gyamfi-Bannerman C, et al. Associations between built environment, neighborhood socioeconomic status, and SARS-CoV-2 infection among pregnant women in New York City. JAMA. 2020 Jul 28;324(4):390–2.

14. Badr DA, Mattern J, Carlin A, Cordier A-G, Maillart E, El Hachem L, et al. Are clinical outcomes worse for pregnant women at ≥20 weeks' gestation infected with coronavirus disease 2019? A multicenter case-control study with propensity score matching. Am J Obstet Gynecol. 2020 Nov;223(5):764–8.

15. Knight M, Bunch K, Vousden N, Morris E, Simpson N, Gale C, et al. Characteristics and outcomes of pregnant women admitted to hospital with confirmed SARS-CoV-2 infection in UK: national population based cohort study. BMJ. 2020 Jun 8;369:m2107.

16. Galang RR, Newton SM, Woodworth KR, Griffin I, Oduyebo T, Sancken CL, et al. Risk factors for illness severity among pregnant women with confirmed severe acute respiratory syndrome coronavirus 2 infection-surveillance for emerging threats to mothers and babies network, 22 state, local, and territorial health departments, 29 March 2020–5 March 2021. Clin Infect Dis. 2021 Jul 15;73(Suppl 1):S17–23.

17. Kasehagen L, Byers P, Taylor K, Kittle T, Roberts C, Collier C, et al. COVID-19-associated deaths after SARS-CoV-2 infection during pregnancy–Mississippi, March 1, 2020–October 6, 2021. MMWR Morb Mortal Wkly Rep. 2021 Nov 26;70(47):1646–8.

18. Centers for Disease Control and Prevention. COVID 19: how to protect yourself & others. 2022 [updated 2023 May 11; cited 2023 Jun 7]. Available from: https://www.cdc.gov/ coronavirus/2019-ncov/prevent-getting-sick/prevention. html.

19. Miller, Emily, Leffert, Lisa, Landau, Ruth. Society for Maternal-Fetal Medicine and Society for Obstetric and Anesthesia and Perinatology. Labor and delivery COVID-19 considerations. 2020 Oct [cited 2023 Jun 7]. Available from: https://s3.amazonaws.com/cdn.smfm.org/media/2542/SMFM-SOAP_ COVID_LD_Considerations_-_revision_10-9-20_(final).pdf.

20. Abuhamad, Alfred, Stone, Joanne. Society for Maternal-Fetal Medicine COVID-19 ultrasound clinical practice suggestions. 2020 Oct [cited 2023 Jun 7]. Available from: https://s3.amazonaws.com/cdn.smfm.org/media/2550/Ultrasound_ Covid19_Suggestions_10-20-20_(final).pdf.

21. Centers for Disease Control and Prevention. COVID-19 vaccines while pregnant or breastfeeding. 2021 [updated 2022 Oct. 20; cited 2023 Jun 7]. Available from: https://www.cdc. gov/coronavirus/2019-ncov/vaccines/recommendations/ pregnancy.html.

22. Society for Maternal-Fetal Medicine (SMFM) statement: SARS-CoV-2 vaccination in pregnancy. 2020 Dec 1 [cited 2021 Nov 22]. Available from: https://s3.amazonaws.com/ cdn.smfm.org/media/2591/SMFM_Vaccine_Statement_12-1-20_(final).pdf.

23. Polack FP, Thomas SJ, Kitchin N, Absalon J, Gurtman A, Lockhart S, et al. Safety and efficacy of the BNT162b2 mRNA COVID-19 vaccine. N Engl J Med. 2020 Dec 31;383(27):2603–15.

24. Baden LR, El Sahly HM, Essink B, Kotloff K, Frey S, Novak R, et al. Efficacy and safety of the mRNA-1273 SARS-CoV-2 vaccine. N Engl J Med. 2021 Feb 4;384(5):403–16.

25. Sadoff J, Gray G, Vandebosch A, Cárdenas V, Shukarev G, Grinsztejn B, et al. Safety and efficacy of single-dose Ad26.COV2.S vaccine against COVID-19. N Engl J Med. 2021 Jun 10;384(23):2187–201.

26. Collier A-RY, McMahan K, Yu J, Tostanoski LH, Aguayo R, Ansel J, et al. Immunogenicity of COVID-19 mRNA vaccines in pregnant and lactating women. JAMA. 2021 Jun 15;325(23):2370–80.

27. Gray KJ, Bordt EA, Atyeo C, Deriso E, Akinwunmi B, Young N, et al. Coronavirus disease 2019 vaccine response in pregnant and lactating women: a cohort study. Am J Obstet Gynecol. 2021 Sep;225(3):303.e1–17.

28. Kugelman N, Nahshon C, Shaked-Mishan P, Cohen N, Sher ML, Gruber M, et al. Maternal and neonatal SARS-CoV-2 immunoglobulin G antibody levels at delivery after receipt of the BNT162b2 messenger RNA COVID-19 vaccine during the second trimester of pregnancy. JAMA Pediatr. 2022 Mar 1;176(3):290–5.

29. Shanes ED, Otero S, Mithal LB, Mupanomunda CA, Miller ES, Goldstein JA. Severe acute respiratory syndrome coronavirus 2 (SARS-CoV-2) vaccination in pregnancy: measures of immunity and placental histopathology. Obstet Gynecol. 2021 Aug 1;138(2):281–3.

30. Theiler RN, Wick M, Mehta R, Weaver AL, Virk A, Swift M. Pregnancy and birth outcomes after SARS-CoV-2 vaccination in pregnancy. Am J Obstet Gynecol MFM. 2021 Nov;3(6):100467.

31. Dagan N, Barda N, Biron-Shental T, Makov-Assif M, Key C, Kohane IS, et al. Effectiveness of the BNT162b2 mRNA COVID-19 vaccine in pregnancy. Nat Med. 2021 Oct;27(10):1693–5.

32. Tseng HF, Ackerson BK, Luo Y, Sy LS, Talarico CA, Tian Y, et al. Effectiveness of mRNA-1273 against SARS-CoV-2 Omicron and Delta variants. Nat Med. 2022 May;28(5):1063–71.

33. Thompson MG, Natarajan K, Irving SA, Rowley EA, Griggs EP, Gaglani M, et al. Effectiveness of a third dose of mRNA vaccines against COVID-19-associated emergency department and urgent care encounters and hospitalizations among adults during periods of Delta and Omicron variant predominance–VISION Network, 10 states, August 2021–January 2022. MMWR Morb Mortal Wkly Rep. 2022 Jan 21;71(4):139–45.

34. Beharier O, Plitman Mayo R, Raz T, Nahum Sacks K, Schreiber L, Suissa-Cohen Y, et al. Efficient maternal to neonatal transfer of antibodies against SARS-CoV-2 and BNT162b2 mRNA COVID-19 vaccine. J Clin Invest. 2021 Jul 1;131(13): e150319.

35. Rottenstreich A, Zarbiv G, Oiknine-Djian E, Zigron R, Wolf DG, Porat S. Efficient maternofetal transplacental transfer of anti-severe acute respiratory syndrome coronavirus 2 (SARS-CoV-2) spike antibodies after antenatal SARS-CoV-2 BNT162b2 messenger RNA vaccination. Clin Infect Dis. 2021 Nov 16;73(10): 1909–12.

36. Nir O, Schwartz A, Toussia-Cohen S, Leibovitch L, Strauss T, Asraf K, et al. Maternal-neonatal transfer of SARS-CoV-2 immunoglobulin G antibodies among parturient women treated with BNT162b2 messenger RNA vaccine during pregnancy. Am J Obstet Gynecol MFM. 2021 Sep 20;4(1):100492.

37. Mithal LB, Otero S, Shanes ED, Goldstein JA, Miller ES. Cord blood antibodies following maternal coronavirus disease 2019 vaccination during pregnancy. Am J Obstet Gynecol. 2021 Aug;225(2):192–4.

38. Prabhu M, Murphy EA, Sukhu AC, Yee J, Singh S, Eng D, et al. Antibody response to coronavirus disease 2019 (COVID-19) messenger RNA vaccination in pregnant women and transplacental passage into cord blood. Obstet Gynecol. 2021 Aug 1;138(2):278–80.

39. Halasa NB, Olson SM, Staat MA, Newhams MM, Price AM, Boom JA, et al. Effectiveness of maternal vaccination with mRNA COVID-19 vaccine during pregnancy against COVID-19-associated hospitalization in infants aged <6 months–17 states, July 2021–January 2022. MMWR Morb Mortal Wkly Rep. 2022 Feb 18;71(7):264–70.

40. Bookstein Peretz S, Regev N, Novick L, Nachshol M, Goffer E, Ben-David A, et al. Short-term outcome of pregnant women vaccinated with BNT162b2 mRNA COVID-19 vaccine. Ultrasound Obstet Gynecol. 2021 Sep;58(3):450–6.

41. Shimabukuro TT, Kim SY, Myers TR, Moro PL, Oduyebo T, Panagiotakopoulos L, et al. Preliminary findings of mRNA Covid-19 vaccine safety in pregnant persons. N Engl J Med. 2021 Jun 17;384(24):2273–82.

42. Kharbanda EO, Haapala J, DeSilva M, Vazquez-Benitez G, Vesco KK, Naleway AL, et al. Spontaneous abortion following COVID-19 vaccination during pregnancy. JAMA. 2021 Oct 26;326(16):1629–31.

43. Kachikis A, Englund JA, Singleton M, Covelli I, Drake AL, Eckert LO. Short-term reactions among pregnant and lactating individuals in the first wave of the COVID-19 vaccine rollout. JAMA Netw Open. 2021 Aug 2;4(8):e2121310.

44. Kiefer MK, Mehl R, Costantine MM, Johnson A, Cohen J, Summerfield TL, et al. Characteristics and perceptions associated with COVID-19 vaccination hesitancy among pregnant and postpartum individuals: a cross-sectional study. BJOG. 2022 Jul;129(8):1342–51.

45. Metz TD, Clifton RG, Hughes BL, Sandoval G, Saade GR, Grobman WA, et al. Disease severity and perinatal outcomes of pregnant patients with coronavirus disease 2019 (COVID-19). Obstet Gynecol. 2021 Apr 1;137(4):571–80.

46. Villar J, Ariff S, Gunier RB, Thiruvengadam R, Rauch S, Kholin A, et al. Maternal and neonatal morbidity and mortality among pregnant women with and without COVID-19 infection: The INTERCOVID Multinational Cohort Study. JAMA Pediatr. 2021 Aug 1;175(8):817–26.

47. Stock SJ, Carruthers J, Calvert C, Denny C, Donaghy J, Goulding A, et al. SARS-CoV-2 infection and COVID-19 vaccination rates in pregnant women in Scotland. Nat Med. 2022 Mar;28(3):504–2.

48. Cavalcante MB, de Melo Bezerra Cavalcante CT, Cavalcante ANM, Sarno M, Barini R, Kwak-Kim J. COVID-19 and miscarriage: from immunopathological mechanisms to actual clinical evidence. J Reprod Immunol. 2021 Nov;148:103382.

49. Wang M, Yang Q, Ren X, Hu J, Li Z, Long R, et al. Investigating the impact of asymptomatic or mild SARS-CoV-2 infection on female fertility and in vitro fertilization outcomes: a retrospective cohort study. EClinicalMedicine. 2021 Aug;38: 101013.

50. Patel DP, Punjani N, Guo J, Alukal JP, Li PS, Hotaling JM. The impact of SARS-CoV-2 and COVID-19 on male reproduction and men's health. Fertil Steril. 2021 Apr;115(4):813–23.

51. Ko JY, DeSisto CL, Simeone RM, Ellington S, Galang RR, Oduyebo T, et al. Adverse pregnancy outcomes, maternal complications, and severe illness among US delivery

hospitalizations with and without a coronavirus disease 2019 (COVID-19) diagnosis. Clin Infect Dis. 2021 Jul 15;73(Suppl 1):S24–31.

52. Allotey J, Stallings E, Bonet M, Yap M, Chatterjee S, Kew T, et al. Clinical manifestations, risk factors, and maternal and perinatal outcomes of coronavirus disease 2019 in pregnancy: living systematic review and meta-analysis. BMJ. 2020 Sep 1;370:m3320.

53. Wei SQ, Bilodeau-Bertrand M, Liu S, Auger N. The impact of COVID-19 on pregnancy outcomes: a systematic review and meta-analysis. CMAJ. 2021 Apr 19;193(16):E540–8.

54. Son M, Gallagher K, Lo JY, Lindgren E, Burris HH, Dysart K, et al. Coronavirus disease 2019 (COVID-19) pandemic and pregnancy outcomes in a U.S. population. Obstet Gynecol. 2021 Oct 1;138(4):542–51.

55. Blumberg DA, Underwood MA, Hedriana HL, Lakshminrusimha S. Vertical transmission of SARS-CoV-2: what is the optimal definition? Am J Perinatol. 2020 Jun;37(8):769–72.

56. Shah PS, Diambomba Y, Acharya G, Morris SK, Bitnun A. Classification system and case definition for SARS-CoV-2 infection in pregnant women, fetuses, and neonates. Acta Obstet Gynecol Scand. 2020 May;99(5):565–8.

57. World Health Organization. Definition and categorization of the timing of mother-to-child transmission of SARS-CoV-2. 2021 Feb 7 [cited 2023 Jun 7]. Available from: https://www.who.int/publications/i/item/WHO-2019-nCoV-mother-to-child-transmission-2021.1.

58. Vivanti AJ, Vauloup-Fellous C, Prevot S, Zupan V, Suffee C, Do Cao J, et al. Transplacental transmission of SARS-CoV-2 infection. Nat Commun. 2020 Jul 14;11(1):3572.

59. Edlow AG, Li JZ, Collier A-RY, Atyeo C, James KE, Boatin AA, et al. Assessment of maternal and neonatal SARS-CoV-2 viral load, transplacental antibody transfer, and placental pathology in pregnancies during the COVID-19 pandemic. JAMA Netw Open. 2020 Dec 1;3(12):e2030455.

60. Ouyang Y, Bagalkot T, Fitzgerald W, Sadovsky E, Chu T, Martínez-Marchal A, et al. Term human placental trophoblasts express SARS-CoV-2 entry factors ACE2, TMPRSS2, and furin. mSphere. 2021 Apr 14;6(2):e00250–21.

61. Pique-Regi R, Romero R, Tarca AL, Luca F, Xu Y, Alazizi A, et al. Does the human placenta express the canonical cell entry mediators for SARS-CoV-2? Elife. 2020 Jul 14;9.

62. Halscott T, Vaught, Jason, Society for Maternal Fetal Medicine COVID-19 Taskforce. Management considerations for pregnant patients with COVID-19. 2021 Feb 2 [cited 2023 Jun 7]. Available from: https://s3.amazonaws.com/cdn.smfm.org/media/2734/SMFM_COVID_Management_of_COVID_pos_preg_patients_2-2-21_(final).pdf.

63. National Institutes of Health. COVID-19 treatment guidelines: special considerations in pregnancy. 2021 [updated 2023 Apr 20; cited 2023 Jun 7]. Available from: https://www.covid19treatmentguidelines.nih.gov/special-populations/pregnancy/.

64. National Institutes of Health. COVID-19 treatment guidelines: therapeutic management of hospitalized adults with COVID 19. 2021 [updated 2023 Apr 20; cited 2023 Jun 7]. Available from: https://www.covid19treatmentguidelines.nih.gov/management/clinical-management/hospitalized-adults-therapeutic-management/.

65. Prabhu M, Cagino K, Matthews KC, Friedlander RL, Glynn SM, Kubiak JM, et al. Pregnancy and postpartum outcomes in a universally tested population for SARS-CoV-2 in New York City: a prospective cohort study. BJOG. 2020 Nov;127(12):1548–56.

66. Gee S, Chandiramani M, Seow J, Pollock E, Modestini C, Das A, et al. The legacy of maternal SARS-CoV-2 infection on the immunology of the neonate. Nat Immunol. 2021 Dec;22(12):1490–502.

67. Krogstad P, Contreras D, Ng H, Tobin N, Chambers CD, Bertrand K, et al. No infectious SARS-CoV-2 in breast milk from a cohort of 110 lactating women. Pediatr Res. 2022 Oct;92(4):1140–5.

68. Salvatore CM, Han J-Y, Acker KP, Tiwari P, Jin J, Brandler M, et al. Neonatal management and outcomes during the COVID-19 pandemic: an observation cohort study. Lancet Child Adolesc Health. 2020 Oct;4(10):721–7.

69. Raschetti R, Vivanti AJ, Vauloup-Fellous C, Loi B, Benachi A, De Luca D. Synthesis and systematic review of reported neonatal SARS-CoV-2 infections. Nat Commun. 2020 Oct 15;11(1):5164.

Chapter 32
Recurrent Pregnancy Loss

Claudio V. Schenone and Stephanie T. Ros
Department of Obstetrics and Gynecology, Division of Maternal-Fetal Medicine, University of South Tampa, FL, USA

Approximately one in five clinically recognized pregnancies is expected to result in pregnancy loss, with the number of cases increasing over time by approximately 2% per year from 1990 to 2011 across all age groups [1]. These numbers do not consider the background rate of pregnancy loss in the general population which exceeds 50% when losses from conception through discernible embryonic development are included [2]. In a review of 3.5 million pregnancies, about 4% of patients had experienced two or more pregnancy losses [3].

The nomenclature of pregnancy loss and recurrent spontaneous abortion (SAB) remains a topic of debate, and during recent years important changes have been made to their definitions. Despite efforts to come up with a unique criterion for diagnosis, significant taxomic heterogeneity exists among leading societal guidelines. There are four main components in the definition of recurrent pregnancy loss (RPL): defining pregnancy (biochemical, sonographic visualization, intrauterine), gestational age cutoff, defining recurrence, and deciding whether those pregnancy losses must be consecutive. A comparison of proposed definitions by different societal guidelines is summarized in Table 32.1 [4,5].

Factors contributing to recurrent pregnancy loss

Genetic abnormalities
The advent of new genetic testing modalities and research in the field has led to a significant rise in the diagnostic accuracy of these tests. Chromosomal microarray is preferred to karyotype, given a higher detection rate of abnormalities while avoiding the issue of maternal contamination and need for cell culture. Whole exome and genome sequencing also has the potential to identify novel genetic causes and risk factors for pregnancy loss. However, this approach will require systematic evaluation of large numbers of cases that are well characterized regarding gestational age, developmental stage, and correlative placental, embryonic and fetal abnormalities. In turn, identification of genes relevant to pregnancy loss may provide novel therapeutic targets in hopes of improving outcomes [6].

Aneuploidy
Aneuploidy of the embryo is an important maternal age-related genetic cause of pregnancy loss. Using standard karyotyping methods, investigators have found that the earlier in gestation the loss occurs, the more likely there is to be a genetic abnormality. A small subset of patients with RPL have recurrent cytogenetically abnormal losses; these individuals may have a yet unidentified abnormality in genes regulating meiosis. Nonetheless, evidence has shown that, in most cases, the prevalence of chromosomal abnormalities in pregnancy loss tissue does not differ between patients with a history of RPL when compared to controls. In fact, some studies report lower rates of cytogenetic abnormalities in cases of RPL, likely owing to an increased proportion of losses due to some underlying parental factors [6].

Parental cytogenetic abnormalities explain approximately 2–5% of cases of RPL, with higher detection rates of chromosomal aberrations as the number of prior SABs increases. Reciprocal and balanced Robertsonian chromosomal translocation represent the most common parental cytogenetic alterations, followed by mosaicism, small supernumerary marker chromosomes, and interstitial microdeletions [7]. Regardless, for these patients, there is about a 60% to 70% chance of live birth of a healthy baby without treatment, similar to those without carrier status, although outcomes vary based on the specific abnormality and other factors such as maternal age [6,8,9]. Thus, the importance of assessing parental karyotype in couples with RPL remains uncertain.

In vitro fertilization (IVF) with preimplantation genetic screening (PGS) has been proposed as theoretically

Queenan's Management of High-Risk Pregnancy: An Evidence-Based Approach, Seventh Edition. Edited by Catherine Y. Spong and Charles J. Lockwood.

Table 32.1 Comparison of the elements of RPL by international guidelines

Comparison of the elements of RPL definitions

Professional society	Pregnancy	Weeks of gestation	Recurrence	Pattern
ESHRE (2017)	Serum or urine hCG; ectopic and molar pregnancies not included in definition	Up to 24 wk	2	Consecutive or nonconsecutive
ASRM (2012–2013)	Clinical pregnancy documented by ultrasonography or histopathological examination	Only mentions that majority lost prior to 10th wk	2	Consecutive
RCOG (2011)	All pregnancy losses	Up to 24 wk	3	Consecutive
CNGOF (2016)	Positive hCG test not further specified	Up to 22 wk gestation (up to 14 wk for RPL)	3	Consecutive

ASRM, American Society for Reproductive Medicine; CNGOF, Collège National des Gynécologues et Obstétriciens Français; ESHRE, European Society of Human Reproduction and Embryology; hCG, human chorionic gonadotrophin; RCOG, Royal College of Obstetricians and Gynaecologists; RPL, recurrent pregnancy loss.

beneficial, although clear proof of efficacy is lacking [6]. Several case series report good outcomes with the use of PGS in couples with parental translocations. For example, one series of 192 couples with at least three prior losses and either reciprocal or Robertsonian translocations noted a live birth rate per cycle of 22% and an overall pregnancy loss rate of 13%. In this regard, Franssen et al. conducted a systematic review comparing outcomes in couples with RPL and balanced translocations after natural conception vs. IVF with PGS. The median rate of live birth after natural conception was higher than in the IVF-PGS group. They concluded that data are insufficient to recommend IVF-PGS to improve live birth rates in couples with RPL and parenteral structural chromosome abnormality [6,10].

Single-gene defects

Numerous single-gene disorders are associated with RPL [7]. These may be X-linked, autosomal recessive or germline mutations involving loss of heterozygosity for developmentally lethal genes. Some of these abnormalities are more commonly associated with second-trimester miscarriage, such as lethal multiple pterygium syndromes, a collection of autosomal recessive and X-linked recessive disorders that are associated with fetal death at 14–20 weeks [11], and incontinentia pigmenti, an X-linked disorder usually lethal in males [12]. Amino acid metabolism abnormalities, peroxisomal storage disorders, and alpha thalassemia major, among many others, are also part of this group. IVF-PGS may be useful for some of these disorders. Gene therapy has also been proposed as a promising tool; however, this technology is not ready for routine clinical use yet [7].

Genetic variants

Different chromosomal alterations not detected by traditional cytogenetic techniques such as the length of telomeres, skewed X inactivation, sperm DNA fragmentation, and microdeletions in the Y chromosome have also been found to be associated with risk of recurrent SAB [7].

Furthermore, a genetic predisposition to obesity has been reported as associated with a greater probability of RPL [13]. Several other studies have investigated additional specific gene variants that can predispose couples to RPL that affect essential processes in pregnancy such as implantation, placentation, blood vessel formation, maintenance of hemostasis, and immune tolerance [14]. However, published literature for these variations is still controversial due to a significant degree of heterogeneity among studies [7].

Uterine abnormalities

Several studies have described a high prevalence of uterine factor abnormalities in patients with RPL. It has been reported as the causative factor in up to 50% of cases [15–18]. A recent meta-analysis estimated the overall prevalence of these abnormalities to be 5.5% in an unselected population vs. 24.5% in those with miscarriage and infertility [19,20]. For this reason, they should be systematically assessed in patients with RPL [15].

Uterine abnormalities may be congenital (Müllerian) or acquired (submucous myomas, endometrial polyps, and uterine synechiae). Septate, bicornuate, and arcuate uterus represent the most common Müllerian anomalies, followed by uterus didelphys, and unicornuate uterus [17,18,20]. Cervical insufficiency also plays a major role [16]. A systematic review of women with congenital uterine abnormalities reported that those with canalization defects, such as septate and partial septate uteri, appeared to have the poorest reproductive performance [19], with significantly increased late first-trimester miscarriages compared with women with unexplained RPL [17,20]). Patients with bicornuate uteri also have an increased risk of second-trimester pregnancy loss [17]. The definite etiology and pathophysiological processes underlying infertility and miscarriage in these patients remain uncertain. Various hypotheses have been put forward, such as endometrium overlying the septum being abnormal thus providing a suboptimal site for implantation, disorderly and decreased blood supply that is insufficient to support placentation and embryo growth, uncoordinated uterine contractions, and reduced uterine capacity [19].

Retrospective and case-control studies have shown that submucosal myomas that cause endometrial cavity distortion are associated with decreased pregnancy and implantation rates. Proposed mechanisms include chronic endometrial inflammation, abnormal vascularization, increased uterine contractility, and abnormal local endocrine patterns. In contrast, an association between pregnancy loss and intramural or subserosal myomas is less clear. Some studies suggest that myomectomy for submucosal myomas improves the chances of pregnancies, but evidence is insufficient to support a true decrease of pregnancy losses and even less for the possible cure of RPL. No clear benefit of surgery has been demonstrated for intramural myomas with no impact on the uterine cavity. Similarly, endometrial polyps have been found in women with RPL but there is no clear evidence showing an association with pregnancy loss [17,18]. According to the European Society of Human Reproduction and Embryology (ESHRE) and American Society for Reproductive Medicine (ASRM), evidence is also insufficient to recommend hysteroscopic removal of polyps to reduce the risk of RPL. Hence, the lack of universally accepted recommendations to guide management in these cases [21,22].

Intrauterine adhesions (IUA) have been reported in up to 84% of patients with infertility, and 15% in those with RPL; however, prevalence varies based on the study, and the overall prevalence is estimated to be between 1% and 10%. There is also no consensus about the proper management of IUA. Similar pregnancy outcomes have been reported following conservative, medical, and surgical treatment. Furthermore, a lack of agreement also exists regarding the optimal surgical method, instruments, or indication for physical barriers for preventing recurrence. Therefore, ESHRE and ASRM guidelines conclude that there is insufficient evidence of a benefit for surgical removal of IUAs in women with RPL [18,21,22].

In a recent consensus publication, ESHRE and the European Society for Gynecological Endoscopy investigated the diagnostic accuracy of different imaging modalities to diagnose Müllerian anomalies. The pooled analysis of 38 studies showed that 3D ultrasound had the highest overall diagnostic accuracy (97.6%), followed by hysterosalpingogram (86.9%), and 2D ultrasound (86.6%). Magnetic resonance imaging (MRI) had a diagnostic accuracy of over 90%. The authors suggested that this modality may be used as needed in complicated cases associated with complex anatomical defects [18]. Combined hysteroscopy and laparoscopy has been considered the gold standard as it offers a simultaneously internal and external view of the uterus and allows concurrent treatment of many intrauterine lesions during the procedure. However, due to cost and invasiveness, this approach is typically reserved for patients in whom intrauterine pathology is suspected, or those with a nondiagnostic evaluation of RPL [17,18,21,23]. Table 32.2 summarizes management guidelines of uterine anomalies for patients with RPL [18].

Immunologic factors

Disruption of maternal immune tolerance has been invoked as one possible cause of RPL. Maternal–fetal tolerance and vascular remodeling is achieved by decidual cell type redistribution and a myriad of complex cellular interactions mediated by factors such as maternal uterine natural killer cell receptors, Killer Ig-like receptors (KIRs), and the embryo's human leukocyte antigen (HLA-C)

Table 32.2 Management guidelines summary of uterine anomalies for patients with RPL

Management guidelines summary of uterine anomalies for patients with RPL			
Society	Anatomical assessment	Congenital anomalies	Acquired anomalies
ESHRE (2017)	2D ultrasound	Resection of uterine septum as part of randomized controlled trials only	Insufficient evidence to make management recommendations
ASRM (2012–2013)	Sonohysterogram, hysteroscopy	Resection of uterine septum	Insufficient evidence to make management recommendations
RCOG (2011)	Pelvic ultrasound, followed by hysteroscopy, laparoscopy or 3D pelvic ultrasound if suspected anomalies	Insufficient evidence to make management recommendations	Insufficient evidence to make management recommendations
CNGOF (2016)	2D or 3D ultrasound, sonohysterogram, hysteroscopy, or MRI depending on availability	Resection of uterine septum	Resection of endometrial polyps, submucosal myomas. Lysis of IUAs

ASRM, American Society for Reproductive Medicine; CNGOF, Collège National des Gynécologues et Obstétriciens Français; ESHRE, European Society of Human Reproduction and Embryology; IUA, intrauterine adhesions; MRI, magnetic resonance imaging; RCOG, Royal College of Obstetricians and Gynaecologists; RPL, recurrent pregnancy loss.

ligand, expressed by extravillous trophoblast cells. Absence of this maternal immune activation, which is observed in KIR AA (inhibitory receptor) carriers, is associated with poor embryo invasion and poor placentation. This is particularly the case when the fetus has more HLAC2 genes than the mother and when additional fetal HLAC2 alleles are of paternal or oocyte donor origin. These patients have increased miscarriage rates and lower live birth rates when compared to those with KIR AB or BB genotypes [24]. Maternal immune response via class I antibodies production against the fetal HLA-C is yet another potential causative of RPL. Specifically, the frequency of HLA-C* 07, one of the most immunogenic HLA-C alleles, was significantly higher in partners of women with recurrent miscarriage, as also were the rates of parental mismatch, and presence of antibodies compared to controls [25]. Some practitioners have advocated therapies including intravenous immunoglobulin (IVIG) or steroids such as prednisone, or other infusions such as intralipid. There is no consistent improvement in live birth rate in the published literature, and these interventions are not widely recommended.

Maternal serum autoantibodies have also been looked at as potential contributors to RPL. An increased prevalence of antinuclear antibodies (ANA) in women with RPL has also been described. In fact, studies have shown that women with RPL have up to threefold higher prevalence of ANA positivity and higher serum titers compared to fertile women. These autoantibodies might impair embryo quality and development, leading to reduced pregnancy and implantation rates. However, further randomized controlled trials are needed to investigate a possible role for ANA testing in the identification of a subset of women eligible for various forms of immunotherapy. Similarly, previous studies in patients with RPL showed a significantly higher frequency of serological markers of celiac disease (anti-transglutaminase and anti-endomysial antibodies) compared to controls. The proposed pathogenic mechanism was both deficiency of nutrients and the ability of anti-transglutaminase antibodies to bind to both trophoblast and human endometrial endothelial cells. However, follow-up studies were not able to confirm this association. Furthermore, evidence comparing the effect of a gluten-free diet on the risk of miscarriage are lacking, and the effect of diet on the recurrence risk remains unclear [26].

Hematologic factors

Antiphospholipid antibody syndrome

Antiphospholipid antibodies (APA) are immunoglobulins directed against proteins bound to negatively charged (anionic) phospholipids [27]. In a review by the members of the Obstetric Task Force of the 14th International Congress on Antiphospholipid Antibodies, an association

between the presence of APA and RPL was shown in 27 out 42 reviewed studies [26,28,29]. Furthermore, their prevalence among women with RPL is estimated to be three times higher compared to fertile women. Specifically, differences were noted for APA in the IgG and IgM, but not IgA isotypes [30].

Antiphospholipid antibody syndrome (APS) is defined by the combination of a prior deep venous or arterial thrombosis or characteristic obstetric complications, associated with laboratory confirmation of APA. Obstetric complications include at least one unexplained fetal death at 10 weeks or more gestation, at least one premature birth before 34 weeks due to pre-eclampsia, eclampsia or placental insufficiency, or at least three consecutive SABs before 10 weeks not explained by other causes. Laboratory criteria include the presence of medium-to-high titer IgG/IgM anticardiolipin antibodies (ACA), IgG/IgM anti-β2-glycoprotein-I antibodies (anti-β2GPI) at levels ≥99th percentile, or presence of a lupus anticoagulant (LAC); any of these laboratory findings need to be positive on ≥two occasions at least 12 weeks apart in order to meet the laboratory criteria for diagnosis [31]. Within this group, ACA is the most often found (61%), and anti-β2GPI antibodies are associated with the lowest live birth rates and highest incidences of obstetric complications compared to ACA or LAC alone. It has also been shown that poorer pregnancy outcomes occur in women with more than one antibody. Accordingly, triple-positive women carry a significantly higher risk of obstetric complications compared to double-positive women. In fact, the chance of a liveborn neonate is approximately 30% for triple-positive, compared to about 80% for women with positivity to LAC alone.

Other nonconventional APA-like antibodies directed against phosphatidylethanolamine, annexin V, and prothrombin, have also been described [26]. Among this group, levels of IgG class of antiphosphatidylserine have been found to be significantly higher in RPL patients by multiple authors [28]. Others have described an increased frequency of antiphosphatidylcholine among women with unexplained infertility, recurrent implantation failure, and RPL in the IgM isotype when compared with controls. Nevertheless, available clinical data regarding these less frequently studied antibodies have shown controversial results, and the clinical utility of testing and treatment warrants further investigation [26].

Six features appeared to be more common in the placentae of women with APS including placental infarction, impaired spiral artery remodeling, decidual inflammation, increased syncytial knots, decreased vasculosyncytial membranes, and deposition of complement split product C4d [26,29,30,32].

Treatment includes low molecular weight heparin (LMWH) and low-dose aspirin (ASA). This combination therapy was proven more effective than ASA alone.

The use of IVIG has had conflicting results from two randomized trials that compared its use with combined LMWH and ASA [29,33–37]. More recent animal studies have suggested that pretreatment with a synthetic peptide, called TIFI, able to mimic the binding site of β2GPI, protects mice from APA-mediated fetal loss [26], which may prove useful in the clinical arena in the future.

In summary, in the event of RPL and other complications of pregnancy as defined by the APS classification criteria, affected women should be screened for APS. For women with a confirmed or presumptive diagnosis, the recommendation is to administer ASA and a prophylactic dose of LMWH from the time of the positive pregnancy test until at least 6 weeks post partum [36].

Inherited thrombophilias

Congenital thrombophilias include inhibitor deficiencies (antithrombin, protein C and protein S deficiency), activated protein C resistance (factor V Leiden mutation [FVL] and prothrombin gene G20210A mutation [PGM]), mutations of fibrinolysis factors (tissue plasminogen activator, plasminogen activator inhibitor-1, and factor VII activating protease), and hyperhomocysteinemia caused by the MTHFR C677T mutation. Up to 15% of the White population has one of the aforementioned thrombophilic disorders, of which MTHFR mutation is the most common, followed by FVL and PGM, respectively [36, 38].

Ulas Barut et al. found a rate of almost 50% of thrombophilia-associated mutations in a population with history of RPL [39]. A meta-analysis carried out in 2010, which included only prospective studies, calculated the pooled odds ratio for all pregnancy losses of women with FVL compared to healthy controls as 1.5 times higher. Patients with antithrombin, protein C deficiency, and homozygous MTHFR C677T mutation did not appear to have an increased risk of RPL. There are almost no data available for significantly rarer and highly thrombophilic constellations such as homozygous mutations (both FVL mutation and PGM G20210A) or complex combined hereditary thrombophilias. The current body of evidence on the association between late miscarriages (after 24 weeks gestation) and the presence of antithrombin or protein C deficiency is also insufficient [36].

The first studies on the prophylactic administration of heparin to women with hereditary thrombophilia and RPL appeared to be promising based on the rate of live births. But these results, which were predominantly obtained from observational studies, were not confirmed by recently carried out prospective randomized controlled studies and metanalyses. In these studies, no difference was found regarding the reduction of late pregnancy losses or recurrent early pregnancy losses between women who received LMWH and those who did not. Therefore, current guidelines recommend against the use of prophylactic administration of LMWH for the management of RPL in patients with thrombophilia [32,36].

Endocrinopathies

Hyperandrogenism

Hyperandrogenism has been linked with miscarriage by way of retardation of endometrial development in the luteal phase leading to reduction in oocyte and embryo viability [40]. Alternative pathways such as indirect effect via insulin-like growth factors have also been suggested [41]. The most recent large-scale study with measurement of the free androgen index (FAI) in the early follicular phase demonstrated a significantly increased risk of miscarriage with increasing FAI [40,41]. Thus, hyperandrogenemia seems to contribute to the pathology of RPL. However, the presence of an independent link between hyperandrogenemia and RPL remains contentious, and further studies are needed to determine whether interventions to reduce the FAI are associated with a reduction in rates of miscarriage in this population [41].

Thyroid dysfunction

A systematic review and meta-analysis by D'Ippolito et al. suggested that the presence of thyroid autoantibodies tripled the odds of miscarriage [26]. The presence of antithyroid antibodies might belong to a wider innate and humoral immunity dysfunction associated with changes in endometrial T-cell, polyclonal B-cell, and cytotoxic natural killer cell levels, as well as vitamin D deficiency [41]. Cross-reactivity of antithyroid antibodies with extrathyroid sites has also been proposed. Accordingly, ESHRE issued a recommendation for thyroid screening in women with RPL [21]. In this regard, two randomized studies evaluated the effect of treatment with levothyroxine on miscarriage rates in patients with positive thyroid autoantibodies without overt hypo- or hyperthyroidism. Both studies, as well as a subsequent metanalysis, revealed a fall in miscarriage rates in the treatment group [26]. However, despite these results, there is no consensus regarding treatment of thyroid autoimmunity in patients with RPL, and further studies are needed to investigate both the role of antithyroid Ab in the pathogenesis of this condition, and potential treatment modalities to improve reproductive outcomes in this subset of patients [42].

Results from studies looking at a potential link between overt hypothyroidism and RPL are conflicting at best [40,43]. Rao et al. reported an increased prevalence of hypothyroidism in nonpregnant patients with RPL, as compared to nonpregnant women with no history of miscarriage and a history of at least one successful pregnancy [44]. However, the design for this and other available studies is suboptimal. Studies on subclinical hypothyroidism are no different, with some reporting an increased prevalence in RPL patients but others reporting similar miscarriage rates across groups [43]. Even if an association exists between low thyroid function and pregnancy loss, there is no direct evidence for a causal role. Regardless, treatment has not proven to modify outcomes [41].

Similarly, multiple systematic reviews have looked at whether hyperthyroidism increases the rate of pregnancy loss. Although one study suggested that excess exogenous thyroid hormone is associated with an elevated rate of fetal loss. Thus far, hyperthyroidism has not commonly been reported as an independent cause of RPL [41,43].

Prolactin

Recent research on rodents has revealed that prolactin receptors are involved not only in generating but also in maintaining pregnancy. Progesterone secretion by cultured granulosa cells obtained from human ovarian follicles is almost completely inhibited by high prolactin concentrations (100 ng/ml). Transient hyperprolactinemia, defined as a rise of 200% over mid-follicular baseline levels at the time of peak follicular maturity has been linked to unexplained infertility and repeated miscarriages [40,41]. An elevated prolactin level was found to increase miscarriage risk in women with RPL in a randomized trial by Hirahara et al. [45]. Rates of successful pregnancy were higher in hyperprolactinemic women with RPL treated with bromocriptine [40,43]. Furthermore, Li et al. evaluated prolactin levels in 174 patients with recurrent miscarriage, 109 of these patients conceived again during the study period, and those who had a spontaneous abortion in the index pregnancy had significantly lower prolactin levels during the follicular phase prior to conception, suggesting that low prolactin levels may also be associated with subsequent pregnancy loss in women with a history of RPL [46]. Based on these findings, normal prolactin levels may play an important role in establishing early pregnancies [43].

Diabetes

Nondiabetic women with RPL have higher rates of insulin resistance when compared to age-matched nondiabetic controls based on fasting glucose, fasting insulin, fasting glucose-to-insulin ratios, and increased Homeostatic Model Assessment of Insulin Resistance. However, to our knowledge, no studies have elucidated whether the relationship between insulin resistance and RPL is causative [43]. Studies have suggested ovarian androgen excess might promote miscarriage by increasing circulating testosterone concentration, hyperhomocysteinemia, and the increased risk of polycystic ovary syndrome (PCOS) [40].

Patients diagnosed with diabetes mellitus (DM) run a significantly increased risk of spontaneous abortion with the main underlying cause being hyperglycemia-induced lethal embryonic malformations, the prevalence of which increases in the case of poorly controlled DM during the periconceptional period [40,41]. In contrast, well-controlled DM is not a risk factor for RPL. Attention should therefore be given to ensuring optimal metabolic control of diabetic women during the preconceptional period [41].

Luteal phase deficiency

Progesterone production triggers morphological and physiological changes in the endometrium creating a suitable environment for the embryo during the implantation window. Progesterone also helps in maintaining early pregnancy, by affecting proliferation and differentiation of stromal cells, augmenting uterine receptivity through the modulation of locally acting growth factors, and regulation of cytokine production in maternal–fetal interface [40]. Luteal phase deficiency (LPD) has been historically reported to occur in up to 35% of women with RPL. However, the actual presence of such deficiency and its relation to miscarriage remains controversial, and there is no consensus on the best method of diagnosis. Progesterone levels can fluctuate during measurements due to pulsatile secretion, therefore the interpretation of progesterone levels becomes difficult [41]. Hence, conclusions regarding the relationship between LPD and RPL are difficult to ascertain due to the heterogeneity in the definitions, as well as the lack of controlled trials [43].

The subject of progesterone administration in patients with RPL is also a topic of debate. Daya's meta-analysis suggested that hormonal treatment was associated with increased rates of a term pregnancy in women with RPL [47]. However, a follow-up Cochrane review by Oates-Whitehead [48], and subsequent 2015 randomized trial [49] demonstrated no improvement in live birth rates when progesterone therapy was initiated after a positive pregnancy test in RPL patients. In contrast, the latter research group did show improved rates of live births when using vaginal progesterone in patients with history of pregnancy loss and vaginal bleeding early in pregnancy [50]. There remains some opportunity for study of progesterone initiated during the luteal phase, prior to measurable human chorionic gonadotrophin levels.

Vitamin D deficiency

Vitamin D has been shown to modulate the immune reaction in the feto-maternal interface, and to contribute to the creation of a more favorable environment for pregnancy development, whereas deficiency has been associated with pregnancy loss [51]. Specifically, in vitro vitamin D3 reduced NK cytotoxicity, suppressed secretion of type 1 cytokines (tumor necrosis factor-α, interferon-γ), reduced interleukin (IL)-23 cytokine levels, and increased type 2 cytokines (IL-10), promoting a shift from type 1 to type 2 immunity response, among other changes that have been linked with those occurring in successful pregnancies [52]. Women with vitamin D deficiency also have increased levels of many serum autoantibodies like anti-β2GPI antibodies, anti-thyroid peroxidase antibodies, ANA, and anti-ssDNA, which also translates into higher levels of disease activity [43,51–53]. Furthermore, vitamin D supplementation was associated with reversal of these profiles both in vitro and in vivo in a study done by Chen et al. [54]. This regulatory role contributes to the association between low levels of vitamin D and RPL, given the association between high levels of autoantibodies with increased frequency of pregnancy loss [43,51,52]. Nonetheless, it is still unclear whether laboratory changes induced by vitamin D in women with RPL are associated with fewer miscarriages, because the reported randomized controlled trials failed to show a significant correlation between vitamin D supplementation and incidence of spontaneous abortion. In practice, it remains uncertain if vitamin D supplementation should be recommended to women with RPL who are pregnant or desire to be pregnant [52].

Polycystic ovary syndrome

Prevalence of PCOS in patients with RPL is extremely variable due to inconsistencies in diagnostic criteria and methodology among studies [55]. It remains unclear whether PCOS per se is predictive of pregnancy loss in women with RPL [41]. Some evidence suggests higher fasting insulin and lower Quantitative Insulin Sensitivity Check Index (QUICKI) scores in patients with RPL and history of PCOS in comparison to controls [43]. However, results from studies that looked at the link between insulin resistance and RPL are inconclusive [55]. Rather, patients with PCOS may have several underlying contributing and confounding factors, which have been reported in women with RPL, regardless of PCOS status, including obesity, hyperinsulinemia, insulin resistance, hyperhomocysteinemia, high levels of plasminogen activator inhibitor-1 factor, hyperandrogenemia, and poor endometrial receptivity [41]. Evidence is also lacking regarding potential benefit of using metformin in patients with RPL and PCOS [55].

Obesity and other social factors

Maternal obesity has been reported as an independent risk factor for miscarriage. It is believed to act on female reproductive function through hyperinsulinemia and androgen production [40]. Two studies demonstrated a significant improvement in the overall rate of miscarriage for a group of obese women following weight loss [56]. In cost-effectiveness analysis, this group showed that a 6-month weight loss and exercise program resulted in a considerable reduction in the cost per live birth compared with traditional interventional treatments. Because programmed weight loss is a simple, safe and inexpensive option, it is crucially important that this is recommended as the first treatment for patients with this condition [55].

An additional number of social and anthropomorphic factors are modestly associated with the occurrence of isolated and recurrent miscarriage. These include cigarette smoking, and heavy caffeine use. Thus, smoking cessation and reduction in caffeine use also seem prudent interventions in affected patients.

Male factor

Decreased sperm global methylation levels and aberrant sperm methylation patterns in the imprinted genes like the IGF2-H19 DMR, IG-DMR, MEST, ZAC, KvDMR, PEG10, and PEG3 were found to be associated with RPL in a study done by Khambata et al. [57]. RPL has also been linked to significantly higher sperm DNA Fragmentation Index than those in whom another identifiable cause was found [58,59]. Y-chromosome polymorphisms have also been studied in this population and suggested as an independent risk factor in patients with unexplained pregnancy loss [60].

Infections

In a study by Cao et al., the rate of bacterial infections with *Ureaplasma urealyticum* or *Mycoplasma hominis* in chorion and decidual tissues, as well as the gene copy numbers for these entities, were significantly higher in the RPL group than in the control group [61,62]. However, there are no unequivocal data establishing an association between chronic genital tract carriage of bacteria and recurrent SAB, and further studies are needed in this area [63].

Evidence-based evaluation of couples experiencing recurrent pregnancy loss

The focus of the evaluation of a patient with recurrent first trimester SAB should be on the identification of genetic factors. Chromosomal microarray is preferred to karyotype and should be offered to couples with RPL, and genetic counseling is advised in case of abnormalities. Genetic evaluation of the conceptus using chromosomal microarray may also be considered in cases of recurrent early losses. IVF with PGS may be useful for some single gene disorders.

Uterine abnormalities should be systematically assessed in patients with history of RPL starting with ultrasound (3D and sonohysterogram) and/or MRI and reserving the use of combined hysteroscopy/laparoscopy for patients in whom intrauterine pathology is suspected or those with a nondiagnostic evaluation of uterine anatomy. In the event of RPL or other complications of pregnancy consistent with APS classification criteria, affected women should be screened for laboratory criteria of APS. For women with a confirmed or presumptive diagnosis of APS, the recommendation is to administer low-dose ASA and a prophylactic dose of LMWH from the time of the positive pregnancy test until at least 6 weeks postpartum.

Assessing prolactin levels, screening for antithyroid antibodies, and providing appropriate treatment with bromocriptine and levothyroxine, respectively, for those found affected may also be reasonable strategies but these approaches require further study. Attention should also be given to ensuring optimal metabolic control of diabetic women during the preconception period.

Programmed weight loss for obese patients, smoking cessation, and reduction in caffeine use also seem prudent interventions in affected patients. Finally, couples experiencing recurrent miscarriage should be screened for depression and posttraumatic stress disorder, and appropriate psychological support should be provided.

CASE PRESENTATION 1

A 33-year-old gravida 4, para 1031, with history of three clinically recognized early pregnancy losses presents to your clinic for evaluation of recurrent pregnancy loss. Laboratory evaluation, including thyroid-stimulating hormone levels, antiphospholipid antibody panel, parental karyotype, and hemoglobin A1C are unremarkable. Hysterosalpingography and three-dimensional saline ultrasonography revealed a midline filling defect. The best next step in management of this patient is

(A) Cervical cerclage in next pregnancy

(B) Diagnostic laparoscopy

(C) Computed tomography of kidneys and pelvis

(D) Hysteroscopic metroplasty

Correct answer: D

Explanation: Patient meets criteria for RPL diagnosis based on her history. Hysterosalpingography and three-dimensional saline sonogram revealed a midline filling defect, which is consistent with a uterine septum. Based on recommendations from societal guidelines, resection of these would be the best next step as evidence has shown that doing so improves outcomes for future pregnancies in this cohort of patients.

CASE PRESENTATION 2

A 30-year-old gravida 3, para 0030, with noncontributory family history, and otherwise unremarkable past medical and surgical history presents with her husband for follow-up visit after her third first-trimester miscarriage. Products of conceptions were analyzed and deemed unremarkable following cytogenetic analysis, and she already underwent hysterosalpingography, which did not show any abnormalities. She and her partner have been anxiously waiting for the results of RPL workup sent during previous visit. Thyroid panel, glycated hemoglobin (HbA1c), antiphospholipid antibodies, and parental karyotypes are all unremarkable. What is the best next step in management?

(A) Expectant management

(B) Hyperhomocysteinemia testing

(C) Levothyroxine

(D) Low-dose aspirin therapy

Correct answer: A

Explanation: This couple with a history of RPL has undergone recommended workup for this condition with unremarkable results. Couples with unexplained RPL should be counseled that, even though a clear etiology has not been identified, successful outcomes may still be achieved with expectant management. Hyperhomocysteinemia is not definitively linked to RPL based on available evidence; therefore, testing for this condition is not warranted. Treatment with levothyroxine or low-dose aspirin is not indicated in a patient with unremarkable past medical history and normal thyroid panel.

References

1. Rossen LM, Ahrens KA, Branum AM. Trends in risk of pregnancy loss among US women, 1990-2011. Paediatr Perinat Epidemiol. 2018 Jan;32(1):19–29.

2. Rai R, Regan L. Recurrent miscarriage. Lancet. 2006;368: 601–11.

3. Lidegaard Ø, Mikkelsen AP, Egerup P, Kolte AM, Rasmussen SC, Nielsen HS. Pregnancy loss: a 40-year nationwide assessment. Acta Obstet Gynecol Scand. 2020;99(11):1492–6.

4. Youssef A, Vermeulen N, Lashley EELO, Goddijn M, van der Hoorn MLP. Comparison and appraisal of (inter)national recurrent pregnancy loss guidelines. Reprod Biomed Online. 2019 Sep;39(3):497–503.

5. Huchon C, Deffieux X, Beucher G, Capmas P, Carcopino X, Costedoat-Chalumeau N, et al. Pregnancy loss: French clinical practice guidelines. Eur J Obstet Gynecol Reprod Biol. 2016 Jun;201:18–26.

6. Page JM, Silver RM. Genetic causes of recurrent pregnancy loss. Clin Obstet Gynecol. 2016 Sep;59(3):498–508.

7. Arias-Sosa LA, Acosta ID, Lucena-Quevedo E, Moreno-Ortiz H, Esteban-Pérez C, Forero-Castro M. Genetic and epigenetic variations associated with idiopathic recurrent pregnancy loss. J Assist Reprod Genet. 2018 Mar;35(3):355–66.

8. Smits MAJ, van Maarle M, Hamer G, Mastenbroek S, Goddijn M, van Wely M. Cytogenetic testing of pregnancy loss tissue: a meta-analysis. Reprod Biomed Online. 2020 Jun 1;40(6):867–79.

9. Elhady GM, Kholeif S, Nazmy N. Chromosomal aberrations in 224 couples with recurrent pregnancy loss. J Hum Reprod Sci. 2020;13(4):340–8.

10. Franssen MTM, Musters AM, van der Veen F, Repping S, Leschot NJ, Bossuyt PMM, et al. Reproductive outcome after PGD in couples with recurrent miscarriage carrying a structural chromosome abnormality: a systematic review. Hum Reprod Update. 2011 Aug;17(4):467–75.

11. Lockwood C, Irons M, Troiani J, Kawada C, Chaudhury A, Cetrulo C. The prenatal sonographic diagnosis of lethal multiple pterygium syndrome: a heritable cause of recurrent abortion. Am J Obstet Gynecol. 1988;159:474–6.

12. Odent S, Le Marec B, Smahi A, Hors-Cayla C, Milon J, Jouan H, et al. Spontaneous abortion of male fetuses with incontinentia pigmenti (apropos of a family). J Gynecol Obstet Biol Reprod (Paris). 1997;26: 633–6.

13. Kacprzak M, Chrzanowska M, Skoczylas B, Moczulska H, Borowiec M, Sieroszewski P. Genetic causes of recurrent miscarriages. Ginekologia Polska. 2016;87(10):722–6.

14. Moghbeli M. Genetics of recurrent pregnancy loss among Iranian population. Mol Genet Genomic Med. 2019 Sep;7(9):e891.

15. Guimarães Filho HA, Mattar R, Pires CR, Araujo Júnior E, Moron AF, et al. Prevalence of uterine defects in habitual abortion patients attended on at a University Health Service in Brazil. Arch Gynecol Obstet. 2006 Oct 1;274(6):345–8.

16. Medrano-Uribe FA. Prevalencia de las alteraciones anatómicas uterinas en mujeres mexicanas con pérdida gestacional recurrente (PGR). Gac Med Mex. 2016;152(2):4.

17. Turocy JM, Rackow BW. Uterine factor in recurrent pregnancy loss. Semin Perinatol. 2019 Mar;43(2):74–9.

18. Carbonnel M, Pirtea P, de Ziegler D, Ayoubi JM. Uterine factors in recurrent pregnancy losses. Fertil Steril. 2021 Mar;115(3):538–45.

19. Akhtar M, Saravelos S, Li T, Jayaprakasan K, the Royal College of Obstetricians and Gynaecologists. Reproductive implications and management of congenital uterine anomalies. BJOG. 2020;127(5):e1–13.

20. Saravelos SH, Cocksedge KA, Li T-C. The pattern of pregnancy loss in women with congenital uterine anomalies and recurrent miscarriage. Reprod Biomed Online. 2010 Mar;20(3):416–22.

21. The ESHRE Guideline Group on RPL, Bender Atik R, Christiansen OB, Elson J, Kolte AM, Lewis S, et al. ESHRE guideline: recurrent pregnancy loss. Hum Reprod Open. 2018 Apr 1;2018(2):hoy004.

22. Evaluation and treatment of recurrent pregnancy loss: a committee opinion. Fertil Steril. 2012 Nov;98(5):1103–11.

23. Grimbizis GF, Di Spiezio Sardo A, Saravelos SH, Gordts S, Exacoustos C, Van Schoubroeck D, et al. The Thessaloniki ESHRE/ESGE consensus on diagnosis of female genital anomalies. Gynecol Surg. 2016 Feb 1;13(1):1–16.

24. Alecsandru D, Klimczak AM, Garcia Velasco JA, Pirtea P, Franasiak JM. Immunologic causes and thrombophilia in recurrent pregnancy loss. Fertil Steril. 2021 Mar;115(3):561–6.

25. Meuleman T, Haasnoot GW, van Lith JMM, Verduijn W, Bloemenkamp KWM, Claas FHJ. Paternal HLA-C is a risk factor in unexplained recurrent miscarriage. Am J Reprod Immunol. 2018;79(2):e12797.

26. D'Ippolito S, Ticconi C, Tersigni C, Garofalo S, Martino C, Lanzone A, et al. The pathogenic role of autoantibodies in recurrent pregnancy loss. Am J Reprod Immunol. 2020 Jan;83(1):e13200.

27. Galli M, Barbui T. Antiphospholipid antibodies and thrombosis: strength of association. Hematol J. 2003;4:180–6.

28. Santos T da S, Ieque AL, de Carvalho HC, Sell AM, Lonardoni MVC, Demarchi IG, et al. Antiphospholipid syndrome and recurrent miscarriage: A systematic review and meta-analysis. J Reprod Immunol. 2017 Sep;123:78–87.

29. Wong L, Porter T, Jesús G de. Recurrent early pregnancy loss and antiphospholipid antibodies: where do we stand? Lupus. 2014 Oct 1;23(12):1226–8.

30. Sauer R, Roussev R, Jeyendran RS, Coulam CB. Prevalence of antiphospholipid antibodies among women experiencing unexplained infertility and recurrent implantation failure. Fertil Steril. 2010 May;93(7):2441–3.

31. Miyakis S, Lockshin MD, Atsumi T, Branch DW, Brey RL, Cervera R, et al. International consensus statement on an update of the classification criteria for definite antiphospholipid syndrome (APS). J Thromb Haemost. 2006;4:295–306.

32. Motha MBC, Palihawadana TS. Recurrent pregnancy loss and thrombophilia. Ceylon Medical Journal. 2014 Mar 25;59(1):1–3.

33. Song Y, Wang H-Y, Qiao J, Liu P, Chi H-B. Antiphospholipid antibody titers and clinical outcomes in patients with recurrent miscarriage and antiphospholipid antibody syndrome: a prospective study. Chin Med J (Engl). 2017 Feb 5;130(3):267–72.

34. Field SL, Brighton TA, McNeil HP, Chesterman CN. Recent insights into antiphospholipid antibody-mediated thrombosis. Baillière's Best Pract Res Clin Haematol. 1999;12:407–22.

35. Rand JH, Wu XX, Andree HA, Lockwood CJ, Guller S, Scher J, et al. Pregnancy loss in the antiphospholipid-antibody syndrome: a possible thrombogenic mechanism. N Engl J Med. 1997;337:154–60.

36. Stefanski A-L, Specker C, Fischer-Betz R, Henrich W, Schleussner E, Dörner T. Maternal thrombophilia and recurrent miscarriage - is there evidence that heparin is indicated as prophylaxis against recurrence? Geburtshilfe Frauenheilkd. 2018 Mar;78(3):274–82.

37. Yang Z, Shen X, Zhou C, Wang M, Liu Y, Zhou L. Prevention of recurrent miscarriage in women with antiphospholipid syndrome: A systematic review and network meta-analysis. Lupus. 2021 Jan 1;30(1):70–9.

38. Liew S-C, Gupta ED. Methylenetetrahydrofolate reductase (MTHFR) C677T polymorphism: epidemiology, metabolism and the associated diseases. Eur J Med Genet. 2015 Jan;58(1):1–10.

39. Barut MU, Bozkurt M, Kahraman M, Yıldırım E, İmirzalioğlu N, Kubar A, et al. Thrombophilia and recurrent pregnancy loss: the enigma continues. Med Sci Monit. 2018 Jun 22;24: 4288–94.

40. Kaur R, Gupta K. Endocrine dysfunction and recurrent spontaneous abortion: An overview. Int J Appl Basic Med Res. 2016; 6(2):79–83.

41. Pluchino N, Drakopoulos P, Wenger JM, Petignat P, Streuli I, Genazzani AR. Hormonal causes of recurrent pregnancy loss (RPL). Hormones. 2014 Jul 1;13(3):314–22.

42. Dal Lago A, Galanti F, Miriello D, Marcoccia A, Massimiani M, Campagnolo L, et al. Positive impact of levothyroxine treatment on pregnancy outcome in euthyroid women with thyroid autoimmunity affected by recurrent miscarriage. J Clin Med. 2021 May 13;10(10):2105.

43. Amrane S, McConnell R. Endocrine causes of recurrent pregnancy loss. Semin Perinatol. 2019 Mar;43(2):80–3.

44. Rao VRC, Lakshmi A, Sadhnani MD. Prevalence of hypothyroidism in recurrent pregnancy loss in first trimester. Indian J Med Sci. 2008 Sep;62(9):357–61.

45. Hirahara F, Andoh N, Sawai K, Hirabuki T, Uemura T, Minaguchi H. Hyperprolactinemic recurrent miscarriage and results of randomized bromocriptine treatment trials. Fertil Steril. 1998 Aug;70(2):246–52.

46. Li W, Ma N, Laird SM, Ledger WL, Li TC. The relationship between serum prolactin concentration and pregnancy outcome in women with unexplained recurrent miscarriage. J Obstet Gynaecol. 2013 Apr;33(3):285–8.

47. Daya S. Efficacy of progesterone support for pregnancy in women with recurrent miscarriage. A meta-analysis of controlled trials. Br J Obstet Gynaecol. 1989 Mar;96(3):275–80.

48. Oates-Whitehead RM, Haas DM, Carrier JAK. Progestogen for preventing miscarriage. Cochrane Database Syst Rev. 2003;(4):CD003511. doi: 10.1002/14651858.CD003511. Update in: Cochrane Database Syst Rev. 2008;(2):CD003511. PMID: 14583982.

49. Coomarasamy A, Williams H, Truchanowicz E, Seed PT, Small R, Quenby S, et al. A randomized trial of progesterone in women with recurrent miscarriages. N Engl J Med. 2015 Nov 26;373(22):2141–8.

50. Coomarasamy A, Williams H, Truchanowicz E, Seed PT, Small R, Quenby S, et al. PROMISE: first-trimester progesterone therapy in women with a history of unexplained recurrent miscarriages–a randomised, double-blind, placebo-controlled, international multicentre trial and economic evaluation. Health Technol Assess. 2016 May;20(41):1–92.

51. Sharif K, Sharif Y, Watad A, Yavne Y, Lichtbroun B, Bragazzi NL, et al. Vitamin D, autoimmunity and recurrent pregnancy loss: more than an association. Am J Reprod Immunol. 2018;80(3):e12991.

52. Gonçalves DR, Braga A, Braga J, Marinho A. Recurrent pregnancy loss and vitamin D: A review of the literature. Am J Reprod Immunol. 2018;80(5):e13022.

53. Zhao H, Wei X, Yang X. A novel update on vitamin D in recurrent pregnancy loss (Review). Mol Med Rep. 2021 May;23(5):382.

54. Chen X, Yin B, Lian R-C, Zhang T, Zhang H-Z, Diao L-H, et al. Modulatory effects of vitamin D on peripheral cellular immunity in patients with recurrent miscarriage. Am J Reprod Immunol. 2016 Dec;76(6):432–8.

55. Cocksedge KA, Li T-C, Saravelos SH, Metwally M. A reappraisal of the role of polycystic ovary syndrome in recurrent miscarriage. Reprod Biomed Online. 2008 Jan;17(1):151–60.

56. Clark AM, Thornley B, Tomlinson L, Galletley C, Norman RJ. Weight loss in obese infertile women results in improvement in reproductive outcome for all forms of fertility treatment. Hum Reprod. 1998 Jun;13(6):1502–5.

57. Khambata K, Raut S, Deshpande S, Mohan S, Sonawane S, Gaonkar R, et al. DNA methylation defects in spermatozoa of male partners from couples experiencing recurrent pregnancy loss. Hum Reprod. 2021 Jan 1;36(1):48–60.

58. Leach M, Aitken RJ, Sacks G. Sperm DNA fragmentation abnormalities in men from couples with a history of recurrent miscarriage. Aust N Z J Obstet Gynaecol. 2015;55(4):379–83.

59. McQueen DB, Zhang J, Robins JC. Sperm DNA fragmentation and recurrent pregnancy loss: a systematic review and meta-analysis. Fertil Steril. 2019 Jul;112(1):54–60.e3.

60. Wang Y, Li G, Zuo M-Z, Fang J-H, Li H-R, Quan D-D, et al. Y chromosome polymorphisms may contribute to an increased risk of male-induced unexplained recurrent miscarriage. Biosci Rep. 2017 Mar 27;37(2):BSR20160528.

61. Cao C-J, Wang Y-F, Fang D-M, Hu Y. Relation between mycoplasma infection and recurrent spontaneous abortion. Eur Rev Med Pharmacol Sci. 2018 Apr;22(8):2207–11.

62. Naessens A, Foulon W, Breynaert J, Lauwers S. Serotypes of ureaplasma urealyticum isolated from normal pregnant women and patients with pregnancy complications. J Clin Microbiol. 1988;26:319–22.

63. Matovina M, Husnjak K, Milutin N, Ciglar S, Grce M. Possible role of bacterial and viral infections in miscarriages. Fertil Steril. 2004;81:662–9.

Further reading

Akhtar M, Saravelos S, Li T, Jayaprakasan K, the Royal College of Obstetricians and Gynaecologists. Reproductive implications and management of congenital uterine anomalies. BJOG. 2020;127(5):e1–13.

American College of Obstetricians and Gynecologists. ACOG Practice Bulletin No. 197: inherited thrombophilias in pregnancy. Obstet Gynecol. 2018;132(1):17.

American College of Obstetricians and Gynecologists. ACOG Practice Bulletin No. 132: antiphospholipid syndrome. Obstet Gynecol. 2012;120:1514–21.

D'Ippolito S, Ticconi C, Tersigni C, Garofalo S, Martino C, Lanzone A, et al. The pathogenic role of autoantibodies in recurrent pregnancy loss. Am J Reprod Immunol. 2020 Jan;83(1):e13200.

ESHRE Guideline Group on RPL, Bender Atik R, Christiansen OB, Elson J, Kolte AM, Lewis S, et al. ESHRE guideline: recurrent pregnancy loss. Hum Reprod Open. 2018 Apr 1;2018(2):hoy004.

Grimbizis GF, Di Spiezio Sardo A, Saravelos SH, Gordts S, Exacoustos C, Van Schoubroeck D, et al. The Thessaloniki ESHRE/ESGE consensus on diagnosis of female genital anomalies. Gynecol Surg. 2016 Feb 1;13(1):1–16.

Porter TF, LaCoursiere Y, Scott JR. Immunotherapy for recurrent miscarriage. Cochrane Database Syst Rev. 2006;2:CD000112. doi: 10.1002/14651858.CD000112.pub3.

Practice Committee of the American Society for Reproductive Medicine. Evaluation and treatment of recurrent pregnancy loss: a committee opinion. Fertil Steril. 2012 Nov;98(5):1103–11.

Chapter 33
Cervical Insufficiency

Rachel Sinkey and John Owen

Department of Obstetrics and Gynecology, Division of Maternal-Fetal Medicine, The University of Alabama, Birmingham, AL, USA

Although the term "cervical incompetence" was first used in *The Lancet* in 1865, the contemporary concept was not widely accepted until the mid-20th century, after Palmer [1] in 1948 and Lash [2] in 1950 independently described interval mechanical repair and support of anatomic cervical defects associated with recurrent midtrimester birth. Thereafter, Shirodkar [3] in 1955, McDonald [4] in 1957, and Benson and Durfee [5] in 1965 described the cerclage procedures still used in today's obstetric practice. Nevertheless, the literature on cervical *insufficiency* (the preferred term) has largely been a chronicle of surgical methods to correct *posttraumatic* anatomic disruption of the internal os, in women who had experienced recurrent painless dilation and midtrimester birth. Since anatomic disruption of the cervix or intrinsic congenital abnormal cervical stromal extracellular matrix (ECM) composition appears to be decreasing in incidence and/or biological plausibility, increasingly cervical insufficiency is viewed as a consequence of early manifestation of the pathologic causes of preterm birth occurring while the myometrium is still refractory to labor contractions.

Syndrome of spontaneous preterm birth

Spontaneous preterm birth (sPTB) is a syndrome involving several anatomic components [6]. These include the uterus and its contractile function (i.e. preterm labor), loss of chorio-amnion integrity (i.e. premature preterm rupture of membranes [PPROM]), and finally, diminished cervical structural integrity, either from an anatomic cervical defect or more commonly from acquired pathologic cervical ECM changes, a functional deficit. In any given pregnancy, a single feature may appear to dominate, even though it is more likely that most cases of sPTB result from an interaction of multiple poorly understood pathological stimuli and functional-anatomic pathways. Importantly, the manifestation and relative contributions of each of these components may vary, not only among different women, but also in successive pregnancies of the same woman. The observed variance in the clinical presentation of cervical insufficiency further challenges the notion that abnormal cervical anatomy is the primary genesis of clinical cervical insufficiency. Pathologic cervical ripening in the mid-trimester may actually be an early indication that the process of parturition has begun.

How can we make the clinical diagnosis of cervical insufficiency, and how effective is cerclage for a history indication?

The incidence of cervical insufficiency in the general obstetric population varies between approximately 1:100 and 1:2000 [7–9]. This large variance is likely due to differences among study populations, reporting bias, and the diagnostic criteria used to establish the diagnosis. Most of what is known about the history of cervical insufficiency and its treatment indicates that it is a *clinical diagnosis*, characterized by recurrent painless dilation and spontaneous midtrimester birth, usually of a living fetus. Associated characteristics, such as antecedent fetal demise, painful uterine contractions, hemorrhage, overt infection (e.g. chorioamnionitis), or PPROM, tend to shift the cause of the birth away from cervical insufficiency and support other anatomic components of the syndrome.

Because cervical insufficiency is likely part of a broader sPTB syndrome, the clinical diagnosis is usually retrospective and suggested only after poor obstetric outcomes have occurred (or, sometimes, in acute settings). Women

Queenan's Management of High-Risk Pregnancy: An Evidence-Based Approach, Seventh Edition. Edited by Catherine Y. Spong and Charles J. Lockwood.

with cervical insufficiency often have some premonitory symptoms such as increased pelvic pressure, vaginal discharge, bleeding, and urinary frequency. Although these symptoms are neither specific nor uncommon in a normal pregnancy, they should not be ignored, particularly in women with risk factors for sPTB. Because there are no proven objective criteria (other than a rare, gross cervical malformation), a careful history and review of the past obstetric records are crucial to making the clinical diagnosis. However, records may be unavailable, and many patients cannot provide an accurate history. Even with excellent records and complete history, clinicians might reasonably disagree on the diagnosis in all but the most classic presentations. Confounding factors in the history, variable descriptions in medical records, or current physical assessment might be used to either support or refute the diagnosis, based on their perceived importance. *It is essential for the physician managing a patient who experiences a spontaneous midtrimester birth to assess and document whether and which clinical criteria for cervical insufficiency were present.*

Most of what is known about the management of the cervical insufficiency is based on case series that reported surgical correction of the presumed underlying mechanical defect in the cervical stroma. In total, over 2000 patients have been reported in these historic cohort comparisons [10,11]. However, interpretation of these data is problematic because:

• Diagnostic criteria were not consistently reported.
• Definitions of treatment success were inconsistent (generally recorded as perinatal survival, as opposed to gestational age at birth).
• Treatments were not always detailed and might include combinations of surgery, medication, bed rest, and other uncontrolled interventions.
• Cases were not subcategorized according to etiology (i.e. anatomic defects versus a presumed functional cause).

Nevertheless, based on compelling but biased efficacy data, placement of a history-indicated cerclage in women with clinically defined cervical insufficiency has become common practice. Because of its unproven efficacy in randomized clinical trials [12], and the attendant surgical risks [13], the recommendation for *history-indicated* cerclage should be limited to women with prior midtrimester sPTB, after a careful history, record review and physical examination suggest a dominant cervical component.

Unless the physical examination confirms a significant, rare, cervical anatomic defect, consistent with disruption of its circumferential integrity, the clinician should assess the history for other components of the sPTB syndrome. Subclinical intrauterine infections are often associated with advanced premature cervical ripening (see *acute cervical insufficiency* section) [14] and contractions, or some bleeding may accompany and complicate the clinical picture of otherwise "painless" cervical dilation. This might predispose to PPROM or ascending genital tract infection with intact membranes, either of which might lead to overt labor and be used to refute the diagnosis. Conversely, it is also plausible that preexisting subclinical intrauterine infection could incite the local effects responsible for the pathologic ripening and dilation.

Should insufficiency be a sonographic diagnosis?

Numerous investigators have asserted that cervical insufficiency can be diagnosed by midtrimester sonographic evaluation of the cervix. Various sonographic findings, including shortened cervical length (CL), funneling at the internal os, and dynamic response to provocative maneuvers (e.g. fundal pressure), have been used to select women for treatment, generally cerclage. In these earlier reports, sonographic evaluations were not blinded, leading to uncontrolled interventions and difficulty determining effectiveness. In many instances, sonographic criteria for cervical insufficiency were only qualitatively described and thus, not reproducible.

A large, randomized trial, performed by a consortium of 15 US centers [15], included only women who had at least one prior sPTB at 17–34 weeks gestation, and were followed with serial transvaginal scans beginning at 16 weeks. If the CL remained at least 30 mm, scans were repeated every 2 weeks, but these increased to weekly if the length was 25–29 mm. Those who developed a shortened CL <25 mm between 16 and 22+6 weeks were randomized to (McDonald) cerclage or no cerclage. These investigators observed a statistically significant decrease in previable birth <24 weeks (6% vs. 14%), perinatal mortality (9% vs. 16%), and birth <37 weeks (45% vs. 60%), but a nonsignificant decrease in rates of PTB <35 weeks (32% vs. 42%), the trial's primary outcome. Cerclage benefit was closely linked to the severity of cervical shortage, and women with CL <15 mm at randomization accrued a much greater benefit than those with a length of 15–24 mm, suggesting that shorter lengths are more amenable to mechanical support.

The generalizability of this clinical trial was expanded by the findings of a 2011 meta-analysis [16]. that investigated whether cerclage prevents preterm birth and perinatal morbidity/mortality in women with a prior sPTB, a singleton gestation and a midtrimester CL <25 mm. Five randomized trials met inclusion criteria. The rate of PTB <35 in women with prior PTB, singleton and CL <25 mm was 28% in patients with a cerclage and 41% in the no cerclage group (relative risk [RR] 0.70, 95% CI 0.55–0.89). Preterm birth reduction in patients with cerclage was found at each gestational age cutoff studied, including PTB <37, <32, <28, and <24 weeks. Importantly, perinatal mortality was also reduced by 51% in these high-risk patients with CL <25 prior to 20 weeks gestation who had a cerclage placed (RR 0.49, 95% CI 0.27–0.87). This meta-analysis established the utility of sonographic screening and ultrasound-indicated cerclage in selected women based on their *obstetric history*. Although determining the "optimal" CL for cerclage in women with a prior sPTB and short cervix was not a primary goal of the Cerclage trial, a secondary analysis demonstrated efficacy across the entire spectrum of shortened CL <25 mm [17]. Collectively, these data make serial cervical surveillance and cerclage for a CL <25 mm a logical choice for nonclassic or confusing cases of prior sPTB.

Can ultrasound replace the history indication?

Although clinicians might be reluctant to withhold cerclage based on history of typical cervical insufficiency, a meta-analysis of four randomized trials (467 women) found similar rates of PTB <37 weeks (31% vs. 32%) and <34 weeks (17% vs. 23%) as well as perinatal mortality (5% vs. 3%) in women who were assigned to ultrasound screening vs. cerclage, respectively [18]. Moreover, less than half of the women assigned to ultrasound screening (42%) underwent ultrasound-indicated cerclage. A multicenter observational study investigated the outcomes of patients with a prior ultrasound-indicated cerclage who were followed subsequently with either a "history-indicated" cerclage or repeat CL surveillance. Of patients followed with sonography, 47% underwent cerclage placement for a CL <25mm. Primary and secondary outcomes between groups were similar [19]. In summary, when evaluating a patient with a prior sPTB history, and especially when the history indication for cerclage is debated, ultrasound surveillance appears to decrease surgical interventions while yielding outcomes similar to a history-indicated cerclage.

What is acute cervical insufficiency and how effective is a physical exam-indicated cerclage?

Uncommonly, a woman will present with symptoms and physical findings that support an antepartum diagnosis of cervical insufficiency. However, this syndrome comprises a wide spectrum of clinical expression. Women with *acute cervical insufficiency*, generally defined as (1) midtrimester cervical dilation of at least 1–2 cm, (2) visible membranes prolapsing to or beyond the internal os, and (3) no other clinically defined cause (e.g. labor, infection, abruption), may be considered for *physical examination-indicated* cerclage. A systematic review and meta-analysis published in 2015 studied the efficacy of physical exam-indicated cerclage, however, of 10 included studies, only 1 small study of 23 patients was a randomized trial.

The authors concluded that physical exam-indicated cerclage was associated with an increase in neonatal survival (RR 1.65, 95% CI 1.19–2.28) and pregnancy prolongation (mean 34 days 95% CI 18–50). Limited and low-quality data were noted as weaknesses [20]. An updated 2020 meta-analysis reached similar conclusions, reporting pregnancy prolongation and neonatal benefit from physical exam-indicated cerclage [21].

Thus, given the lack of well-designed randomized trials, the optimal management of women who present with acute cervical insufficiency remains unknown. Although physical-exam-indicated cerclage may confer some benefit, patient selection remains somewhat empirical and clinical judgment should focus on the presence or absence of perceived contraindications, such as advanced gestational age, advanced cervical dilation, uterine contractions, subclinical infection, bleeding, or membrane prolapse beyond the external os.

Interestingly, women who present with acute cervical insufficiency and undergo amniocentesis have an appreciable (50%) rate of bacterial colonization of their amniotic fluid, including other markers of subclinical chorioamnionitis [22] or proteomic markers of inflammation or bleeding [23]. Women with pathologic amniotic fluid markers have a much shorter presentation-to-delivery interval, regardless of whether they receive cerclage or are managed expectantly (i.e. bed rest). Although not standard care, the evaluation of amniotic fluid for markers of subclinical infection and inflammation appears to have important prognostic value, although it is unclear whether and which fluid analyses should be used to direct patient management.

Can acute cervical insufficiency be predicted and managed?

Another uncommon clinical scenario arises when a low-risk patient who has undergone routine CL screening is diagnosed with a short cervix on ultrasound, is started on vaginal progesterone, and then is found to have progressive cervical shortening; this is a possible harbinger of acute cervical insufficiency.

A systematic review and meta-analysis of randomized controlled trials using individual patient-level data (N=419) concluded that overall, low-risk singletons with no prior sPTB with CL <25 mm do not experience PTB reduction with a cerclage. However, there was benefit among a subset of patients with length <10 mm who underwent cerclage (RR 0.68, 95% CI 0.47–0.98). Tocolytics and antibiotics also conferred some benefit, though the level of evidence was low [24]. Additionally, a secondary analysis of a Maternal-Fetal Medicine Units Network trial was performed among women with a CL ≤25 mm without a prior PTB (n=119). Those with a length ≤11 mm had a significant risk for PTB <37 weeks compared to those

>11 mm (77% vs. 31%, P<0.001). The authors concluded that a physical exam should be performed on patients with a CL ≤11 mm to assess cervical dilation and that additional research is needed to define management [25]. In a separate retrospective series, patients with progressive cervical shortening <10 mm despite vaginal progesterone benefited from a cerclage (and continuation of vaginal progesterone) with improvements in birth gestational age, PTB rate, neonatal intensive care unit (NICU) admissions, and neonatal death [26]. Other investigators reached a similar conclusion regarding cerclage benefit in patients with a CL <10 mm [27]. Although the quality of these data does not support a recommendation for or against continued cervical surveillance after starting progesterone for short cervix, if serial surveillance is chosen, cerclage may be considered in patients whose CL shortens to <10 mm.

When should cerclage be placed in a twin gestation?

A 2005 meta-analysis of trials using individual patient-level data paradoxically found an increased risk for PTB <35 weeks in patients with twins undergoing cerclage placement for an asymptomatic short cervix (RR 2.15, 95% CI 1.15–4.01) [28]. This may have contributed to the American College of Obstetricians and Gynecologists recommending against placement of cerclage for twin gestations outside of a clinical trial [29]. Indeed, an updated systematic review and meta-analysis of randomized trials using individual patient-level data published in 2015 (N = 49) reached a similar conclusion as the 2005 meta-analysis and recommended against cerclage placement in patients with a short cervix and twin gestation. Specifically, neither PTB (<37, <35, <34, <32, <28, <24 weeks), nor perinatal death was reduced in twin gestations in the cerclage group. Furthermore, cases of low birthweight, very low birthweight, and respiratory distress syndrome were higher with a cerclage [30].

Conversely, a 2019 systematic review and meta-analysis suggested that patients with a twin pregnancy and CL <15 mm experienced a reduction of PTB <34 weeks (RR 0.57, 95% CI (0.43–0.75) with cerclage and treated patients with previable cervical dilation and twins also remained pregnant 6.8 weeks longer than controls (95% CI 5.32–8.24) [31]. Another 2021 systematic review and meta-analysis, which also concluded that there was no overall benefit with cerclage in twin gestations, found that a subset of patients with CL <15 mm who underwent cerclage experienced a reduction in PTB at <37, <34, and <32 weeks gestation [32].

Studies focused on physical exam-indicated cerclage in twins have also demonstrated benefit. Among 38 twin gestations with cervical dilation ≥1 cm at 16–24 weeks who underwent cerclage compared to 38 who did not, the interval from diagnosis to delivery was 10.5 ± 5.6 weeks vs. 3.7 ± 3.2 weeks, for a mean difference of 6.8 weeks (95% CI 4.7–8.8) [33]. A clinical trial randomizing 34 patients with twins and previable cervical dilation at 16 to 23+6 weeks gestation was halted by the Data Safety Monitoring Board because a significantly higher rate of perinatal mortality was observed in the no-cerclage group: 76.9% (20/26) vs. 17.6 % (6/34) (RR 0.22, 95% CI 0.1–0.49) [34]. These data suggest a potential cerclage benefit for twin gestations with acute cervical insufficiency.

In summary, cerclage may be considered in selected twin gestations. Emerging data support placement of ultrasound-indicated cerclages in twins with CL<15 mm and in patients with acute cervical insufficiency.

How should women with a prior failed vaginal cerclage be managed?

The International Federation of Gynecology and Obstetrics defines a failed vaginal cerclage as a "delivery before 28 weeks after a history or ultrasound-indicated (but not physical exam-indicated) cerclage" [35]. A patient with a prior failed vaginal cerclage occasionally presents for subsequent obstetric care or preconception counseling. If the prior cerclage had been placed for cervical insufficiency (as opposed to other components of the sPTB syndrome), the patient might be considered a candidate for a cervicoisthmic procedure (placed vaginally or abdominally).

Both vaginal and abdominal approaches to cervicoisthmic cerclages have been well described. Observational data suggest similar neonatal survival between techniques with less maternal morbidity via vaginal approach [36]. However, the most robust evidence supports transabdominal cerclage placement for women with recurrent pregnancy loss attributable to cervical insufficiency. Specifically, Multicentre Abdominal vs Vaginal Randomised Intervention of Cerclage (MAVRIC) was a multicenter trial randomizing 133 women with a prior mid-trimester loss with a "low vaginal" cerclage to one of three arms: transabdominal, high vaginal (i.e. placed higher on the cervix by mobilizing the bladder), or low vaginal cerclage [37]. Rates of PTB <32 weeks gestation were 8% (3/39), 38% (15/39), and 33% (11/39) in the transabdominal, high vaginal and low vaginal cerclage groups, respectively. Women undergoing abdominal cerclage placement had a 77% risk reduction for PTB <32 weeks (RR 0.23, 95% CI 0.07–0.76) compared to those undergoing a low vaginal cerclage. The number needed to treat was 5.3 women to prevent one fetal loss. There was no difference in PTB rates between the high and low vaginal cerclage groups (RR 1.15, 95% CI 0.62–2.16). The MAVRIC authors subsequently reported follow-up on patients in the trial who were randomized to a vaginal cerclage but who experienced yet another failed cerclage defined as a PTB <32 weeks (n=26). Eleven of these 26 patients underwent abdominal cerclage, 9 conceived, and all 9 delivered ≥32 weeks gestation [38]. Because few patients are appropriate candidates, and few physicians have surgical experience with the cervicoisthmic procedure, based on the results of the MAVRIC trial, we suggest referral to a tertiary center for consultation regarding risks and benefits of abdominal cerclage for patients with prior failed vaginal cerclage.

Do cervical procedures cause insufficiency?

Although the historic concept of the diagnosis and treatment of cervical insufficiency often includes women with past cervical trauma from birth-associated lacerations, forced dilation, operative injury, or cervical amputation, the prevalence of these antecedent events appears to be decreasing in contemporary US practice. More common in contemporary practice are patients with current or a history of abnormal cervical cytology and women who have undergone treatment of cervical dysplasia using cold-knife cone, laser cone, or a loop electrosurgical excision procedure (LEEP). Procedures to treat abnormal cervical cells are plausible risk factors for insufficiency. A Cochrane Review including 6.3 million pregnancies concluded that women with cervical intraepithelial neoplasia have an increased risk for PTB. A total of 69 studies were included for a total of 6.38 million pregnancies; 65 098 of these pregnancies received treatment and nearly 6.3 million did not. The rate of extreme prematurity <28–30 weeks gestation (which may be due to a component of cervical insufficiency), was higher in patients who received treatment compared to those who did not: 1% vs. 0.3% (RR 2.23, 95% CI 1.55–3.22). Additionally, excisional procedures, ablative procedures, and increasing depth of excision were associated with increasing rates of prematurity [39].

A systematic review and meta-analysis of interventions to prevent PTB in women with a history of cervical conization that included nine studies, sought to determine whether PTB interventions, progesterone, cerclage, and pessary decrease PTB compared to no intervention in singleton or twin gestations. The evidence did not support cerclage or other interventions to reduce PTB. Specifically, the pooled odds ratio for PTB <34 weeks for patients with singletons and a prior cervical conization who received a cerclage compared to those who did not was 3.99 (95% CI 0.67–23.62) [40]. Available clinical trial data do not suggest a benefit from history-indicated cerclage in women with these risk factors [41]. Surprisingly, a recent systematic review evaluating "prophylactic" transvaginal cerclage after conization included 3560 cases and suggested that cerclage increases the risk of PTB (RR 1.85, 95% CI 1.22–2.80) [42].

What surgical techniques are used for history or ultrasound-indicated vaginal cerclage?

Most obstetricians offer a McDonald cerclage as first-line intervention to patients with adequate cervical tissue and a prior mid-trimester loss or high-risk patients with sonographic short cervix. However, observational data are conflicting regarding whether McDonald or Shirodkar is more effective. A 2006 meta-analysis comparing outcomes between women with Shirodkar (n = 127) and McDonald (n = 150) found no difference in PTB <33 weeks [43]. An updated systematic review and meta-analysis suggested that Shirodkar is more effective than McDonald, prolonging gestation by approximately 2 weeks [44]; but there was no difference in perinatal survival. Shirodkar may have a slight gestational age advantage at the potential cost of some increased surgical morbidity and the requirement for more advanced skills.

To place a McDonald cerclage, the anesthetized patient is placed in the dorsal lithotomy position. At least one assistant is required to provide exposure using right angle or medium-sized Deaver retractors. After an antiseptic vaginal prep, the anterior ectocervix is grasped with a sponge forceps or similar nontraumatic instrument, which is used to provide countertraction.

For right-handed surgeons, the first tissue bite is taken at the 1200–1300 o'clock position on the cervix, exiting at around the 1000–1100 position. When placing the anterior stitch, the surgeon must avoid the bladder mucosa that can be identified by moving the cervix in and out, noting where the vaginal mucosa folds in as it reflects off the ectocervix, similar to starting a vaginal hysterectomy. *However, during the procedure, the axis of the needle driver must be held parallel to the axis of the uterus and cervical canal to avoid having the needle exit further than desired from the bladder reflection (and internal os).* As the descending branches of the uterine artery are found at 0300 and 0900 o'clock, this area should also be avoided when placing the stitches high near the lateral fornices. A total of 4–5 tissue bites are generally taken, and the last bite should exit near the original entry site. The suture is then tied down firmly but should not cause visible blanching of the surrounding tissue. To facilitate later identification and removal, a long tag should be left above the knot. After placement, a digital examination will confirm a closed endocervical canal that is not overly constricted. However, it should not admit a gloved finger. It is necessary to record how many stitches were placed and where the knots were tied to facilitate their later removal. Figure 33.1 shows a short cervix by ultrasound before ultrasound-indicated cerclage placement, and Figure 33.2 shows the visible postoperative suture.

Most surgeons use a permanent synthetic material such as # 1 or # 2 Prolene or Mersilene 5 mm tape. The latter is more difficult to pull through the stroma and requires more tissue traction and manipulation.

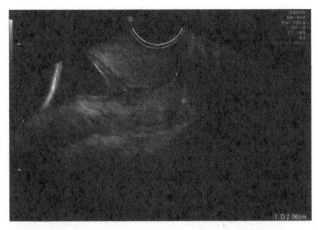

Figure 33.1 Short cervix, measured before cerclage (2.06 cm).

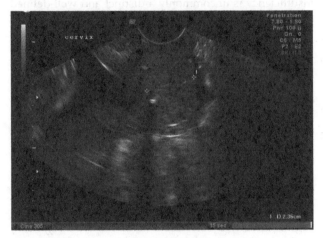

Figure 33.2 Short cervix, with suture visible, measured after ultrasound-indicated cerclage (2.36 cm).

Should postcerclage activity restrictions be recommended?

Empiric recommendations regarding post-cerclage physical activity include a limited interval (24–48 hours) of postoperative bed rest with pelvic rest and sexual abstinence for the remainder of gestation. Because the use of bed rest in pregnancy as an effective therapy has been questioned [45], it seems reasonable to individualize this recommendation based on a patient's symptoms and postcerclage physical findings. However, because women with cerclage indications are still at appreciable risk for sPTB, physically demanding occupations or prolonged standing should probably be curtailed.

When should a cerclage be removed?

In the absence of indications for earlier removal, the stitch should be removed around 37 weeks gestation in the outpatient setting, but it may be complicated by difficulty locating the embedded suture or by hemorrhage.

Generally buried under the bladder reflection, removal of a Shirodkar cerclage may be particularly troublesome and is often performed in the operating room, where light conscious sedation may be required.

Because many women with cervical insufficiency and cerclage remain at high risk for developing other components of the sPTB syndrome, indications for cerclage removal remote from term may develop. Patients with cerclage should be instructed on symptoms of preterm labor and PPROM and present early for evaluation. Preterm labor can be managed with tocolytic medications and corticosteroids according to guidelines. Nevertheless, if labor is progressive, based on serial examination, the cerclage is removed. Preterm prelabor rupture of membranes complicates 25–30% of pregnancies managed with cerclage [9,46]. A multicenter randomized clinical trial in 27 centers studied whether cerclage removal vs. nonremoval prolonged gestation or increased perinatal infection. The study was stopped for futility after 56 were enrolled. This underpowered study showed no difference in pregnancy prolongation or infection. However, the authors noted "a numerical trend in the direction of less infectious morbidity with immediate removal" [47]. In the absence of a well-controlled trial confirming harm from leaving the stitch in situ, individualization should be permitted. One compromise is to retain the cerclage until the corticosteroids are completed.

Cerclage complications

The perceived simplicity and safety of transvaginal cerclage have made this treatment subject to empiric use, despite the risk of associated complications [48]. The most commonly reported complications associated with cerclage are membrane rupture and intrauterine infection. Bleeding may occur, but serious hemorrhage is generally limited to the cervicoisthmic procedures. Essentially all transvaginal cerclage procedures are performed under regional anesthesia, which has a low complication rate. To what extent cerclage *causes* infection or preterm labor may be difficult to ascertain because it is recognized that sPTB, of which cervical insufficiency may be a *forme fruste*, has an appreciable *association* with infection and uterine activity. This is especially true in cases of physical exam-indicated cerclage where preexisting subclinical infection is not uncommon. The most common iatrogenic complication from physical exam-indicated cerclage is intraoperative membrane rupture, although various adjunctive surgical strategies have been suggested to reduce the risk. The incidence of this complication varies by the clinical presentation (i.e. degree of dilation and membrane prolapse), surgical skill and the use of adjunctive intraoperative strategies (e.g. membrane replacement using a Foley catheter). Cervical lacerations from preterm labor with cerclage in situ can also occur.

Overall, complication rates for abdominal cerclage appear to be appreciably higher than rates for vaginal cerclage, including the need for a mandatory cesarean delivery, although fetal death or anomaly discovered at <16 weeks may generally be managed via a vaginal procedure. Potential complications should be included as part of a consultation at a referral center.

Adjunctive management strategies for cervical insufficiency

Alternative therapies for cervical insufficiency can be broadly classified as either providing mechanical support or administering medications to reduce inflammation and infection and maintain uterine quiescence. Two systematic reviews synthesizing the available literature concluded that addition of progesterone, tocolytics, antibiotics, or pessary demonstrated no benefit over cerclage alone [49,50]. However, the authors cautioned that the included studies were small, of low quality, and that properly designed trials were needed. Subsequent to these publications, the benefit of adjunctive antibiotics and tocolytics in patients undergoing exam-indicated cerclage was also documented in a randomized trial of 53 patients by Miller and colleagues. Eligible participants were randomized to exam-indicated cerclage alone verses exam-indicated cerclage plus perioperative indomethacin and antibiotics. The outcome of attaining at least 28 days post cerclage was significantly higher in the adjunctive cohort: 92% compared to 63% ($P=0.01$) [51]. The 2020

Cochrane Review on this topic included Miller's study but concluded that there is insufficient evidence (owing to small numbers) to recommend perioperative tocolytics and antibiotics [52]. The available evidence suggests the following: (1) adjunctive medical therapies are not warranted for patients undergoing a history- or ultrasound-indicated cerclage, and (2) indomethacin and perioperative antibiotics may be considered for patients undergoing exam-indicated cerclage, acknowledging that data supporting this practice are limited.

Conclusion

Contemporary lines of evidence indicate that cervical insufficiency is uncommonly a distinct and well-defined clinical entity but rather only one anatomic component of a larger and more complex syndrome of sPTB. The original paradigm of obstetric and gynecologic trauma as a common antecedent of cervical insufficiency has been replaced by the recognition of *functional*, as opposed to *anatomic* deficits as the more prevalent etiology. Functional cervical *competence* is influenced by both endogenous and exogenous factors that interact through various pathways with other recognized components of the sPTB syndrome: uterine contractions and decidual activation/membrane rupture. Functional cervical insufficiency as manifested by progressive mid-trimester cervical shortening and ripening may also suggest that preterm parturition has begun. Thus, the convenient term *cervical insufficiency* may represent an oversimplified, incomplete description of the more complex and poorly understood pathophysiologic processes.

CASE PRESENTATION

A 24-year-old para 0200 is seen for preconception counseling. Her obstetric history includes two prior sPTB at 22 and 20 weeks gestation. In her first pregnancy she presented at 21 weeks gestation reporting increased vaginal discharge. A sterile speculum exam revealed a 4 cm dilated cervix. She was admitted for observation and experienced membrane rupture at 21+3 weeks gestation. Multidisciplinary counseling with neonatology and maternal-fetal medicine consultants was performed, and she declined fetal/neonatal intervention until 23 weeks gestation. She spontaneously labored at 22 weeks gestation and the infant died at 3 hours of life. The diagnosis assigned by the treating physicians was (acute) cervical insufficiency. Three months after delivery she underwent a uterine cavity evaluation that was normal. In her subsequent pregnancy she was counseled regarding the option of ultrasound surveillance but underwent placement of a

history-indicated cerclage at 12 weeks. Despite this she experienced PPROM at 19 weeks. The cerclage was removed, and her cervix was visually 4 cm dilated. She was admitted for observation and 48 hours later experienced spontaneous labor. The infant died at 1 hour of life.

Interval physical examination revealed normal cervical anatomy with no palpable defect around the circumference. The CL to palpation was 1.5 cm. The external os appeared parous but the internal os was firmly closed. She was referred to a tertiary center for consideration of an abdominal cerclage. After a discussion of the risks and benefits, she underwent abdominal cerclage prior to her next conception, which occurred 6 months later. At 29 weeks she experienced PPROM followed by regular, painful contraction. Corticosteroids for lung maturation were begun, but she required cesarean delivery. The infant had a 10-week NICU course but survived with no long-term sequelae.

References

1. Palmer R, Lacomme M. La béance de l'orifice interne, cause d'avortements à répétition? Une observation de déchrure cervico-isthmique répareeé chirurgicalement, avec gestation à terme consécutive. Gynecol Obstet. 1948;47:905–6.

2. Lash AF, Lash SR. Habitual abortion; the incompetent internal os of the cervix. Am J Obstet Gynecol. 1950;59:68–76.

3. Shirodkar VJA. A new method of operative treatment for habitual abortions in the second trimester of pregnancy. Antiseptic. 1955;52:299–300.

4. McDonald IA. Suture of the cervix for inevitable miscarriage. J Obstet Gynaecol Br Emp. 1957;12:673–4.

5. Benson RC, Durfee RB. Transabdominal cervicouterine cerclage during pregnancy for the treatment of cervical incompetency. Obstet Gynecol. 1965;25:145–55.

6. Romero R, Espinoza J, Kusanovic JP, Gotsch F, Hassan S, Erez O, et al. The preterm parturition syndrome. BJOG. 2006; 113:17–42.

7. Barter RH, Riva HL, Parks J, Dusbabek JA. Surgical closure of the incompetent cervix during pregnancy. Am J Obstet Gynecol. 1958;75:511–21; discussion 521-4.

8. Jennings CL, Jr. Temporary submucosal cerclage for cervical incompetence: report of forty-eight cases. Am J Obstet Gynecol. 1972;113:1097–102.

9. Kuhn R, Pepperell R. Cervical ligation: a review of 242 pregnancies. Aust NZ J Obstet Gynaecol. 1977;17:79–83.

10. Branch DW. Operations for cervical incompetence. Clin Obstet Gynecol. 1986;29:240–54.

11. Cousins L. Cervical incompetence, 1980: a time for reappraisal. Clin Obstet Gynecol. 1980;23:467–79.

12. Medley N, Vogel JP, Care A, Alfirevic Z. Interventions during pregnancy to prevent preterm birth: an overview of Cochrane systematic reviews. Cochrane Database Syst Rev. 2018; 11(11):CD012505. doi: 10.1002/14651858.CD012505.pub2.

13. Dahlke JD, Sperling JD, Chauhan SP, Berghella V. Cervical cerclage during periviability: can we stabilize a moving target? Obstet Gynecol. 2016;127:934–40.

14. Burdet J, Rubio AP, Salazar AI, Ribeiro ML, Ibarra C, Franchi AM. Inflammation, infection and preterm birth. Curr Pharm Des. 2014;20:4741–8.

15. Owen J, Hankins G, Iams JD, Berghella V, Sheffield JS, Perez-Delboy A, et al. Multicenter randomized trial of cerclage for preterm birth prevention in high-risk women with shortened midtrimester cervical length. Am J Obstet Gynecol. 2009;201:375.e1–8.

16. Berghella V, Rafael TJ, Szychowski JM, Rust OA, Owen J. Cerclage for short cervix on ultrasonography in women with singleton gestations and previous preterm birth: a meta-analysis. Obstet Gynecol. 2011;117:663–71.

17. Szychowski JM, Owen J, Hankins G, Iams JD, Sheffield JS, Perez-Delboy A, et al. Can the optimal cervical length for placing ultrasound-indicated cerclage be identified? Ultrasound Obstet Gynecol. 2016;48:43–7.

18. Berghella V, Mackeen AD. Cervical length screening with ultrasound-indicated cerclage compared with history-indicated cerclage for prevention of preterm birth: a meta-analysis. Obstet Gynecol. 2011;118:148–55.

19. Suhag A, Reina J, Sanapo L, Martinelli P, Saccone G, Simonazzi G, et al. Prior ultrasound-indicated cerclage: comparison of cervical length screening or history-indicated cerclage in the next pregnancy. Obstet Gynecol. 2015;126:962–8.

20. Ehsanipoor RM, Seligman NS, Saccone G, Szymanski LM, Wissinger C, Werner EF, et al. Physical examination-indicated cerclage: a systematic review and meta-analysis. Obstet Gynecol. 2015;126:125–35.

21. Chatzakis C, Efthymiou A, Sotiriadis A, Makrydimas G. Emergency cerclage in singleton pregnancies with painless cervical dilatation: a meta-analysis. Acta Obstet Gynecol Scand. 2020;99:1444–57.

22. Romero R, Gonzalez R, Sepulveda W, Brandt F, Ramirez M, Sorokin Y, et al. Infection and labor. VIII. Microbial invasion of the amniotic cavity in patients with suspected cervical incompetence: prevalence and clinical significance. Am J Obstet Gynecol. 1992;167:1086–91.

23. Weiner CP, Lee KY, Buhimschi CS, Christner R, Buhimschi IA. Proteomic biomarkers that predict the clinical success of rescue cerclage. Am J Obstet Gynecol. 2005;192:710–8.

24. Berghella V, Ciardulli A, Rust OA, To M, Otsuki K, Althuisius S, et al. Cerclage for sonographic short cervix in singleton gestations without prior spontaneous preterm birth: systematic review and meta-analysis of randomized controlled trials using individual patient-level data. Ultrasound Obstet Gynecol. 2017;50:569–77.

25. Boelig RC, Dugoff L, Roman A, Berghella V, Ludmir J. Predicting asymptomatic cervical dilation in pregnant patients with short mid-trimester cervical length: A secondary analysis of a randomized controlled trial. Acta Obstet Gynecol Scand. 2019;98:761–8.

26. Enakpene CA, DiGiovanni L, Jones TN, Marshalla M, Mastrogiannis D, Della Torre M. Cervical cerclage for singleton pregnant patients on vaginal progesterone with progressive cervical shortening. Am J Obstet Gynecol. 2018;219:397.e1–10.

27. Gulersen M, Bornstein E, Domney A, Blitz MJ, Rafael TJ, Li X, et al. Cerclage in singleton gestations with an extremely short cervix (≤10 mm) and no history of spontaneous preterm birth. Am J Obstet Gynecol MFM. 2021;3:100430.

28. Berghella V, Odibo AO, To MS, Rust OA, Althuisius SM. Cerclage for short cervix on ultrasonography: meta-analysis of trials using individual patient-level data. Obstet Gynecol. 2005;106:181–9.

29. ACOG Practice Bulletin No.142: cerclage for the management of cervical insufficiency. Obstet Gynecol. 2014;123:372–9.

30. Saccone G, Rust O, Althuisius S, Roman A, Berghella V. Cerclage for short cervix in twin pregnancies: systematic review and meta-analysis of randomized trials using individual patient-level data. Acta Obstet Gynecol Scand. 2015;94:352–8.

31. Li C, Shen J, Hua K. Cerclage for women with twin pregnancies: a systematic review and metaanalysis. Am J Obstet Gynecol. 2019;220:543–57.e1.

32. Liu Y, Chen M, Cao T, Zeng S, Chen R, Liu X. Cervical cerclage in twin pregnancies: an updated systematic review and meta-analysis. Eur J Obstet Gynecol Reprod. Biol 2021;260:137–49.

33. Roman A, Rochelson B, Martinelli P, Saccone G, Harris K, Zork N, et al. Cerclage in twin pregnancy with dilated cervix

between 16 to 24 weeks of gestation: retrospective cohort study. Am J Obstet Gynecol. 2016;215:98.e1–11.

34. Roman A, Zork N, Haeri S, Schoen CN, Saccone G, Colihan S, et al. Physical examination-indicated cerclage in twin pregnancy: a randomized controlled trial. Am J Obstet Gynecol. 2020;223:902.e1–11.

35. Shennan A, Story L, Jacobsson B, Grobman WA. FIGO good practice recommendations on cervical cerclage for prevention of preterm birth. Int J Gynaecol Obstet. 2021;155:19–22.

36. Witt MU, Joy SD, Clark J, Herring A, Bowes WA, Thorp JM. Cervicoisthmic cerclage: transabdominal vs transvaginal approach. Am J Obstet Gynecol. 2009;201:105.e1–4.

37. Shennan A, Chandiramani M, Bennett P, David AL, Girling J, Ridout A, S et al. MAVRIC: a multicenter randomized controlled trial of transabdominal vs transvaginal cervical cerclage. Am J Obstet Gynecol. 2020;222:261.e1–9.

38. Suff N, Carter J, Chandiramani M, Shennan A. Pregnancy outcomes following transabdominal cerclage after recurrent failed vaginal cerclage. Eur J Obstet Gynecol Reprod Biol. 2021;258:469–70.

39. Kyrgiou M, Athanasiou A, Kalliala IEJ, Paraskevaidi M, Mitra A, Martin-Hirsch PP, et al. Obstetric outcomes after conservative treatment for cervical intraepithelial lesions and early invasive disease. Cochrane Database Syst Rev. 2017;11(11): CD012847. doi: 10.1002/14651858.CD012847.

40. Grabovac M, Lewis-Mikhael AM, McDonald SD. Interventions to try to prevent preterm birth in women with a history of conization: a systematic review and meta-analyses. J Obstet Gynaecol Can. 2019;41:76–88.e7.

41. Final report of the Medical Research Council/Royal College of Obstetricians and Gynaecologists: multicentre randomised trial of cervical cerclage. MRC/RCOG Working Party on Cervical Cerclage. Br J Obstet Gynaecol. 1993;100:516–23.

42. Wang T, Jiang R, Yao Y, Huang X. Can prophylactic transvaginal cervical cerclage improve pregnancy outcome in patients receiving cervical conization? A meta-analysis. Ginekologia Polska. 2021;92:704–13.

43. Odibo AO, Berghella V, To MS, Rust OA, Althuisius SM, Nicolaides KH. Shirodkar versus McDonald cerclage for the prevention of preterm birth in women with short cervical length. Am J Perinatol. 2007;24:55–60.

44. Hessami K, Kyvernitakis I, Cozzolino M, Moisidis-Tesch C. McDonald versus Shirodkar cervical cerclage for prevention of preterm birth: a systematic review and meta-analysis of pregnancy outcomes. J Matern Fetal Neonatal Med. 2021:1–8.

45. Biggio JR, Jr. Bed rest in pregnancy: time to put the issue to rest. Obstet Gynecol. 2013;121:1158–60.

46. Treadwell MC, Bronsteen RA, Bottoms SF. Prognostic factors and complication rates for cervical cerclage: a review of 482 cases. Am J Obstet Gynecol. 1991;165:555–8.

47. Galyean A, Garite TJ, Maurel K, Abril D, Adair CD, Browne P, et al. Removal versus retention of cerclage in preterm premature rupture of membranes: a randomized controlled trial. Am J Obstet Gynecol. 2014;211:399.e1–7.

48. Harger JH. Cerclage and cervical insufficiency: an evidence-based analysis. Obstet Gynecol. 2002;100:1313–27.

49. Smith J, DeFranco EA. Tocolytics used as adjunctive therapy at the time of cerclage placement: a systematic review. J Perinatol. 2015;35:561–5.

50. Defranco EA, Valent AM, Newman T, Regan J, Smith J, Muglia LJ. Adjunctive therapies to cerclage for the prevention of preterm birth: a systematic review. Obstet Gynecol Int. 2013;2013:528158.

51. Miller ES, Grobman WA, Fonseca L, Robinson BK. Indomethacin and antibiotics in examination-indicated cerclage: a randomized controlled trial. Obstet Gynecol. 2014;123:1311–16.

52. Eleje GU, Eke AC, Ikechebelu JI, Ezebialu IU, Okam PC, Ilika CP. Cervical stitch (cerclage) in combination with other treatments for preventing spontaneous preterm birth in singleton pregnancies. Cochrane Database Syst Rev. 2020;9(9):CD012871. doi: 10.1002/14651858.CD012871.pub2.

Chapter 34
Gestational Hypertension, Preeclampsia, and Eclampsia

Michal Fishel Bartal[1,2] and Baha M. Sibai[1]

[1] Department of Obstetrics, Gynecology and Reproductive Sciences, McGovern Medical School,
The University of Texas Health Science Center, Houston, TX, USA
[2] Department of Obstetrics and Gynecology, Sheba Medical Center, Tel Hashomer, Sackler School of Medicine, Tel Aviv, Israel

Hypertension complicates 7–10% of pregnancies; of cases, 70% are due to gestational hypertension/preeclampsia, and 30% are due to essential chronic hypertension [1]. Risk factors include:

- Nulliparity
- Advanced maternal age (greater than 35 years)
- Obesity (body mass index greater than 30 kg/m²)
- Multifetal gestation
- Assisted reproductive technology
- Preexisting hypertension or renal disease
- Preeclampsia in a previous pregnancy
- Diabetes mellitus or gestational diabetes
- Antiphospholipid antibody syndrome
- Systemic lupus erythematosus
- Molar or partial molar pregnancy.
- Family history of preeclampsia or eclampsia

Preeclampsia rarely develops before 20 weeks of gestation. However, one should rule out underlying renal disease, molar pregnancy, and other medical disorders in this early stage.

Pathophysiology

Preeclampsia is a disorder of unknown etiology that is peculiar to human pregnancy. The pathophysiological abnormalities in preeclampsia include inadequate maternal vascular response to placentation, endothelial dysfunction, abnormal angiogenesis, and exaggerated inflammatory response with resultant generalized vasospasm, activation of platelets, and abnormal hemostasis. These abnormalities result in pathophysiological vascular lesions in peripheral vessels, uteroplacental vascular beds, and various organ systems, including the kidneys, liver, lungs, and brain. Consequently, these pregnancies, particularly those with preeclampsia and severe features, are associated with increased maternal and perinatal mortality and morbidity due to reduced uteroplacental blood flow, placental abruption, and preterm delivery. However, recent evidence indicates that preeclampsia is an endothelial disorder. Thus, in some patients, the disease may manifest itself in either a capillary leak, fetal growth restriction, reduced amniotic fluid, or a spectrum of abnormal laboratory tests with multiple organ dysfunction (Figure 34.1).

Diagnosis

Gestational hypertension

- Systolic blood pressure (BP) at least 140 mmHg, but less than 160 mmHg or/and diastolic BP at least 90 mmHg, but less than 110 mmHg.
- Blood pressure was noted to be abnormal after 20 weeks of gestation.
- These pressures were observed on at least two occasions 4 hours apart.
- BP readings can vary with the type of equipment used, cuff size, the position of the arm, position of the patient, duration of the rest period, obesity, smoking, anxiety, and the Korotkoff sound used to assess diastolic BP. Only Korotkoff sound V should be used to establish diastolic BP.

Severe gestational hypertension

- Sustained elevations in systolic BP to at least 160 mmHg and/or diastolic BP to at least 110 mmHg for at least 4 hours apart.
- Individuals with severe gestational hypertension should be managed like individuals with preeclampsia with severe features.

Queenan's Management of High-Risk Pregnancy: An Evidence-Based Approach, Seventh Edition. Edited by Catherine Y. Spong and Charles J. Lockwood.

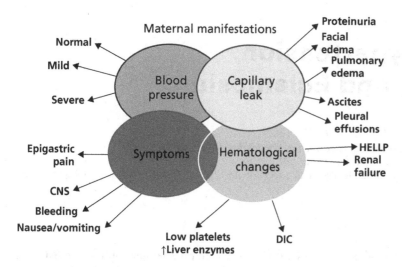

Figure 34.1 Signs and symptoms of preeclampsia and organ dysfunction. CNS, central nervous system; DIC, disseminated intravascular coagulation; HELLP, hemolysis, elevated liver enzymes, and low platelet count.

Proteinuria

• Protein excretion in the urine increases in normal pregnancy from approximately 5 mg/dL in the first and second trimesters to 15 mg/dL in the third trimester. These low levels are not detected by dipstick. The urinary protein concentration is influenced by contamination with vaginal secretions, blood, bacteria, or amniotic fluid. It also varies with urine-specific gravity and pH, exercise, and posture.

• Proteinuria is defined as 300 mg or more in a 24-hour urine collection or a protein/creatinine ratio of 0.3 mg/mg or more.

• Proteinuria usually appears after hypertension in the disease process, but it could occur before the rise in blood pressure in some individuals.

Edema

• Excessive weight gain greater than 4 lb/week (greater than 1.8 kg/week) in the second or third trimester may be the first sign of the potential development of preeclampsia.

• Up to 40% of women with preeclampsia do not have edema.

Preeclampsia

• The American College of Obstetricians and Gynecologists (ACOG) practice bulletin on gestational hypertension and preeclampsia classifies preeclampsia with or without severe features. The term mild preeclampsia has been removed and should not be used [2].

• Preeclampsia is defined as gestational hypertension with proteinuria (≥300 mg per 24 hours urine collection or protein/creatinine ratio ≥0.3, or dipstick reading 1+ if other methods are unavailable).

• In the absence of proteinuria, preeclampsia is defined as new-onset hypertension with the new onset of any severe features (described later).

Preeclampsia with severe features

Any of the following:

• Systolic BP at least 160 mmHg or diastolic BP at least 110 mmHg on two occasions at least 4 hours apart or sustained severe BP for more than 15 minutes requiring intravenous therapy.

• New-onset persistent cerebral symptoms (headaches) unresponsive to medications or persistent visual disturbances.

• Impaired liver function as indicated by abnormally elevated liver enzymes (twice-normal levels), severe persistent right upper quadrant or epigastric pain unresponsive to medications and not accounted by alternative diagnosis, or both.

• Thrombocytopenia (platelet count less than 100 000/μL).

• Progressive renal insufficiency (serum creatinine greater than 1.1 mg/dL or a doubling of the serum creatinine concentration).

• Pulmonary edema.

• The amount of proteinuria, presence of oliguria, and fetal growth restriction have been removed from the diagnosis of severe disease.

Eclampsia

• The convulsive manifestation of hypertensive disorders of pregnancy.

• Defined as new-onset tonic–clonic, focal, or multifocal seizures in the absence of other causative conditions (such as cerebral arterial ischemia, intracranial hemorrhage, drug use, or epilepsy) in women with hypertensive disorder of pregnancy [3].

HELLP

• Hemolysis: abnormal peripheral blood smear; increased bilirubin 1.2 mg/dL or higher; low haptoglobin levels.

- Elevated liver enzymes: increased lactic dehydrogenase (LDH), alanine aminotransferase (ALT), or aspartate aminotransferase (AST) greater than twice the upper limit of normal.
- Low platelets: less than 100 000/μL.
- It occurs in 10% to 20% of individuals with preeclampsia with severe features.
- More frequent in White women and multiparas.
- Complaints of nausea and vomiting (50%), malaise of a few days' duration (90%), epigastric or right upper quadrant pain (65%), or swelling. Others will have vague abdominal pain, flank or shoulder pain, jaundice, hematuria, gastrointestinal bleeding, or gum bleeding [4].
- Onset antepartum in 70% of the cases and postpartum in 30% of the cases.
- In the postpartum period, the onset of the clinical manifestations may range from a few hours to one week, with the majority developing within 48 hours.
- Hypertension may be absent in 20% and mild in 30% of the cases.
- Proteinuria may be absent in 5% of cases.

Management

Delivery is the only available cure for preeclampsia. The ultimate goals of any management plan must be the mother's safety first and then the delivery of a live mature newborn that will not require intensive and prolonged neonatal care. The decision between immediate delivery and expectant management will depend on one or more of the following: maternal and fetal conditions at the time of evaluation, fetal gestational age, presence of labor or rupture of membranes, the severity of the disease process, and maternal desire.

Initial evaluation
- Initial evaluation includes clinical maternal and fetal assessment.
- A complete blood count, serum creatinine, LDH, AST, ALT.
- Fetal evaluation includes ultrasound for estimated fetal weight and amniotic fluid and antepartum testing, including a nonstress test (NST) or biophysical profile (BPP).

Gestational hypertension and preeclampsia without severe features
Figure 34.2 provides a management algorithm for gestational hypertension and preeclampsia without severe features.

37 weeks or more
- At 37 weeks or more of gestation, induction of labor is indicated.
- In a randomized control study for women with gestational hypertension and preeclampsia without severe

Maternal and fetal evaluation

Indication for delivery:
- ≥ 37 wk of gestation
- ≥ 34 wk of gestation with PPROM or active labor
- Eclampsia
- Pulmonary edema
- DIC
- Acute renal failure
- Placental abruption
- Abnormal fetal testing

If these conditions are absent, patient is a candidate for expectant management

Expectant management:
- Inpatient/outpatient
- At least 1 visit/wk in clinic
- Laboratory testing once a week (CBC, CMP)
- Serial ultrasound for fetal growth (every 3–4 wk) and weekly antepartum testing

Deliver at 37 wk

Figure 34.2 Recommended management of gestational hypertension or preeclampsia without severe features. CBC, complete blood count; CMP, comprehensive metabolic panel; DIC, disseminated intravascular coagulation; PPROM, preterm premature rupture of the membranes.

features after 36 weeks of gestation (HYPITAT trial), induction of labor was associated with a reduction of composite adverse maternal outcomes, including new-onset severe preeclampsia, hemolysis, elevated liver enzymes, and low platelet count (HELLP) syndrome, eclampsia, pulmonary edema, or placental abruption compared to expectant management. There was no difference in the rate of cesarean deliveries or neonatal outcomes between the groups [5].
- Delivery may also be indicated earlier for any signs of maternal–fetal distress (suspected abruption, confirmed fetal growth restriction, labor, or rupture of membranes).

Less than 37 weeks
- In all patients, the maternal and fetal conditions should be evaluated.

• Outpatient management is possible if the patient's systolic BP is less than 160 mmHg and/or diastolic BP is less than 110 mmHg, with a platelet count of more than 100,000/mL, normal liver enzymes and reassuring fetal testing. The patient should also have no subjective symptoms and be compliant and reliable.

• Whether the patient is in the hospital or being managed at home, the following should be observed:

– Salt restriction, diuretics, antihypertensive drugs, and sedatives are not used.

– The patient should have at least one clinic visit per week, laboratory evaluation of hematocrit, platelets, liver function tests, serum creatinine once a week, and serial ultrasound to determine fetal growth (every 3–4 weeks) weekly antepartum testing.

– Patients should be educated about preeclampsia warning signs, such as severe headache, visual disturbances, epigastric pain, nausea and vomiting, and shortness of breath. In addition, the patient should be instructed about daily kick counts and labor signs or vaginal bleeding.

– No additional measuring of proteinuria.

– Weekly NST or BPP for patients with gestational hypertension or preeclampsia without severe features.

• Prompt hospitalization is needed for disease progression: severe acute hypertension, development of new symptoms or abnormal laboratory findings, outpatient management unsatisfactory for the specific patient, or abnormal fetal testing.

Preeclampsia with severe features or severe gestational hypertension

• Preeclampsia with severe features or severe gestational hypertension is associated with significant maternal and fetal complications, including pulmonary edema, stroke, coagulopathy, renal failure, placental abruption, and fetal death.

• Beyond 34 weeks: induction and delivery. There is no need to assess fetal lung maturity, and delivery should not be delayed for the administration of steroids for fetal lung maturity.

• Less than 34 weeks with stable maternal and fetal conditions consider expectant management. Expectant management is intended to provide neonatal benefits but is associated with increased maternal risks.

• Figure 34.3 provides a management algorithm for preeclampsia with severe features or severe gestational hypertension.

• Patients eligible for expectant management should receive antenatal steroids for fetal lung maturity.

• Less than 23 weeks: Given the high maternal morbidity and extremely low perinatal survival in expectant management at <23 weeks, termination of pregnancies may be offered in some centers after extensive counseling.

1. Admit to the hospital
2. Monitor for symptoms, labs
3. Ultrasound, FHR tracing
4. Corticosteroids, MgSo4 prophylaxis, antihypertensive treatment

Contraindication to continued expectant management
• Uncontrolled severe range blood pressure
• Persistent headache not responsive to treatment
• Eclampsia
• Pulmonary edema
• HELLP syndrome
• Acute renal failure
• Placental abruption
• Abnormal fetal testing
• Extreme prematurity/ IUFD/lethal anomalies
• Fetal growth restriction with reversed end diastolic flow in the umbilical artery >32 wk

Offer expectant management
• Inpatient management
• D/C MgSo4
• Monitor for symptoms
• Daily maternal and fetal testing
• Twice weekly labs

Figure 34.3 Recommended management of preeclampsia with severe features or severe gestational hypertension <34 weeks. D/C, discontinue; FHR, fetal heart rate; HELLP, hemolysis, elevated liver enzymes, and low platelet count; IUFD, intrauterine fetal demise; MgSo4, magnesium sulfate.

Management of preeclampsia with severe features or severe gestational hypertension

• A patient with preeclampsia with severe features or severe gestational hypertension should be admitted to the hospital until delivery.

• The main objectives for those patients are controlling their blood pressure and preventing seizures [6].

• Seizure prophylaxis: magnesium sulfate has been shown to reduce the risk of eclampsia by more than one half compared to placebo.

• We recommend initial intravenous magnesium sulfate for 24 hours.

• If the patient is offered expectant management, magnesium will be restarted when the patient is delivered.

• The recommended dose is administering a 4–6 g loading dose over 20–30 minutes, followed by a 2 g/hour maintenance dose.

Blood pressure control

- Antihypertensive should be started for severe hypertension (sustained elevations in systolic BP to at least 160 mmHg and/or in diastolic BP to at least 110 mmHg).
- Intravenous hydralazine, labetalol, or oral nifedipine can be used for initial treatment (Tables 34.1, 34.2).
- Following the initial blood pressure control, the patient can be transitioned to an oral regimen (Table 34.1).
- The aim is diastolic BP 90 to 100 mmHg and systolic BP 140 to 150 mmHg. Avoid lowering BP to values below 130 mmHg systolic or 80 mmHg diastolic because of the risk of decreased uteroplacental perfusion.
- All patients with expectant management should receive antenatal steroids.

Table 34.1 Drugs used to treat hypertension in pregnancy

Drug	Starting dose	Maximum dose
Acute treatment of severe hypertension		
Hydralazine	5–10 mg IV every 20 min	25 mg*
Labetalol*	20–40 mg IV every 10–15 min	300 mg*
Nifedipine	10–20 mg oral every 20–30 min	50 mg*
Long-term treatment of hypertension		
Labetalol	100–200 mg bid	2400 mg/day
Nifedipine	30 mg daily	120 mg/day
Thiazide diuretic	12.5 mg daily	50 mg/day

* If desired blood pressure levels are not achieved, switch to another drug.
IV, intravenous.

Table 34.2 Protocols for treatment of severe hypertension (SBP ≥160 or DP ≥110 mmHg)

Time Min	Labetalol IV (mg)	Hydralazine IV (mg)	Nifedipine Oral (mg)
0	20	5-10	10
10	SBP ≥160 or DBP ≥ 110 40	Check BP	Check BP
20	SBP ≥160 or DBP ≥110 80	SBP ≥160 or DBP ≥110 10	SBP ≥160 or DBP ≥110 20
30	SBP ≥160 or DBP ≥110 Give IV hydralazine 10		Check BP
40	Check BP	SBP ≥160 or DBP ≥110 Give IV labetalol 40	SBP ≥160 or DBP ≥110 20
50	SBP ≥160 or DBP ≥110 Consult	SBP ≥160 or DBP ≥110 Consult	SBP ≥160 or DBP ≥110 IV labetalol 40 Consult

DBP, diastolic blood pressure; IV, intravenous; SBP, systolic blood pressure.

- Most patients with preeclampsia with severe features will require delivery in the next 2 weeks.
- Indications for delivery are:
    1. Uncontrolled severe BP defined as maximum dosing of oral labetalol (2400 mg daily) and extended-release nifedipine (120 mg daily) or not responding to maximum intravenous medications to control BP (Table 34.2)
    2. Persistent headaches, epigastric pain, or visual changes
    3. Eclampsia
    4. Pulmonary edema
    5. HELLP syndrome
    6. New or worsening renal dysfunction
    7. Placental abruption
    8. A nonreassuring fetal heart tracing
    9. Fetal death/ lethal anomaly
    10. Severe fetal growth restriction with reverse end-diastolic flow in the umbilical artery after 32 weeks of gestation

HELLP

- Expectant management of HELLP for 48 hours (for the administration of steroids) is only possible in the absence of disseminated intravascular coagulation (DIC) and a stable patient.
- All patients with HELLP syndrome should be delivered after administration of steroids or earlier if not stable.

Eclampsia

- Initial management–call for help and stabilize a patient.
- Delay delivery until maternal status is stable.
- The patient should be given a loading dose of magnesium sulfate IM/IV [7].
- If the seizures recur, another dose of magnesium 2 g can be given.
- Once the patient is stable, proceed with delivery. Mode of delivery will depend on gestational age (GA) and Bishop score. If the cervix is unfavorable and GA is <30 weeks, consider elective cesarean delivery [3].

Complications of preeclampsia and HELLP

Complications include placental abruption, pulmonary edema, acute renal failure, liver hematoma with possible rupture, postpartum hemorrhage, wound or intra-abdominal hematomas, DIC, and multiorgan failure, including liver, kidneys, and lungs (adult respiratory distress syndrome). Neurologic-like eclampsia, hypertensive encephalopathy, ischemia, infarcts, edema, and hemorrhage can also occur as a cardiorespiratory arrest [8–10].

Intrapartum management of preeclampsia with severe features

- The priority is to assess and stabilize the maternal condition and evaluate fetal well-being. Finally, a decision must be made as to whether immediate delivery is indicated.
- Intravenous magnesium sulfate should be started.
- Accurate measurement of fluid input and output: Foley catheter, restrict total intake to 100 mL/h to avoid pulmonary edema.
- If pulmonary edema is suspected, give 40 mg IV Lasix and obtain chest X-ray and maternal echocardiography if needed.
- Frequent monitoring of pulse, BP, urine output, and respiration.
- Continuous fetal monitoring.
- Monitor for signs of magnesium toxicity and have a magnesium level drawn if needed.
- In case of suspected magnesium toxicity, give 10 mL of 10% calcium gluconate intravenously and intubate if the patient develops respiratory arrest.
- For HELLP patients, type and crossmatch with two units of blood. Have platelets available if the platelet count is below 50,000/μL.
- Routine obstetric considerations should determine the mode of delivery
- If the cervix is unfavorable and GA is <30 weeks, consider elective cesarean delivery.
- Epidural anesthesia is preferred to general anesthesia in case of abdominal delivery if personnel skilled in obstetric anesthesia are available.
- Regional anesthesia is contraindicated in women with coagulopathy or women with platelet count less than 70000/μL as it might result in hematoma formation [11].
- If thrombocytopenia is present, it should be corrected before surgery: Transfuse with 6–10 units of platelets in all patients with a platelet count less than 40000/μL.

Postpartum management

- Adequate observation of the mother in the recovery room for 12 to 24 hours under magnesium sulfate coverage. Remember that 25–30% of the eclampsia cases and 30% of the HELLP cases occur in the postpartum period.
- In addition, some women will develop new-onset hypertension or preeclampsia for the first time postpartum. The majority will occur at 3–7 days postpartum. Therefore, patients with hypertensive disorders should have a BP recording at 3 days postpartum and again at 5–7 days after discharge [12].

- Most patients will show evidence of resolution of the disease process within 24 hours after delivery. Some, especially those with severe disease in the mid-trimester, HELLP, or eclampsia, require close monitoring for 2–3 days.
- By the time of discharge, most patients will be normotensive. However, if hypertension persists, antihypertensive medications are prescribed for 1 week, after which the patient is reevaluated. In addition, all patients should be given written instructions about signs and symptoms to report and a phone number to call in case of the development of new symptoms or severe hypertension. In addition, follow-up BP recordings can be done at home or in an office.
- Patients with preeclampsia with severe features and those with superimposed preeclampsia may receive nonsteroidal anti-inflammatory agents for pain.

Follow up and maternal counseling

- Women who develop preeclampsia in their first pregnancy are at increased risk (20%) for the development of preeclampsia in subsequent pregnancies. The risk of preeclampsia in the sister of a patient with preeclampsia is 14%.
- With severe disease in a first pregnancy, recurrence is about 30%. With severe disease in the second trimester, the risk of recurrent preeclampsia is 50%. In 21% of cases, the disease also occurs in the second trimester. HELLP recurs in about 5% of cases [13].
- There is an increased risk of chronic hypertension and undiagnosed renal disease. This is especially true in patients with two episodes of preeclampsia in the second trimester [14].
- There is also an increased risk of fetal growth restriction in a subsequent pregnancy.
- Finally, women who develop hypertensive disorders in pregnancy are at increased risk for cardiovascular disease and metabolic syndrome later in life. Therefore, they should receive close monitoring for these complications [14].
- For women who developed preeclampsia in their previous pregnancy, aspirin is recommended in their subsequent pregnancy. Aspirin should be started between 12 and 28 weeks, the earliest as possible [2].
- ACOG recommends a low dose of aspirin (80–120 mg per day) should also be given for all women with chronic hypertension, multiple gestations, and pregestational diabetes or women with two or more risk factors such as body mass index >30 and nulliparity [2].

CASE PRESENTATION

A healthy 35-year-old, G2P0010, presented to the clinic for prenatal care at 25 weeks. She denies any history of chronic hypertension or other comorbidities. Her blood pressure is 140/95; she denies any other symptoms such as headache, blurry vision, or epigastric pain. The physical exam in the clinic is within normal limits. Repeat blood pressure is 143/92. Laboratory studies showed normal hematocrit, platelet count, and liver transaminase levels. The urine protein creatinine ratio is 0.25. On ultrasound, the estimated fetal weight is ninth percentile with normal amniotic fluid. The patient is diagnosed with gestational hypertension and fetal growth restrictions. Weekly follow-up in the clinic are planned with weekly labs.

At 34 weeks 5 days during the clinic visit, the patient reported headaches, and her blood pressure was 162/102; she was sent to triage for evaluation. Her repeat blood pressure is 165/100. Her laboratory studies, including complete blood count, creatinine, and liver enzymes, are within normal limits. Fetal heart tracing is reassuring with a normal biophysical profile. Intravenous labetalol 20 mg is given to manage severe hypertension with a repeat blood pressure check-in 15 minutes. The patient is diagnosed with gestational hypertension with severe features and is admitted to labor and delivery for labor induction. On admission, magnesium is started for seizure prophylaxis with a 6 g loading dose over 20–30 minutes, followed by a 2 g/hour maintenance dose. Induction of labor is started with close monitoring of blood pressure and symptoms. The patient progresses in labor and has a spontaneous vaginal delivery without complications. Following delivery, magnesium is continued for 24 hours for seizure prophylaxis. On postpartum day 2, her blood pressure was 158/100, and her repeat blood pressure was 156/102; she was started on oral nifedipine 30mg for blood pressure control. Blood pressures following starting the medication were within normal limits. She was discharged home on postpartum day 3 with a follow-up in the clinic within 7 days from delivery for a blood pressure check.

References

1. Hutcheon JA, Lisonkova S, Joseph KS. Epidemiology of preeclampsia and the other hypertensive disorders of pregnancy. Best Pract Res Clin Obstet Gynaecol. 2011;25(4):391–403.

2. ACOG Practice Bulletin No. 222: gestational hypertension and preeclampsia. Obstet Gynecol. 2020;135(6):e237–60.

3. Fishel Bartal M, Sibai BM. Eclampsia in the 21st century. Am J Obstet Gynecol. 2022;226(2S):S1237–53.

4. Sibai BM. Diagnosis, controversies, and management of the syndrome of hemolysis, elevated liver enzymes, and low platelet count. Obstet Gynecol. 2004;103(5 Pt 1):981–91.

5. Koopmans CM, Bijlenga D, Groen H, Vijgen SM, Aarnoudse JG, Bekedam DJ, et al. Induction of labour versus expectant monitoring for gestational hypertension or mild preeclampsia after 36 weeks' gestation (HYPITAT): a multicentre, open-label randomised controlled trial. Lancet. 2009;374(9694):979–88.

6. Sibai BM, Barton JR. Expectant management of severe preeclampsia remote from term: patient selection, treatment, and delivery indications. Am J Obstet Gynecol. 2007;196(6):514.e1–9.

7. Sibai BM, Graham JM, McCubbin JH. A comparison of intravenous and intramuscular magnesium sulfate regimens in preeclampsia. Am J Obstet Gynecol. 1984;150(6):728–33.

8. Abalos E, Cuesta C, Carroli G, Qureshi Z, Widmer M, Vogel JP, et al. Pre-eclampsia, eclampsia and adverse maternal and perinatal outcomes: a secondary analysis of the World Health Organization Multicountry Survey on Maternal and Newborn Health. BJOG. 2014;121 Suppl 1:14–24.

9. MacKay AP, Berg CJ, Atrash HK. Pregnancy-related mortality from preeclampsia and eclampsia. Obstet Gynecol. 2001;97(4):533–8.

10. Sibai BM, Sarinoglu C, Mercer BM. Eclampsia. VII. Pregnancy outcome after eclampsia and long-term prognosis. Am J Obstet Gynecol. 1992;166(6 Pt 1):1757–61; discussion 1761-53.

11. Lee LO, Bateman BT, Kheterpal S, Klumpner TT, Housey M, Aziz MF, et al. Risk of epidural hematoma after neuraxial techniques in thrombocytopenic parturients: a report from the Multicenter Perioperative Outcomes Group. Anesthesiology. 2017;126(6):1053–63.

12. Matthys LA, Coppage KH, Lambers DS, Barton JR, Sibai BM. Delayed postpartum preeclampsia: an experience of 151 cases. Am J Obstet Gynecol. 2004;190(5):1464–6.

13. Sibai BM, Mercer B, Sarinoglu C. Severe preeclampsia in the second trimester: recurrence risk and long-term prognosis. Am J Obstet Gynecol. 1991;165(5 Pt 1):1408–12.

14. Ackerman CM, Platner MH, Spatz ES, Illuzzi JL, Xu X, Campbell KH, et al. Severe cardiovascular morbidity in women with hypertensive diseases during delivery hospitalization. Am J Obstet Gynecol. 2019;220(6):582.e1–11.

Chapter 35
Postpartum Hemorrhage

David B. Nelson

Division of Maternal-Fetal Medicine, Department of Obstetrics and Gynecology, University of Texas Southwestern Medical Center at Dallas, Dallas, TX, USA

Postpartum hemorrhage (PPH) continues to be the leading preventable cause of maternal illness and death worldwide [1,2]. In the United States, 10.7% of all pregnancy-related deaths during 2014 to 2017 were associated with PPH [1,3]. When maternal death is considered within the time frame up to 1 year after delivery, PPH is responsible for approximately one in nine maternal deaths with up to one third of cases likely preventable [3,4]. Obstetric hemorrhage also results in significant morbidity. Severe maternal morbidities (SMMs) are unexpected outcomes of labor and delivery that result in significant short- or long-term consequences to a pregnant individual's health [5]. These rates are now chronicled by organizations such as the Centers for Disease Control and Prevention, using administrative codes. Blood transfusion is a substantial contributor to the SMM rate accounting for more than 80% of the rate nationally [5].

Because of the importance of PPH contributing to maternal morbidity and mortality, national organizations now recommend that a multidisciplinary approach with safety bundles, staged-based protocols, and standardized checklists be used to resolve maternal hemorrhage at the earliest stage possible [6–8]. The Joint Commission (TJC) has also implemented elements of performance standards under the Provision of Care, Treatment, and Services chapter for obstetrical hemorrhage [9]. All of these platforms emphasize the need for recognition and timely response for early resuscitation, escalation of care, and if necessary, deployment of a massive transfusion protocol to prevent hypoperfusion that can lead to multiorgan dysfunction and coagulopathy [1,6–9]. These principles are paramount in management to reduce adverse maternal consequences from PPH.

Hematologic parameters

An understanding of coagulation–both in normal hemostasis and pathologic processes–is critical in managing PPH. Coagulation is the process by which thrombin is activated and soluble plasma fibrinogen is converted into insoluble fibrin. For years, coagulation was described as a "cascade" with two pathways: the extrinsic, or tissue factor, pathway and the intrinsic, or contact activation, pathway [10–12]. Both converge to a common pathway converting fibrinogen into an insoluble cross-linked fibrin clot. This traditional description of clotting was useful in teaching concepts and interpreting coagulation studies but are now considered to be physiologically inaccurate [12]. It is now proposed that coagulation is normally initiated through tissue factor (TF) exposure and activation through the classic extrinsic pathway but with amplification through elements of the classic intrinsic pathway (11). *Specifically, the current theory is that coagulation is primarily initiated by TF that forms complexes with factor VII/VIIa* [11]. The development of TF-FVIIa complexes ultimately generates activated factor X to initiate clotting whereas the previously labeled "intrinsic" pathway is responsible for the amplification of this process [11]. The product of this process is fibrin formation, which is then counterbalanced by the fibrinolytic system [11]. The use of viscoelastic testing discussed later leverages these principles by identifying both the timing and strength of clot formation as well as fibrinolysis.

Normal pregnancy is associated with marked changes in the hematologic system to accommodate the demands of the enlarging uterus, support the growing placenta and fetus, and protect the pregnant patient against adverse

Queenan's Management of High-Risk Pregnancy: An Evidence-Based Approach, Seventh Edition. Edited by Catherine Y. Spong and Charles J. Lockwood.

effects of blood loss with delivery. Of these, one important change is the increase in maternal blood volume that averages 45–50% above the nonpregnant state [11]. This expansion results from an increase in both plasma and erythrocytes with the most rapid increase during the second trimester. Along with the substantive increase in plasma volume, there is augmented production of most procoagulants [11]. Fibrinogen concentration, for example, increases approximately 50% above nonpregnant values, and during late pregnancy, it ranges from approximately 375 to 620 mg/dL [13]. At the same time, there is a reduction in levels of natural anticoagulants, such as protein C and S [11]. The net result is that pregnancy is a procoagulant state. Table 35.1 displays pregnancy-related hematologic indices relative to nonpregnant values [13]. The impact of these changes on the interpretation of referent ranges for laboratory measures is obvious [14]. *Importantly, "normal values," as indicated by the electronic medical record – often using nonpregnant reference ranges – may be profoundly abnormal in the pregnant patient and postpartum patient.* Fibrinogen levels are one example. Thus, pregnancy-related laboratory alterations should be appreciated in management of PPH

Defining excessive blood loss

Beginning in 2017, the American College of Obstetricians and Gynecologists (ACOG) adopted the definition of PPH as cumulative blood loss greater than or equal to 1000 mL or blood loss accompanied by signs or symptoms of hypovolemia within 24 hours after the birth process regardless of the route of delivery [6]. This differs from previous definitions that used blood loss greater than 500 mL after vaginal birth and 1000 mL for cesarean birth. Defining an incidence of PPH is difficult given these varying definitions. In a study of more than 115,000 deliveries,

the incidence of PPH with vaginal delivery was 5.3%, and it was 10.5% for cesarean delivery when defined using the historical precepts (e.g. more than 500 mL for vaginal birth) or explicitly documented treatment measures [15]. Alternatively, a decrease in hematocrit of 10% had been proposed as an alternative marker to define PPH; however, determinations of hemoglobin or hematocrit concentrations are often delayed, may not reflect current hematologic status, and are not clinically useful in the setting of acute postpartum hemorrhage beyond establishing a baseline measure [6]. From the National Hospital Discharge Summary database, PPH incidence between 2001 and 2005 was only 2.6% [16]. Thus, PPH rates appear to be underreported when comparing administrative data to clinical research studies, and these variations have obvious impact on reported SMM rates and quality measures [17]. Beyond definition differences, comparison among reports is also difficult given case mix variations – vis-à-vis risk profile – of population studied [18].

Use of quantitative blood loss (QBL), rather than visual estimation, has recently been suggested as it is more accurate for defining blood loss at delivery [19]. Several QBL methods are available including weighing blood-soaked items, calibrated collection drapes and devices, and more recently, tablet-devices with colorimetric analysis. Despite improved accuracy, definitive clinical effectiveness for one method over the other has not yet been demonstrated [19,20]. Regardless of assessment method, PPH should be considered when blood loss is more than expected and any accompanying evidence of hypovolemia should serve as an indication to investigate promptly. Importantly, in a patient with tachycardia and hypotension, considerable blood loss, usually representing 25% of the total blood volume (or approximately 1500 mL or more), has occurred [6]. Awaiting vital sign alterations to begin responding during a PPH can be fatal because the morbidity and mortality associated with hemorrhage

Table 35.1 Normal reference ranges in pregnant women compared to nonpregnant adults

	Nonpregnant adult	First trimester	Second trimester	Third trimester
Hematology				
Hemoglobin (g/dL)	12–15.8	11.6–13.9	9.7–14.8	9.5–15.0
Hematocrit (%)	35.4–44.4	31.0–41.0	30.0–39.0	28.0–40.0
Platelets (x10^9/L)	165–415	174–391	155–409	146–429
Coagulation				
D-dimer (µg/mL)	0.22–0.74	0.05–0.95	0.32–1.29	0.13–1.7
Fibrinogen (mg/dL)	233–496	244–510	291–538	373–619
International Normalized Ratio	0.9–1.04	0.89–1.05	0.85–0.97	0.80–0.94
Partial thromboplastin time, activated (sec)	26.3–39.4	24.3–38.9	24.2–38.1	24.7–35.0
Prothrombin time (sec)	12.7–15.4	9.7–13.5	9.5–13.4	9.6–12.9
Protein C, functional (%)	70–130	78–121	88–133	67–135
Protein S, functional activity (%)	65–140	57–95	42–68	16–42

Adapted from [13].

is often due to delayed recognition and inadequate restoration of circulating blood volume. Because of this, nursing-provider communication strategies with "urgent request to the bedside" have been encouraged within maternity services to record time interval for response to such emergencies.

Prevention

Active management of the third stage of labor is recommended by several organizations, including the World Health Organization, to reduce the incidence of PPH [6]. Active management includes (1) oxytocin administration, (2) uterine massage, and (3) umbilical cord traction. Prophylactic oxytocin, by dilute intravenous infusion, or intramuscular injection (10 units), remains the most effective medication with the fewest adverse effects [6]. The timing of oxytocin administration–after delayed umbilical cord clamping, with delivery of the anterior shoulder, or with placental delivery – has not been adequately studied but it is recommended after all births for PPH prevention [6]. Oxytocin has specific uterine receptors and intravenous administration results in immediate onset of action [21]. The mean plasma half-life is 3 minutes and continuous intravenous infusion is needed to ensure sustained contraction. The usual concentration is 20–40 units per liter of crystalloid, with the infusion rate titrated to response. Steady-state concentration is reached after 30 minutes. Intramuscular injection has a time to onset of 3–7 minutes. Oxytocin is metabolized by both the liver and kidneys. Because it has approximately 5% of the antidiuretic effect of vasopressin, if given in large volumes of electrolyte-free solution, oxytocin can cause water toxicity (headache, vomiting, drowsiness, and convulsions), and symptoms that may be mistakenly attributed to other causes. Rapid administration of an intravenous bolus of oxytocin (5–10 U) results in relaxation of vascular smooth muscle. Hypotension with a reflex tachycardia may occur, followed by a small but sustained increase in blood pressure. In addition, bolus doses have been associated with electrocardiogram (ECG) abnormalities (e.g. ST-depression) as reduction in cerebral perfusion pressure. Oxytocin is stable at temperatures up to 25°C, but refrigeration may prolong shelf-life.

Risk factors and etiologies

In most cases, the source of PPH can and should be determined. When evaluating a patient who is bleeding, it may be helpful to consider "the 4 Ts" mnemonic device: tone, trauma, tissue, and thrombin [6]. Selected risk factors for PPH are listed in Table 35.2, and TJC requires accredited delivery services to evaluate for PPH risk on admission to

Table 35.2 Selected risk factors for postpartum hemorrhage

Obesity	General anesthesia
Nulliparity	Labor induction
High parity	Rapid labor
Previous postpartum hemorrhage	Prolonged labor
Anticoagulation	Augmented labor
Preeclampsia/eclampsia	Chorioamnionitis
Acute fatty liver of pregnancy	Operative vaginal delivery
Large fetus	Breech extraction
Multiple gestation	Excessive cord traction
Hydramnios	Intrauterine manipulation
Uterine fibroids	Episiotomy

labor and delivery and postpartum [9]. Several tools for risk assessment are available from national organizations (eg. Association of Women's Health, Obstetric and Neonatal Nurses) and state-based quality collaborative groups (e.g. California Maternal Quality Care Collaborative); however, these risk scoring systems only modestly predict PPH, so vigilance for all patients is paramount [22].

PPH within 24 hours of birth is defined as primary (or early) and after 24 hours is secondary (or late). Etiologies of primary PPH include uterine atony, uterine inversion, genital tract lacerations, uterine rupture, retained placenta, placenta accreta spectrum disorder (PAS), placental abruption, and coagulation defects. Secondary PPH may be caused by infection (endomyometritis), retained products of conception, inherited coagulation defects, and subinvolution of the placental site.

Uterine atony

Despite preventative measures, uterine atony occurs in approximately 5% of pregnancies and accounts for 80% of primary PPH. Many evidence-based resources exist to assist in optimizing the outcome in obstetrical hemorrhage and two of the most important are checklist-based protocols and multidisciplinary team drills. The fundamental principles of these programs are to establish a standardized response to PPH. An example of the Parkland hemorrhage response checklist that shares similar principles to the ACOG Obstetric Hemorrhage checklist and state programs, such as in Texas with partnership from the Alliance for Innovation on Maternal Health, is shown in Figure 35.1. Within this checklist are uterotonic agents, including oxytocin given as prophylaxis, to treat PPH and measures discussed in foregoing text.

Methylergonovine/ergometrine

Methylergonovine (methylergometrine) and its parent compound ergometrine result in sustained tonic contraction of uterine smooth muscle by stimulation of α-adrenergic myometrial receptors [1,21]. The dose of methylergonovine is 0.2 mg, and doses may be repeated in 2–4 hours if needed. Plasma levels do not correlate with

POST PARTUM HEMORRHAGE (PPH) CHECKLIST

Initial Actions
- ☐ Call for assistance
- ☐ Response team to the bedside
  - • Delivering attending MD/CNM
  - • Primary RN
  - • Anesthesiologist
- ☐ Brief: appoint leader, recorder, nursing roles
- ☐ Identify hemorrhage stage and document EBL & interventions

Normal vital signs and lab values:
Blood loss > 500 mL vaginal - OR - blood loss > 1000 mL cesarean

- ☐ Record VS/O₂ saturation every 5 minutes
- ☐ Monitor cumulative blood loss
- ☐ Insert foley catheter
- ☐ Ensure IV access: 18 gauge if possible
- ☐ Increase IV fluid (crystalloid: estimated blood loss in 2:1 ratio <u>without</u> oxytocin)
- ☐ Fundal massage
- ☐ Determine and treat etiology (4 T's - Tone, Trauma, Tissue, Thrombin)
- ☐ Contact blood bank: type and crossmatch 2 units PRBCs

Medications for Uterine Atony

Oxytocin (Pitocin)	10-40 international units/liter intravenously, or 10 units IM if no IV access
Methylergonovine (Methergine)	0.2 milligrams intramuscularly (may be repeated every 2-4 hours)
15-methyl PGF₂ₐ (Hemabate, Carboprost)	250 micrograms intramuscularly (may repeat every 15 minutes, maximum 8 doses)
Misoprostol (Cytotec)	800-1000 micrograms rectally

Normal vital signs and lab values:
Continued bleeding with EBL up to 1500 mL **OR** any patient requiring ≥ 2 uterotonics

- ☐ Obtain 2nd IV access (18 gauge if possible)
- ☐ STAT labs, with coags & fibrinogen
- ☐ Medications: continue medications from Stage 1
- ☐ Transfuse per clinical signs/symptoms
  - • Notify blood bank of OB hemorrhage, bring 2 units PRBCs to bedside, thaw 2 units FFP. **DO NOT wait for labs!**
- ☐ For uterine atony → Consider uterine balloon or packing, possible surgical interventions
- ☐ Consider moving patient to OR (better exposure, potential D&C)
- ☐ Mobilize additional team members as necessary
- ☐ Warming blanket

Abnormal vital signs/labs/oliguria:
Continued bleeding with EBL > 1500 mL **OR** > 2 units PRBCs given **OR** patient at risk for occult bleeding (post-cesarean) & DIC

- ☐ Outline management plan → Serial re-evaluation → Communicate plans with hemorrhage team
- ☐ Transfusion → RBC-FFP-Platelets in a 6:4:1 ratio (active Massive Transfusion Protocol - MTP) → If coagulopathic, add cryoprecipitate. Consider consultation for alternative agents
- ☐ Identify etiology for bleeding (if still unclear)
- ☐ Rule out lacerations (exam), coagulopathy (labs), occult bleeding (imaging)
- ☐ Achieve hemostasis immediately, interventions based on etiology
- ☐ Adopt additional measure (if poor response)

Cardiovascular Collapse:
For patients with cardiovascular collapse in setting of massive hemorrhage consider the following etiologies:

- ☐ Profound hypovolemic shock (blood loss not replaced)
- ☐ AFE (sudden CV collapse followed by heavy uterine bleeding from uterine relaxation and associated coagulopathy)

> • Immediate surgical interventions to ensure hemostasis (hysterectomy) may be necessary.
> • Simultaneous aggressive blood and factor replacement & medical interventions initiated regardless of the patient's coagulation status.
> • Expeditious hemostasis is the only step that will maximize survival rates for these critical patients.

Post-Hemorrhage Management
- ☐ Debrief with entire care team
- ☐ Document after team debrief
- ☐ Discuss interventions with patient/family members

Figure 35.1 Parkland Hospital postpartum hemorrhage checklist. Used with permission from Parkland Hospital, Michael Malaise, SVP Corp Affairs/Ext Com.

uterine effect. The onset of action is within 2–5 minutes when given intramuscularly and is sustained for 3 hours or more. These drugs are extensively metabolized in the liver and the mean plasma half-life is approximately 30 minutes. When oxytocin and ergometrine derivatives are used together, two different mechanisms are active, oxytocin producing an immediate response and ergometrine a more sustained action. Nausea and vomiting are common side effects. Vasoconstriction of vascular smooth muscle also occurs as a consequence of their α-adrenergic action. This can result in elevation of central venous pressure and systemic blood pressure. Contraindications include heart disease, autoimmune conditions associated with Raynaud phenomenon, peripheral vascular disease, arteriovenous shunts even if surgically corrected, and hypertension. Women with preeclampsia-eclampsia are particularly at risk of severe and sustained hypertension. These agents should not be used intravenously except perhaps in individualized extreme circumstances (moribund, shocked patient with no other alternative).

Prostaglandins

Prostaglandin F2α results in contraction of smooth muscle cells [21]. Hemabate® (carboprost) or 15-methyl prostaglandin F2α is an established second-line treatment for postpartum hemorrhage unresponsive to oxytocic agents. It is available in single-dose vials of 0.25 mg and is given by deep intramuscular injection or by direct injection into the myometrium under direct vision at cesarean section. It is not licensed for the latter route and caution should be exercised to prevent direct injection into a uterine sinus [23]. Repeat intramuscular doses may be given every 15 minutes to a maximum of eight doses. This class of prostaglandins causes bronchoconstriction, venoconstriction, and constriction of gastrointestinal smooth muscle. Associated side effects include nausea, vomiting, diarrhea, pyrexia, and bronchospasm. There are case reports of hypotension and intrapulmonary shunting with arterial oxygen desaturation, and prostaglandin F2α is contraindicated in patients with known cardiac or pulmonary disease.

Prostaglandin E2 (dinoprostone) is generally a vasodilatory prostaglandin; however, it causes contraction of smooth muscle in the pregnant uterus [21]. Vaginal administration is possible but in the setting of active bleeding with compression maneuvers access and placement is difficult such that rectal administration (2 mg) is advisable. Due to its vasodilatory effect, this drug should be avoided in hypotensive and hypovolemic patients; however, it may be useful in patients with heart or lung disease in whom carboprost is contraindicated [24].

Misoprostol

Misoprostol is a synthetic analog of prostaglandin E1 and is metabolized in the liver. The tablet(s) can be given orally, vaginally, or rectally. As prophylaxis for postpartum hemorrhage, an international multicenter randomized trial reported that oral misoprostol is less successful than parenteral oxytocin administration [25]. Furthermore, recent reviews and meta-analyses have questioned the usefulness as a second-line agent [26]. If used to treat atony, doses of 600 to 1000 µg are recommended [6].

Mechanical and surgical control of bleeding

If bleeding continues despite uterotonics, exploration of the genital tract is necessary to detect other causes such as trauma (uterine, cervical, or vaginal tears) or retained placental tissue, particularly in cases where risk factors were present (i.e. operative delivery). Persisting with the exclusive use of manual uterine compression and oxytocic administration in the face of continuous hemorrhage is not advised. Progressively invasive, and sometimes surgical, solutions may be required.

Uterine tamponade

Historically, uterine packing was performed by inserting sterile gauze into the uterus either using a specific packing instrument or long forceps [27]. Packs are generally left in situ for 12–24 hours and prophylactic antibiotics are advised. Currently, several inflatable mechanical devices are used for uterine tamponade. These temporizing devices may allow for correction of coagulopathy in anticipation of, or during, surgical intervention. Insertion requires several team members to act in concert with one performing transabdominal sonography, and the second placing the deflated balloon and inflating the device. Inflation occurs with rapid infusion of 150 mL followed by further instillation over a few minutes to a total of 300 to 500 mL. A continuous oxytocin infusion (with or without other uterotonic agents) and prophylactic antibiotic coverage (e.g. cefazolin, 1 g every 8 hours) are advised when using these devices to reduce risk of endometritis [28]. It is possible that balloon tamponade acts by direct pressure on the open venous channels, stretching and compression of the atonic myometrium, increasing intramuscular vascular resistance, and direct compression of the arteries supplying the uterus [29]. Failure of uterotonic agents and tamponade requires more invasive measures, including uterine compression sutures, angiographic embolization, and hysterectomy.

Uterine compression sutures

There are a number of uterine compression sutures that are variants of the B-Lynch suture, which was designed to vertically compress the uterine body in cases of uterine atony [30]. Because they give the appearance of suspenders, they are also called braces. In order to assess whether the suture will be effective, bimanual compression is applied to the uterus. Most commonly, a number 2 Chromic Catgut suture is used. Normal uterine anatomy has been demonstrated on follow-up, and in most cases, subsequent pregnancies are uneventful if compression sutures had previously been used. Complications from compression sutures include uterine ischemic necrosis, occlusion of the uterine cavity with subsequent development of infection (pyometria), and later development of uterine cavity synechiae, but these are rare.

Uterine devascularization

Uterine devascularization has been used for stepwise management of PPH due to atony, abnormal placentation, and trauma. Uterine artery ligation may be unilateral or bilateral; however, in our experience it is most helpful for management of lacerations at hysterotomy rather than atony. Internal iliac artery ligation may also be unilateral or bilateral and has been shown to decrease distal arterial pulse pressure by 85%, with a 24% reduction in mean arterial pressure [31]. This converts the arterial pressures into pressures approaching the venous system which creates vessels more amenable to hemostasis via pressure and clot formation. Ligation of the internal iliac artery at a point 5 cm distal to the common iliac bifurcation will usually avoid the posterior division branches, and care must be taken not to perforate the contiguous large veins [32]. For years, this has been used to reduce pelvic hemorrhage; however, the procedure may be technically difficult and is successful in only half of cases.

Arterial embolization

Uterine devascularization by selective arterial embolization using pledgets of absorbable gelatin sponge can effect a temporary blockade with resorption within approximately 10 days [33]. If the site of bleeding cannot be identified, embolization of the anterior branch of the internal iliac artery or the uterine artery is performed. Fever, contrast media renal toxicity, and leg ischemia are rare but reported complications of this procedure. A variation on this theme is the prophylactic placement of inflatable balloon catheters in the internal iliac arteries of patients who are expected to bleed excessively at the time of surgery, for example cesarean delivery in a patient with placenta accreta spectrum disorder. *It should be clearly understood that arterial embolization should not be used in a critically unstable and profusely bleeding patient.* This technique is best suited to those patients with persistent bleeding amenable to embolization who are hemodynamically stable and who, it is anticipated, can be maintained that way for at least a few hours with transfusion and support. Severe hemorrhage uncontrolled by medical means and tamponade procedures requires decisive and definitive surgical treatment in an operating room setting.

Hysterectomy

Peripartum hysterectomy is frequently considered the definitive procedure for obstetric hemorrhage but is not without complications. The procedure can be complicated by ongoing blood loss and grossly distorted pelvic anatomy due to edema, abnormal vascularization and dilated vessels, retroperitoneal and other hematoma formation, and trauma. Adequate hemostasis is not always easily achieved, and further procedures may be necessary. The incidence of febrile morbidity is high, with rates of 5–85% in different series. The interval between delivery and successful surgery is a very important prognostic factor, and if a primary procedure (such as brace suture or devascularization) fails, hysterectomy should be undertaken promptly. A supracervical (subtotal) hysterectomy can be performed if bleeding is from the uterine body, and it is generally simpler than a total hysterectomy. The cervix and vaginal angles can be difficult to identify in patients who have labored to full dilation, and a subtotal hysterectomy has less risk of injury to the ureters (0.5%) and bladder (7.2%) compared with total hysterectomy [34]. In almost all cases, general endotracheal anesthesia is best because of prolonged surgical time, need for abdominal packing, extensive dissection and manipulation, and anticipated massive blood transfusion. Further details of hysterectomy methods and complications can be found in Chapter 43.

Pelvic packing

For significant bleeding refractory to medical and surgical maneuvers, pelvic packing with gauze and termination of operation may be necessary as "damage control" [35]. Rolls of gauze are packed to provide constant local pressure to serve as either a temporizing measure to embolization or to treat refractory bleeding. A similar concept can be used with a pelvic pressure pack, also known as the "parachute" or "umbrella" pack, which involves the use of a sterile radiology plastic bag filled with gauze bandages tied together. The bag is inserted abdominally and the open end is passed through the vaginal cuff and out of the vagina. It is then placed on traction to fit the pack snugly into the pelvic bowl and compress the pelvic structures. Once bleeding has abated, the bandage can be gradually removed from the bag which is then pulled out of the vagina. Packing may be left for 24 hours in most cases before removal or replacement, and in some cases, up to 72 hours.

Uterine inversion

Uterine inversion is the folding of the fundus into the uterine cavity in varying degrees:
• First degree: wall extends as far as, but not through the cervix
• Second degree: fundus prolapsed through the cervix but not out of the vagina
• Third degree: prolapse of the fundus outside the vagina
• Fourth degree: complete prolapse of both uterus and vagina

Acute inversion occurs within the first 24 hours after delivery; subacute refers to inversion between 24 hours and 30 days after delivery, and chronic inversion is inversion after 30 days.

Predisposing factors include alone on in combination: fundal placenta, intrapartum fundal pressure, short umbilical cord, inappropriate cord traction, uterine atony, placenta accreta spectrum disorder (Chapter 43), intrinsic myometrial weakness/damage, acute tocolysis with potent uterine relaxant or anesthetic drug, and idiopathic factors [36]. It is unknown if active management of third stage of labor raises the likelihood [37]. The incidence of uterine inversion ranges from 1 in 2000 to 1 in 20,000 vaginal deliveries. In approximately 60–70% of cases, the placenta is still attached at the moment of inversion. Extent of the bleeding is variable and depends on the degree of prolapse. Frequently, the degree of shock is reported to be out of proportion to that attributable to the observed blood loss, and this may be neurogenic shock due to a parasympathetic outflow from stretching peritoneum or reproductive organs. Underestimation of blood loss at the time of delivery may, however, be an important confounder. The physical examination in cases of partial inversion (first degree) can be misleading. Examination often reveals a mass suggestive of a uterine myoma or pelvic tumor. The cervix is still palpable and can be visualized (if the bleeding is not too excessive), and sonography can aid in the diagnosis. In second-degree inversion, the inverted portion of the fundus remains in the vagina, having passed through the cervix, and the examiner is unable to palpate the uterine fundus on abdominal examination, and cannot see or feel the cervix during pelvic examination. Due to the potential complexities of presentation, ultrasound can be helpful, however, the diagnosis may only be established at laparotomy in some cases.

Management

Immediate recognition improves chances of a resolution and avoids increased edema, blood loss, and associated morbidities. Once recognized, several steps must be implemented urgently and simultaneously: (1) aggressive blood product and fluid replacement, (2) replacement of the uterus, and (3) administration of potent uterotonics to keep the uterus contracted and prevent reinversion. The placenta should not generally be removed before replacement because this can exacerbate blood loss. Replacement can usually be accomplished manually by placing a hand in the vagina with the fingers placed circumferentially around the prolapsed fundus. The last region of the uterus that inverted should be the first to be replaced. Care is taken to not apply so much force with the fingertips as to perforate the uterine fundus. Uterine relaxation may be necessary, with 250 μg subcutaneous terbutaline or 50 to 100 μg intravenous nitroglycerine [38]. General anesthesia and use of halogenated gases may be needed to provide full uterine relaxation.

In most cases, the inversion can be resolved using the maneuvers described. If there is a tightly contracted cervical ring that prohibits vaginal replacement of the fundus, surgical options may be necessary. These include incising the ring via a vaginal approach, or more likely, emergent laparotomy. There several abdominal procedures described at laparotomy: (1) stepwise traction on the funnel of the inverted uterus or the round ligaments, using ring or Allis forceps reapplied progressively as the fundus emerges (Huntington procedure); (2) longitudinal incision posteriorly through the cervix, relieving cervical constriction and allowing traction on the round ligaments (as in the Huntington procedure) combined with stepwise replacement of the uterus from below with subsequent repair of the incision from inside the abdomen (Haultain procedure); and (3) dissection of the bladder off the cervix and entry into the vagina with a longitudinal incision. Uterotonic drugs are then given immediately to maintain uterine contraction and to prevent reinversion. Recurrent uterine inversion may be prevented by placement of a balloon catheter.

Once the uterus has been replaced, all uterine relaxant drugs should be stopped, manual removal of the placenta, and uterotonic agents are given. In some cases, the uterus will again invert after repositions requiring uterine compression sutures.

Most authorities recommend antibiotic use after manual replacement although specific evidence of the utility of this is lacking.

Genital tract lacerations

Childbirth is invariably associated with trauma to pelvic structures ranging from minor mucosal tears to severe lacerations leading to life-threatening hemorrhage either by compounding blood loss or hematomas. Lacerations may lie proximally or distally along lower genital tract. Careful inspection for cervical, vaginal, perineal, or rectovaginal lacerations is important, and these should be promptly repaired with absorbable sutures [1]. Exposure, visualization, and good surgical technique are paramount [39]. Deep cervical lacerations generally require surgical repair with suture placement above angle of apex taking care to avoid injury to bladder anteriorly. For persistent bleeding from diffuse points with edematous tissue, vaginal packing for 12–24 hours may be useful.

A serious consequence of lacerations are the development of hematomas which can manifest in the vulvar, vulvovaginal, paravaginal, or rectovaginal areas. Often, these may be resultant from operative vaginal deliveries. Findings include perineal, vulvar, and rectal pain with a mass distorting normal anatomy. Some may be undetected until findings of hypovolemia are present with extension into the pelvis. Imaging with sonography or computed tomography may be indicated. Small, nonexpanding hematomas may be managed with conservative measures including cool packs, analgesics, and observation. For expanding hematomas or with evidence of hypovolemia, surgical exploration at point of maximal distention may be indicated. Often distinct bleeding points may not be identified, and thus, the goal is to obliterate the cavity with layered absorbable sutures. Transfusion may be indicated as blood loss often exceeds clinical estimates with large hematomas. Embolization, similar to atony management, can be used primarily for hemodynamically stable patients, or for secondary measures if local measures fail.

Uterine rupture
This subject has been dealt with elsewhere (Chapter 47) but the general principles addressed here and in blood transfusion in foregoing text apply in this situation.

Retained placenta
Inspection of the placenta after delivery is important to rule out retained placental tissue or a succenturiate lobe [1]. When retained placental tissue is suspected, manual exploration or a banjo (blunt) curette under ultrasound guidance is recommended. With such maneuvers, antibiotic treatment should be instituted. Potential PAS should always be considered, especially with excessive bleeding.

Placenta accreta spectrum disorder
The prevalence of PAS has been steadily increasing alongside the number of cesarean deliveries [40]. Over the past decade, the rate of peripartum hysterectomy has nearly doubled and the indication has changed from predominantly uterine atony to now placental invasion [41]. Chapter 43 outlines assessment and management of PAS.

Treatment

Once the diagnosis of PPH is established, evaluation, initiation of treatment, and a call for assistance should occur simultaneously in a multidisciplinary approach. The level of intervention is based upon the classification of hemorrhage and the maternal condition. Unless there is another obvious etiology, empiric treatment for uterine atony should be initiated. If the bleeding continues, then activation of a predefined obstetric emergency response team should be initiated when PPH is diagnosed or when there are clinical signs of hypovolemia (Figure 35.1). At a minimum the team should consist of sufficient nursing personnel to complete all necessary tasks, an anesthesia provider team, transfusion services, the laboratory, and obstetric assistants.

A standard approach for laboratory testing for coagulopathy during PPH response is to obtain a panel of hematologic studies with five tests: hematocrit, platelet count, international normalized ratio/prothrombin time, activated partial thromboplastin time, and fibrinogen [14]. These tests have been incorporated into various scoring systems for disseminated intravascular coagulation; however, the clinical application in the midst of an active obstetric hemorrhage remain challenging. These tests, however, do not necessarily assess the quality and strength of the clot, and turnaround time for results may be 30–60 minutes rendering the results irrelevant in a rapidly evolving hemorrhage. Because of these challenges, viscoelastic testing with thromboelastography and rotational thromboelastometry is being increasingly used as adjunct point-of-care tests during an obstetric hemorrhage to assess multiple facets of hemostasis: coagulation, platelet function, and fibrinolysis [14]. These tests work by analyzing both clot formation and breakdown with information displayed as a graphical report with indices for time to clot formation, clot strength, and fibrinolysis. Two important caveats in use of these point-of-care tests are that these should not be interpreted by inadequately trained personnel, and these tests should not be applied in the setting of active, large-volume hemorrhage [14]. Regardless of testing modality, a key analyte for management of PPH is fibrinogen, which often becomes depleted after ongoing bleeding and selected replacement of only packed red blood cells. This is especially true with PPH in the setting of placental abruption where fibrinogen levels may be dangerously low before delivery. A surrogate for fibrinogen may be quickly obtained by drawing a red top tube for a clot test. If the red top tube clots and does not lyse within 30 minutes, the fibrinogen level may be assumed to be greater than 150 mg/dL, and conversely, lack of clot development or early clot dissolution may suggest coagulopathy.

The provider should vigorously perform bimanual uterine massage, expel clots from the uterus, and empty the urinary bladder by placing a Foley catheter. Indeed, use of urine output is a critical vital sign for hypovolemia in the management of PPH. The perineum, vagina, cervix, and uterus are assessed for lacerations, hematomas, and retained products of conception. The uterine decidua should be wiped clean with a sponge or bluntly curetted with a large curette. This requires adequate anesthesia, lighting, instruments, assistance, and proper patient positioning. Ultrasound may be useful for examining the uterus. Early transfer to the operating room may facilitate establishing the diagnosis and facilitate management. Hemorrhage carts with additional supplies often needed in the management of PPH have also been encouraged. These carts contain additional sponges, retractors, sponge count bags, Foley catheter, transfusion tubing, and laboratory collection materials that are often needed in the setting of PPH. Uterine atony should only be diagnosed once other etiologies have been excluded.

Volume resuscitation, and treatment by medical, conservative surgical, and definitive (i.e. hysterectomy) surgical techniques, must be concurrent. Aggressive volume resuscitation is normally appropriate unless the patient has an underlying condition such as a cardiomyopathy, which would contradict a large volume infusion. Initially a volume of isotonic crystalloid, such as lactated Ringers solution, should be given. Colloid solutions such as albumin have not been demonstrated to be superior to crystalloid. If there is not an immediate cessation of the bleeding, preparation for blood product replacement should begin, and consideration given to initiating a massive transfusion protocol (MTP) as development of coagulopathy can be fatal [42]. MTPs are standardized protocols that transfuse preemptively with blood products using a balanced ratio of plasma and platelets to red blood cells. The intent of MTP is twofold: (1) to effectively replace blood and clotting factors to avoid dilutional coagulopathy, and (2) remove barriers from transfusion services to administration at the bedside. These protocols have effectively replaced the traditional approach of delaying replacement of plasma and platelets until deficiencies were demonstrated by laboratory analysis. Upon admission for delivery, a blood type and antibody screen is performed on all pregnant individuals at Parkland given that any patient is at significant risk for hemorrhage and the aforementioned limitations of risk prediction tools. If type and screen is not available, it may be necessary to transfuse blood that is either type O negative or only type specific while the transfusion protocol is being instituted.

In addition to MTPs, other agents are being explored for use in obstetrics to mitigate PPH. These include recombinant Factor VII and tranexamic acid; as well as topical hemostatic agents such as topical thrombin, fibrin sealant, gelatin matrix, chitosan-covered gauze, and oxidized regenerated cellulose. Use of Factor VII in obstetrics is controversial, and there is a concern with associated arterial–and to a lesser degree venous–thrombosis. At this time, it is not recommended to be used as a first-line agent and is currently deployed as part of MTP in response to profound hemorrhage [6]. Evidence supporting tranexamic acid use as an adjunct in obstetrical hemorrhage is currently evolving. Routine use for prophylaxis is not currently recommended [43]. It may be considered in the setting of PPH when initial medical therapy fails [6]. The benefit, particularly reduction in mortality, appears to be primarily in patients treated sooner than 3 hours from time of delivery. Intraoperative blood salvage with reinfusion has also become an intervention considered in obstetric patients. Theoretical concerns of safety with risk of amniotic fluid embolism have been disproven; however, resources and cost may also be prohibitive for some centers given the unpredictable nature of PPH.

Preservation of fertility is the main advantage of conservative surgical intervention. Also, the likelihood of surgical morbidity will be less if hysterectomy can be avoided. However, fertility preservation must always come second to preservation of life. Therefore, when there is ongoing significant hemorrhage and the patient exhibits signs of hypovolemic shock, it is imperative that hysterectomy not be delayed. When to proceed with a hysterectomy is a judgment decision and it is generally best to err on the side of early hysterectomy.

Complications

Transfusion-related acute lung injury (TRALI) and transfusion-associated circulatory overload (TACO) are the most common causes of transfusion-related mortality [44]. Affected patients characteristically have severe dyspnea, hypoxia, and pulmonary edema that develop within 6 hours of transfusion. Of the two, TACO is more common, and its incidence nears 1%, and TRALI is estimated to complicate at least 1 in 12 000 transfusions. TACO is suspected to be due to pulmonary edema related to circulatory overload whereas TRALI is thought to be injury to the pulmonary capillaries from human leukocyte antigen antibodies and human neutrophil antibodies in donor plasma. In general, TRALI is more likely to be associated with fever, hypotension, and exudative pulmonary infiltrates. In contrast, TACO is more likely to be associated with findings suggesting volume overload. Management includes stopping the transfusion, assessment with chest imaging, supportive care with possible mechanical ventilation, and in the case of TACO diuresis.

Conclusion

Postpartum hemorrhage remains one of the major contributors to maternal mortality, and in many cases, that mortality may have been prevented by the institution of prophylactic and interventional measures. Recognition of risk factors, institution of standard procedures and protocols, and a team approach to this problem will almost certainly result in drastically decreased morbidity and mortality. Recently, there has been a significant effort in obstetric units to encourage team-based training to better respond to PPH emergencies given its frequency and associated maternal consequences. Obstetric simulation that includes multidisciplinary team members has been particularly useful in training for such emergencies. Components of a simulation program include standardized lectures to provide the necessary background, clinical checklists for reference during the course, a simulated event, and team debriefing following the scenario. This provides hands-on opportunities to improve individual skills and the critical teamwork and communication skills necessary to care for patients during obstetric emergencies. Data on improved clinical performance in response to PPH with simulation have found faster response to treatment and reduced blood loss [45]. Both ACOG and SMFM (Society for Maternal-Fetal Medicine) have developed courses for such training. Through improved recognition, enhanced timeliness of response, and system-based protocols with team-based training, maternal morbidity and mortality from PPH can be reduced.

CASE PRESENTATION

A 26-year-old gravida 5, para 4 patient with gestational diabetes presented at term with polyhydramnios. Following a labor course, complicated by chorioamnionitis, the patient was delivered vaginally with forceps with a third-degree laceration. The baby weighed 4.3 kg and did well. After delivery of the infant, the umbilical cord avulsed, and the placenta was removed manually in pieces. Heavy vaginal bleeding ensued within minutes, and in addition to a routine oxytocin infusion (20 U in 1 L Ringer's lactate at 250 mL/h), an intramuscular 0.2 mg methylergonovine was provided because the uterus was felt to be atonic. At this time, blood loss was 750 mL. Manual compression of the uterus was initiated, Foley catheter inserted, and a second intravenous line (18 gauge) was started. Because of the piecemeal placental removal, an ultrasound unit was brought to the bedside and transabdominal scanning revealed retained placental fragments. Curettage was performed with a wide-diameter curette. Continued bleeding and persistent uterine atony were noted with blood loss now 1000 mL. Emergent studies were drawn to include a complete blood count and coagulation profile. Two units of packed red blood cells (PRBCs) were ordered. The patient was given an intramuscular injection of 0.25mg carboprost tromethamine and a second obstetric physician and the anesthesiologist were summoned.

The patient continued to bleed heavily with estimated blood loss of 1500mL. An additional two PRBC and two units of fresh frozen plasma (FFP) were ordered with tranexamic acid 1 g intravenously given over 10 minutes. When blood loss was estimated to be in excess of 2000 mL it was noted that vital signs indicated incipient collapse (decreasing systolic pressure with narrowed pulse pressure, tachycardia, increased respiratory rate, and restlessness). Both intravenous lines were opened fully and crystalloid (2 L of Ringer's lactate solution) was rapidly infused while the patient was taken to the operating room and massive transfusion protocol activated.

In the operating room, the patient was placed in lithotomy position and a tamponade balloon was placed through her cervix into the uterus and filled with 500 mL of normal saline. A second intramuscular injection of 0.25 carboprost tromethamine was given, and 1000 mcg of misoprostol was placed in the patient's rectum. The first MTP cooler of 5 PRBC and 5 FFP arrived and were administered. At this point the bleeding diminished significantly. The patient was monitored closely in the operating room until it was determined that the bleeding was controlled and viscoelastic testing was ordered. The patient was moved to the intensive care unit (ICU) with serial hematologic testing and a team debrief was conducted. The tamponade balloon was removed after 18 hours when her coagulation profile was normal and there was no further significant vaginal bleeding. Three additional units of PRBCs were given in the ICU. The patient was discharged in stable condition 4 days postpartum.

References

1. Bienstock JL, Eke AC, Hueppchen NA. Postpartum hemorrhage. N Engl J Med. 2021 Apr 29;384(17):1635–45.
2. Say L, Chou D, Gemmill A, Tunçalp Ö, Moller AB, Daniels J, et al. Global causes of maternal death: a WHO systematic analysis. Lancet Glob Health. 2014 Jun;2(6):e323–33.
3. Centers for Disease Control and Prevention. Pregnancy Mortality Surveillance System. [last reviewed 2023 Mar 23; cited 2023 Jun 7]. Available from: https://www.cdc.gov/reproductivehealth/maternal-mortality/pregnancy-mortality-surveillance-system.htm.
4. Lepine SJ, Geller SE, Pledger M, Lawton B, MacDonald EJ. Severe maternal morbidity due to obstetric haemorrhage: potential preventability. Aust N Z J Obstet Gynaecol. 2020;60(2):212–17.
5. Centers for Disease Control and Prevention. Severe maternal morbidity in the United States. [last reviewed 2021 Feb 2; cited 2022 Feb 17]. Available from: https://www.cdc.gov/reproductivehealth/maternalinfanthealth/severematernal-morbidity.html.
6. American College of Obstetricians and Gynecologists. Practice Bulletin No. 183: postpartum hemorrhage. Obstet Gynecol. 2017;130:e168–86.
7. Alliance for Innovation on Maternal Health. Obstetric hemorrhage patient safety bundle. 2021 [cited 2023 Jun 7]. Available from: https://saferbirth.org/psbs/obstetric-hemorrhage.
8. California Maternal Quality Care Collaborative. OB Hemorrhage Toolkit V3.0 Errata 2022 Jul 18 [cited 2023 Jun 7]. Available from: https://www.cmqcc.org/resources-tool-kits/toolkits/ob-hemorrhage-toolkit.

9. The Joint Commission. Provision of care, treatment, and services standards for maternal safety. The Joint Commission R3 report. 2019 Aug 19 [cited 2022 Jan 17]. Available from: https://www.jointcommission.org/-/media/tjc/documents/standards/r3-reports/r3-issue-24-maternal-12-7-2021.pdf.

10. Arruda VR, High KA. Coagulation disorders. In: Jameson J, Fauci AS, Kasper DL, Hauser SL, Longo DL, Loscalzo J, editors. Harrison's principles of internal medicine. 20th ed. New York: McGraw-Hill; 2018 [cited 2022 Feb 17]. Available from: https://accessmedicine.mhmedical.com/content.aspx?bookid=2129&sectionid=192018684.

11. Cunningham FG, Nelson DB. Disseminated intravascular coagulation syndromes in obstetrics. Obstet Gynecol. 2015 Nov;126(5):999–1011.

12. Konkle BA. Bleeding and thrombosis. In: Jameson J, Fauci AS, Kasper DL, Hauser SL, Longo DL, Loscalzo J, editors. Harrison's principles of internal medicine. 20th ed. New York: McGraw-Hill; 2018 [cited 2022 Feb 17]. Available from: https://accessmedicine.mhmedical.com/content.aspx?bookid=2129&sectionid=192014303.

13. Abbassi-Ghanavati M, Greer LG, Cunningham FG. Pregnancy and laboratory studies: a reference table for clinicians. Obstet Gynecol. 2009;114(6):1326–31.

14. Nelson DB, Ogunkua O, Cunningham FG. Point-of-care viscoelastic tests in the management of obstetric hemorrhage. Obstet Gynecol. 2022;139(3):463–72.

15. Yee LM, McGee P, Bailit JL, Reddy UM, Wapner RJ, Varner MW, et al. Daytime compared with nighttime differences in management and outcomes of postpartum hemorrhage. Obstet Gynecol. 2019;133(1):155–62.

16. Berg CJ, MacKay AP, Qin C, Callaghan WM. Overview of maternal morbidity during hospitalization for labor and delivery in the United States: 1993–1997 and 2001–2005. Obstet Gynecol. 2009;13(5):1075–81.

17. Fridman M, Korst LM, Reynen DJ, Nicholas LA, Greene N, Saeb S, et al. Severe maternal morbidity in California hospitals: performance based on a validated multivariable prediction model. Jt Comm J Qual Patient Saf. 2021;47(11):686–95.

18. Nelson DB, Spong CY. Look before leaping: the value of understanding a quality measure before adoption to public reporting. Jt Comm J Qual Patient Saf. 2021;47(11):681–3.

19. American College of Obstetricians and Gynecologist. ACOG Committee Opinion No. 794. quantitative blood loss in obstetric hemorrhage: Obstet Gynecol. 2019;134(6):e150–6.

20. Diaz V, Abalos E, Carroli G. Methods for blood loss estimation after vaginal birth. Cochrane Database Syst Rev. 2018;9(9):CD010980. doi: 10.1002/14651858.CD010980.pub2.

21. Chelmow C, O'Brien B. Postpartum haemorrhage: prevention. Clin Evid. 2006:1932–50.

22. Chu T, Rodriguez AN, Kleinmann W, Patel S, Horsager R, Bird A, et al. Correlation of postpartum hemorrhage risk stratification with calculated blood loss greater than 1000 millimeters. Am J Obstet Gynecol. 2020;222(1):S673.

23. Hayashi R, Castillo M, Noah M. Management of severe postpartum hemorrhage with a prostaglandin F2 alpha analogue. Obstet Gynecol. 1984;63:806–8.

24. Barrington J, Roberts A. The use of gemeprost pessaries to arrest postpartum haemorrhage. Br J Obstet Gynaecol. 1993;100:691–2.

25. Gülmezoglu A, Villar J, Ngoc N, Piaggio G, Carroli G, Adetoro L, et al. WHO Collaborative Group to Evaluate Misoprostol in the Management of the Third Stage of Labour. WHO multicentre randomised trial of misoprostol in the management of the third stage of labour. Lancet. 2001;358:689–95.

26. Gallos ID, Papadopoulou A, Man R, Merriel A, Gee H, Lissauer D, et al. Uterotonic agents for preventing postpartum haemorrhage: a network meta-analysis. Cochrane Database Syst Rev. 2018;12(12):CD011689. doi: 10.1002/14651858.CD011689.pub3.

27. Katesmark M, Brown R, Raju K. Successful use of a Sengstaken-Blakemore tube to control massive postpartum haemorrhage. Br. J Obstet Gynaecol. 1994;101(3):259–60.

28. Martingano D, Mitrofanova A, Kim AF, Ulfers A, Mersch M, Stevenson R, et al. Antibiotic prophylaxis during intrauterine balloon tamponade following vaginal deliveries with postpartum hemorrhage. AJOG. 2020;222(1 Suppl):S253 [cited 2022 Feb 19]. Available from: https://www.ajog.org/article/S0002-9378(19)31767-3/fulltext.

29. Belfort MA, Dildy GA, Garrido J, White GL. Intraluminal pressure in a uterine tamponade balloon is curvilinearly related to the volume of fluid infused. Am J Perinatol. 2011;28(8):659–66. Epub 2011 April 15.

30. B-lynch C, Coker A, Lawal AH, Abu J, Cowen MJ. The B-Lynch surgical technique for the control of massive postpartum haemorrhage: an alternative to hysterectomy? Five cases reported. Br J Obstet Gynaecol. 1997;104:372–5.

31. Burchell R, Olson G. Internal iliac artery ligation: aortograms. Am J Obstet Gynecol. 1966;94:117–24.

32. Bleich AT, Rahn DD, Wieslander CK, Wai CY, Roshanravan SM, Corton MM. Posterior division of the interal iliad artery: anatomic variations and clinical applications. Am J Obstet Gynecol. 2007;197(6):658.e1–5.

33. Hansch E, Chitkara U, McAlpine J, El-Sayed Y, Dake M, Razavi M. Pelvic arterial embolization for control of obstetric hemorrhage: a five-year experience. Am J Obstet Gynecol. 1999;180:1454–60.

34. Wright JD, Devine P, Shah M, et al. Morbidity and mortality of peripartum hysterectomy. Obstet Gynecol. 2010;115:1187–93.

35. Pacheco LD, Lozada MJ, Saade GR, Hankins GDV. Damage-control surgery for obstetric hemorrhage. Obstet Gynecol. 2018;132(2):423–7.

36. Wendel MP, Shnaekel KL, Magann EF. Uterine inversion: a review of a life-threatening obstetrical emergency. Obstet Gynecol Surv. 2018;73(7):411–17.

37. Deneux-Tharauz C, Sentilhes L, Maillard F, Closset E, Vardon D, Lepercq J, et al. Effect of routine controlled cord traction as part of the active management of the third stage of labour on postpartum haemorrhage: multicentre randomised controlled trial (TRACOR). BMJ. 2013;346:f1541.

38. Dayan S, Schwalbe S. The use of small-dose intravenous nitroglycerine in a case of uterine inversion. Anesth Analg. 1996;82:1091–3.

39. American College of Obstetricians and Gynecologists. ACOG Practice Bulletin No. 198: prevention and management of obstetric lacerations at vaginal delivery. Obstet Gynecol. 2018;132:e87–102.

40. Pinas Carrilo A, Chandraharan E. Placenta accrete spectrum: risk factors, diagnosis and management with special reference to the Triple P procedure. Womens Health (Lond.) 2019;15:1745506519878081.

41. Fleming ET, Yule CS, Lafferty AK, Happe SK, McIntire DD, Spong SY. Changing patterns of peripartum hysterectomy over time. Obstet Gynecol. 2021;138(5):799–801.

42. Cunningham FG, Nelson DB. Disseminated intravascular coagulation syndromes in obstetrics. Obstet Gynecol. 2015;126(5):999–1011.

43. Pacheco LD. Tranexamic acid for the prevention of obstetrical hemorrhage after cesarean delivery: a randomized controlled trial. AJOG. 2022;226(1 Suppl): S779–S780 [cited 2022 Feb 19].

Available from: https://www.ajog.org/article/S0002-9378(21)02663-6/fulltext.

44. Semple JW, Rebetz J, Kapur R. Transfusion-associated circulatory overload and transfusion-related acute lung injury. Blood. 2019;133(17):1840–53.

45. Dillon SJ, Kleinmann W, Fomina Y, Werner B, Schultz S, Klucsarits S, et al. Does simulation improve clinical performance in management of postpartum hemorrhage? Am J Obstet Gynecol. 2021;225(4):435.e1–8.

Chapter 36
Emergency Care

Sarah Rae Easter

Division of Maternal-Fetal Medicine, Department of Obstetrics and Gynecology; Division of Critical Care Medicine, Department of Anesthesiology, Perioperative and Pain Medicine, Brigham and Women's Hospital, Harvard Medical School, Boston, MA, USA

Obstetrics is a field characterized by high-acuity low-frequency events most often involving an otherwise healthy group of individuals. These features of the obstetric population mirror those of patients encountered in a trauma or acute care setting which may explain the similarities in the approach to management. Whether in the trauma bay or on labor and delivery principles of emergent care for all patients center on timely and dynamic assessment, stabilization and resuscitation, and appropriate resource use. These tenets should be championed for pregnant persons as well with the additional challenges of accounting for the physiologic modifications of pregnancy and the well-being of the fetus. This protocol reviews fundamental principles of acute care through the lens of trauma and cardiac arrest in pregnancy highlighting key strategies that can be translated to other emergent scenarios encountered in obstetrics.

Timely and dynamic assessment of trauma

The Advanced Trauma Life Support (ATLS) Guidelines from the American College of Surgeons popularized the protocolized approach to initial and subsequent assessment characterized as the primary, secondary, and tertiary survey. The primary survey focuses on identifying and addressing life-threatening injuries on arrival to care and represent the minimum assessment required before intervening in the care of an unstable patient. For hemodynamically stable patients the protocol progresses to a secondary survey characterized by a more detailed but targeted history, physical exam, and complement of diagnostic studies to detect additional significant injuries or clinical conditions. The tertiary survey is essentially the secondary survey repeated later. This reassessment not only increases the rate of detection of injuries overlooked on presentation, but it also provides time for subclinical injuries to evolve to clinical manifestations.

These frameworks may appear to complicate what is clinically intuitive for the seasoned clinician, but the protocolized nature of these surveys serve two key roles. First, a systematic approach reduces the risk of undiscovered injuries–a key feature in the setting of pregnancy where concerns about the fetus may distract the nonobstetric care provider from a typical approach. The emergent care of a pregnant person is likely to require multidisciplinary involvement that underscores another key benefit of protocolized approach to care–ensuring that team members share the same mental model. These protocols optimize the ability of providers to share a similar care process in high-acuity scenarios where timeliness improves outcomes. This imperative for a shared mental model informs the need for obstetric care providers to be familiar with principles of emergency care. A basic understanding of the standard of care allows the obstetric care provider to ensure this is not compromised due to pregnancy and to offer clinical insights into pertinent modifications should they exist.

Primary survey

The primary survey focused on assessment and stabilization of life-threatening injuries follows the mnemonic ABCDE representing Airway, Breathing, Circulation, Disability, and Exposure. Table 36.1 provides an overview of the components of the primary survey noting caveats in the setting of pregnancy.

In most settings the trauma team will consist of a sufficient number of team members to perform this assessment in parallel, but it is worth noting that in the absence of cardiac arrest, airway, and breathing supersede circulation for more than just alphabetical convenience. Injury to the airway is

Queenan's Management of High-Risk Pregnancy: An Evidence-Based Approach, Seventh Edition. Edited by Catherine Y. Spong and Charles J. Lockwood.

Table 36.1 Primary survey with considerations for the pregnant trauma patient

	Components	Obstetric considerations
Airway	Evaluate airway and consider intubation if concern for neurologic injury compromising ability to protect airway, penetrating chest trauma, or hemodynamic instability.	Assume "difficult airway" and ensure most experienced provider available for intubation. Decreased functional residual capacity will precipitate earlier hypoxemia during apneic ventilation and may lower intubation threshold.
Breathing	Assess oxygenation and ventilation with vital signs with low threshold for chest radiography	Provide oxygen targeting SpO_2 ≥95% Place thoracostomy tube 1–2 spaces higher
Circulation	Check pulses, establish adequate IV access, control hemorrhage, and use FAST to evaluate for hemorrhagic or traumatic causes of shock (e.g. tamponade, tension pneumothorax)	Ensure IV placement above the diaphragm Consider left uterine displacement Assess for obstetric causes of hemorrhage or hypotension Evaluate fetal heart rate with ultrasound
Disability	Assess for neurologic injury and quantify with Glasgow Coma Scale[a] and ensure immobilization with any concern for spinal cord injury.	Provide reassurance about safety of ionizing radiation in this setting (e.g. CT) to avoid delay in diagnosis associated with studies not associated with radiation (e.g. MRI).
Exposure	Undress patient for full visual assessment for injuries while avoiding or correcting hypothermia	Visual assessment for vaginal bleeding or leakage of fluid

[a]Glasgow Coma Scale assigns points for eye opening (spontaneous = 4, response to verbal command = 3, response to pain = 2, no eye opening = 1), best verbal response (oriented = 5, confused = 4, inappropriate words = 3, incomprehensible sounds = 2, no verbal response = 1), and best motor response (obeys commands = 6, localizing response to pain = 5, withdrawal response to pain = 4, flexion to pain = 3, extension to pain = 2, no motor response = 1) and is reported as aggregate score out of 15 possible points.
CT, computed tomography; FAST, Focused Assessment with Sonography for Trauma; IV, intravenous; MRI, magnetic resonance imaging; SpO_2, oxygen saturation.

not only a leading cause of death in trauma patients but a leading cause of preventable death in this setting. Although unconscious patients warrant intubation for airway protection the decision to intubate a patient who is able to respond to simple questions–demonstrating their ability to speak and sufficient mental status to protect the airway–can be more challenging. The presence of head or neck injuries, penetrating chest trauma, as well as comorbid hemodynamic instability may motivate elective intubation even in the presence of an otherwise reassuring assessment in anticipation of the clinical course.

The *physiologic changes of pregnancy characterized by airway edema and increased aspiration risk* due to progesterone-mediated lower esophageal sphincter relaxation challenge intubation. The anticipated "difficult airway" coupled with reduced functional residual capacity predisposing to hypoxemia during apneic ventilation *lowers the threshold for intubation in the setting of pregnancy.* Per Advanced Cardiac Life Support (ACLS) Guidelines this intubation should be performed by the most experienced operator, which would suggest involvement of anesthesiologists experienced with obstetrics as a part of the trauma team.

Assessment of breathing characterized by both oxygenation and ventilation may happen in parallel with airway assessment but should become the priority once the airway is secured or the exam provides enough reassurance to determine intubation is not warranted. In addition to routine vital signs assessing for hypoxemia or tachypnea physical examination with or without supplemental diagnostic imaging (e.g. chest radiography [CXR] or lung

ultrasound) provides additional information. Screening chest imaging should be sought for any patient with hemodynamic instability, but needle decompression in cases of suspected tension pneumothorax (characterized by dyspnea, hypotension, and decreased breath sounds) should not be delayed for diagnostic studies. Obstetric care providers can aid in management by *providing reassurance about the safety of CXR and fetal benefits of maternal stabilization in this setting.* Additional physiologic and anatomic modifications in the setting of pregnancy include the need to provide supplemental oxygen to maintain saturations at 95% and guidelines supporting *placement of thoracostomy tube 1 to 2 intercostal spaces higher* than the standard approach. Although assessment of arterial blood gas is not a part of the primary survey, reminding the trauma team of the *compensated respiratory alkalosis of pregnancy* may be another relevant contribution.

Management of circulation is characterized by assessment of pulses, establishing adequate intravenous (IV) access, and management of hemorrhage. The Focused Assessment with Sonography for Trauma (FAST) exam employs standardized views with point of care ultrasound to assess for intraperitoneal and pericardial blood and is a critical component of the primary survey in the hemodynamically unstable patient (Figure 36.1). Though not all shock is hemorrhagic in nature it is the most likely etiology of hypotension in the setting of both trauma and obstetrics. The obstetric care provider can offer critical insights into diagnostic considerations and management approach at this juncture. Reminding the team of the

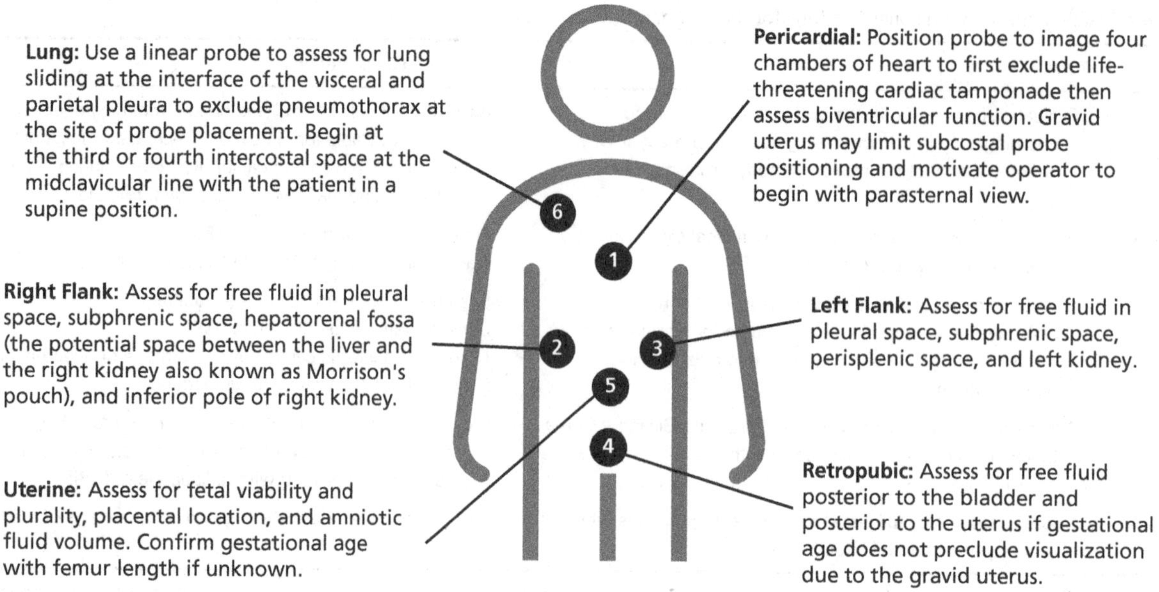

Lung: Use a linear probe to assess for lung sliding at the interface of the visceral and parietal pleura to exclude pneumothorax at the site of probe placement. Begin at the third or fourth intercostal space at the midclavicular line with the patient in a supine position.

Right Flank: Assess for free fluid in pleural space, subphrenic space, hepatorenal fossa (the potential space between the liver and the right kidney also known as Morrison's pouch), and inferior pole of right kidney.

Uterine: Assess for fetal viability and plurality, placental location, and amniotic fluid volume. Confirm gestational age with femur length if unknown.

Pericardial: Position probe to image four chambers of heart to first exclude life-threatening cardiac tamponade then assess biventricular function. Gravid uterus may limit subcostal probe positioning and motivate operator to begin with parasternal view.

Left Flank: Assess for free fluid in pleural space, subphrenic space, perisplenic space, and left kidney.

Retropubic: Assess for free fluid posterior to the bladder and posterior to the uterus if gestational age does not preclude visualization due to the gravid uterus.

Figure 36.1 Focused assessment with sonography for trauma.

impact of aortocaval compression on hemodynamics and supporting manual left uterine displacement to optimize cardiac output is essential. The impact of the gravid uterus on return of blood to the heart also informs the need to *ensure IV placement is above the diaphragm* as emphasized in guidelines for the management of cardiac arrest in pregnancy.

Assessment of fetal heart rate (FHR) is considered a vital sign for obstetric patients but, like measurement of blood pressure, should not interfere with stabilization of airway and breathing. A primary assessment of FHR will often occur during circulatory assessment during the FAST exam. FAST may be delayed until the secondary survey for hemodynamically stable patients, but logic would suggest a sonographic assessment of FHR should occur at this juncture. Clinical guidelines and principles emphasize that *fetal assessment should not interfere with maternal stabilization* but assessment for the presence or absence of a normal FHR serves two roles. First, it confirms the presence of a living fetus. Although the priority should be placed on maternal well-being at this stage diagnosis of a demise may affect clinical management, provide anticipatory guidance for the patient's support network, and provide psychological and medicolegal protection for the clinical team. Second, it can lend insights into the impact of maternal hemodynamics on fetal perfusion–a particularly relevant concern in settings where permissive hypotension is being considered.

Assessment of disability occurs next and is commonly communicated using the Glasgow Coma Scale (GCS) score through assessment of eye opening, verbal response, and motor response (Table 36.1). GCS may be confounded in the setting of administration of sedatives or intoxication and does not predict long-term neurocognitive

outcomes, but it does standardize communication about neurologic status and can be easily reproduced over time. Assessment for spinal cord injury can occur at this juncture though all patients with potential for spinal cord injury should receive appropriate immobilization of the spine. Obstetric care providers can offer reassurance about the *safety of neuroimaging* in pregnancy to ensure indicated diagnostic studies that require ionizing radiation such as computed tomography (CT) are not delayed in favor of magnetic resonance imaging (MRI). For patients who are "found down" without a witnessed insult the obstetric care provider can offer insights to broaden the differential diagnosis to ensure obstetric diagnoses like eclampsia are not missed.

The final component of the primary survey is exposure and environmental control, which includes completely undressing the patient to examine for signs of injury while avoiding and/or correcting hypothermia. A visual assessment for the presence of amniotic fluid or vaginal bleeding is a critical part of this step and may provide insights into injury burden though sterile vaginal examination is typically deferred until the secondary survey and after assessment of the stability of the bony pelvis.

Secondary survey

Hemodynamically unstable trauma patients may require advanced imaging or procedural intervention before a secondary survey can be performed. Resuscitation or intervention to address issues identified in the primary survey is a critical intervening step between the primary and secondary survey. If a patient is deemed stable after the assessment and interventions of the primary survey, the secondary survey focuses on obtaining an adequate history, performing an efficient physical examination, and executing targeted diagnostic studies.

The history should be detailed enough to provide safe care and provide insights into the mechanism of injury and may be obtained from the patient, support persons, or emergency personnel from the scene. The mnemonic AMPLE is often used as a cognitive aid focusing on Allergies, Medications, Past illnesses and surgery, Last oral intake, and Events leading to injury. The obstetric care provider can work to obtain relevant obstetric history in a parallel fashion. The word CODE has been proposed as a cognitive aid for the key components of this history representing Complications of pregnancy, Obstetric history and provider, Dating of pregnancy, and Event details.

Establishing reliable dating is of the utmost importance but may be challenged in the confused or intubated patient. In these settings history can be supplemented by physical exam as a part of the secondary survey. Measurement of fundal height may provide a gross estimate of weeks of pregnancy with the gravid uterus at the level of the umbilicus indicating 20 weeks of pregnancy in most settings. Fundal height may be unreliable in the setting of obesity, multiple gestation, or uterine pathology (e.g. fibroids) but can provide a gross estimate while assessing the potential for the gravid uterus to provide aortocaval compression and impact hemodynamics. Although traditional biometry may provide an estimate of gestational age the time required to perform this assessment may detract from other indicated care. In the absence of reliable dating a femur length at or above 4 cm is often considered consistent with a viable gestational age (i.e. 22 to 24 weeks of pregnancy) and can be easily obtained during the routine FAST exam while assessing for free fluid in the pelvis.

Table 36.2 outlines the components of the secondary survey to aid the obstetric care provider in sharing the same mental model with other members of the trauma team. Additional components of the secondary survey relevant to the obstetric care provider include abdominal exam and vaginal exam. Abdominal exam should focus on uterine tone and presence of contractions or palpation of abnormalities to the uterine contour that may portend obstetric injury. Vaginal examination should focus on evaluation for evidence of amniotic fluid, bleeding, and labor. Sonographic evaluation for placental location (to exclude the presence of placenta previa), evidence of placental abruption (acknowledging the low sensitivity of ultrasound for this finding), amniotic fluid volume, and cervical length can be helpful adjuncts after initial stabilization.

Table 36.2 Components of secondary survey with associated diagnostic testing and management consideration

Area of exam	Components of exam	Role of imaging
Head and face	Assess for lacerations, skeletal deformities, and damage to anatomy or function of eye	Obtain CT for eye injury or facial fractures with low threshold for CTA
Neck	Assume cervical spine injury in all patients with blunt trauma	Use clinical decision tools to dictate need for radiography
Chest	Inspect skin for changes to suggest high-risk mechanism that may increase risk of blunt cardiac injury or aortic injury; palpate thoracic skeleton assessing for tenderness or crepitus; consider lung ultrasound if not performed in primary survey	Lung US superior to CXR for detection of pneumothorax; consider chest CT if abnormal findings. ECG; consideration of CTA or TEE for aortic injury
Abdomen	Perform FAST exam if not done during the primary survey; inspection and palpation may provide insights but are unreliable in pregnancy due to anatomic changes	CT or CTA of abdomen and pelvis should not be avoided or exchanged for MRI in cases with positive FAST exam or hemodynamic instability
Genitourinary	Vaginal examination to assess for injury, bleeding, leakage of amniotic fluid, or labor	Bleeding and contractions should prompt fetal monitoring to evaluate for placental abruption
Musculoskeletal	Inspect and palpate all long bones for evidence of injury; evaluate for pulses to assess neurovascular status; palpate pelvis for stability prior to pelvic examination	Evaluate any areas of tenderness with targeted plain radiograph; monitor pulses in injured extremities for evidence of compartment syndrome
Neurologic	Serial examination for evolving injury including reassessment of GCS	Low threshold for noncontrast head CT to exclude neurologic injury if any clinical concern for preeclampsia and to assess for safety of neuraxial analgesia
Skin	Examine entirety of skin for lacerations, ecchymosis, or other lesions	Consider imaging fetus with radiography if concern for penetrating trauma

CT, computed tomography; CTA, computed tomography with angiography; CXR, chest X-ray or radiography; ECG, electrocardiogram; FAST, Focused Assessment with Sonography for Trauma; GCS, Glasgow Coma Scale; MRI, magnetic resonance imaging; TEE, transesophageal echocardiogram; US, ultrasound.

Diagnostic studies

Basic laboratory studies for every trauma patient include a type and screen, a pregnancy test, and a fingerstick glucose with additional studies dictated by the clinical scenario. For example, patients with blunt thoracic injury warrant an electrocardiogram as well as assessment of troponin levels as the cardiac biomarker not altered in pregnancy. A basic or comprehensive metabolic panel is low yield in most trauma patients with normal fingerstick blood glucose levels. Assessment of renal and hepatic function as well as electrolytes may be warranted in obstetrics if the clinical history includes altered mental status or raises concern for diagnoses like preeclampsia.

In the absence of anticoagulation the assessment of the complete blood count and coagulation studies are likely to be low yield during stabilization as lab results are likely to lag the dynamic clinical scenario. That said, baseline coagulation studies including fibrinogen can be helpful to evaluate for contributing obstetric diagnoses and assess baseline coagulation status for monitoring for placental abruption. Obstetric care providers should remind members of the trauma team about the anticipated elevation of fibrinogen in pregnancy and potential obstetric causes for consumptive coagulopathy such as placental abruption. Intoxicated patients or those with altered mental status warrant an alcohol level or toxicology screen. These results are unlikely to dictate care in the moment but can be helpful to better understand contributing factors and ongoing needs.

Most obstetric care providers will be familiar with existing protocols to monitor for evolving placental *abruption* as a consequence of trauma, which consist of an *initial 4 hours of continuous electronic FHR monitoring and tocometry.* Any clinical concern for abruption based on hemodynamics (hemorrhagic shock or abnormal fetal heart rate in fetus), symptoms (including abdominal pain, vaginal bleeding, or skin changes signifying significant abdominal trauma), or diagnostic studies (ultrasound, abnormal coagulation profile, or the presence of 1 or more contractions every 10 minute on initial monitoring) will warrant an additional 24 hours of continuous monitoring to monitor for changes that may signify evolving placental abruption. A type and screen will be sent on every trauma patient but is of paramount importance in the obstetric patient to ensure empiric administration of rho-D immune globulin for the prevention of alloimmunization. For patients with Rh-negative blood type a Kleihauer-Betke should be sent to determine dosing requirements but not as an indicator of the presence or absence of abruption.

Cardiac arrest in pregnancy

Cardiac arrest in pregnancy is the extreme example of a high-acuity low-frequency event with population-level prevalence estimated at 1 in 25,000. With a prevalence of 1 in 12,000 delivery hospitalizations an obstetric care provider could practice their entire career without experiencing this event. However, the 60% survival after in-hospital cardiac in this setting (compared to roughly 5–20% survival in the overall population) underscores the potential to meaningfully impact outcomes in this uniquely resilient group of patients. The most common etiologies of the arrests during delivery hospitalization are obstetric including hemorrhage, and amniotic fluid embolism, as well as sepsis suggesting that the obstetric care provider may be tasked with managing the initial critical minutes of in-hospital cardiac arrest until further support is available. This protocol therefore focuses on key principles in the management of the first 5 minutes of cardiac arrest in pregnancy through the lens of obstetrics.

Circulation

The only two factors demonstrated to improve survival in the setting of cardiac arrest are high-quality chest compressions and short interval between arrest and defibrillation. Their impact on survival places them at the top of all basic and advanced cardiac life support (BLS and ACLS, respectively) guidelines making them of critical importance for the obstetric care provider tasked with responding to a cardiac arrest. Obstetric care providers should also note three key modifications to the provision of BLS and ACLS in the setting of pregnancy as outlined next and in Figure 36.2.

High-quality chest compressions are those occurring at a rate of 100–120 beats per minute compressing to a depth of 2 cm and allowing adequate time for chest recoil. The physiologic importance of these characteristics can be understood by the need to perfuse the cerebral and coronary vasculature–the latter of which happens in diastole. Unlike prior guidelines specific to cardiac arrest in pregnancy Contemporary recommendations recommend *providing manual left uterine displacement* (LUD) by a dedicated member of the resuscitation team. This is a change from earlier guidelines that suggested tilting the backboard to relieve aortocaval compression, a technique that has fallen out of favor due to its interference with high-quality chest compressions. LUD can be provided manually by pushing or pulling the gravid uterus from the right to the left to ensure adequate venous return and relieve the hemodynamic impact of aortocaval compression. Avoiding interruptions in chest compressions is highlighted in all guidelines with interruption for defibrillation as the only notable exception in the case of shockable rhythms.

There are no modifications to defibrillation for so-called shockable rhythms–ventricular fibrillation (VF) or pulseless ventricular tachycardia (VT)–in the setting of pregnancy. ACLS guidelines recommend use of the biphasic defibrillator at initial dose of energy recommended by the manufacturer ranging between 120 and

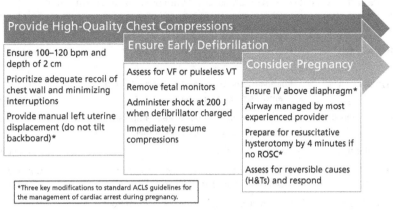

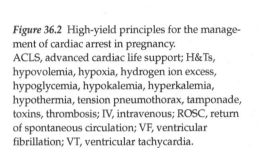

Figure 36.2 High-yield principles for the management of cardiac arrest in pregnancy.
ACLS, advanced cardiac life support; H&Ts, hypovolemia, hypoxia, hydrogen ion excess, hypoglycemia, hypokalemia, hyperkalemia, hypothermia, tension pneumothorax, tamponade, toxins, thrombosis; IV, intravenous; ROSC, return of spontaneous circulation; VF, ventricular fibrillation; VT, ventricular tachycardia.

200 joules (J). If this is not known to the operator delivery of a shock at maximal energy of 200 J is a safe and reasonable strategy. Placement of defibrillator pads should not be modified for pregnancy. However, evidence suggesting that change in position from anterior-lateral to anterior-posterior positioning may increase the rate of successful cardioversion in VF and VT coupled with the potential of the gravid uterus to interfere with placement may motivate some providers to try this approach if initial defibrillation fails to achieve return of spontaneous circulation (ROSC). Removal of FHR monitors is recommended at the onset of cardiac arrest to both avoid fetal concerns detracting from maternal resuscitation and to facilitate rapid defibrillation by removal of extraneous material.

Most medications previously recommended in the setting of cardiac arrest have little evidentiary support and have been removed from guidelines over time. Epinephrine remains a key component of ACLS algorithms that recommend administration of 1 mg of epinephrine as soon as feasible but certainly by 3–5 minutes of the resuscitation. A second key modification of the ACLS algorithm in the setting of pregnancy is the imperative to *ensure IV access above the diaphragm to ensure aortocaval compression does not interfere with circulation of medications to the heart.* Additional medication administration will be dictated by the etiology of the arrest—a particularly salient consideration in the setting of pulseless electrical activity (PEA) arrest or asystole. The differential diagnosis for reversible causes of PEA arrest with considerations for management and pregnancy is outlined in Table 36.3.

The third key change recommends *pursuing delivery at 4 minutes of cardiac arrest if unable to achieve ROSC.* For most patients this will be via a hysterotomy or cesarean delivery. It is prudent to remember that this resuscitative hysterotomy is for *maternal* benefit to decrease hemodynamic demands and increase preload with hopes of achieving ROSC. Although this may also optimize fetal outcome depending on the gestational age of the fetus,

the recommendation to pursue this intervention beginning at 20 weeks–well before the limits of viability–emphasize its role in maternal resuscitation.

Airway and breathing

As opposed to ATLS guidelines that prioritize airway, *circulation* takes the priority spot in evidence-based ACLS guidelines. This reflects the importance of circulatory support in optimizing outcomes as well as the lack of benefit from advanced airway in available trials. Current guidelines recommend provision of either bag mask ventilation (BVM) supported by an oropharyngeal or nasopharyngeal airway or blindly inserted extraglottic airway (e.g. laryngeal mask airway or laryngeal tube) with the latter offering additional protection against aspiration. For patients whose airway is managed with BVM the recommendation is for synchronized ventilation at a ratio of 2 breaths for every 30 chest compressions (i.e. 30:2) to ensure adequate delivery of ventilation. For those with an extraglottic airway or endotracheal tube (ETT) delivery of 6 to 10 nonsynchronized breaths per minute with tidal volume of 600 ccs is recommended in ACLS guidelines. *Avoiding hyperventilation is of critical importance to ensure excess intrathoracic pressure does not impact venous return and cardiac output.*

A few caveats about these guidelines and the evidence informing them must be noted when considered through the lens of pregnancy. The majority of randomized controlled trial data failing to show benefit with advanced airway placement were all in the prehospital environment limiting their application to in-hospital cardiac arrest–particularly in the setting of pregnancy. *Pregnancy-specific guidelines support placement of an advanced airway by the most experienced provider, which reflects some of the unique considerations in the gravid airway.* As noted, edematous tissue, the decreased functional residual capacity, and the progesterone-mediated decrease in lower esophageal tone both challenge safe intubation and increase the risk of aspiration, respectively. These physiologic realities

Table 36.3 Reversible causes of cardiac arrest with pulseless electrical activity

Cause[a]	Obstetric scenarios	Management considerations
Hypovolemia	Hemorrhage, sepsis, severe dehydration	Provide crystalloid while awaiting blood products for balanced transfusion; prioritize source control
Hypoxia	Pulmonary edema, aspiration, amniotic fluid embolism, cardiomyopathy	Prioritize airway with high PEEP >10 Early TTE and consider vasopressors +/- MCS in cardiac dysfunction
Hypo/hyperkalemia	Acute kidney injury (due to preeclampsia, hemorrhage, sepsis); consider magnesium toxicity	Administer calcium chloride 1 g in suspected magnesium toxicity
Hypothermia	Trauma, intraoperative	Hypothermia associated with fetal bradycardia and DIC
H+ Ions	Sepsis, ketosis due to diabetes or starvation, profound hypovolemic shock	Consider sodium bicarbonate therapy (50–100 mEq IV) in the setting of acidosis (pH <7.2)
Thrombosis	Pulmonary embolism, amniotic fluid embolism, coronary artery disease	Use TTE to narrow differential and direct interventions and support Early cardiothoracic surgery consult
Toxins	Total spinal anesthesia, anaphylaxis, local anesthetic toxicity, opioid overdose	Targeted antidote such as intralipid for local toxicity, naloxone for opioid, or epinephrine for anaphylaxis
Tension pneumothorax	Trauma, connective tissue disease	Rare causes but easily excluded with point of care ultrasound
Tamponade	Trauma, pericarditis	

DIC, disseminated intravascular coagulation; IV, intravenous; MCS, mechanical circulatory support; PEEP, positive end expiratory pressure; TTE, transthoracic echocardiogram.

[a]Additional mnemonic proposed for pregnancy-specific cause of cardiac arrest with ABCDEFGH corresponding to **A**nesthetic complications, **B**leeding, **C**ardiovascular, **D**rugs, **E**mbolic, **F**ever, **G**eneral nonobstetric, **H**ypertension.

coupled with the knowledge that intubation may be on the pathway to achieving ROSC in cases of hypoxia-mediated PEA arrest inform this approach.

Postarrest care

The care of all patients who achieve ROSC after cardiac arrest should focus on understanding and addressing the underlying cause for the arrest and prevention of long-term sequelae–the most concerning of which are neurologic sequelae due to anoxia. The role of therapeutic hypothermia for prevention of adverse neurologic sequelae has been replaced by a concept of targeted temperature management using adjunctive therapies to maintain normothermia (<36 ° Celsius) as opposed to the hypothermia previously endorsed. Pregnancy is not a contraindication to these therapies *though obstetric care providers should anticipate associated fetal bradycardia with lower maternal temperatures and interpret this as a physiologic vagal response and not a sign of fetal distress.*

Stabilization and resuscitation

The emergent care of all patients often demands that evaluation and management be performed in parallel and the patient's response to an intervention can offer insights into the underlying etiology. The concept of using an intervention for both therapy and diagnosis is pervasive throughout acute care settings but is most salient when considering the management of shock. Shock is divided

into four subtypes–hypovolemic, cardiogenic, distributive, and obstructive–but these rarely exist in isolation. Table 36.4 outlines physiologic parameters associated with each including those obtained with invasive hemodynamic monitoring and point of care ultrasound. Although these offer a conceptual framework, the rarity of invasive hemodynamic monitoring in obstetrics coupled with the overlap of shock states makes this less helpful in a clinical setting.

A more relevant way to think of shock is to integrate clinical history with an assessment of fluid responsiveness. Evidence-based guidelines emphasize initial use of crystalloids in bolus form with evaluation of the response to dictate the next interventions. From a practical standpoint administration of a 500 ml bolus of a balanced crystalloid and evaluation of subsequent hemodynamics can offer insights. Patients with hemorrhagic or distributive shock will be expected to be fluid responsive whereas fluids in the setting of cardiogenic shock may worsen hypotension. Patients with obstructive shock due to tamponade or tension pneumothorax are unlikely to respond to volume due to mechanical barriers to venous return to the heart. These conditions are rare in obstetrics in the absence of risk factors such as trauma or cardiothoracic surgery. The aforementioned ATLS guidelines and those related to hemodynamic instability after cardiac surgery target the early diagnosis and management of these life-threatening conditions. Therefore, subsequent discussion of fluid responsiveness will emphasize the stabilization of patients with hemorrhagic shock and septic shock as the hallmark

Table 36.4 Anticipated hemodynamic parameters according to type of shock

Parameter	Hypovolemic	Distributive	Cardiogenic
Systolic blood pressure	Low	Varies	Low
Diastolic blood pressure	High	Low	High
Pulse pressure	Narrow	Wide	Narrow
Straight leg raise	BP increases	BP increases	BP decreases
Inferior vena cava diameter[a]	Collapsible (<2 cm)	Collapsible (<2 cm)	Plethoric (>2 cm)
Left ventriclular filling[a]	Low volume	Low volume	Normal volume
Left ventricular contractility[a]	Normal	Hyperdynamic	Low
Stroke volume variation[b]	High	Varies	Low
Central venous pressure[b]	Low	Varies	High
Wedge pressure[b]	High	Low	High
Systemic vascular resistance[b]	Normal	Normal/high	Low
Mixed venous oxygen[b]	Normal	Normal/high	Low
Cardiac output[b]	Normal	High	Low

[a] Parameters obtained through point-of-care ultrasound.

[b] Parameters obtained through invasive hemodynamic monitoring including arterial line (stroke volume variation), central venous catheter (central venous pressure), or pulmonary artery catheter (wedge pressure, systemic vascular resistance, mixed venous oxygen, cardiac output).

BP, blood pressure.

subtypes of hypovolemic and distributive shock encountered in obstetrics. In many ways the final common pathway for all types of shock is cardiogenic shock. A complete discussion of the management of cardiogenic shock is beyond the scope of this protocol but clinical pearls in the use of vasopressors can also be used in combination with diuresis to stabilize those with concern for cardiogenic shock.

Principles of resuscitation in hemorrhagic shock

Resuscitation of the bleeding patient with crystalloids should be restricted to 500 ml boluses targeting a systolic blood pressure of 90 mmHg while awaiting arrival of blood products. The concept of permissive hypotension – in which a systolic blood pressure of 70 is targeted – is one approach employed in trauma patients to minimize blood product requirements and iatrogenic volume overload. This strategy also provides the theoretical benefit of reducing ongoing bleeding by lowering perfusion pressure to the bleeding organ. The presence of comorbid neurologic injury including spinal injury are contraindications to this approach in trauma patients and has not been evaluated in the setting of pregnancy in a rigorous manner. That said, *this strategy should be abandoned in the pregnant patient with an abnormal fetal heart rate tracing with the assumption that permissive hypotension is failing to provide adequate placental perfusion.*

Contemporary guidelines emphasize the importance of having a massive transfusion protocol for the management of obstetric hemorrhage. In cases of hemorrhagic shock with ongoing bleeding a balanced transfusion strategy emphasizing repletion of each of the components of whole blood (assuming whole blood transfusion products are not available) should be prioritized. The key components of this approach including the role of tranexamic acid and other adjuncts are outlined in Table 36.5. In the presence of active bleeding hemodynamics, as opposed to labs, should guide resuscitation. Once bleeding has been addressed attention should then shift to optimizing the approach to resuscitation.

Although point-of-care ultrasound was designed to narrow the differential and determine next steps in management, it can also provide tremendous insights into the need for resuscitation. Point of care ultrasound assessment of inferior vena cava diameter or left ventricular filling may help provide additional insights into need for additional transfusion (Table 36.4). In the absence of ongoing bleeding or hemodynamic stability evidence-based guidelines suggest targeting a hemoglobin of 7 g/dL based on evidence demonstrating a mortality benefit with a more restrictive transfusion strategy when compared to targeting the historic standard of 10 g/dL. Point-of-care viscoelastic coagulation studies such as rotational thromboelastometry or thromboelastography can offer insights into clot formation, stability, and fibrinolysis that may provide faster feedback on transfusion needs than traditional clotting studies. Regardless of the parameters used to guide ongoing resuscitation the point of each of these tools is to target euvolemia with the goal of providing adequate end-organ perfusion while avoiding iatrogenic complications such as transfusion-associated lung injury or transfusion-associated circulatory overload.

Principles of resuscitation in septic shock

Sepsis is the most commonly encountered cause of distributive shock in pregnancy with anaphylaxis and hypotension associated with neuraxial analgesia as other notable etiologies. Each may be exacerbated by hypovolemia but share the underlying physiology of a decrease in systemic vascular resistance leading to inadequate preload

Table 36.5 Therapies for resuscitation in hemorrhagic shock

Therapy	Indication	Hemodynamic target	Laboratory target
Red blood cells	Increase oxygen carrying capacity and intravascular volume	Systolic blood pressure = 90 mmHg in active bleeding	Hgb 7 g/dL once bleeding controlled (1 unit increases Hgb by 1 g/dL)
Fresh frozen plasma	Increase clotting factors, fibrinogen, and volume	Transfuse 1 unit for every 1 unit RBCs in active bleeding	Target INR <1.5, normal R[a] or CT[b], or absence of clinical bleeding
Platelets	Replace platelets in active bleeding or to facilitate neuraxial analgesia	Transfuse 1 unit[c] for every 5-6 units RBCs in active bleeding	Target >50K in settings of recent bleeding, >70K for neuraxial analgesia, or normal MA[a] or MCF[b]
Cyroprecipitate	Replace fibrinogen; factors V, VIII, XIII; and von Willebrand factor	Transfuse 1 unit (pooled from donors) for every 4–6 units RBCs	Target fibrinogen >150, normal K[a] or CFT[b], and normal R[a] or CT[b]
Fibrinogen concentrate	Replaces only fibrinogen with more reliable concentration (1 g/vial)	Transfuse 1 unit for every 4–6 units RBCs without additional volume of cryoprecipitate	Target fibrinogen >150, normal K[a] or CFT[b]; will not affect factor levels and associated labs
Tranexamic acid	Binds 5-lysine spot on plasminogen to inhibit conversion to plasmin and fibrin split products worsening coagulopathy	Dose 1 g for bleeding >500 ml; not typically given >3 hours after postpartum hemorrhage	Hyperfibrinolysis detected by thrombin time, LY30[a] or CL30[b]. Redosing not anticipated to impact labs.
Calcium	Replace calcium bound by citrate in blood products	Replete 1 g calcium gluconate/5 units RBCs transfused; empirically in hypotension	Empirically in refractory hypotension, target ionized calcium >1.1 mmol/L

[a] Parameters detected via thromboelastography (TEG). Reaction time (or R value) is time required to initiate fibrin clot. K value is time required to achieve a stable clot representing thrombin (required to convert fibrinogen into fibrin) and platelet interaction. Maximum amplitude captures strength of the clot and relies on platelet quantity and function (corresponds to maximum amplitude of curve on the thromboelastogram). LY30 captures the percentage of clot lysis 30 minutes after MA a higher number raising concern for hyperfibrinolysis as seen in disseminated intravascular coagulation.
[b] Parameters detected via rotational thromboelastometry (ROTEM) with corresponding value in TEG nomenclature in parentheses. Clotting time refers to time required to initiate fibrin clot (reaction time) with ability to distinguish between deficiencies in intrinsic and extrinsic pathway with ROTEM and not TEG. Clot formation time refers to the time required to achieve a stable clot in the assay representing thrombin and platelet interaction (K value). Maximum clot firmness captures strength of the clot (MA). CL30 captures the percentage of clot lysis 30 min after the MCF (LY30).
[c] Platelets typically available as 350–400 cc single-donor unit achieved via apheresis in contemporary transfusion medicine. Historically this same volume was achieved by pooling the platelets of six donors therefore achieving the ratio of 1:1:1 units of RBCs:FFP:platelets.
CL30, clot lysis 30 min after MCF; CFT, clot formation time; CT, clotting time; FFP, fresh frozen plasma; Hgb, hemoglobin; INR, international normalized ratio; K, K value; LY30, lysis at 30 min after MA; MA, maximum amplitude; MCF, maximum clot firmness; Plts, platelets; R, reaction time; RBC, red blood cells.

and cardiac output. The multidisciplinary Surviving Sepsis Campaign (SSC) Guidelines emphasize the need for early recognition of this life-threatening medical emergency including the recommendation of providing 30 ml/kg of IV crystalloid within the first 3 hours of the resuscitation. Other key management include the imperative to initiate broad spectrum antibiotics within an hour of presentation, obtain cultures prior to initiation of antibiotics, and to conduct active reevaluation of the resuscitation after the initial 3-hour period.

These guidelines emphasize the use of hemodynamics to guide the resuscitation and preference for dynamic variables (such as passive leg raise or stroke volume variation) as opposed to more traditional static variables (such as central venous pressure or mixed venous oxygen saturation). The need to assess lactic acid levels on admission and at 3-hour intervals until stabilization is a key feature of contemporary guidelines. Normalization of lactate is a target of the resuscitation in septic shock but evolving data suggest that ongoing administration of IV fluids may

not portend the mortality benefit suggested by older trials in support of early goal-directed therapy in septic shock.

Prioritization of vasopressors after the restoration of circulating volume is achieved addresses both distributive and cardiogenic shock encountered in sepsis. The SSC guidelines recommend the use of norepinephrine as the first-line vasopressor based on available evidence with addition of vasopressin if higher doses are required to achieve a mean arterial pressure of 65 mmHg. While there is often hesitation to initiate vasopressors outside of the intensive care unit (ICU) setting it is important to note that all vasopressors can be safely given for a short period of time through peripheral IV access. Though guidelines recommend placement of arterial catheter as an invasive monitor of blood pressure, the absence of this therapy or central venous access should not deter clinicians from pursuing the standard of care while awaiting transfer to a higher-acuity setting.

The physiology of distributive shock underscores the need to use vasopressors once euvolemia is achieved

Table 36.6 Vasopressors and inotropes for use in shock

Medication	Mechanism	Indication	Dosing strategy
Norepinephrine	Alpha agonist: ↑ SVR to ↑ BP and ↑ preload Beta-1: ↑ HR (minor effect)	First-line vasopressor in undifferentiated shock and preferred agent in septic shock (with vasopressin)	1–30 mcg/kg/min
Vasopressin	V1a agonist: Peripheral vasoconstriction (oxytocin analogue)	Addition to norepinephrine in septic shock; sedation-associated decrease in SVR as etiology of shock	0.03 units/min (add on after norepinephrine 5–10)
Epinephrine	Alpha and beta: ↑ SVR, ↑ HR, ↑ cardiac contractility	Anaphylaxis Cardiogenic Shock	1–10 mcg/kg/min
Dobutamine	Beta 1: ↑ cardiac contractility Some beta 2: ↓ SVR without impacting BP	Inodilator for cardiogenic shock to increase cardiac output and decrease afterload	1–5 mcg/kg/min
Milrinone	Phosphodiesterase III inhibitor: Increased calcium in heart, dilation of arteries and veins elsewhere	Increased contractility and improved relaxation; concern for arrhythmias, renal clearance	0.375–0.75 mcg/kg/min (typically with loading dose)

BP, blood pressure; HR, heart rate; SVR, systemic vascular resistance.

based not only on the decrease in systemic vascular resistance but recognizing the high likelihood of a cardiogenic contribution to hypotension. Comorbid cardiogenic shock should be presumed in common causes of distributive shock in obstetrics including septic shock and amniotic fluid embolism. Table 36.6 presents commonly used vasopressors and inotropes for use in cardiogenic and other shock states. Contemporary guidelines outlining evidence-based practice would suggest that patients with this degree of illness have improved outcomes when managed by a multidisciplinary team. Recognizing there is tremendous variability in the timely availability of additional personnel also suggest that the obstetric care provider should have some baseline familiarity with these medications, their indications, and an approach to initiating these therapies when indicated.

Optimizing resource use in emergency care

Contemporary medicine is best practiced as a team—especially in acute care settings. Although a multidisciplinary team-based approach to emergency care improves outcomes in many diseases, it is also not without challenges. Integrating the collective knowledge and experience of team members with different backgrounds and skill sets in low-frequency high-acuity events is subject to a number of cognitive and communication errors. Premature diagnosis, reliance on early negative results, downgrading findings, and succumbing to distractions or fixation are some notable cognitive pitfalls from the trauma literature that are relevant to the emergent care of the pregnant patient. The low frequency of adverse outcomes in the generally young and healthy obstetric population dictates that the least concerning diagnosis is most likely

the correct one. The remarkable physiologic reserve of most pregnant patients also suggests that probability-based decision making can delay the diagnosis of a life-threatening condition and cause the patient to suffer from increased morbidity or even death. This mathematical and physiologic reality coupled with the a priori distraction of the fetus underscore the importance of cognitive rigor and optimized team dynamics in emergent care in pregnancy.

Most contemporary obstetric care providers have some exposure to crisis resource management—the set of principles designed to optimize teamwork in dynamic high-acuity environments. These principles are reviewed in Figure 36.3 and, in many cases, highlight the practice patterns that have

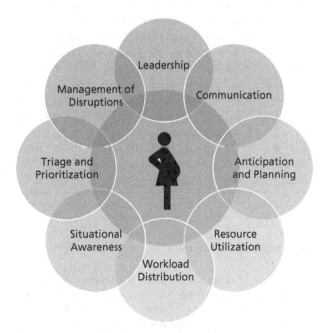

Figure 36.3 Principles of crisis resource management to optimize outcomes for the emergent care of the pregnant patient.

become standard of care in modern obstetrics. High-yield and specific applications of these principles relevant to emergent care of the pregnant patient include establishing a strategy for communication of obstetric concerns with the team leader with a dedicated obstetric team leader, prioritization of maternal status, adherence to existing guidelines including the reliance on checklists when available, contingency planning for delivery, and establishing criteria for notification of the obstetric care team after initial stabilization. The obstetric care provider may be as unfamiliar with trauma guidelines as the trauma surgeon is with pregnancy they still share a common understanding of these principles of effective teamwork. Ensuring that these principles are the foundation of the approach to care will optimize the timely risk assessment, targeted resuscitation, and downstream outcomes for the pregnant patient.

CASE PRESENTATION

A 22-year-old gravida 1, para 0 at 28 weeks of pregnancy is brought to the emergency department (ED) by ambulance after a relative found her unconscious in the floor of her bathroom and called 911. The transporting paramedics placed a cervical-spine collar and backboard and placed a 20-gauge antecubital IV to administer 2 liters of crystalloid for BP of 90/40 mmHg. The obstetrics team joins the trauma team with an ED physician as team leader and OB physician as checklist whisperer. The primary survey reveals a tachypneic patient responding slowly to questions, oxygen saturation 92% on room air improved to 96% on 4 liters nasal cannula, BP 80/40 mmHg and sinus tachycardia with heart rate (HR) 120 beats per minute (bpm) prompting an additional 1 L bolus of crystalloid, Glasgow Coma Score (GCS) 14 (3 eye, 5 verbal, 6 motor), temperature 102.0 degrees Fahrenheit, and no obvious injuries. Extended focused assessment with sonography for trauma (E-FAST) exam is negative and confirms singleton fetus with FHR of 170 bpm.

Secondary survey reveals a 3 cm hemostatic laceration over the left occipital bone, a closed long cervix, a localizing response to pain at the costovertebral angles bilaterally, and GCS 12 (E3, V4, M5). After a quick huddle the team elects to intubate the patient with concern for altered mental status and worsening tachypnea. An uncomplicated rapid sequence intubation is performed by an obstetric anesthesiologist using propofol and succinylcholine. The patient develops worsening hypotension unresponsive to left uterine displacement and passive leg raise and norephinephrine is started at 5 mcg/minute to achieve a mean arterial pressure of 65. A chest X-ray demonstrates appropriate placement of the endotracheal tube with pulmonary edema and bilateral pleural effusions not seen on initial E-FAST. The patient is taken for computed tomography of head with extension of imaging to include the chest, abdomen, and pelvis given shock and respiratory failure. The computed tomography scan reveals no acute intracranial findings, diffuse bilateral ground glass opacities of the lungs, and right perinephric stranding. Labs sent during the secondary survey are notable for white blood cell count 22,000 with 10% bands, potassium 5.1, creatinine 1.2, lactate 4.1, anion gap 22, fibrinogen 460, B+ blood type, urinalysis with nitrites. The fetus is placed on continuous monitoring notable for a baseline FHR in the 170s with minimal variability and recurrent late decelerations in response to irregular contractions every 12 to 15 minutes.

The next huddle highlights clinical concern for urosepsis and shock with comorbid altered mental status, acute respiratory distress syndrome, and acute kidney injury. The emergency room team takes responsibility for ensuring collection of blood and urine cultures, initiation of vancomycin, cefepime, and antenatal corticosteroids; placement of a urinary catheter, arterial line and additional IV access; requesting admission to the ICU; and optimizing volume status and ventilatory parameters. The obstetrics team dedicates a nurse to stay at the bedside for continuous fetal monitoring, notifies the neonatal ICU team of the admission in case delivery ensues, and updates the family. The debrief concludes by reviewing relevant hemodynamic targets through the lens of pregnancy physiology, exchanging contact information for relevant updates, and planning another update in 2 hours after repeat lactate and outstanding labs are reviewed.

Suggested readings

1. American College of Surgeons Committee on Trauma. Advanced trauma life support: student course manual. 10th ed. Chicago, IL: American College of Surgeons; 2018.
2. Levitov A, Frankel HL, Blaivas M, Kirkpatrick AW, Su E, Evans D, et al. Guidelines for the appropriate use of bedside general and cardiac ultrasonography in the evaluation of critically ill patients–part II: cardiac ultrasonography. Crit Care Med. 2016 Jun;44(6):1206–27.
3. Jeejeebhoy FM, Zelop CM, Lipman S, Carvalho B, Joglar J, Mhyre JM, et al.; American Heart Association Emergency Cardiovascular Care Committee, Council on Cardiopulmonary, Critical Care, Perioperative and Resuscitation, Council on Cardiovascular Diseases in the Young, and Council on Clinical Cardiology. Cardiac arrest in pregnancy: a scientific statement

from the American Heart Association. Circulation. 2015 Nov 3;132(18):1747–73.

4. Pacheco LD, Clark SL, Klassen M, Hankins GD. Amniotic fluid embolism: principles of early clinical management. Am J Obstet Gynecol. 2020 Jan;222(1):48–52.

5. Dankiewicz J, Cronberg T, Lilja G, Jakobsen JC, Levin H, Ullén S, et al.; TTM2 Trial Investigators. Hypothermia versus normothermia after out-of-hospital cardiac arrest. N Engl J Med. 2021 Jun 17;384(24):2283–94.

6. WOMAN Trial Collaborators. Effect of early tranexamic acid administration on mortality, hysterectomy, and other morbidities in women with post-partum haemorrhage (WOMAN): an international, randomised, double-blind, placebo-controlled trial. Lancet. 2017 May 27; 389(10084):2105–16.

7. Brill JB, Brenner M, Duchesne J, Roberts D, Ferrada P, Horer T, et al. The role of TEG and ROTEM in damage control resuscitation. Shock. 2021 Dec;56(1S):52–61.

8. Rhodes A, Evans LE, Alhazzani W, Levy MM, Antonelli M, Ferrer R, et al. Surviving Sepsis Campaign: international guidelines for management of sepsis and septic shock: 2016. Crit Care Med. 2017 Mar;45(3):486–552.

9. Brown RM, Semler MW. Fluid management in sepsis. J Intensive Care Med. 2019 May;34(5):364–73.

Chapter 37
Rh and Other Blood Group Alloimmunizations

Kenneth J. Moise Jr.

Department of Women's Health, Dell Medical School–University of Texas at Austin and the Comprehensive Fetal Care Center at Dell Children's Medical Center, Austin, TX, USA

The time-honored concept that the placenta is relatively impervious to cell trafficking between the fetus and its mother is no longer accepted. Flow cytometry can detect fetal red cell and red cell precursors in the maternal circulation in virtually all pregnancies [1].

In some patients, this exposure to fetal red cell antigens produces an antibody response that can be harmful to future offspring. The process is known as red cell alloimmunization (formerly isoimmunization). Active transplacental transport of these antibodies leads to their attachment to fetal red cells and sequestration in the fetal spleen. The quantity of the maternal antibody, the subclass of immunoglobulin G (IgG), and even the response of the fetal reticuloendothelial system have roles in the development of fetal anemia–a disease state known as hemolytic disease of the fetus and newborn (HDFN). In extreme cases, this severe anemia is associated with the accumulation of extracellular fluid in the form of ascites, pleural effusions, and scalp edema, a condition termed hydrops fetalis.

Prophylaxis

Prevention of maternal alloimmunization is almost uniformly successful in the case of exposure to the RhD or "rhesus" antigen. Prophylactic immunoglobulin (rhesus immunoglobulin; RhIg) is now available in the United States in the form of four commercial preparations–two can be administered only intramuscularly and two can be given either intramuscularly or intravenously. RhIg is not effective once the patient has developed endogenous antibodies. Immunoglobulins to prevent sensitization to other red cell antigens are not available.

All pregnant patients should undergo an antibody screen to red cell antigens at the first prenatal visit. In the case of a negative screen in the RhD-negative patient, further testing is unnecessary until 28 weeks gestation. Unless the patient's partner is documented to be RhD negative, a 300 μg dose of RhIg should be administered at 28 weeks. In addition, a repeat antibody screen should also be obtained at that time as recommended by the American College of Obstetricians and Gynecologists [2]. The intramuscular RhIg injection can be administered before the patient is sent for venipuncture because the short time interval between procedures will not affect the results of the antibody screen.

At delivery, a cord blood sample should be tested for neonatal RhD typing. If the neonate is determined to be RhD positive, a second dose of 300 μg RhIg should be administered to the mother within 72 hours of delivery. Approximately 0.1% of deliveries will be associated with a fetomaternal hemorrhage (FMH) in excess of 30 mL. More than the standard dose of RhIg will be required in these cases. Because risk factor assessment will identify only 50% of patients who have an excessive FMH at delivery, the routine screening of all postpartum women is now recommended. Typically, this involves a sheep rosette test that is read qualitatively as positive or negative. If negative, one vial of RhIg (300 μg) is given. If positive, the bleed is quantitated with a Kleihauer–Betke stain or fetal cell stain by flow cytometry. Blood bank consultation should then be undertaken to determine the number of doses of RhIg to administer.

The mechanism by which RhIg prevents sensitization is not well understood. Biochemical studies have revealed that the standard dose is insufficient to block all of the antigenic sites on the fetal red cells in the maternal circulation [3]. Therefore, if RhIg is inadvertently omitted after delivery, some protection has been proven with administration within 13 days. It should not be withheld as late as 28 days after delivery if the need arises [4].

Queenan's Management of High-Risk Pregnancy: An Evidence-Based Approach, Seventh Edition. Edited by Catherine Y. Spong and Charles J. Lockwood.

Table 37.1 Indications for administration of Rhesus immunoglobulin

Indication	Level of evidence
Spontaneous abortion	A
Elective abortion	A
Threatened abortion	C
Ectopic pregnancy	A
Hydatidiform mole	B
Genetic amniocentesis	A
Chorion villus biopsy	A
Fetal blood sampling	A
Placenta previa with bleeding	C
Suspected abruption	C
Intrauterine fetal demise	C
Blunt trauma to the abdomen (includes motor vehicle accidents)	C
At 28 wk gestation, unless father of fetus is RhD negative	A
Amniocentesis for fetal lung maturity	A
External cephalic version	C
Within 72 h of delivery of an RhD-positive infant	A
After administration of RhD-positive blood components	C

Level A evidence (good and consistent scientific evidence) [3].
Level B evidence (Fairly strong evidence. Based on evidence from case-control or cohort studies) [3]
Level C evidence (consensus and expert opinion) [3].
Reproduced with permission from Moise KJ. Red cell alloimmunization. In: Gabbe S, Niebyl J, J Simpson et al. editors. Obstetrics: normal and abnormal pregnancies. 5th ed. Philadelphia: Elsevier Saunders; 2007.

Additional indications for RhIg are listed in Table 37.1. Although a 50 μg dose of RhIg has been recommended for clinical situations up to 13 weeks gestation, most hospitals no longer stock this preparation, and the cost is comparable to the standard 300 μg dose.

Methods of surveillance

In recent years, techniques for fetal surveillance in cases of RhD alloimmunization have evolved to a more noninvasive approach. Many of these have led to a reduction in the rate of enhanced maternal immunization due to associated invasive procedures as well as a reduction in the rate of perinatal loss. Consultation with a maternal–fetal specialist should be considered in these cases to offer the patient the latest advancements in the field.

Antibody titer
In the first affected pregnancy, the maternal antibody titer continues to be used as the first level of surveillance in the United States. Once the maternal antibody screen indicates the presence of an anti-D antibody, a titer should be ordered. A critical titer has been defined as the value for a particular institution that is associated with a risk for fetal hydrops. An anti-D titer of 16 in the first affected pregnancy is often used. However, one must be cautious in the interpretation of antibody titers as they are crude estimates of the amount of circulating antibody.

In the past the indirect Coombs titer was performed as serial dilutions in glass tubes. Many labs today have changed to gel technology which may yield results that are two or more dilutions higher than expected with older tube technology [5].

Ultrasound
Ultrasound has revolutionized the surveillance of the anemic fetus. The peak systolic velocity in the middle cerebral artery (MCA-PSV) is now considered the standard of care for the detection of fetal anemia [6]. Color Doppler is used to locate the vessel and then pulsed Doppler is used to measure the peak systolic velocity just distal to its bifurcation from the internal carotid artery. Enhanced fetal cardiac output and a decrease in blood viscosity contribute to an increased blood flow velocity in fetal anemia. Because the general trend is for the MCA-PSV value to increase with advancing gestational age, results are converted to multiples of the median (MoM), much like maternal serum α-fetoprotein values. The actual value can be plotted on standard curves (Table 37.2) or entered into a website that will calculate the MoM value (www.perinatology.com). A value greater than 1.5 MoM is suggestive of moderate-to-severe fetal anemia and requires further investigation through direct ultrasound-guided fetal blood sampling (cordocentesis).

MCA-PSV measurements are usually initiated at 18 weeks gestation and should be repeated every

Table 37.2 Peak systolic middle cerebral artery values

Weeks of gestation	1.29 MoM (mild anemia) (cm/s)	1.50 MoM (moderate–severe anemia) (cm/s)
18	29.9	34.8
20	32.8	38.2
22	36.0	41.9
24	39.5	46.0
26	43.3	50.4
28	47.6	55.4
30	52.2	60.7
32	57.3	66.6
34	62.9	73.1
36	69.0	80.2
38	75.7	88.0
40	83.0	96.6

MoM, multiples of the mean.
Adapted from [6].

1–2 weeks as the clinical situation warrants. In some situations where there has been an early onset of fetal anemia in a previous pregnancy, MCA-PSV can be started as early as 15 weeks gestation (calculator: https://portal.medicinafetalbarcelona.org/calc/; anemia). After 35 weeks gestation, the false-positive rate for the prediction of fetal anemia is increased probably due to fetal heart rate accelerations. Serial MCA-PSV measurements result in an 80% reduction in the need for invasive diagnostic procedures such as amniocentesis and cordocentesis.

Fetal blood typing through DNA analysis

Paternal testing should begin early in the evaluation process of the alloimmunized patient. An RhD-negative result with assurance of paternity requires no further maternal testing after proper documentation of the paternity discussion with the patient in the medical record. Because more than 50% of RhD-positive partners are heterozygous, testing using DNA analysis can be undertaken to determine zygosity. Serologic testing can be used to detect paternal zygosity in the case of other Rh antibodies (C, c, E, e) or other irregular anti-red cell antibodies such as Kell in consultation with the blood bank.

An exciting new development in fetal RhD typing involves the isolation of free fetal DNA in maternal serum [7]. In many European countries, this technique has replaced amniocentesis for fetal typing in the case of a heterozygous paternal phenotype. A free fetal DNA test for RHD, RHE, RHc, Kell (K1) and FyA is now commercially available in the United States.

Overall clinical management

First sensitized pregnancy

• Follow maternal titers every 4 weeks up to 24 weeks gestation; repeat every 2 weeks thereafter.
• Assess paternal zygosity.
• Once a critical maternal titer value (usually 16) is reached in cases of a heterozygous paternal phenotype, perform free fetal DNA as early as 10–12 weeks gestation to determine the fetal genotype status.
• If an antigen-negative fetus is found, no further testing is warranted.
• If a there is homozygous paternal phenotype or antigen-positive fetus by DNA analysis, begin serial MCA-PSVs as early as 18 weeks gestation. Repeat weekly three times and assess trend. If not rising rapidly, consider MCA-PSVs every 2 weeks.

• If the MCA-PSV is >1.5 MoM, perform cordocentesis with blood readied for intrauterine transfusion (IUT; discussed later) for a fetal hematocrit of <30%.
• Begin weekly antenatal testing at 32 weeks with biophysical profiles or nonstress testing.
• If repeat the MCA-PSV remains <1.5 MoM, consider induction by 38 weeks gestation.
• In the case of an elevated MCA-PSV after 35 weeks gestation, consider repeating the study the following day. If the value remains elevated, induction of labor should be undertaken.
• If normal MCA-PSV values, induce by 38 weeks gestation.

Previous severely affected fetus or infant (previous child requiring intrauterine or neonatal transfusion)

• Maternal titers are less useful in predicting the onset of fetal anemia after the first affected gestation. However, an initial titer should still be obtained to see if the patient is a candidate for immunomodulation (see subsequent section).
• In cases of a heterozygous paternal phenotype, analyze free fetal DNA from maternal blood to determine the fetal genotype. If an antigen-negative fetus is found, no further testing is warranted.
• If fetus is antigen positive, begin MCA-PSV assessments at 15–18 weeks gestation. Repeat every week.
• When an MCA-PSV is >1.5 MoM is noted, perform cordocentesis with blood readied for IUT for fetal hematocrit of <30%. Prior to 18–20 weeks gestation, intravascular intrauterine transfusions (IVT) may not be technically possible and are often associated with a higher rate of perinatal loss. Prior to this gestational age, intraperitoneal transfusions have been employed as a bridging therapy until an IVT can be undertaken (see subsequent section).
• If the MCA-PSV does not become elevated, follow the same protocol after 35 weeks as for the first affected pregnancy (discussed previously).

Intrauterine transfusion

First introduced in 1963 by Sir William Liley, IUT of red cells has withstood the test of time as the most successful fetal therapy [8]. Initially the peritoneal cavity was used as the site of transfusion; however, hydropic fetuses were found to exhibit poor absorption of transfused red blood cells. Today the direct IVT of donor red blood cells into the fetal umbilical vein at its placental insertion is the most common method of IUT. The red cells prepared for transfusion should be negative for the offending red cell antigen, cytomegalovirus negative, irradiated with 25 Gy to prevent graft-vs.-host reaction and concentrated to a final hematocrit of 75–85%. Online calculators are available to determine the volume of blood to infuse (https://www.mdcalc.com/intrauterine-rbc-transfusion-dosage). Variations in the standard IVT approach include the inclusion of additional transfused cells into the peritoneal cavity at the same setting to prolong the interval between procedures [9]. Additionally, the intrahepatic portion of the umbilical vein is used as the access site for IVT in many centers in Europe [10].

Limited visualization of the umbilical cord insertion precludes successful IVT prior to 18 weeks gestation. However, in cases of severe HDFN in the early second trimester, serial intraperitoneal transfusions have been used until IVTs are technically possible [11]. After the first IVT, the second procedure is usually planned 7–10 days later with an expected decrement in the fetal hematocrit of approximately 1% per day. Subsequent procedures are repeated at 2- to 3-week intervals based on fetal response and suppression of fetal erythropoiesis. Most centers will not perform an IUT after 35 weeks.

After the last procedure, the patient is scheduled for induction of labor at 38–39 weeks gestation to allow for fetal liver maturity. The addition of oral maternal phenobarbital (30 mg orally three times daily) may further enhance the ability of the fetal liver to conjugate bilirubin, thereby potentially preventing the need for neonatal exchange transfusions [12]. Currently, the typical neonatal course for the fetus treated successfully with serial IUTs includes minimal need for phototherapy and discharge to home with the mother at the end of a routine postpartum stay.

Outcome

In experienced centers, the overall perinatal survival with IUT exceeds 95% [13]. Hydropic fetuses fare more poorly, with a 15% decrease in survival compared to nonhydropic counterparts [14]. Suppression of fetal erythropoiesis secondary to serial IUTs can be associated with profound anemia in the first few months of newborn life. Weekly hematocrit and reticulocyte counts should be followed until there is evidence of renewed production of red cells. Top-up red cell transfusions may be required in as many as 50% of cases [15].

Neurodevelopmental follow-up studies of neonates transfused by IVT are limited in number. Most point to over a 90% chance of intact survival [16]. Sensorineural hearing loss may be slightly increased due to prolonged exposure of the fetus to high levels of bilirubin. A hearing screen should be performed during the early neonatal course and repeated by 2 years of life.

Immunomodulation

Patients with a history of a previous fetal demise or failed IUT prior to 20–24 weeks gestation are considered to have early-onset HDFN (EOS-HDFN). In these cases, a similar or more severe clinical course can be expected in the following pregnancy if the fetus is determined to be antigen positive. In addition, first time alloimmunized cases with a maternal RhD titer of ≥1024 or a Kell titer of ≥512 are at significant risk for EOS-HDFN.

Despite improvements in ultrasound imaging, challenging technical issues at a gestational age of 20–24 weeks limit the success of IUTs. In one series, the perinatal loss rate when IUTs were undertaken prior to 20 weeks gestation was increased threefold as compared to procedures performed after 20 weeks [17].

Weekly intravenous immune globulin (1 g/kg) has been proposed in these pregnancies as a means to prolong the interval until the first IUT is necessary. In an international registry, patients with a previous history of EOS-HDFN that received intravenous immunoglobulin prior to 13 weeks gestation developed fetal anemia 21 days later than in their previous pregnancies. There was also a 31% reduction in the onset of fetal anemia prior to 20 weeks gestation [18].

Therapies that target the transplacental passage of anti-red cell antibodies represent the future of immunomodulation. A new monoclonal antibody (nipocalimab) is currently being investigated in EOS-HDFN in a phase II clinical trial (clinicaltrials.gov: NCT03842189).

Hemolytic disease of the fetus and newborn caused by non-RhD antibodies

Antibodies to the red cell antigens Lewis, I, and P are often encountered through antibody screening during prenatal care. Because these antibodies are typically of the IgM class, they do not cross the placenta and are not associated with HDFN.

Antibodies to more than 50 other red cell antigens have been reported to be associated with HDFN (Table 37.3). However, only four of these antibodies cause significant hemolytic disease where treatment with IUT is necessary: anti-RhD, anti-Rhc, anti-E, and anti-Kell (K1). Most centers use a maternal titer of 16 in cases of non-RhD antibodies to initiate fetal surveillance. Because the Kell antibody affects the fetus both at the level of the bone marrow to suppress erythropoiesis as well as causing the destruction of circulating red cells, a critical titer of 4 is used in the case of Kell antibodies [19].

Table 37.3 Red blood cell antibodies associated with hemolytic disease of the fetus and newborn

Antigen group	Specific antigen(s)	Disease severity
ABO	A, B	Mild
Chido-Rodgers	Ch1, Ch2, Ch3, Ch4, Ch5, Ch6, WH, Rg1, Rg2	None
Colton	Co^a	Moderate
	Co^b, Co^3	Mild
Cromer	Cr^a, Tc^a, Tc^b, Tc^c, Dr^a, Es^a, IFC, WES^a, WES^b, UMC, GUTI, SERF, ZENA, CROV, CRAM	None
Diego	Di^a, Di^b, Wr^a, ELO	Moderate
	Wr^b, Wd^a, Rb^a, WARR, Wu, Bp^a, Mo^a, Hg^a, Vg^a, Sw^a, BOW, NFLD, Jn^a, KREP, Tr^a, Fr^a, SW1	None
Dombrock	Do^a, Do^b, Gy^a, Hy, Jo^a, DOYA	None
Duffy	Fy^a	Moderate
	Fy^b	Mild
	Fy^3, Fy^4, Fy^5, Fy^6	None
Forssman	FOR	None
Gerbich	Ge3	Moderate
	Ge2, Ge4, Wb, Ls^a, An^a, Dh^a, GEIS	None
Gill	Gil	None
Globoside	PP_1P_k	Severe
H	H	Moderate
I	I, i	None
Indian	In^a, In^b, INFI, INJA	None
John Milton Hagen	JMH, JMHK, JMHL, JMHG, JMHM	None
Junior	Jr^a	Mild (rare: severe)
Kell	K, k, Ku, Js^b	Severe
	Kp^b	Moderate
	Kp^a, Js^a, Ul^a	Mild
	K11, K12, K13, K14, K15, K16, K17, K18, K19, K20, K21, K22, K23, K24, VLAN, TOU, RAZ, KUCI, KANT, KASH, VONG, KALT, KTIM, KYO	None
Kidd	Jk^a, Jk^b	Mild (rare: severe)
	Jk3	Mild
Knops	Kn^a, Kn^b, McC^a, Sl1, Yka, Sl2, Sl3, KCAM	None
Kx	Kx	None
Langereis	Lan	Mild (rare: moderate)
Landsteiner-Weiner	LW^a, LW^{ab}, LW^b	None
Lewis	Le^a, Le^b, Le^{ab}, Le^{bH}, Ale^b, Ble^b	None
Lutheran	Lu^a	Mild
	Lu^b, Lu3, Lu4, Lu5, Lu6, Lu7, Lu8, Lu9, Lu10, Lu11, Lu12, Lu13, Lu14, Lu15, Lu16, Lu17, Au^a, Au^b, Lu20, Lu21	None
Mittenberger	Mi^a	Severe
	Mi^b	None
MNSs	Vw, Mur, MUT	Severe
	U	Moderate (rare: severe)
	M	Mild (rare: severe)
	S, s, Mt^a, M^v	Moderate
	N, Hil, Or	Mild
	He, Mi^a, M^c, M^g, Vr, M^e, St^a, Ri^a, Cl^a, Ny^a, Hut, Far, s^D, Mit, Dantu, Hop, Nob, En^a, En^aKT, 'N', DANE, TSEN, MINY, SAT ERIK, Os^a, ENEP, ENEH, HAG, ENAV, MARS, ENDA, ENEV, MNTD	None
Ok	Ok^a	None
P1Pk	P, P1, pk	None
Raph	MER2	None
RHAG	Duclos, Ol^a, Duclos-like	None
Rhesus	D, c, f, Ce, C^w, cE	Severe
	E, Hr_0	Moderate (rare: severe)
	E^W, hr^S, Tar, Rh32, Hr^B	Moderate
	C	Mild (rare: severe)
	G	Mild (rare: moderate)
	e, C^x, VS, CE, Be^a, JAL	Mild
	V, Hr, C^G, D^W, c-like, hr^H, Rh29, Go^a, Rh33, hr^B, Rh35, Evans, Rh39, Rh41, Rh42, Crawford, Nou, Riv, Sec, CELO, Dav, STEM, FPTT, MAR, BARC, JAHK, DAK, LOCR, CENR, CEST	None

Table 37.3 (*Continued*)

Antigen group	Specific antigen(s)	Disease severity
Scianna	Rd	Mild (rare: moderate)
	SC2	Mild
	SC1, SC3, STAR, SCER, SCAN	None
Vel	Vel	Severe
Xg	Xgᵃ	Mild
	CD99	None
Yt(Cartwright)	Ytᵃ, Ytᵇ	None
Antigens not classified to a blood group		
Cost	Csᵃ, Csᵇ	None
Er	Erᵃ, Erᵇ, ABTI	None
High-prevalence antigens	Atᵃ	Mild
	AnWj, Emm, MAM, PEL, Sdᵃ	None
Low-prevalence antigens	HJK	Severe
	Kg, Sara	Moderate
	Chrᵃ, Bi, Bxᵃ, Toᵃ, Ptᵃ, Reᵃ, Jeᵃ, Liᵉ, Milne, RASM, JFV, JONES, HOFM, REIT	None

Mild: Neonatal therapy only: phototherapy or simple transfusion.
Moderate: Neonatal exchange transfusion.
Severe: Significant fetal disease possible with need for intrauterine transfusion.
Reproduced with permission from Moise KJ Jr., Kennedy MS, Management of non-Rhesus (D) red blood cell alloantibodies during pregnancy. In: Post TW, ed. *UpToDate*. Waltham, MA: UpToDate Inc. Copyright © 2022 UpToDate Inc. [cited 2022 Jan 15]. For more information visit www.uptodate.com.

CASE PRESENTATION 1: SURVEILLANCE OF A FIRST AFFECTED GESTATION

A 30-year-old gravida 2, para 1001 was noted to have a positive antibody screen for anti-D at her first prenatal visit at 8 weeks gestation. The patient had not received Rh immunoglobulin after her previous delivery in Mexico 3 years earlier. Her titer was 32 for anti-D. Paternal DNA testing revealed a heterozygous state. The patient was scheduled for amniocentesis at 16 weeks gestation but elected to undergo free fetal DNA testing instead. Results indicated an RHD-positive fetus. At 24 weeks gestation the anti-D titer remained stable at 32. Serial MCA Doppler studies were initiated each week. After 3 weeks, these remained at 1.1–1.2 MoM so the testing interval was lengthened to every 2 weeks. The MCA-PSV values remained normal. Induction of labor was undertaken at 38 weeks gestation. A healthy 3713 g (8 lb 3 oz) female fetus was born vaginally. Cord blood revealed the child to be A, RHD positive, the direct Coombs was 1+, and the total bilirubin was 2.1 mg/dL. The infant required 3 days of phototherapy therapy with a peak bilirubin of 10 mg/dL. The infant was discharged on the fourth day of life and required no further treatment.

CASE PRESENTATION 2: SURVEILLANCE OF A SUBSEQUENTLY AFFECTED GESTATION

The patient in case 1 returned 2 years later with her third pregnancy. The current pregnancy had been fathered by the same partner as her previous gestation. At 10 weeks gestation, the maternal anti-D titer was 128. Free fetal DNA testing at that time indicated an RHD-positive fetus. Serial MCA Dopplers were initiated each week starting at 18 weeks gestation. At 25 weeks, the MCA-PSV was 1.45 MoM. One week later it had risen to 1.7 MoM. The following day, an IUT was scheduled. Initial fetal blood at the time of cordocentesis revealed blood type O, RhD positive, with a 3+ direct Coombs test. The fetal hematocrit was 25% with 15% reticulocytes. An intravascular transfusion of 45 mL raised the fetal hematocrit to 50%. The patient returned for five additional IUTs, the last one being performed at 35 weeks gestation. Oral phenobarbital was prescribed to the patient 10 days prior to her planned induction date to enhance the neonatal capability to conjugate bilirubin.

She was induced at 38 weeks gestation and delivered a healthy 3004 g (6 lb 10 oz) male fetus. Cord blood testing revealed a hematocrit of 45% with a Kleihauer–Betke stain consisting of 100% adult hemoglobin-containing red cells, indicating complete suppression of the fetal bone marrow. The infant was discharged on the second day of life and did not require phototherapy. He was followed with weekly hematocrit and reticulocyte counts by his pediatrician. At 4 weeks of age he was noted to be feeding poorly; the hematocrit had declined to 23%. He was admitted overnight for a "top-up" red cell transfusion. Subsequent weekly testing revealed a rising reticulocyte count 3 weeks later. The infant required no further therapy.

References

1. Medearis AL, Hensleigh PA, Parks DR, Herzenberg LA. Detection of fetal erythrocytes in maternal blood post partum with the fluorescence-activated cell sorter. Am J Obstet Gynecol. 1984;148(3):290–5.

2. American College of Obstetricians and Gynecologists. Practice Bulletin No. 181: prevention of RhD alloimmunization. Obstet Gynecol. 2017;181:1–13.

3. Kumpel BM. On the mechanism of tolerance to the Rh D antigen mediated by passive anti-D (Rh D prophylaxis). Immunol Lett. 2002;82(1-2):67–73.

4. Bowman JM. Controversies in Rh prophylaxis. Who needs Rh immune globulin and when should it be given? Am J Obstet Gynecol. 1985;151(3):289–94.

5. Novaretti MC, Jens E, Pagliarini T, Bonifacio SL, Dorlhiac-Llacer PE, Chamone DA. Comparison of conventional tube test with diamed gel microcolumn assay for anti-D titration. Clin Lab Haematol. 2003;25(5):311–5.

6. Mari G, for the Collaborative Group for Doppler Assessment of the Blood Velocity in Anemic Fetuses. Noninvasive diagnosis by Doppler ultrasonography of fetal anemia due to maternal red-cell alloimmunization. N Engl J Med. 2000;342:9–14.

7. Finning KM, Martin PG, Soothill PW, Avent ND. Prediction of fetal D status from maternal plasma: introduction of a new noninvasive fetal RHD genotyping service. Transfusion. 2002;42(8):1079–85.

8. Liley AW. Intrauterine transfusion of foetus in haemolytic disease. BMJ. 1963;2:1107–9.

9. Moise KJ, Jr., Carpenter RJ, Jr., Kirshon B, Deter RL, Sala JD, Cano LE. Comparison of four types of intrauterine transfusion: effect on fetal hematocrit. Fetal Ther. 1989;4(2-3):126–37.

10. Nicolini U, Santolaya J, Ojo OE, Fisk NM, Hubinont C, Tonge M, et al. The fetal intrahepatic umbilical vein as an alternative to cord needling for prenatal diagnosis and therapy. Prenat Diagn. 1988;8(9):665–71.

11. Yinon Y, Visser J, Kelly EN, Windrim R, Amsalem H, Seaward PG, et al. Early intrauterine transfusion in severe red blood cell alloimmunization. Ultrasound Obstet Gynecol. 2010;36(5):601–6.

12. Trevett TN, Jr., Dorman K, Lamvu G, Moise KJ, Jr. Antenatal maternal administration of phenobarbital for the prevention of exchange transfusion in neonates with hemolytic disease of the fetus and newborn. Am J Obstet Gynecol. 2005;192(2):478–82.

13. Zwiers C, Lindenburg ITM, Klumper FJ, de Haas M, Oepkes D, Van Kamp IL. Complications of intrauterine intravascular blood transfusion: lessons learned after 1678 procedures. Ultrasound Obstet Gynecol. 2017;50(2):180–6.

14. van Kamp IL, Klumper FJ, Bakkum RS, Oepkes D, Meerman RH, Scherjon SA, et al. The severity of immune fetal hydrops is predictive of fetal outcome after intrauterine treatment. Am J Obstet Gynecol. 2001;185(3):668–73.

15. Ree IMC, Lopriore E, Zwiers C, Bohringer S, Janssen MWM, Oepkes D, et al. Suppression of compensatory erythropoiesis in hemolytic disease of the fetus and newborn due to intrauterine transfusions. Am J Obstet Gynecol. 2020;223(1):119. e1–e10.

16. Lindenburg IT, Smits-Wintjens VE, van Klink JM, Verduin E, van Kamp IL, Walther FJ, et al. Long-term neurodevelopmental outcome after intrauterine transfusion for hemolytic disease of the fetus/newborn: the LOTUS study. Am J Obstet Gynecol. 2012;206(2):141.e1–e8.

17. Lindenburg IT, van Kamp IL, van Zwet EW, Middeldorp JM, Klumper FJ, Oepkes D. Increased perinatal loss after intrauterine transfusion for alloimmune anaemia before 20 weeks of gestation. BJOG. 2013;120(7):847–52.

18. Zwiers C, van der Bom JG, van Kamp IL, van Geloven N, Lopriore E, Smoleniec J, et al. Postponing Early intrauterine Transfusion with Intravenous immunoglobulin Treatment; the PETIT study on severe hemolytic disease of the fetus and newborn. Am J Obstet Gynecol. 2018;219(3):291.e1–e9.

19. Slootweg YM, Lindenburg IT, Koelewijn JM, Van Kamp IL, Oepkes D, De Haas M. Predicting anti-Kell-mediated hemolytic disease of the fetus and newborn: diagnostic accuracy of laboratory management. Am J Obstet Gynecol. 2018;219(4):393.e1–e8.

Chapter 38
Multiple Gestations

Maria Andrikopoulou and Mary E. D'Alton

Department of Obstetrics and Gynecology, Columbia University Medical Center and Columbia Presbyterian Hospital, New York, NY, USA

An epidemic of multiple gestations has occurred over the past 2 decades, attributed largely to an older patient population secondary to delayed childbearing and the rise in the use of assisted reproductive technology (ART) and ovulation induction. According to the National Vital Statistics Report for 2019, the twin birth rate was 32.1 twin births per 1000 total live births, and the triplet or higher order birth rate: 87.7 per 100 000 live births [1]. Maternal and neonatal outcomes have been strongly affected by the widespread prevalence of multiple gestations as these pregnancies account for a disproportionate share of adverse outcomes.

The most profound implication of multiple gestations is preterm delivery, the leading cause of hospitalization among pregnant women and the leading cause of infant death [2]. In addition to prematurity, multiple pregnancy is known to be associated with a greater number of other maternal and fetal complications including preeclampsia, fetal anomalies, placental abruption, gestational diabetes, operative delivery, low birthweight, and adverse neurologic outcomes [3]. The overall increased perinatal risks associated with multiple gestations compared with singleton pregnancies are well documented, and these high-risk pregnancies have a profound effect on medical expenditures and public health [1]. This chapter reviews multiple gestations and the current strategies for managing these complex pregnancies.

Impact on perinatal outcomes

The two largest contributors to increased perinatal morbidity and mortality in multiple gestations are increased rates of prematurity and complications of monochorionicity. In the United States, the mean age at delivery is 35 weeks for twins, 31.7 weeks for triplets, and 30.0 weeks for quadruplets, compared to 38.5 weeks for singletons and 19.5% of twin gestations, 63% of triplets and 82.6% of quadruplets are delivered prior to 34 weeks [4]. Multiple gestations are associated with increased risk for intrauterine fetal demise and neonatal death [3].

Offspring of multiple pregnancies also have lower birthweights than singletons; 55.4% of twins and 95% of triplets are low birthweight [4]. In addition, neonates from multiple gestations currently comprise a disproportionate share of neonatal intensive care admissions. Although the offspring of multiple gestations may be born earlier than singletons, preterm twin and triplet neonates appear to have similar birthweights, morbidities, and mortalities as gestational age-matched singleton controls [5–7].

Patients with multiples are also at increased risk for adverse perinatal outcomes resulting from complications unique to the twinning process. Monochorionic placentation accounts for 20% of all twin pregnancies and carries a worse prognosis than dichorionicity. Complications from monochorionicity such as twin–twin transfusion syndrome (TTTS) continue to place these offspring at higher risk for long-term adverse outcomes. Cases of single intrauterine fetal death (IUFD) in twins sharing a single placenta can be associated with a coincident insult leading to demise or white matter damage in the surviving twin. Other unique but rare complications that occur in monochorionic pregnancies include cord entanglement in monoamniotic twins, conjoined twins, and twin reversed arterial perfusion sequence, also known as a cardiac twinning.

Multiple gestation is an independent risk factor for long-term neurologic impairment. In various studies, children from a multiple pregnancy have a 4–17 times higher risk of developing cerebral palsy compared to their singleton counterparts [3,8–10]. Because this correlation holds for higher birthweights, the risk may not simply be related to an increased preterm delivery rate [9,10]. One epidemiologic study reported that the risk of producing one child with cerebral palsy in twin, triplet, and

Queenan's Management of High-Risk Pregnancy: An Evidence-Based Approach, Seventh Edition. Edited by Catherine Y. Spong and Charles J. Lockwood.

quadruplet gestations was 15 per 1000 twins, 80 per 1000 triplets, and 429 per 1000 quadruplets [10]. Although many previous studies investigating this association were not optimally designed, the prevalence of cerebral palsy in multiple pregnancies reported in these studies is similar and ranges from 6.7 to 12.6 per 1000 surviving infants [9]. In addition to prematurity, other risk factors for cerebral palsy seen with higher frequency in multiples include maternal hypertensive disease, bleeding in pregnancy, low birthweight infants, congenital anomalies, and complications specific to monochorionicity [9,11].

Zygosity and chorionicity

Embryology
Zygosity refers to the genetic constitution of a twin pregnancy, and chorionicity indicates the pregnancy's membrane composition. In dizygotic twins, chorionicity is determined by the mechanism of fertilization, whereas in monozygotic twins it is determined by the timing of embryonic division. The vast majority of dizygotic twins have separate dichorionic diamniotic placentas (each fetus has its own placental disk with a separate amnion and chorion). This is because dizygotic twins result from the fertilization of two different ova by two separate sperm. The type of placenta that develops in a monozygotic pregnancy is determined by the timing of cleavage of the fertilized ovum. If twinning is accomplished during the first 2–3 days, it precedes the separation of cells that eventually become the chorion. In that case, two chorions and two amnions will be formed. After approximately 3 days, twinning cannot split the chorionic cavity and from that time forward, a monochorionic placenta results. If the split occurs between the third and eighth days, a diamniotic monochorionic placenta develops. Between the 8th and 13th days, the amnion has already formed, thus, splitting in this interval results in a monoamniotic and monochorionic placenta. Embryonic cleavage between the 13th and 15th days results in conjoined twins within a single amnion and chorion; beyond that point, the process of twinning does not occur [12]. Interestingly, rare cases of dizygotic monochorionic twins conceived following ART have been reported [13,14].

Ultrasound diagnosis of chorionicity
The determination of chorionicity is important in the management of multiple gestations as monochorionic twins are at increased risk for adverse outcomes. Antenatal knowledge of chorionicity can be critical for determining optimal management of a variety of pregnancy complications, including growth disorders. Precise knowledge of chorionicity is imperative when contemplating the selective termination of one abnormal twin or when performing elective first-trimester multifetal pregnancy reduction.

If the gestation is monochorionic, a shared placental circulation could result in death or injury to a surviving fetus, depending on the technique used for the termination procedure.

Chorionicity is most accurately determined in the first trimester. From 6 to 10 weeks, counting the number of gestational sacs with evaluation of the thickness of the dividing membrane is the optimal method. Two separate gestational sacs, each containing a fetus and a thick dividing membrane, suggests a dichorionic diamniotic pregnancy, whereas one gestational sac with a thin dividing membrane and two fetuses suggests a monochorionic diamniotic pregnancy [15]. The number of yolk sacs can also be used as an indirect method of determining amnionicity. Identification of two yolk sacs in monochorionic twins may enable the diagnosis of diamniotic twins early in the first trimester, before the amniotic membrane can be seen; however, when there is presence of one yolk sac, a follow up ultrasound is needed to definitely assign amnionicity [16]. After 9 weeks, the dividing membranes become progressively thinner in monochorionic pregnancies. In dichorionic pregnancies, they remain thick and easy to identify at their attachment to the placenta as a triangular projection (lambda or twin peak sign) (Figure 38.1) [17–19]. Thus, in the late first trimester, sonographic examination of the base of the intertwin membrane for the presence or absence of the lambda sign provides a reliable distinction between dichorionic and monochorionic pregnancies [20].

Later in pregnancy, determination of chorionicity and amnionicity becomes less accurate and requires different techniques. The sonographic prediction of chorionicity and amnionicity should be systematically approached by determining the number of placentas visualized and the sex of each fetus and then by assessing the membranes that divide the sacs. If two separate placental disks are seen, the pregnancy is dichorionic. Likewise, if the twins are different genders, the pregnancy is most likely dichorionic. When a single placenta is present and the twins are

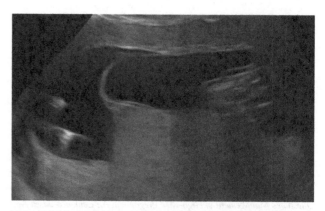

Figure 38.1 Lambda or twin peak sign in dichorionic diamniotic pregnancy.

of the same sex, careful sonographic examination of the dividing membrane will typically result in a correct diagnosis. Evaluation of three features in the intertwin membrane will provide an almost certain diagnosis about the chorionicity of a twin pregnancy:
• thickness of the intertwin membrane
• number of layers visualized in the membrane
• assessment of the junction of the membrane with the placenta for the "twin peak" sign [21].

It should be mentioned that the absence of the twin peak sign does not guarantee that the pregnancy is monochorionic.

In some pregnancies with monochorionic diamniotic placentation, the dividing membranes may not be sonographically visualized because they are very thin. In other cases, they may not be seen because severe oligohydramnios causes them to be closely apposed to the fetus in that sac. This results in a "stuck twin" appearance, where the trapped fetus remains firmly held against the uterine wall despite changes in maternal position. Diagnosis of this condition confirms the presence of a diamniotic gestation, which should be distinguished from a monoamniotic gestation with an absent dividing membrane. In the latter situation, free movement of both twins, and entanglement of their umbilical cords, can be identified [22].

Fetal complications and multiple gestations

The offspring of a multiple gestation are at risk for many complications in utero that may lead to long-term adverse outcomes, including growth abnormalities, fetal loss, and complications unique to the twinning process (Box 38.1).

Box 38.1 Multiple gestation: fetal and neonatal risks

• Fetal loss
• Chromosomal abnormalities
• Congenital malformations
• Monochorionicity:
  – TTTS
  – Monoamnionicity
  – TRAP
• Growth discordance/FGR
• Amniotic fluid volume abnormalities
• Prematurity
• Low birthweight
• Perinatal mortality
• Cerebral palsy

FGR, fetal growth restriction; TRAP, twin reversed arterial perfusion; TTTS, twin–twin transfusion syndrome.

Intrauterine growth restriction and growth discordance

Birthweight is linked to many factors, including gestational age, rate of fetal growth, ethnicity, and genetic composition. Two important antenatal markers for growth abnormalities for multiple pregnancies are fetal growth restriction (FGR) and growth discordance. FGR remains a sonographic and statistical diagnosis consisting of an estimated fetal weight (EFW) <10th percentile for gestational age or abdominal circumference <10%. Growth discordance is generally defined as >20% difference in EFW between fetuses of the same pregnancy expressed as a percentage of the larger EFW [23]. Both growth abnormalities are seen with increased frequency in multiple gestations.

FGR has long been known to be associated with adverse perinatal outcomes. Neonatal morbidity (such as meconium aspiration syndrome, hypoglycemia, polycythemia, and pulmonary hemorrhage) may be present in up to 50% of FGR neonates. Long-term studies show a twofold increased incidence of cerebral dysfunction (ranging from minor learning disabilities to cerebral palsy) in FGR infants delivered at term and an even higher incidence if the infant was born preterm [9]. Multiple gestations present a dilemma both in diagnosis and management of FGR. For example, fetuses suspected to be normally grown may be affected by iatrogenic preterm delivery secondary to interventions for a growth-restricted twin. Current management of FGR is aimed at timely diagnosis and fetal surveillance to aid in timing delivery. Growth discordance may be associated with an increased risk for adverse perinatal outcomes [24]. Approximately 15% of twins are diagnosed with this condition [24]. Risk factors include monochorionicity, velamentous cord insertion, antenatal bleeding, uteroplacental insufficiency, and gestational hypertensive disease [24]. Growth discordance has different implications depending on chorionicity and is more concerning in monochorionic twinning. Although FGR can complicate a pregnancy with growth discordance, the second does not necessarily imply the first. Although some studies have demonstrated an increased risk for perinatal morbidity in growth discordant twins, others have not. In approximately two thirds of discordant twin pairs, the smaller twin has a birthweight of less than 10% [25]. In a study of more than 10 000 discordant twins, the neonatal mortality rates were 29 vs. 11 per 1000 live births when the smaller twin weighed l<10th percentile, compared with those who were above it [25]. Conversely, another study suggests that 20% growth discordance may result in an increased risk for some adverse outcomes but not for serious sequelae [26]. After adjusting for chorionicity, administration of antenatal corticosteroids, oligohydramnios, preeclampsia, and gestational age at delivery, discordant twins were at increased risk for low or very low birthweight, neonatal intensive care unit (NICU) admission, neonatal oxygen requirement, and hyperbilirubinemia but did not seem to be at increased risk for serious neonatal morbidity and mortality. It is not clear whether growth discordance in the setting of fetuses that are appropriate for gestational age, is associated with adverse perinatal outcomes [4].

Fetal loss

The incidence of early pregnancy loss in multiple gestations is higher than previously thought. The routine use of ultrasound has shown that early fetal loss is common in multiple gestations. In patients with twin gestations scanned in the first trimester, rates of demise ranged from 13% to 78% [27]. This phenomenon has been termed the *vanishing twin.* Explanations for this occurrence include physiologic resorption, artifact, and sonographic error. Although this condition has been associated with first-trimester bleeding and spotting, it has not been associated with adverse pregnancy outcomes.

During the second and third trimester, IUFD occurs more commonly in multiple gestations than in singletons, with IUFD of one fetus occurring in approximately 2–5% of twin pregnancies. In patients with high-order multiples, however, death of a single fetus may be more common with single IUFD rates up to 17% in triplet pregnancies [28]. Data suggest that the risk of intrauterine death of one or both twins is higher in monochorionic than dichorionic pregnancies. In a study of 1000 consecutive twin-pairs, monochorionic-diamniotic twins had a higher risk of stillbirth compared with dichorionic-diamniotic twins, both overall and at each gestational age after 24 weeks [29]; this increased risk of fetal loss persisted in "apparently normal" monochorionic-diamniotic twins unaffected by growth abnormalities, congenital anomalies, or TTTS.

Death of one twin in the second or third trimesters can adversely affect the surviving fetus or fetuses in two ways:
• risk for multicystic encephalomalacia and multiorgan damage in the surviving twin in monochorionic pregnancies; and
• preterm labor and delivery in both dichorionic and monochorionic twins resulting in prematurity.

Although multiorgan damage in surviving monochorionic twins was once thought to be due to disseminated intravascular coagulation in the surviving twin caused by transfer of thromboplastic materials from the dead fetus [30], a more recent and widely accepted theory suggests that the surviving twin may rapidly "back-bleed" into the dead twin through placental anastomoses (a capacitance effect), resulting in profound hypovolemia and anemia in the surviving twin [31]. Decreased circulatory tone in the dead twin causing blood to flow from the viable to the dead twin may be the underlying pathophysiology [32]. If the hypotension is severe enough, the surviving twin is at risk for ischemic damage to vital organs. Most evidence in the literature now suggests that "back-bleeding" and subsequent hemodynamic changes are the cause of multiorgan injury in surviving twins. As a result, immediate delivery of the twin following diagnosis of an unwitnessed single IUFD in a monochorionic pregnancy does not improve outcome but rather adds to the additional risk of prematurity. Most cases are managed expectantly with close fetal surveillance. Normal fetal heart rate patterns and antenatal testing cannot rule out multicystic encephalomalacia. Normal fetal magnetic resonance imaging, while investigational, may be reassuring [33]. In addition to multiorgan ischemic damage in monochorionic pregnancies, IUFD of one twin can result in preterm delivery. Both dichorionic and monochorionic pregnancies are at risk for preterm delivery following a single fetal demise. In a study of 17 twin pregnancies complicated by a single IUFD, 76% of these pregnancies were delivered before 37 weeks. Eighty-six percent of the patients delivering prematurely presented in active labor [34].

When IUFD occurs in a multiple pregnancy, baseline maternal hematologic laboratory investigation is suggested, including prothrombin time, partial thromboplastin time, fibrinogen level, and platelet count, because of the theoretical risk of maternal consumptive coagulopathy in the setting of a single IUFD. Of note, mothers with IUFD in one twin do not appear to be at increased risk of infection from a retained twin [34]. Dystocia secondary to the demised fetus has been reported infrequently. Cesarean delivery rates appear increased in patients with single IUFD complicating a twin gestation because of higher rates of nonreassuring fetal status in the surviving twin [34].

Discordant congenital anomalies

There is general agreement that anomalies occur more frequently in twins than in singletons, but controversy exists regarding the degree of difference [35–38]. Monochorionic twin gestations are associated with higher risk for congenital anomalies [3]. The diagnosis of discordance for major genetic disorders or anatomic abnormalities in the second trimester places parents in a difficult position. Management choices include:
• expectant management
• termination of the entire pregnancy
• selective termination of the anomalous fetus

The term "selective termination" refers to terminating a specific fetus that is known to have a fetal abnormality. In contrast, the term multifetal pregnancy reduction (MPR) refers to reduction in the number of fetuses a woman is carrying to reduce her risk of preterm delivery and other pregnancy complications. For dichorionic pregnancies, intracardiac injection with potassium chloride can be used. Because of the placental anastomoses between monochorionic fetuses, however, cord occlusive procedures are employed in monochorionic pregnancies to reduce the risk to the surviving twin [39]. Cord occlusion techniques include suture ligation, bipolar or laser coagulation, or radiofrequency ablation.

Several issues should be considered when counseling patients about the management of a multiple pregnancy complicated by a discordant anomaly:

• Severity of the anomaly and prognosis
• Chorionicity
• Effect of the anomalous fetus on the remaining fetus or fetuses
• The parents' personal, moral, and ethical beliefs

It is important to counsel patients that conservative management may result in adverse outcomes for the healthy twin. Several studies have demonstrated that the nonaffected fetus in a twin pregnancy discordant for major fetal anomalies may be at increased risk for preterm delivery, low birthweight, and perinatal morbidity and mortality [40–42].

Complications unique to monochorionicity

Monoamnionicity

Less than 1% of monozygotic twins are monoamniotic [43]. Monoamniotic twins have a high rate of perinatal mortality. Previous studies report a fetal mortality rate of greater than 50% but more recent studies indicate a perinatal mortality rate ranging from 10% to 21% [44–46]. Preterm delivery, FGR, congenital anomalies, cord entanglement, and cord accidents remain common in monoamniotic pregnancies. The management of these pregnancies is controversial, particularly regarding the optimal protocol for antenatal surveillance and the optimal timing for delivery. Because IUFD can occur at any gestational age, some experts suggest early delivery in the late preterm period [47]. However, this decision should take into consideration the risk of prematurity [48]. Although the optimal management and timing of delivery for monoamniotic twins remain uncertain, our current practice includes routine hospitalization beginning at 24–26 weeks, with close fetal monitoring, and, if uncomplicated, delivery at 32–34 weeks [49].

Twin–twin transfusion syndrome

Monochorionic twins occur spontaneously in 0.4% of the general population. However, studies have reported that monozygotic twinning may be greater than 10 times higher in pregnancies following fertility treatment [50]. The primary concerns about monochorionic placentation include complications such as TTTS. Although all monochorionic twins share a portion of their vasculature, only approximately 15–20% will develop this condition [43].

Left untreated, there is up to 60–100% mortality rate for both twins.

Antenatal diagnosis of TTTS is made sonographically. The diagnosis requires the presence of a monochorionic diamniotic gestation and the presence of amniotic fluid discordance between the twins with diagnosis of oligohydramnios (defined as a maximal vertical pocket [MVP] of <2 cm) in one sac, and of polyhydramnios (MVP of >8 cm) in the other sac [51]. Growth discordance and FGR are not included in the diagnostic criteria. However, these entities are common findings in cases of TTTS. The recipient twin may have signs of heart failure and hydrops and the donor may demonstrate IUGR and a "stuck" appearance. Umbilical artery Doppler studies can be variable [52]. TTTS may be chronic or acute. A staging system devised by Quintero et al. [53] is commonly used to categorize disease severity and standardize comparison of different therapies. The system has five stages, ranging from early and mild disease with isolated amniotic fluid volume discordance to severe disease with demise of one or both twins [51] (Table 38.1). Although the exact etiology has not been clearly delineated, the mechanism is likely to involve shunting of arteriovenous anastomoses [54]. Even though cases with stage I disease can progress to more advanced stages, the natural history of TTTS is not always predictable [51]. Thus, serial ultrasound surveillance is recommended for monochorionic diamniotic twin gestations starting at 16 weeks, every 2 weeks to screen for TTTS.

Management of TTTS include expectant management, amnioreduction, fetoscopic laser photocoagulation, and selective reduction [51]. Amnioreduction involves the removal of amniotic fluid from the sac of recipient twins with polyhydramnios. Fetoscopic laser photocoagulation is coagulation of the communicating vessels. Selective fetal reduction involves interruption of umbilical flow of one twin, resulting in fetal demise of the twin, to improve the outcomes for the other twin [51]. Treatment depends on gestational age at diagnosis and stage of disease.

Patients with mild TTTS (Quintero stage I) are generally followed expectantly with serial ultrasound examinations given that in most cases the disease process remains stable or improve. Compared to amnioreduction, some studies have shown improved perinatal outcomes with

Table 38.1 Staging of twin–twin transfusion syndrome

Stage I	MVP <2 in donor sac, MVP >8 in recipient sac
Stage II	No visualization of fetal bladder for over 60 min
Stage III	At least one of the following is present in either twin: Absent or reversed umbilical artery diastolic flow, reversed ductus venosus a-wave flow, pulsatile umbilical vein flow
Stage IV	Signs of hydrops in one or both twins
Stage V	Fetal demise in one or both twins

MVP, maximal vertical pocket.
Adapted from [51].

fetoscopic laser coagulation [55–59]. Based on the published literature and expert reviews, fetoscopic laser coagulation of placental anastomoses is considered the best approach for Quintero stages II–IV TTTS prior to 26 weeks of gestation, whereas amnioreduction can be used severe TTTS beyond 26 weeks or when laser ablation is not available.

Maternal obstetric complications

Antepartum complications develop in over 80% of multiple pregnancies compared to 25% of singleton gestations. Examples include anemia, urinary tract infections, gestational diabetes, abnormal placentation, thromboembolism, preterm prelabor rupture of membranes, abruption, and postpartum hemorrhage (Box 38.2) [3,60–62]. Pulmonary embolism, the leading cause of maternal death in the United States and around the world, and thromboembolism are about five times more likely during pregnancy or the puerperium than in the nonpregnant state [63]. Women with multiple gestation are believed to be at increased risk for both.

Preeclampsia and its related spectrum of diseases occur in approximately 5–8% of singleton pregnancies but the incidence is higher in multiples [64,65]. Hypertensive diseases during pregnancy may manifest as hemolysis, elevated liver enzymes, and low platelet (HELLP) syndrome or eclampsia and can be associated with adverse sequelae including FGR, placental abruption, disseminated intravascular coagulation, renal failure, and IUFD [64]. Currently, low dose aspirin is recommended in multifetal gestations for preeclampsia prevention [66]. Other interventions such as calcium supplementation have not been shown to prevent or reduce the incidence of preeclampsia in these high-risk pregnancies [67]. Both gestational hypertension and preeclampsia are more common in

women carrying multiples, with the rates estimated to be 2–2.6 times higher in twins compared to singletons [65]. Rates of preeclampsia seem to be the same for both monozygotic and dizygotic twins [68]. When preeclampsia occurs in triplets and higher order multiples, it often occurs earlier, can be more severe and have atypical presentation [60,69]. Additionally, another complication that can arise in women carrying multifetal pregnancies is acute fatty liver of pregnancy, one of the most serious maternal obstetric complications [70]. This disease process is characterized by hepatic dysfunction, severe coagulopathy, hypoglycemia, and hyperammonemia and can result in fetal and/or maternal death.

Antepartum management of multiple gestations

The antepartum management of multiple pregnancies warrants attention to ensure adequate nutrition, increased frequency of prenatal visits and mitigation of risks associated with multiple gestations. Patients should be counseled regarding the increased risk of maternal, fetal, and obstetric complications associated with multiple gestations. Women with multifetal pregnancies are currently recommended to increase their daily caloric intake approximately 300 kcal more than women with singletons. Iron and folic acid supplementation is also advised. Although the optimal weight gain for women with multiples has not been determined, it has been suggested that women with twins gain 16.8–24.5 kg (37–54 lb) for women of normal weight [3,71]. Patients with multiple gestations should be followed with serial growth scans because clinical examination is inadequate in assessing growth of individual fetuses and because of the increased risk of fetal growth abnormalities in these pregnancies.

Multifetal pregnancy reduction

Ovulation induction and ART have greatly contributed to the increasing number of high-order multiples. The purpose of first trimester MPR is to improve perinatal outcomes by decreasing maternal complications secondary to multiple gestations and by decreasing adverse fetal outcomes associated with preterm delivery. Reducing a high-order multiple gestation to a lower-order pregnancy lowers the risk of pregnancy loss, preterm labor and delivery and increases the chances of higher birthweight and gestational age at delivery. Additionally, it reduced the risk of medical complications during pregnancy. Thus, nondirective counseling should be offered to all women with high-order multifetal pregnancies. The risks of the pregnancy should be discussed in detail and all options, including continuation and multifetal reduction [72]. The procedure is most commonly performed transabdominally under ultrasound guidance between 10 and

---

Box 38.2 Multiple gestation: maternal risks

- Hyperemesis
- Threatened miscarriage
- Anemia
- Gestational hypertension
- Preterm labor/delivery:
  - Tocolysis complications
  - Long-term bed rest
- Placental abnormalities:
  - Abruption
  - Abnormal placentation
- Urinary tract infection
- Gestational diabetes
- Postpartum hemorrhage
- Operative delivery
- Thromboembolism

13 weeks gestation. Potassium chloride is injected into the fetal heart until asystole is achieved. If selective fetal reduction, the fetus with genetic anomaly or abnormal ultrasound findings, is targeted. At multifetal reduction, the fetus most easily accessible is chosen. In monochorionic pregnancies, selectively reducing one fetus using intracardiac potassium chloride is contraindicated because of the presence of communicating placental anastomoses. Selective reduction in these cases involves more technically challenging procedures.

There are several studies documenting pregnancy loss rates associated with MPR. With extensive experience, the current loss rate is approximately 6% [73]. There are also some maternal risks associated with the procedure. The terminated fetus is usually resorbed or becomes a small papyraceous fetus. There have been no reports of coagulation disorders following this procedure [74]. Maternal serum α-fetoprotein (MSAFP) is elevated following MPR and selective termination and therefore cannot be used as a screening tool in these pregnancies.

Prenatal diagnosis

Prenatal diagnosis and genetic counseling are important in the management of patients with a multiple gestation because these pregnancies are at increased risk for both chromosomal and structural anomalies. All women, regardless of age, should be counseled about the option for either screening or diagnostic testing for fetal aneuploidy [75]. Many known chromosomal anomalies have been reported in twins. The maternal age-related risk for chromosomal abnormalities for each twin in dizygotic pregnancies is the same as in singleton pregnancies and, because each fetus has its own independent risk of aneuploidy, the chance of at least one chromosomally abnormal fetus is increased. Reports suggest that the risk of having one fetus with Down syndrome is similar for a woman between the ages of 31 and 33 carrying dizygotic twins and a 35-year-old woman with a singleton [76,77]. In monozygotic twins, the risk for chromosomal abnormalities is the same as in singletons, and in the vast majority of cases both fetuses are affected or both are unaffected [78]. However, there are occasional case reports of monozygotic twins discordant for abnormalities of autosomal or sex chromosomes [79,80].

Screening for fetal aneuploidy

Both first- and second-trimester serum markers are approximately twice as high in twin pregnancies as in singleton pregnancies [81]. Interpretation of abnormal serum screening results is difficult because it is not possible to determine which of the fetuses is responsible for the abnormal analyte concentration. In cases discordant for abnormalities, altered serum levels from the affected fetus will be brought closer to the mean by the unaffected twin. Methods of aneuploidy screening that includes a serum sample in twin gestations are not as accurate or reliable as for singleton pregnancies; Patients should be counseled on the limitations of the available test in multiple gestations.

First-trimester nuchal translucency ultrasound measurement, which assesses each fetus independently, is a promising method for aneuploidy screening in patients with multiples. Because the nuchal translucency distribution does not differ significantly in singletons compared to twins, the trisomy 21 detection rate in multiples using nuchal translucency measurement together with maternal age is similar to that of singletons [82]. Nuchal translucency appears to be higher in patients with monochorionic pregnancies and it has been suggested that this may reflect an early manifestation of TTTS in a proportion of cases [83]. Nuchal translucency can also be performed in triplet and higher-order multiple pregnancies with similar accuracy as in singletons.

In singletons, first-trimester combined screening, including maternal age and nuchal translucency combined with maternal serum free β-human chorionic gonadotropin (β-hCG) and pregnancy-associated plasma protein A, has been shown to detect approximately 82% of cases of Down syndrome for a 5% false-positive rate [84]. A meta-analysis showed that first-trimester combined screening in twins has a detection rate of 89% with a false-positive rate of 5.4%, which is similar to singleton gestations; In dichorionic twins, sensitivity and specificity were 0.862 and 0.952 respectively and in monochorionic twins, the sensitivity and specificity were 0.874 (95% confidence interval [CI] 0.526–0.977) and 0.954 (95% CI 0.943–0.963), respectively [85]. A prospective study of second-trimester maternal serum markers (alphafetoprotein and free β-hCG in 11 040 twin pregnancies showed that second-trimester serum screening of twin gestations can identify approximately 63% of fetuses affected with trisomy 21 with false-positive rate of 10.8% [86]. Cell-free DNA screening can be performed in twin gestations; It has been reported that sensitivity for trisomy 21 in twin pregnancies may be comparable to singleton gestations; however, it may be associated with higher risk for test failure [87].

Diagnostic testing for fetal aneuploidy

The accurate assessment of chorionicity is important when counseling patients regarding diagnostic testing. Diagnostic testing should be performed on one fetus only if monozygosity is certain. Otherwise, diagnostic testing should be done on all fetuses given the individual risk of aneuploidy in each fetus.

Genetic amniocentesis in multiples is performed using an ultrasound-guided multiple-needle approach. Indigo carmine dye may be used to confirm proper needle placement. Chorionic villus sampling (CVS) offers the advantage of earlier diagnosis and can be performed between

10 and 13 weeks. A systematic review of pregnancy loss after CVS or amniocentesis for twin gestations showed similar overall pregnancy-loss rates for both with the excess risk of around 1% above the background risk [88].

Screening for neural tube defects in multiples
In singletons, a second-trimester MSAFP of greater than 2.5 multiples of the median (MoM) has been used to screen for neural tube defects. Different MSAFP cutoffs are needed for twin pregnancies because the MSAFP level in a twin pregnancy is approximately double that of a singleton pregnancy. A cutoff of 4.5 MoM is often used for twins because it has a detection rate of 50–85% for a 5% false-positive rate. If an abnormal MSAFP is found, ultrasound is required for further evaluation. It is important to note that like maternal serum screening for aneuploidy, maternal serum screening for neural tube defects in a twin pregnancy will always be limited because it is impossible to confirm which fetus is affected without performing an ultrasound examination. As a result, many centers do not offer this type of serum screening for twin pregnancies.

Screening for anatomic abnormalities
As noted, fetuses of multiple gestations seem to be at increased risk for anatomic abnormalities. Careful sonographic, anatomic evaluation of each fetus should be obtained. No large-scale studies of ultrasound for fetal anatomy in multiples have been performed. Small studies have attempted to determine the predictive value of ultrasound in the detection of fetal anomalies in multiples and found it effective [89]. Studies have also demonstrated that monochorionic-diamniotic twins, both with and without TTTS, appear to be at increased risk of congenital heart disease, suggesting that screening fetal echocardiography may be considered in these pregnancies [90].

Prevention of preterm delivery
No therapy has proven to be efficacious in decreasing the adverse outcomes from prematurity except the administration of corticosteroids and surfactant to improve fetal lung maturity and antibiotics to lengthen the latency period for patients with preterm prelabor rupture of membranes [91–93]. This therapy does not treat the primary problem of preterm labor. Management strategies aimed at reducing the rate of preterm delivery that have not proven beneficial include prophylactic cervical cerclage, routine bed rest, prophylactic tocolytics, progesterone supplementation, or home uterine monitoring.

Prophylactic cervical cerclage in patients with a multiple gestation has not been consistently proven to prevent prematurity. A systematic review of five small studies showed that for unselected multiple gestations, there is no evidence that cerclage is an effective

intervention for preventing preterm births and reducing perinatal deaths or neonatal morbidity [94]. Thus, prophylactic cervical cerclage is not recommended based solely on the indication of multiple gestation [95–97]. However, a recent randomized trial that included women with twin gestation and cervical dilation between 1 to 5 cm, between 16–23 weeks, who were randomized to cerclage vs. no cerclage placement, showed that combination of physical examination-indicated cerclage, indomethacin, and antibiotics significantly decreased preterm birth; in this cohort of women cerclage placement was associated with a 50% decrease in early preterm birth at <28 weeks gestation and with a 78% decrease in perinatal mortality [98].

Restriction of physical activity has not been shown to reduce the risk for preterm birth and there is increased evidence that it is associated with adverse maternal outcomes. The literature does not support any significant benefit from routine bed rest or hospitalization in multiples [99]. A Cochrane database review of six randomized trials involving over 600 multiples demonstrated a trend toward a decrease in low birthweight infants and a paradoxical increased risk of delivery at less than 34 weeks gestation with inpatient bed rest [100]. In addition, prophylactic bed rest may be associated with adverse complications such as thromboembolic disease.

Administration of prophylactic tocolytic agents has been attempted but has not been beneficial. Women with multifetal pregnancies appear to be particularly prone to developing pulmonary edema and cardiovascular complications after administration of β-adrenergic agents because of their higher blood volume and lower colloid osmotic pressure [101]. As such, it seems prudent to restrict the use of those agents when indicated.

Ambulatory home monitoring of uterine contractions with a tocodynamometer in an attempt to predict preterm labor has not been shown to be useful. A meta-analysis of six randomized trials was unable to demonstrate a significant benefit of home uterine activity monitoring to reduce the risk of preterm delivery in patients with twins [102]. Furthermore, a prospective trial of 2422 patients (including 844 twins) randomized women to weekly nurse contact, daily nurse contact, or daily nurse contact in addition to home uterine activity monitoring and demonstrated no difference in preterm delivery prior to 35 weeks gestation [103].

Several studies have investigated the role of 17-hyrdoxy progesterone caproate in multiple gestations to prevent preterm birth. However, these studies have showed no evidence of benefit; thus, it is currently not recommended on the indication of multiple gestation [104]. Similarly, vaginal progesterone administration for unselected twin gestations have not been proved to be beneficial [105]. Cervical pessary has not been proven to prevent preterm birth in unselected twin pregnancies [106–108].

Antenatal surveillance

Although it is prudent to follow fetal growth with serial ultrasound scans, it is unclear if routine antenatal testing in patients with an uncomplicated multiple gestation improves outcomes. Antenatal testing is suggested in all patients with multiple gestations complicated by FGR, discordant growth, abnormal amniotic fluid volumes, TTTS, monoamnionicity, fetal anomalies, single IUFD, and other medical or obstetric complications (Box 38.3). For women with uncomplicated twin gestation, antenatal testing can be considered at 36 weeks weekly, and for uncomplicated monochorionic twin gestation at 32 weeks weekly [109]. When patients with a multiple gestation present for antenatal testing or labor monitoring, each fetal heart rate should be independently identified to ensure precision. Monitoring of triplets and high-order multiples may require frequent sonographic identification of the appropriate fetus.

Box 38.3 Ultrasound management of patients with twins

- Ideally, ultrasound is performed in the first trimester to determine the number of fetuses, amnionicity, and chorionicity. Patients are also offered nuchal translucency ultrasound at 10–14 wk gestation.
- A detailed ultrasound is scheduled at 18–20 wk gestation. This includes standard biometry, assessment of amniotic fluid volume in each sac, and an anatomic survey of each fetus. If the patient did not have a first-trimester ultrasound, an attempt is made to determine chorionicity by examining fetal gender, the number of placentas, the thickness as well as number of layers in the membrane separating the sacs, and the presence or absence of the lambda or twin peak sign.
- If a dichorionic pregnancy, fetal growth is performed every 3–4 wk if an uncomplicated gestation, as long as fetal growth and amniotic fluid volume in each sac remain normal.
- If the initial scan is suggestive of a monochorionic diamniotic pregnancy, subsequent scans are repeated every 2 wk to follow for signs of TTTS. Fetal echocardiography is offered to patients with monochorionic twins because these pregnancies may be at increased risk for congenital heart defects.
- In either dichorionic or monochorionic pregnancies, if there is evidence of FGR, discordant fetal growth, or discordant fluid volumes, fetal surveillance is intensified and includes frequent nonstress tests along with biophysical profile and Doppler velocimetry studies in cases of FGR.
- Antenatal testing can be considered for uncomplicated dichorionic diamniotic twins starting at 36 wk at weekly intervals
- Antenatal testing can be considered for uncomplicated monochorionic diamniotic twins starting at 32 wk at weekly intervals
- Antenatal testing for dichorionic diamniotic twins or monochorionic diamniotic twins complicated by fetal or maternal disorders, or monochorionic monoamniotic twins should be individualized.

FGR, fetal growth restriction; IUFD, intrauterine fetal death; TTTS, twin–twin transfusion syndrome.

Routine Doppler studies have not been found to be helpful in the management of women with multiple gestations [110]. However, when FGR or growth discordance is suspected in one or more fetuses, Doppler velocimetry of the umbilical artery is a useful adjunct in assessing and following these pregnancies. Furthermore, in cases of monochorionic twins with FGR, discordant growth, or amniotic fluid volume abnormalities, Doppler studies of the ductus venosus may be helpful in identifying the possible overlapping pathologies of uteroplacental insufficiency and cardiac dysfunction.

Intrapartum period

A number of factors must be considered when determining the mode of delivery for patients with multiple gestations. These variables include the gestational age and estimated weights of the fetuses, their positions, the availability of real-time ultrasound on the labor floor and in the delivery room, the capability of monitoring each twin independently during the entire intrapartum period, and the health care provider experience. When both twins are vertex, vaginal delivery is possible. During the time period between the delivery of the first and second twin, it is important to demonstrate reassuring status of the undelivered twin as evidenced by continuous fetal heart rate monitoring or by ultrasound. If the presenting twin is nonvertex, cesarean delivery is suggested. Management of vertex/nonvertex twins is variable. Vaginal delivery of a breech second twin with an EFW of 1500–3500 g in a patient with an adequate pelvis is reasonable. Cesarean delivery may be the preferred route of delivery if there is significant growth discordance between the twins or if the provider does not have adequate experience with such deliveries. Some obstetricians have had favorable experiences delivering triplets vaginally. Nonetheless, most providers deliver triplets and higher-order multiples by cesarean because continuous fetal heart rate monitoring of triplets and higher order multiples in labor is challenging [3,71].

Conclusion

Advances in fertility treatment and delayed childbearing have resulted in a substantial increase in the incidence of multiple gestations. The high perinatal morbidity and mortality rates associated with multiple gestations are the result of a variety of factors, some of which cannot be altered. Nonetheless, technologic advances in recent years have given us new insights into problems particular to multifetal pregnancies as well as tools with which to detect and try to mitigate these risks. Early diagnosis of multiple gestations, serial ultrasound surveillance and close prenatal care are important steps in the management of these high-risk pregnancies.

CASE PRESENTATION

A 38-year-old gravida 1 with twins in the moderate preterm gestation presented to a routine prenatal care visit and reported an "upset stomach" the previous weekend. Her prenatal course was significant for a history of polycystic ovarian syndrome and an initial quadruplet pregnancy conceived with ovulation induction and intrauterine insemination. She had elected to have CVS and subsequent MPR to a dichorionic twin gestation. During a routine anatomic ultrasound survey at 20 weeks, the patient was noted to have a short cervix measuring 24 mm. Preterm labor precautions were reviewed, and serial cervical length measurements were scheduled. At 28 weeks gestation, the patient was diagnosed with gestational diabetes which subsequently required insulin for glycemic control.

At her office visit at 30w 6d gestation, the patient's blood pressure was 150/92 mmHg and a urine dipstick revealed 2+ proteinuria. She was admitted and corticosteroids were administered to assist fetal lung maturation. After 72 hours of hospitalization, a 24-hour urine collection revealed 6 g protein and the patient developed unremitting epigastric pain. Laboratory evaluation revealed a platelet count of 70, liver enzymes of 530 and 478, and a lactic dehydrogenase of 990; the findings were consistent with HELLP syndrome. A bedside ultrasound revealed the fetal presentations to be cephalic/breech. The cervix was 3 cm dilated with a Bishop score of 8. However, a 38% twin weight discordance had been estimated during a routine scan at 30 weeks, with a higher EFW for twin B.

Immediate delivery was recommended, and the risks and benefits of attempted vaginal delivery and cesarean were discussed. The patient underwent an uncomplicated, primary low transverse cesarean delivery. Vigorous male and female infants were born. Although each neonate spent a brief period in the NICU, they were both discharged home after 2 weeks. There were no postpartum maternal complications, and the patient was discharged home on postoperative day 4.

This case highlights many of the common features of multiple pregnancy, including assisted conception, MPR, medical and obstetric complications, and preterm delivery. While the outcome for the majority of multiple gestations is favorable, these high-risk pregnancies can be associated with maternal and neonatal morbidity and mortality and thus warrant increased vigilance.

References

1. Hamilton BE, Martin JA, Osterman MJ. Births: provisional data for 2019. Vital Statistics Rapid Release, no. 8. Hyattsville, MD: National Center for Health Statistics; 2020 [cited 2023 Jun 8]. Available from: https://www.cdc.gov/nchs/data/vsrr/vsrr-8-508.pdf.

2. Beato CV. Healthy People 2010 progress report: maternal, infant, and child health. Washington, DC: US Department of Health and Human Services; 2003.

3. American College of Obstetricians and Gynecologists. ACOG Practice Bulletin No. 231; multiple gestation: complicated twin, triplet, and high-order multifetal pregnancy. Obstet Gynecol. 2021;137:e145–62.

4. Martin JA, Hamilton BE, Osterman MJ, Driscoll AK. Births: final data for 2019. Natl Vital Stat Rep. 2021 Apr 1;70(2):1–51.

5. Martin JA, Hamilton BE, Ventura SJ, Menacker F, Park MM, Sutton PD. Births: final data for 2001. Natl Vital Stat Rep. 2001;51:1–102.

6. Nielson HC, Harvey-Wilkes K, MacKinnon B, Hung S. Neonatal outcome of very premature infants from multiple and singleton gestations. Am J Obstet Gynecol. 1997; 177:653–9.

7. Kaufman GE, Malone FD, Harvey-Wilkes KB, Chelmow D, Penzias AS, D'Alton ME. Neonatal morbidity and mortality associated with triplet pregnancy. Obstet Gynecol. 1998; 91:342–8.

8. Topp M, Huusom LD, Langhoff-Roos J, Delhumeau C, Hutton JL, Dolk H; SCPE Collaborative Group. Multiple birth and cerebral palsy in Europe: a multicenter study. Acta Obstet Gynecol Scand. 2004;83:548–53.

9. American College of Obstetricians and Gynecologists. Neonatal encephalopathy and cerebral palsy: defining the pathogenesis and pathophysiology. Washington, DC: American College of Obstetricians and Gynecologists; 2003.

10. Yokoyama Y, Shimizu T, Hayakawa K. Prevalence of cerebral palsy in twins, triplets and quadruplets. Int J Epidemiol. 1995;24:943–8.

11. Russell EM. Cerebral palsied twins. Arch Dis Child. 1961;36:328–36.

12. Benirschke K. The biology of the twinning process: how placentation influences outcome. Semin Perinatol. 1995; 19:342–50.

13. Souter VL, Kapur RP, Nyholt DR, Skogerboe K, Myerson D, Ton CC, et al. A report of dizygous monochorionic twins. N Engl J Med 2003;349:154–8.

14. Miura K, Niikawa NJ. Do monochorionic dizygotic twins increase after pregnancy by assisted reproductive technology? Hum Genet. 2005;50:1–6.

15. Barth RA, Crowe HC. Ultrasound evaluation of multifetal gestations. In: Callen PW, editor. Ultrasonography in obstetrics and gynecology. 4th ed. Philadelphia: WB Saunders; 2000. p.171.

16. Bromley B, Benacerraf B. Using the number of yolk sacs to determine amnionicity in early first trimester monochorionic twins. J Ultrasound Med. 1995;14:415–19.

17. Bessis R, Papiernik E. Echographic imagery of amniotic membranes in twin pregnancies. In: Gedda L, Parisi P, editors.

Twin research 3: twin biology and multiple pregnancy. New York: Alan R. Liss, 1981. p.183.

18. Finberg HJ. The "twin peak" sign: reliable evidence of dichorionic twinning. J Ultrasound Med. 1992;11:571–7.

19. Monteagudo A, Timor-Tritsch IE, Sharma S. Early and simple determination of chorionic and amniotic type in multifetal gestations in the first fourteen weeks by high-frequency transvaginal ultrasonography. Am J Obstet Gynecol. 1994; 170:824–9.

20. Sepulveda W, Seibre NJ, Hughes K, Odibo A, Nicolaides KH. The lambda sign at 10–14 weeks of gestation as a predictor of chorionicity in twin pregnancies. Ultrasound Obstet Gynecol. 1996;7:421–3.

21. Egan JFX, Borgida AF. Multiple gestations: the importance of ultrasound. Obstet Gynecol Clin North Am. 2004;31:141–58.

22. Nyberg DA, Filly RA, Golbus MS, Stephens JD. Entangled umbilical cords: a sign of monoamniotic twins. J Ultrasound Med. 1984;3:29–32.

23. Breathnach FM, McAuliffe FM, Geary M, Daly S, Higgins JR, Dornan J, et al. Definition of intertwin birth weight discordance. Obstet Gynecol. 2011 Jul 1;118(1):94–103.

24. Demissie K, Ananth CV, Martin J, Hanley ML, MacDorman MF, Rhoads GG. Fetal and neonatal mortality among twin gestations in the United States: the role of intrapair birth weight discordance. Obstet Gynecol 2002;100:474–80.

25. Blickstein I, Keith LG. Neonatal mortality rates among growth-discordant twins, classified according to the birth weight of the smaller twin. Am J Obstet Gynecol. 2004;190:170–4.

26. Amaru RC, Bush MC, Berkowitz RL, Lapinski RH, Gaddipati S. Is discordant growth in twins an independent risk factor for adverse neonatal outcome? Obstet Gynecol. 2004;103:71–6.

27. Landy HJ, Keith L, Keith D. The vanishing twin. Acta Genet Med Gemellol (Roma). 1982;31:179–94.

28. Cleary-Goldman J, D'Alton M. Management of single fetal demise in a multiple gestation. Obstet Gynecol Surv. 2004; 59:285–98.

29. Lee YM, Wylie BJ, Simpson LL, D'Alton ME. Twin chorionicity and the risk of stillbirth. Obstet Gynecol. 2008;111:301–8.

30. Landry HJ, Weingold AB. Management of a multiple gestation complicated by antepartum fetal demise. Obstet Gynecol Surv. 1989;44:171–6.

31. Okamura K, Murotsuki J, Tanigawara S, Uehara S, Yajima A. Funipuncture for evaluation of hematologic and coagulation indices in the surviving twin following co-twins death. Obstet Gynecol. 1994;83:975–8.

32. Fusi L, McParland P, Fisk N, Wigglesworth J. Acute twin–twin transfusion: a possible mechanism for brain-damaged survivors after intrauterine death of a monochorionic twin. Obstet Gynecol. 1991;78:517–20.

33. Weiss JL, Cleary-Goldman J, Budorick N, Tanji K, D'Alton ME. Multicystic encephalomalacia after first trimester intrauterine fetal demise in monochorionic twins. Am J Obstet Gynecol. 2004;190:563–5.

34. Carlson N, Towers C. Multiple gestation complicated by the death of one fetus. Obstet Gynecol. 1989;73:685–9.

35. Onyskowova A, Dolezal A, Jedlicka V. The frequency and the character of malformations in multiple birth (a preliminary report). Teratology. 1971;4:496.

36. Hendricks CH. Twinning in relation to birth weight, mortality, and congenital anomalies. Obstet Gynecol. 1966;27:47–53.

37. Kohl SG, Casey G. Twin gestation. Mt Sinai J Med. 1975; 42:523–39.

38. Benirschke K, Kim CK. Multiple pregnancy [first of two parts]. N Engl J Med. 1973;288:1276–84.

39. Spadola AC, Simpson LL. Selective termination procedures in monochorionic pregnancies. Semin Perinatol. 2005;29:330–7.

40. Malone FD, Craigo SD, Chelmow D, D'Alton ME. Outcome of twin gestations complicated by a single anomalous fetus. Obstet Gynecol. 1996;88:1–5.

41. Sebire NJ, Sepulveda W, Hughes KS, Noble P, Nicolaides KH. Management of twin pregnancies discordant for anencephaly. Br J Obstet Gynaecol. 1997;107:216–19.

42. Gul A, Cebecia A, Aslan H, Polat I, Sozen I, Ceylan Y. Perinatal outcomes of twin pregnancies discordant for major fetal anomalies. Fetal Diagn Ther. 2005;20:244–8.

43. D'Alton ME, Simpson LL. Syndromes in twins. Semin Perinatol. 1995;19:375–86.

44. Carr SR, Aronson MP, Coustan DR. Survival rates of monoamniotic twins do not decrease after 30 weeks' gestation. Am J Obstet Gynecol. 1990;163:719–22.

45. Rodis JF, McIlveen PF, Egan JF, Borgida AF, Turner GW, Campbell WA. Monoamniotic twins: improved perinatal survival with accurate prenatal diagnosis and antenatal fetal surveillance. Am J Obstet Gynecol. 1997;177:1046–9.

46. Allen VM, Windrim R, Barrett J, Ohlsson A. Management of monoamniotic twin pregnancies: a case series and systematic review of the literature. Br J Obstet Gynaecol. 2001;108:931–6.

47. Rogue H, Gillen-Goldstein J, Funai E, Young BK, Lockwood CJ. Perinatal outcomes in monoamniotic gestations. J Mat Fetal Neonatal Med. 2003;13:414–21.

48. Tessen JA, Zlatnik FJ. Monoamniotic twins: a retrospective controlled study. Obstet Gynecol. 1991;77:832–4.

49. American College of Obstetricians and Gynecologists. ACOG Committee Opinion No. 831: medically indicated late-preterm and early-term deliveries. Obstet Gynecol. 2021;138(1):e35–9.

50. Blickstein I. Estimation of iatrogenic monozygotic twinning rate following assisted reproduction: pitfalls and caveats. Am J Obstet Gynecol. 2005;192:365–8.

51. Simpson LL, Society for Maternal-Fetal Medicine. Twin–twin transfusion syndrome. Am J Obstet Gynecol. 2013 Jan 1;208(1):3–18.

52. Malone FD, D'Alton ME. Anomalies peculiar to multiple gestations. Clin Perinatol. 2000;27:1033–46.

53. Quintero RA, Morales WJ, Allen MH, Bornick PW, Johnson PK, Kruger M. Staging of twin–twin transfusion syndrome. J Perinatol. 1999;19:550–5.

54. Bajoria R, Wigglesworth J, Fisk NM. Angioarchitecture of monochorionic placentas in relation to the twin–twin transfusion syndrome. Am J Obstet Gynecol. 1995;172:856–63.

55. De Lia JE, Cruikshank DP, Keye WR Jr. Fetoscopic neodymium:YAG laser occlusion of placental vessels in severe twin–twin transfusion syndrome. Obstet Gynecol. 1990;75:1046.

56. Hecher K, Plath H, Bregenzer T, Hansmann M, Hackeloer BJ. Endoscopic laser surgery versus serial amniocenteses in the treatment of severe twin–twin transfusion syndrome. Am J Obstet Gynecol. 1999;180:717–24.

57. Quintero RA, Dickinson JE, Morales WJ, Bornick PW, Bermúdez C, Cincotta R, et al. Stage-based treatment of twin–twin transfusion syndrome. Am J Obstet Gynecol, 2003;188: 1333–40.

58. Senat MV, Deprest J, Boulvain M, Paupe A, Winer N, Ville Y. Endoscopic laser surgery versus serial amnioreduction for severe twin-to-twin transfusion syndrome. N Engl J Med. 2004;351:136–44.

59. Rossi AC, D'Addario V. Laser therapy and serial amnioreduction as treatment for twin-twin transfusion syndrome: a metaanalysis and review of literature. Am J Obstet Gynecol. 2008;198:147.

60. Devine PC, Malone FD, Athanassiou A, Harvey-Wilkes K, D'Alton ME. Maternal and neonatal outcome of 100 consecutive triplet pregnancies. Am J Perinatol. 2001;18:225–35.

61. Graham G, Simpson LL. Diagnosis and management of obstetrical complications unique to multiple gestations. Clin Obstet Gynecol. 2004;47:163–80.

62. Campbell DM, Templeton A. Maternal complications of twin pregnancy. Int J Gynaecol Obstet. 2004;84:71–3.

63. American College of Obstetricians and Gynecologists. ACOG Practice Bulletin No. 19: thromboembolism in pregnancy. Obstet Gynecol. 2000;96(2).

64. American College of Obstetricians and Gynecologists. ACOG Practice Bulletin No. 33: diagnosis and management of preeclampsia and eclampsia. Obstet Gynecol. 2002;99:159–67.

65. Sibai BM, Hauth J, Caritis S, Lindheimer MD, MacPherson C, Klebanoff M, et al. Hypertensive disorders in twin versus singleton gestations. National Institute of Child Health and Human Development Network of Maternal-Fetal Medicine Units. Am J Obstet Gynecol. 2000;182:938–42.

66. Caritis S, Sibai B, Hauth J, Lindheimer MD, Klebanoff M, Thom E, et al. Low-dose aspirin to prevent preeclampsia in women at high risk. National Institute of Child Health and Human Development Network of Maternal-Fetal Medicine Units. N Engl J Med. 1998;338:701–5.

67. American College of Obstetricians and Gynecologists. ACOG Committee Opinion No. 743: low-dose aspirin use during pregnancy. Obstet Gynecol. 2018;132:e44–52.

68. Levine RJ, Hauth JC, Curet LB, Sibai BM, Catalano PM, Morris CD, et al. Trial of calcium to prevent preeclampsia. N Engl J Med. 1997;337:69–76.

69. Hardardottir H, Kelly K, Bork MD, Cusick W, Campbell WA, Rodis JF. Atypical presentation of preeclampsia in high-order multifetal gestations. Obstet Gynecol. 1996;87:370–4.

70. Davidson KM, Simpson LL, Knox TA, D'Alton ME. Acute fatty liver of pregnancy in triplet gestation. Obstet Gynecol. 1998;91:806–8.

71. American College of Obstetricians and Gynecologists. ACOG Committee opinion no. 548: weight gain during pregnancy. Obstet Gynecol. 2013 Jan;121(1):210–2.

72. American College of Obstetricians and Gynecologists. ACOG Committee Opinion No. 719: multifetal pregnancy reduction. Obstet Gynecol. 2017;130:e158–63.

73. Stone J, Eddleman K, Lynch L, Berkowitz RL. A single center experience with 1000 consecutive cases of multifetal pregnancy reduction. Am J Obstet Gynecol. 2002;187:1163–7.

74. Malone FD, D'Alton ME. Anomalies peculiar to multiple gestations. Clin Perinatol. 2000;27:1033–46.

75. American College of Obstetricians and Gynecologists. ACOG Practice Bulletin No. 88: invasive prenatal testing for aneuploidy. Obstet Gynecol. 2007;110:1459–67.

76. Meyers C, Adam R, Dungan J, Prenger V. Aneuploidy in twin gestations: when is maternal age advanced? Obstet Gynecol. 1997;89:248–51.

77. Odibo AO, Elkousy MH, Ural SH et al. Screening for aneuploidy in twin pregnancies: maternal age- and race-specific risk assessment between 9–14 weeks. Twin Res. 2003;6:251–6.

78. Cleary-Goldman J, D'Alton ME, Berkowitz RL. Prenatal diagnosis and multiple pregnancy. Semin Perinatol. 2005;29:312–20.

79. Rogers JG, Voullaire L, Gold H. Monozygotic twins discordant for trisomy 21. Am J Med Genet. 1982;11:143–6.

80. Dallapiccola B, Stomeo C, Ferranti B, Di Lecce A, Purpura M. Discordant sex in one of three monozygotic triplets. J Med Genet. 1985;22:6–11.

81. Graham G, Simpson LL. Diagnosis and management of obstetrical complications unique to multiple gestations. Clin Obstet Gynecol. 2004;47:163–80.

82. Odibo AO, Lawrence-Cleary K, Macones GA. Screening for aneuploidy in twins and higher-order multiples: is first-trimester nuchal translucency the solution? Obstet Gynecol Surv. 2003;58:609–14.

83. Sebire NJ, D'Ercole C, Hughes K, Carvalho M, Nicolaides KH. Increased nuchal translucency thickness at 10–14 weeks of gestation as a predictor of severe twin-to-twin transfusion syndrome. Ultrasound Obstet Gynecol. 1997;10:86–9.

84. Malone FD, D'Alton ME, Society for Maternal-Fetal Medicine. First-trimester sonographic screening for Down syndrome. Obstet Gynecol. 2003;102:1066–79.

85. Prats P, Rodriguez I, Comas C, Puerto B. Systematic review of screening for trisomy 21 in twin pregnancies in first trimester combining nuchal translucency and biochemical markers: a meta-analysis. Prenat Diagn. 2014 Nov;34(11):1077–83.

86. Garchet-Beaudron A, Dreux S, Leporrier N, Oury JF, Muller F. Second-trimester Down syndrome maternal serum marker screening: a prospective study of 11040 twin pregnancies. Prenat Diagn. 2008 Dec;28(12):1105–9.

87. Galeva S, Gil MM, Konstantinidou L, Akolekar R, Nicolaides KH. First-trimester screening for trisomies by cfDNA testing of maternal blood in singleton and twin pregnancies: factors affecting test failure. Ultrasound Obstet Gynecol. 2019 Jun;53(6):804–9.

88. Agarwal K, Alfirevic Z. Pregnancy loss after chorionic villus sampling and genetic amniocentesis in twin pregnancies: a systematic review. Ultrasound Obstet Gynecol. 2012 Aug;40(2):128–34.

89. Edwards MS, Ellings JM, Newman RB, Menard MK. Predictive value of antepartum ultrasound examination for anomalies in twin gestations. Ultrasound Obstet Gynecol. 1995;6:43–9.

90. Bahtiyar MO, Dulay AT, Weeks BP, Friedman AH, Copel JA. Prevalence of congenital heart defects in monochorionic/diamniotic twin gestations: a systematic literature review. J Ultrasound Med. 2007;26(11):1491–8.

91. National Institutes of Health. National Institutes of Health Consensus Development Conference Statement: effect of corticosteroids for fetal maturation on perinatal outcomes, February 28–March 2, 1994. Am J Obstet Gynecol. 1995;173:246–52.

92. Mercer BM, Miodovnik M, Thurnau GR, Goldenberg RL, Das AF, Ramsey RD, et al. Antibiotic therapy for reduction of infant morbidity after preterm premature rupture of the membranes: a randomized controlled trial. JAMA. 1997;278:989–95.

93. Lovett SM, Weiss JD, Diogo MJ, Williams PT, Garite TJ. A prospective double-blind, randomized, controlled clinical trial of ampicillin-sulbactam for preterm premature rupture of membranes in women receiving antenatal corticosteroid therapy. Am J Obstet Gynecol. 1997;176:1030–8.

94. Rafael TJ, Berghella V, Alfirevic Z. Cervical stitch (cerclage) for preventing preterm birth in multiple pregnancy. Cochrane Database Syst Rev.2014 Sep 10;(9):CD009166. doi: 10.1002/14651858.CD009166.pub2.

95. Rust OA, Atlas RO, Reed J, van Gaalen J, Balducci J. Revisiting the short cervix detected by transvaginal ultrasound in the second trimester: why cerclage therapy may not help. Am J Obstet Gynecol. 2001 Nov 1;185(5):1098–105.

96. Althuisius SM, Dekker GA, Hummel P, Bekedam DJ, van Geijn HP. Final results of the Cervical Incompetence Prevention Randomized Cerclage Trial (CIPRACT): therapeutic cerclage with bed rest versus bed rest alone. Am J Obstet Gynecol. 2001 Nov 1;185(5):1106–12.

97. Berghella V, Odibo AO, Tolosa JE. Cerclage for prevention of preterm birth in women with a short cervix found on transvaginal ultrasound examination: a randomized trial. Am J Obstet Gynecol. 2004 Oct 1;191(4):1311–7.

98. Roman A, Zork N, Haeri S, Schoen CN, Saccone G, Colihan S, et al. Physical examination-indicated cerclage in twin pregnancy: a randomized controlled trial. Am J Obstet Gynecol. 2020 Dec 1;223(6):902–e1.

99. Saunders MC, Dick JS, Brown IM, McPherson K, Chalmers I. The effects of hospital admission for bed rest on the duration of twin pregnancy: a randomized trial. Lancet. 1985;2:793–5.

100. Crowther CA. Hospitalisation and bed rest for multiple pregnancy. Cochrane Database Syst Rev. 2001;(1):CD000110. doi: 10.1002/14651858.CD000110. Update in: Cochrane Database Syst Rev. 2010;(7):CD000110. doi: 10.1002/14651858.CD000110.pub2.

101. Katz M, Robertson PA, Creasy RK. Cardiovascular complications associated with terbutaline treatment for preterm labor. Am J Obstet Gynecol. 1981;139:605–8.

102. Colton T, Kayne HL, Zhang Y, Heeren TA. A metaanalysis of home uterine activity monitoring. Am J Obstet Gynecol. 1995; 173:1499–505.

103. Dyson DC, Danbe KH, Bamber JA, Crites YM, Field DR, Maier JA, et al. Monitoring women at risk for preterm labor. N Engl J Med. 1998;338:15–19.

104. Dodd JM, Grivell RM, OBrien CM, Dowswell T, Deussen AR. Prenatal administration of progestogens for preventing spontaneous preterm birth in women with a multiple pregnancy. Cochrane Database Syst Rev. 2017 Oct 31;10(10):CD012024. doi: 10.1002/14651858.CD012024.pub2. Update in: Cochrane Database Syst Rev. 2019 Nov 20;2019(11):CD012024. doi: 10.1002/14651858.CD012024.pub3.

105. Rehal A, Benkő Z, Matallana CD, Syngelaki A, Janga D, Cicero S, et al. Early vaginal progesterone versus placebo in twin pregnancies for the prevention of spontaneous preterm birth: a randomized, double-blind trial. Am J Obstet Gynecol. 2021 Jan 1;224(1):86–e1.

106. Conde-Agudelo A, Romero R, Nicolaides KH. Cervical pessary to prevent preterm birth in asymptomatic high-risk women: a systematic review and meta-analysis. Am J Obstet Gynecol. 2020;223(1): 42–65.

107. Goya M, De La Calle M, Pratcorona L, Merced C, Rodó C, Muñoz B, et al. Cervical pessary to prevent preterm birth in women with twin gestation and sonographic short cervix: a multicenter randomized controlled trial (PECEP-Twins). Am J Obstet Gynecol. 2016 Feb 1;214(2):145–52.

108. Liem S, Schuit E, Hegeman M, Bais J, De Boer K, Bloemenkamp K, et al. Cervical pessaries for prevention of preterm birth in women with a multiple pregnancy (ProTWIN): a multicentre, open-label randomised controlled trial. Lancet. 2013 Oct 19; 382(9901):1341–9.

109. American College of Obstetricians and Gynecologists. ACOG Committee Opinion No. 828. indications for outpatient antenatal fetal surveillance. Obstet Gynecol. 2021 Jun 1;137(6): e177–97.

110. Giles W, Bisits A, O'Callahan S, Gill A, DAMP Study Group. The Doppler assessment in multiple pregnancy randomised controlled trial of ultrasound biometry versus umbilical artery Doppler ultrasound and biometry in twin pregnancy. Br J Obstet Gynaecol. 2003;110:593–7.

Chapter 39
Polyhydramnios and Oligohydramnios

Ron Beloosesky[1] and Michael G. Ross[2]

[1] Department of Obstetrics and Gynecology, Rambam Health Care Campus and Ruth and Bruce Rappaport Faculty of Medicine, Technion, Haifa, Israel

[2] Department of Obstetrics, Gynecology and Public Health, UCLA School of Medicine and Public Health and Harbor-UCLA Medical Center, Torrance, CA, USA

All that fluid which is contained in the ovum is called by the general name of the waters. The quantity, in proportion to the size of the different parts of the ovum, is greatest by far in early pregnancy. At the time of parturition, in some cases, it amounts to or exceeds four pints. In others, it is scarcely equal to as many ounces. It is usually in the largest quantity when the child has been some time dead, or is born in a weakly state. (T. Denman, 1815)

In 1815, Denman recognized the great variation in amniotic fluid (AF) volume and associated polyhydramnios with congenital malformations, fetal death, and fetal disease [1]. Although our current knowledge of the intrauterine environment has expanded many fold, we have affirmed the majority of Denman's concepts (1). Polyhydramnios and oligohydramnios are pathologic conditions representing excess AF and diminished AF, respectively. Numerous serious clinical conditions are associated with polyhydramnios and oligohydramnios. An understanding of the normal AF parameters and the AF turnover is necessary before embarking on the pathologic considerations.

Normal amniotic fluid composition and volume

During the first trimester, AF is isotonic with maternal plasma [2] but contains minimal protein. It is thought that the fluid arises either from a transudate of fetal plasma through nonkeratinized fetal skin or maternal plasma across the uterine decidua and/or placenta surface [3]. Thus, fetuses with renal agenesis may demonstrate normal first-trimester AF volumes. With advancing gestation, AF osmolality and sodium concentration decrease, a result of the mixture of dilute fetal urine and isotonic fetal lung liquid production. In comparison with the first half of pregnancy, AF osmolality decreases by 20–30 mOsm/kg with advancing gestation to levels approximately 85–90% of maternal serum osmolality [4]. Concentrations of AF urea, creatinine, and uric acid increase during the second half of pregnancy, resulting in AF concentrations of these urinary byproducts two to three times higher than found in fetal plasma [4]. Investigators have long been intrigued with the concept of quantitating the volume of AF. In 1972, Queenan et al., using dye dilution technique, measured the AF volumes in 187 samples from 115 patients with normal pregnancies [5]. The volumes varied widely for the various weeks of gestation. The mean volumes were 239 mL at 25–26 weeks, 984 mL at 33–34 weeks (the peak volume), 836 mL at term, and 544 mL at 41–42 weeks (Figure 39.1).

Brace and Wolf analyzed AF volumes in 12 published studies including 705 normal pregnancies at 8–43 weeks gestation [6]. They found that average AF volume rises linearly from early gestation until 32 weeks, whereupon it remains relatively constant until term, ranging between 700 and 800 mL. After 40 weeks, AF volume declines at a rate of 8% a week, to an average of 400 mL at 42 weeks. At 30 weeks gestation, the 95% confidence intervals about the mean (817 mL) are 318 to 2100 mL. Thus, a volume <318 mL may be considered oligohydramnios and >2100 mL polyhydramnios. The wide biologic variability in the AF volume with advancing gestational age, especially before 32–35 weeks, as well as the difficulty in measuring volume make absolute volume criteria for oligohydramnios and polyhydramnios inappropriate. Accordingly, AF volume abnormalities are best defined as a volume < 5th percentile or > 95th percentile for gestational age.

Dynamics of amniotic fluid turnover

Amniotic fluid is produced and resorbed in a dynamic process with large volumes of water circulated between the AF and fetal compartments. During the latter half of

Queenan's Management of High-Risk Pregnancy: An Evidence-Based Approach, Seventh Edition. Edited by Catherine Y. Spong and Charles J. Lockwood.

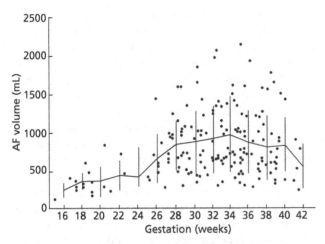

Figure 39.1 Normal amniotic fluid (AF) volumes are plotted against weeks of gestation. The mean values ± 1 SD are calculated for each 2-wk period. Adapted from [5].

gestation, the primary sources of AF include fetal urine excretion and fetal lung secretion. The primary pathways for water exit from the AF include removal by fetal swallowing and intramembranous absorption across the fetal membranes into fetal blood. If the balance of fluid exchange is disturbed, polyhydramnios or oligohydramnios develops. For instance, if a pathologic condition increased the AF volume by 1 oz or 30 mL/day, 1 L of excess AF would accumulate in a month.

Fetal urine

Fetal micturition is known to be the major source of AF. Chez et al. [7] studied fetal urine production with indwelling catheters in rhesus monkeys and reported a rate of 5 mL/kg/h, which correlates with the rate of swallowing observed in human fetuses by Pritchard [8]. In humans, fetal urine production changes with increasing gestation. The amount of urine produced by the human fetus has been estimated by the use of ultrasound measurements of fetal bladder volume [9], although the accuracy of these measurements has been called into question. Exact human fetal urine production rates across gestation are not established but appear to be in the range of 25% of body weight per day or nearly 1000 mL/day near term [7,9].

Kurjak et al. studied fetal renal function in 255 normal singleton pregnancies and 133 complicated pregnancies between 22 and 41 weeks gestation [10]. They evaluated the hourly fetal urine production rate (HFUPR), fetal glomerular filtration rate (GFR), fetal tubular water reabsorption (TWR), and the effect of furosemide on fetal micturition by sonography and biochemical tests. In normal pregnancies, the HFUPR increased from 2.2 mL/h at 22 weeks to 26.3 mL/h at 40 weeks gestation. The fetal GFR was 2.66 mL/min at term and the percentage of TWR was 78%. In growth-restricted fetuses, the HFUPR

was below the 10th percentile in 59% and above normal in only 6% of cases. The diuretic effect of furosemide was the same in growth-restricted and normal fetuses. In diabetic pregnancies, HFUPR values varied considerably and correlated with fetal size. In 90% of pregnancies with polyhydramnios, the HFUPR was normal.

Oligohydramnios is associated with severe malformations of the fetal urinary system (e.g. renal agenesis), which is incompatible with urine production. In a review of 295 fetuses with renal agenesis, Jeffcoate and Scott found sufficient clinical data in 100 cases to establish a diagnosis of oligohydramnios [11]. From these data, the investigators inferred that conditions affecting fetal urine production would alter the AF volume. On the other hand, they also reported renal agenesis in a fetus with polyhydramnios. Others have reported renal agenesis and normal AF volume [12,13] suggesting that fluid arises from other sites.

Fetal lung fluid

All mammalian fetuses normally secrete fluid from their lungs. In the human, AF clearly contains phospholipids, such as lecithin and sphingomyelin derived from type II alveolar cells; thus, at least some tracheal fluid contributes to AF volume. Liley described some 800 mothers who had radiologic contrast media injected into the AF and noted that only four had media demonstrated in fetal or neonatal lungs [14].

The absolute rate of fluid production by the human fetal lungs has not been determined, although animal studies suggest that the respiratory tract has a major role in AF production. Goodlin and Lloyd demonstrated that the fetal lamb produces 50–80 mL/day of tracheal fluid [15]. Adamson et al. reported that the near term lamb has tracheal secretions of 200–400 mL/day [16]. Tracheal ligation in animals leads to overdistension of the lungs, suggesting a relatively large outflow of fluid from the lungs. This knowledge has been used in the development of therapeutic approaches to the in utero treatment of diaphragmatic hernia; tracheal occlusion results in pulmonary distension despite the presence of a thoracic mass. Under physiologic conditions, half of the fluid exiting the lungs enters the AF and half is swallowed [17]; therefore, an average of approximately 165 mL/day lung liquid enters the AF near term.

Fetal lung fluid production is affected by physiologic and endocrine factors, but nearly all these factors have been demonstrated to reduce fetal lung liquid production, with no evidence of factors that stimulate production or induce nominal changes in fluid composition. Increased arginine vasopressin [18], catecholamines [19], and cortisol [20] decrease lung fluid production. The marked increase in fetal plasma levels of these hormones during labor results in a cessation of lung fluid production, after which lung liquid is resorbed into pulmonary lymphatics to prepare for the newborn for physiologic respiration.

Fetal swallowing

Swallowing is the major pathway for AF removal. Evidence of fetal swallowing of AF was established many years ago by amniography. Studies of near-term pregnancies suggest that the human fetus swallows an average of 210–760 mL/day [21], which is considerably less than the volume of urine produced each day. However, fetal swallowing may be reduced beginning a few days before delivery [22], so the rate of human fetal swallowing is probably underestimated. Fetal swallowing is increased during active (i.e. rapid eye movement [REM] sleep) as compared with quiet sleep states. Furthermore, the near-term fetus develops functional ingestive responses such that fetal swallowing may increase in response to thirst or appetite stimulation. Of note, fetal swallowing decreases with acute arterial hypotension [23] or hypoxia [17,24], indicating that oligohydramnios associated with fetal hypoxia is not caused by increased AF resorption via swallowing.

The effect of fetal swallowing can be demonstrated by studying mothers who have delivered babies with tracheo-esophageal fistulas. Of 228 such cases, 25 fetuses had complete obstruction between the mouth and the stomach and 19 (76%) of these had polyhydramnios [25]. In a study of 169 cases of polyhydramnios, 54 (32%) of the fetuses were unable to swallow [11].

Anencephaly is also associated with a high incidence of polyhydramnios. Although swallowing has been demonstrated in some of these fetuses, it is reasonable to believe that the swallowing capability is reduced or absent in many. The exposed meninges in anencephaly have been described as the source of the production of the excess AF [26]. Other authors disagree [27], noting that the rudimentary and distorted brain is almost always covered with a collagen membrane. They proposed that fetal polyuria may contribute to the observed polyhydramnios because anencephalic fetuses lack antidiuretic hormone. Naeye et al. also suggested that polyuria of the anencephalic fetus causes polyhydramnios [28].

The importance of swallowing in controlling AF volume remains undefined. An inability to swallow in the setting of esophageal atresia but not in anencephaly appears to result in polyhydramnios in some cases.

Intramembranous flow

The amount of fluid swallowed by the fetus does not equal the amount of fluid produced by both the kidneys and the lungs in either human or ovine gestation. As the volume of AF does not greatly increase during the last half of pregnancy, another route of fluid absorption is needed. The intramembranous (IM) pathway refers to the route of absorption between the fetal circulation and the amniotic cavity directly across the amnion. Although the contribution of the IM pathway to overall regulation and maintenance of AF volume and composition has yet to be completely understood, results from in vivo and in vitro studies of ovine membrane permeability suggest that permeability of the fetal chorioamnion is important in determining AF composition and volume [29–31]. This IM flow, recirculating AF water to the fetal compartment, is thought to be driven by the significant osmotic gradient between the hypotonic AF and isotonic fetal plasma [32]. In addition, electrolytes (e.g. Na^+) may diffuse down a concentration gradient from fetal plasma into the AF while peptides (e.g., arginine vasopressin) and other electrolytes (e.g. Cl^-) may be recirculated to the fetal plasma. Studies have demonstrated the expression of aquaporins (AQP; 1, 3, 8, and 9), which are cell membrane proteins that serve as water channels, in human chorioamniotic membranes and placenta. The expression of AQP8 and AQP9 mRNA and protein was significantly increased in the amnion and placenta of patients with polyhydramnios, suggesting that aquaporins may play an important role in the regulation of amniotic fluid resorption via the IM pathway [33–36]. In contrast, when measured in amniotic fluid of patients with polyhydramnios, AQP-3 levels tended to be decreased whereas AQP-8 levels were decreased from midgestation [37].

Although never directly measured in humans, indirect evidence supports the presence of IM flow. Studies of intraamniotic ^{51}Cr injection demonstrated appearance of the tracer in the circulation of fetuses with impaired swallowing [38]. Additionally, alterations in IM flow may contribute to AF clinical abnormalities, as membrane ultrastructure changes are noted with polyhydramnios or oligohydramnios [39]. Experimental estimates of the net IM flow average 200–250 mL/day in fetal sheep and likely this balances the flow of urine and lung liquid with fetal swallowing under homeostatic conditions.

Amniotic fluid turnover

The AF is constantly recirculating. When diffusion of water is measured, approximately 500 mL water enters and leaves the amniotic sac each hour [40], with little effect on the total AF volume. However, estimates of actual bulk flow of water suggest that approximately 1000 mL/day enter and leave the amniotic cavity at term [41]. This results in a turnover of the entire volume of AF each day.

Clinical measurement of amniotic fluid

A few decades ago, AF volume was estimated in crude ways such as measurement of fundal height, roentgenographic, or direct measurement at the time of delivery. The para-aminohippuric dye dilution technique provides an accurate measurement but is an invasive technique and therefore limited to research settings [42].

Ultrasound examination is the only practical clinical means of assessing the AF volume. Several ultrasound methods have been used to estimate the AF volume; each has limitations in the detection of abnormal AF volumes. These methods can better identify true normal AF volumes than the presence of abnormal AF volumes (oligohydramnios and polyhydramnios), which they all detect poorly.

The single deepest pocket (SDP) measurement refers to the vertical dimension of the largest pocket of AF not containing umbilical cord or fetal extremities and measured at a right angle to the uterine contour. The horizontal component of this vertical dimension must be at least 1 cm. A normal SDP measurement is 2.1–8 cm, with oligohydramnios defined as <2.0 cm and polyhydramnios as >8.0 cm. In a comparison of SDP with dye-determined AF volume, SDP identifies patients with oligohydramnios poorly [43,44].

The amniotic fluid index (AFI) is measured by first dividing the uterus into four quadrants using the linea nigra for the right and left divisions and the umbilicus for the upper and lower quadrants. The maximum vertical AF pocket diameter in each quadrant not containing cord or fetal extremities is measured in centimeters; the sum of these measurements is the AFI. A normal AFI is 5 to <24 cm [45], with oligohydramnios defined as ≤5.0 cm and polyhydramnios as 24 cm or more. Borderline low normal values are 5.1–8.0 cm. The accuracy of the AFI has been examined in several studies [43,46–49]. In comparison to dye dilution technique, the sonographic AFI overestimated actual volumes by 89% at low volumes and underestimated actual volumes by 54% at high volumes. Chauhan et al. demonstrated that the sensitivity, specificity, positive, and negative predictive values of AFI ≤5 for prediction of oligohydramnios were 5%, 98%, 80%, and 49%, respectively; these same characteristics for AFI >24 for prediction of polyhydramnios were 30%, 98%, 57%, and 93%, respectively [48]. Notably, AFI standards have been demonstrated using grayscale ultrasound. When color flow Doppler is used for AFI determination, oligohydramnios may be overdiagnosed due to more frequent visualization of umbilical cord [50–52].

The two-diameter AF pocket is the product of the vertical depth multiplied by the horizontal diameter of the largest pocket of AF not containing umbilical cord or extremities (with the transducer held at a right angle to the uterine contour). A normal two-dimensional measurement is 15.1–50 cm^2, with oligohydramnios defined as <15 cm^2 and polyhydramnios as >50 cm^2. Two series compared the two-diameter pocket to dye-determined AF volume and found the former identified 81–94% of dye-determined normal volumes and about 60% of pregnancies with low volumes [39,47]. Receiver operator curve analysis showed that for any specific two-diameter pocket, the 95% confidence range was so wide that ultrasonographic assessment was not a reasonable reflection of actual AF volume, and thus was not clinically useful [48].

Subjective assessment of AF volume refers to visual interpretation without sonographic measurements [53]. The ultrasonographer scans the uterine contents and subsequently reports the AF volume as oligohydramnios, normal, or polyhydramnios. One study involving 63 pregnancies compared the subjective assessment of AF volume with semiquantitative measurement of AFI, the SDP technique, and the two-diameter pocket method in estimating dye-determined AF volume [53]. The subjective assessment of AF volume by an experienced examiner had similar sensitivity to other techniques in identifying dye-determined AF volumes. Thus, although a qualitative assessment of mild, moderate, or severe polyhydramnios can be made initially, we recommend a quantitative approach because it provides a measurement that can be compared over serial examinations. Both SDP and AFI are accepted standards for diagnosis and clinical management. Although these tests perform relatively poorly against quantitative measurements using dye dilution (research studies), they correlate with adverse outcomes and thus have clinical utility. It appears that the SDP overdiagnoses polyhydramnios compared with AFI whereas AFI may overdiagnose oligohydramnios when compared with SDP [54].

All obstetric ultrasound examinations should include an assessment of AF volume. Although the ultrasonographer may elect to use only a subjective assessment, we recommend use of an objective measure (e.g. AFI) if the subjective assessment is abnormal, in patients at increased risk of pregnancy complications, and in all patients examined in the third trimester.

Polyhydramnios

Definition

Historically, polyhydramnios has been characterized by an excessive accumulation of AF, usually >2000 mL. However, this definition does incorporate normal physiologic changes in the volume of AF as gestational weeks change. There is a progressive increase in AF volume from a mean of 30 mL at 10 weeks to 190 mL at 16 weeks, peaking at 780 mL at 32–35 weeks gestation; thereafter, AF volume progressively decreases to approximately 550 mL at 42 weeks [6]. The wide biologic variability in AF volume with advancing gestation makes an absolute volume criterion for oligohydramnios or polyhydramnios inappropriate. Accordingly, AF volume abnormalities are best defined as a volume < 5th percentile or > 95th percentile for gestational age, respectively.

Diagnosis

Polyhydramnios generally presents in the late second to early third trimester. The clinician may notice that the uterus is consistently larger than expected for gestation, or there may be a sudden increase in uterine size. The fetal parts may be difficult to palpate, and the fetal heart may be difficult to hear with Doppler ultrasound if the fetus moves about in the large volume of AF.

The diagnosis of polyhydramnios can be confirmed by sonography by quantifying AF volume. As noted, it is possible to make a qualitative judgment as to the presence or absence of polyhydramnios. At 16 weeks gestation, when genetic amniocentesis is commonly performed, the fetus and placenta each weigh approximately 100 g and the AF volume is 200 mL. Therefore, AF volume constitutes approximately 50% of the sonographic uterine image. At 28 weeks, when the fetus weighs 1000 g and the placenta weighs 200 g, AF volume is approximately 1000 mL and comprises approximately 45% of the image of the uterus. At term, when the fetus and placenta weigh 3300 and 500 g respectively, AF volume is approximately 800 mL and makes up only approximately 17% of the image of the uterus. Keeping these guidelines in mind will facilitate making a judgment about the normality of AF volume vs. the presence of polyhydramnios or oligohydramnios. In severe cases, the mere ultrasound image confirms the diagnosis because the findings are dramatic. Nonetheless, it is useful to have a quantifiable value such as the AFI. The diagnosis of polyhydramnios is established by an AFI ≥24 cm or vertical pocket ≥8 cm [45].

Polyhydramnios may have both maternal and fetal sequelae. In mild cases, there are minimal maternal symptoms, generally consisting of abdominal discomfort and slight dyspnea. In moderate-to-severe polyhydramnios (e.g. AF volume greater than 4000 mL), there may be marked respiratory distress: dyspnea and orthopnea and often edema of the lower extremities.

The increased AF volume and overstretched myometrium place the patient with polyhydramnios at risk of certain complications. Spontaneous labor with intact membranes usually produces contractions that are of poor quality because of the excessive uterine size. There is an increased incidence of abnormal fetal presentations and therefore more operative deliveries. Spontaneous rupture of the membranes causes a sudden decompression of the uterus, which increases the incidence of abruptio placentae and cord prolapse. There is a marked increase in the incidence of postpartum hemorrhage because of uterine overdistension, resulting in uterine atony. Fetal complications include myriad congenital anomalies or abnormalities that result in increased fluid production or reduced fluid resorption.

Associations

Clinically detectable polyhydramnios occurs in 0.4–0.5% of pregnancies. Most cases (35–66%) of mild polyhydramnios (e.g. AFI 25–30 cm) are idiopathic, and have a good prognosis, although the risks of preterm labor and fetal malpresentation remain. After birth an abnormality can be diagnosed in up to 25% of cases considered idiopathic [55]. With increasing degrees of AF volume, the rate of fetal anomalies approaches 50%. Polyhydramnios may be associated with diabetes mellitus, structural congenital malformations (usually of the central nervous system or gastrointestinal tract) impairing fetal swallowing, chromosomal abnormalities, multiple pregnancy (especially twin–twin transfusion syndrome or acardiac twinning), or maternal–fetal blood group incompatibilities. When associated with fetal hydrops, polyhydramnios may be a result of fetal cardiac abnormalities (structural and arrhythmias), aneuploidy, discrete genetic syndromes (e.g. inborn errors of metabolism, Pena–Shokeir, arthrogyposis syndromes), thoracic anomalies, skeletal dysplasias (e.g. thanatophoric dysplasia, short-rib polydactyly syndrome), lymphatic maldevelopment, anemia, infections (e.g. parvovirus B19, syphilis, toxoplasmosis, cytomegalovirus) or hypoproteinemia (e.g Finnish nephrosis). Once polyhydramnios is diagnosed, a systematic maternal workup is necessary to determine the cause. Management is determined by the underlying cause. The clinician should rule out such conditions as diabetes mellitus, erythroblastosis fetalis, and multiple pregnancy (e.g. twin–twin transfusion) by performing a glucose tolerance test, indirect Coombs test, and sonography, respectively.

In Queenan and Gadow's 1970 series of 358 patients with polyhydramnios, the major associated conditions were diabetes mellitus (25%), congenital malformations (20%), and erythroblastosis fetalis (11%) (Table 39.1) [56]. By 1987, the causes had changed considerably, according to Hill et al. [57]. The representation of diabetes mellitus was lower, reflecting stricter blood glucose control, and the occurrence of polyhydramnios resulting from rhesus (Rh) incompatibility was markedly decreased because of Rh immunoglobulin prophylaxis. Idris et al. recently reported an 18.8% incidence of polyhydramnios among patients with pregestational diabetes, with the AF excess associated with poor diabetes control [58]. Panting-Kemp et al. reported a 66% incidence of idiopathic polyhydramnios, with 4% of patients demonstrating a fetal congenital malformation and 28% with maternal diabetes mellitus [59]. In contrast Adams demonstrated 42% of polyhydramnios cases were idiopathic, whereas diabetes was

Table 39.1 Polyhydramnios: associated conditions

Causes	1970 [56]	1987 [57]	1999 [59]	2017 [61]	2020 [60]
Idiopathic (%)	35	66	66	80	42
Diabetes mellitus (%)	25	15	28	9	25
Congenital malformations (%)	21	13	4	11	23
Rh incompatibility (%)	11	1	-	-	-
Multiple pregnancy (%)	8	5	-	-	-
Macrosomia (%)					10

present in 25% of cases [60]. A recent study of 1545 patients with polyhydramnios found that only 8.5% of cases could be attributed to diabetes, and those patients usually had mild polyhydramnios [61]. The reduction in the rate of fetal malformations associated with polyhydramnios over time may represent a higher detection rate of the malformation by first and second-trimester ultrasound and termination of severe cases before reaching viability.

Evaluation

Following the diagnosis of polyhydramnios a detailed medical history should be obtained and screening for maternal diabetes, if not previously performed. A comprehensive sonographic evaluation should be undertaken for fetal anomalies. The likelihood of identifying the etiology of polyhydramnios prenatally correlates with severity of fluid accumulation. Measurement of peak systolic blood flow in the fetal middle cerebral artery is a sensitive test for the diagnosis of associated fetal anemia [62]. Genetic counseling and amniocentesis for fetal microarray should be offered to patients with a congenital anomaly or severe polyhydramnios. In pregnancies with a male fetus and unexplained severe polyhydramnios in the second trimester, especially with previous history of severe polyhydramnios, genetic studies for identification of mutations in *MAGED2*, which causes antenatal Bartter syndrome, should be offered [63].

Management

Treatment of polyhydramnios depends on the etiology and prognosis. Therapeutic amniocentesis is an option for the treatment of twin–twin transfusion syndrome. However, recent studies have indicated that fetoscopic laser ablation of the communicating blood vessels is of greater efficacy in severe cases presenting prior to fetal viability [64].

Conservative management includes modified bed rest and assessment of uterine activity and fetal well-being. Diuretics are generally contraindicated because they deplete maternal vascular volume with little effect on the total AF volume. If moderate-to-severe polyhydramnios results in pronounced maternal distress, and sonographic study reveals a normal-appearing fetus, a more aggressive approach becomes necessary. If the fetus is nearly

mature, delivery may be indicated. If the fetus is too immature for delivery, amniocentesis with drainage to normalize AF volume may be indicated. Complications of rapid removal of AF occur in 2–3% of procedures and include placental abruption and premature rupture of membranes [65–67]. Reaccumulation of AF may rapidly occur, and the procedure may need to be repeated every 2–3 days. A tocolytic agent should be considered to decrease the occurrence of uterine contractions. For severe symptomatic polyhydramnios at <32 weeks gestation because of shortness of breath, abdominal discomfort or increased uterine contractions we also consider a short course (48 hours) of indomethacin before and/or after the amnioreduction procedure to use both its tocolytic properties and antidiuretic effect to maintain normal AF volume without exposing the fetus to the risks of serial invasive procedures. Prostaglandin synthetase inhibitors may stimulate fetal secretion of arginine vasopressin and facilitate vasopressin-induced renal antidiuretic responses and reduced renal blood flow, thereby reducing fetal urine flow. These agents may also impair production or enhance reabsorption of lung liquid [68]. Indomethacin is started at 25 mg orally four times daily for 48 hours [69]. Maternal side effects, such as nausea, esophageal reflux, gastritis, and emesis, are seen in approximately 4% of patients treated with indomethacin for preterm labor. The primary fetal concern with use of indomethacin is constriction of the ductus arteriosus and recent information suggests an increased risk of intraventricular hemorrhage. Although the Society for Maternal-Fetal Medicine (SMFM) has recommended not using indomethacin for the sole purpose of decreasing amniotic fluid in these cases because of concerns about medication-related neonatal complications [45], we believe a short course with careful fetal observation may be considered.

If the fetus is found to have major malformations incompatible with life, delivery may be considered. For patients <34 weeks with severe symptoms due to recurrent polyhydramnios after an initial amnioreduction, we may perform repeat amnioreduction. For patients with severe symptomatic polyhydramnios at ≥34 weeks in whom amnioreduction has been unsuccessful because of reaccumulation of fluid, we discuss preterm delivery for relief of maternal discomfort and make this shared decision on a case-by-case basis. For all cases timing of delivery depends upon the etiology and severity of polyhydramnios. In accordance with the SMFM [45] and the American College of Obstetricians and Gynecologists (ACOG) [70] we recommend that delivery occur by 39 0/7 to 40 6/7 weeks of gestation for women with mild idiopathic polyhydramnios in the absence of other indications with mode of delivery determined on usual obstetric indications. In patients with severe idiopathic polyhydramnios, we offer induction of labor at 37 weeks to minimize the risk of umbilical cord prolapse and/or abruption in the event of spontaneous prelabor rupture of membranes.

Future therapies

Future therapeutic approaches for polyhydramnios include the use of intraamniotic pharmacologic agents to reduce fetal fluid production. In ovine pregnancy, intraamniotic administration of either arginine vasopressin or deamino arginine vasopressin results in rapid fetal plasma absorption and a marked decrease in fetal urine flow, although there is no effect on fetal swallowing [71].

The recent discovery of the AQPs and their differential expression in hydramnios may facilitate novel therapeutic approaches, targeting those cell membrane proteins that serve as water channels.

Oligohydramnios

Definition

Oligohydramnios is a pathologic condition characterized by a decrease in AF volume. Although it can occur in the first half of pregnancy, it is generally a problem of the second half. Oligohydramnios occurs in <1% of preterm pregnancies and is more common in pregnancies that reach term. In a study of 3050 uncomplicated pregnancies with singleton nonanomalous fetuses between 40 and 41.6 weeks oligohydramnios was observed in 11% [72].

Diagnosis

Oligohydramnios is suspected when the uterus is smaller than the date of gestation would suggest, and the diagnosis is made by sonography. The clinician relies on a quantifying method such as depth of the SDP or the AFI. An AFI of 5.0–8.0 cm indicates borderline AF, whereas an AFI of <5.0 or SDP <2 cm indicates oligohydramnios. The time in pregnancy when it develops has a bearing on the prognosis as oligohydramnios occurring in the second trimester has a very poor prognosis [73]. Moore et al. demonstrated the reliability and predictive value of a scoring system for oligohydramnios in the second trimester [74]. Sixty-two cases of oligohydramnios were diagnosed sonographically between 13 and 28 weeks gestation. Three experienced sonographers used a subjective scale to rate the oligohydramnios as mild, moderate, severe, or anhydramniotic. Intraobserver reliability was excellent (intraclass correlation coefficient, 0.81). The overall perinatal mortality was 43% and the incidence of pulmonary hypoplasia was 33%. One third had lethal congenital anomalies. The frequency of adverse outcomes strongly correlated with the most severe oligohydramnios or anhydramnios; 88% of the fetuses with severe oligohydramnios or anhydramnios had lethal outcomes, compared with 11% in the mild and moderate oligohydramnios group. The presence of an anuric urinary tract anomaly

was associated with the most severe grades of oligohydramnios and was uniformly fatal. Pulmonary hypoplasia was diagnosed in 60% of the severe oligohydramnios group vs. 6% of the moderate group. The investigators concluded that subjective grading of oligohydramnios by experienced observers in the second trimester is both reliable and predictive of outcome. The finding of severe oligohydramnios in the second trimester is highly predictive of a poor fetal outcome and should stimulate an extensive search for the etiology and consideration of intervention.

Clinical significance

Oligohydramnios occurring in first trimester is an ominous finding, and the pregnancy usually aborts [75]. Oligohydramnios occurring as early as the second trimester is also associated with a poor prognosis. Mercer and Brown reported 39 cases of oligohydramnios in the second trimester, diagnosed by sonography [76]. Nine of the pregnancies were associated with fetal malformations: Potter syndrome (5), atrioventricular disassociation (39), congenital absence of the thyroid (1), and multiple anomalies (5). There were 10 unexplained stillbirths, one death resulting from abruptio placentae, eight with perinatal mortality and morbidity after premature labor or abruptio placentae, and six live-born term infants. Although oligohydramnios in the second trimester is associated with a marked increase in perinatal mortality, it is not uniformly associated with a poor outcome.

Although oligohydramnios can be idiopathic, commonly it is associated with a specific clinical condition. The clinical conditions most associated with oligohydramnios are discussed below.

Premature rupture of membranes

Premature rupture of membranes (PROM) occurs in 2–4% of preterm gestations. The clinical implications for oligohydramnios in the setting of PROM are as follows. If PROM occurs before 24 weeks, there is an 80% chance of labor, infection, or both. The rate of perinatal mortality is 54% and the risk of permanent handicap in survivors is 40% [77]. It is not unusual for a pregnancy complicated by PROM to present initially as oligohydramnios with a normally functioning fetal bladder. Further workup reveals a slow leak of AF resulting from PROM.

The earlier in pregnancy that PROM occurs, the more likely the risk of fetal pulmonary hypoplasia. If the PROM occurs at 16–24 weeks gestation, the threat of pulmonary hypoplasia is great. A recent review emphasized that the benefits of amnioinfusion for periviable PROM are unproven and the risks remain undetermined [78].

Oligohydramnios occurring secondary to PROM later in pregnancy creates a risk of umbilical cord compression. If compression occurs during labor, variable decelerations may become problematic. This can be treated with amnioinfusion to create a cushion to relieve the cord compression.

Congenital malformation

When managing oligohydramnios, the clinician should always rule out structural malformations and consider chromosome abnormalities. Malformations of the urogenital system are the most commonly associated with oligohydramnios. The classic is Potter syndrome, with renal agenesis, low-set ears, and facial pressure deformities. With little or no AF, it is very difficult to image the fetus and adrenal glands may be mistaken for kidneys. Fetal magnetic resonance imaging may be of value in cases in which ultrasound is inconclusive. Transabdominal amnioinfusion can help in providing fluid contrast for proper imaging. Additional urogenital problems can be encountered in the form of obstructive uropathy, such as posterior urethral valve syndrome, ureteropelvic junction syndrome, or ureterocystic junction obstruction. The obstructive uropathies can be detected as early as 14–16 weeks gestation. Bilateral cystic dysplasia of the fetal kidneys may be detected as early as 12 weeks gestation. If the problem is unilateral, oligohydramnios is not likely. Cystic kidneys and renal pelvis dilation are found with trisomy 21 and trisomy 18, so karyotype should be determined.

Intrauterine growth restriction

Between 3% and 7% of all pregnancies are complicated by intrauterine growth restriction (IUGR). These fetuses have a considerably higher incidence of problems including hypoxia, acidosis, meconium aspiration, and polycythemia. After birth, potential complications include hypoglycemia, necrotizing enterocolitis, and impaired growth and development.

Approximately 60% of fetuses with IUGR have decreased AF volume discernible on sonographic examination. This feature may be very useful in differentiating the pathologically growth-restricted fetus from the one that is merely constitutionally small. Generally, oligohydramnios in the IUGR fetus is a sign of potential fetal jeopardy and a thorough evaluation of fetal well-being is indicated.

Postdate pregnancy

Approximately 3–7% of pregnancies extend beyond 42 completed weeks of gestation, dated from the first day of the last normal menstrual period. These pregnancies have a higher incidence of perinatal mortality, perinatal morbidity, and macrosomia. Postdate pregnancies are a leading cause of obstetric malpractice litigation, with most of the cases involving neurologically impaired babies [79].

The incidence of oligohydramnios increases in postdate pregnancies, in part as a result of normal shifts in the rates of fluid production and resorption (e.g. increased fetal swallowing) as well as a potential response to relative fetal hypoxia or nutrient restriction secondary to placental aging. The significance of oligohydramnios and spontaneous fetal heart rate decelerations during antepartum testing of postdate pregnancies was evaluated by Small et al. [80]. The occurrence of oligohydramnios or spontaneous decelerations during testing necessitates consideration of prompt delivery. Fetuses with decreased AF volume are at increased risk for umbilical cord compression, meconium aspiration, and fetal compromise.

Twin pregnancy

Seventy-five percent of twin pregnancies are dichorionic and 25% are monochorionic. The fetal loss rate is much higher in monochorionic pregnancies because of twin–twin transfusion syndrome. Monochorionic twin pregnancies may be identified by the telltale "T sign" at the base of the intertwin membrane. The first manifestation of twin–twin transfusion syndrome may be an increased nuchal translucency in one or both fetuses at 10–14 weeks gestation. Subsequently, at 15–17 weeks gestation there may be intertwin disparity of AF volume manifested by folding of the intertwin membrane [81].

In multiple pregnancies where polyhydramnios and oligohydramnios occur in separate sacs, there is a danger to the fetus with oligohydramnios. Chescheir and Seeds reported on seven such twins with twin–twin transfusion syndrome resulting in a perinatal mortality rate of 71% [82]. The occurrence of the complication before 26 weeks gestation resulted in death of all fetuses despite a variety of attempted therapies. In twin–twin transfusion syndrome, the donor twin becomes anemic and, over time, growth restricted, and develops oligohydramnios. When the oligohydramnios is severe, the fetus becomes immobilized, generally against the uterine wall because of pressure from the sac with polyhydramnios. The fetus does not move despite changing of maternal position. This has been called the trapped twin syndrome.

Endoscopic laser ablation of the intercommunicating placental vessels is recommended for severe twin–twin transfusion syndrome presenting prior to fetal viability [83]. Following viability, drainage of AF from the twin with polyhydramnios may improve the AF volume of the donor twin with oligohydramnios [81].

Management

Amnioinfusion may be considered in pregnancies complicated by oligohydramnios when the physician feels that augmenting the AF volume will provide diagnostic or therapeutic benefit. Amnioinfusion may be performed therapeutically, prophylactically, or as a diagnostic intervention. Maternal hydration via oral hydration or intravenous hypotonic fluid is a means of transiently increasing amniotic fluid volume and is less invasive than amnioinfusion [84–86]. Hydration with oral water reduces maternal plasma osmolality and sodium concentration, resulting in an osmotically driven maternal-to-fetal water flux. Increased placental blood flow volume, fetal urine output, and possibly decreased reabsorption of amniotic fluid via swallowing or intramembranous flow increases the amniotic fluid volume [87].

For women with idiopathic oligohydramnios one small, randomized trial tried to evaluate outcomes with expectant management vs. intervention. In this trial 54 pregnancies with isolated oligohydramnios beyond 40 weeks were randomly assigned to either expectant management or induction of labor [88]. No differences were found for any important maternal or neonatal outcome. In accord with ACOG policies, we recommend delivery at 36 0/7 to 37 6/7 weeks of gestation for isolated oligohydramnios [70].

Conclusion

Recent clinical and laboratory studies have provided an ever-increasing understanding of the dynamics of amniotic fluid volume, the clinical importance of oligo- and polyhydramnios, and the potential use of the amniotic cavity as a route for the administration of therapeutic agents to the fetus. AF is a dynamic body of water that provides essential functions for appropriate fetal growth and development. The extremes of volume–too much or too little–may be associated with an unfavorable prognosis. Appropriate diagnosis and management of polyhydramnios and oligohydramnios are essential to optimize fetal outcome.

CASE PRESENTATION

A 26-year-old gravida 2, para 1 with a history of one prior term vaginal delivery presented for prenatal care in the first trimester. The patient's fundal height was slightly greater than her dates, and a subsequent ultrasound revealed a twin gestation with a dividing membrane consistent with diamniotic monochorionic placentation. Repeat ultrasounds demonstrated symmetric growth until a 26-week scan revealed a 20% weight discordance. A repeat ultrasound 2 weeks later demonstrated marked oligohydramnios (i.e. stuck twin) in the smaller twin, associated with an absence of bladder filling and polyhydramnios in the larger twin. A diagnosis of twin–twin transfusion syndrome was made. As the gestation was beyond fetal viability, laser ablation of placental anastomoses was not entertained. An amnioreduction procedure was performed with withdrawal of 2 L fluid from the polyhydramnios sac. Subsequent ultrasound confirmed a reduction in amniotic fluid in the polyhydramnios sac, and reaccumulation of fluid in the oligohydramnios sac, although still subjectively reduced. A repeat amnioreduction was performed 1 week later. Shortly thereafter, the

patient progressed into spontaneous labor and was operatively delivered at 29 weeks gestation. Twins demonstrated a 25% discordancy in weight, with evidence of polycythemia and anemia in the larger and smaller twin, respectively.

This case represents an example of twin–twin transfusion syndrome. The donor twin's anemia reduced intravascular volume, and mild hypoxemia result in relative oliguria. Continued fetal swallowing, despite reduced amniotic fluid (e.g. urine) production, contributes to the oligohydramnios. Conversely, the recipient twin develops polycythemia, increased intravascular volume, and elevated plasma atrial natriuretic factor levels. Markedly increased urine production contributes to the polyhydramnios state. Amnioreduction reduces intraamniotic volume and pressure, potentiating increased maternal-to-fetal placental water flow, and facilitating intravascular volume repletion and urine output in the donor twin. However, the twin–twin transfusion pathophysiology continues, with continued transfer of plasma and red cells, and polyhydramnios/oligohydramnios recurs.

References

1. Denman T. An introduction to the practice of midwifery. London: Bliss and White; 1825.
2. Campbell J, Wathen N, Macintosh M, Cass P, Chard T, Mainwaring BR. Biochemical composition of amniotic fluid and extraembryonic coelomic fluid in the first trimester of pregnancy. Br J Obstet Gynaecol. 1992;99(7):563–5.
3. Faber JJ, Gault CF, Green TJ, Long LR, Thornburg KL. Chloride and the generation of amniotic fluid in the early embryo. J Exp Zool. 1973;183(3):343–52.
4. Gillibrand PN. Changes in the electrolytes, urea and osmolality of the amniotic fluid with advancing pregnancy. J Obstet Gynaecol Br Commonw. 1969;76(10):898–905.
5. Queenan JT, Thompson W, Whitfield CR, Shah SI. Amniotic fluid volumes in normal pregnancies. Am J Obstet Gynecol. 1972;114(1):34–8.
6. Brace RA, Wolf EJ. Normal amniotic fluid volume changes throughout pregnancy. Am J Obstet Gynecol. 1989;161(2):382–8.
7. Chez RA, Smith RG, Hutchinson DL. Renal function in the intrauterine primate fetus. I. Experimental technique: rate of formation and chemical composition of urine. Am J Obstet Gynecol. 1964;90:128–31.
8. Pritchard JA. Deglutition by normal and anencephalic fetuses. Obstet Gynecol. 1965;25:289–97.
9. Rabinowitz R, Peters MT, Vyas S, Campbell S, Nicolaides KH. Measurement of fetal urine production in normal pregnancy

by real-time ultrasonography. Am J Obstet Gynecol. 1989; 161(5):1264–6.

10. Kurjak A, Kirkinen P, Latin V, Ivankovic D. Ultrasonic assessment of fetal kidney function in normal and complicated pregnancies. Am J Obstet Gynecol. 1981;141(3):266–70.

11. Jeffcoate TN, Scott JS. Polyhydramnios and oligohydramnios. Can Med Assoc J. 1959;80(2):77–86.

12. Shiller W, Toll CM. An inquiry into the cause of oligohydramnios. Am J Obstet Gynecol.1927;12:689.

13. Sylvester PE, Hughes DR. Congenital absence of both kidneys; a report of four cases. BMJ. 1954;4853:77–9.

14. Liley AW. Disorders of amniotic fluid. In: Assali NS, editor. Pathophysiology of gestation. New York: Academic Press; 1972.

15. Goodlin R, Lloyd D. Fetal tracheal excretion of bilirubin. Biol Neonat. 1968;12(1):1–12.

16. Adamsons TM, Brodecky V, Lambert V, Maloney JE, Ritchie BC, Walker A. The production and composition of lung liquid in the in utero foetal lamb. In: Dawes GS, editor. Foetal and neonatal physiology. Cambridge, UK: Cambridge University Press; 1973.

17. Brace RA, Wlodek ME, Cock ML, Harding R. Swallowing of lung liquid and amniotic fluid by the ovine fetus under normoxic and hypoxic conditions. Am J Obstet Gynecol. 1994; 171(3):764–70.

18. Ross MG, Ervin G, Leake RD, Fu P, Fisher DA. Fetal lung liquid regulation by neuropeptides. Am J Obstet Gynecol. 1984; 150(4):421–5.

19. Lawson EE, Brown ER, Torday JS, Madansky DL, Taeusch HW Jr. The effect of epinephrine on tracheal fluid flow and surfactant efflux in fetal sheep. Am Rev Respir Dis. 1978;118(6): 1023–6.

20. Dodic M, Wintour EM. Effects of prolonged (48 h) infusion of cortisol on blood pressure, renal function and fetal fluids in the immature ovine foetus. Clin Exp Pharmacol Physiol. 1994; 21(12):971–80.

21. Pritchard JA. Fetal swallowing and amniotic fluid volume. Obstet Gynecol. 1966;28(5):606–10.

22. Bradley RM, Mistretta CM. Swallowing in fetal sheep. Science. 1973;179(77):1016–17.

23. El-Haddad MA, Ismail Y, Guerra C, Day L, Ross MG. Effect of oral sucrose on ingestive behavior in the near-term ovine fetus. Am J Obstet Gynecol. 2002;187(4):898–901.

24. Sherman DJ, Ross MG, Day L, Humme J, Ervin MG. Fetal swallowing: response to graded maternal hypoxemia. J Appl Physiol. 1991;71(5):1856–61.

25. Carter CO. Congenital malformation. Ciba Foundation Symposium. 1960;264.

26. Gadd RL. Liquor amnii. In: Phillipp EE, Barnes J, Newton M, editors. Scientific foundations of obstetrics and gynaecology. London: Butterworth Heinemann; 1987. p.254.

27. Benirschke K, McKay DG. The antidiuretic hormone in fetus and infant: histochemical observations with special reference to amniotic fluid formation. Obstet Gynecol. 1953;1(6):638–49.

28. Naeye RL, Milic AM, Blanc W. Fetal endocrine and renal disorders: clues to the origin of hydramnios. Am J Obstet Gynecol. 1970;108(8):1251–6.

29. Lingwood BE, Wintour EM. Amniotic fluid volume and in vivo permeability of ovine fetal membranes. Obstet Gynecol. 1984;64(3):368–72.

30. Gilbert WM, Newman PS, Eby-Wilkens E, Brace RA. Technetium Tc 99m rapidly crosses the ovine placenta and intramembranous pathway. Am J Obstet Gynecol. 1996;175(6): 1557–62.

31. Lingwood BE, Wintour EM. Permeability of ovine amnion and amniochorion to urea and water. Obstet Gynecol. 1983;61(2): 227–32.

32. Gilbert WM, Brace RA. The missing link in amniotic fluid volume regulation: intramembranous absorption. Obstet Gynecol. 1989;74(5):748–54.

33. Huang J, Qi HB. [Expression of aquaporin 8 in human fetal membrane and placenta of idiopathic polyhydramnios]. Zhonghua Fu Chan Ke Za Zhi. 2009;44(1):19–22.

34. Zhu XQ, Jiang SS, Zou SW, Hu YC, Wang YH. [Expression of aquaporin 3 and aquaporin 9 in placenta and fetal membrane with idiopathic polyhydramnios.]. Zhonghua Fu Chan Ke Za Zhi. 2009;44(12):920–3.

35. Mann SE, Dvorak N, Gilbert H, Taylor RN. Steady-state levels of aquaporin 1 mRNA expression are increased in idiopathic polyhydramnios. Am J Obstet Gynecol. 2006;194(3):884–7.

36. Wang S, Chen J, Huang B, Ross MG. Cloning and cellular expression of aquaporin 9 in ovine fetal membranes. Am J Obstet Gynecol. 2005;193(3):841–8.

37. Guibourdenche J, Bonnet-Serrano F, Younes Chaouch L, Sapin V, Tsatsaris V, Combarel D, et al. Amniotic aquaporins (AQP) in normal and pathological pregnancies: interest in polyhydramnios. Reprod Sci. 2021 Oct;28(10):2929–38.

38. Queenan JT, Allen FH Jr, Fuchs F, Stakemann G, Freisleben E, Fogh J, et al. Studies on the method of intrauterine transfusion. I. Question of erythrocyte absorption from amniotic fluid. Am J Obstet Gynecol. 1965;92:1009–13.

39. Hebertson RM, Hammond ME, Bryson MJ. Amniotic epithelial ultrastructure in normal, polyhydramnic, and oligohydramnic pregnancies. Obstet Gynecol. 1986;68(1):74–9.

40. Gillibrand PN. The rate of water transfer from the amniotic sac with advancing pregnancy. J Obstet Gynaecol Br Commonw. 1969 Jun;76(6):530–3.

41. Ross MG, Nijland MJ. Development of ingestive behavior. Am J Physiol. 1998 Apr;274(4):R879–93.

42. Charles D, Jacoby HE. Preliminary data on the use of sodium aminohippurate to determine amniotic fluid volumes. Am J Obstet Gynecol. 1966;95(2):266–9.

43. Magann EF, Nolan TE, Hess LW, Martin RW, Whitworth NS, Morrison JC. Measurement of amniotic fluid volume: accuracy of ultrasonography techniques. Am J Obstet Gynecol. 1992; 167(6):1533–7.

44. Horsager R, Nathan L, Leveno KJ. Correlation of measured amniotic fluid volume and sonographic predictions of oligohydramnios. Obstet Gynecol. 1994;83(6):955–8.

45. Society for Maternal-Fetal Medicine (SMFM). Dashe JS, Pressman EK, Hibbard JU. SMFM Consult Series #46: evaluation and management of polyhydramnios. Am J Obstet Gynecol. 2018 Oct;219(4):B2–B8. doi:10.1016/j.ajog.2018.07.016. Epub 2018 Jul 23.

46. Dildy GA III, Lira N, Moise KJ Jr, Riddle GD, Deter RL. Amniotic fluid volume assessment: comparison of ultrasonographic estimates versus direct measurements with a dyedilution technique in human pregnancy. Am J Obstet Gynecol. 1992;167(4 Pt 1):986–94.

47. Magann EF, Morton ML, Nolan TE, Martin JN Jr, Whitworth NS, Morrison JC. Comparative efficacy of two sonographic measurements for the detection of aberrations in the amniotic fluid volume and the effect of amniotic fluid volume on pregnancy outcome. Obstet Gynecol. 1994;83(6):959–62.

48. Chauhan SP, Magann EF, Morrison JC, Whitworth NS, Hendrix NW, Devoe LD. Ultrasonographic assessment of amniotic fluid does not reflect actual amniotic fluid volume. Am J Obstet Gynecol. 1997;177(2):291–6.

49. Magann EF, Doherty DA, Chauhan SP, Busch FW, Mecacci F, Morrison JC. How well do the amniotic fluid index and single deepest pocket indices (below the 3rd and 5th and above the 95th and 97th percentiles) predict oligohydramnios and hydramnios? Am J Obstet Gynecol. 2004;190(1):164–9.

50. Magann EF, Chauhan SP, Barrilleaux PS, Whitworth NS, McCurley S, Martin JN. Ultrasound estimate of amniotic fluid volume: color Doppler overdiagnosis of oligohydramnios. Obstet Gynecol. 2001;98(1):71–4.

51. Goldkrand JW, Hough TM, Lentz SU, Clements SP, Bryant JL, Hodges JA. Comparison of the amniotic fluid index with gray-scale and color Doppler ultrasound. J Matern Fetal Neonatal Med. 2003;13(5):318–22.

52. Zlatnik MG, Olson G, Bukowski R, Saade GR. Amniotic fluid index measured with the aid of color flow Doppler. J Matern Fetal Neonatal Med. 2003;13(4):242–5.

53. Magann EF, Nevils BG, Chauhan SP, Whitworth NS, Klausen JH, Morrison JC. Low amniotic fluid volume is poorly identified in singleton and twin pregnancies using the 2 x 2 cm pocket technique of the biophysical profile. South Med J. 1999;92(8):802–5.

54. Hughes DS, Magann EF, Whittington JR, Wendel MP, Sandlin AT, Ounpraseuth ST. Accuracy of the ultrasound estimate of the amniotic fluid volume (amniotic fluid index and single deepest pocket) to identify actual low, normal, and high amniotic fluid volumes as determined by quantile regression. J Ultrasound Med. 2020 Feb;39(2):373–8.

55. Abele H, Starz S, Hoopmann M, Yazdi B, Rall K, Kagan KO. Idiopathic polyhydramnios and postnatal abnormalities. Fetal Diagn Ther. 2012;32(4):251–5.

56. Queenan JT, Gadow EC. Polyhydramnios: chronic versus acute. Am J Obstet Gynecol. 1970;108(3):349–55.

57. Hill LM, Breckle R, Thomas ML, Fries JK. Polyhydramnios: ultrasonically detected prevalence and neonatal outcome. Obstet Gynecol. 1987;69(1):21–5.

58. Idris N, Wong SF, Thomae M, Gardener G, McIntyre DH. Influence of polyhydramnios on perinatal outcome in pregestational diabetic pregnancies. Ultrasound Obstet Gynecol. 2010;36(3):338–43.

59. Panting-Kemp A, Nguyen T, Chang E, Quillen E, Castro L. Idiopathic polyhydramnios and perinatal outcome. Am J Obstet Gynecol. 1999;181(5 Pt 1):1079–82.

60. Adam MJ, Enderle I, Le Bouar G, Cabaret-Dufour AS, Tardif C, Contin L, et al. Performance of diagnostic ultrasound to identify causes of hydramnios. Prenat Diagn. 2021 Jan;41(1):111–22.

61. Moore LE. Amount of polyhydramnios attributable to diabetes may be less than previously reported. World J Diabetes. 2017 Jan 15;8(1):7–10.

62. Tanaka K, Hosoi K, Yoshiike S, Nagahama K, Tanigaki S, Shibahara J, et al. Mirror syndrome due to anti-Jra alloimmunization. Taiwan J Obstet Gynecol. 2020 May;59(3):456–9.

63. Laghmani K, Beck BB, Yang SS, Seaayfan E, Wenzel A, Reusch B, et al. Polyhydramnios, transient antenatal Bartter's syndrome, and MAGED2 mutations. N Engl J Med. 2016 May 12;374(19):1853–63.

64. Bamberg C, Hecher K. Update on twin-to-twin transfusion syndrome. Best Pract Res Clin Obstet Gynaecol. 2019 Jul;58:55–65.

65. Queenan JT. Recurrent acute polyhydramnios. Am J Obstet Gynecol. 1970;106(4):625–6.

66. Elliott JP, Sawyer AT, Radin TG, Strong RE. Large-volume therapeutic amniocentesis in the treatment of hydramnios. Obstet Gynecol. 1994;84(6):1025–7.

67. Leung WC, Jouannic JM, Hyett J, Rodeck C, Jauniaux E. Procedure-related complications of rapid amniodrainage in the treatment of polyhydramnios. Ultrasound Obstet Gynecol. 2004;23(2):154–8.

68. Kramer WB, van den Veyver, I, Kirshon B. Treatment of polyhydramnios with indomethacin. Clin Perinatol. 1994;21(3):615–30.

69. Cabrol D, Landesman R, Muller J, Uzan M, Sureau C, Saxena BB. Treatment of polyhydramnios with prostaglandin synthetase inhibitor (indomethacin). Am J Obstet Gynecol. 1987;157(2):422–6.

70. American College of Obstetricians and Gynecologists' Committee on Obstetric Practice, Society for Maternal-Fetal Medicine. Medically indicated late-preterm and early-term deliveries: ACOG Committee Opinion, Number 831. Obstet Gynecol. 2021 Jul 1;138(1):e35–9.

71. Gilbert WM, Cheung CY, Brace RA. Rapid intramembranous absorption into the fetal circulation of arginine vasopressin injected intraamniotically. Am J Obstet Gynecol. 1991;164(4):1013–18.

72. Locatelli A, Zagarella A, Toso L, Assi F, Ghidini A, Biffi A. Serial assessment of amniotic fluid index in uncomplicated term pregnancies: prognostic value of amniotic fluid reduction. J Matern Fetal Neonatal Med. 2004 Apr;15(4):233–6.

73. Moore TR. Oligohydramnios. In: Queenan JT, Hobbins JC, editors. Protocols in high-risk pregnancies. Cambridge, MA: Blackwell Science; 1996. p.488.

74. Moore TR, Longo J, Leopold GR, Casola G, Gosink BB. The reliability and predictive value of an amniotic fluid scoring system in severe second-trimester oligohydramnios. Obstet Gynecol. 1989;73(5 Pt 1):739–42.

75. Bromley B, Harlow BL, Laboda LA, Benacerraf BR. Small sac size in the first trimester: a predictor of poor fetal outcome. Radiology. 1991 Feb;178(2):375–7.

76. Mercer LJ, Brown LG. Fetal outcome with oligohydramnios in the second trimester. Obstet Gynecol. 1986;67(6):840–2.

77. Ghidini A, Romero R. Prelabor rupture of the membranes. In: Queenan JT, Hobbins JC, editors. Protocols in high-risk pregnancies. Cambridge, MA: Blackwell Science; 1996. p.547.

78. Waters TP, Mercer BM. The management of preterm premature rupture of the membranes near the limit of fetal viability. Am J Obstet Gynecol 2009;201(3):230–40.

79. Quilligan EJ. Postdate pregnancies. In: Queenan JT, Hobbins JC, editors. Protocols in high-risk pregnancies. Cambridge, MA: Blackwell Science; 1996. p. 633.

80. Small ML, Phelan JP, Smith CV, Paul RH. An active management approach to the postdate fetus with a reactive nonstress test and fetal heart rate decelerations. Obstet Gynecol. 1987;70(4):636–40.

81. Nicolaides K, Sebire N, d'Ercole C. Prediction, diagnosis and management of twin-to-twin transfusion syndrome. In: Cockburn F, editor. Advances in perinatal medicine. New York: Parthenon Publishing; 1997. p. 200.

82. Chescheir NC, Seeds JW. Polyhydramnios and oligohydramnios in twin gestations. Obstet Gynecol. 1988;71(6 Pt 1):882–4.

83. Ville Y, Hecher K, Gagnon A, Sebire N, Hyett J, Nicolaides K. Endoscopic laser coagulation in the management of severe twin-to-twin transfusion syndrome. Br J Obstet Gynaecol. 1998;105(4):446–53.

84. Ghafarnejad M, Tehrani MB, Anaraki FB, Mood NI, Nasehi L. Oral hydration therapy in oligohydramnios. J Obstet Gynaecol Res. 2009;35(5):895–900.

85. Yan-Rosenberg L, Burt B, Bombard AT, Callado-Khoury F, Sharett L, Julliard K, et al. A randomized clinical trial comparing the effect of maternal intravenous hydration and placebo on the amniotic fluid index in oligohydramnios. J Matern Fetal Neonatal Med. 2007;20(10):715–18.

86. Doi S, Osada H, Seki K, Sekiya S. Effect of maternal hydration on oligohydramnios: a comparison of three volume expansion methods. Obstet Gynecol. 1998;92(4 Pt 1):525–9.

87. Hofmeyr GJ, Gulmezoglu AM. Maternal hydration for increasing amniotic fluid volume in oligohydramnios and normal amniotic fluid volume. Cochrane Database Syst Rev. 2002;(1):CD000134. doi: 10.1002/14651858.CD000134.

88. Ek S, Andersson A, Johansson A, Kublicas M. Oligohydramnios in uncomplicated pregnancies beyond 40 completed weeks. A prospective, randomised, pilot study on maternal and neonatal outcomes. Fetal Diagn Ther. 2005 May–Jun;20(3):182–5.

Chapter 40
Pathogenesis and Prediction of Preterm Delivery

Anthony M. Kendle[1], Catalin S. Buhimschi[2], and Charles J. Lockwood[1]

[1]Department of Obstetrics and Gynecology, Morsani College of Medicine, University of South Florida, Tampa, FL, USA
[2]Department of Obstetrics and Gynecology, University of Illinois College of Medicine, Chicago, IL, USA

Preterm delivery (PTD) is defined as a birth before 37 weeks gestation. In the United States, the preterm birth rate increased from 9.57% in 2014 to 10.49% in 2021, marking the highest PTD rate since 2007 [1]. Increased rates were observed for both early preterm (less than 34 weeks) and late preterm (34–36 weeks) delivery with increases from 2.70% to 2.81% and from 7.40% to 7.67%, respectively, from 2020 to 2021. Increased rates were registered for almost all age, race, and ethnic categories. The PTD rate among Black women remains disparately high compared to their White counterparts at 14.75% vs. 9.50%, respectively. Unfortunately, Black women deliver low birthweight and very low birthweight infants at more than twice the rate of their White counterparts (14.66% vs. 7.03% and 2.91% vs. 1.02%, respectively). The medical relevance of this observation is that it is these latter newborns who are at the highest risk of early death or disability.

Over the past 3 decades much of the increase in prematurity has been attributed to the epidemic of multifetal gestations and to generally later PTDs, necessitated by deteriorating maternal or fetal health [2]. Although consistent declines in rates of multifetal gestations since 2015 help explain the recent downward trends, PTD remains a leading cause of infant morbidity and mortality [3].

Etiology and pathogenesis of spontaneous preterm delivery

Proximate causes of PTD include medically indicated PTDs (18.7–35.2% of cases) and spontaneous PTDs resulting from either preterm labor (PTL) with intact fetal membranes (23.2–64.1%) or preterm premature rupture of membranes (PPROM) (7.1–51.2%) [4]. There is compelling evidence to suggest that spontaneous PTD results from multiple pathogenic pathways and/or etiologic factors [5–7]. At least four distinct pathways have been defined: idiopathic or stress-associated premature activation of the maternal, placental and/or fetal hypothalamic–pituitary–adrenal (HPA) axis; decidual-amnion-chorion inflammation; decidual hemorrhage (abruption); and pathological uterine-myometrial stretch [8]. Genome-wide association studies have identified an association between gestational duration and genetic variations (EBF1, EEFSEC, AGTR2, WNT4, ADCY5, and RAP2C) in loci associated with uterine development, maternal nutrition, and vascular control [9]. However, because of the diverse pathways leading to prematurity and complex interactions among putative effectors, no single genetic factor accounts for more than a fraction of PTD cases. Moreover, there is obviously intense evolutionary pressure against mutations that lead to potentially lethal early PTD.

Regardless of the initial pathogenic and etiologic stimulus and genetic predisposition, all spontaneous PTDs use a common final biochemical pathway characterized by increased genital tract inflammation and neutrophil infiltration, enhanced net prostaglandin (PG) release, altered cervical extracellular matrix (ECM) components and enhanced protease production in the cervix, decidua, myometrium, and fetal membranes coupled with alterations in progesterone receptor (PR) levels or the relative expression of PR isoforms in the cervix, decidua, and myometrium [10–12]. This final common pathway is employed by each of the main four major pathogenic pathways.

Idiopathic and stress-associated premature activation of the maternal-placental–fetal hypothalamic–pituitary–adrenal axis

Human parturition involves complex maternal, fetal, and placental interactions. Stress can be a common element

---

activating a series of physiologic adaptive responses in each of these compartments [13]. Periconceptional maternal stress and anxiety are associated with modestly increased rates of spontaneous PTD with odds ratios (ORs) of 1.16 (95% confidence interval [CI] 1.05–1.29) [14]. Data derived from registry-linked births to mothers with posttraumatic stress disorder noted higher odds of PTD (adjusted OR 2.48, 95% CI 1.05–5.84) [15]. Depression among women of African descent is associated with an adjusted OR for PTD of 1.96 (95% CI 1.04–3.72) [16]. Meta-analysis of pregnancies complicated by maternal anxiety found an increased association with PTD with a risk ratio of 1.50 (95% CI 1.33–1.70) [17]. Thus, women with depression and other mood disorders are at increased risk for PTD, although the magnitude of the effect varies as a function of the method of ascertainment of depression and socioeconomic status [18].

Placental abnormalities may also prompt stress-induced changes implicated in PTD. Placental pathologic changes consistent with shallow placentation, inflammation, and ischemia-induced fetal stress are 3–7 times more common in patients with spontaneous PTD compared with term controls [19,20]. Additionally, pregnancies affected by both spontaneous and medically indicated PTD are 4–7 times more likely to have histologic evidence of placental vascular damage, altered blood vessel integrity, or derangement in maternal spiral artery development [21]. Both elevated maternal stress and aberrant placentation are more common with first pregnancies. Based on large registry-based cohorts, nulligravidas who deliver preterm have a 6.12-fold increase (95% CI 5.84–6.42) in subsequent PTD in a second pregnancy compared to those who deliver at term in their first pregnancy [22]. In addition, there appears to be a genetic predisposition to both maternal mood disorders [23] and impaired placentation [24].

Placental corticotropin-releasing hormone (CRH) and accelerated HPA activation

Corticotropin-releasing hormone (CRH), a 41-amino acid peptide initially discovered in the hypothalamus but also expressed by placental, chorionic, amnionic, and decidual cells, may have a role in stress-associated PTDs [25]. In uncomplicated (physiologic) pregnancies maternal plasma-free CRH concentrations, which are almost entirely placental derived, rise during the second half of pregnancy and peak during labor [26]. The CRH concentration curve across gestation in women with subsequent PTD runs parallel to the CRH curve of normal pregnancy, but the absolute CRH level for a given week of gestation is displaced significantly upward and to the left [27]. In contrast to the hypothalamus, where glucocorticoids inhibit CRH release, cortisol enhances placental production of CRH [28]. This positive feed-forward system is a unique biologic feature causing progressive increases in placental CRH production as pregnancy advances to

term. Both maternal and fetal stress (i.e. fetal growth restriction) are associated with elevated maternal and/or fetal cortisol levels [29–31].

Lockwood and colleagues [32] examined paired maternal and fetal HPA axis hormone levels in patients undergoing cordocentesis across the second half of gestation and noted that placental-derived maternal serum CRH values correlated best with fetal cortisol (r = 0.40, $P = 0.0002$) but also modestly correlated with maternal cortisol levels (r = 0.28, $P = 0.01$). Thus, rising maternal and/or fetal cortisol levels likely establish a positive feedback loop (i.e. placental-derived CRH stimulates the release of fetal pituitary adrenocorticotropin [ACTH] to enhance fetal adrenal cortisol production), which further stimulates placental CRH release [32].

Despite the evidence described here, it is unclear whether precocious elevation of plasma CRH levels is an epiphenomenon or consequence of maternal or fetal stress vs. a trigger for PTD mechanisms [33]. For example, there is evidence for a myometrial relaxing effect of CRH, favoring uterine quiescence, in contrast to its indirect uterotonic effect documented in vitro [34]. Conversely, output of $PGF_2\alpha$ and/or PGE_2 is increased by addition of CRH to cultured amnionic, chorionic, decidual, and placental cells [35,36]. Both $PGF_2\alpha$ and/or PGE_2 bind to uterotonic receptors, F-prostanoid, and EP-1/3, respectively, in the fundus and corpus of the uterus to mediate calcium flux, which triggers effective contractions and increases myometrial expression of oxytocin receptor, connexin 43 (gap junctions), and cyclooxygenase (COX)-2 [37–40]. In turn, the latter augments additional PG production. In addition, CRH-induced PG synthesis can promote PROM and cervical change by enhancing the synthesis of matrix metalloproteinases (MMPs) in the fetal membranes and cervix [38,41]. Moreover, PGs increase cervical expression of interleukin (IL)-8, which recruits and activates neutrophils, releasing additional MMPs and elastases that can promote cervical ECM dissolution and weakening of the fetal membranes [42].

At term, cortisol released into the amniotic fluid can directly stimulate fetal membrane PG production by increasing amnionic COX-2 expression and inhibiting the chorionic PG metabolizing enzyme, 15-hydroxyprostaglandin dehydrogenase (PGDH) [43,44]. Both PGE_2 and $PGF_2\alpha$ have been reported to increase the proinflammatory PR-A isoform and decrease the anti-inflammatory PR-B isoform in myometrium, cervix, and decidua [45–47]. Because PR-A antagonizes the classic PR-mediated genomic effects of PR-B, PGs appear to induce a functional progesterone (P4) withdrawal. Merlino et al. have reported that in contrast to the intense nuclear PR mRNAs and proteins expression observed in decidual cells, PR expression is barely detectable in amnion and chorion [48]. The authors suggest that decidual cells, and not amnion and chorion cells, are the direct target of P4 during human pregnancy.

With the development of the fetal adrenal zone of the fetal adrenal after 28–30 weeks gestation, stress-associated activation of the placental–fetal HPA axis also mediates PTD by enhancing placental estrogen production. This is because increased fetal adrenal zone production of dehydroepiandrosterone sulfate (DHEAS) accompanies ACTH-induced fetal adrenal cortisol production. In addition, CRH can directly augment fetal adrenal DHEAS production [49]. Placental sulfatases cleave the sulfate conjugates of DHEAS and its 16-hydroxy hepatic derivative, allowing their conversion to estradiol (E2) and estrone (E1), as well as estriol (E3), respectively. These estrogens increase myometrial expression of contraction-associated proteins such as oxytocin receptor and connexin-43 [50,51]. Because reductions in PR-B expression lead to increased expression of the active form of the estrogen receptor-β (ER-β), rising placental estrogen production would be matched to PG-induced increases in myometrial ER-β expression [35,52].

FK506-binding protein 51 and intracellular functional progesterone (P4) withdrawal

The immunophilin co-chaperone FK506-binding protein 51 (FKBP51) appears to play an important role in glucocorticoid-mediated functional withdrawal of P4 at time of parturition. FKBP51 is present in decidual cells and binds to both unliganded PR and glucocorticoid receptor (GR) with the net effect of decreasing receptor-mediated transcription [53]. Glucocorticoids upregulate FKBP51, which in turn downregulates GR activity as part of an intracellular negative feedback loop [54]. Although this mechanism may protect against deleterious effects of excess glucocorticoid [55], in decidual cells glucocorticoid-mediated enhancement of FKBP51 simultaneously reduces PR activity [56]. Guzeloglu-Kayisli and colleagues have shown enhanced in situ FKBP51 protein expression and increased nuclear FKBP51-PR binding in decidual cells of women with idiopathic PTD vs. gestational age-matched controls [57]. *Fkbp5*-deficient (*Fkbp5⁻/⁻*) mice are highly resistant to stress-induced depressive and anxiety-like behaviors. In wild type *Fkbp5⁺/⁺* mice, maternal restraint stress increased *Fkbp5*, decreased PR, and elevated expression of the P4 metabolizing enzyme, AKR1C18, in uteri at E17.25 days (of 20-day gestation). This was followed by reduced P4 levels and increased oxytocin receptor (*Oxtr*) expression at 18.25 in uteri resulting in PTD. These changes correlate with inhibition of uterine PR function by maternal stress-induced FKBP51. In contrast, *Fkbp5⁻/⁻* (knock out) mice exhibit prolonged gestation and are completely resistant to maternal stress-induced PTD and labor-inducing uterine changes detected in stressed *Fkbp5⁺/⁺* mice. These results suggest a functional intracellular P4 withdrawal mechanism mediated by stress-induced enhanced uterine FKBP51 expression and FKPB51-PR binding, resulting in PTD.

These compelling data suggest that pathological maternal and/or fetal stress, and both physiological term and idiopathic preterm activation of the fetal HPA axis, as well as enhanced intracellular FKBP51 expression, permit the fetus to actively participate in the timing of delivery via production of adrenal hormonal precursors [58]. From an evolutionary perspective this pathway links birth with fetal organ maturation and facilitates removal of a prematurely mature fetus from a hostile intrauterine environment. This thesis is also supported by the evidence that at term, prior to the onset of labor, the weight and volume of the fetal adrenal gland is equal to those of the adult [59]. Interestingly, in the setting of intraamniotic inflammation, the fetal cortisol-to-DHEAS ratio was low, with no direct correlation between the adrenal gland volume and either cortisol or DHEAS [60]. This suggests that infection-mediated PTD may act via a different pathway (discussed later).

Decidual-amnion-chorion inflammation

Systemic inflammation resulting from pneumonia, sepsis, pancreatitis, acute cholecystitis, pyelonephritis, and asymptomatic bacteriuria as well as genital tract inflammatory states such as deciduitis, chorioamnionitis, periodontal infection, and intraamniotic infections are all associated with PTD [61–68]. Genital tract inflammation is recognized as the most common antecedent of very early PTDs, accounting for more than half of cases [64,65].

The vaginal microbiome and preterm delivery

Bacterial vaginosis (BV) is the most common lower genital tract microbial-related syndrome among women of reproductive age [69]. Multiple prospective cohort studies have established a modest association between BV and spontaneous PTD (OR 1.4–2.2), with the strongest association noted for BV detected at less than 16 weeks (OR 7.55, 95% CI 1.80–31.65) [70–72]. BV facilitates overgrowth of upper genital tract facultative bacteria such as *Mycoplasma* species and *Gardnerella vaginalis*, gram-negative bacteria such as *Escherichia coli*, and gram-positive cocci [73,74], as well as urinary tract colonization and infections [75]. Several studies report that asymptomatic bacteriuria and vaginal *E. coli* colonization are linked to a twofold increase in PTD [76–78].

The mechanism(s) by which BV affects PTD risk remain unknown. Moreover, the most recent report from the US Preventive Services Task Force recommends against routine screening for BV in pregnancies at low risk for PTD though there is insufficient evidence to guide screening for BV in pregnancies at increased risk for PTD [79]. A subgroup of high-risk women may still benefit from BV screening and treatment. However, there may also be a subgroup for whom BV treatment with metronidazole could increase the occurrence of PTD [80].

The absence of clear evidence that treatment of BV reduces the risk of PTD [81] suggests that it is the broader abnormal vaginal flora that contributes to prematurity. Normally the vaginal microbiome shifts in pregnancy toward a *Lactobacillus*-dominated profile [82]. In a longitudinal study of vaginal microbiome profiles among women mostly of African ancestry, Fettweis and colleagues noted that women with PTD had significantly lower levels of *Lactobacillus crispatus* and higher levels of BVAB1, *Sneathia amnii*, TM7-H1, *Prevotella* species, and nine additional taxa that correlated with increased proinflammatory cytokines in vaginal fluid [83]. A nested case–control study comparing cervicovaginal microbiota among patients with and without spontaneous PTD also found seven distinct bacterial taxa to be associated with increased risk of PTD [84]. *Mobiluncus curtisii/mulieris* was the only taxon associated with increased PTD among all participants; however, five distinct taxa were identified among Black women with PTD. The presence of *Lactobacillus*-poor vaginal community state type 4 microbiome has been significantly associated with early gestational age at delivery [85]. Several other studies have also demonstrated that African American populations have a higher prevalence of vaginal microbiome deficient in *Lactobacillus* species [86]. Although this may contribute to increased rates of PTD, there are still many Black women lacking *Lactobacillus* who deliver at term. Thus, these findings suggest a complex interplay of cervicovaginal microbiome with immune and inflammatory modulators in the setting of PTD.

Maternal genital tract inflammation and preterm delivery

Two complementary inflammatory networks have been described: the innate and adaptive immune systems. Innate immunity is an evolutionarily preserved defense mechanism, designed to provide a first line of resistance against exogenous and endogenous pathogens. Genetically programmed "modules" of the innate immune system respond rapidly, nonspecifically and without memory to pathogens [86,87]. The best characterized inflammatory response is that elicited by microbial pathogens which trigger a vast array of transcriptional events following engagement of Toll-like receptors (TLRs). The TLRs are transmembrane receptors that participate in host defense mechanisms through engagement of pathogen-associated molecular patterns [88].

Owing to their strategic positioning at the maternal/fetal interface and cervical mucosa, TLRs are considered key operative agents of the response to infection. Gram-negative, bacteria-derived endotoxins bind to cervical and fetal membrane TLR-4 and gram-positive bacteria-derived exotoxins bind to TLR-2 on decidual cells and leukocytes to elicit production of tumor necrosis factor-α (TNF-α) and IL-1β [89–91]. In turn, TNF-α, IL-1β, and/or endotoxins such as lipopolysaccharide induce expression of the transcription factor NFκB, which enhances MMP-1, 3, and 9 as well as COX-2 expression while promoting apoptosis in amnion epithelial cells. These biochemical cascades underline the central role of inflammation in promoting ECM remodeling processes linked to PPROM and to early cervical ripening and dilation [92–101].

It was shown that PG metabolizing PGDH activity and PGDH mRNA were significantly lower in membranes of women with infection-induced chorioamnionitis compared to women with idiopathic PTD or at term [94]. This NFκB-mediated effect may allow passage of the unmetabolized PG to the decidua and myometrium and contribute to premature activation of myometrial contractility and PTD. In addition, TNF-α, IL-1β, and endotoxin stimulate IL-6 production in amniochorion and decidua [102,103], which further augments amnionic and decidual PG production [104]. Using specific inhibitors of NFκB activation, Lockwood et al. were able to demonstrate that inhibition of IL-1β enhanced IL-6 expression levels in cultured decidual cells [105].

Inflammation is also associated with functional P4 withdrawal in the reproductive tract. Immunohistochemistry has revealed that chorioamnionitis-associated PTD is accompanied by reduced decidual PR expression and IL-1β decreases decidual cell expression of PR and increases expression of PGE$_2$, PGF$_2$α, and COX-2 [106]. Although addition of PGF$_2$α to decidual cell cultures also suppressed PR expression, the COX inhibitor, indomethacin, failed to reverse IL-1β suppression of PR expression in these cells. The PR inhibitory effects of IL-1β are mediated by ERK1/2 MAPK signaling, and inhibition of this pathway reverses IL-1β suppression of PR levels. Finally, TNF-α and IL-1β induce IL-8 production in the fetal membranes, decidua, and cervix, effects that are potentiated by IL-6 [101,107]. Given that IL-8 causes recruitment and activation of neutrophils that release additional MMPs and elastases, it further exacerbates the PTD-enhancing effects of genital tract inflammation.

The biologic activity of the TLRs is dependent not only on the presence of bacterial pathogen-associated molecular patterns but also on a palette of intracellular signaling adaptors (e.g. MyD88) and coreceptor molecules (e.g. CD14) that associate with TLRs in complex supramolecular arrangements [108]. Equally important is that TLR signaling can be elicited by endogenous damage-associated molecular pattern molecules (DAMPs) [109]. Released by activated or damaged cells under inflammatory conditions, DAMPs are endogenous proinflammatory molecules. Acting through TLR2, TLR4, and the receptor for advanced glycation end-products (RAGE), DAMPs recruit inflammatory cells, which in turn amplify innate immune responses and enhance levels of cytokine activation [107]. Buhimschi et al. reported that the DAMP-RAGE system is present in women with PTD and intraamniotic infection and its activation correlates with the degree of inflammation in amnion epithelial, decidual, and extravillous cells [110]. Lastly, the roles of soluble receptor modulators (soluble TLR2, soluble TNF receptor-1, soluble IL-6 receptor, soluble gp130, and soluble RAGE) in fine-tuning human trophoblast TLR-mediated signaling have been well studied and demonstrated [111–114].

Abruption-associated preterm delivery

Decidual hemorrhage (placental abruption) originates in damaged spiral arteries or arterioles and presents clinically as vaginal bleeding or either a retroplacental or retrochorionic hematoma formation noted on ultrasound. The incidence ranges from 0.5% to 2% depending on the clinical definition and criteria used to characterize abruption intensity [115]. Abruption-associated PTDs are more common in older, White, married, parous, college-educated patients presenting a demographic profile distinct from that associated with patients with stress-induced PTDs (nulliparous, anxious, or depressed patients) or inflammation-associated PTDs (young, minority, poor socioeconomic status) [116]. Large prospective studies reported that vaginal bleeding during the first half of pregnancy increases the relative risk (RR) of spontaneous PTD (RR of 1.4, 95% CI 1.2–1.5), PPROM (RR 2.1, 95% CI 1.2–2.3), and placental abruption (RR 1.1, 95% CI 1.01–1.2) [117]. When vaginal bleeding occurs in more than one trimester, it is associated with a nearly 50% risk of PPROM (OR 7.4, 95% CI 2.2–25.6) [118]. That inherited or acquired thrombophilias are associated with adverse pregnancy outcomes such as placental abruption is controversial [119–121] and testing for inherited thrombophilias in women who have experienced placental abruption is not recommended [119].

The key histologic finding in placental abruption is hemorrhage in the decidua basalis. Decidual hemosiderin deposition and retrochorionic hematoma formation is present in 38% of patients with PTD between 22 and 32 weeks gestation resulting from PPROM and 36% of patients experiencing PTD after preterm labor with intact membranes (PTL) compared with only 0.8% following term delivery [122]. As with stress-associated PTD, uteroplacental vascular lesions associated with abruption include spiral artery vascular thrombosis and failed physiologic transformation of uteroplacental vessels. Placental abruption is generally regarded as an acute event. This assertion is supported by the histologic evidence that acute lesions of chorioamnionitis and funisitis can be associated with decidual bleeding [123]. However, histological evaluation of the vasculopathy accompanying decidual hemorrhage suggests a chronic process. Chronic deciduitis and villitis, infarcts, necrosis, blood vessels with absent physiologic changes, vascular thrombosis,

and increased numbers of circulating nucleated erythrocytes are the most frequently encountered histopathologic lesions co-associated with chronic decidual bleeding leading to PTD [120]. Trauma, hypertension, heavy cigarette smoking, and cocaine use may induce or exacerbate the acute and chronic vasculopathies attendant upon placental abruption [124]. The association of abruption with increasing maternal age may reflect increased myometrial artery sclerosis present in 11% of spiral arteries at ages 17–19 years but in 83% after age 39 [125].

Dysregulation of the molecular mechanisms responsible for vascular and decidual penetration by extravillous trophoblasts increases the risk of hemorrhage leading to abruption [126]. The decidua is a rich source of tissue factor, the primary initiator of clotting through thrombin generation [127], and decidual hemorrhage results in intense local thrombin generation and, in severe cases, systemic effects that include hypofibrinogenemia and disseminated intravascular coagulation. Studies examining thrombin-antithrombin (TAT) complexes in amniotic fluid of second trimester pregnancies have demonstrated that higher TAT concentrations are associated with increased incidence of PTD [128]. Abruption-induced PTD is associated with reduced decidual PR expression and, similar to the role of IL-1β in inflammation-associated PTD, thrombin binds to its protease-activated receptor (PAR-1) to inhibits PR protein and mRNA expression in decidual cells via activation of ERK1/2 MAP kinase [129]. Thus abruption is also associated with functional P4 withdrawal.

The expression of MMP-1 and MMP-3 protein and mRNA output by cultured term decidual cells is significantly enhanced by thrombin binding to PAR-1 [130,131]. Lockwood et al. [132] reported that abruption-associated PPROM is accompanied by dense decidual neutrophil infiltration in the absence of infection. Decidual neutrophils co-localized with areas of thrombin-induced fibrin deposition and thrombin–PAR-1 interactions enhance IL-8 mRNA and protein expression in cultured term decidual cells [130]. Neutrophils are a rich source of elastase and MMP-9 [133] that contribute to PPROM and cervical effacement. Stephenson et al. [134] have shown that thrombin also enhances MMP-9 expression in cultured amniochorion. These studies suggest a mechanism linking abruption-associated PPROM to decidual thrombin–PAR interactions. A link between thrombin and PTL has been described by Phillippe and Chien [135] who reported that thrombin–PAR interactions directly trigger myometrial contractions. In either case, abruption can be accompanied by a robust intraamniotic inflammatory process in the absence of infection [136]. Proteomics-based studies demonstrated that coagulation proteases and free hemoglobin chains control different modules of the innate immunity and a feed-forward mechanism reinforces a "sterile" inflammatory process leading to PPROM, PTL, and PTD [134].

Mechanical stretching of the uterus

Pregnancy transforms the thick uterus into a thin-walled muscular organ to accommodate the fetus, placenta, and amniotic fluid [137]. These changes facilitate uterine adaptation to stretch such that a state of myometrial contractile quiescence can be maintained. Buhimschi and associates showed that in singleton gestations there is significant and widespread ultrasonographic thinning of the myometrium during active labor whether this occurs at term or preterm [135,138]. Various mathematical models indicate that wall stress (applied force per unit of cross-sectional area) is directly proportional to intracavitary pressure and the radius of curvature but inversely proportional to the thickness of the muscle [139]. Thus, the thinner the myometrium during contraction, the greater will be the generated uterine wall stress.

There is a decrease in the gestational age at delivery with increasing numbers of fetuses. For example, the average gestational age of delivery with twins is 35.3 weeks compared with 29.9 weeks for quadruplets [140], implicating mechanical stretching directly in the PTD process. Twin pregnancy was characterized by a significant, selective and gradual thinning of the lower uterine segment during gestation. Thinning of the lower uterine segment occurred earlier in twin pregnancies destined to deliver preterm [139].

Excessive myometrial stretch and wall stress alter gene expression pathways that orchestrate a transition from quiescence to active myometrial contractions. In vitro, mechanical stretch increases MMP-1 secretion from human uterine cervical fibroblasts [41]. Similarly, stretching of the human uterine myocytes induces oxytocin receptor, COX-2, IL-8, and connexin-43 expression [141–144]. In vivo, mechanical dilation of the cervix promoted cervical ripening through the induction of endogenous PGs [145] and increased MMP-1 expression [146]. Polyhydramnios and multifetal gestation-induced mechanical stretch increases amnion COX-2 expression and related PG production [147,148]. These data consolidate the argument that mechanical stretch contributes to the massive increase in the expression of procontractile molecules with central roles in premature activation of the myometrial contractile machinery leading to PTD.

Final common pathway of preterm delivery

The generation of PGs, proteases, and a large array of pro-inflammatory cytokines reflects the final common pathway of both term and all spontaneous preterm deliveries. Levels of PGs increase in reproductive tract tissues, maternal plasma, and amniotic fluid immediately before and during parturition [149–152]. Concomitant with

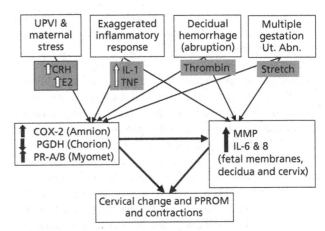

Figure 40.1 Pathogenesis of preterm delivery (PTD). COX-2, cyclooxygenase 2; CRH, corticotropin-releasing hormone; IL, interleukin; MMP, metalloproteinase; Myomet, myometrium; PGDH, 15-hydroxy-prostaglandin dehydrogenase; PR-A/B progesterone receptor isoform A to B ratio; PPROM, preterm premature rupture of the membranes; TNF, tumor necrosis factor; UPVI, uteroplacental vascular insufficiency; Ut Abn, uterine abnormality.

rising PG levels is the upregulation of myometrial PG receptors prior to the onset of labor [153,154]. Moreover, all the pathways of prematurity described above also directly trigger MMP and IL-8 expression to mediate cervical change and fetal membrane rupture. Prior to 20 weeks gestation, the myometrium is quiescent because of the high P4 levels and PR-B expression, coupled with low circulating estrogen levels and ER-β expression which inhibit expression of contraction-associated genes. Thus, activation of this pathway before 20 weeks causes incompetent cervix to be the *forme fruste* of the PTD process in the first half of gestation. Figure 40.1 presents a schematic of the discrete pathogenic processes leading to prematurity and their final common biochemical pathway.

Prediction of preterm delivery: interpretation of test results

The four PTD pathogenic processes outlined here present unique biochemical or biophysical signatures. Efforts to exploit these "signatures" to identify patients at risk for PTD from a given pathway have met with only modest success. The final common pathway of cervical and fetal membrane proteolysis can be discerned by assessment of cervicovaginal levels of fetal fibronectin (fFN) derived from the chorion or cervical length determination by ultrasound. In addition, high-throughput, high-dimensional proteomics technologies provide early detection of the pathophysiologic conditions leading to PTD. Unfortunately, studies examining the efficacy of various putative biomarkers continue to be marked by heterogeneous patient populations with varying distributions of pathogenic mechanisms and prevalence of PTD, as well as by diverse assay strategies, inconsistent cutoff values, and varying definitions of PTD.

Comparison of marker efficacy therefore requires conversion of their predictive estimates to positive and negative likelihood ratios (LR) [155]. The LR is a measure of the predictive accuracy of a diagnostic test independent of disease prevalence. The LR expresses how many more times (LR positive [+]) or fewer times (LR negative [-]) a test result is to be identified in subjects with the outcome of interest compared with those without the outcome. Interpretation of LRs is intuitive. The higher the LR(+) and the lower the LR(−), the better the diagnostic test performance. A LR(+) is calculated by dividing the sensitivity by the false-positive rate. An LR(−) is calculated by dividing the false-negative rate by specificity. An LR of 1.0 indicates no change from pretest probability, suggesting a useless test. As general guidelines, a LR(+) >2 corresponds to the probability of disease of approximately 67% [156,157]. Values of LR(+) >5 argue strongly for presence of the disease, whereas values of LR(−) <0.2 strongly militate against the presence of a disease.

Pathway-specific markers

Inflammatory biomarkers

Interleukins

Lockwood et al. [158] conducted a prospective cohort study in 161 high-risk asymptomatic patients. Sampling of the cervicovaginal secretions every 3–4 weeks between 24 and 36 weeks revealed a 4.2-fold increase in maximal cervical IL-6 concentrations among patients with subsequent PTDs <37 weeks compared with those with subsequent term deliveries [159]. A single cervical IL-6 value >250 pg/mL identified patients with subsequent PTD compared with those having term deliveries with LR(+) of 3.33 and LR(−) of 0.59. Multiple logistic regression indicated that a cervical IL-6 level >250 pg/mL was an independent predictor of spontaneous PTD with an adjusted OR of 4.8 (95% CI 1.7–14.3). The National Institute of Child Health and Human Development (NICHD) Maternal-Fetal Medicine Units (MFMU) Network conduced a nested case–control study in an asymptomatic high-risk population and noted that while IL-6 concentrations were significantly higher in cases compared with controls (212 ± 339 vs. 111 ± 186 pg/mL, P <0.008), only 20% of cases had IL-6 values >90th percentile [160]. Moreover, regression analysis suggested that after adjusting for other PTD risk factors, including a positive fFN test result, body mass index (BMI) <19.8 kg/m^2, vaginal bleeding in the first or second trimester, previous spontaneous PTD and short cervix, elevated cervical IL-6 levels were not independently associated with spontaneous

PTD. Among symptomatic patients, the published LRs for cervical IL-6 for the prediction of PTD were 1.82–3.63 for LR(+) and 0.3–0.8 for LR(−) [104,161–164].

Holst and associates [107] found higher cervical IL-8 levels among women who subsequently delivered preterm compared with those delivering at term (median 11.3 ng/mL, range 0.15–98.1 ng/mL vs. 4.9 ng/mL, range 0.15–41.0 ng/mL, P <0.002). The presence of cervical IL-8 values >7.7 ng/mL predicted PTD <7 days with LR(+) of 2.38 and LR(−) of 0.51. Kurkinen-Raty and colleagues [162] observed LR(+) of 1.4 (95 % CI 0.9–2.4) for a cervical IL-8 value >3.74 µg/L among symptomatic patients sampled between 22 and 32 weeks. Rizzo et al. [163] observed that cervical IL-8 values >450 pg/mL were comparable with fFN values >50 ng/mL in predicting PTD and that a cervical IL-8 level >860 pg/mL predicted a positive amniotic fluid culture with LR(+) of 2.4 and LR(−) of 0.28. In contrast, Coleman et al. [164] were not able to confirm any PTD predictive value for cervical IL-8 determinations. Other markers of lower genital tract infection including cervical lactoferrin, sialidase, defensins, follistatin-free activin, serum β2-microglobulin, latex C-reactive protein, intracellular adhesion molecule-1, elevated vaginal pH, and cervical neutrophils are not predictive of PTD [165–171].

Proteomic-based markers

Identification of relevant cervicovaginal protein biomarkers that can lead to early diagnosis and treatment of PTD is theoretically possible through application of proteomics high-throughput technologies that directly interrogate differences in protein biomarkers [172]. Based on previous studies, the cervicovaginal proteome of pregnant women is rich in innate immunity proteins [173]. Several immunoregulatory proteins, such as lactotransferin, neutrophil gelatinase, S100 A8 (calgranulin A), S100A9 (calgranulin B), haptoglobin, defensins, lactoferrin, azurocidin, annexins, and transferrin, were previously linked to PTD [174–176]. However, the presence of these proteins in cervicovaginal secretions does not appear to necessarily result from an inflammatory response but rather these proteins are normal components of the cervical innate immune system [177].

Advances in proteomics have spurred investigation into maternal serum markers of PTD. The Proteomic Assessment of Preterm Risk study enrolled 5501 pregnancies from 2011–2013 from 11 sites in the United States [178]. A predictor score was calculated based on ratio of insulin-like growth factor-binding protein 4 (IBP4) and sex-hormone binding globulin (SHBG). Within this cohort, there were 217 spontaneous PTDs. After stratification by BMI, the IBP4/SHBG predictor had an OR of 5.04 (95% CI 1.4–18) for spontaneous PTD. The utility of this model was recently confirmed in an independent cohort of 847 pregnancies. The IBP4/SHBG ratio was able to predict PTD <32 week's gestation with an area under the curve (AUC) of 0.76 (95% CI 0.59–0.93) [179].

Several studies focused on identification of amniotic fluid protein biomarkers that could accurately predict PTD in women with intraamniotic inflammation [180–182]. Buhimschi and associates used surface-enhanced laser desorption ionization time-of-flight mass spectrometry and named the analysis method mass restricted (MR) scoring. Proteomic identification techniques established that presence of four protein biomarkers (defensin-2, defensin-1, S100A12, S100A8) in the amniotic fluid was diagnostic of intraamniotic inflammation [183]. The MR score was reproducible and maintained its highly accurate signature when tested prospectively in women with intraamniotic fluid inflammation/infection [184]. A key finding of this study was that women with "severe amniotic fluid inflammation" (MR score with three or four proteomic biomarkers present) had shorter amniocentesis-to-delivery intervals than women with "no inflammation" (MR 0, all four markers absent) or even "minimal inflammation" (MR score with one or two markers present). Nonetheless, a "minimal" degree of inflammation was associated with PTD regardless of membrane status. This is relevant because in this population, biochemical tests such as amniotic fluid glucose and lactate dehydrogenase levels and white blood cell count traditionally used to diagnose intraamniotic inflammation were reported as normal.

Studies have also examined the role of amniotic fluid biomarkers to predict risk of PTD in asymptomatic women. In a case-control study of singleton pregnancies who underwent genetic amniocentesis in the second trimester, MMP-8 was positive in 42.2% of patients who went on to have PTD <30 weeks gestation. No patient delivering at term had a positive amniotic MMP-8 [185]. Owing to its high specificity, MMP-8 is a promising marker for PTD. Other amniotic proteins such as vascular endothelial growth factor, placental growth factor, and soluble fms-like tyrosine kinase-1 have been linked with an increased risk of PTD in asymptomatic women [186–188]. Currently, amniocentesis is not recommended for the sole indication of assessing risk of PTD.

Biomarkers of decidual hemorrhage and dysregulation in coagulation pathways

Given the high concentrations of tissue factor in the decidua [125], abruption leads to excess thrombin generation, explaining the consumptive coagulopathy noted in severe cases. Thus, thrombin would appear to be an ideal marker for the detection of abruption-associated PTDs. Rosen et al. [189] noted that TAT >3.9 µg/L predict subsequent PPROM in asymptomatic patients with LR(+) of 2.75 and LR(−) of 0.18. Among symptomatic patients, TAT complex levels >6.3 µg/L between 24 and 33 weeks predict PTD within 3 weeks with LR(+) of 5.5 and LR(−) of

0.55 [190]. Chaiworapongsa et al. [191] observed that TAT complex levels >20 µg/L predict PTD <37 weeks with LR(+) of 2.9 and LR(−) of 0.6.

Markers of the final preterm delivery common pathway

Fetal fibronectin (fFN)

Fibronectins are large ECM and plasma proteins. A heavily glycosylated form, termed fFN, is present in the amniotic fluid, placental, and fetal membranes [192]. It is produced by extravillous cytotrophoblasts in the anchoring villi and cytotrophoblastic shell as well as the chorion; it is released into cervicovaginal secretions when the chorionic–decidual ECM is disrupted prior to labor [193]. It is also produced by amnion epithelium and released into amniotic fluid [190]. Thus, fFN is positioned to be deported into the cervicovaginal secretions following occult or overt PPROM [191].

Lockwood et al. [192] first described the association between cervicovaginal fFN (>50 ng/mL) between 22 and 37 weeks and an increased risk of PTD among symptomatic patients with LR(+) of 4.67 and LR(−) of 0.22. Given evidence that fFN determinations retained their predictive value for only 2–3 weeks, Peaceman et al. [194] assessed the value of fFN for predicting PTD within 7–14 days in symptomatic patients and noted LR(+) of 4.9 and 4.9, respectively, and LR(−) of 0.15 and 0.21, respectively. Of note, the corresponding negative predictive values in this population-based study were 99.5% and 99.2%, respectively. A meta-analysis of 14 studies examining the accuracy of fFN reported pooled LRs for the prediction of PTD within 7–14 days in symptomatic patients of 5.43 (95% CI 4.36–6.74) for LR(+) and 0.25 (95% CI 0.2–0.31) for LR(−). The comparable values for predicting PTD prior to 34 weeks were 3.64 (95% CI 3.32–5.73) and 0.32 (95% CI 0.16–0.66), respectively, among eight studies [195]. A meta-analysis of 32 pooled studies confirmed these results with LRs for a positive and negative fFN test of 4.20 (95% CI 3.53–4.99) and 0.29 (95% CI 0.22–0.38), respectively [196].

Lockwood et al. [197] also initially assessed the utility of serial cervicovaginal fFN determinations in the prediction of subsequent PTD among high-risk asymptomatic patients sampled every 2–4 weeks between 24 and 37 weeks gestation. A vaginal fFN value >50 ng/mL predicted PTD with LR(+) of 3.4 and LR(−) of 0.4. Vaginal fFN predicted PTDs resulting from PTL and PPROM with equal efficiency. The NICHD MFMU Network subsequently assessed the value of cervicovaginal fFN obtained at 22–24 weeks among nearly 3000 asymptomatic women and found an even more robust LR(+) of 6.3 but less strong LR(−) of 0.84 [198]. A meta-analysis of studies among high-risk asymptomatic patients has demonstrated a pooled LR(+) for the prediction of PTD <34 weeks of 4.01 (95% CI 2.93–5.49) and a LR(–) of 0.78 (95% CI 0.72–0.84) [195].

The fFN test appears equally valid in patients with twins, cervical cerclage, and prior multifetal reduction procedures [199–201]. Although its principal utility lies in its high negative predictive value (>99% for delivery within 2 weeks), most studies suggest a positive predictive value for PTD of >50%, suggesting that fFN-positive patients beyond 23 completed weeks of gestation should receive corticosteroids. Several attempts have been made to investigate the value of quantitative assessment of fFN in predicting PTB as an aid to the cervical length [202,203]. Following completion of these studies, controversy remains if quantitative fFN carries an important role in predicting PTB based on parity, because data suggest this biomarker performs better quantitatively in nulliparous women. However, there is consensus that the clinical value of fFN remains in its high NPV. A speculum exam need not be used to obtain a vaginal specimen [204]. At this point fFN remains the cervical biomarker with the greatest clinical usefulness [196,205].

Sonographic cervical length measurements

Between 22 and 30 weeks gestation, the length of the cervix assumes a Gaussian distribution with the 5th percentile at 20 mm, 10th percentile at 25 mm, 50th percentile at 35 mm, and 90th percentile at 45 mm [206]. The relative risk of PTD increases as the length of the cervix decreases. When women with shorter cervixes at 24 weeks were compared with women with values above the 75th percentile, the relative risks of PTD among the women with shorter cervixes were as follows: 1.98 for cervical lengths ≤40 mm, 2.35 for lengths ≤35 mm, 3.79 for lengths ≤30 mm, 6.19 for lengths ≤26 mm, 9.49 for lengths ≤22 mm, and 13.99 for lengths ≤13 mm [207].

Among symptomatic women who go on to deliver preterm, 80–100% have a cervical length ≤30 mm when initially evaluated because of contractions. As a rule, a subsequent PTD is highly unlikely in symptomatic women when the cervix is longer than 30 mm, unless an acute abruption is the cause of their contractions [206]. Conversely, PTD is quite likely when a cervix measures <15 mm. In one study of 216 women, in 173 cases the cervical length was ≥15 mm and only one of these women delivered within 7 days, while in the 43 patients with cervical lengths <15 mm, delivery within 7 days occurred in 37% [208]. Vendittelli and Volumenie [209] conducted a meta-analysis of the utility of cervical sonographic length determination for the prediction of PTD among symptomatic patients. Nine articles met their inclusion criteria, the optimal predictive cutoff varied from 18 to 30 mm, and the prevalence of PTD was 37.3%. The authors found that relative risk for the occurrence of PTD when the cervical length was ≤18 mm was 3.9 (95% CI 1.8–8.5) and that sensitivities for predicting PTD ranged from 68% to 100%, and the specificity ranged from 30% to 78%.

In asymptomatic women with a history of PTD, the gestational age at PTD in the previous pregnancy correlates with the cervical length in the subsequent gestation [210]. Cervical length measurements in the second trimester in asymptomatic women with a history of prior spontaneous PTD predict recurrent spontaneous PTD. The MFMU Network examined the value of cervical ultrasound in predicting PTD <35 weeks among high-risk asymptomatic patients [211]. Patients underwent cervical sonography every 2 weeks and lengths <25 mm noted at any time were associated with a relative risk for spontaneous PTD of 4.5 (95% CI 2.7–7.6) but LR(+) of only 1.5 and LR(–) of 0.39. The efficacy of cervical length in predicting PTD in asymptomatic low-risk women is quite low. In a series of 3694 unselected Finnish women scanned at 18–24 weeks, a 25 mm cutoff yielded insignificant LR(+) and LR(–) [212]. Similar results were found in a large US cohort [213].

Ultrasound cervical elastography

There is recent interest in evaluating additional sonographic parameters of the uterine cervix in the context of PTD prediction. Ultrasound elastography is a noninvasive method of assessing tissue stiffness, and it is already employed to assess liver, breast, thyroid, and prostate pathologies [214]. As such, its application to the dynamic tissue of the uterine cervix is of increasing interest, especially as it relates to prediction of PTD. Strain elastography and shear wave are the two principal methods used to assess cervical tissue elasticity [215]. Strain elastography measures elasticity by comparing tissue characteristics before and after a manually applied external force. Thus, it is useful for measuring differences in tissue stiffness. On the other hand, shear wave elastography relies on measuring propagation of transverse waves in tissue and does not rely on application of external deforming forces. As such, it can measure absolute values of tissue stiffness. A systematic review and meta-analysis calculated a sensitivity of 0.81 (95% CI 0.64–0.92) and specificity of 0.88 (95% CI 0.78–0.94) of cervical elastography to predict PTD with an AUC of 0.90 (95% CI 0.87–0.93) [216]. These findings suggest that cervical elastography is not only useful to predict PTD but may be better than cervical length measurement alone. However, successful implementation of such screening modality for PTD requires additional training of ultrasound technicians. Furthermore, due to its operator-dependent nature, standardized methods for cervical strain elastography have not been established, and use of cervical shear wave elastography requires specialized transducers [217].

Additional novel sonographic methods of the cervix are under investigation. The cervical consistency index (CCI) is a ratio of the anterior-posterior diameter of the cervix measured before and after application of pressure with a transvaginal probe [218]. Cervical texture (CTx) is a quantitative assessment of the anterior cervical stroma that processes digital images of greyscale speckle patterns to equate cervical microstructure [219]. In prospective case–control trials, both CCI and CTx better predicted PTD than cervical length alone in asymptomatic women.

Combining sonographic cervical length and fFN

The optimal PTD diagnostic accuracy occurs when combining vaginal fFN with cervical length determinations. Hincz et al. [220] prospectively evaluated 82 symptomatic patients with cervical sonography and fFN if the cervical length was between 2.0 and 3.1 cm. Defining positive patients as those with either a cervical length <2.1 cm or a positive fFN, they predicted delivery within 28 days with LR(+) of 8.6 and LR(−) of 0.16. The sensitivity of this two-step method was 86%, with a specificity of 90%, positive predictive value of 63%, and negative predictive value of 97%. Interestingly, among patients with a cervical length of 2.0–3.1 mm, 71.4% of those with a positive fFN delivered within 28 days whereas only 7.4% of those with negative fFN delivered within 28 days. Figure 40.2 describes an algorithm for evaluating symptomatic patients with both fFN and cervical sonography. Patients found at risk qualify for antenatal steroids when ≥24 weeks, as well as short-term tocolysis, and antibiotic therapy for urinary

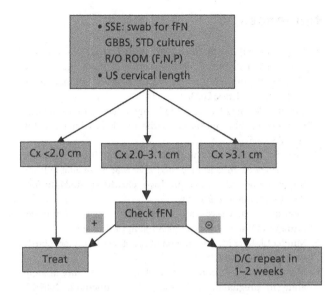

Figure 40.2 Algorithm for using fetal fibronectin (fFN) and/or cervical ultrasound in symptomatic patients. Cx, cervix; D/C, discharge patient; GBBS, group B β-streptococcus; R/O ROM, rule out rupture of fetal membranes; SSE, sterile speculum exam; STD, sexually transmitted disease; US, ultrasound.

tract infections, or group B β-streptococcus if present or while cultures are pending.

CASE PRESENTATION 1

A 37-year-old primigravida at 31 weeks notes sudden onset of intermittent abdominal tightening and back pain. She contacts the on-call obstetrician who instructs her to go to the hospital. At presentation, she is noted to have a category I fetal heart rate tracing and contractions occurring three times every 10 min for 30 min. Intravenous fluids are administered. An ultrasonographic cervical length of 2.2 cm is noted. A vaginal swab was obtained prior to the ultrasound and was sent for fFn determination. The fFN returns positive. The patient is admitted, tocolysis commenced, penicillin given for group B β-streptococcus prophylaxis after rectovaginal cultures were obtained and steroids administered. After 72 hours of observation, uterine contractions subside. She is discharged home with specific instructions including reduced physical effort. At 36 weeks she enters spontaneous labor and delivers a healthy infant.

CASE PRESENTATION 2

A 38-year-old gravida 1, para 0, at 32 weeks, presents to labor and delivery with sudden onset of abdominal pain and vaginal bleeding. The pregnancy had been complicated by vaginal bleeding of uncertain etiology in the first trimester and at 20 weeks. The fetal heart rate tracing remains category 1 with rare contractions, her fibrinogen level is stable at 345 and 338 mg/dL over 4 h and she is observed for 24 h without cervical change or increasing contractions. Vaginal spotting continues intermittently for 1 week and she re-presents 7 days later with frank PPROM. The patient is admitted, given intravenous fluids, antibiotics, and two doses of corticosteroids. After 72 h of observation, she develops sudden onset of heavy vaginal bleeding, fetal bradycardia and uterine hypertonus, prompting intensive resuscitation with blood and crystalloids and an emergency cesarean delivery. A Couvelaire uterus and a large retroplacental hematoma are noted.

References

1. Osterman MJK, Hamilton BE, Martin JA, Driscoll AK, Valenzuela CP. Births: Final data for 2021. National Vital Statistics Reports; vol 72 no 1. Hyattsville, MD: National Center for Health Statistics; 2023.

2. Ananth CV, Vintzileos AM. Medically indicated preterm birth: recognizing the importance of the problem. Clin Perinatol. 2008;35:53–67.

3. Centers for Disease Control and Prevention. Infant mortality. [last reviewed 2022 Jun 22; cited 2022 Mar 6]. Available from: https://www.cdc.gov/reproductivehealth/maternalinfanthealth/infantmortality.htm.

4. Moutquin JM. Classification and heterogeneity of preterm birth. Br J Obstet Gynaecol. 2003;10(Suppl 20):30–3.

5. Muglia LJ, Katz M. The enigma of spontaneous preterm birth. N Engl J Med. 2010;362:529–35.

6. Mendelson CR. Minireview: fetal-maternal hormonal signaling in pregnancy and labor. Mol Endocrinol. 2009;23:947–54.

7. Buhimschi CS, Rosenberg VA, Dulay AT, Thung S, Sfakianaki AK, Bahtiyar MO, et al. Multidimensional system biology: genetic markers and proteomic biomarkers of adverse pregnancy outcome in preterm birth. Am J Perinatol. 2008;25:175–87.

8. Lockwood CJ, Kuczynski E. Risk stratification and pathological mechanisms in preterm delivery. Paediatr Perinat Epidemiol. 2001;2:78–89.

9. Zhang G, Feenstra B, Bacelis J, Liu X, Muglia LM, Juodakis J, et al. Genetic Associations with Gestational Duration and Spontaneous Preterm Birth. N Engl J Med. 2017 Sep 21;377(12):1156–67.

10. Anum EA, Springel EH, Shriver MD, Strauss JF 3rd. Genetic contributions to disparities in preterm birth. Pediatr Res. 2009;65:1–9.

11. Zakar T, Hertelendy F. Progesterone withdrawal: key to parturition. Am J Obstet Gynecol. 2007;196:289–96.

12. Lockwood CJ, Stocco C, Murk W, Kayisli UA, Funai EF, Schatz F. Human labor is associated with reduced decidual cell expression of progesterone, but not glucocorticoid, receptors. J Clin Endocrinol Metab. 2010;95:2271–5.

13. Petraglia F, Imperatore A, Challis JR. Neuroendocrine mechanisms in pregnancy and parturition. Endocr Rev. 2010;31(6):783–816.

14. Copper RL, Goldenberg RL, Das A, Elder N, Swain M, Norman G, et al. The preterm prediction study: maternal stress is associated with spontaneous preterm birth at less than thirty-five weeks' gestation. National Institute of Child Health and Human Development Maternal-Fetal Medicine Units Network. Am J Obstet Gynecol. 1996;175:1286–92.

15. Lipkind HS, Curry AE, Huynh M, Thorpe LE, Matte T. Birth outcomes among offspring of women exposed to the September 11, 2001, terrorist attacks. Obstet Gynecol. 2010;116:917–25.

16. Orr ST, James SA, Blackmore Prince C. Maternal prenatal depressive symptoms and spontaneous preterm births among African-American women in Baltimore, Maryland. Am J Epidemiol. 2002;156:797–802.

17. Ding XX, Wu YL, Xu SJ, Zhu RP, Jia XM, Zhang SF, et al. Maternal anxiety during pregnancy and adverse birth outcomes: a systematic review and meta-analysis of prospective cohort studies. J Affect Disord. 2014 Apr;159:103–10.

18. Grote NK, Bridge JA, Gavin AR, Melville JL, Iyengar S, Katon WJ. A meta-analysis of depression during pregnancy and the risk of preterm birth, low birth weight, and intrauterine growth restriction. Arch Gen Psychiatry. 2010;67:1012–24.

19. Germain AM, Carvajal J, Sanchez M, Valenzuela GJ, Tsunekawa H, Chuaqui B. Preterm labor: placental pathology and clinical correlation. Obstet Gynecol. 1999;94:284–9.

20. Arias F, Rodriquez L, Rayne SC, Kraus FT. Maternal placental vasculopathy and infection: two distinct subgroups among patients with preterm labor and preterm ruptured membranes. Am J Obstet Gynecol. 1993;168:585–91.

21. Kelly R, Holzman C, Senagore P, Wang J, Tian Y, Rahbar MH, et al. Placental vascular pathology findings and pathways to preterm delivery. Am J Epidemiol. 2009 Jul 15;170(2):148–58.

22. Lykke JA, PAidas MJ, Langhoof-Roos J. Recurring complications in second pregnancy. Obstet Gynecol. 2009; 113:1217.

23. Craddock N, Forty L. Genetics of affective (mood) disorders. Eur J Hum Genet. 2006;14:660–8.

24. Svensson AC, Pawitan Y, Cnattingius S, Reilly M, Lichtenstein P. Familial aggregation of small-for-gestational-age births: the importance of fetal genetic effects. Am J Obstet Gynecol. 2006;194:475–9.

25. Challis JR, Lye SJ, Gibb W, Whittle W, Patel F, Alfaidy N. Understanding preterm labor. Ann N Y Acad Sci. 2001;943:225–34.

26. McLean M, Bisits A, Davies J, Woods R, Lowry P, Smith R. A placental clock controlling the length of human pregnancy. Nat Med. 1995;1:460–3.

27. Wolfe CD, Patel SP, Linton EA, Campbell EA, Anderson J, Dornhorst A, et al. Plasma corticotrophinreleasing factor (CRF) in abnormal pregnancy. Br J Obstet Gynaecol. 1988;95:1003–6.

28. Jones SA, Brooks AN, Challis JR. Steroids modulate corticotropin-releasing hormone production in human fetal membranes and placenta. J Clin Endocrinol. Metab 1989;68:825–30.

29. Sandman CA, Glynn L, Schetter CD, Wadhwa P, Garite T, Chicz-DeMet A, et al. Elevated maternal cortisol early in pregnancy predicts third trimester levels of placental corticotropin releasing hormone (CRH): priming the placental clock. Peptides. 2006;27:1457–63.

30. Economides DL, Nicolaides KH, Linton EA, Perry LA, Chard T. Plasma cortisol and adrenocorticotropin in appropriate and small for gestational age fetuses. Fetal Ther. 1988;3:158–64.

31. Amiel-Tison C, Cabrol D, Denver R, Jarreau PH, Papiernik E, Piazza PV. Fetal adaptation to stress. Part I: acceleration of fetal maturation and earlier birth triggered by placental insufficiency in humans. Early Hum Dev. 2004;78:15–27.

32. Lockwood CJ, Radunovic N, Nastic D, Petkovic S, Aigner S, Berkowitz GS. Corticotropin-releasing hormone and related pituitary-adrenal axis hormones in fetal and maternal blood during the second half of pregnancy. J Perinat Med. 1996;24:243–51.

33. Florio P, Zatelli MC, Reis FM, degli Uberti EC, Petraglia F. Corticotropin releasing hormone: a diagnostic marker for behavioral and reproductive disorders? Front Biosci. 2007;12:551–60.

34. Challis JRG, Matthews SG, Gibb W, Lye SJ. Endocrine and paracrine regulation of birth at term and preterm. Endocr Rev. 2000;21:514–50.

35. Jones SA, Challis JR. Effects of corticotropin-releasing hormone and adrenocorticotropin on prostaglandin output by human placenta and fetal membranes. Gynecol Obstet Invest. 1990;29:165–8.

36. Jones SA, Challis JR. Steroid, corticotrophin-releasing hormone, ACTH and prostaglandin interactions in the amnion and placenta of early pregnancy in man. J Endocrinol. 1990;125:153–9.

37. Myatt L, Lye SJ. Expression, localization and function of prostaglandin receptors in myometrium. Prostaglandins Leukot Essent Fatty Acids. 2004;70:137–48.

38. Garfield RE, Sims S, Daniel EE. Gap junctions: their presence and necessity in myometrium during parturition. Science. 1977;198:958–60.

39. Olson DM. The role of prostaglandins in the initiation of parturition. Best Pract Res Clin Obstet Gynaecol. 2003;17:717–30.

40. Cook JL, Zaragoza DB, Sung DH, Olson DM. Expression of myometrial activation and stimulation genes in a mouse model of preterm labor: myometrial activation, stimulation, and preterm labor. Endocrinology. 2000;141:1718–28.

41. Yoshida M, Sagawa N, Itoh H, Yura S, Takemura M, Wada Y, et al. Prostaglandin F(2alpha), cytokines and cyclic mechanical stretch augment matrix metalloproteinase-1 secretion from cultured human uterine cervical fibroblast cells. Mol Hum Reprod. 2002;8:681–7.

42. Denison FC, Calder AA, Kelly RW. The action of prostaglandin E2 on the human cervix: stimulation of interleukin 8 and inhibition of secretory leukocyte protease inhibitor. Am J Obstet Gynecol. 1999;180:614–20.

43. Zakar T, Hirst JJ, Mijovic JE, Olson DM. Glucocorticoids stimulate the expression of prostaglandin endoperoxide H synthase-2 in amnion cells. Endocrinology. 1995;136:1610–19.

44. Patel FA, Clifton VL, Chwalisz K, Challis JR. Steroid regulation of prostaglandin dehydrogenase activity and expression in human term placenta and chorio-decidua in relation to labor. J Clin Endocrinol Metab. 1999;84:291–9.

45. Madsen G, Zakar T, Ku CY, Sanborn BM, Smith R, Mesiano S. Prostaglandins differentially modulate progesterone receptor-A and -B expression in human myometrial cells: evidence for prostaglandin-induced functional progesterone withdrawal. J Clin Endocrinol Metab. 2004;89:1010–13.

46. Stjernholm-Vladic Y, Wang H, Stygar D, Ekman G, Sahlin L. Differential regulation of the progesterone receptor A and B in the human uterine cervix at parturition. Gynecol Endocrinol. 2004;18:41–6.

47. Oh SY, Kim CJ, Park I et al. Progesterone receptor isoform (A/B) ratio of human fetal membranes increases during term parturition. Am J Obstet Gynecol. 2005;193:1156–60.

48. Merlino A, Welsh T, Erdonmez T, Madsen G, Zakar T, Smith R, et al. Nuclear progesterone receptor expression in the human fetal membranes and decidua at term before and after labor. Reprod Sci. 2009;16:357–63.

49. Parker CR Jr, Stankovic AM, Goland RS. Corticotropinreleasing hormone stimulates steroidogenesis in cultured human adrenal cells. Mol Cell Endocrinol. 1999;155:19–25.

50. Di WL, Lachelin GC, McGarrigle HH, Thomas NS, Becker DL. Oestriol and oestradiol increase cell to cell communication and connexin43 protein expression in human myometrium. Mol Hum Reprod. 2001;7:671–9.

51. Richter ON, Kubler K, Schmolling J, Kupka M, Reinsberg J, Ulrich U, et al. Oxytocin receptor gene expression of estrogen-stimulated human myometrium in extracorporeally perfused non-pregnant uteri. Mol Hum Reprod. 2004;10:339–46.

52. Mesiano S, Chan EC, Fitter JT, Kwek K, Yeo G, Smith R. Progesterone withdrawal and estrogen activation in human parturition are coordinated by progesterone receptor A expression in the myometrium. J Clin Endocrinol Metab. 2002;87:2924–30.

53. Schatz F, Guzeloglu-Kayisli O, Basar M, Buchwalder LF, Ocak N, Guzel E, et al. Enhanced human decidual cell-expressed FKBP51 may promote labor-related functional progesterone withdrawal. Am J Pathol. 2015 Sep;185(9):2402–11.

54. Storer CL, Dickey CA, Galigniana MD, Rein T, Cox MB. FKBP51 and FKBP52 in signaling and disease. Trends Endocrinol Metab. 2011 Dec;22(12):481–90.

55. Stechschulte LA, Sanchez ER. FKBP51 – a selective modulator of glucocorticoid and androgen sensitivity. Curr Opin Pharmacol. 2011 Aug;11(4):332–7.

56. Hubler TR, Denny WB, Valentine DL, Cheung-Flynn J, Smith DF, Scammell JG. The FK506-binding immunophilin FKBP51 is transcriptionally regulated by progestin and attenuates progestin responsiveness. Endocrinology. 2003 Jun;144(6):2380–7.

57. Guzeloglu-Kayisli O, Semerci N, Guo X, Larsen K, Ozmen A, Arlier S, et al. Decidual cell FKBP51-progesterone receptor binding mediates maternal stress-induced preterm birth. Proc Natl Acad Sci U S A. 2021 Mar 16;118(11):e2010282118.

58. Challis JR. CRH, a placental clock and preterm labour. Nat Med. 1995;1:416.

59. Langlois D, Li JY, Saez JM. Development and function of the human fetal adrenal cortex. J Pediatr Endocrinol 2002;15(Suppl 5):1311–22.

60. Buhimschi CS, Turan OM, Funai EF, Azpurua H, Bahtiyar MO, Turan S, et al. Fetal adrenal gland volume and cortisol/dehydroepiandrosterone sulfate ratio in inflammation-associated preterm birth. Obstet Gynecol 2008;111:715–22.

61. Offenbacher S, Boggess KA, Murtha AP et al. Progressive periodontal disease and risk of very preterm delivery. Obstet Gynecol 2006;107:29–36.

62. Locksmith G, Duff P. Infection, antibiotics, and preterm delivery. Semin Perinatol. 2001;25:295–309.

63. Richey SD, Roberts SW, Ramin KD, Ramin SM, Cunningham FG. Pneumonia complicating pregnancy. Obstet Gynecol. 1994;84:525–8.

64. Goldenberg RL, Hauth JC, Andrews WW. Intrauterine infection and preterm delivery. N Engl J Med. 2000;342:1500–7.

65. Mueller-Heubach E, Rubinstein DN, Schwarz SS. Histologic chorioamnionitis and preterm delivery in different patient populations. Obstet Gynecol. 1990;75:622–6.

66. Andrews WW, Hauth JC, Goldenberg RL, Gomez R, Romero R, Cassell GH. Amniotic fluid interleukin-6: correlation with upper genital tract microbial colonization and gestational age in women delivered after spontaneous labor versus indicated delivery. Am J Obstet Gynecol. 1995;173:606–12.

67. Han YW. Oral health and adverse pregnancy outcomes -what's next? J Dent Res. 2011;90(3):289–93.

68. Polyzos NP, Polyzos IP, Mauri D, Tzioras S, Tsappi M, Cortinovis I, et al. Effect of periodontal disease treatment during pregnancy on preterm birth incidence: a metaanalysis of randomized trials. Am J Obstet Gynecol. 2009;200:225–32.

69. Pirotta M, Fethers KA, Bradshaw CS. Bacterial vaginosis – more questions than answers. Aust Fam Physician. 2009;38:394–7.

70. Meis PJ, Goldenberg RL, Mercer B, Moawad A, Das A, McNellis D, et al. The preterm prediction study: significance of vaginal infections. National Institute of Child Health and Human Development Maternal-Fetal Medicine Units Network. Am J Obstet Gynecol. 1995;173:1231–5.

71. Hillier SL, Nugent RP, Eschenbach DA, Krohn MA, Gibbs RS, Martin DH, et al. Association between bacterial vaginosis and preterm delivery of a low-birth-weight infant. The Vaginal Infections and Prematurity Study Group. N Engl J Med. 1995;333:1737–42.

72. Leitich H, Bodner-Adler B, Brunbauer M, Kaider A, Egarter C, Husslein P. Bacterial vaginosis as a risk factor for preterm delivery: a meta-analysis. Am J Obstet Gynecol. 2003;189:139–47.

73. Jeffcoat M, Parry S, Sammel M, Clothier B, Catlin A, Macones G. Periodontal infection and preterm birth: successful periodontal therapy reduces the risk of preterm birth. Br J Obstet Gynaecol. 2011;118(2):250–6.

74. Hillier SL. The complexity of microbial diversity in bacterial vaginosis. N Engl J Med. 2005;353:1886–7.

75. Hillebrand L, Harmanli OH, Whiteman V, Khandelwal M. Urinary tract infections in pregnant women with bacterial vaginosis. Am J Obstet Gynecol. 2002;186:916–17.

76. Romero R, Oyarzun E, Mazor M, Sirtori M, Hobbins JC, Bracken M. Meta-analysis of the relationship between asymptomatic bacteriuria and preterm delivery/low birth weight. Obstet Gynecol. 1989;73:576–8.

77. Villar J, Gulmezoglu AM, de Onis M. Nutritional and antimicrobial interventions to prevent preterm birth: an overview of randomized controlled trials. Obstet Gynecol. Surv 1998; 53:575–85.

78. Krohn MA, Thwin SS, Rabe LK, Brown Z, Hillier SL. Vaginal colonization by Escherichia coli as a risk factor for very low birth weight delivery and other perinatal complications. J Infect Dis. 1997;175:606–10.

79. Kahwati LC, Clark R, Berkman ND, Urrutia R, Patel SV, Zeng J, et al. Screening for bacterial vaginosis in pregnant adolescents and women to prevent preterm delivery. Evidence synthesis, No. 191. Rockville (MD): Agency for Healthcare Research and Quality (US); 2020 Apr [cited 2023 Jun 7]. Available from: https://www.ncbi.nlm.nih.gov/books/NBK555831/.

80. Shennan A, Crawshaw S, Briley A, Hawken J, Seed P, Jones G, et al. A randomised controlled trial of metronidazole for the prevention of preterm birth in women positive for cervicovaginal fetal fibronectin: the PREMET Study. Br J Obstet Gynaecol. 2006;113:65–74.

81. Carey JC, Klebanoff MA, Hauth JC, Hillier SL, Thom EA, Ernest JM, et al. Metronidazole to prevent preterm delivery in pregnant women with asymptomatic bacterial vaginosis. National Institute of Child Health and Human Development Network of Maternal-Fetal Medicine Units. N Engl J Med. 2000 Feb 24;342(8):534–40.

82. Serrano MG, Parikh HI, Brooks JP, Edwards DJ, Arodz TJ, Edupuganti L, et al. Racioethnic diversity in the dynamics of the vaginal microbiome during pregnancy. Nat Med. 2019 Jun;25(6):1001–11.

83. Fettweis JM, Serrano MG, Brooks JP, Edwards DJ, Girerd PH, Parikh HI, et al. The vaginal microbiome and preterm birth. Nat Med. 2019 Jun;25(6):1012–21.

84. Elovitz MA, Gajer P, Riis V, Brown AG, Humphrys MS, Holm JB, et al. Cervicovaginal microbiota and local immune response modulate the risk of spontaneous preterm delivery. Nat Commun 2019;10(1):1305. Published 2019 Mar 21.

85. DiGiulio DB, Callahan BJ, McMurdie PJ, Costello EK, Lyell DJ, Robaczewska A, et al. Temporal and spatial variation of the human microbiota during pregnancy. Proc Natl Acad Sci U S A. 2015 Sep 1;112(35):11060–5.

86. Kapetanovic R, Cavaillon JM. Early events in innate immunity in the recognition of microbial pathogens. Expert Opin Biol Ther. 2007;7:907–18.

87. Medzhitov R. Inflammation 2010: new adventures of an old flame. Cell. 2010;140:771–6.

88. Brodsky IE, Medzhitov R. Targeting of immune signalling networks by bacterial pathogens. Nat Cell Biol. 2009;11:521–6.

89. Pioli PA, Amiel E, Schaefer TM, Connolly JE, Wira CR, Guyre PM. Differential expression of Toll-like receptors 2 and 4 in tissues of the human female reproductive tract. Infect Immunol. 2004;72:5799–806.

90. Kim YM, Romero R, Chaiworapongsa T, Kim GJ, Kim MR, Kuivaniemi H, et al. Toll-like receptor-2 and -4 in the chorioamniotic membranes in spontaneous labor at term and in preterm parturition that are associated with chorioamnionitis. Am J Obstet Gynecol. 2004;191:1346–55.

91. Holmlund U, Cebers G, Dahlfors AR, Sandstedt B, Bremme K, Ekström ES, et al. Expression and regulation of the pattern recognition receptors Toll-like receptor-2 and Toll-like receptor-4 in the human placenta. Immunology. 2002;107:145–51.

92. Belt AR, Baldassare JJ, Molnar M, Romero R, Hertelendy F. The nuclear transcription factor NF-κB mediates interleukin-1 β-induced expression of cyclooxygenase-2 in human myometrial cells. Am J Obstet Gynecol. 1999;181:359–66.

93. Yan X, Wu Xiao C, Sun M, Tsang BK, Gibb W. Nuclear factor κB activation and regulation of cyclooxygenase type-2 expression in human amnion mesenchymal cells by interleukin-1β. Biol Reprod. 2002;66:1667–71.

94. Lee Y, Allport V, Sykes A, Lindstrom T, Slater D, Bennett P. The effects of labour and of interleukin 1 beta upon the expression of nuclear factor κB related proteins in human amnion. Mol Hum Reprod. 2003;9:213–18.

95. Arechavaleta-Velasco F, Ogando D, Parry S, Vadillo-Ortega F. Production of matrix metalloproteinase-9 in lipopolysaccharidestimulated human amnion occurs through an autocrine and paracrine proinflammatory cytokine-dependent system. Biol Reprod. 2002;67:1952–8.

96. Van Meir CA, Sangha RK, Walton JC, Mathews SG, Keirse MJ, Challis JR. Immunoreactive 15-hydroxyprosta-glandin dehydrogenase (PGDH) is reduced in fetal membranes from patients at preterm delivery in the presence of infection. Placenta. 1996;17:291–7.

97. McLaren J, Taylor DJ, Bell SC. Prostaglandin E(2)-dependent production of latent matrix metalloproteinase-9 in cultures of human fetal membranes. Mol Hum Reprod. 2000;6:1033–40.

98. Ito A, Nakamura T, Uchiyama T, Hirose K, Hirakawa S, Sasaguri Y, et al. Stimulation of the biosynthesis of interleukin 8 by interleukin 1 and tumor necrosis factor alpha in cultured human chorionic cells. Biol Pharm Bull. 1994; 17:1463–7.

99. So T, Ito A, Sato T, Mori Y, Hirakawa S. Tumor necrosis factoralpha stimulates the biosynthesis of matrix metalloproteinases and plasminogen activator in cultured human chorionic cells. Biol Reprod. 1992;46:772–8.

100. Fortunato SJ, Menon R, Lombardi SJ. Role of tumor necrosis factor-alpha in the premature rupture of membranes and preterm labor pathways. Am J Obstet Gynecol. 2002;187:1159–62.

101. Lei H, Furth EE, Kalluri R, et al. A program of cell death and extracellular matrix degradation is activated in the amnion before the onset of labor. J Clin Invest. 1996;98:1971–8.

102. Dudley DJ, Trautman MS, Araneo BA, Edwin SS, Mitchell MD. Decidual cell biosynthesis of interleukin-6: regulation by inflammatory cytokines. J Clin Endocrinol Metab. 1992;74:884–9.

103. Fortunato SJ, Menon RP, Swan KF, Menon R. Inflammatory cytokine (interleukins 1, 6 and 8 and tumor necrosis factoralpha) release from cultured human fetal membranes in response to endotoxic lipopolysaccharide mirrors amniotic fluid concentrations. Am J Obstet Gynecol. 1996;174:1855–61.

104. Mitchell MD, Dudley DJ, Edwin SS, Schiller SL. Interleukin-6 stimulates prostaglandin production by human amnion and decidual cells. Eur J Pharmacol. 1991;192:189–91.

105. Lockwood CJ, Murk WK, Kayisli UA, Buchwalder LF, Huang SJ, Arcuri F, et al. Regulation of interleukin-6 expression in human decidual cells and its potential role in chorioamnionitis. Am J Pathol. 2010;177:1755–64.

106. Guzeloglu-Kayisli O, Kayisli UA, Semerci N, Basar M, Buchwalder LF, Buhimschi CS, et al. Mechanisms of chorioamnionitis-associated preterm birth: interleukin-1β inhibits progesterone receptor expression in decidual cells. J Pathol. 2015 Dec;237(4):423–34.

107. Holst RM, Mattsby-Baltzer I, Wennerholm UB, Hagberg H, Jacobsson B. Interleukin-6 and interleukin-8 in cervical fluid in a population of Swedish women in preterm labor: relationship to microbial invasion of the amniotic fluid, intra-amniotic inflammation, and preterm delivery. Acta Obstet Gynecol Scand. 2005;84:551–7.

108. Miyake K. Innate immune sensing of pathogens and danger signals by cell surface Toll-like receptors. Sem Immunol. 2007;19:3–10.

109. Lotze MT, Zeh HJ, Rubartelli A, Sparvero LJ, Amoscato AA, Washburn NR, et al. The grateful dead: damage-associated molecular pattern molecules and reduction/oxidation regulate immunity. Immunol Rev. 2007;220:60–81.

110. Buhimschi IA, Zhao G, Pettker CM, Bahtiyar MO, Magloire LK, Thung S, et al. The receptor for advanced glycation end products (RAGE) system in women with intraamniotic infection and inflammation. Am J Obstet Gynecol. 2007;196:181.

111. Dulay AT, Buhimschi CS, Zhao G, Oliver EA, Mbele A, Jing S, et al. Soluble TLR2 is present in human amniotic fluid and modulates the intraamniotic inflammatory response to infection. J Immunol 2009;182:7244–53.

112. Menon R, Velez DR, Morgan N, Lombardi SJ, Fortunato SJ, Williams SM. Genetic regulation of amniotic fluid TNF-alpha and soluble TNF receptor concentrations affected by race and preterm birth. Hum Genet. 2008;124:243–53.

113. Buhimschi CS, Baumbusch MA, Dulay AT, Oliver EA, Lee S, Zhao G, et al. Characterization of RAGE, HMGB1, and S100beta in inflammation-induced preterm birth and fetal tissue injury. Am J Pathol. 2009;175:958–75.

114. Lee S, Buhimschi IA, Zhao G, Ali UA, Zhao G, Abdel-Razeq SS et al. The interleukin-6 (IL-6) Trans-signaling system: evidence for presence and activation in pregnancies complicated by intra-amniotic infection. Am J Obstet Gynecol. 2008;199:S141.

115. Elsasser DA, Ananth CV, Prasad V, Vintzileos AM, New Jersey-Placental Abruption Study Investigators. Diagnosis of placental abruption: relationship between clinical and histopathological findings. Eur J Obstet Gynecol Reprod Biol. 2010;148:125–30.

116. Strobino B, Pantel-Silverman J. Gestational vaginal bleeding and pregnancy outcome. Am J Epidemiol. 1989;129:806–15.

117. Dadkhah F, Kashanian M, Eliasi G. A comparison between the pregnancy outcome in women both with or without threatened abortion. Early Hum Dev. 2010;86:193–6.

118. Harger JH, Hsing AW, Tuomala RE, Gibbs RS, Mead PB, Eschenbach DA, et al. Risk factors for preterm premature rupture of fetal membranes: a multicenter case–control study. Am J Obstet Gynecol. 1990;163:130–7.

119. Roque H, Paidas MJ, Funai EF, Kuczynski E, Lockwood CJ. Maternal thrombophilias are not associated with early pregnancy loss. Thromb Haemost. 2004;91:290–5.

120. Nurk E, Tell GS, Refsum H, Ueland PM, Vollset SE. Associations between maternal methylenetetrahydrofolate reductase polymorphisms and adverse outcomes of pregnancy: the Hordaland Homocysteine Study. Am J Med. 2004;117:26–31.

121. American College of Obstetricians and Gynecologists. Practice Bulletin No. 113: inherited thrombophilias in pregnancy. Obstet Gynecol. 2010;116:212–22.

122. Salafia CM, Lopez-Zeno JA, Sherer DM, Whittington SS, Minior VK, Vintzileos AM. Histologic evidence of old intrauterine bleeding is more frequent in prematurity. Am J Obstet Gynecol. 1995;173:1065–70.

123. Ferrand PE, Parry S, Sammel M, Macones GA, Kuivaniemi H, Romero R, et al. A polymorphism in the matrix metalloproteinase-9 promoter is associated with increased risk of preterm premature rupture of membranes in African Americans. Mol Hum Reprod. 2002;8:494–501.

124. Misra DP, Ananth CV. Risk factor profiles of placental abruption in first and second pregnancies: heterogeneous etiologies. J Clin Epidemiol. 1999;52:453–61.

125. Naeye RL. Maternal age, obstetric complications, and the outcome of pregnancy. Obstet Gynecol. 1983;61:210–16.

126. Buhimschi CS, Schatz F, Krikun G, Buhimschi IA, Lockwood CJ. Novel insights into molecular mechanisms of abruption-induced preterm birth. Expert Rev Mol. Med 2010;12:e35.

127. Lockwood C, Krikun G, Schatz F. The decidua regulates hemostasis in the human endometrium. Semin Reprod Endocrinol. 1999;17:45–51.

128. Vidaeff AC, Monga M, Ramin SM, Saade G, Sangi-Haghpeykar H. Is thrombin activation predictive of subsequent preterm delivery? Am J Obstet Gynecol. 2013 Apr;208(4):306.e1–7.

129. Lockwood CJ, Kayisli UA, Stocco C, Murk W, Vatandaslar E, Buchwalder LF, et al. Abruption-induced preterm delivery is associated with thrombin-mediated functional progesterone withdrawal in decidual cells. Am J Pathol. 2012 Dec;181(6):2138–48.

130. Mackenzie AP, Schatz F, Krikun G, Funai EF, Kadner S, Lockwood CJ. Mechanisms of abruption-induced premature rupture of the fetal membranes: thrombin enhanced decidual matrix metalloproteinase-3 (stromelysin-1) expression. Am J Obstet Gynecol. 2004;191:1996–2001.

131. Rosen T, Schatz F, Kuczynski E, Lam H, Koo AB, Lockwood CJ. Thrombin-enhanced matrix metalloproteinase-1 expression: a mechanism linking placental abruption with premature rupture of the membranes. J Matern Fetal Neonatal Med. 2002;11:11–17.

132. Lockwood CJ, Toti P, Arcuri F, Paidas M, Buchwalder L, Krikun G, et al. Mechanisms of abruption- induced premature rupture of the fetal membranes: thrombin-enhanced interleukin-8 expression in term decidua. Am J Pathol 2005;167:1443–9.

133. Lathbury LJ, Salamonsen LA. In vitro studies of the potential role of neutrophils in the process of menstruation. Mol Hum Reprod. 2000;6:899–906.

134. Stephenson CD, Lockwood CJ, Ma Y, Guller S. Thrombin-dependent regulation of matrix metalloproteinase (MMP)-9 levels in human fetal membranes. J Matern Fetal Neonatal Med. 2005;18:17–22.

135. Phillippe M, Chien EK. Intracellular signaling and phasic myometrial contractions. J Soc Gynecol Invest. 1998;5: 169–77.

136. Buhimschi IA, Zhao G, Rosenberg VA, Abdel-Razeq S, Thung S, Buhimschi CS. Multidimensional proteomics analysis of amniotic fluid to provide insight into the mechanisms of idiopathic preterm birth. PLoS One. 2008;3:e2049.

137. Buhimschi CS, Buhimschi IA, Malinow AM, Weiner CP. Myometrial thickness during human labor and immediately postpartum. Am J Obstet Gynecol. 2003;188:553–9.

138. Buhimschi CS, Buhimschi IA, Norwitz ER, Sfakianaki AK, Hamar B, Copel JA, et al. Sonographic myometrial thickness predicts the latency interval of women with preterm premature rupture of the membranes and oligohydramnios. Am J Obstet Gynecol. 2005;193:762–70.

139. Veille JC, Hosenpud JD, Morton MJ, Welch JE. Cardiac size and function in pregnancy induced hypertension. Am J Obstet Gynecol. 1984;150:443–9.

140. Martin JA, Hamilton BE, Sutton PD, Ventura SJ, Menacker F, Munson ML. Births: final data for 2002. Natl Vital Stat Rep. 2003 Dec 17;52(10):1–113.

141. Terzidou V, Sooranna SR, Kim LU, Thornton S, Bennett PR, Johnson MR. Mechanical stretch up-regulates the human oxytocin receptor in primary human uterine myocytes. J Clin Endocrinol Metab. 2005;90:237–46.

142. Sooranna SR, Engineer N, Loudon JA, Terzidou V, Bennett PR, Johnson MR. The mitogen-activated protein kinase dependent expression of prostaglandin H synthase-2 and interleukin-8 messenger ribonucleic acid by myometrial cells: the differential effect of stretch and interleukin-1β. J Clin Endocrinol Metab. 2005;90:3517–27.

143. Loudon JA, Sooranna SR, Bennett PR, Johnson MR. Mechanical stretch of human uterine smooth muscle cells increases IL-8 mRNA expression and peptide synthesis. Mol Hum Reprod. 2004;10:895–9.

144. Ou CW, Orsino A, Lye SJ. Expression of connexin-43 and connexin-26 in the rat myometrium during pregnancy and labor is differentially regulated by mechanical and hormonal signals. Endocrinology. 1997;138:5398–407.

145. Levy R, Kanengiser B, Furman B, Ben Arie A, Brown D, Hagay ZJ. A randomized trial comparing a 30-mL and an 80-mL Foley catheter balloon for preinduction cervical ripening. Am J Obstet Gynecol. 2004;191:1632–6.

146. Olund A, Jonasson A, Kindahl H, Fianu S, Larsson B. The effect of cervical dilatation by laminaria on the plasma levels of 15-keto-13,14-dihydro-PGF2 alpha. Contraception. 1984; 30:23–7.

147. Leguizamon G, Smith J, Younis H, Nelson DM, Sadovsky Y. Enhancement of amniotic cyclooxygenase type 2 activity in women with preterm delivery associated with twins or polyhydramnios. Am J Obstet Gynecol. 2001;184:117–22.

148. Terakawa K, Itoh H, Sagawa N, Yura S, Yoshida M, Korita D, et al. Site-specific augmentation of amnion cyclooxygenase-2 and decidua vera phospholipase-A2 expression in labor: possible contribution of mechanical stretch and interleukin-1 to amnion prostaglandin synthesis. J Soc Gynecol Invest. 2002;9:68–74.

149. Husslein P, Sinzinger H. Concentration of 13,14-dihydro-15-k eto-prostaglandin E2 in the maternal peripheral plasma during labour of spontaneous onset. Br J Obstet Gynaecol. 1984;91:228–31.

150. Sellers SM, Hodgson HT, Mitchell MD, Anderson AB, Turnbull AC. Raised prostaglandin levels in the third stage of labor. Am J Obstet Gynecol. 1982;144:209–12.

151. Keirse MJNC, Turnbull AC. Prostaglandins in amniotic fluid during late pregnancy and labour. J Obstet Gynaecol Br Commonw. 1973;80:970–3.

152. Casey ML, MacDonald PC. Biomolecular processes in the initiation of parturition: decidual activation. Clin Obstet Gynecol. 1988;31:533–52.

153. Matsumoto T, Sagawa N, Yoshida M, Mori T, Tanaka I, Mukoyama M, et al. The prostaglandin E2 and F2 alpha receptor genes are expressed in human myometrium and are down-regulated during pregnancy. Biochem Biophys Res Commun. 1997;238:838–41.

154. Brodt-Eppley J, Myatt L. Prostaglandin receptors in lower uterine segment myometrium during gestation and labor. Obstet Gynecol. 1999;93:89–93.

155. Attia J. Moving beyond sensitivity and specificity: using likelihood ratios to help interpret diagnostic tests. Aust Prescr. 2003; 26:111–13.

156. Foy R, Warner P. About time: diagnostic guidelines that help clinicians. Qual Saf Health Care. 2003;12:205–9.

157. Want ST, Pizzolato S, Demshar HP. Receiver operating characteristic plots to evaluate Guthrie, Wallac, and Isolab phenylalanine kit performance for newborn phenylketonuria screening. Clin Chem. 1997;43:1838–42.

158. Lockwood CJ, Ghidini A, Wein R, Lapinski R, Casal D, Berkowitz RL. Increased interleukin-6 concentrations in cervical secretions are associated with preterm delivery. Am J Obstet Gynecol. 1994;171:1097–102.

159. Turan OM, Turan S, Funai EF, Buhimschi IA, Copel JA, Buhimschi CS. Fetal adrenal gland volume: a novel method to identify women at risk for impending preterm birth. Obstet Gynecol. 2007;109:855–62.

160. Goepfert AR, Goldenberg RL, Andrews WW, Hauth JC, Mercer B, Iams J, et al., National Institute of Child Health and Human Development Maternal-Fetal Medicine Units Network. The Preterm Prediction Study: association between cervical interleukin 6 concentration and spontaneous preterm birth. National Institute of Child Health and Human Development Maternal-Fetal Medicine Units Network. Am J Obstet Gynecol. 2001;184:483–8.

161. Trebeden H, Goffinet F, Kayem G, Maillard F, Lemoine E, Cabrol D, et al. Strip test for bedside detection of interleukin-6 in cervical secretions is predictive for impending preterm delivery. Eur Cytokine Netw. 2001;12:359–60.

162. Kurkinen-Raty M, Ruokonen A, Vuopala S, Koskela M, Rutanen EM, Kärkkäinen T, et al. Combination of cervical interleukin-6 and -8, phosphorylated insulin-like growth factor-binding protein-1 and transvaginal cervical ultrasonography in assessment of the risk of preterm birth. Br J Obstet Gynaecol. 2001;108:875–81.

163. Rizzo G, Capponi A, Vlachopoulou A, Angelini E, Grassi C, Romanini C. The diagnostic value of interleukin-8 and fetal fibronectin concentrations in cervical secretions in patients with preterm labor and intact membranes. J Perinat Med. 1997;25:461–8.

164. Coleman MA, Keelan JA, McCowan LM, Townend KM, Mitchell MD. Predicting preterm delivery: comparison of cervicovaginal interleukin (IL)-1β, IL-6 and IL-8 with fetal fibronectin and cervical dilatation. Eur J Obstet Gynecol Reprod Biol. 2001;95:154–8.

165. Lange M, Chen FK, Wessel J, Buscher U, Dudenhausen JW. Elevation of interleukin-6 levels in cervical secretions as a predictor of preterm delivery. Acta Obstet Gynecol Scand. 2003;82:326–9.

166. Goldenberg RL, Andrews WW, Guerrant RL, Newman M, Mercer B, Iams J, et al. The Preterm Prediction Study: cervical lactoferrin concentration, other markers of lower genital tract infection, and preterm birth. National Institute of Child Health and Human Development Maternal-Fetal Medicine Units Network. Am J Obstet Gynecol. 2000;182:631–5.

167. Andrews WW, Tsao J, Goldenberg RL, Hauth JC, Mercer B, Iams J, et al. The Preterm Prediction Study: failure of midtrimester cervical sialidase level elevation to predict subsequent spontaneous preterm birth. Am J Obstet Gynecol. 1999;180:1151–4.

168. Wang EY, Woodruff TK, Moawad A. Follistatin-free activin A is not associated with preterm birth. Am J Obstet Gynecol. 2002;186:464–9.

169. Moawad AH, Goldenberg RL, Mercer B, Meis PJ, Iams JD, Das A, et al. The Preterm Prediction Study: the value of serum alkaline phosphatase, alpha-fetoprotein, plasma corticotropin-releasing hormone, and other serum markers for the prediction of spontaneous preterm birth. Am J Obstet Gynecol 2002;186:990–6.

170. Simhan HN, Caritis SN, Krohn MA, Hillier SL. Elevated vaginal pH and neutrophils are associated strongly with early spontaneous preterm birth. Am J Obstet Gynecol. 2003; 189:1150–4.

171. Simhan HN, Caritis SN, Krohn MA, Hillier SL. The vaginal inflammatory milieu and the risk of early premature preterm rupture of membranes. Am J Obstet Gynecol. 2005;192:213–18.

172. Buhimschi CS, Baumbusch MA, Campbell KH, Dulay AT, Buhimschi IA. Insight into innate immunity of the uterine cervix as a host defense mechanism against infection and preterm birth. Expert Rev Obstet Gynecol. 2009;4:9–15.

173. Klein LL, Jonscher KR, Heerwagen MJ, Gibbs RS, McManaman JL. Shotgun proteomic analysis of vaginal fluid from women in late pregnancy. Reprod Sci. 2008;15:263–73.

174. Shaw JL, Smith CR, Diamandis EP. Proteomic analysis of human cervico-vaginal fluid. J Proteome Res. 2007;6:2859–65.

175. Pereira L, Reddy AP, Jacob T, Thomas A, Schneider KA, Dasari S, et al. Identification of novel protein biomarkers of preterm birth in human cervical–vaginal fluid. J Proteome Res. 2007;6:1269–76.

176. Hitti J, Lapidus JA, Lu X, Reddy AP, Jacob T, Dasari S, et al. Noninvasive diagnosis of intraamniotic infection: proteomic biomarkers in vaginal fluid. Am J Obstet Gynecol. 2010;203:32.

177. Buhimschi IA, Buhimschi CS, Weiner CP, Kimura T, Hamar BD, Sfakianaki AK, et al. Proteomic but not enzyme-linked immunosorbent assay technology detects amniotic fluid monomeric calgranulins from their complexed calprotectin form. Clin Diagn Lab Immunol. 2005;12:837–44.

178. Saade GR, Boggess KA, Sullivan SA, Markenson GR, Iams JD, Coonrod DV, et al. Development and validation of a spontaneous preterm delivery predictor in asymptomatic women. Am J Obstet Gynecol. 2016 May;214(5):633.e1–24.

179. Markenson GR, Saade GR, Laurent LC, Heyborne KD, Coonrod DV, Schoen CN, et al. Performance of a proteomic preterm delivery predictor in a large independent prospective cohort. Am J Obstet Gynecol MFM. 2020 Aug;2(3):100140.

180. Rüetschi U, Rosén A, Karlsson G, Zetterberg H, Rymo L, Hagberg H, et al. Proteomic analysis using protein chips to detect biomarkers in cervical and amniotic fluid in women with intra-amniotic inflammation. J Proteome Res 2005;4: 2236–42.

181. Buhimschi IA, Christner R, Buhimschi CS. Proteomic biomarker analysis of amniotic fluid for identification of intraamniotic inflammation. Br J Obstet Gynaecol. 2005;112:173–81.

182. Gravett MG, Novy MJ, Rosenfeld RG, Reddy AP, Jacob T, Turner M, et al. Diagnosis of intraamniotic infection by proteomic profiling and identification of novel biomarkers. JAMA. 2004;292:462–9.

183. Gabay C, Kushner I. Acute-phase proteins and other systemic responses to inflammation. N Engl J Med. 1999;340:448–54.

184. Buhimschi CS, Bhandari V, Hamar BD, Bahtiyar MO, Zhao G, Sfakianaki AK, et al. Proteomic profiling of the amniotic fluid to detect inflammation, infection, and neonatal sepsis. PLoS Med. 2007;4:e18.

185. Kim SM, Romero R, Lee J, Chaemsaithong P, Lee MW, Chaiyasit N, et al. About one-half of early spontaneous preterm deliveries can be identified by a rapid matrix metalloproteinase-8 (MMP-8) bedside test at the time of mid-trimester genetic amniocentesis. J Matern Fetal Neonatal Med. 2016; 29(15):2414–22.

186. Lee SE, Kim SC, Kim KH, Yoon MS, Eo WK, Kim A, et al. Detection of angiogenic factors in midtrimester amniotic fluid and the prediction of preterm birth. Taiwan J Obstet Gynecol. 2016 Aug;55(4):539–44.

187. Hong SN, Joo BS, Chun S, Kim A, Kim HY. Prediction of preterm delivery using levels of vascular endothelial growth factor and leptin in amniotic fluid from the second trimester. Arch Gynecol Obstet. 2015 Feb;291(2):265–71.

188. Lee H, Kwon JY, Lee S, Kim SJ, Shin JC, Park IY. Elevated placenta growth factor levels in the early second-trimester amniotic fluid are associated with preterm delivery. J Matern Fetal Neonatal Med. 2016 Oct;29(20):3374–8.

189. Rosen T, Kuczynski E, O'Neill LM, Funai EF, Lockwood CJ. Plasma levels of thrombin–antithrombin complexes predict preterm premature rupture of the fetal membranes. J Matern Fetal Med. 2001;10:297–300.

190. Elovitz MA, Baron J, Phillippe M. The role of thrombin in preterm parturition. Am J Obstet Gynecol. 2001;185:1059–63.

191. Chaiworapongsa T, Espinoza J, Yoshimatsu J, Kim YM, Bujold E, Edwin S, Yoon BH, et al. Activation of coagulation system in preterm labor and preterm premature rupture of membranes. J Matern Fetal Neonatal Med. 2002;11:368–73.

192. Lockwood CJ, Senyei AE, Dische MR, Casal D, Shah KD, Thung SN, et al. Fetal fibronectin in cervical and vaginal secretions as a predictor of preterm delivery. N Engl J Med. 1991;325:669–74.

193. Feinberg RF, Kliman HJ, Lockwood CJ. Is oncofetal fibronectin a trophoblast glue for human implantation? Am J Pathol. 1991;138:537–43.

194. Peaceman AM, Andrews WW, Thorp JM, Cliver SP, Lukes A, Iams JD, et al. Fetal fibronectin as a predictor of preterm birth in patients with symptoms: a multicenter trial. Am J Obstet Gynecol. 1997;177:13–18.

195. Honest H, Bachmann LM, Gupta JK, Kleijnen J, Khan KS. Accuracy of cervicovaginal fetal fibronectin test in predicting risk of spontaneous preterm birth: systematic review. BMJ. 2002;325:301–4.

196. Sanchez-Ramos L, Delke I, Zamora J, Kaunitz AM. Fetal fibronectin as a short-term predictor of preterm birth in symptomatic patients: a meta-analysis. Obstet Gynecol. 2009;114:631–40.

197. Lockwood CJ, Wein R, Lapinski R, Casal D, Berkowitz G, Alvarez M, et al. The presence of cervical and vaginal fetal fibronectin predicts preterm delivery in an inner-city obstetric population. Am J Obstet Gynecol. 1993;169:798–804.

198. Goldenberg RL, Mercer BM, Meis PJ, Copper RL, Das A, McNellis D. The Preterm Prediction Study: fetal fibronectin testing and spontaneous preterm birth. NICHD Maternal Fetal Medicine Units Network. Obstet Gynecol. 1996;87:643–8.

199. Goldenberg RL, Iams JD, Miodovnik M, Van Dorsten JP, Thurnau G, Bottoms S et al. The Preterm Prediction Study: risk factors in twin gestations. National Institute of Child Health and Human Development Maternal-Fetal Medicine Units Network. Am J Obstet Gynecol. 1996;175:1047–53.

200. Roman AS, Rebarber A, Sfakianaki AK, Mulholland J, Saltzman D, Paidas MJ, et al. Vaginal fetal fibronectin as a predictor of spontaneous preterm delivery in the patient with cervical cerclage. Am J Obstet Gynecol 2003;189:1368–73.

201. Roman AS, Rebarber A, Lipkind H, Mulholland J, Minior V, Roshan D. Vaginal fetal fibronectin as a predictor of spontaneous preterm delivery after multifetal pregnancy reduction. Am J Obstet Gynecol. 2004;190:142–6.

202. Levine LD, Downes KL, Romero JA, Pappas H, Elovitz MA. Quantitative fetal fibronectin and cervical length in symptomatic women: results from a prospective blinded cohort study. J Matern Fetal Neonatal Med. 2019 Nov;32(22):3792–800.

203. Esplin MS, Elovitz MA, Iams JD, Parker CB, Wapner RJ, Grobman WA, et al.; nuMoM2b Network. Predictive accuracy of serial transvaginal cervical lengths and quantitative vaginal fetal fibronectin levels for spontaneous preterm birth among nulliparous women. JAMA. 2017 Mar 14;317(10):1047–56.

204. Roman AS, Koklanaris N, Paidas MJ, Mulholland J, Levitz M, Rebarber A. "Blind" vaginal fetal fibronectin as a predictor of spontaneous preterm delivery. Obstet Gynecol. 2005;105:285–9.

205. Audibert F, Fortin S, Delvin E, Djemli A, Brunet S, Dubé J, et al. Contingent use of fetal fibronectin testing and cervical length measurement in women with preterm labour. J Obstet Gynaecol Can. 2010;32:307–12.

206. Iams JD. Prediction and early detection of preterm labor. Obstet Gynecol. 2003;10:402–12.

207. Iams JD, Goldenberg RL, Meis PJ, Mercer BM, Moawad A, Das A, et al. The length of the cervix and the risk of spontaneous premature delivery. National Institute of Child Health and Human Development Maternal Fetal Medicine Unit Network. N Engl J Med. 1996;334:567–72.

208. Tsoi E, Akmal S, Rane S, Otigbah C, Nicolaides KH. Ultrasound assessment of cervical length in threatened preterm labor. Ultrasound Obstet Gynecol. 2003;21:552–5.

209. Vendittelli F, Volumenie J. Transvaginal ultrasonography examination of the uterine cervix in hospitalised women undergoing preterm labour. Eur J Obstet Gynecol Reprod Biol. 2000;90:3–11.

210. Iams JD, Johnson FF, Sonek J, Sachs L, Gebauer C, Samuels P. Cervical competence as a continuum: a study of ultrasonographic cervical length and obstetric performance. Am J Obstet Gynecol. 1995;172:1097–1103.

211. Owen J, Yost N, Berghella V, Thom E, Swain M, Dildy GA 3rd, et al. National Institute of Child Health and Human Development, Maternal-Fetal Medicine Units Network. Midtrimester endovaginal sonography in women at high risk for spontaneous preterm birth. JAMA. 2001;286:1340–8.

212. Taipale P, Hiilesmaa V. Sonographic measurement of uterine cervix at 18–22 weeks' gestation and the risk of preterm delivery. Obstet Gynecol. 1998;92:902–7.

213. Iams JD, Goldenberg RL, Mercer BM, Moawad AH, Meis PJ, Das AF, et al. The Preterm Prediction Study: can low-risk women destined for spontaneous preterm birth be identified? Am J Obstet Gynecol. 2001;184:652–5.

214. Ozturk A, Grajo JR, Dhyani M, Anthony BW, Samir AE. Principles of ultrasound elastography. Abdom Radiol (NY). 2018;43(4):773–85. doi: 10.1007/s00261-018-1475-6.

215. Shiina T, Nightingale KR, Palmeri ML, Hall TJ, Bamber JC, Barr RG, et al. WFUMB guidelines and recommendations for clinical use of ultrasound elastography. Part 1: basic principles and terminology. Ultrasound Med Biol. 2015;41:1126–47.

216. Wang B, Zhang Y, Chen S, Xiang X, Wen J, Yi M, et al. Diagnostic accuracy of cervical elastography in predicting preterm delivery: A systematic review and meta-analysis. Medicine (Baltimore). 2019;98(29):e16449.

217. Fruscalzo A, Mazza E, Feltovich H, Schmitz R. Cervical elastography during pregnancy: a critical review of current approaches with a focus on controversies and limitations. J Med Ultrason (2001). 2016 Oct;43(4):493–504.

218. Parra-Saavedra M, Gómez L, Barrero A, Parra G, Vergara F, Navarro E. Prediction of preterm birth using the cervical consistency index. Ultrasound Obstet Gynecol. 2011 Jul;38(1):44–51.

219. Baños N, Perez-Moreno A, Julià C, Murillo-Bravo C, Coronado D, Gratacós E, et al. Quantitative analysis of cervical texture by ultrasound in mid-pregnancy and association with spontaneous preterm birth. Ultrasound Obstet Gynecol. 2018 May;51(5):637–43.

220. Hincz P, Wilczynski J, Kozarzewski M, Szaflik K. Two-step test: the combined use of fetal fibronectin and sonographic examination of the uterine cervix for prediction of preterm delivery in symptomatic patients. Acta Obstet Gynecol Scand. 2002;81:58–63.

Chapter 41
Preterm (Prelabor) Premature Rupture of Membranes

Brian M. Mercer and Kelly S. Gibson
Department of Reproductive Biology, Case Western Reserve University and The MetroHealth System, Cleveland, OH, USA

Rupture of fetal membranes before the onset of labor (premature rupture of membranes, prelabor rupture of membranes, PROM) complicates 8–10% of pregnancies, and is responsible for nearly one third of preterm births. PROM, especially preterm PROM (PPROM), has been associated with brief latency from membrane rupture to delivery, an increased risk of chorioamnionitis, and umbilical cord compression. As such, PPROM is associated with increased risk of perinatal complications. An understanding of gestational age-dependent risks of delivery, the risks and potential benefits of conservative management, and opportunities to reduce complications of preterm birth will help clinicians improve outcomes after this frequent pregnancy complication.

Mechanisms

Spontaneous membrane rupture at term results from progressive weakening of the membranes because of collagen remodeling and cellular apoptosis and from increased intrauterine pressure with uterine contractions when membrane rupture occurs subsequent to the onset of labor. Although PPROM near term likely results in many cases from these same physiologic processes, PPROM remote from term has been associated with several pathologic processes, especially infection and inflammation. Reported clinical risk factors predisposing to intrauterine infection, inflammation, membrane stretch, and local tissue hypoxia have included low socioeconomic status, maternal undernutrition, cigarette smoking, uterine bleeding and work in pregnancy; cervical cerclage, prior preterm labor and acute pulmonary disease in the current pregnancy; and bacterial vaginosis in addition to other urogenital infections [1–6]. It has been proposed that there could be a genetic predisposition to PPROM in some people, either through inheritance of polymorphisms for proinflammatory cytokines and matrix metalloproteinases [7,8] or through heritable connective tissue disorders of collagen metabolism.

Among the strongest risk factors for PPROM is a history of preterm birth in a previous gestation, particularly one resulting from PPROM (odds ratio [OR] 3.3–6.3) [6]. The role of ascending infection in the pathogenesis of PPROM is particularly plausible as bacterial proteases (collagenases and phospholipases) can cause membrane weakening. Ascending bacterial colonization can also cause a maternal inflammatory response including production of cytokines, prostaglandins, and metalloproteinases locally, which cause membrane degradation and weakening. Preterm contractions can lead to separation of the amnion and choriodecidua with an overall reduction in membrane tensile strength [9], and cervical dilation can result in exposure of the membranes to vaginal microorganisms and reduce underlying tissue support.

Prediction and prevention

Although the aforementioned clinical risk factors have been associated with PPROM, most gravidas with these characteristics do not develop PPROM and the majority of cases of PPROM lack these risk factors. This has led to interest in ancillary testing for prediction of PPROM. Both short cervical length on transvaginal ultrasound (<25 mm; relative risk [RR] 3.2) and the presence of fetal fibronectin (fFN) in cervicovaginal secretions (RR 2.5) in the later second trimester are associated with an increased risk of preterm birth resulting from PPROM [6]. However, like clinical risk factors, these modalities also fail to identify the majority of those destined to have PPROM and are not recommended as routine screening tests for low-risk gravidas.

Those who suffer PPROM are at increased risk for recurrence in a future pregnancy. Although general guidance directed against factors associated with spontaneous preterm birth (e.g. adequate nutrition, smoking cessation, avoidance of heavy lifting and prolonged standing without breaks, early treatment of urogenital infections) may reduce the risk of PPROM, direct benefit from these has not been demonstrated. Identification and treatment of sexually transmitted urogenital infections such as *Chlamydia trachomatis* and *Neisseria gonorrhoeae* can reduce the risks of PPROM and preterm birth. Although treatment of symptomatic bacterial vaginosis and *Trichomonas vaginalis* infection is appropriate, treatment of gravidas with asymptomatic vaginal infections is controversial and may even promote preterm birth [10,11].

While it is biologically plausible that progestogen administration could play a role prevention of PPROM through inhibition of tumor necrosis factor-alpha (TNFα) and thrombin-induced fetal membrane weakening and TNFα-induced apoptosis in human fetal membranes [12,13]. The Food and Drug Administration (FDA) recently withdrew its approval of intramuscular and subcutaneous 17-alpha hydroxyprogesterone caproate (17-OHPC) for prevention of recurrent spontaneous preterm birth [14]. Both the American College of Obstetricians and Gynecologists (ACOG) and the Society for Maternal Fetal Medicine (SMFM) subsequently advised against the use of intramuscular and subcutaneous 17-OHPC for prevention of recurrent preterm birth and that vaginal progesterone be reserved for those with a short cervical length [15,16]. Though vitamin C deficiency has been linked to PPROM, data are conflicting regarding the potential risks and benefits of treatment with vitamin C supplementation and this treatment is not recommended to prevent recurrent PPROM [17–19].

Diagnosis

Diagnosis of membrane rupture is best made by sterile speculum examination of those presenting with a suspicious clinical history or who are found to have oligohydramnios on ultrasonography. Evident fluid passing through the cervical os is diagnostic. An alkaline vaginal pH (>6.0–6.5) with nitrazine paper and the presence of a "ferning" pattern on microscopic examination of dried secretions obtained from the vaginal side wall are supportive when visual inspection is equivocal. These tests are subject to false-positive findings because of the presence of cervical mucus, blood, semen, alkaline antiseptics, or bacterial vaginosis and can be falsely negative with prolonged leakage and oligohydramnios. Repeat speculum examination after prolonged bed rest may provide needed diagnostic information if initial testing is negative despite a suspicious history. In the absence of fetal growth restriction or urogenital abnormalities, ultrasound evidence of oligohydramnios is suggestive but not diagnostic of

membrane rupture. The diagnosis can be confirmed unequivocally by indigo carmine amnio-infusion with observation for passage of dye *per vaginam*. Alternatives such as sodium fluorescein, phenolsulfonphthalein, and indocyanine green can be considered. However, the fetal and maternal risks related to intraamniotic instillation of these agents have not been thoroughly studied. Phenazopyridine, Evans blue, and methylene blue dyes are not recommended due to potential fetal and maternal risks.

Although a variety of substances, including fFN, α-fetoprotein, total T4 and free T4, prolactin, human chorionic gonadotropin, interleukin-6, placental α-microglobulin (PAMG)-1, and insulin-like growth factor binding protein (IGFBP)-1, among others, have been evaluated for their ability to assist in the diagnosis of membrane rupture, these have not generally been studied for their diagnostic ability among those in whom the diagnosis of membrane rupture remains unclear after clinical examination. Further, some of these markers do not require membrane rupture to be found in cervicovaginal secretions [20–22]. In a comparative study of two rapid tests, PAMG-1 identified lower concentrations of amniotic fluid than IGFBP-1 [23]. PAMG-1 in cervicovaginal secretions can confirm PROM in nearly 99% of cases where the diagnosis is evident on traditional testing [20]. But it has also been found to be positive among 30.9% of laboring patients and in 4.8% of nonlaboring gravidas without suspected membrane rupture, raising questions regarding its utility when membrane rupture is not clinically evident [24]. In 2018, the Food and Drug Administration advised that biochemical tests for fetal membrane rupture should be part of an overall clinical evaluation [25]. Confirmation of membrane rupture with these ancillary tests is rarely needed and should not replace a thorough clinical assessment.

Clinical course

Brief latency from membrane rupture to delivery, increased risk of intrauterine and neonatal infection, and oligohydramnios have been considered hallmarks of PPROM. Each can affect pregnancy outcomes, and each has implications regarding clinical management of patients with PPROM.

Although it is true that mean and median latency from membrane rupture to delivery increase with decreasing gestational age at membrane rupture, the clinical importance of this finding is overstated. The likelihood that a conservatively managed patient with PPROM at 24–31 weeks will deliver within 1 week is approximately 50% [26]. Approximately one quarter of those with membrane rupture near the limit of viability will remain pregnant for 1 month or more. Alternatively, those with PROM at or near term are rarely given the opportunity to remain pregnant for an extended time and the most will enter active labor within 24 hours after membrane rupture. Benefits of conservative management of PPROM include additional time for induction of fetal pulmonary maturity and prevention of intraventricular hemorrhage through administration of antenatal corticosteroids (24–48 hour latency required), and reduction of gestational age-dependent morbidity through extended latency (more than approximately 1 week latency required).

Chorioamnionitis complicates 13–60% of pregnancies with PROM and is increasingly common with decreasing gestational age at membrane rupture [27]. Abruptio placentae, amnionitis, and endometritis complicate 4–12%, 13–60%, and 2–13% of pregnancies, respectively, when membrane rupture occurs remote from term [27–31]. Amniotic fluid cultures from amniocentesis specimens are positive in 25–35% of asymptomatic gravidas after PPROM [32]. Maternal sepsis is uncommon (approximately 1%) but is a serious complication of PROM remote from term. Conservative management of PROM at any gestational age increases the risk of chorioamnionitis. Fetal demise after PPROM is believed to result in most cases from umbilical cord compression. Fetal infection, placental abruption, and umbilical cord prolapse can also lead to fetal death. Overall, fetal death complicates approximately 1–2% of pregnancies conservatively managed after PPROM. This risk increases in the face of chorioamnionitis, and when PPROM occurs near the limit of potential viability (periviable).

Therefore, expeditious delivery should be considered if the fetus is considered to be at low risk for gestational age-dependent morbidity, if antenatal corticosteroids are not going to be administered when only brief pregnancy prolongation is anticipated, or after antenatal corticosteroid treatment has been completed if continued attempts to extend latency more than approximately 1 week are not planned.

Evaluation

In general, gravidas with PROM at term do not require specific evaluations unless additional complications occur. Initial evaluation of the gravida presenting with PPROM includes (Box 41.1):

• maternal uterine activity and fetal heart rate monitoring for labor, umbilical cord compression, and for fetal well-being if the limit of potential viability has been reached
• clinical assessment for chorioamnionitis (fever ≥38.0° C [100.4° F] with uterine tenderness, maternal or fetal tachycardia, vaginal discharge)
• ultrasound to confirm gestational age and to identify fetal malformations associated with PROM and oligohydramnios if not previously performed, to determine fetal presentation, and to estimate fetal weight and amniotic fluid volume

Box 41.1 Considerations for initial evaluation of the gravida with preterm premature rupture of membranes

• Maternal uterine activity monitoring for labor
• Fetal heart rate monitoring for umbilical cord compression (and fetal well-being if the limit of viability has been reached)
• Clinical assessment for chorioamnionitis
• Ultrasound to confirm gestational age, estimate fetal growth, and amniotic fluid volume, identify fetal malformations associated with PROM/oligohydramnios if not previously carried out, and to determine fetal presentation
• Visual inspection of cervical dilation and effacement if not in active labor
• Cervical cultures for *Neisseria gonorrhoeae* and *Chlamydia trachomatis* if not recently performed
• Vaginal-rectal swab for group B streptococcus culture if not recently performed
• Urinalysis with urine culture if not recently performed
• Baseline maternal blood white blood cell count

PROM, premature rupture of membranes.

Digital cervical examination should be avoided if possible until the diagnosis of PPROM has been excluded or a decision to deliver has been made. Digital examination in this setting shortens latency and increases the risk of chorioamnionitis while adding little information over that obtained by visual examination [33]. Cervical cultures for *Neisseria gonorrhoeae* and *Chlamydia trachomatis*, vaginal-rectal culture for group B β-hemolytic streptococci (GBS) and urinalysis with urine culture should be considered if not recently performed.

If the diagnosis of chorioamnionitis is suspected but not clear, maternal blood white blood cell (WBC) count and ultrasound-guided amniocentesis can sometimes be helpful (Box 41.2). A maternal blood WBC count >16 000/mm³ is supportive of suspicious clinical findings. It is helpful to obtain a baseline blood WBC count on presentation after PPROM to be used during initial assessment and for subsequent comparison if needed during conservative management. It is important to remember that there is significant variation in WBC count between patients and that the WBC count is elevated in pregnancy and for 5–7 days after administration of antenatal corticosteroids. As such, this test should not be used in isolation. Amniotic fluid gram stain, WBC count (≥30 cells/μL considered abnormal), and glucose concentration (less than 16–20 mg/dL considered abnormal) can also provide rapid supportive information regarding the presence of intraamniotic infection [34,35]. Elevated amniotic fluid and vaginal fluid cytokine levels have also been associated with intrauterine infection after PPROM; however, tests for these markers are not generally available for clinical use. Amniotic fluid culture for aerobic and anaerobic bacteria and for mycoplasma can be helpful, but results are generally not available before a management decision is needed.

Box 41.2 Adjuncts to the evaluation of the gravida with equivocal findings of intraamniotic infection

- Maternal blood white blood cell count: rising values and a value >16 000/mm³ are supportive of the diagnosis if antenatal corticosteroids not administered within 5–7 d
- Ultrasound-guided amniocentesis:
  - Positive gram stain supportive but may be falsely positive as a result of contamination
  - White blood cell count ≥30 cells/µL considered abnormal
  - Glucose concentration <16–20 mg/dL considered abnormal
  - Positive culture considered abnormal, but result typically not available in time for acute management

Management

Delivery after PPROM is required in the presence of clinical chorioamnionitis, nonreassuring fetal testing, significant vaginal bleeding, and advanced labor (Box 41.3). In the absence of these conditions, conservative management may be appropriate. If conservative management of the patient with PPROM is being considered, initial extended monitoring followed by intermittent monitoring at least daily is appropriate if testing remains reassuring. Biophysical profile testing can be helpful if fetal heart rate testing is nonreactive. A non-reactive fetal heart rate or a nonreassuring biophysical profile score can be a sign of intrauterine infection, particularly if testing had previously been reassuring [36,37]. In the stable patient, gestational age is important in determining whether conservative management or expeditious delivery should be pursued [32].

Intrapartum GBS prophylaxis should be given to those with a recent (<6 weeks) positive anovaginal GBS culture regardless of intervening antibiotic treatments [38]. Intrapartum GBS prophylaxis should also be given to gravidas delivering preterm without a recent anovaginal recent culture result, to all patients with GBS bacteriuria at any time in the current pregnancy, and to all patients with a previously affected infant regardless of culture results in the current pregnancy.

Preterm premature rupture of membranes at 32 to 36 weeks of gestation

Infants born at 34 to 36 weeks gestation (i.e. late preterm birth) have a higher risk of complications than term infants but are unlikely to suffer severe acute or chronic complications related to preterm birth [39,40]. Antenatal corticosteroids for fetal lung maturation may be administered, but magnesium sulfate for neuroprotection is not recommended in this gestational age range. Reports in the United States have shown that conservative management of PPROM at 34 to 36 weeks prolongs pregnancy by only

days, significantly increases the risk for chorioamnionitis (16% vs. 2%; $P = .001$), without improving newborn outcomes [40–42]. Similarly, a multicenter European PPROMEXIL study found conservative management of PPROM at 34 through 36 weeks to increase average latency by only 3 days, while increasing the frequencies of clinical and histologic chorioamnionitis, and funisitis [43]. Conversely, active delivery resulted in more frequent newborn hypoglycemia and hyperbilirubinemia., and longer hospital stay, but shorter neonatal intensive care unit stay. A follow-up study of similar design – The PPROMEXIL-2 trial had similar findings but no improvements in newborn outcomes with conservative management [44]. Both studies included patients who had suffered PPROM before 34 weeks gestation. A third study, the PPROMT trial, also evaluated induction vs. conservative management of PPROM at 34 to 36 weeks and also included women with PPROM onset before 34 weeks [45]. Antenatal steroids were administered in 40% of cases. In this study, conservative management led to less frequent respiratory distress syndrome (RDS), less need for mechanical ventilation, and shorter newborn hospital and neonatal intensive care unit stays. Again, pregnancy prolongation was brief and maternal intrapartum fever was more common with conservative management. An individual patient data meta-analysis of these studies reported that immediate delivery results in comparable rates of the composite of adverse neonatal outcomes to conservative management, but is associated with more frequent RDS, hyperbilirubinemia, and neonatal intensive care unit (NICU) admissions [46]. Taken together, these data suggest that conservative management of PPROM near term is associated with only brief pregnancy prolongation, increased intrauterine infection, and prolonged maternal stay. Newborn benefits have not been consistently demonstrated but conservative management near term may be associated with less frequent RDS, hyperbilirubinemia, and NICU admissions. For these reasons, delivery after presentation with PPROM at 34–36 weeks is appropriate, but conservative management may be acceptable if there is considered to be a low likelihood of intrauterine infection and significant potential for fetal maturation. Administration of antenatal corticosteroids to accelerate fetal maturation and antibiotics to reduce intrauterine infection should be considered if conservative management is pursued. Delivery after completion of antenatal steroid administration is acceptable.

In the past, assessment of fetal pulmonary maturity, with delivery for a mature result has been suggested. But fetal pulmonary maturity testing is now unavailable in many institutions. In settings where laboratory support for fetal pulmonary maturity testing is available, the presence of documented fetal pulmonary maturity at 34 to 36 weeks should lead to consideration of active delivery.

Box 41.3 Options for management of the gravida with preterm premature rupture of membranes according to gestational age at membrane rupture

PROM at 32–36 weeks of gestation

- Consider expeditious delivery by labor induction or cesarean delivery as indicated
- *Consider assessment of fetal pulmonary maturity with delivery for documented maturity, if testing is available at the institution*
- If managed conservatively, administer antenatal steroids for fetal maturation and antibiotics to reduce infection followed by:
  - delivery 24–48 hours after antenatal corticosteroids if latency of 1 or more weeks not anticipated after completion antenatal steroid treatment
  - delivery at 34 weeks gestation
- Tocolytic therapy for labor to facilitate antenatal corticosteroids administration or maternal transport before 34 0/7 weeks of gestation is acceptable, but should not be administered if there is suspicion of intrauterine infection, fetal compromise, or placental abruption
- Intrapartum GBS prophylaxis**
- Broad-spectrum intrapartum antibiotics for suspected chorioamnionitis

PROM before 32 weeks of gestation

- Conservative inpatient management
- Antenatal corticosteroids for fetal maturation if not previously administered
- Broad-spectrum antibiotics to prolong pregnancy and reduce neonatal morbidity
- Magnesium sulfate for fetal neuroprotection
- Transfer to a tertiary care facility if adequate facilities for neonatal care not available
- At least daily assessment for labor, amnionitis, placental abruption, and fetal well-being
- Leg exercises, antiembolic stockings, and/or prophylactic heparin
- Fetal growth assessment by ultrasound every 3–4 weeks
- Tocolytic therapy for labor to facilitate antenatal corticosteroids administration or maternal transport before 34 0/7 weeks of gestation

is acceptable, but should not be administered if there is suspicion of intrauterine infection, fetal compromise, or placental abruption
- Consider elective delivery at 34 weeks gestation if remains pregnant to this time
- Intrapartum GBS prophylaxis**
- Broad-spectrum intrapartum antibiotics for suspected chorioamnionitis

PROM before viability

- Counsel regarding:
  - potential for previable, periviable, and preterm birth
  - impact of oligohydramnios on pulmonary development and risk of lethal pulmonary hypoplasia and restriction deformities
  - risks of adverse fetal, neonatal, and long-term infant outcomes with early preterm birth
  - risks of maternal morbidities with conservative management
- Deliver by labor induction or dilation and evacuation according to individual circumstances
  or
- Manage conservatively with:
  - initial evaluation for intrauterine infection, labor, fetal death, or placental abruption
  - strict pelvic rest and modified bed/couch rest
  - serial ultrasound for fetal pulmonary growth and amniotic fluid volume with additional counseling as appropriate for persistent oligohydramnios or suspected pulmonary hypoplasia
  - serial ultrasound for estimated fetal weight and pulmonary growth, and amniotic fluid volume
  - broad-spectrum antibiotics to prolong pregnancy and reduce neonatal morbidity may be helpful but no specific data are available for this gestational age
  - treat as for PPROM at 23–31wk 6 d once the limit of viability has been reached

GBS, group B streptococcus; PPROM, preterm premature rupture of membranes.
*Delivery is indicated for the presence of chorioamnionitis, nonreassuring fetal testing/fetal death, significant vaginal bleeding, and for advanced labor.
**Once the limit of viability has been reached, intrapartum GBS prophylaxis should be given to those with a recent positive GBS culture regardless of intervening antibiotic treatments. Intrapartum GBS prophylaxis should also be given to those delivering preterm without a recent culture result, to all patients with GBS bacteriuria at any time in the current pregnancy, and to all with a previously affected infant regardless of culture results in the current pregnancy.

When PPROM occurs at 32 to 33 weeks of gestation there is greater potential for newborn complications of preterm birth. Conservative management for induction of fetal pulmonary maturation with antenatal corticosteroids followed by delivery at 24–48 hours or at 34 weeks gestation is appropriate. If antenatal corticosteroid administration is complete and continued conservative management for 1 or more weeks is not anticipated, delivery is recommended before complications ensue. Alternatively, if fetal pulmonary maturity testing is available and maturity is documented, expeditious delivery without antenatal corticosteroid administration is also

appropriate. If conservative management is pursued, evaluation and treatment should be as described next for PPROM before 32 weeks.

Premature rupture of membranes before 32 weeks of gestation

Delivery before 32 weeks of gestation is associated with significant risks of neonatal morbidity and mortality resulting from prematurity. These patients are generally best served by conservative inpatient management after

PPROM to prolong pregnancy and reduce gestational age-dependent morbidity in the absence of chorioamnionitis, placental abruption, advanced labor, or nonreassuring fetal testing. Because the latency is frequently brief and clinical findings can change over a short period of time, transfer to a tertiary care facility before acute complications occur should be considered if adequate facilities are not available at the initial institution.

During conservative management, patients should have at least daily assessment for evidence of labor, chorioamnionitis, placental abruption, and fetal well-being. Leg exercises, antiembolic stockings, and/or prophylactic doses of subcutaneous heparin may be of value in preventing thromboembolic complications. Fetal growth should be assessed with ultrasound every 3–4 weeks. Although the extent of oligohydramnios is inversely related to latency, low amniotic fluid volume is an inaccurate predictor of latency and neonatal outcome and should not be used to determine clinical management other than as a tool to confirm resealing of the membranes with restoration of a normal amniotic fluid index. The patient who remains stable is generally delivered at 34 weeks gestation because of the ongoing but low risk of fetal loss with conservative management and the high likelihood of survival without long-term complications after delivery at this gestational age.

Several adjunctive therapies have been proposed during conservative management of PPROM remote from term. A single course of antenatal corticosteroids for fetal maturation is recommended to reduce the risks of neonatal respiratory distress and intraventricular hemorrhage, without increasing the risk of neonatal infection [47,48]. Either 12 mg betamethasone intramuscular (IM) every 24 hours for two doses, or 6 mg dexamethasone IM every 12 hours for four doses is appropriate. Broad-spectrum antibiotic therapy should be administered to treat or prevent ascending subclinical decidual infection to prolong pregnancy and to reduce neonatal infectious and gestational age-dependent morbidity [49,50]. Intravenous (IV) therapy (48 hours) with ampicillin (2 g intravenous [IV] every 6 hours) and erythromycin (250 mg IV every 6 hours) followed by limited-duration oral therapy (5 days) with amoxicillin (250 mg PO every 8 hours) and enteric-coated erythromycin base (333 mg PO every 8 hours) has been recommended by the National Institute of Child Health and Human Development and the Maternal-Fetal Medicine Units (NICHD-MFMU) Network. Therapy for shorter periods has not been studied with adequate numbers, has not been shown to offer equivalent neonatal benefits [51,52], and is not recommended.

Antibiotic shortages have led to the need for substitution of alternative agents. Oral ampicillin, erythromycin,

and azithromycin are likely appropriate substitutions, as needed. The optimal broad-spectrum therapy for those who are penicillin allergic has not been determined. The Oracle trial [53] suggested that single-agent erythromycin may be appropriate but also raised concern that broad-spectrum amoxicillin-clavulanate therapy might increase the risk of necrotizing enterocolitis. This latter finding is not consistent with the NICHD-MFMU trial in which broad spectrum antibiotic therapy in a higher risk population reduced the risk of stage 2–3 necrotizing enterocolitis [49]. Of note, despite conflicting results from a concurrent study of antibiotics for preterm labor with intact membranes, the Oracle trial for gravidas with PPROM revealed no increases or decreases in long-term morbidities for infants exposed to antepartum antibiotics [54].

Management of GBS carriers after the initial 7 days of antibiotic therapy has not been well studied. Options include:
• subsequent intrapartum prophylaxis only,
• continued narrow-spectrum GBS prophylaxis from completion of the initial 7-day course through delivery, or
• follow-up anovaginal culture after completion of the 7-day course, with continued narrow-spectrum therapy against GBS until delivery for those with persistently positive cultures.

Regardless of antepartum antibiotic treatments, intrapartum prophylaxis should be given to all known GBS carriers.

Magnesium sulfate infusion is also recommended when preterm PPROM occurs before 32 weeks of gestation regardless of whether conservative management is pursued [55,56]. In the NICHD-funded BEAM (Beneficial Effects of Antenatal Magnesium Sulfate) study, 87% of participants had PPROM [56]. Magnesium sulfate was administered as a 6-g bolus followed by an infusion at 2 g/hour for 12 hours if imminent delivery was not anticipated. Retreatment was attempted for those subsequently delivering before 34 weeks gestation if circumstances allowed. Treatment reduced the frequencies of moderate to severe cerebral palsy from 3.9 to 1.9% ($P = 0.03$) and total cerebral palsy from 7.3% to 4.2% ($P = 0.004$).

Tocolytic therapy for gravidas with PPROM has been shown to reduce the likelihood of delivery at 24–48 hours in some studies [57–60]. However, a meta-analysis of such treatment did not find evidence of benefit from the use of tocolysis in this setting [61]. Despite this, ACOG has suggested that tocolytic agents can be considered for steroid benefit or maternal transport before 34 0/7 weeks absent evidence of infection or abruption [62]. Tocolytic therapy should not be administered after PPROM if there is suspicion of intrauterine infection, fetal compromise, or placental abruption.

Previable premature rupture of membranes before the limit of viability

Preterm premature rupture of membranes before the limit of viability is particularly concerning as it can lead to previable delivery with no potential for survival, periviable delivery near the limit of viability where the majority of survivors are at risk for acute and long-term complications, or to delivery after extended latency with pulmonary hypoplasia and restriction deformities resulting from severe oligohydramnios at the time of critical pulmonary and skeletal development. Alternatively, some conservatively managed patients will have extended latency with survival of a healthy infant, and some may have spontaneous resealing of the membranes with reaccumulation of amniotic fluid.

Gestational age should be estimated based on the earliest available ultrasound and menstrual history. These patients should be counseled realistically regarding potential fetal and neonatal outcomes after early preterm birth [32]. The risk of stillbirth during conservative management and delivery is approximately 15%. Most of these pregnancies will deliver before or near the limit of viability, where neonatal death is either assured or common. The risk of long-term sequelae will depend on the gestational age at delivery. Persistent oligohydramnios is a prognostic indicator of poor outcomes after PPROM before 20 weeks, with a high risk of lethal pulmonary hypoplasia regardless of extended latency. Conservative management is also associated with frequent chorioamnionitis (39%), endometritis (14%), retained placenta/postpartum hemorrhage necessitating curettage (12%), and placental abruption (3%).

Should the patient desire delivery after counseling, options for labor induction include high-dose intravenous oxytocin, intravaginal prostaglandin E_2, and oral or intravaginal prostaglandin E_1 (misoprostol) according to clinical circumstances. Dilation and evacuation can be an option for caregivers with experience in this technique. Placement of intracervical laminaria before labor induction or dilation and evacuation may be helpful. Patients undergoing conservative management should be initially evaluated for evidence of intrauterine infection, labor, or placental abruption. Although supportive data are lacking, it is prudent to advise the patient managed in an ambulatory setting to pursue strict pelvic rest to reduce the potential for ascending infection and it may be helpful to maintain modified bed or couch rest to enhance the potential for membrane resealing. In the absence of data supporting either approach, inpatient or outpatient monitoring after initial evaluation may be considered appropriate with consideration given to individual clinical

circumstances. Serial ultrasound can be helpful to evaluate for persistent oligohydramnios and to estimate fetal pulmonary growth (e.g. measurement of thoracic/abdominal circumference ratio or chest circumference) [63–65]. Information from such testing is useful in counseling and ongoing care of the patient with PPROM before the limit of viability.

A number of small studies have evaluated the potential to reseal the fetal membranes after previable PPROM. Some techniques have included transabdominal/transcervical amnio-infusion and Gelfoam or fibrin platelet-cryoprecipitate instillation [66–68]. Data regarding efficacy and safety of these techniques are too limited currently to warrant their incorporation into clinical practice.

Once the limit of viability has been reached, many clinicians will admit the patient with PPROM for ongoing bed rest to allow early diagnosis and intervention for infection, abruption, labor, and nonreassuring fetal heart rate patterns (see the section on management of PPROM before 32 weeks of gestation). Administration of antenatal corticosteroids for fetal maturation is appropriate at this time. Patients with PPROM before the limit of viability have been included in some studies of broad-spectrum antibiotic therapy after PPROM. However, the numbers of these are too small to know if treatment is effective for this subgroup. It is also unknown if antibiotic administration at the time of readmission at viability will improve pregnancy outcomes for those who have already had a prolonged latency without evident infection.

Special circumstances

Cerclage

Cerclage is a well-described risk factor for PPROM [69, 70]. When the cerclage is removed after PPROM occurs, the risk of perinatal complications is comparable to patients with PPROM who had no cerclage [70,71]. Contemporary retrospective studies comparing cerclage retention or removal after PPROM have suggested variably increased latency with conservative management but no improvements in newborn outcomes and inconsistent findings regarding chorioamnionitis [72–74]. The only prospective trial regarding this issue was discontinued for futility after randomization of 56 patients [75]. This study found no statistically significant differences in pregnancy or newborn outcomes though the authors suggested that there was a numerical trend towards less infectious morbidity with immediate cerclage removal (25% vs. 42%). In the absence of newborn benefits, cerclage should generally be removed when PPROM occurs. If the cerclage is retained concurrent to antenatal corticosteroid treatment for fetal maturation, broad-spectrum antibiotic administration should be given to reduce the risk of infection and the cerclage should generally be removed after steroid benefit has been achieved (24–48 hours).

Herpes simplex virus

Typically, gravidas with active primary or secondary herpes simplex virus (HSV) infection should be delivered expeditiously by cesarean delivery when PROM occurs at or near term. Alternatively, when PPROM complicates HSV infection before 32 weeks gestation and the mother shows no evidence of systemic infection, conservative management may be appropriate [76]. During conservative management, treatment with acyclovir (200 mg PO five times a day or 500 mg IV every 6 hours) would be appropriate to reduce viral shedding and the likelihood of recurrences before delivery.

Human immunodeficiency virus (HIV)

There are not adequate data to make evidence-based recommendations for treatment of the HIV-infected gravida with PPROM. Given the poor prognosis of perinatally acquired HIV infection and increasing risk of vertical transmission with increasing duration of membrane rupture, expeditious cesarean delivery is generally recommended when PROM occurs after the limit of fetal viability. Conservative management to prolong pregnancy may be appropriate for selected patients with an undetectable viral load at the time of PPROM remote from term, but the gestational age limit, risks, and benefits or this approach have not been studied. If conservative management is undertaken, multiagent antiretroviral therapy with serial monitoring of maternal viral load and CD4 counts should be initiated.

Resealing of the membranes

A small number of gravidas will have cessation of leakage with resealing of the membranes, particularly those with PPROM after amniocentesis [77,78]. In the absence of data in this regard, we empirically continue inpatient observation for approximately 1 week after cessation of leakage and normalization of the amniotic fluid index to encourage healing of the membrane rupture site. They are subsequently discharged with instructions for modified bed rest and pelvic rest and are advised to return should labor, vaginal bleeding, abdominal tenderness or fever, or recurrent membrane rupture ensue.

CASE PRESENTATION

A 23-year-old, gravida 2, para 0101, with singleton gestation, presented at 23 weeks with perineal wetness for approximately 4 hours. She denied contractions, abdominal pain, vaginal bleeding, fever, or chills. She had a prior 32-week preterm birth resulting from preterm labor, but no other pregnancy complications. Past medical and allergy histories were negative. Specific clinical findings included temperature 37.2° C, pulse 92 beats/min, respiratory rate 18/min, symphysis-fundal height 22 cm, with no fundal tenderness. A catheterized urine specimen revealed no leukocytes and culture was subsequently negative. Sterile speculum examination revealed moist vaginal side walls but no fluid pool in the posterior fornix. A sterile swab of the vaginal side walls revealed a complex arborized ferning pattern and nitrazine paper applied to this site turned blue, confirming the clinical suspicion of membrane rupture. Visual inspection suggested an undilated cervix with approximately 1.5 cm of intravaginal cervical length. Endocervical swabs for *Neisseria gonorrhoeae* and *Chlamydia trachomatis*, and distal vagina/anal swabs for GBS were obtained. Ultrasound revealed appropriate fetal growth, a longitudinal cephalic lie, and oligohydramnios (amniotic fluid index = 2.4 cm). The fetal bladder was normal in size and position, and no hydronephrosis was evident. Monitoring revealed a fetal heart rate of 150 beats/min with moderate variability, and

no recurrent decelerations or contractions. Maternal WBC count was 12000/mm^3.

After counseling regarding the risks of preterm birth at 23 weeks and of conservative management, and the potential benefits of conservative management, antibiotics (NICHD-MFMU protocol), corticosteroid treatment (12 mg betamethasone IM every 24 hours for two doses) and magnesium sulfate for neuroprotection (6-g bolus followed by an infusion at 2 g/hour for 12 hours) were initiated, and neonatology consultation was obtained. The patient was transferred to the antepartum unit after 6 hours of reassuring continuous fetal/contraction monitoring, for continued bed rest with bathroom privileges. Daily assessments revealed no clinically evident chorioamnionitis, abruption, or contractions. Fetal testing remained appropriate to gestational age, without concern for metabolic acidemia or umbilical cord compression. Cultures were negative.

On hospital day 31, at 27 weeks gestation, the patient reported mild lower abdominal cramping. External monitoring revealed irregular brief contractions with moderate variable-type decelerations. Speculum examination revealed umbilical cord at the external os. There was not time to reinitiate magnesium sulfate therapy or to give a rescue course on antenatal corticosteroids. With the patient in knee–chest position and a vaginal hand elevating the presenting part, the patient was taken for immediate cesarean delivery, resulting in a liveborn infant with Apgar scores of 4 and 7 at 1 and 5 minutes. Newborn resuscitation and intubation were performed before transfer to the neonatal ICU. Cord blood pH was within normal limits and placental evaluation revealed no chorioamnionitis. The mother was discharged home on postoperative day 3 for outpatient postoperative evaluation and for counseling regarding her risk of another spontaneous preterm birth. The infant suffered respiratory distress syndrome and hyperbilirubinemia requiring phototherapy but no sepsis or intraventricular hemorrhage, and is gaining weight at 3 weeks of life.

References

1. Skinner SJM, Campos GA, Liggins GC. Collagen content of human amniotic membranes: effect of gestation length and premature rupture. Obstet Gynecol. 1981;57:487–9.

2. Lavery JP, Miller CE, Knight RD. The effect of labor on the rheologic response of chorioamniotic membranes. Obstet Gynecol. 1982;60:87–92.

3. Taylor J, Garite T. Premature rupture of the membranes before fetal viability. Obstet Gynecol. 1984;64:615–20.

4. Naeye RL. Factors that predispose to premature rupture of the fetal membranes. Obstet Gynecol. 1992;60:93.

5. Harger JH, Hsing AW, Tuomala RE, Gibbs RS, Mead PB, Eschenbach DA, et al. Risk factors for preterm premature rupture of fetal membranes: a multicenter case–control study. Am J Obstet Gynecol. 1990;163:130.

6. Mercer BM, Goldenberg RL, Meis PJ, Moawad AH, Shellhaas C, Das A, et al. NICHD-MFMU Network. The Preterm Prediction Study: prediction of preterm premature rupture of the membranes using clinical findings and ancillary testing. Am J Obstet Gynecol. 2000;183:738–45.

7. Roberts AK, Monzon-Bordonaba F, van Deerlin PG, Holder J, Macones GA, Morgan MA, et al. Association of polymorphism within the promoter of the tumor necrosis factor alpha gene with increased risk of preterm premature rupture of the fetal membranes. Am J Obstet Gynecol. 1999;180:1297–1302.

8. Ferrand PE, Parry S, Sammel M, Macones GA, Kuivaniemi H, Romero R, et al. A polymorphism in the matrix metalloproteinase-9 promoter is associated with increased risk of preterm premature rupture of membranes in African Americans. Mol Hum Reprod. 2002;8:494–501.

9. Strohl A, Kumar D, Novince R, Shaniuk P, Smith J, Bryant K, et al. Decreased adherence and spontaneous separation of fetal membrane layers–amnion and choriodecidua–a possible part of the normal weakening process. Placenta. 2010;31(1):18–24.

10. Klebanoff MA, Carey JC, Hauth JC, Hillier SL, Nugent RP, Thom EA, et al.; National Institute of Child Health and Human Development Maternal-Fetal Medicine Units Network. Failure of metronidazole to prevent preterm delivery among pregnant women with asymptomatic Trichomonas vaginalis infection. N Engl J Med. 2001;345:487–93.

11. Carey JC, Klebanoff MA, Hauth JC, Hillier SL, Thom EA, Ernest JM, et al.; National Institute of Child Health and Human Development Maternal-Fetal Medicine Units Network. Metronidazole to prevent preterm delivery in pregnant women with asymptomatic bacterial vaginosis. N Engl J Med. 2000; 342:534–40.

12. Kumar D, Springel E, Moore RM, Mercer BM, Philipson E, Mansour JM, et al. Progesterone inhibits in vitro fetal membrane weakening. Am J Obstet Gynecol. 2015;213:520.e1–9.

13. Wang Y, Abrahams VM, Luo G, Norwitz NG, Snegovskikh VV, Ng SW, et al. Progesterone inhibits apoptosis in fetal membranes by altering expression of both pro- and antiapoptotic proteins. Reprod Sci. 2018;25:1161–7.

14. U.S. Food and Drug Administration. FDA Commissioner and Chief Scientist announce decision to withdraw approval of Makena. FDA; 2023. Accessed April 6, 2023. Available at: https://www.fda.gov/news-events/press-announcements/fda-commissioner-and-chief-scientist-announce-decision-withdraw-approval-makena.

15. American College of Obstetricians and Gynecologists. Practice Advisory: Updated Clinical Guidance for the Use of Progesterone Supplementation for the Prevention of Recurrent Preterm Birth. April 2023. Available at: https://www.acog.org/clinical/clinical-guidance/practice-advisory/articles/2023/04/updated-guidance-use-of-progesterone-supplementation-for-prevention-of-recurrent-preterm-birth.

16. SMFM Statement: Response to the Food and Drug Administration's withdrawal of 17-alpha hydroxyprogesterone caproate. Available at: https://www.smfm.org/publications/467-smfm-special-statement-response-to-the-food-and-drug-administrations-withdrawal-of-17-alpha-hydroxyprogesterone-caproate.

17. Spinnato JA, Freire S, Pinto e Silva JL, Rudge MV, Martins-Costa S, Koch MA, et al. Antioxidant supplementation and premature rupture of the membranes: a planned secondary analysis. Am J Obstet Gynecol. 2008;199:433.

18. Mercer BM, Abdelrahim A, Moore RM, Novak J, Kumar D, Mansour JM, et al. The impact of vitamin C supplementation in pregnancy and in vitro upon fetal membrane strength and remodeling. Reprod Sci. 2010;17:685–95.

19. Casanueva E, Ripoll C, Tolentino M, et al. Vitamin C supplementation to prevent premature rupture of the chorioamniotic membranes: a randomized trial. Am J Clin Nutr 2005; 81:859–863.

20. Lee SE, Park JS, Norwitz ER, Kim KW, Park HS, Jun JK. Measurement of placental alpha-microglobulin-1 in cervicovaginal discharge to diagnose rupture of membranes. Obstet Gynecol. 2007;109:634–40.

21. Lockwood CJ, Wein R, Chien D, Ghidini A, Alvarez M, Berkowitz RL. Fetal membrane rupture is associated with the presence of insulin-like growth factor-binding protein-1 in vaginal secretions. Am J Obstet Gynecol. 1994;171:146–50.

22. Gaucherand P, Guibaud S, Awada A, Rudigoz RC. Comparative study of three amniotic fluid markers in premature rupture of membranes: fetal fibronectin, alpha-fetoprotein, diaminooxydase. Acta Obstet Gynecol Scand. 1995;74:118–21.

23. Chen FC, Dudenhausen JW. Comparison of two rapid strip tests based on IGFBP-1 and PAMG-1 for the detection of amniotic fluid. Am J Perinatol. 2008;25:243–6.

24. Lee SM, Lee J, Seong HS, Lee SE, Park JS, Romero R, et al. The clinical significance of a positive Amnisure test in women with term labor with intact membranes. J Matern Fetal Neonatal Med. 2009;22:305–10.

25. U.S. Food and Drug Administration. Risks associated with use of rupture of membranes tests - letter to health care providers | FDA Silver Spring, MD: FDA; 2018 Aug 8 [cited 2022 Apr 23]. Available from: https://www.fda.gov/news-events/press-announcements/fda-alerts-healthcare-providers-women-about-risks-associated-improper-use-rupture-membranes-tests.

26. Mercer BM, Goldenberg RL, Das AF, Thurnau GR, Bendon RW, Miodovnik M, et al.; National Institute of Child Health and Human Development Maternal-Fetal Medicine Units Network. What have we learned regarding antibiotic therapy for the reduction of infant morbidity? Semin Perinatol. 2003;27:217–30.

27. Hillier SL, Martius J, Krohn M, Kiviat N, Holmes KK, Eschenbach DA. A case-control study of chorioamnionic infection and histologic chorioamnionitis in prematurity. N Engl J Med. 1988;319:972–8.

28. Gunn GC, Mishell DR, Morton DG. Premature rupture of the fetal membranes: a review. Am J Obstet Gynecol. 1970; 106:469–82.

29. Garite TJ, Freeman RK. Chorioamnionitis in the preterm gestation. Obstet Gynecol. 1982;59:539–45.

30. Vintzileos AM, Campbell WA, Nochimson DJ, Weinbaum PJ. Preterm premature rupture of the membranes: a risk factor for the development of abruptio placentae. Am J Obstet Gynecol. 1987;156:1235–8.

31. Mercer BM, Moretti ML, Prevost RR, Sibai BM. Erythromycin therapy in preterm premature rupture of the membranes: a prospective, randomized trial of 220 patients. Am J Obstet Gynecol. 1992;166:794–802.

32. Mercer BM. Preterm premature rupture of the membranes. Obstet Gynecol. 2003;101:178–93.

33. Alexander JM, Mercer BM, Miodovnik M, Thurnau GR, Goldenberg RL, Das AF, et al. The impact of digital cervical examination on expectantly managed preterm rupture of membranes. Am J Obstet Gynecol. 2000;183:1003–7.

34. Broekhuizen FF, Gilman M, Hamilton PR. Amniocentesis for gram stain and culture in preterm premature rupture of the membranes. Obstet Gynecol. 1985;66:316–21.

35. Romero R, Yoon BH, Mazor M, Gomez R, Gonzalez R, Diamond MP, et al. A comparative study of the diagnostic performance of amniotic fluid glucose, white blood cell count, interleukin-6, and Gram stain in the detection of microbial invasion in patients with preterm premature rupture of membranes. Am J Obstet Gynecol. 1993;169:839–51.

36. Vintzileos AM, Campbell WA, Nochimson DJ, Weinbaum PJ. Fetal breathing as a predictor of infection in premature rupture of the membranes. Obstet Gynecol. 1986;67:813–17.

37. Vintzileos AM, Campbell WA, Nochimson DJ, Connolly ME, Fuenfer MM, Hoehn GJ. The fetal biophysical profile in patients with premature rupture of the membranes: an early predictor of fetal infection. Am J Obstet Gynecol. 1985; 152:510–16.

38. American College of Obstetricians and Gynecologists. ACOG Committee Opinion No. 797: prevention of group B streptococcal early-onset disease in newborns. Obstet Gynecol. 2020;135: e51–72.

39. Escobar GJ, Clark RH, Greene JD. Short-term outcomes of infants born at 35 and 36 weeks' gestation: we need to ask more questions. Semin Perinatol. 2006;30:28–33.

40. Neerhof MG, Cravello C, Haney EI, Silver RK. Timing of labor induction after premature rupture of membranes between 32 and 36 weeks' gestation. Am J Obstet Gynecol. 1999;180:349–52.

41. Naef RW 3rd, Allbert JR, Ross EL, Weber BM, Martin RW, Morrison JC. Premature rupture of membranes at 34 to 37 weeks' gestation: aggressive versus conservative management. Am J Obstet Gynecol. 1998;178:126–30.

42. Mercer BM, Crocker L, Boe N, Sibai B. Induction versus expectant management in PROM with mature amniotic fluid at 32-36 weeks: a randomized trial. Am J Obstet Gynecol. 1993; 82:775–82.

43. Van der Ham DP, Vijgen SM, Nijhuis JG, van Beek JJ, Opmeer BC, Mulder AL, et al.; PPROMEXIL trial group. Induction of labor versus expectant management in women with preterm prelabor rupture of membranes between 34 and 37 weeks: a randomized controlled trial. PLoS Med. 2012;9:e1001208.

44. van der Ham DP, van der Heyden JL, Opmeer BC, Mulder AL, Moonen RM, van Beek JH, et al. Management of late-preterm premature rupture of membranes: the PPROMEXIL-2 trial. Am J Obstet Gynecol. 2012;207:276.e1–10.

45. Morris JM, Roberts CL, Bowen JR, Patterson JA, Bond DM, Algert CS, et al.; PPROMT Collaboration. Immediate delivery compared with expectant management after preterm prelabour rupture of the membranes close to term (PPROMT trial): a randomised controlled trial. Lancet. 2016;387:444–52.

46. Quist-Nelson J, de Ruigh AA, Seidler AL, van der Ham DP, Willekes C, Berghella V, et al.; Preterm Premature Rupture of Membranes Meta-analysis (PPROMM) Collaboration. Immediate delivery compared with expectant management in late preterm prelabor rupture of membranes: an individual participant data meta-analysis. Obstet Gynecol 2018;131(2):269–79.

47. Harding JE, Pang J, Knight DB, Liggins GC. Do antenatal corticosteroids help in the setting of preterm rupture of membranes? Am J Obstet Gynecol. 2001;184:131–9.

48. American College of Obstetricians and Gynecologists' Committee on Obstetric Practice; Society for Maternal-Fetal Medicine. Committee Opinion No. 677: antenatal corticosteroid therapy for fetal maturation. Obstet Gynecol. 2016;128(4):e187–94.

49. Mercer B, Miodovnik M, Thurnau G, Goldenberg RL, Das AF, Ramsey RD, et al.; National Institute of Child Health and Human Development Maternal-Fetal Medicine Units Network. Antibiotic therapy for reduction of infant morbidity after preterm premature rupture of the membranes: a randomized controlled trial. JAMA. 1997;278:989–95.

50. Kenyon S, Boulvain M, Neilson J. Antibiotics for preterm rupture of the membranes: a systematic review. Obstet Gynecol. 2004;104:1051–7.

51. Lewis DF, Adair CD, Robichaux AG, Jaekle RK, Moore JA, Evans AT, et al. Antibiotic therapy in preterm premature rupture of membranes: are seven days necessary? A preliminary, randomized clinical trial. Am J Obstet Gynecol. 2003;188:1413–16; discussion 1416-17.

52. Segel SY, Miles AM, Clothier B, Parry S, Macones GA. Duration of antibiotic therapy after preterm premature rupture of fetal membranes. Am J Obstet Gynecol. 2003;189:799–802.

53. Kenyon SL, Taylor DJ, Tarnow-Mordi W, Oracle Collaborative Group. Broad spectrum antibiotics for preterm, prelabor rupture of fetal membranes: the Oracle I randomized trial. Lancet. 2001;357:979–88.

54. Kenyon S, Pike K, Jones DR, Brocklehurst P, Marlow N, Salt A, et al. Childhood outcomes after prescription of antibiotics to pregnant women with preterm rupture of the membranes: 7-year follow-up of the ORACLE I trial. Lancet. 2008;372:1310–18.

55. Doyle LW, Crowther CA, Middleton P, Marret S, Rouse D. Magnesium sulphate for women at risk of preterm birth for neuroprotection of the fetus. Cochrane Database Syst Rev. 2009;(1):CD004661. doi: 10.1002/14651858.CD004661.pub3.

56. Rouse DJ, Hirtz DG, Thom E, Varner MW, Spong CY, Mercer BM, et al.; Eunice Kennedy Shriver NICHD Maternal-Fetal Medicine Units Network. A randomized, controlled trial of magnesium sulfate for the prevention of cerebral palsy. N Engl J Med. 2008;359:895–905.

57. Christensen KK, Ingemarsson I, Leideman T, Solum T, Svenningsen N. Effect of Ritodrine on labor after premature rupture of the membranes. Obstet Gynecol. 1980;55:187–90.

58. Weiner CP, Renk K, Klugman M. The therapeutic efficacy and cost-effectiveness of aggressive tocolysis for premature labor associated with premature rupture of the membranes. Am J Obstet Gynecol. 1988;159:216–22.

59. Garite TJ, Keegan KA, Freeman RK, Nageotte MP. A randomized trial of Ritodrine tocolysis versus expectant management in patients with premature rupture of membranes at 25 to 30 weeks of gestation. Am J Obstet Gynecol. 1987;157:388–93.

60. How HY, Cook CR, Cook VD, Miles DE, Spinnato JA. Preterm premature rupture of membranes: aggressive tocolysis versus expectant management. J Matern Fetal Med. 1998;7:8–12.

61. Mackeen AD, Seibel-Seamon J, Muhammad J, Baxter JK, Berghella V. Tocolytics for preterm premature rupture of membranes. Cochrane Database Syst Rev. 2014;(2):CD007062. doi: 10.1002/14651858.CD007062.pub3.

62. American College of Obstetricians and Gynecologists. ACOG Practice Bulletin No. 217: Prelabor Rupture of Membranes: Obstet Gynecol. 2020;135:e80–e97.

63. Lauria MR, Gonik B, Romero R. Pulmonary hypoplasia: pathogenesis, diagnosis, and antenatal prediction. Obstet Gynecol. 1995;86:466–75.

64. D'Alton M, Mercer B, Riddick E, Dudley D. Serial thoracic versus abdominal circumference ratios for the prediction of pulmonary hypoplasia in premature rupture of the membranes remote from term. Am J Obstet Gynecol. 1992;166:658–63.

65. Vintzileos AM, Campbell WA, Rodis JF, Nochimson DJ, Pinette MG, Petrikovsky BM. Comparison of six different ultrasonographic methods for predicting lethal fetal pulmonary hypoplasia. Am J Obstet Gynecol. 1989;161:606–12.

66. Sciscione AC, Manley JS, Pollock M, et al. Intracervical fibrin sealants: a potential treatment for early preterm premature rupture of the membranes. Am J Obstet Gynecol. 2001;184:368–73.

67. Quintero RA, Morales WJ, Bornick PW, Allen M, Garabelis N. Surgical treatment of spontaneous rupture of membranes: the amniograft–first experience. Am J Obstet Gynecol. 2002;186:155–7.

68. O'Brien JM, Barton JR, Milligan DA. An aggressive interventional protocol for early midtrimester premature rupture of the membranes using gelatin sponge for cervical plugging. Am J Obstet Gynecol. 2002;187:1143–6.

69. Treadwell MC, Bronsteen RA, Bottoms SF. Prognostic factors and complication rates for cervical cerclage: a review of 482 cases. Am J Obstet Gynecol. 1991;165:555–8.

70. Blickstein I, Katz Z, Lancet M, Molgilner BM. The outcome of pregnancies complicated by preterm rupture of the membranes with and without cerclage. Int J Gynaecol Obstet. 1989;28:237–42.

71. Yeast JD, Garite TR. The role of cervical cerclage in the management of preterm premature rupture of the membranes. Am J Obstet Gynecol. 1988;158:106–10.

72. Vitner D, Melamed N, Elhadad D, Phang M, Ram M, Asztalos E, et al. Removal vs. retention of cervical cerclage in pregnancies complicated by preterm premature rupture of membranes: a retrospective study. Arch Gynecol Obstet. 2020;302(3):603–9.

73. Suff N, Kunitsyna M, Shennan A, Chandiramani M. Optimal timing of cervical cerclage removal following preterm premature rupture of membranes; a retrospective analysis. Eur J Obstet Gynecol Reprod Biol. 2021;259:75–80.

74. Jenkins TM, Berghella V, Shlossman PA, McIntyre CJ, Maas BD, Pollock MA, et al. Timing of cerclage removal after preterm premature rupture of membranes: maternal and neonatal outcomes. Am J Obstet Gynecol. 2000;183(4):847–52.

75. Galyean A, Garite TJ, Maurel K, Abril D, Adair CD, Browne P, et al.; Obstetrix Perinatal Collaborative Research Network. Removal versus retention of cerclage in preterm premature rupture of membranes: a randomized controlled trial. Am J Obstet Gynecol. 2014;211(4):399.e1–7.

76. Major CA, Towers CV, Lewis DF, Garite TJ. Expectant management of preterm premature rupture of membranes complicated by active recurrent genital herpes. Am J Obstet Gynecol. 2003;188:1551–4.

77. Johnson JWC, Egerman RS, Moorhead J. Cases with ruptured membranes that "reseal." Am J Obstet Gynecol. 1990;163:1024–32.

78. Gold RB, Goyer GL, Schwartz, Evans MI, Seabolt LA. Conservative management of second trimester postamniocentesis fluid leakage. Obstet Gynecol. 1989;74:745–7.

Chapter 42
Management of Preterm Labor

Georgios Doulaveris[1] and Vincenzo Berghella[2]

[1]Department of Obstetrics & Gynecology and Women's Health, Albert Einstein College of Medicine, Montefiore Medical Center, Bronx, NY, USA

[2]Department of Obstetrics and Gynecology, Thomas Jefferson University, Philadelphia, PA, USA

Evaluation: history, physical exam, and screening tests

At a minimum, a patient's history should include a review of specific symptoms, such as menstrual-like cramps, abdominal "tightening," low backache, pelvic pressure, increased vaginal discharge, spotting or bleeding. It is paramount to obtain the exact determination of gestational age, ideally by ultrasound performed at <22 weeks. To assess prognosis, specific risk factors for preterm birth (PTB) should be carefully reviewed. These are listed in Box 42.1.

The physical exam should include an assessment of vital signs, cardiotocography, an abdominal exam for uterine tenderness, contractions, fetal size and position, a cervical exam by speculum for pooling of amniotic fluid, nitrazine and ferning testing, visual examination of cervix (especially if preterm prelabor rupture of membranes [PPROM] is suspected), collection for fetal fibronectin (fFN), group B streptococci (GBS), *Chlamydia*, and gonorrhea DNA tests. If PPROM is suspected and there is no evidence of pooling, commercial tests that detect amniotic fluid in the vagina may be used to confirm or exclude the diagnosis. If PPROM is ruled out, a manual cervical exam can be performed for dilation, cervical length and/or effacement, station, and presentation.

Laboratory tests that should be considered include rapid plasma reagin to rule out syphilis, rapid HIV (if status unknown), cervicovaginal fFN, vaginorectal GBS, urinary drug screen, urinalysis, and urine culture. In women without specific symptoms of these infections, there is no evidence that screening for bacterial vaginosis, *Trichomonas*, *Mycoplasma*, or *Ureaplasma* is beneficial.

In addition, an ultrasound should be performed to assess for fetal demise, major anomaly, polyhydramnios, placenta previa, placental abruption, fetal presentation, and estimated fetal weight. A transvaginal ultrasound (TVU) can be performed for cervical length (CL) evaluation. Amniocentesis may be considered to check for intraamniotic infection (IAI) if equivocal signs of chorioamnionitis are present. If the diagnosis of IAI is made clinically (maternal fever ≥ 39.0° C [102.2° F] once or 38–38.9° C [100.4–102.1° F] on two occasions 30 minutes apart in the absence of other infection, *plus* fetal tachycardia or maternal leukocytosis or purulent cervical discharge), delivery is recommended without amniocentesis. The rates of IAI (documented by amniotic fluid culture) by pregnancy status at <37 weeks are approximately 5–15% for preterm labor (PTL; intact membranes), 20–30% for PPROM (no labor), 30–40% for PPROM (labor), and 50% for women with cervical dilation (cervix ≥2 cm/80%) without active PTL in the second trimester. The rates of infection are indirectly proportional to gestational age, as well as CL. There is insufficient evidence to recommend amniocentesis in all cases of PTL.

Initial assessment

Diagnosis of preterm labor

Most women who present with symptoms of PTL do not deliver preterm even without intervention. Therefore, it is important to establish the diagnosis of PTL before any treatment is considered. One of the most used signs of PTL diagnoses is the presence of uterine contractions (≥4/20 min or ≥8/hour) *and* documented cervical change (cervical dilation ≥3 cm) *or* CL <20 mm on TVU *or* CL 20–29 mm on TVU with a positive fFN, with intact membranes at 20–36 weeks 6 days of gestation. In fact, 70–80% of women even with this diagnosis of PTL do not deliver preterm. The presence of uterine contractions in the absence of documented cervical change does not meet

Queenan's Management of High-Risk Pregnancy: An Evidence-Based Approach, Seventh Edition. Edited by Catherine Y. Spong and Charles J. Lockwood.
© 2024 John Wiley & Sons Ltd. Published 2024 by John Wiley & Sons Ltd.

Box 42.1 Risk factors for preterm birth

- Obstetric and gynecologic history: prior spontaneous PTB; prior STL; prior surgical uterine evacuation; prior cone biopsy; uterine malformations; myomata; extremes of interpregnancy intervals; ART
- Extremes of maternal prepregnancy weight or BMI, poor nutritional status
- Maternal age extremes (<19 y; >35 y)
- Race and ethnicity (especially non-Hispanic Black)
- Education (<12th grade)
- Maternal medical conditions (e.g. DM, HTN, anemia, periodontal disease)
- Low socioeconomic status; unmarried; physical or psychological abuse
- Limited prenatal care
- Family history of spontaneous PTB
- Multiple gestation
- Fetal disease (e.g. anomalies, growth restriction)
- Working conditions and physically demanding work (e.g. >80 h/week; standing >8 h; shift work, fixed night shifts)
- Vaginal bleeding (especially during second trimester)
- Maternal substance use (e.g. use of tobacco, alcohol, cocaine, heroin, etc.)
- Antenatal stress (including post-traumatic stress disorder), depression, exposure to selective serotonin reuptake inhibitors
- Maternal infections
- Short cervical length between 14–28 wk
- Positive fetal fibronectin
- Uterine contractions

ART, assisted reproductive technologies; BMI, body mass index; DES, diethylstilbestrol; DM, diabetes mellitus; HTN, hypertension; PTB, preterm birth; STL, second trimester loss.

criteria for PTL and should therefore not receive treatment.

Fetal fibronectin and cervical length

Because so many women with a diagnosis of PTL do not deliver preterm, two predictive tests, fFN and TVU CL, can be used, where available, in the initial assessment of the chance of delivering preterm. In symptomatic women with threatened PTL, knowledge of TVU CL results is associated with significantly lower rate of PTB <37 weeks [1]. Similarly, PTL management based on knowledge of fFN results may reduce PTB <37 weeks [2]. Women with suspected PTL but TVU CL ≥30 mm have a less than 2% chance of delivering within 1 week, more than 95% chance of delivering ≥35 weeks without therapy [3] and should therefore not receive treatment. Women with TVU CL 20–29 mm and positive fFN, or especially those with TVU CL less than 20 mm, are at highest risk of PTB and should receive intervention. Management of threatened PTL based on fFN and TVU CL (Figure 42.1) has been associated with a significant reduction in PTB <37 weeks in a randomized controlled trial (RCT) [4].

Management

The main interventions for a woman with PTL at high risk for delivering preterm are aimed at increasing fetal maturation and stopping uterine contractions to delay PTB. In addition, it is important to consider referral to a tertiary care center if the neonatal intensive care unit (NICU) is not adequate to care for an infant delivering at that gestational age. The woman and her family members should be counseled regarding morbidity and mortality for the possible preterm infant. Current (2018) survival is 0% at 21 weeks, 11% at 22 weeks, 50% at 23 weeks, 79% at 25 weeks, and more than 95% at 29 weeks, whereas intact survival at 18 months is >50% after 25 weeks [5]. Disabilities in mental and psychomotor development, neuromotor function (including cerebral palsy), or sensory and communication function are present in at least 50% of fetuses born ≤25 weeks gestation [6]. A neonatology consult for affected women at 22–34 weeks should always be obtained to discuss neonatal prognosis and management. Obstetric counseling should review the principles and progress of management of PTL. Specific interventions should aim to treat any positive tests or infections, such as urinary tract infections, sexually transmitted diseases, GBS, and HIV.

Women with multiple gestations should not be treated differently from those with singletons, except for caution in that their risk of pulmonary edema is greater when exposed to β-mimetics or magnesium sulfate [7].

Prophylaxis to prevent neonatal morbidity/mortality from preterm birth (fetal maturation)

Betamethasone and dexamethasone are the only two corticosteroids that cross the placenta reliably and have been shown to benefit the fetus. Both choices are acceptable, as there is no clear evidence that one type is superior to the other. The regimen for one course of betamethasone is 12 mg IM every 24 hours for two doses and for dexamethasone is 6 mg IM every 6 hours for four doses. Antenatal administration of betamethasone or dexamethasone to women expected to give PTB (either spontaneous or indicated) is associated with a 15% reduction in perinatal death, 22% reduction in neonatal death, 29% reduction in respiratory distress syndrome (RDS), 42% reduction in intraventricular hemorrhage (IVH) and 49% reduction in developmental delay in childhood [8]. There is a trend for a 50% reduction in necrotizing enterocolitis (NEC). Corticosteroid administration is also associated with decreased needs for surfactant, oxygen, and mechanical ventilation in the neonatal period.

These benefits apply to at least 23–33 weeks 6 days and are not limited by fetal gender or race. At 22 to 22 weeks 6 days, corticosteroids may be considered if delivery is anticipated within 7 days and the patient desires neonatal

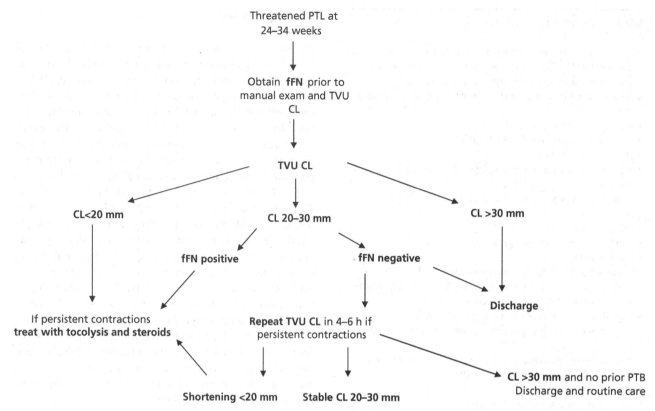

Figure 42.1 Preterm labor management algorithm. Adapted from [4]. CL, cervical length; fFN, fetal fibronectin; PTB, preterm birth; PTL, preterm labor; TVU CL, transvaginal ultrasound cervical length.

resuscitation. Between 34 and 36 weeks 6 days, antenatal corticosteroids are associated with 26% reduction in RDS, 44% reduction in transient tachypnea of the newborn, as well as decreased needs for surfactant, oxygen supplementation and mechanical ventilation [9]. Thus, between 34 and 36 weeks 6 days, a single course of corticosteroids should be considered in women with a singleton gestation who are at risk for PTB within 7 days (symptomatic and cervix is ≥3 cm or ≥75%). Late preterm administration of corticosteroids is not indicated in women with infection, chorioamnionitis, multiple gestations, or pregestational diabetes and those who have previously received a course of corticosteroids prior to 34 weeks as they were not included in the late preterm RCTs. After 34 weeks, tocolytics should not be administered to delay delivery for completion of corticosteroids course. Use of corticosteroids after 34 weeks increases the risk for neonatal hypoglycemia [9].

The effects of corticosteroid treatment are significant mostly at 48 hours to 7 days from the first dose, but treatment should not be withheld even if delivery appears imminent, and effects even for babies delivered more than 7 days later have been reported [10]. Corticosteroids should therefore be administered to any woman at these gestational ages at significant PTB risk upon identification of that risk. Published results are mostly from singleton gestations, with fewer data on multiple gestations. There are no absolute contraindications to corticosteroids; however, they should be used with caution in cases of systemic maternal infection (e.g. pyelonephritis, pneumonia) and women with chorioamnionitis should be delivered promptly without delay for corticosteroid therapy. There is no evidence that treatment with antenatal corticosteroids increases risk of maternal death, infection or sepsis or fetal/neonatal infection. When used for only one course, no significant side effects have been reported. No adverse consequences of corticosteroids for PTB in either the mothers or, most important, the infants, even at 10 years follow-up, have been identified.

One single additional (rescue) course of antenatal corticosteroids should be considered in women at <34 weeks who are still pregnant 14 days after the initial course and are deemed to be at imminent risk for PTB within seven days. A repeat course of betamethasone, when administered prior to 30 weeks, has been associated with decreased risk of RDS, surfactant use, mechanical ventilation, and composite neonatal morbidity [11,12]. More than two repeated courses of steroids should NOT be administered [13]. Although weekly repeated courses in women who remain at risk for PTB have been associated with reduced risk of RDS and serious infant outcomes, if repeated courses, especially four or more, are used, there is a possible association with decreased birthweight, length, and head circumference. At early childhood, no differences are seen between infants exposed and unexposed to repeat courses, regarding death, disability, and growth assessment [13].

Thyrotropin-releasing hormone, phenobarbital, vitamin K, and ambroxol have not been shown to be beneficial for fetal maturation and PTL management.

Neuroprotection

Antenatal magnesium sulfate given to women at immediate risk for PTB because of PTL or PPROM is associated with a 32% decrease in the incidence of cerebral palsy and 39% reduction in rates of substantial gross motor reduction, with no other significant benefits or detriments [14]. In arecent RCT, administration of magnesium sulfate prior to PTB between 30–34 weeks, did notdecrease the incidence of death or cerebral palsy at 2 years, however the study was underpoweredto detect small differences between groups [15]. Magnesium sulfate therapy should be administered to women with either singleton or multiple gestations between 23–31 weeks 6 days when PTB is deemed to be imminent. An intravenous 4–6 g loading dose of magnesium sulfate is administered over 20–30 minutes, followed by maintenance infusion of 1–2 g/hour. Magnesium sulfate should not delay the delivery and it should be discontinued if PTB is no longer deemed imminent.

Nontocolytic interventions

Bed rest

Activity restriction has not been shown to be beneficial in preventing PTB in singleton or multiple gestations [16,17]. Extended bed rest increases the risk of thromboembolic events.

Hydration

Intravenous hydration is not beneficial in preventing PTB, even during the period of evaluation soon after admission for PTL [18]. No studies have evaluated oral hydration.

Prophylactic antibiotics

There is no evidence of benefit from prophylactic antibiotic treatment for women with PTL with intact membranes on neonatal outcomes, and there are concerns about a trend for 52% increase in neonatal mortality for those who received antibiotics [19]. Rates of PTB <36–37 weeks are similar in antibiotic and placebo groups, as is perinatal mortality. In the largest trial, with the longest (7 years) follow-up, both amoxicillin/clavulanic acid (co-amoxiclav) and erythromycin were associated with significant increases in cerebral palsy and erythromycin with an increase in functional impairment [20]. Therefore,

antibiotics should not be used for prophylaxis in women with PTL.

Group B streptococcus prophylaxis

Antibiotics should be used for GBS prophylaxis only in those pregnancies deemed at high risk to deliver preterm within 2–3 days, such as those with TVU CL <20 mm. Until GBS maternal status is known, these women should receive penicillin (or ampicillin if penicillin is not available) to prevent GBS neonatal infections, unless allergic [21].

Progesterone

Progesterone has been associated with prevention of PTB in certain asymptomatic women, that is, those with prior PTB and/or with short CL before 24 weeks. In women presenting with PTL, there is insufficient evidence that progestational agents prevent PTB when used in addition to tocolytics or solely for this purpose [22].

Tocolysis

The principles of tocolytic therapy are listed in Box 42.2, and contraindications are listed in Box 42.3.

Primary tocolysis–single agent

β-mimetics

Terbutaline is the most used β-mimetic.

Dose. Terbutaline: 0.25 mg SQ every 20 minutes at first, then 2–3 hours, or 5–10 µg/minute IV, max 80 µg/minute;

Box 42.2 Principles of tocolytic therapy

- At 23–33 wk 6 d, steroids for fetal maturation should always be given if tocolysis is initiated. Tocolytics should not be used without concomitant use of steroids for fetal maturation
- Tocolysis is typically used for 48 h to allow steroid effect. Given side effects, stop tocolytic therapy at 48 h after steroids given.
- No tocolytic agent has been shown to improve perinatal mortality
- No tocolytic agent has been proven safer or more efficacious. COX inhibitors are the only class of primary tocolytics shown to decrease PTB <37 weeks compared with placebo, whereas COX inhibitors and ORA have been shown to significantly prolong pregnancy at 48 h and 7 d compared with placebo. COX inhibitors, CCB, and ORA, when properly used, have significantly fewer side effects than β-mimetics. CCB and COX inhibitors are the tocolytic agents best supported by evidence for safety and effectiveness.
- There is no *maintenance* tocolytic agent that has been proven to prevent PTB or perinatal morbidity/mortality.
- There is insufficient evidence to evaluate multiple tocolytic agents for primary tocolysis, refractory (primary agent is failing, so another is started) tocolysis, or repeated tocolysis (after successful primary tocolysis)

CCB, calcium channel blocker; COX, cyclooxygenase; ORA, oxytocin receptor antagonist; PTB, preterm birth; PTL, preterm labor.

Box 42.3 Contraindications to tocolytic therapy

Maternal

- Chorioamnionitis
- Severe vaginal bleeding/abruption
- Preeclampsia
- Medical contraindications to specific tocolytic agent
- Other maternal medical condition that makes continuing the pregnancy inadvisable

Fetal

- Fetal death
- Major (especially lethal) fetal anomaly or chromosome abnormality
- Other fetal conditions in which prolongation of pregnancy is inadvisable
- Documented fetal maturity

or 2.5–5 mg PO every 2–4 hours (hold if maternal heart rate over 120 beats/minute).

Mechanism of action. Stimulate Beta$_2$ receptor through cyclic adenosine monophosphate, decreases free calcium needed for myometrial contractions.

Evidence for effectiveness. β-mimetics decrease the number of women in PTL giving birth within 48 hours and within 7 days by 32% and 20% respectively, compared with placebo, but are not associated with a significant decrease in PTB <37 weeks [23]. No benefit is demonstrated for β-mimetics on RDS or perinatal death. A few trials reported no difference detected in cerebral palsy, infant death, and NEC. There is no sufficient evidence to support the use of any particular β-mimetic, though terbutaline is the most commonly used such agent in the United States.

Specific contraindications. Cardiac arrhythmia or other significant cardiac disease; diabetes mellitus; poorly controlled thyroid disease.

Side effects. Maternal: withdrawal from treatment due to adverse effects, chest pain, dyspnea, tachycardia, palpitation, tremor, headaches, hypokalemia (K <3 mEq/L in 50%), hyperglycemia (140–200 mg/dL glucose in 20–50%), nausea/vomiting, nasal stuffiness. Fetal/neonatal: tachycardia, hypoglycemia.

Calcium channel blockers

Nifedipine (most commonly used) and nicardipine have been the calcium channel blocker (CCB) agents studied for tocolysis.

Dose. Nifedipine 20–30 mg once, then 10–20 mg every 4–8 hours (max. 90 mg/day) (nicardipine dose similar).

Mechanism of action. Impair calcium channels, so inhibit influx of calcium into cell, and therefore impede myometrial contraction.

Evidence for effectiveness. When compared with placebo, CCB reduce PTB within 48 hours by 70%, with insufficient

evidence to assess effect on PTB within 7 days, and <37 weeks [24]. When compared with other tocolytic agents, there is no difference in PTB within 48 hours, but CCB increase the interval from initiation of treatment to delivery and decrease PTB, RDS, NEC, IVH, hyperbilirubinemia, and NICU admission. CCB also have fewer adverse drug reactions resulting in treatment cessation. CCB should therefore be preferred to β-mimetics for tocolysis. There are insufficient data regarding the effects of different dosage regimens and formulations of CCB on maternal and neonatal outcomes; the most studied is nifedipine, at the dosage shown here.

Specific contraindications. Cardiac disease; hypotension (<90/50 mmHg); concomitant use of magnesium; caution in renal disease.

Side effects. Maternal: flushing, headache, dizziness, nausea, transient hypotension. Caution in women with hypotension and renal disease, as well as those on magnesium (cardiovascular collapse). Fetal/neonatal: none.

Cyclooxygenase inhibitors

Nonselective cyclooxygenase (COX) inhibitors: indomethacin (Indocin). Selective COX inhibitors (preferential COX-2 inhibitors): sulindac (Clinoril); rofecoxib (Vioxx); celecoxib (Celebrex); ketorolac (Toradol); nimesulide.

Dose. Indomethacin: 50–100 mg loading dose (rectal or vaginal route preferred, oral otherwise), then 25–50 mg every 6 hours for 48 hours maximum. Sulindac: 200 mg PO every 12 hours for 48 hours. Ketorolac: 60 mg IM, then 30 mg IM every 6 hours for 48 hours. All COX inhibitors should be used only at <32 weeks.

Mechanism of action. Inhibit prostaglandin synthesis, therefore inhibit myometrial contraction.

Evidence for effectiveness. The nonselective COX inhibitor indomethacin was used in most trials. When compared with placebo, COX inhibition (indomethacin only) results in a 79% reduction in PTB <37 weeks, an increase in gestational age of 3.5 weeks, and an increase in birthweight of approximately 700 g [25]. There is no difference in PTB within 48 hours and 7 days. No differences are detected in any other reported outcomes including perinatal morbidity and mortality.

Compared with β-mimetics, COX inhibitors reduce PTB within 48 hours and <37 weeks by 73% and 47% respectively and should therefore be preferred over β-mimetics for tocolysis. There is no difference between COX inhibitors and magnesium sulfate or CCB [25].

Comparisons of nonselective COX 1 and 2 inhibitors (indomethacin and sulindac) vs. selective (rofecoxib and nimesulide) COX-2 inhibitors do not demonstrate differences in maternal or neonatal outcomes. Because of the small numbers, all estimates of effect are imprecise and need to be interpreted with caution.

Specific contraindications. Renal or hepatic disease, active peptic ulcer disease, poorly controlled hypertension, nonsteroidal anti-inflammatory drug (NSAID)-sensitive asthma, coagulation disorders/thrombocytopenia.

Side effects. When used for only 48 hours at < 32 weeks, no serious maternal or fetal/neonatal side effects occur, and fetal surveillance is not indicated. Usually, COX inhibitors are better tolerated by the mother than other tocolytics such as magnesium and β-mimetics. Maternal: as with any NSAID, mild gastrointestinal upset – nausea, heartburn (take with some food/milk) (COX-1). Gastrointestinal bleeding (COX-1), coagulation and platelet abnormalities (COX-1), asthma if aspirin sensitive. NSAIDs may obscure elevation in temperature. Long-term rofecoxib use in adults has been associated with stroke, so this drug is now not available in many countries. Fetal/neonatal: in RCTs, 403 women received short-term tocolysis (up to 48 hours) with COX inhibitors (mainly indomethacin) and there was only one case of antenatal constriction of the ductus arteriosus (incidence <0.3%). There was no increase in the incidence of patent ductus arteriosus postnatally [26]. Use for >48 hours, especially ≥32 weeks, is associated with significant fetal effects such as constriction of the ductus arteriosus, which can lead to hydrops, pulmonary hypertension, and death, and renal insufficiency, manifested in utero by oligohydramnios. Antenatal indomethacin use has also been linked to neonatal IVH, NEC and periventricular leucomalakia [27]. Selective COX-2 inhibitors have not been shown consistently to be any safer for the fetus/neonate than nonselective COX inhibitors. Therefore, continuous use of COX inhibitors for more than 48 hours and ≥32 weeks is contraindicated.

Magnesium sulfate (MgSO₄)

Dose. 40 g MgSO₄ in 1 L 5% dextrose in half normal saline (d5½NS). Initial: 4–6 grams/30 minute, then 2 g/hour. A dose of 5 g/hour has not been shown to be beneficial in perinatal outcome compared with a dose of 2 g/hour and is associated with significant side effects [28]. Weaning MgSO₄ tocolysis has no benefits and a few harmful side effects compared with stopping MgSO₄ abruptly [29].

Mechanism of action. Intracellular calcium antagonist.

Evidence for effectiveness. Compared with placebo, there is insufficient evidence to show if magnesium sulfate reduces the incidence of PTB or perinatal morbidity and mortality [30]. Compared with all controls (including other tocolytics), magnesium sulfate does not prevent PTB at 48 hours, PTB <37 weeks or <32 weeks. Perinatal death is higher (but very rare), and perinatal morbidities are similar. Dosage of magnesium does not affect efficacy.

Specific contraindications. Myasthenia gravis.

Management. Goal: MgSO₄ levels of 4–7 mEq/L. Monitor urinary output. Follow deep tendon reflexes: decrease reflexes observed at ≥8 mEq/L, absent reflexes at ≥10 mEq/L, respiratory depression at ≥10 mEq/L, and cardiac arrest at ≥15 mEq/L.

Side effects. Maternal: flushing, lethargy, headache, muscle weakness, diplopia, dry mouth, pulmonary edema (1%; mechanism: intravenous overhydration), cardiac arrest. Fetal/neonatal: lethargy, hypotonia, hypocalcemia, respiratory depression. Prolonged use: demineralization.

Oxytocin receptor antagonists

Atosiban (Tractocile in Europe) is not Food and Drug Administration approved, and therefore not available in the United States.

Dose. Atosiban 6.75 mg bolus, then 300 µg/minute IV for 3 hours, then 100 µg/minute (for a maximum of 45 hours).

Mechanism of action. Competitive inhibitor of oxytocin via blockade of oxytocin receptor.

Evidence for effectiveness. Compared with placebo, atosiban does not reduce incidence of PTB or improve neonatal outcome [31]. In one trial, atosiban was associated with an increase in PTB <28 weeks and infant deaths at 12 months of age compared with placebo [31]. However, this trial randomized significantly more women to atosiban before 26 weeks gestation. Use of atosiban results in lower infant birthweight and more maternal adverse drug reactions. Compared with β-mimetics, atosiban has similar incidences of PTB and perinatal morbidity/mortality and has fewer maternal drug reactions requiring treatment cessation.

Side effects. Minimal to none.

There is currently insufficient evidence to support the administration of nitric oxide donors [32] for prevention of PTB in women with PTL.

Additional tocolysis and antibiotics used simultaneously

Indomethacin and ampicillin-sulbactam do not prevent PTB compared with placebo in women in PTL already receiving MgSO₄ tocolysis [33].

Refractory tocolysis–primary agent is failing

In a small RCT, indomethacin was similar to sulindac in delaying delivery for 48 hours or 7 days in women failing primary MgSO₄ tocolysis [34].

Maintenance tocolysis–after successful primary tocolysis

There is evidence that all agents used so far for maintenance tocolysis do not prevent PTB, recurrent PTL, recurrent hospitalizations, or perinatal morbidity and mortality. These include oral β-mimetics [35], terbutaline pump [36], CCB [37], COX inhibitors [38], magnesium [39], or atosiban [40].

Mode of delivery

There is insufficient evidence to evaluate the use of a policy for uniform planned cesarean delivery compared with expectant management and selective cesarean for preterm babies (approximately 24–36 weeks) [41]. Mothers in the planned cesarean delivery group have higher morbidity, whereas babies in the planned cesarean delivery group show no significant differences in perinatal morbidity/mortality or abnormal childhood follow-up. In cases of preterm breech presentation, cesarean delivery is the preferred mode of delivery as it results in a 37% risk reduction for neonatal mortality [42].

CASE PRESENTATION

A 25-year-old, non-Hispanic Black, gravida 6, para 0141 calls her obstetrician at 28 weeks 6 days gestation with complaints of vaginal pressure. Upon questioning, she states that she might have intermittent cramps. Based on this history, the attending physician asks her to come to labor and delivery to be evaluated.

Her past obstetric history is significant for two spontaneous abortions, two surgical uterine evacuations for elective terminations, and one PTB at 30 weeks the year before preceded by PTL unsuccessfully treated with magnesium sulfate. She received steroids for fetal maturation and delivered a 1484 g (3 lb 4 oz) infant currently doing well. She denies any other risk factors for PTB. Her prenatal course has been uneventful. Her expected date of delivery has been confirmed by an 18-week ultrasound. Her prenatal laboratory tests were within normal limits, including a negative HIV test.

On physical exam, her blood pressure is 110/74 mmHg, pulse 86 beats/minute, temperature 36.9° C (98.4° F), respiratory rate 20. No tenderness or contractions are identified. On speculum exam, pooling, ferning, and nitrazine are negative, and so rupture of membranes is ruled out. Tests for fFN, GBS, gonorrhea, and *Chlamydia* are collected. Her cervical exam is 2 cm dilated, 1 cm long, -2 station. The clinical impression is vertex presentation and size less than dates. Cardiotocography is initiated.

Twenty minutes after arrival, the fetal heart appears reassuring and appropriate for gestational age. On tocography, she is contracting every 4 minutes. An ultrasound is performed and reveals an appropriate for gestational age estimated fetal weight (1498 g), vertex presentation, no placenta previa, and amniotic fluid index of 10. TVU reveals a cervical length of 19 mm.

Based on contraction frequency and cervical exam findings, especially the short CL <20 mm, a diagnosis of PTL is made. Betamethasone 12 mg IM is given with a plan to give a second dose at 24 hours. A dose of 100 mg indomethacin is given *per rectum*, with a plan for continuing with 50 mg every 6 hours for 48 hours. Extensive counseling is given regarding safety and effectiveness of all interventions, prognosis, and possible complications. A neonatal consult is ordered. The Neonatal Intensive Care Unit is a level III facility, and there is availability for care in case of a 28-week PTB.

An hour later, contractions are diminishing in frequency and intensity. Regular nutrition is allowed. Later, the contractions resolve, the fFN result returns as positive, and GBS, gonorrhea, *Chlamydia*, and urine culture are negative. Antibiotics for GBS prophylaxis are discontinued. Hospitalization is continued as planned for a total of 48 hours, with tocography for 1 hour every shift and at the patient's request if she feels symptoms of PTL.

Forty-eight hours after initial assessment, she is discharged home with PTL precautions and close follow-up, aware of her high chance of PTB at <35 weeks and its consequences.

References

1. Berghella V, Palacio M, Ness A, Alfirevic Z, Nicolaides KH, Saccone G. Cervical length screening for prevention of preterm birth in singleton pregnancy with threatened preterm labor: systematic review and meta-analysis of randomized controlled trials using individual patient-level data. Ultrasound Obstet Gynecol. 2017 Mar;49(3):322–9.

2. Berghella V, Saccone G. Fetal fibronectin testing for reducing the risk of preterm birth. Cochrane Database Syst Rev. 2019 Jul 29;7(7):CD006843. doi: 10.1002/14651858.CD006843.pub3.

3. Berghella V, Ness A, Bega G, Berghella M. Cervical sonography in women with symptoms of preterm labor. Obstet Gynecol Clin North Am. 2005;32:383–96.

4. Ness A, Visintine J, Ricci E, Berghella V. Does knowledge of cervical length and fetal fibronectin affect management of women with threatened preterm labor? A randomized trial. Am J Obstet Gynecol. 2007;197(4):426.

5. Bell EF, Hintz SR, Hansen NI, Bann CM, Wyckoff MH, DeMauro SB, et al.; Eunice Kennedy Shriver National Institute of Child Health and Human Development Neonatal Research Network. Mortality, in-hospital morbidity, care practices, and 2-year outcomes for extremely preterm infants in the US, 2013–2018. JAMA. 2022 Jan 18;327(3):248–63.

6. Larson JE, Desai SA, McNett W. Perinatal care and long-term implications. In: Berghella V, editor. Preterm birth. Oxford: Blackwell Publishing; 2010.

7. American College of Obstetricians and Gynecologists. Practice Bulletin No. 171: management of preterm labor. Obstet Gynecol. 2016 Oct;128(4):e155–64.

8. McGoldrick E, Stewart F, Parker R, Dalziel SR. Antenatal corticosteroids for accelerating fetal lung maturation for women at risk of preterm birth. Cochrane Database Syst Rev. 2020 Dec 25;12(12):CD004454. doi: 10.1002/14651858. CD004454.pub3.

9. Saccone G, Berghella V. Antenatal corticosteroids for maturity of term or near term fetuses: systematic review and meta-analysis of randomized controlled trials. BMJ. 2016 Oct 12;355:i5044. doi: 10.1136/bmj.i5044.

10. Melamed N, Shah J, Soraisham A, Yoon EW, Lee SK, Shah PS, et al. Association between antenatal corticosteroid administration-to-birth interval and outcomes of preterm neonates. Obstet Gynecol. 2015 Jun;125(6):1377–84.

11. Garite TJ, Kurtzman J, Maurel K, Clark R. Impact of a "rescue course" of antenatal cortocosteroids: a multicenter randomized placebo-controlled trial. Am J Obstet Gynecol. 2009;248:e1–9.

12. McEvoy C, Schilling D, Peters D, Tillotson C, Spitale P, Wallen L, et al. Respiratory compliance in preterm infants after a single rescue course of antenatal steroids: a randomized controlled trial. Am J Obstet Gynecol. 2010;202:544:e1–9.

13. Crowther CA, McKinlay CJ, Middleton P, Harding JE. Repeat doses of prenatal corticosteroids for women at risk of preterm birth for improving neonatal health outcomes. Cochrane Database Syst Rev. 2015 Jul 5;2015(7):CD003935. doi: 10.1002/14651858.CD003935.pub4.

14. Doyle LW, Crowther CA, Middleton P, Marret S, Rouse D. Magnesium sulphate for women at risk of preterm birth for neuroprotection of the fetus. Cochrane Database Syst Rev. 2009;1:CD004661. doi: 10.1002/14651858.CD004661.pub3.

15. Crowther CA, Ashwood P, Middleton PF, et al. Prenatal Intravenous Magnesium at 30-34 Weeks' Gestation and Neurodevelopmental Outcomes in Offspring: The MAGENTA Randomized Clinical Trial. JAMA. 2023;330(7):603–614. doi:10.1001/jama.2023.12357.

16. Sosa CG, Althabe F, Belizán JM, Bergel E. Bed rest in singleton pregnancies for preventing preterm birth. Cochrane Database Syst Rev. 2015 Mar 30;2015(3):CD003581. doi: 10.1002/14651858. CD003581.pub3.

17. Crowther CA, Han S. Hospitalisation and bed rest for multiple pregnancy. Cochrane Database Syst Rev. 2010 Jul 7;2010(7): CD000110. doi: 10.1002/14651858.CD000110.pub2.

18. Stan CM, Boulvain M, Pfister R, Hirsbrunner-Almagbaly P. Hydration for treatment of preterm labour. Cochrane Database Syst Rev. 2013 Nov 4;(11):CD003096. doi: 10.1002/14651858. CD003096.

19. Flenady V, Hawley G, Stock OM, Kenyon S, Badawi N. Prophylactic antibiotics for inhibiting preterm labour with intact membranes. Cochrane Database Syst Rev. 2013 Dec 5;(12):CD000246. doi: 10.1002/14651858.CD000246.pub2.

20. Kenyon S, Pike K, Jones DR, Brocklehurst P, Marlow N, Salt A, et al. Childhood outcomes after prescription of antibiotics to pregnant women with spontaneous preterm labor: 7-year follow-up of the ORACLE II trial. Lancet. 2008; 372:1319–27.

21. Gibbs RS, Schrag S, Schuchat A. Perinatal infections due to group B streptococci. Obstet Gynecol. 2004;104: 1062–76.

22. Su LL, Samuel M, Chong YS. Progestational agents for treating threatened or established preterm labour. Cochrane Database Syst Rev. 2014 Jan 31;(1):CD006770. doi: 10.1002/14651858. CD006770.pub3.

23. Neilson JP, West HM, Dowswell T. Betamimetics for inhibiting preterm labour. Cochrane Database Syst Rev. 2014 Feb 5;(2):CD004352. doi: 10.1002/14651858.CD004352.pub2.

24. Flenady V, Wojcieszek AM, Papatsonis DN, Stock OM, Murray L, Jardine LA, et al. Calcium channel blockers for inhibiting preterm labour and birth. Cochrane Database Syst Rev. 2014 Jun 5;2014(6):CD002255. doi: 10.1002/14651858.CD002255.pub2.

25. Reinebrant HE, Pileggi-Castro C, Romero CL, Dos Santos RA, Kumar S, Souza JP, et al. Cyclo-oxygenase (COX) inhibitors for treating preterm labour. Cochrane Database Syst Rev. 2015 Jun 5;2015(6):CD001992. doi: 10.1002/14651858.CD001992.pub3.

26. Sawdy RJ, Lye S, Fisk NM, Bennett PR. A double-blind randomized study of fetal side effects during and after the short-term maternal administration of indomethacin, sulindac, and nimesulide for the treatment of preterm labor. Am J Obstet Gynecol. 2003 Apr;188(4):1046–51.

27. Hammers AL, Sanchez-Ramos L, Kaunitz AM. Antenatal exposure to indomethacin increases the risk of severe intraventricular hemorrhage, necrotizing enterocolitis, and periventricular leukomalacia: a systematic review with metaanalysis. Am J Obstet Gynecol. 2015 Apr;212(4):505.e1–13.

28. Terrone DA, Rinehart BK, Kimmel ES, May WL, Larmon JE, Morrison JC. A prospective randomized controlled trial of high and low maintenance doses of magnesium sulfate for acute tocolysis. Am J Obstet Gynecol. 2000;182:1477–82.

29. Lewis DF, Bergstedt S, Edwards MS et al. Successful magnesium sulfate tocolysis: is "weaning" the drug necessary? Am J Obstet Gynecol. 1997;177:742–5.

30. Crowther CA, Brown J, McKinlay CJ, Middleton P. Magnesium sulphate for preventing preterm birth in threatened preterm labour. Cochrane Database Syst Rev. 2014 Aug 15;(8):CD001060. doi: 10.1002/14651858.CD001060.pub2.

31. Flenady V, Reinebrant HE, Liley HG, Tambimuttu EG, Papatsonis DN. Oxytocin receptor antagonists for inhibiting preterm labour. Cochrane Database Syst Rev. 2014 Jun 6;(6):CD004452. doi: 10.1002/14651858.CD004452.pub3.

32. Duckitt K, Thornton S, O'Donovan OP, Dowswell T. Nitric oxide donors for treating preterm labour. Cochrane Database Syst Rev. 2014 May 8;2014(5):CD002860. doi: 10.1002/14651858. CD002860.pub2.

33. Newton ER, Shields L, Rigway LE, Berkus MD, Elliott BD. Combination antibiotics and indomethacin in idiopathic preterm labor: a randomized double-blind study. Am J Obstet Gynecol. 1991;165:1753–9.

34. Carlan S, O'Brien WF, O'Leary TD, Mastrogiannis D. Randomized comparative trial of indomethacin and sulindac for the treatment of refractory preterm labor. Obstet Gynecol. 1992;79:223–8.

35. Dodd JM, Crowther CA, Middleton P. Oral betamimetics for maintenance therapy after threatened preterm labour. Cochrane Database Syst Rev. 2012 Dec 12;12:CD003927. doi: 10.1002/14651858.CD003927.pub3.

36. Nanda K, Cook LA, Gallo MF, Grimes DA. Terbutaline pump maintenance therapy after threatened preterm labour for preventing preterm birth. Cochrane Database Syst Rev. 2002;4:CD003933. doi: 10.1002/14651858.CD003933.

37. Naik Gaunekar N, Raman P, Bain E, Crowther CA. Maintenance therapy with calcium channel blockers for preventing preterm birth after threatened preterm labour. Cochrane Database Syst Rev. 2013 Oct 31;(10):CD004071. doi: 10.1002/14651858. CD004071.pub3.

38. Humprey RG, Bartfield MC, Carlan SJ, O'Brien WF, O'Leary TD, Triana T. Sulindac to prevent recurrent preterm labor: a randomized controlled trial. Obstet Gynecol. 2001;98:555–62.

39. Han S, Crowther CA, Moore V. Magnesium maintenance therapy for preventing preterm birth after threatened preterm labour. Cochrane Database Syst Rev. 2013 May 31; 2013(5):CD000940. doi: 10.1002/14651858.CD000940.pub3.

40. Valenzuela GJ, Sanchez-Ramos L, Romero R, Silver HM, Koltun WD, Millar L, et al. Maintenance treatment of preterm labor with the oxytocin antagonist atosiban. Am J Obstet Gynecol. 2000;182:1184–90.

41. Alfirevic Z, Milan SJ, Livio S. Caesarean section versus vaginal delivery for preterm birth in singletons. Cochrane Database Syst Rev. 2013 Sep 12;2013(9):CD000078. doi: 10.1002/14651858. CD000078.pub3.

42. Bergenhenegouwen LA, Meertens LJ, Schaaf J, Nijhuis JG, Mol BW, Kok M, et al. Vaginal delivery versus caesarean section in preterm breech delivery: a systematic review. Eur J Obstet Gynecol Reprod Biol. 2014 Jan;172:1–6.

Chapter 43
Placenta Previa and Related Disorders

Yinka Oyelese

Obstetric Imaging, Beth Israel Deaconess Medical Center, Boston, MA, USA

Placenta previa and the related placental disorders, placenta accreta spectrum and vasa previa, are important causes of obstetric hemorrhage that may threaten the well-being and life of fetus and/or mother [1, 2]. The key to achieving good outcomes in these conditions lies in prenatal diagnosis with ultrasound, and subsequent appropriate management, usually with cesarean delivery in the late preterm or early term period [1,2].

Placenta previa

In normal pregnancy, the placenta implants into the fundus or corpus of the uterus and separates only after the child is born. In placenta previa, the placenta overlies the cervix. When the cervix dilates, as occurs in labor, the placenta separates from the cervix and profuse bleeding occurs.

Definitions

Placenta previa occurs when the placenta covers the internal cervical os to any degree (Figure 43.1), and a low-lying placenta is one that lies within 2 cm from the internal os (Figure 43.2) [3,4]. These definitions are an important change from the prior classification of placenta previa into "complete," "partial," "marginal," and "low-lying," which were made prior to wide availability of transvaginal ultrasound. Transvaginal ultrasound has made it possible to accurately assess the relationship between the placenta and the internal os, and hence those previously used terms should be abandoned [2–6].

Clinical significance

Placenta previa is a leading cause of maternal hemorrhage in the late third trimester [1,2,7]. Labor leads to separation of the placenta from the cervix and lower uterine segment with resultant torrential and life-threatening hemorrhage. Placenta previa may be associated with significant maternal and perinatal morbidity, and in severe cases, mortality [7–9].

Incidence, pathophysiology, and risk factors

Placenta previa complicates approximately 0.5% (1 in 200) pregnancies at term [1,2,10]. The strongest risk factor for placenta previa is a history of prior cesarean delivery, with the risk of previa increasing with the number of prior cesarean deliveries in a dose–response manner [11,12]. Other risk factors for placenta previa include prior placenta previa, history of intrauterine surgery (such as dilation and curettage, myomectomy, and hysteroscopic surgery), smoking, multifetal gestation, cocaine use, increasing parity, and increasing maternal age [11–14]. It is likely that scarring of the endometrium because of prior cesarean delivery or intrauterine surgery significantly increases the risk of implantation in the lower uterus and hence leads to placenta previa [1,2].

Clinical presentation

Prior to widespread use of ultrasound, late mid- or early third-trimester bleeding was the most common presentation of placenta previa. Placenta previa is now most often diagnosed at the time of the second trimester anatomy scan [1,2,5]. The terms "placenta previa" and "low-lying placenta" should not be used prior to 18 weeks of gestation because most of these will resolve [15]. Over 90% of cases of placenta previas diagnosed in the second trimester will no longer cover the cervix by the time of delivery [1,2,15–17]. The greater the extent to which the placenta overlies the internal os in the second trimester, the less the chance of resolution. Becker et al., in a study of placental location in 8560 pregnancies at 20–23 weeks, found resolution did not occur if the lower edge of the placenta covered the cervix by more than 2.5 cm [16]. The later in gestation that placenta previa is seen, the less likely resolution is to occur [17].

Approximately two thirds of patients diagnosed with placenta previa will have some bleeding [18]. The first episode of bleeding is typically painless and occurs at a gestational age approximately between 24 and 28 weeks [1,2]. However, bleeding may be accompanied by pain or

Queenan's Management of High-Risk Pregnancy: An Evidence-Based Approach, Seventh Edition. Edited by Catherine Y. Spong and Charles J. Lockwood.

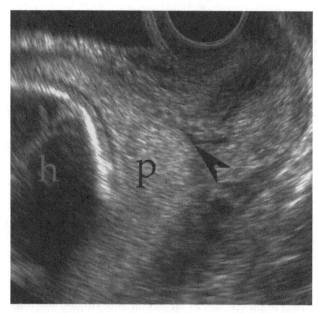

Figure 43.1 Transvaginal sonogram of a placenta previa (placenta marked "p"). The placenta can be seen completely overlying the internal os (indicated by the arrow). The fetal head is marked "h."

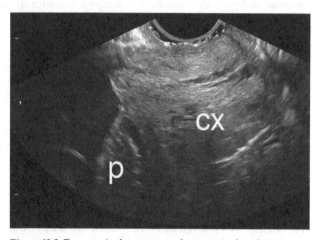

Figure 43.2 Transvaginal sonogram of a posterior low-lying placenta previa (placenta marked "p"). The lower placenta margin is 0.57 cm from the internal os (indicated by the calipers). The cervix is marked "cx."

contractions. As such, when bleeding occurs in the second half of pregnancy, whether or not accompanied by pain, placenta previa must be ruled out. Not infrequently, there is a fetal malpresentation or unstable lie, because the placenta lies in the lower uterine segment, preventing engagement of the fetal head. It is therefore prudent to evaluate placental location in cases of fetal malpresentation or unstable lie in the third trimester. In all cases of vaginal bleeding after 20 weeks of gestation, an ultrasound should be performed to rule out placenta previa prior to performing a digital examination. Digital examinations may provoke torrential vaginal bleeding when a placenta previa is present.

Diagnosis

Placenta previa is usually diagnosed by ultrasound in one of two scenarios. In the first, the diagnosis is made in asymptomatic women on routine sonography; the second is when sonography is performed in women who present with vaginal bleeding in the late second or early third trimester. Transabdominal sonography will detect the majority of cases of placenta previa. However, transabdominal sonography will also produce false-positive or false-negative diagnoses of placenta previa in 10–20% of cases [19]. Numerous studies have consistently demonstrated that transvaginal sonography is more accurate in the diagnosis of placenta previa than transabdominal sonography [20,21]. Furthermore, the technique has consistently been demonstrated to be safe and not associated with an increase in vaginal bleeding [20,21]. Transvaginal sonography avoids the false positive diagnoses of placenta previa that would occur with transabdominal ultrasound; thus, the reported incidence of placenta previa using transvaginal sonography is considerably lower than that obtained by transabdominal sonography [19]. This has several potential benefits, the main one being that women who do not actually have a placenta previa do not have unnecessary lifestyle restrictions and interventions [1].

Management

In the past, patients with placenta previa were frequently delivered after the first heavy bleed for fear of life-threatening hemorrhage. However, McAfee in 1945 showed that there was high perinatal mortality due to preterm delivery and that expectant management led to significantly improved outcomes for the baby [22]. The contemporary antepartum management of placenta previa is conservative, with the goal of prolonging the pregnancy until the early term period [1,2,22–24].

Asymptomatic patients with placenta previa or low-lying placenta should be managed as outpatients in the absence of bleeding. There is no evidence that activity limitation is beneficial. Patients are often advised to avoid intercourse, although there are no data to support that recommendation. In most cases, when bleeding occurs, the patient is admitted to hospital for observation for at least 24–48 hours or until bleeding stops [1,2]. Transvaginal ultrasound should be performed to accurately determine placental location. Bed rest is not beneficial and has risks and therefore is not recommended. In cases in which bleeding has occurred, corticosteroids should be administered to promote fetal lung maturation if the gestational age is between 24 and 34 weeks, and the patient should have at least one wide bore intravenous line placed. Rh immune globulin should be administered to Rh negative women. Blood pressure, pulse, and urine output should be monitored closely. At least initially, continuous fetal heart rate monitoring should be performed. Fetal sonography should be performed to rule out fetal anomalies and to evaluate fetal growth and amniotic fluid volume.

In women who are having contractions, cautious use of tocolytics is reasonable to allow administration of corticosteroids. Frequently, the contractions cause more placental separation, which causes further bleeding, which in turn causes more contractions, and thus a vicious cycle is set up. Studies of tocolytic usage in women with placenta previa have demonstrated that they may safely be used with caution and are associated with significant prolongation of gestation and increased birthweight [25,26].

The subsequent management depends on gestational age, fetal and maternal status, and the presence of any other coexisting conditions. At a gestational age of <36 weeks, conservative management, rather than immediate delivery, is desirable, because prematurity is the cause of most of the perinatal mortality associated with placenta previa. Blood transfusions may be given as required. Cotton et al. found that delivery could be deferred with conservative management in two thirds of patients with symptomatic placenta previa and that half of patients with an initial hemorrhagic episode exceeding 500 mL did not require immediate delivery [23]. These authors achieved a mean prolongation of pregnancy of 16.8 days in women with symptomatic previas. Similarly, Silver and colleagues showed that conservative aggressive management with multiple transfusions, volume expansion, and tocolytics prolonged gestation by at least 4 weeks in 50% of patients with a symptomatic previa [24].

Following initial evaluation in hospital, most patients with placenta previa who have experienced bleeding that resolves may be safely managed as outpatients if they have access to telephones, have a responsible adult at home, and live close to and have ready access to the hospital. However, when the patient lives in a remote region, and cannot reach the hospital promptly, inpatient management may be considered.

Outpatient management has been compared with inpatient management in a few studies [27,28]. These studies have found that stable patients with placenta previa can be safely managed as outpatients with substantial savings in hospital costs and no worse outcomes (assessed by gestational age at delivery, birthweights, blood transfusions, and neonatal outcomes) compared with women managed as inpatients [27,28]. A retrospective study by Stafford and colleagues found that the cervical length was predictive of bleeding; patients with a cervical length of <3 cm were at increased risk for bleeding, contractions, and preterm delivery [29]. In another study, cervical lengths were not associated with bleeding, but women with shorter cervices had higher rates of emergency cesarean delivery at <34 weeks [30]. However, the Society for Maternal Fetal Medicine does not recommend routine cervical length screening in patients with placenta previa [31].

Traditionally, patients are admitted to hospital after their third bleeding episode and kept in hospital until delivery. However, this approach has no scientific basis. A heavy bleed, in which the patient loses significant amounts of blood, may be more clinically important than recurrent light bleeds. Conversely, a significant proportion of placenta previa cases diagnosed in the early third trimester will resolve prior to delivery. For this reason, decisions regarding inpatient vs. outpatient management should be individualized based on risk factors, severity of bleeding, availability of resources, and patient's proximity to the hospital. Final decisions regarding mode or timing of delivery should be deferred until the late third trimester. It would be prudent to perform a transvaginal ultrasound evaluation of placental location within 2 weeks of planned delivery.

Timing and mode of delivery

When placenta previa persists until the late third trimester, it is preferable to have a delivery under controlled circumstances than to deliver an unstable patient who had presented with life-threatening bleeding as an emergency. For this reason, early term scheduled cesarean delivery at 36 to 37+6 weeks is recommended [31]. Amniocentesis to assess fetal lung maturation prior to delivery is no longer recommended [31]. Patients should be delivered in centers with adequate blood bank facilities.

The minimum distance from the lower placental edge to the internal os at which a vaginal delivery may safely be undertaken is the subject of debate. Oppenheimer and colleagues were among the first to show that when the lower placental edge is ≥ 2 cm from the internal cervical os, women may safely deliver vaginally [6]. Subsequently, this 2 cm distance was confirmed by Bhide et al. and Dawson and colleagues [32]. More recent studies have suggested that approximately 75% of patients with lower placental edges >1 cm from the internal os may safely undergo vaginal delivery without an increase in bleeding when compared with those in whom the lower placental edge is >2 cm from the internal os [33–36]. It must be pointed out that in these studies, the delivering obstetricians were not blinded to the ultrasound results, and thus these results may be significantly biased. Nonetheless, based on newer data, it does appear reasonable to offer a trial of labor to women with a placental edge-to-os distance of 11 mm or greater by transvaginal sonography, and who have no other contraindications to vaginal delivery. Regardless, patients who have placentas that lie to any degree within the lower uterine segment and even those in whom second trimester low-lying placentas have resolved have increased risks for postpartum hemorrhage and should be delivered in centers with adequate surgical and blood bank facilities [37]. This may be because some of the placental bed lies within the noncontractile lower uterine segment.

In women with an anterior placenta previa, the surgeon usually has to either incise through the placenta or separate the placenta prior to delivery of the fetus or make an incision that avoids the placenta, such as a vertical fundal incision. Generally, a lower segment transverse incision can be used, but it may be beneficial to determine placental location by sonography prior to the operation and preferably to avoid the placenta.

Vasa previa

In this condition, fetal vessels run through the membranes over the cervix, unprotected by placental tissue or umbilical cord (Plate 43.1), and are subject to compression by the fetal presenting part [1,2,38]. Vasa previa presents a great hazard to the fetus, because undiagnosed prenatally, these vessels frequently rupture at the time of spontaneous or artificial rupture of the membranes, as often occurs during labor [38]. Rupture of these vessels frequently results in rapid fetal exsanguination. As such, approximately 56% of babies die when vasa previa is not diagnosed prenatally and the vessels rupture [39]. Survivors in cases not diagnosed prenatally typically have low Apgar scores; a large study found median Apgar scores of 1 and 4 at 1 and 5 minutes, respectively, in cases of vasa previa not diagnosed prenatally [39]. Furthermore, a systematic review and meta-analysis found a 25-fold increase in death and a 50-fold increase in neonatal asphyxia in vasa previa not diagnosed prenatally [40]. The only effective way to prevent this high perinatal mortality is making the diagnosis prenatally with ultrasound and scheduled cesarean delivery prior to rupture of the membranes [41].

Pathophysiology

Vasa previa may occur due to a velamentous cord insertion (Type 1); when unprotected vessels run between placental lobes in a bilobed placenta or placentas with succenturiate lobes (Type 2); or when there is a normal umbilical cord insertion, and unprotected fetal vessels run through the membranes from one placental edge to another (Type 3). It is thought that most cases of vasa previa start off as a placenta previa. As the placenta grows preferentially toward the better vascularized fundus of the uterus, the placental tissue over the cervix atrophies leaving exposed vessels that run through the membranes.

Incidence and risk factors

It has been estimated that vasa previa complicates approximately 1 in 1666 pregnancies at term [42]. Risk factors for vasa previa include second-trimester placenta previa or low-lying placenta (even if the placenta resolves with advancing gestational age), multifetal gestations, and pregnancies resulting from in-vitro fertilization [1,2,42,43].

Diagnosis

Vasa previa is diagnosed prenatally by ultrasound [1,2,41,43–45]. The ideal way to make the diagnosis is with transvaginal ultrasound with color and pulse wave Doppler [41,44,45]. A policy of routinely identifying the placental cord insertion and performing a Doppler sweep of the lower uterine segment is highly effective in diagnosing vasa previa [41]. In patients with risk factors such as a second-trimester low-lying placenta or placenta previa, transvaginal ultrasound with Doppler should be performed to rule out vasa previa.

The sonographic findings in vasa previa include hypoechoic circular or linear structures overlying the cervix (Figure 43.3) [45]. Color Doppler confirms flow through these structures (Figure 43.4). Pulse wave Doppler should be used to confirm a fetal arterial or venous signal through

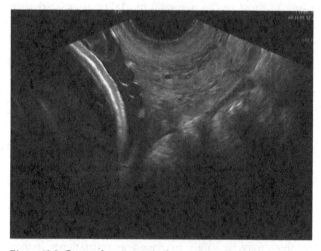

Figure 43.3 Grayscale transvaginal sonogram showing circular hypoechoic structures (fetal vessels) running over the cervix.

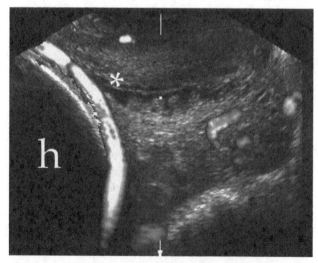

Figure 43.4 Color Doppler of vasa previa showing flow through a vessel running over the internal os (marked by the asterisk). The fetal head is marked "h."

these structures to confirm the diagnosis of vasa previa (Plate 43.2) [45].

Approximately 20% of cases of vasa previa diagnosed in the second trimester will resolve prior to 36 weeks [46,47]. For this reason, it would be prudent to confirm the diagnosis with transvaginal ultrasound with Doppler at 32 weeks [41]. Importantly, in the third trimester, the presenting part may be well applied to the cervix and may compress fetal vessels making it appear that there is no vasa previa [45]. In evaluating vasa previa after 32 weeks, it is important to mobilize the fetal presenting part cephalad away from the cervix. It is only then that one can conclusively rule out vasa previa.

The differential ultrasound diagnoses for vasa previa include funic presentation, chorioamniotic membrane separation, placenta previa, maternal vessels, and Doppler artifact [45]. In the case of funic presentation, the fetal vessels will move away from the cervix with changes in maternal position and with repeated ultrasound examinations. Neither chorioamniotic separation nor color Doppler artifact due to motion in the amniotic fluid will demonstrate a fetal vessel waveform with pulse wave Doppler. Maternal vessels will not lie within the membranes and will not demonstrate a fetal waveform.

In the past, tests examining vaginal blood for fetal cells such as the Apt test were used to help make a diagnosis of vasa previa in bleeding patients [38]. These tests are no longer widely used in the United States. In cases that are not diagnosed prenatally, very rarely, fetal vessels may be palpated running through the intact membranes in a dilated cervix [38]. Even more rarely, when there is cervical dilation with intact membranes, these vessels may be visualized on speculum examination. The more common presentation in patients without prenatal diagnosis with ultrasound is of vaginal bleeding following spontaneous

or artificial rupture of the membranes, followed by dramatic changes in the fetal heart rate tracing, such as a sinusoidal fetal heart tracing (Figure 43.5) or fetal bradycardia [38]. Often, very quickly, the fetal heart rate can no longer be detected. The diagnosis is confirmed based on a dead baby and ruptured velamentous vessels seen on placental examination.

Management
Once a diagnosis of vasa previa is made, the patient should be counseled about the implications of the condition. It is important to reassure the patient that outcomes in prenatally diagnosed cases are excellent and that the risk is almost entirely at the time of rupture of the membranes or in labor. The patient should have regular growth ultrasound examinations every 4–6 weeks. Transvaginal ultrasound evaluation should be performed at about 32 weeks of gestation to confirm the diagnosis [41]. Delivery should occur in centers with adequate neonatal facilities, and the neonatologists should be informed of the potential for neonatal anemia and hypovolemia.

Patients are often admitted to hospital at about 32 weeks. The primary reason for the admission is for proximity to the operating room should unexpected rupture of the membranes occur [41,43]. However, outpatient management may be considered in carefully selected asymptomatic patients [41]. It is important that these patients be thoroughly counseled and informed consent for outpatient management be obtained. Furthermore, the patients should have quick access to the hospital if symptoms of labor, bleeding, or rupture of membranes were to occur. In women managed as inpatients, corticosteroids to promote fetal lung maturity should be administered on admission. Delivery should be considered if the patient has significant bleeding, regular painful contractions, nonreassuring fetal testing, or ruptures her membranes. Although the

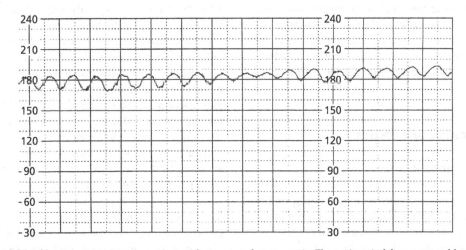

Figure 43.5 Sinusoidal fetal heart rate tracing in a patient with a ruptured vasa previa. The patient, in labor, ruptured her membranes and had bleeding at the same time. Emergency cesarean delivery was performed. The infant was born extremely pale, was immediately transfused, and did well.

role of cervical length in vasa previa has not been studied, a cervical length of less than 2.5 cm should be considered an indication for inpatient management [41].

Mode and timing of delivery

When vasa previa is diagnosed prenatally, the patient should be delivered by scheduled cesarean in the late preterm period, before rupture of the membranes or labor occur [1,2,41,43]. It remains unclear how far fetal vessels should be from the internal cervical os to be termed "vasa previa." The Society for Maternal Fetal Medicine defines vasa previa as exposed fetal vessels within 2 cm from the internal cervical os [43]. However, this was likely extrapolated from low-lying placentas in which placentas that are >2 cm from the internal cervical os may safely deliver vaginally. In the case of exposed fetal vessels, given that the cervix dilates to 10 cm, any exposed fetal vessels within a radius of 5 cm of the internal os are theoretically at risk of rupture [41]. Given that the consequences of rupture of a vasa previa are so catastrophic, it would be prudent to discuss the potential risk of rupture with the patient and involve the patient in the decision regarding mode of delivery rather than to assume that the risk is low and recommend a vaginal delivery.

Women diagnosed with vasa previa should be delivered by scheduled cesarean at 35–36 weeks [1,2,41]. A decision analysis recommended delivery at 34 weeks [48]. More recent data suggest that delivery at 36 weeks in stable asymptomatic patients without risk factors may improve neonatal outcomes without an observed increase in adverse outcomes [41]. Earlier delivery may be performed in women who have regular painful contractions, those with bleeding, rupture of the membranes, or other risk factors for preterm delivery. At delivery the fetal membranes are at risk of laceration, which could lead to significant fetal blood loss and need for neonatal blood transfusions. We have used a technique of carefully incising the uterus down to the level of the membranes and then exposing the membranes with the vessels running through them. Following this, the membranes may be incised under direct visualization, avoiding the blood vessels; this may reduce the chance for lacerating these vessels and may prevent fetal blood loss [41].

Placenta accreta spectrum

Clinical significance

The placenta accreta spectrum (PAS) disorders include placenta accreta, increta, and percreta, depending on the degree to which the placenta "invades" the uterine wall. In PAS there is no clear plane of cleavage between the placenta and the myometrium [1,2,49]. In a normal pregnancy, after delivery of the baby, the placenta peels off the wall of the uterus and is delivered. In PAS, the placenta is abnormally attached to the uterine wall and does not separate. Trying to remove the placenta leads to tearing of both placenta and uterine wall with resultant torrential and potentially life-threatening hemorrhage, disseminated intravascular coagulopathy, and in severe cases, maternal death [49]. PAS is also associated with significant surgical morbidity and a high risk for intensive care unit admission. A study of 292 patients with PAS found that urologic morbidity, defined as cystotomy, ureteral injury, or bladder fistula, occurred in 58 patients (19.9%) [50].

Pathophysiology

The current consensus is that most cases of PAS are the result of implantation in a decidua deficient cesarean scar rather than due to true placental invasion of the myometrium [1,2,49]. A retrospective study by Comstock and colleagues, of first-trimester ultrasound images of patients who later ended up with PAS, found that the gestational sac was implanted abnormally low and in the anterior part of the uterus [51]. Observations such as these have led to the hypothesis that placenta accreta generally starts off as pregnancy implantation in the decidua deficient scar of a prior cesarean and that the placenta does not actually pathologically invade the myometrium. This implantation in the scar leads to abnormal angiogenesis and adhesion formation [2,49].

Incidence and risk factors

The incidence of PAS has risen significantly in recent years due to the increase in cesarean deliveries, now complicating approximately 1 in 300 pregnancies [49,52]. PAS has become a leading reason for peripartum hysterectomy. Most cases of PAS occur in the presence of a placenta previa coexisting with a history of one or more prior cesarean deliveries. Although multiple prior cesarean deliveries and placenta previa are both independent risk factors for PAS, the two together greatly amplify that risk. The risk of PAS in patients with prior cesarean deliveries without coexistent placenta previa increases from 0.3% in women with one prior cesarean delivery to 6.7% in women with five or more prior cesarean deliveries [53]. More than 80% of patients with placenta accreta have a placenta previa. The risk of placenta accreta in women with a placenta previa without a history of prior cesarean delivery was 3% [49]. A large study found that the risks of placenta accreta in women with placenta previa were 11%, 40%, 61%, and 67% in women with one, two, three, and four or more prior cesarean deliveries, respectively [54].

In a study of 4146 pregnant women, of whom 87 (2.1%) had PAS, Imafuku and colleagues performed multivariable analyses that revealed risk factors for PAS included prior histories of cesarean delivery, dilation and curettage, hysteroscopic surgery, or uterine artery embolization, pregnancy conceived via assisted reproductive technology, and the presence of placenta previa in the current pregnancy [55].

Diagnosis

Ultrasound is highly sensitive and specific in the diagnosis of PAS [56,57]. The highest detection of PAS is in women with placenta previa and prior cesarean deliveries. In women without these risk factors, the accuracy of ultrasound is much more limited and has not been adequately studied. Both ultrasound and magnetic resonance imaging (MRI) have poor predictive value in determining the degree of invasion [58].

Ultrasound findings suspicious for PAS include multiple irregular hypoechoic spaces (lacunae) in the placenta, loss of the retroplacental hypoechoic clear zone (Figure 43.6), turbulent "tornado" blood flow in the lacunae on Doppler, thinning or absence of the myometrium, irregularity and hypervascularity of the uterovesical region, and bulging of the placenta into the bladder, lower uterine segment, or serosa [56,57]. Other Doppler signs include bridging vessels from the placenta to the uterine margin and gaps in myometrial blood flow [57]. These signs individually vary in their sensitivity and specificity and have limited predictive value for PAS, and the likelihood of PAS increases with the number of signs [56,57]. A systematic review of 23 studies and 3707 pregnancies found a mean sensitivity of ultrasound for PAS of 90.72% (95% confidence interval [CI] 87.2–93.6) and a specificity of 96.4% (95% CI 96.3–97.5%) [59]. More recently, first-trimester ultrasound has shown promise in prenatal screening for PAS [51,60].

Although ultrasound is highly sensitive for diagnosing PAS, in women with high risk for PAS whose imaging does not show clear evidence of PAS, the condition cannot be excluded with certainty. Therefore, although these women may not necessarily require a hysterectomy, all women at high risk for PAS should be managed in experienced centers by a multidisciplinary team even if imaging is negative [61].

MRI may be used in the diagnosis of PAS. A systematic review compared ultrasound and MRI for the diagnosis of PAS and found that both tests performed similarly [62]. Ultrasound sensitivity and specificity were 0.833 (95% CI, 0.7776–0.877) and 0.834 (95% CI 0.77–0.897), respectively, compared with MRI sensitivity of 0.838 (95% CI 0.786–0.879) and specificity of 0.831 (95% CI 0.77–0.878) [62]. Given that prenatal ultrasound is universally used and accessible, and that obstetric imaging experience with ultrasound is generally much greater than with MRI, in most circumstances, ultrasound should be the imaging of choice for suspected PAS. Although some studies have found elevated maternal serum alpha-fetoprotein to be associated with increased risk of PAS, this test is neither sensitive nor specific for PAS.

Management

The key to preventing the high maternal morbidity and mortality associated with PAS lies in making the diagnosis prenatally and making adequate preparation for delivery by a multidisciplinary team in a center with adequate resources (including an adequately staffed blood bank with protocols for massive blood transfusion) and with experience in the management of the condition [1,2,49,63]. Thus, patients in whom PAS is suspected should be delivered in a Level III or IV center, with subspecialist level care [49]. The specifics of the multidisciplinary team depend on the particular center but may include such specialists as maternal fetal medicine, blood bank/hematology, anesthesia, urology, interventional radiology, intensive care, neonatology, nursing, and gynecologic oncology. The standard management of PAS in most cases is scheduled cesarean delivery and then hysterectomy without attempting to remove the placenta [49]. It has been proposed that there should be regionalization of care of PAS with cases delivered in "Centers of Excellence" [64].

Once placenta accreta is diagnosed prenatally, patients should be counseled on the clinical significance of the condition and a plan be made for the management of the pregnancy. Serial ultrasound examinations should be performed every 4–6 weeks to evaluate fetal growth and to assess the placenta. A multidisciplinary team meeting should be convened in the early third trimester to lay out plans for delivery, preparing both for scheduled delivery and for unplanned delivery as an emergency if necessary. The patient's hemoglobin levels should be optimized prior to delivery. Routine hospitalization is not recommended nor is bed rest. It may be prudent to avoid intercourse. Hospitalization should be considered when bleeding occurs.

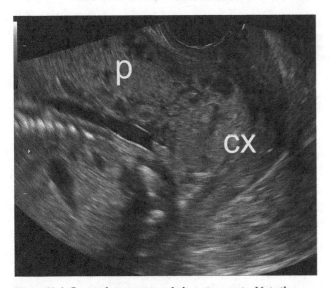

Figure 43.6 Grayscale sonogram of placenta accreta. Note the prominent lacunae in the placenta (p), giving a "moth-eaten" appearance. The retroplacental clear space is not seen. The cervix (cx) is not well defined and also shows prominent lacunae.

Conservative management without hysterectomy, leaving the placenta in situ, has been used as a management option for selected patients with PAS [49]. The potential benefits include preservation of future fertility, possible decrease in blood loss, and avoiding a hysterectomy. Risks include massive uncontrolled hemorrhage, sepsis, possible need for later hysterectomy, and prolonged period of waiting for placental involution, during which complications may occur [49]. This technique is employed mainly in Europe but is not favored in the United States.

Timing and mode of delivery

It is preferable to perform a scheduled delivery for patients in whom there is a prenatal diagnosis of PAS rather than to have to deliver them as emergencies when significant bleeding has occurred. For this reason, scheduled delivery by cesarean is recommended at 34 0/7 to 37+0 weeks [31,49]. Adequate intravenous access should be achieved prior to delivery and at least four units of blood should be available in the operating room. The patient should be delivered by cesarean, avoiding incision of the placenta, and following delivery of the baby, a hysterectomy should be performed, with no attempts to remove the placenta (i.e. leaving it in situ) [49]. This will often require a vertical classical uterine incision. Although a vertical skin incision is often used, the skin incision should be individualized. Importantly, surgery for PAS may be extremely difficult and carries significant risk for sudden life-threatening hemorrhage. Because PAS often involves the cervix, in most cases a total rather than supracervical hysterectomy is necessary.

A variety of techniques have been used to minimize blood loss including uterine or internal iliac vessel ligation, intra-aortic balloons and balloon catheterization or embolization of the internal iliac arteries [49]. Although some of these techniques may lead to reduced blood loss, data are conflicting as to their benefit when done prophylactically. These techniques also carry significant risk for serious complications, especially when performed in centers without adequate experience and skill in their usage. For this reason, the use of these techniques should be individualized. Cell salvage may be used to reduce the need for transfusion. Tranexamic acid has been shown to significantly reduce blood loss and should be used prophylactically in cases of PAS [49]. Anesthesia may be regional or general, depending on local expertise and resources.

In some cases, previously unsuspected PAS will be encountered at the time of delivery. If PAS is discovered at the time of cesarean delivery, and there is no life-threatening hemorrhage, it would be prudent to close the uterus and to summon adequately skilled surgical and anesthesiology personnel and mobilize blood resources. It may be necessary to delay proceeding with the surgery until these resources are available. It is important to avoid further placental manipulation and to perform a hysterectomy as expeditiously as possible. In cases of minimal or focal PAS in stable patients, local resection of the uterus with the adherent placenta may be performed.

Conclusion

The key to good outcomes in most placental disorders lies in prenatal diagnosis with ultrasound and then planned delivery. This requires high index of suspicion.

CASE PRESENTATION

A 37-year-old gravida 6 para 4014 woman had a routine fetal anatomy survey ultrasound at 20 weeks. She had a history of four prior cesarean deliveries. The fetus was appropriately grown, and no fetal anomalies were noted. There was an anterior placenta previa. The placenta was noted to have several large irregular echolucent areas (lacunae), absence of the retroplacental clear space, thinning of the myometrium in the lower segment, hypervascularity of the lower uterine wall, and the cervix also appeared to contain irregular lacunae. Based on her history of four prior cesarean deliveries coexisting with the placenta previa, and the ultrasound findings, a diagnosis of PAS was made. The patient was informed of the findings and was counseled that the recommended treatment would be an elective cesarean at about 34–35 weeks with hysterectomy. A multidisciplinary team meeting was held in the third trimester to plan her delivery. The patient was delivered by scheduled cesarean at 35 weeks. A course of corticosteroids was administered 4 days prior to delivery. A vertical fundal incision was made in the uterus, through which the baby was delivered. The lower uterine segment was noted to be ballooned out with the placenta seen through the serosa. There were prominent blood vessels all over the anterior lower uterine segment. Following this, a cesarean hysterectomy was performed. The quantitative blood loss was 2500 ml. The patient was transfused with three units of packed red blood cells. The patient had an uncomplicated recovery. Pathological examination of the uterus confirmed a diagnosis of placenta increta.

The patient had four prior cesarean deliveries and a placenta previa. The ultrasound examination had several findings consistent with PAS. There should be a high index of suspicion for PAS in all patients who have placenta previa with a history of prior cesarean deliveries. Ultrasound should be performed in the second trimester to carefully examine the lower uterine segment and the placenta for evidence of PAS. Good outcomes depend on a high degree of suspicion and elective delivery by cesarean with immediate hysterectomy in patients with a prenatal diagnosis of PAS. A multidisciplinary team approach in a center with experience in the management of patients with PAS improves outcomes.

The patient was managed conservatively until 35 weeks, and then delivered. Earlier cesarean delivery would have been performed if she had experienced significant bleeding or had gone into labor. The risk of uncontrolled maternal hemorrhage outweighs those of prematurity at 35 weeks. These babies should be delivered in centers with neonatal units and the neonatologists should be informed prior to delivery.

References

1. Oyelese Y, Smulian JC. Placenta previa, accreta, and vasa previa. Obstet Gynecol. 2006;107:927–41.

2. Silver RM. Abnormal placentation: Placenta previa, vasa previa, and placenta accrete. Obstet Gynecol. 2015;126:654–68.

3. Reddy UM, Abuhamad AZ, Leevine D, Saade GR; Fetal Imaging Workshop Invited Participants. Fetal imaging: executive summary of a joint Eunice Kennedy Shriver National Institute of Child Health and Human Development, Society for Maternal-Fetal Medicine, American Institute of Ultrasound in Medicine, American College of Obstetricians and Gynecologists, American College of Radiology, Society for Pediatric Radiology, and Society of Radiologists in Ultrasound Fetal Imaging workshop. Am J Obstet Gynecol. 2014;210:387–97.

4. Oppenheimer LW. Farine D. A new classification of placenta previa: Measuring progress in obstetrics. Am J Obstet Gynecol. 2009;201(3):227–9.

5. Oyelese Y. Placenta previa: the evolving role of ultrasound. Ultrasound Obstet Gynecol. 2009;34:123–6.

6. Oppenheimer LW, Farine D, Ritchie JW, Lewinsky RM, Telford J, Fairbanks LA. What is a low-lying placenta? Am J Obstet Gynecol. 1991;165:1036–8.

7. Crane JM, van den Hof MC, Dodds L, Armson BA, Liston R. Maternal complications with placenta previa. Am J Perinatol. 2000;17:101–5.

8. Crane JM, van den Hof MC, Dodds L, Armson BA, Liston R. Neonatal outcomes with placenta previa. Obstet Gynecol. 1999;93:541–4.

9. Ananth CV, Smulian JC, Vintzileos AM. The effect of placenta previa on neonatal mortality: a population-based study in the United States, 1989 through 1997. Am J Obstet Gynecol. 2003;188:1299–304.

10. Iyasu S, Saftlas AK, Rowley DL, Koonin LM, Lawson HW, Atrash HK. The epidemiology of placenta previa in the United States, 1979 through 1987. Am J Obstet Gynecol. 1993;168:1424–9.

11. Faiz AS, Ananth CV. Etiology and risk factors for placenta previa: an overview and meta-analysis of observational studies. J Matern Fetal Neonatal Med. 2003;13:175–90.

12. Ananth CV, Smulian JC, Vintzileos AM. The association of placenta previa with history of cesarean delivery and abortion: a metaanalysis. Am J Obstet Gynecol. 1997;177:1071–8.

13. Ananth CV, Demissie K, Smulian JC, Vintzileos AM. Placenta previa in singleton and twin births in the United States, 1989 through 1998: a comparison of risk factor profiles and associated conditions. Am J Obstet Gynecol. 2003;188:275–81.

14. Zhang J, Savitz DA. Maternal age and placenta previa: a population-based, case-control study. Am J Obstet Gynecol. 1993;168:641–5.

15. Jain V, Bos H, Bujold E. Guideline No. 402: diagnosis and management of placenta previa. J Obstet Gynaecol Can. 2020;42(7):906–17.

16. Becker BH, Vonk R, Mende BC, Ragosch V, Entezami M. The relevance of placental location at 20-23 gestational weeks for prediction of placenta previa at delivery: evaluation of 8650 cases. Ultrasound Obstet Gynecol. 2001;17: 496–501.

17. Dashe JS, McIntire DD, Ramus RM, Santos-Ramos R, Twickler DM. Persistence of placenta previa according to gestational age at ultrasound detection. Obstet Gynecol.2002;99(5 Pt 1):692–7.

18. Hill DJ, Beischer NA. Placenta praevia without antepartum haemorrhage. Aust N Z J Obstet Gynaecol. 1980;20:21–3.

19. Smith RS, Lauria MR, Comstock CH, Treadwell MC, Kirk JS, Lee W, et al. Transvaginal ultrasonography for all placentas that appear to be low-lying or over the internal cervical os. Ultrasound Obstet Gynecol. 1997;9:22–4.

20. Leerentveld RA, Gilberts EC, Arnold MJ, Wladimiroff JW. Accuracy and safety of transvaginal sonographic placental localization. Obstet Gynecol. 1990;76:759–62.

21. Timor-Tritsch IE, Yunis RA. Confirming the safety of transvaginal sonography in patients suspected of placenta previa. Obstet Gynecol. 1993;81:742–4.

22. MacAfee CHG. Placenta previa: a study of 174 cases. J Obstet Gynecol Br Commonwealth. 1945;52:313–17.

23. Cotton DB, Read JA, Paul RH, Quilligan EJ. The conservative aggressive management of placenta previa. Am J Obstet Gynecol. 1980;137:687–95.

24. Silver R, Depp R, Sabbagha RE, Dooley SL, Socol ML, Tamura RK. Placenta previa: aggressive expectant management. Am J Obstet Gynecol. 1984;150:15–22.

25. Sharma A, Suri V, Gupta I. Tocolytic therapy in conservative management of symptomatic placenta previa. Int J Gynaecol Obstet. 2004;84:109–13.

26. Besinger RE, Moniak CW, Paskiewicz LS, Fisher SG, Tomich PG. The effect of tocolytic use in the management of symptomatic placenta previa. Am J Obstet Gynecol. 1995;172:1770–5.

27. Mouer JR. Placenta previa: antepartum conservative management, inpatient versus outpatient. Am J Obstet Gynecol. 1994;170:1683–5.

28. Wing DA, Paul RH, Millar LK. Management of the symptomatic placenta previa: a randomized, controlled trial of inpatient versus outpatient expectant management. Am J Obstet Gynecol. 1996;175:806–11.

29. Stafford IA, Dashe JS, Shivvers SA, Alexander JM, McIntire DD, Leveno KJ. Ultrasonographic cervical length and risk of hemorrhage in pregnancies with placenta previa. Obstet Gynecol. 2010;116:595–600.

30. Ghi T, Contro E, Martina T et al. Cervical length and risk of antepartum bleeding in women with complete placenta previa. Ultrasound Obstet Gynecol. 2009;33(2):209–12.

31. Society for Maternal-Fetal Medicine (SMFM); Gyamfi-Bannerman C. Society for Maternal-Fetal Medicine (SMFM) Consult Series #44: management of bleeding in the late preterm period. Am J Obstet Gynecol. 2018;218(1):B2–B8.

32. Bhide A, Prefumo F, Moore J, Hollis B, Thilaganathan B. Placental edge to internal os distance in the late third trimester and mode of delivery in placenta praevia. Br J Obstet Gynaecol. 2003;110:860–4.

33. Dawson WB, Dumas MD, Romano WM, Gagnon R, Gratton RJ, Mowbray RD. Translabial ultrasonography and placenta previa: does measurement of the os–placenta distance predict outcome? J Ultrasound Med. 1996;15:441–6.

34. Vergani P, Ornaghi S, Pozzi I, Beretta P, Russo FM, Follesa I, et al. Placenta previa: distance to internal os and mode of delivery. Am J Obstet Gynecol. 2009;201(3):266.

35. Bronsteen R, Valice R, Lee W, Blackwell S, Balasubramaniam M, Comstock C. Effect of a low-lying placenta on delivery outcome. Ultrasound Obstet Gynecol. 2009;33(2):204–8.

36. Ornaghi S. Tessitore IV. Vergani P. Pregnancy and delivery outcomes in women with persistent versus resolved low-lying placenta in the late third trimester. J Ultrasound Med. 2022;41(1):123–33.

37. DeBolt CA, Rosenberg HM, Pruzan A, Goldberger C, Kaplowitz E, Buckley A,et al. Patients with resolution of low-lying placenta and placenta previa remain at increased risk of postpartum hemorrhage. Ultrasound Obstet Gynecol. 2022 Jul;60(1):103–8.

38. Oyelese KO, Turner M, Lees C, Campbell S. Vasa previa: an avoidable obstetric tragedy. Obstet Gynecol Surv. 1999; 54:138–45.

39. Oyelese Y, Catanzarite V, Prefumo F, Lashley S, Schachter M, Tovbin Y, et al. Vasa previa: the impact of prenatal diagnosis on outcomes. Obstet Gynecol. 2004;103:937–42.

40. Zhang W. Geris S. Al-Emara N, Ramadan G, Sotiriadis A, Akolekar R. Perinatal outcome of pregnancies with prenatal diagnosis of vasa previa: systematic review and meta-analysis. Ultrasound Obstet Gynecol. 2021;57:710–19.

41. Oyelese Y. Vasa previa: time to make a difference Am J Obstet Gynecol. 2019;221(6):539–41.

42. Ruiter L, Kok N, Limpens J, Derks JB, deGraaf IM, Mol Bwj, et al. Incidence of and risk indicators for vasa praevia: a systematic review. BJOG. 2016;123:1278–87.

43. Society for Maternal-Fetal Medicine (SMFM) Publications Committee; Sinkey RG, Odibo, AO, Dashe JS. Diagnosis and management of vasa previa. Am J Obstet Gynecol. 2015; 213:615–9.

44. Ruiter L, Kok N, Limpens J, Derks JB, de Graaf IM, Mol BW, et al. Systematic review of accuracy of ultrasound in the diagnosis of vasa previa. Ultrasound Obstet Gynecol. 2015;45(5):516–22.

45. Ranzini A. Oyelese Y. How to screen for vasa previa. Ultrasound Obstet Gynecol. 2021 May;57(5):720–5.

46. Klahr R, Fox NS, Zafman K, Hill MB, Connolly CT, Rebarber A. Frequency of spontaneous resolution of vasa previa with advancing gestational age. Am J Obstet Gynecol. 2019; 221:646.e1–7.

47. Erfani H, Haeri S, Shainker SA, Saad AF, Ruano R, Dunn TN, et al. Vasa previa: a multicenter retrospective cohort study. Am J Obstet Gynecol. 2019 Dec;221(6):644.e1–5.

48. Robinson BK. Grobman WA. Effectiveness of timing strategies for delivery of individuals with vasa previa. Obstet Gynecol. 2011;177:542–9.

49. American College of Obstetricians and Gynecologists, Society for Maternal-Fetal Medicine. Placenta accreta spectrum: obstetric care consensus #7. Am J Obstet Gynecol. 2018;219:B2–B16.3.

50. Erfani H, Salmanian B, Fox KA, Coburn M, Meshinchiasl N, Shamshirsaz AA, et al. Urologic morbidity associated with placenta accreta spectrum surgeries: single-center experience with a multidisciplinary team. Am J Obstet Gynecol. 2022;226(2):245.e1–5.

51. Comstock CH, Lee W, Vettraino IM, Bronsteen RA. The early sonographic appearance of placenta accreta. J Ultrasound Med. 2003;22:19–23.

52. Mogos MF, Salemi JL, Ashley M, Whiteman VE, Salihu HM. Recent trends in placenta accreta in the United States and its impact on maternal-fetal morbidity and healthcare-associated costs,1998–2011. J Matern Fetal Neonatal Med 2016; 29:1077–82.

53. Marshall NE. Fu R. Guise JM. Impact of multiple cesarean deliveries on maternal morbidity: a systematic review. Am J Obstet Gynecol. 2011;205:262.e1–8.

54. Silver RM, Landon MB, Rouse DJ, Leveno KJ, Spong CY, Thom EA, et al.; National Institute of Child Health and Human Development Maternal-Fetal Medicine Units Network. Maternal morbidity associated with multiple repeat cesarean deliveries. Obstet Gynecol. 2006;107(6):1226–32.

55. Imafuku H, Tanimura K, Shi Y, Uchida A, Deguchi M, Terai Y. Clinical factors associated with a placenta accreta spectrum. Placenta. 2021 Sep 1;112:180–4.

56. Comstock CH, Love JJ Jr, Bronsteen RA, Lee W, Vettraino IM, Huang RR, et al. Sonographic detection of placenta accreta in the second and third trimesters of pregnancy. Am J Obstet Gynecol. 2004;190:1135–40.

57. Srinivasan D, Shaw CJ, Dall'Asta A, Papanikoloau K, Yazbek J, Lees CC. Expert opinion: Stepwise ultrasound assessment of suspected placenta accreta spectrum using 2D, Doppler and 3D imaging. Eur J Obstet Gynecol Reprod Biol. 2022 Mar;270:181–9.

58. Morel O, van Beekhuizen HJ, Braun T, Collins S, Pateisky P, Calda P, et al.; International Society for Placenta Accreta Spectrum (IS-PAS). Performance of antenatal imaging to predict placenta accreta spectrum degree of severity. Acta Obstet Gynecol Scand. 2021;100 Suppl 1:21–8.

59. D'Antonio F. Iacovella C. Bhide A. Prenatal identification of invasive placentation using ultrasound: systematic review and meta-analysis. Ultrasound Obstet Gynecol. 2013;42:509–17.

60. Yule CS, Lewis MA, Do QN, Xi Y, Happe SK, Spong CY et al. Color Mapping ultrasound in the first trimester predicts placenta accreta spectrum: a retrospective cohort study. J Ultrasound Med. 2021;40(12):2735–43.

61. Reeder CF, Sylvester-Armstrong KR, Silva LM, Wert EM, Smulian JC, Genc MR. Outcomes of pregnancies at high-risk for placenta accreta spectrum following negative diagnostic imaging. J Perinat Med. 2022 Feb 25;50(5):595–600.

62. Carniello MO, Oliveira Brito LG, Sarian LOZ, Bennini JR. Diagnosis of placenta accreta spectrum in high-risk women using ultrasonography or magnetic resonance imaging: systematic review to compare accuracy of tests. Ultrasound Obstet Gynecol. 2022 Apr;59(4):428–36.

63. Shamshirsaz AA, Fox KA, Salmanian B, Diaz-Arrastia CR, Lee W, Baker BW, et al. Maternal morbidity in patients with morbidly adherent placenta treated with and without a standardized multidisciplinary approach. Am J Obstet Gynecol. 2015;212(2):218.e1–9.

64. Silver RM, Fox KA, Barton JR, Abuhamad AZ, Simhan H, Huls CK, et al. Center of excellence for placenta accreta. Am J Obstet Gynecol. 2015;212(5):561–8.

Chapter 44
Fetal Growth Restriction

Katherine H. Bligard and Anthony O. Odibo
Department of Obstetrics and Gynecology, Washington University School of Medicine in St. Louis, St. Louis, MO, USA

Definition of fetal growth restriction

Terminology used to describe fetuses and neonates that are abnormally small can be inconsistent and confusing. Clear communication among providers and to their patients is of utmost importance to facilitate adequate care for the dyad. The preferred term to convey inadequate fetal growth in utero is fetal growth restriction (FGR), which has replaced the previously used term of intrauterine growth restriction. The term small for gestational age (SGA) should be used to describe a neonate with a birthweight less than expected.

Unfortunately, the criteria for defining FGR and SGA are not universally agreed upon. SGA has been historically defined as neonatal weight of less than 2500 g at term [1]. More recent definitions use an estimated weight <10th percentile for gestational age (GA) or weight that is less than two standard deviations (SD) below the anticipated value for GA [1,2]. Because of its greater clinical relevance, some authors prefer to define SGA as weight below the fifth or even third percentile [3].

Likewise, FGR has multiple proposed definitions worldwide that incorporate absolute sonographically determined estimated fetal weight (EFW), specific biometric measurements (most commonly abdominal circumference [AC]), growth trajectory, and Doppler assessments. Additionally, FGR can further be categorized by severity based on the degree of abnormality of each assessment. For this chapter, we use the definition proposed by the Society for Maternal-Fetal Medicine (SMFM) of EFW or AC <10th percentile for GA [4].

Epidemiology

The prevalence of FGR is dependent on the definition used to diagnose the condition. However, using the SMFM definition, FGR is seen in slightly more than 10% of all pregnancies. The prevalence does vary based on geographic location, with higher rates of FGR occurring in developing countries [5]. Unfortunately, access to prenatal diagnosis and management of FGR is also limited in lower resource settings. When discussing FGR, it is important to note that not all pregnancies affected by FGR reflect a pathologically small fetus, as some fetuses at or below the 10th percentile are simply constitutionally small. Likewise, regardless of the FGR definition used, not all pathologically small fetuses will be detected.

Perinatal morbidity and mortality

It is well known that FGR increases the risk of perinatal morbidity and mortality. The risk of stillbirth increases as the EFW percentile decreases, with a stillbirth rate as high as 2.5% when the EFW falls below the fifth percentile [4,6]. Growth-restricted neonates experience increased need for immediate resuscitation and respiratory support and higher rates of intensive care unit admission, hypoglycemia, and seizures [7]. Perinatal death rates are also higher in neonates with low birthweight compared to those with a normal birthweight. Many growth-restricted fetuses also require preterm delivery, which can further exacerbate the poor neonatal outcomes seen. FGR is also well known to have long-term effects that persist into adolescence. Rates of metabolic syndrome, cardiovascular disease, cerebral palsy, and long-term neurologic impairment are significantly higher in children who at FGR prior to delivery [8]. In fact, the rates of learning disabilities in these cases are estimated to be as high as 40% at school age [9].

Etiologies

The etiology of pathologically impaired growth in utero is frequently due to impaired oxygen and nutrient delivery to the fetus. However, the upstream conditions that ultimately lead to the impaired fetal perfusion vary widely. The etiology of FGR can be used to further refine risk of poor pregnancy outcomes. It also can be helpful in determining the risk of recurrent FGR in future pregnancies. Most generally, the etiology can be categorized as placental, maternal, fetal, or idiopathic. As the placenta mediates transport of oxygen and nutrients from the gravida to the fetus, about 30% of FGR cases are ultimately attributed to placental disorders. A ubiquitous, though poorly defined, term used to describe this phenomenon is placental insufficiency. Increased placental resistance identified by abnormal fetal blood velocity within the umbilical artery is especially important in FGR as abnormal results are known to be associated with higher rates of perinatal morbidity and mortality.

Certain placental disorders including abruption and infarction are well known to predispose to FGR given their disruption of maternal-fetal gas exchange; however, not all placental abnormalities impact fetal growth. In fact, placenta accreta spectrum disorders and placenta previa have not been consistently associated with FGR.

Likewise, some umbilical cord abnormalities may predispose to growth restriction. Single umbilical artery, marginal cord insertion, and velamentous cord insertion have all been implicated in FGR but data are not consistent.

Any maternal condition that is complicated by vascular disease may result in FGR due to impaired uterine perfusion. Chronic hypertension, hypertensive disorders of pregnancy, and preexisting diabetes are among the most common maternal etiologies of FGR seen in pregnancy. Although antiphospholipid antibody syndrome, an acquired immune-mediated thrombotic state, increases the risk of FGR, the underlying mechanism is not understood, especially as other maternal thrombophilias have not been as consistently associated with FGR. Maternal cyanotic cardiac disease or severe lung disease even in the absence of vascular complications can predispose to FGR likely related to decreased oxygen delivery to the uterus.

Maternal exposure to toxins and teratogens, including tobacco, alcohol, marijuana, and illicit drugs, also increases the risk of FGR. In fact, tobacco use is associated with an over three-fold increased risk of SGA [10]. In most cases, the risk of FGR is related to the dosage, timing, and duration of exposure to the teratogen.

Maternal malnutrition has been shown to be associated with SGA, particularly in pregnancies that occur during famine and in the setting of poor protein intake [11]. Although famine is rare in developed countries, food insecurity is unfortunately common and may affect appropriate macronutrient intake. Additionally, maternal eating disorders are underrecognized in pregnancy, and severe caloric restriction has been associated with lower birthweight [12].

Fetal etiologies of FGR include multifetal gestation, genetic and structural abnormalities, and congenital infections. The risk of SGA in multiple gestation has been reported to be as high as 25% in twin pregnancies and 60% in higher order multiples [12]. Although there are some proponents for customized growth nomograms for multiples, the perinatal outcomes appear similar to singletons born at the same gestational age and weight, implying that multifetal gestations do have higher rates of FGR and that this FGR is still pathologic and should be managed as such.

Fetal structural abnormalities are a significant risk factor for FGR, with FGR occurring in up to 25% of anomalous fetuses [13]. Any anomaly that impairs adequate oxygenation can increase the risk for FGR. Although infants with congenital heart defect (CHD) are at a particularly high risk for failure to thrive, the in utero cardiac shunting via the foramen ovale and ductus arteriosus make fetuses with CHD less prone to growth restriction in utero, though still at higher risk than those fetuses without anomaly. Additionally, there are structural abnormalities, like gastroschisis or skeletal dysplasia, that impair our ability to accurately estimate fetal weight in utero by affecting the measurement of standard biometry. Although these cases of FGR may not reflect poor fetal perfusion, they are likely still at increased risk of poor fetal and neonatal outcomes due to their presence.

Certain genetic abnormalities are known to cause FGR in most cases. These include digynic triploidy, trisomy 13, and trisomy 18, though most genetic disorders can affect fetal growth patterns. Additionally, confined placental mosaicism, especially involving chromosome 16 has been implicated in FGR [14]. Presumably this genetic anomaly in the placenta interferes with adequate fetal perfusion in these otherwise normal fetuses.

Intrauterine infection causes up to 10% of FGR cases worldwide, with malaria being the most common [15]. However, even in developed countries, congenital infections with cytomegalovirus, toxoplasmosis, syphilis, and other pathogens can cause FGR and other congenital complications.

Despite the myriad identified risk factors and etiologies for FGR, many times an etiology for FGR is not identified and the FGR can be called idiopathic. In these cases, the pregnancy should be monitored closely for additional signs that may explain the cause. However, we know that not all fetuses with FGR are pathologically small and constitutional smallness may ultimately be the diagnosis made after delivery.

Diagnosis

Accurate estimation of the GA is critical for the diagnosis of FGR. Ultrasound dating is superior to the last menstrual period for this purpose, as approximately 30–50%

of pregnant women cannot recall their last cycle. The accuracy of ultrasound in estimating GA is inversely proportional to GA [16,17]. Specifically, the crown–rump length most accurately predicts the GA in the first trimester of pregnancy [18].

Once the GA is established, the next step is to identify those pregnancies at risk for FGR. Although several screening strategies for FGR have been reported in the literature, none of these are recommended for use clinically [19]. Historically, the distance in centimeters from the pubic symphysis to the fundus (fundal height measurement) is commonly used as a clinical screening for fetal growth, however, the accuracy of this method is limited [20].

Ultrasound remains the gold standard to detect FGR. Detection rate varies according to the ultrasound parameter and the gestational age at which the ultrasound evaluation is performed. The EFW is usually calculated using multiple fetal biometry parameters, such as the head circumference, biparietal diameter, the femur length, and the AC [21,22].

There has been some debate about the best formula or weight chart to use for the EFW, or for assigning growth percentiles. There are proponents of both population-based growth curves as well as customized nomograms that adjust for variations of fetal size based on fetal sex, race, or maternal height or body mass index [23–30]. The argument for more diverse population derived charts is based on studies where differences in fetal growth has been noted among different races and ethnicities. However, there is lack of convincing evidence to support the use of these newly proposed charts when compared with that by Hadlock et al. [22].

Management of FGR

Once a diagnosis of FGR has been established, major goals of management are prevention of stillbirth and optimizing timing of delivery. This involves the use of Doppler, non-stress tests (NSTs), and biophysical profiles (BPPs) for antenatal testing to monitor the well-being of the pregnancy.

Additionally, evaluation into possible etiology of FGR can be considered. Gravidas without prior genetic testing or screening should be offered diagnostic testing via amniocentesis, especially in cases when FGR is diagnosed prior to the third trimester. If diagnostic testing is declined, noninvasive genetic screening with cell-free fetal DNA (cffDNA) can also be considered. However, patients should understand that cffDNA only screens for certain conditions. A full anatomic assessment of the fetus should be performed to evaluate for any major malformations. Gravidas should be questioned about risk factors for congenital infection, such as recent illnesses or exposure; however, serologic screening for congenital infection in all growth-restricted fetuses is not costeffective. In patients undergoing an amniocentesis, cytomegalovirus polymerase chain reaction testing can be considered [4,31]. With the exception of cases in which delivery to avoid stillbirth is not planned, as in previable fetuses or fetuses with lethal anomalies, the management of FGR remains the similar regardless of etiology.

Antenatal surveillance

Umbilical artery (UA) Doppler assessment is recommended to identify those fetuses with FGR at greater risk for adverse outcomes. In addition, the NST alone or as part of the BPP has been used in pregnancies with FGR to further identify those at risk for fetal acidosis or hypoxia and intervene before deterioration of the fetal status.

UA Doppler velocimetry assesses the resistance to blood flow within the fetal portion of the placenta [32]. As placental resistance increases, forward flow during diastole decreases. The pulsatility index (PI), resistance index (RI), and systolic-to-diastolic (S/D) ratio are all options for quantifying these changes seen in diastolic flow. Abnormalities in UA Doppler flow can be seen on a spectrum. Normal UA Doppler assessment is defined as a PI, RI, or S/D ratio ≤95th percentile for gestational age. The earliest change to UA Doppler velocimetry that reflects poor diastolic flow is a PI, RI, or S/D ratio >95th percentile but with persistently forward flow during diastole, which may be referred to as "elevated" Doppler results. As placental resistance increases, we can see absence of blood flow in the umbilical artery at end-diastole, commonly referred to as absent end-diastolic flow or velocity (AEDF/V), and as this process worsens further, reversal of flow in the umbilical artery at the end of diastole, which is referred to as reversed end-diastolic flow or velocity (REDF/V) (Figure 44.1). Since UA Doppler results can progress over the course of a pregnancy, serial UA Doppler assessments are recommended once FGR is diagnosed [4]. However, the ideal frequency of UA Doppler assessments is not agreed upon, but SMFM recommends this testing every 1–2 weeks if normal and more frequently if AEDV or REDV is seen.

There is limited evidence supporting NST as surveillance tool in pregnancies with FGR. Only one trial comparing a regimen of twice weekly NST to fortnightly NST in women with SGA fetuses with normal UA Doppler studies has been conducted. There was no difference in neonatal outcomes between the two groups in this study; and there was an increased incidence of induction of labor in the twice weekly NST group [33]. Despite this paucity of data, the NST is now a routine tool used in the surveillance of pregnancies with FGR.

The BPP includes the evaluation of the amniotic fluid volume, fetal movement, fetal tone, and fetal breathing with or without an NST. When normal, each parameter

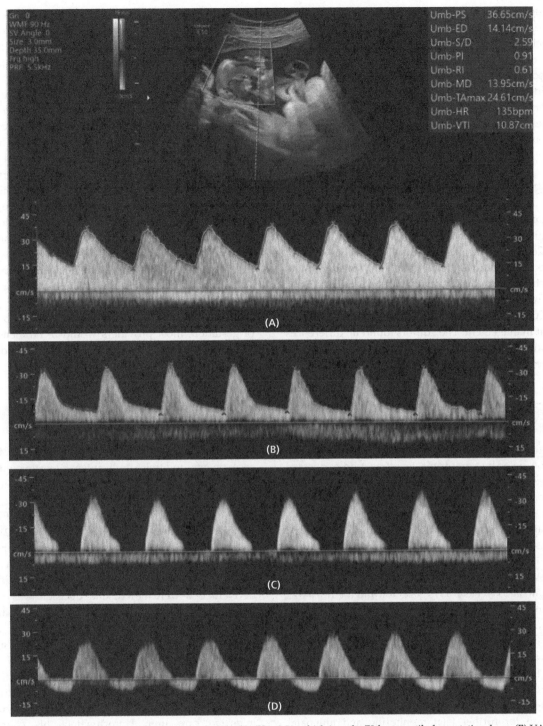

Figure 44.1 (A) UA Dopplers demonstrating normal results. The UA PI is 0.91, which is at the 70th percentile for gestational age. (B) UA Dopplers with decreased forward flow during diastole. The UA PI is 1.44, which is at the 98th percentile for gestational age. (C) UA Dopplers with absent forward flow at end-diastole. (D) UA Dopplers with reversed flow in the UA at end-diastole. PI, pulsatility index; UA, umbilical artery.

receives two points, for a maximum of 10 points [34]. The NST can be excluded, allowing a maximum score of 8/8 [35]. Abnormal BPP scores have been associated with fetal acidosis [36]. However, like the NST, the BPP has a high false-positive rate and lack of trials demonstrating prevention of adverse outcomes. For example, a study on

the use of daily BPPs in preterm fetuses with severe FGR (<1000 g with abnormal UA Doppler indices) reported high false-positive and false-negative rates and concluded that the BPP was not reliable in the evaluation of these pregnancies [37]. Perhaps one of the most important components of the BPP is the assessment of the amniotic fluid, as investigators have documented that oligohydramnios was independent risk factor for perinatal mortality in pregnancies with preterm FGR [38,39].

Further refinement of the risk to the fetus has been attempted with the use of ductus venosus Doppler studies, middle cerebral artery Doppler studies, and even uterine artery Doppler studies. However, the clinical utility of these studies is not well proven, and they should not be routinely adopted at this time [4].

Timing of delivery in FGR

In pregnancies with FGR, GA is the most important factor determining perinatal survival. For instance, the survival rate at 26 weeks exceeds 50% and it reaches 90% at 30 weeks of gestation [40–42]. In the Disproportionate Intrauterine Growth Intervention Trial at Term (DIGITAT), women with singleton gestations ≥36 weeks with suspected FGR were randomized to undergo delivery or expectant management. The authors found no differences in composite neonatal outcome (death before hospital discharge, 5-minute Apgar score of less than 7, umbilical artery pH of less than 7.05, or admission to the intensive care unit) between these two groups, although the study cohort was not large enough to determine if individual outcomes, such as perinatal death, differed between the groups [43].

Based on current evidence, when there are no other clear indications for delivery in the setting of FGR, the accepted practice is to use abnormal UA Doppler findings as a critical element for delivery timing. Those with normal UA can be monitored less closely, and if the UA Doppler waveforms remain normal, delivery can be deferred until 38–39 weeks. In cases where there is elevated UA PI, most institutions will increase surveillance with frequent UA Doppler assessment in conjunction of fetal surveillance testing (BPP or NST) and consider delivery by 37 weeks. Once the UA end-diastolic flow becomes absent or reversed, most maternal–fetal medicine services will admit these patients and initiate steroids for fetal lung maturity. If the UA Doppler waveforms show persistent AEDF or REDF and the pregnancy has reached 32 weeks of gestation, most providers would recommend suggest delivery and not to extend the pregnancy beyond 34 weeks regardless of the BPP or NST result [4].

CASE PRESENTATION

The patient is a 35-year-old gravida 1 at 20 weeks 2 days gestation, dated by a first-trimester ultrasound performed at 11 weeks gestation. Her medical history was notable for chronic hypertension that did not require medications and obesity with a body mass index of 49 kg/m². Cell-free fetal DNA testing had been low risk in the pregnancy. She was seen in the ultrasound suite for a routine fetal anatomic survey that showed no fetal malformations, but the EFW was noted to be at the 7th percentile. She was seen again at 23 weeks 2 days gestation and the EFW was 467 g and plotted at the 5th percentile. After counseling regarding the prognosis of severe growth restriction in the periviable period, she opted to begin UA Doppler testing at 25 weeks 2 days. The UA Dopplers revealed absent flow at end-diastole in some but not all of the cardiac cycles. She was further counseled on risk for poor outcome with this finding and opted for inpatient admission for further fetal monitoring and antenatal corticosteroid administration for fetal lung maturity. The fetus was managed with planned ultrasound growth assessments every 3 weeks, twice weekly UA Doppler assessments, and twice daily antenatal testing with either NST or BPP. At 26 weeks 2 days, the UA Doppler studies worsened, showing reversed end-diastolic flow, and the interval fetal growth was suboptimal with an EFW at the first percentile, measuring 672 g, a gain of only 215g over a 3-week period. BPP performed at the same time revealed normal fluid, breathing, tone, and movement. However, on NST later that night, multiple fetal decelerations were noted, and decision was made to proceed with delivery via primary classical cesarean for breech presentation. Birthweight of the male neonate was 610 g. The APGAR scores were 3 and 7 at 1 and 5 minutes of life, respectively. The UA pH was 7.1 with a base excess of -10 mmol/L and a lactate of 14.2 mmol/L. The infant required intubation in the delivery room at 8 minutes of life and was admitted to the neonatal intensive care unit. Unfortunately, his course was complicated by difficult ventilation and ultimate respiratory decompensation and death on day of life 24.

References

1. World Health Organization. international statistical classification of diseases and related health problems. Geneva: World Health Organization; 1992.

2. Doubilet PM, Benson CB. Ultrasound evaluation of fetal growth. In: Callen PW, edito.r Ultrasonography in obstetrics and gynecology. Philadelphia, WB Saunders, Co.; 2000.

3. McIntire DD, Bloom SL, Casey BM, Leveno KJ. Birth weight in relation to morbidity and mortality among newborn infants. N Engl J Med. 1999;340:1234–8.

4. Society for Maternal-Fetal Medicine (SMFM). Martins JG, Biggio JR, Abuhamad A. Society for Maternal-Fetal Medicine Consult Series #52: diagnosis and management of fetal growth restriction. Am J Obstet Gynecol. 2020 Oct;223(4):B2–B17.

5. de Onis M, Blössner M, Villar J. Levels and patterns of intrauterine growth retardation in developing countries. Eur J Clin Nutr. 1998 Jan;52 Suppl 1:S5–15.

6. Getahun D, Ananth CV, Kinzler WL. Risk factors for antepartum and intrapartum stillbirth: a population-based study. Am J Obstet Gynecol. 2007 Jun;196(6):499–507.

7. Madden JV, Flatley CJ, Kumar S. Term small-for-gestational-age infants from low-risk women are at significantly greater risk of adverse neonatal outcomes. Am J Obstet Gynecol. 2018 May;218(5):525.e1–9.

8. Crispi F, Miranda J, Gratacós E. Long-term cardiovascular consequences of fetal growth restriction: biology, clinical implications, and opportunities for prevention of adult disease. Am J Obstet Gynecol. 2018 Feb;218(2S):S869–79.

9. Leitner Y, Fattal-Valevski A, Geva R, Eshel R, Toledano-Alhadef H, et al. Neurodevelopmental outcome of children with intrauterine growth retardation: a longitudinal, 10-year prospective study. J Child Neurol. 2007 May;22(5):580–7.

10. American College of Obstetricians and Gynecologists' Committee on Practice Bulletins–Obstetrics and the Society for Maternal-Fetal Medicine. ACOG Practice Bulletin No. 204: fetal growth restriction. Obstet Gynecol. 2019 Feb;133(2): e97–e109.

11. Luke B. Nutritional influences on fetal growth. Clin Obstet Gynecol. 1994 Sep;37(3):538–49.

12. Pasternak Y, Weintraub AY, Shoham-Vardi I, Sergienko R, Guez J, Wiznitzer A, et al. Obstetric and perinatal outcomes in women with eating disorders. J Womens Health (Larchmt). 2012 Jan;21(1):61–5.

13. Centofanti SF, Brizot Mde L, Liao AW, Francisco RP, Zugaib M. Fetal growth pattern and prediction of low birth weight in gastroschisis. Fetal Diagn Ther. 2015;38(2):113–8.

14. Grati FR, Ferreira J, Benn P, Izzi C, Verdi F, Vercellotti E, et al. Outcomes in pregnancies with a confined placental mosaicism and implications for prenatal screening using cell-free DNA. Genet Med. 2020 Feb;22(2):309–16.

15. Matteelli A, Caligaris S, Castelli F, Carosi G. The placenta and malaria. Ann Trop Med Parasitol. 1997 Oct;91(7):803–10.

16. Cosmi E, Ambrosini G, D'Antona D, Saccardi C, Mari G. Doppler, cardiotocography, and biophysical profile changes in growth-restricted fetuses. Obstet Gynecol. 2005;106(6):1240–5.

17. Crimmins S, Desai A, Block-Abraham D, Berg C, Gembruch U, Baschat AA. A comparison of Doppler and biophysical findings between liveborn and stillborn growth-restricted fetuses. Am J Obstet Gynecol. 2014;211(6):669 e1–10.

18. Andersen HF, Johnson TR Jr, Flora JD Jr, Barclay ML. Gestational age assessment. II. Prediction from combined clinical observations. Am J Obstet Gynecol. 1981;140(7):770–4.

19. Carbone JF, Tuuli MG, Bradshaw R, Liebsch J, Odibo AO. Efficiency of first-trimester growth restriction and low pregnancy-associated plasma protein-A in predicting small for gestational age at delivery. Prenat Diagn. 2012;32(8):724–9.

20. Lindhard A, Nielsen PV, Mouritsen LA, Zachariassen A, Sorensen HU, Roseno H. The implications of introducing the symphyseal-fundal height-measurement. A prospective randomized controlled trial. Br J Obstet Gynaecol. 1990; 97(8):675–80.

21. Abuhamad A, Martins JG, Biggio JR. Diagnosis and management of fetal growth restriction: the SMFM guideline and comparison with the ISUOG guideline. Ultrasound Obstet Gynecol. 2021 Jun;57(6):880–3.

22. Hadlock FP, Harrist RB, Sharman RS, Deter RL, Park SK. Estimation of fetal weight with the use of head, body, and femur measurements–a prospective study. Am J Obstet Gynecol. 1985;151(3):333–7.

23. Gardosi J, Francis A, Turner S, Williams M. Customized growth charts: rationale, validation and clinical benefits. Am J Obstet Gynecol. 2018;218(2S):S609–18.

24. Sovio U, Smith GCS. The effect of customization and use of a fetal growth standard on the association between birthweight percentile and adverse perinatal outcome. Am J Obstet Gynecol. 2018;218(2S):S738–44.

25. Odibo AO, Francis A, Cahill AG, Macones GA, Crane JP, Gardosi J. Association between pregnancy complications and small-for-gestational-age birth weight defined by customized fetal growth standard versus a population-based standard. J Matern Fetal Neonatal Med. 2011;24(3):411–17.

26. Odibo AO, Cahill AG, Odibo L, Roehl K, Macones GA. Prediction of intrauterine fetal death in small-for-gestational-age fetuses: impact of including ultrasound biometry in customized models. Ultrasound Obstet Gynecol. 2012; 39(3):288–92.

27. Buck Louis GM, Grewal J, Albert PS, Sciscione A, Wing DA, Grobman WA, et al. Racial/ethnic standards for fetal growth: the NICHD Fetal Growth Studies. Am J Obstet Gynecol. 2015;213(4):449.e1–41.

28. Papageorghiou AT, Ohuma EO, Altman DG, Todros T, Cheikh Ismail L, et al. International standards for fetal growth based on serial ultrasound measurements: the Fetal Growth Longitudinal Study of the INTERGROWTH-21st Project. Lancet. 2014;384(9946):869–79.

29. Anderson NH, Sadler LC, McKinlay CJD, McCowan LME. INTERGROWTH-21st vs customized birthweight standards for identification of perinatal mortality and morbidity. Am J Obstet Gynecol. 2016;214(4):509.e1–7.

30. Odibo AO, Nwabuobi C, Odibo L, Leavitt K, Obican S, Tuuli MG. Customized fetal growth standard compared with the INTERGROWTH-21st century standard at predicting small-for-gestational-age neonates. Acta Obstet Gynecol Scand. 2018;97(11):1381–7.

31. Yamamoto R, Ishii K, Shimada M, Hayashi S, Hidaka N, Nakayama M, Mitsuda N. Significance of maternal screening for toxoplasmosis, rubella, cytomegalovirus and herpes simplex virus infection in cases of fetal growth restriction. J Obstet Gynaecol Res. 2013 Mar;39(3):653–7.

32. Trudinger BJ, Stevens D, Connelly A, Hales JR, Alexander G, Bradley L, et al. Umbilical artery flow velocity waveforms and placental resistance: The effects of embolization of the umbilical circulation. Am J Obstet Gynecol. 1987;157:1443–8.

33. McCowan LM, Harding JE, Roberts AB, Barker SE, Ford C, Stewart AW. A pilot randomized controlled trial of two regimens of fetal surveillance for small-for-gestational-age fetuses with normal results of umbilical artery doppler velocimetry. Am J Obstet Gynecol. 2000;182(1 Pt 1):81–6.

34. Manning FA, Platt LD, Sipos L. Antepartum fetal evaluation: development of a fetal biophysical profile. Am J Obstet Gynecol. 1980;136(6):787–95.

35. Manning FA, Morrison I, Lange IR, Harman CR, Chamberlain PF. Fetal biophysical profile scoring: selective use of the non-stress test. Am J Obstet Gynecol. 1987;156(3):709–12.

36. Vintzileos AM, Fleming AD, Scorza WE, Wolf EJ, Balducci J, Campbell WA, et al. Relationship between fetal biophysical activities and umbilical cord blood gas values. Am J Obstet Gynecol. 1991;165(3):707–13.

37. Kaur S, Picconi JL, Chadha R, Kruger M, Mari G. Biophysical profile in the treatment of intrauterine growth-restricted fetuses who weigh <1000 g. Am J Obstet Gynecol. 2008;199(3):264 e261–4.

38. Hecher K, Bilardo CM, Stigter RH, Ville Y, Hackelöer BJ, Kok HJ, et al. Monitoring of fetuses with intrauterine growth restriction: a longitudinal study. Ultrasound Obstet Gynecol. 2001;18(6):564–70.

39. Scifres CM, Stamilio D, Macones GA, Odibo AO. Predicting perinatal mortality in preterm intrauterine growth restriction. Am J Perinatol. 2009;26(10):723–8.

40. Lees C, Marlow N, Arabin B, Bilardo CM, Brezinka C, Derks JB, et al. Perinatal morbidity and mortality in early-onset fetal growth restriction: cohort outcomes of the trial of randomized umbilical and fetal flow in Europe (TRUFFLE). Ultrasound Obstet Gynecol. 2013;42(4):400–8.

41. GRIT Study Group. A randomised trial of timed delivery for the compromised preterm fetus: short term outcomes and Bayesian interpretation. BJOG. 2003;110(1):27–32.

42. Walker DM, Marlow N, Upstone L, Gross H, Hornbuckle J, Vail A, et al. The Growth Restriction Intervention Trial: long-term outcomes in a randomized trial of timing of delivery in fetal growth restriction. Am J Obstet Gynecol. 2011;204(1):34.e31–9.

43. Boers KE, Vijgen SM, Bijlenga D, van der Post JA, Bekedam DJ, Kwee A, et al. Induction versus expectant monitoring for intrauterine growth restriction at term: randomised equivalence trial (DIGITAT). BMJ. 2010;341:c7087.

Chapter 45
Induction of Labor

Emily H. Adhikari

Department of Obstetrics and Gynecology, University of Texas Southwestern Medical Center, Dallas, TX, USA

Labor induction, or iatrogenic stimulation of uterine contractions prior to the onset of spontaneous labor, is one of the most routinely performed obstetric procedures in the United States. Recent rates of labor induction declined to a nadir of 23.2% in 2014 [1], then increased each year to a new high of 31.4% of births in 2020 [2]. Factors likely contributing to this increase include trends such as increasing maternal age at delivery and declining teen births and births per 1000 women in the United States [2]. Additional notable trends in recent years include a decline in preterm (<37 completed weeks) in 2020 for the first time since 2014, and a steady decline in late term (41 completed weeks) and a steady increase in early term (37–38 completed weeks) births since 2014 [2]. The 2018 publication of the ARRIVE (A Randomized Trial of Induction Versus Expectant Management) trial cemented the practice of elective induction at 39 weeks in low-risk women as accepted part of routine obstetric management [3]. Whether and how labor and delivery units can accommodate potentially increased numbers of women scheduled for induction remains to be seen. Importantly, use of standardized protocols for labor management is associated with reduced cesarean delivery and neonatal morbidity among Black women compared to labor management according to provider discretion [4].

Whether elective or indicated, the procedure of labor induction requires an appreciation of the available cervical ripening or induction agents and their appropriate use or contraindications, as well as management of any complications that may result from use of these agents. Although there is no evidence that labor and delivery unit policies on labor induction changed when the COVID-19 pandemic began [5], longitudinal studies to understand the impact of labor induction policies on maternal and neonatal outcomes in the context of the pandemic are still needed.

Indications and contraindications to labor induction

Indications for delivery are classified as either maternal or fetal. In most cases, when the benefits of expeditious delivery to the mother or fetus outweigh the risk of continuing the pregnancy, induction of labor should take place in appropriate candidates. Generally, cesarean delivery is reserved for situations in which vaginal delivery is contraindicated or risks of induction clearly outweigh the benefits of vaginal delivery. Following labor induction, the degree of maternal or fetal risk for morbidities such as cesarean delivery or neonatal respiratory compromise is contingent upon factors such as cervical status, severity of maternal medical comorbidities, diagnosed fetal or placental abnormalities and ongoing fetal status assessment, and gestational age at delivery.

Contraindications to labor induction include those that proscribe spontaneous labor and vaginal delivery (Box 45.1). Other clinical scenarios are not absolute contraindications but require a cautious approach because of the potential for maternal or fetal morbidity during the induction process. These may include nonreactive nonstress testing, fetal growth disorders, multifetal pregnancy, and previous low transverse cesarean delivery. Continuous fetal monitoring and frequent maternal assessment during induction is required in these cases, along with a low threshold for intervention if labor is not progressing or there are signs of fetal intolerance.

Medically indicated delivery timing

The American College for Obstetricians and Gynecologists (ACOG) provides guidance for delivery timing with certain medical or obstetric complications according to available

Queenan's Management of High-Risk Pregnancy: An Evidence-Based Approach, Seventh Edition. Edited by Catherine Y. Spong and Charles J. Lockwood.

Box 45.1 Contraindications to labor induction with a living fetus

Absolute contraindications

- Prior classic uterine incision or transfundal uterine surgery
- Active genital herpes infection
- Placenta or vasa previa
- Umbilical cord prolapse
- Absolute cephalopelvic disproportion (as in women with pelvic deformities)

Relative contraindications

- Cervical carcinoma
- Fetal malpresentation

evidence and expert consensus (Box 45.2) [6]. Common obstetric and medical conditions for which early term or preterm delivery may be indicated include gestational hypertensive disease, fetal growth restriction, and prelabor rupture of membranes. Recommended timing of delivery depends on the specific condition and any additional medical comorbidities that may coexist. For example, high-quality evidence exists to support the maternal benefit of induction of labor after 37 weeks among women with mild pregnancy-related hypertensive disease and show no increase in cesarean delivery [7]. Labor induction is a reasonable approach for women with singleton pregnancies with an indication for delivery, who do not have a contraindication to vaginal delivery, and for whom the fetus is vertex and status is reassuring. Limited observational evidence suggests that medically indicated preterm labor induction is not associated with increased risk for maternal or neonatal adverse outcomes after adjustment for confounders [8].

Box 45.2 Indications for labor induction (timing may differ according to indication and severity of the condition as well as gestational age)

Maternal medical indications

- Hypertensive disorders of pregnancy
  - Chronic hypertension, gestational hypertension, preeclampsia with or without severe features
- Poorly controlled diabetes mellitus and/or vascular complications
- Intrahepatic cholestasis of pregnancy

Obstetric indications

- Prelabor rupture of membranes at or after 34 wk
- Chorioamnionitis
- Fetal demise

Fetal indications

- Fetal growth restriction (depending on fetal status, estimated fetal weight, and umbilical artery Doppler studies)
- Alloimmunization
- Nonreassuring antepartum fetal testing
- Oligohydramnios

Elective induction of labor

The initiation of labor for a pregnancy with no medical or obstetric indication is referred to as elective induction of labor and should be differentiated from induction that is undertaken for an indication but without the presence of endogenous labor. Major concerns associated with elective induction have historically included the potential for iatrogenic neonatal morbidity, increased risk for primary cesarean delivery among women with an unfavorable cervix, and cost associated with additional time in the hospital. Perceived benefits include potentially lower stillbirths or neonatal adverse outcomes, as well as maternal hypertensive disorders. A discerning reader reviews labor induction trial reports with an appreciation of whether the primary outcome of a trial is time to delivery, mode of delivery, or maternal or neonatal outcomes.

A large, randomized trial of labor induction (ARRIVE) among low-risk, nulliparous women at 39 weeks vs. expectant management until 40 weeks 5 days recently addressed unresolved questions about the safety of elective induction [3]. The investigators demonstrated no difference in a composite primary outcome of perinatal death or severe neonatal complications for the two study arms. Additionally, there was a significantly lower rate of cesarean delivery, the principal secondary outcome, in the induction group (18.6% vs. 22.2%). The induction group had a significantly longer stay on the labor and delivery unit compared with the expectant management group (20 vs. 14 hours). Although the participants were recruited from over 50,000 potentially eligible candidates at several large medical centers, 16,000 women declined to participate, and those who agreed were generally younger and more likely to be Black or Hispanic than women who delivered in the United States in the year 2016 [9].

In a trial comparing labor induction at 41 weeks compared with 42 weeks among low-risk Swedish women, Wennerholm et al. found that the rate of an overall adverse perinatal composite outcome did not differ, but there were six perinatal deaths (five stillbirths and one early neonatal death) in the expectant management group compared to none in the induction group [10]. Finally, a population-based cohort study from Sweden demonstrated increased cesarean delivery following labor induction at 38 weeks in a cohort of nulliparous, nondiabetic women with large-for-gestational-age fetuses [11].

Considering the available evidence, the impact of increasing induction numbers on delivery hospitals, and the critical nursing and obstetric care shortages recognized in the United States in recent years [12,13], the decision for routine elective induction between 39 weeks and no later than 41 weeks of gestation is made more logistically complex. However, elective induction within these parameters appears to be reasonable for pregnancies without another indication for delivery.

Predicting a successful induction

Factors associated with successful vaginal delivery following labor induction include prior vaginal delivery, younger maternal age, favorable or open cervix, low body mass index (BMI), and greater maternal height [14–16]. The Bishop score, a composite assessment of cervical dilation, position, effacement, station, and consistency, has historically been used as a tool to predict likelihood of vaginal delivery. Its utility depends on the population being studied. A simplified Bishop score including only cervical dilation, effacement, and fetal station has similar predictive ability to the original score, with use for different populations including patients undergoing labor induction and spontaneous labor [17]. Individualized models have recently been proposed to predict the likelihood of vaginal delivery after elective induction at 39 weeks [18], but the role of this customized tool in clinical obstetrics is unclear.

Longer duration of latent labor is also associated with successful vaginal delivery, discussed in the next section. Although transvaginal sonographic measurement of cervical length or uterocervical angle has been proposed for predicting response to labor induction (such as reaching active labor or achieving vaginal delivery), its utility in clinical obstetrics has not been defined [19].

Defining failed induction

Considerations for defining failed induction have changed in recent years. Historic trials have compared length of labor, morbidity risks, and vaginal delivery rates among women undergoing induction to those in spontaneous labor. However, we now understand that patients undergoing induced labor differ from those in spontaneous labor, and that the two should not be compared; rather, the appropriate comparison is an expectantly managed group. Labor characteristics also differ. ACOG encourages longer duration of latent phase (up to 24 hours or longer) and oxytocin administration for at least 12–18 hours after membrane rupture if maternal and fetal status are reassuring before cesarean delivery is performed for failed induction [20]. This may be particularly beneficial for nulliparous patients [21].

Allowing more time for latent labor is also supported by a multicenter cohort study by the Eunice Kennedy Shriver National Institute of Child Health and Human Development (NICHD) Maternal-Fetal Medicine Units Network. Grobman et al. found that active phase labor (defined as 5 cm cervical dilation) was reached by 15 hours in over 96% of women [22]. Additionally, although maternal adverse outcomes increased with greater time in the latent phase, the absolute frequency was relatively small, and over 40% of women whose latent phase lasted at least 18 hours underwent vaginal delivery. These findings support the practice that if maternal and fetal status remain reassuring, allowing

continued labor induction may be individualized. Importantly, close attention to maternal and fetal status during a prolonged induction is imperative to allow timely intervention when indicated. Colvin et al. demonstrated that in a cohort of 3990 women with hypertensive disorders of pregnancy, after multivariable adjustment, duration of labor induction over 24 hours was associated with increased maternal (adjusted relative risk [aRR] 1.39, 95% confidence interval [CI] 1.20–1.62) and neonatal (aRR 1.32, 95% CI 1.11–1.56) risks [23]. The maternal composite outcome studied included operative vaginal delivery, chorioamnionitis, blood transfusion, intensive care unit admission, placental abruption, third- or fourth-degree perineal laceration, endometritis, postpartum hemorrhage, or venous thromboembolism; the neonatal composite outcome included neonatal intensive care unit (NICU) admission, respiratory distress syndrome, 5-minute Apgar score ≤7, seizure, infection, intrapartum meconium aspiration, intracranial hemorrhage, shoulder dystocia, and neonatal death.

Thus, risks of labor induction are discussed in the context of individual characteristics and balanced with the benefits of indicated delivery where appropriate. When labor induction is undertaken, frequent reassessment of these risks and benefits is critical.

Preinduction considerations

Prior to undergoing labor induction, examination of the maternal and fetal condition is essential to ensure that there are no contradictions to labor or vaginal delivery. Other prerequisites include evaluation of fetal presentation and cervical examination, along with an estimate of fetal weight, and clinical pelvimetry, all of which should be documented. Indications and contraindications for induction should be reviewed, and risks and benefits of labor induction should be discussed with the patient. Verification of pregnancy dating by the obstetric estimate of gestational age is essential prior to elective labor induction. If preterm induction is planned for maternal or fetal indication, consideration is given to administering antenatal corticosteroids if indicated; importantly, a medically indicated preterm delivery should not be delayed for the administration of antenatal corticosteroids [6].

The timing and location of elective induction should be contingent upon the availability of personnel who are familiar with the process and its potential complications in nonemergency settings. Employment of continuous electronic fetal monitoring and uterine activity monitoring are recommended for any gravida receiving uterotonic drugs.

Cervical ripening

Cervical remodeling occurs during normal parturition and involves endogenous prostaglandins, collagen breakdown, changes in glycosaminoglycans, neutrophil infiltration, and increased cytokines. The process may be initiated for patients with an unfavorable cervix (often defined as modified Bishop score <5 or Bishop score <7). Cervical ripening agents include both mechanical and pharmacological agents. They are typically used prior to stimulation of uterine contractions with oxytocin, which is associated with increased cesarean delivery when used alone for women with an unfavorable cervix. Studies frequently compare cervical ripening agents in the context of labor induction, for which the outcomes of interest should be vaginal vs. cesarean delivery and maternal and neonatal safety rather than time to delivery or change in Bishop score. Thus, studies comparing cervical ripening agents are studies of labor induction.

Mechanical cervical ripening methods include laminaria, used more commonly before induction in the second trimester, and transcervical Foley catheter, which may be used in place of or in addition to pharmacologic agents. Of the larger randomized induction trials, the PROBAAT and PROBAAT-II trials demonstrated no difference in cesarean delivery following use of Foley as compared with vaginal prostaglandin E_2 or oral misoprostol as a cervical ripening agent [24,25]. Another trial comparing oral misoprostol with or without placement of transcervical Foley catheter demonstrated no benefit in achieving vaginal delivery, but 30% increased risk for chorioamnionitis in the Foley group [26].

Common pharmacologic cervical ripening agents include oral or buccal prostaglandin E_1 (misoprostol, Cytotec) at doses of 50–100 μg, vaginal misoprostol at doses of 25–50 μg, and vaginal prostaglandin E_2 (dinoprostone) in the form of a gel (Prepidil) or an insert (Cervidil). Compared with oxytocin use alone, prostaglandin use is associated with decreased cesarean delivery in women with an unfavorable cervix. Vaginal misoprostol may be superior to buccal misoprostol for achieving vaginal delivery [27]. Whether vaginal or oral misoprostol is associated with lower cesarean delivery is controversial [28]; vaginal misoprostol may be associated with more uterine tachysystole [29]. A noninferiority randomized trial comparing vaginal misoprostol with slow-release dinoprostone demonstrated similar rates of cesarean delivery (22.1% vs. 19.9%, respectively) and maternal and neonatal morbidities, but higher maternal satisfaction with vaginal misoprostol [30]. As with all clinical trials, understanding the characteristics of the population studied and eligibility and indication(s) for induction are key to determining generalizability.

Risks associated with labor induction

Counseling regarding maternal and fetal risks associated with induction of labor is individualized. Risks depend on the indication for delivery, gestational age, and maternal and fetal complications as well as obstetric complications that occur during the induction process. For example, in a secondary analysis of the ARRIVE trial, increasing BMI was associated with an increased perinatal composite outcome (aRR 1.04/unit increase, 95% CI 1.02–1.05), and risk of postpartum hemorrhage was observed among Hispanic compared with White women studied (6.3% vs 4.0%; aRR 1.64, 95% CI 1.18–2.29) [31]. As previously described, duration of labor induction over 24 hours is associated with increased maternal and neonatal risks [23].

Uterine tachysystole

Uterine overactivity is the most frequent complication of oxytocin or prostaglandin administration. Historic terms commonly used to describe uterine overactivity are tachysystole, hypertonus, and hyperstimulation. A 2008 Eunice Kennedy Shriver NICHD workshop issued revised standardized definitions for fetal heart rate and uterine contraction patterns that have the potential for reducing miscommunication among obstetric care providers [32]. Tachysystole is now the preferred term and defined as more than five contractions in 10 minutes, averaged over a 30-minute window. Any co-existent fetal heart rate abnormality is described separately. Tachysystole following cervical ripening and labor induction is not associated with adverse neonatal outcomes despite increased frequency of nonreassuring fetal heart rate changes when compared to those without tachysystole [33]. In a clinical trial evaluating continuation of oxytocin following active labor diagnosis, there was increased tachysystole and fetal heart rate abnormalities and a nonsignificant decrease in cesarean delivery compared to oxytocin discontinuation [34].

Hyponatremia

Oxytocin has a comparable structure to vasopressin (antidiuretic hormone) and can cross-react with the renal vasopressin receptor. If high doses of oxytocin are administered in large quantities of hypotonic solutions for extended periods of time, excessive water retention can occur and result in severe, symptomatic hyponatremia characterized by abdominal pain, headache, nausea, vomiting, lethargy, anorexia, seizures, and potentially irreversible neurologic injury. Use of standardized oxytocin titration protocols help safeguard against these risks.

Hypotension

Rapid intravenous injection of oxytocin can result in hypotension; however, studies demonstrating this result were performed in men, nonpregnant women, and first trimester patients under general anesthesia. A randomized trial of oxytocin bolus vs. slow infusion in women at delivery of the anterior shoulder did not find clinically significant differences in hemodynamic responses [35]. Nonetheless, oxytocin should be administered by infusion pump or slow drip, since bolus injections of oxytocin can cause tachysystole.

Additional considerations

Immediate vs. delayed pushing

A large randomized trial of immediate vs. delayed pushing following either induction or spontaneous labor among nulliparas receiving neuraxial analgesia demonstrated no difference in the rate of vaginal delivery [36]. Among secondary outcomes, the second stage was longer, and rates of chorioamnionitis and study-defined adverse events were higher in the delayed pushing group. These results call into question perceived benefits of "laboring down" once complete cervical dilation is achieved. Preinduction counseling should address potential questions about second stage labor management with this evidence in mind.

Induction of labor in women with prior cesarean delivery

Allowing a period of either spontaneous or induced labor with the aim of achieving vaginal delivery after a previous cesarean delivery is known as a trial of labor after cesarean (TOLAC). The process carries inherent increased risk because of the enhanced potential for uterine rupture. Nonetheless, the rates of vaginal delivery after cesarean have increased in the United States from 12.4% in 2016 to 13.3% in 2018 [37]. Compared to women undergoing repeat cesarean, women who deliver vaginally after previous cesarean experience lower birth-related morbidity such as blood transfusion, ruptured uterus, unplanned hysterectomy, and ICU admission [38]. Clinical trials of efficacy and safety of labor induction in women with prior cesarean are generally underpowered, and fail to demonstrate differences in rare but potentially catastrophic events such as uterine dehiscence or rupture. Notably, however, at least one clinical trial was stopped for safety concerns following use of vaginal misoprostol for induction [39]. The use of oxytocin for augmentation of labor is considered acceptable, although a dose-response effect exists with higher maximum oxytocin dose associated with higher rates of uterine rupture [40]. ACOG acknowledges that several factors may increase the potential for a failed TOLAC, which in turn is associated with increased maternal and perinatal morbidity compared to spontaneous labor [41]. Induction of labor may be one of these factors, although large, prospective trials comparing induction with expectant management among people with prior cesarean at term have not been conducted. Thus, assessing the likelihood of success or failure as well as individual risks is critical to determining whether any individual is an appropriate candidate for TOLAC.

Conclusion

Induction of labor is one of the most frequently performed obstetric procedures and should be undertaken only after careful consideration of the indication, the likelihood of success and relative risks and benefits for an individual patient. A variety of agents exist for cervical ripening and labor induction, and the use of standardized induction protocols is encouraged. In assessment of the literature, outcomes most relevant to clinical practice include mode of delivery and maternal and neonatal outcomes.

CASE PRESENTATION

A 22-year-old primigravida presents to your office for a routine prenatal care visit at 38 weeks gestation. You have seen her since 8 weeks of gestation and her antepartum course has been uncomplicated. She is anxious about not going into labor but is tired of being pregnant. At this visit, you find that she is in good health, is normotensive, and has an unfavorable cervix that is long and closed. The fetus is in vertex presentation.

You review the risks and benefits of induction vs. expectant management, and the fact that her pregnancy has been low risk. You discuss with her the potential for scheduling induction of labor at 39 weeks of gestation based on the findings from the ARRIVE trial, which demonstrated no increase in a composite adverse outcomes and a secondary outcome of lower cesarean delivery in the group undergoing induction. Additionally, you describe the limitations of the trial, including the characteristics of patients and the longer duration of time on the labor and delivery unit. You discuss the need for cervical ripening should labor induction be indicated or elected. You also discuss how, despite advances in the various mechanical and pharmacologic methods by which to prepare the cervix prior to labor induction, no method has been proven to be universally effective in achieving vaginal delivery for all women. She asks what methods would be used for cervical ripening, and you review the evidence supporting use of prostaglandins and transcervical Foley catheter, and the risks of each. She asks about the possibility of beginning the process of cervical ripening at home, and you explain that protocols at your institution are standardized and that you recommend adhering to the institutional protocol for induction practices.

References

1. Osterman MJK, Martin JA. Recent declines in induction of labor by gestational age. NCHS data brief, no 155. Hyattsville, MD: National Center for Health Statistics; 2014.

2. Osterman MJK, Hamilton BE, Martin JA, Driscoll AK, Valenzuela CP. Births: Final data for 2020. National Vital Statistics Reports; vol 70 no 17. Hyattsville, MD: National Center for Health Statistics; 2022.

3. Grobman WA, Rice MM, Reddy UM, Tita ATN, Silver RM, Mallett G, et al.; Eunice Kennedy Shriver National Institute of Child Health and Human Development Maternal–Fetal Medicine Units Network. Labor induction versus expectant management in low-risk nulliparous women. N Engl J Med. 2018 Aug 9;379(6):513–23.

4. Hamm RF, Srinivas SK, Levine LD. A standardized labor induction protocol: impact on racial disparities in obstetrical outcomes. Am J Obstet Gynecol MFM. 2020 Aug;2(3):100148.

5. Greene NH, Kilpatrick SJ, Wong MS, Ozimek JA, Naqvi M. Impact of labor and delivery unit policy modifications on maternal and neonatal outcomes during the coronavirus disease 2019 pandemic. Am J Obstet Gynecol MFM. 2020 Nov;2(4):100234.

6. ACOG Committee Opinion No. 764: medically indicated late-preterm and early-term deliveries. Obstet Gynecol. 2019 Feb;133(2):e151–5.

7. Koopmans CM, Bijlenga D, Groen H, Vijgen SM, Aarnoudse JG, Bekedam DJ, et al.; HYPITAT Study Group. Induction of labour versus expectant monitoring for gestational hypertension or mild pre-eclampsia after 36 weeks' gestation (HYPITAT): a multicentre, openlabel randomised controlled trial. Lancet. 2009;374(9694):979–88.

8. Kuper SG, Sievert RA, Steele R, Biggio JR, Tita AT, Harper LM. Maternal and neonatal outcomes in indicated preterm births based on the intended mode of delivery. Obstet Gynecol. 2017 Nov;130(5):1143–51.

9. Greene MF. Choices in managing full-term pregnancy. N Engl J Med. 2018 Aug 9;379(6):580–1.

10. Wennerholm UB, Saltvedt S, Wessberg A, Alkmark M, Bergh C, Wendel SB, et al. Induction of labour at 41 weeks versus expectant management and induction of labour at 42 weeks (SWEPIS): multicentre, open label, randomised, superiority trial. BMJ. 2019 Nov 20;367:l6131.

11. Moldéus K, Cheng YW, Wikström AK, Stephansson O. Induction of labor versus expectant management of large-for-gestational-age infants in nulliparous women. PLoS One. 2017 Jul 20;12(7):e0180748.

12. Auerbach DI, Buerhaus PI, Staiger DO. Implications of the rapid growth of the nurse practitioner workforce in the US. Health Aff (Millwood). 2020 Feb;39(2):273–9.

13. Kozhimannil KB, Interrante JD, Tuttle MKS, Henning-Smith C. Changes in hospital-based obstetric services in rural US counties, 2014–2018. JAMA. 2020;324(2):197–9.

14. Tolcher MC, Holbert MR, Weaver AL, McGree ME, Olson JE, El-Nashar SA, et al. Predicting cesarean delivery after induction of labor among nulliparous women at term. Obstet Gynecol. 2015 Nov;126(5):1059–68.

15. Freret TS, Woods GT, James KE, Kaimal AJ, Clapp MA. Incidence of and risk factors for failed induction of labor using

16. Roland C, Warshak CR, DeFranco EA. Success of labor induction for pre-eclampsia at preterm and term gestational ages. J Perinatol. 2017 Jun;37(6):636–40.

17. Laughon SK, Zhang J, Troendle J, Sun L, Reddy UM. Using a simplified Bishop score to predict vaginal delivery. Obstet Gynecol. 2011 Apr;117(4):805–11.

18. Silver RM, Rice MM, Grobman WA, Reddy UM, Tita ATN, Mallett G, et al.; Eunice Kennedy Shriver National Institute of Child Health and Human Development (NICHD) Maternal-Fetal Medicine Units (MFMU) Network. Customized probability of vaginal delivery with induction of labor and expectant management in nulliparous women at 39 weeks of gestation. Obstet Gynecol. 2020 Oct;136(4):698–705.

19. Yang SW, Kim SY, Hwang HS, Kim HS, Sohn IS, Kwon HS. The uterocervical angle combined with Bishop score as a predictor for successful induction of labor in term vaginal delivery. J Clin Med. 2021 May 10;10(9):2033.

20. American College of Obstetricians and Gynecologists. Obstetric Care Consensus No. 1: safe prevention of the primary cesarean delivery. Obstet Gynecol. 2014 Mar;123(3):693–711.

21. Rouse DJ, Owen J, Hauth JC. Criteria for failed labor induction: prospective evaluation of a standardized protocol. Obstet Gynecol. 2000 Nov;96(5 Pt 1):671–7.

22. Grobman WA, Bailit J, Lai Y, Reddy UM, Wapner RJ, Varner MW, et al.; Eunice Kennedy Shriver National Institute of Child Health and Human Development Maternal-Fetal Medicine Units Network. Defining failed induction of labor. Am J Obstet Gynecol. 2018 Jan;218(1):122.e1–8.

23. Colvin Z, Feng M, Pan A, Palatnik A. Duration of labor induction in nulliparous women with hypertensive disorders of pregnancy and maternal and neonatal outcomes. J Matern Fetal Neonatal Med. 2022 Oct;35(20):3964–71.

24. Jozwiak M, Oude Rengerink K, Benthem M, Benthem M, van Beek E, Dijksterhuis MG, et al.; PROBAAT Study Group. Foley catheter versus vaginal prostaglandin E2 gel for induction of labour at term (PROBAAT trial): an open-label, randomised controlled trial. Lancet. 2011 Dec 17;378(9809):2095–103.

25. Ten Eikelder ML, Oude Rengerink K, Jozwiak M, de Leeuw JW, de Graaf IM, van Pampus MG, et al. Induction of labour at term with oral misoprostol versus a Foley catheter (PROBAAT-II): a multicentre randomised controlled non-inferiority trial. Lancet. 2016 Apr 16;387(10028):1619–28.

26. Adhikari EH, Nelson DB, McIntire DD, Leveno KJ. Foley bulb added to an oral misoprostol induction protocol: a cluster randomized trial. Obstet Gynecol. 2020 Nov;136(5):953–61.

27. Haas DM, Daggy J, Flannery KM, Dorr ML, Bonsack C, Bhamidipalli SS, et al. A comparison of vaginal versus buccal misoprostol for cervical ripening in women for labor induction at term (the IMPROVE trial): a triple-masked randomized controlled trial. Am J Obstet Gynecol. 2019 Sep;221(3):259.e1–16.

28. Alfirevic Z, Aflaifel N, Weeks A. Oral misoprostol for induction of labour. Cochrane Database Syst Rev. 2014 Jun 13;2014(6):CD001338. doi: 10.1002/14651858.CD001338.pub3.

29. Hokkila E, Kruit H, Rahkonen L, Timonen S, Mattila M, Laatio L, et al. The efficacy of misoprostol vaginal insert compared with oral misoprostol in the induction of labor of nulliparous

a contemporary definition. Obstet Gynecol. 2021 Mar 1; 137(3):497–504.

women: A randomized national multicenter trial. Acta Obstet Gynecol Scand. 2019 Aug;98(8):1032–9.

30. Gaudineau A, Senat MV, Ehlinger V, Gallini A, Morin M, Olivier P, et al.; Groupe de Recherche en Obstétrique et Gynécologie. Induction of labor at term with vaginal misoprostol or a prostaglandin E2 pessary: a noninferiority randomized controlled trial. Am J Obstet Gynecol. 2021 Nov;225(5):542.e1–8.

31. El-Sayed YY, Rice MM, Grobman WA, Reddy UM, Tita ATN, Silver RM, et al.; Eunice Kennedy Shriver National Institute of Child Health and Human Development (NICHD) Maternal-Fetal Medicine Units (MFMU) Network. Elective labor induction at 39 weeks of gestation compared with expectant management: factors associated with adverse outcomes in low-risk nulliparous women. Obstet Gynecol. 2020 Oct;136(4):692–7.

32. Macones GA, Hankins GD, Spong CY, Hauth J, Moore T. The 2008 National Institute of Child Health and Human Development Research Workshop Report on electronic fetal heart rate monitoring. Obstet Gynecol. 2008;112:661–6.

33. Bofill JA, Darby MM, Castillo J, Sawardecker SU, Magann EF, Morrison JC. Tachysystole following cervical ripening and induction of labor is not associated with adverse outcomes. Gynecol Obstet Invest. 2017;82(5):487–93.

34. Boie S, Glavind J, Uldbjerg N, Steer PJ, Bor P; CONDISOX trial group. Continued versus discontinued oxytocin stimulation in the active phase of labour (CONDISOX): double blind randomised controlled trial. BMJ. 2021 Apr 14;373:n716.

35. Davies GA, Tessier JL, Woodman MC, Lipson A, Hahn PM. Maternal hemodynamics after oxytocin bolus compared with infusion in the third stage of labor: A randomized controlled trial. Obstet Gynecol. 2005;105:294–9.

36. Cahill AG, Srinivas SK, Tita ATN, Caughey AB, Richter HE, Gregory WT, et al. Effect of immediate vs delayed pushing on rates of spontaneous vaginal delivery among nulliparous women receiving neuraxial analgesia: a randomized clinical trial. JAMA. 2018;320(14):1444–54.

37. Osterman MJK. Recent trends in vaginal birth after cesarean delivery: United States, 2016–2018. NCHS data brief, No 359. Hyattsville, MD: National Center for Health Statistics; 2020.

38. Curtin SC, Gregory KD, Korst LM, Uddin SF. Maternal morbidity for vaginal and cesarean deliveries, according to previous cesarean history: New data from the birth certificate, 2013. National Vital Statistics Reports; Vol 64 No 4. Hyattsville, MD: National Center for Health Statistics; 2015.

39. Wing DA, Lovett K, Paul RH. Disruption of prior uterine incision following misoprostol for labor induction in women with previous cesarean delivery. Obstet Gynecol. 1998;91(5 Pt 2):828–30.

40. Cahill AG, Waterman BM, Stamilio DM, Odibo AO, Allsworth JE, Evanoff B, et al. Higher maximum doses of oxytocin are associated with an unacceptably high risk for uterine rupture in patients attempting vaginal birth after cesarean delivery. Am J Obstet Gynecol. 2008;199:32.e1–5.

41. American College of Obstetricians and Gynecologists. ACOG Practice Bulletin No. 205: vaginal birth after cesarean delivery. Obstet Gynecol. 2019 Feb;133(2):e110–27.

Chapter 46
Cesarean Delivery

Elaine L. Duryea

Department of Obstetrics and Gynecology, University of Texas Southwestern Medical Center, Dallas, TX, USA

Cesarean delivery (CD), arguably one of the greatest obstetric interventions to reduce perinatal morbidity and mortality, has been firmly established in Western obstetric practice since the mid-twentieth century. Initially performed to improve maternal outcomes in labor, practice evolved to include fetal indications for CD as electronic fetal monitoring became omnipresent and advances in neonatal medicine occurred.

By 1987 the CD rate in the United States had risen to comprise 24% of all births [1]. The ensuing 15-year interval saw a stabilization of this rate (approximately 21% from 1994 to 1998), in large part due to efforts to encourage vaginal birth following previous CD (VBAC) [2,3,4]. Subsequently CD rates increased, due in part to decrease frequency of VBAC in community hospitals [5], though many other factors contribute including increasing average maternal age, rates of obesity, and occurrence of medical comorbidities and abandonment of trials of labor with fetal breech presentations. The most common indications for primary CD include failure to make adequate progress in labor (35.4%), nonreassuring fetal heart rate tracing (27.3%), and fetal malpresentation (1`8.5%) [6]. An additional factor, the performance of CD on maternal request, is thought to comprise < 3% of all births in the United States, and guidance on counseling women regarding the benefits of vaginal delivery as compared to CD, including the increased risk of complications in future repeat CD such as abnormal placentation and hysterectomy is provided by the American College of Obstetricians and Gynecologists (ACOG) [7]. The most recent US CD rate available at the time of writing is 31.7%, which has remained essentially unchanged over the past 15 years [7].

Maternal and perinatal morbidity and mortality

Maternal mortality rates in the United States have remained relatively low and stable in the first 2 decades of the twenty-first century; however, racial/ethnic disparities in outcomes persist and information on cause of death and contributing factors are limited [8]. Better reporting systems are needed to meaningfully interpret and intervene to reduce disparities and reduce overall maternal mortality. Women undergoing CD are at increased risk for hemorrhage, infection, and venous thromboembolism as compared to women delivering vaginally [9]. A report by Clark and associates suggests that CD increases the maternal mortality ratio from 0.2 per 100 000 for vaginal birth to 2.2 per 100 000 live births for women delivered via CD, though absolute numbers remain low [10]. Put another way, women undergoing CD are more likely to suffer a maternal death as well as experience severe maternal morbidities as measured by the Centers for Disease Control and Prevention [11]. Severe maternal morbidity indications include acute renal failure, myocardial infarction, adult respiratory distress syndrome, and transfusion. Severe maternal morbidity occurs in 0.4–1.0% of pregnancies in developed countries [12].

In contrast, neonatal mortality rates continue to decrease, though whether this is a result of increased CD for fetal distress is not known, given advances in neonatal medicine during the same period. To the contrary, there is evidence that babies delivered by scheduled elective repeat CD at term are at increased risk of developing respiratory problems (adjusted odds ratio [OR] 2.3, 95% confidence interval [CI] 1.4–3.8) [13].

Queenan's Management of High-Risk Pregnancy: An Evidence-Based Approach, Seventh Edition. Edited by Catherine Y. Spong and Charles J. Lockwood.

Evidence-based operative considerations

While debate about indications for CD is ongoing, there has been a substantial body of evidence-based recommendations regarding timing, preoperative, intraoperative, and postoperative management. Guidelines regarding indications for late preterm and early term delivery exist, based predominantly on expert opinion [14]. Uncomplicated repeat cesarean deliveries should not be considered prior to 39 weeks gestation to optimize neonatal outcomes.

Enhanced recovery after surgery (ERAS) is an evidence-based, multidisciplinary approach to improving surgical care in the perioperative period. ERAS aims to minimize the pathophysiologic perturbations during surgery, optimizing patient outcomes without increasing postoperative complications. Enhanced recovery after cesarean (ERAC) expands ERAS principles to apply to obstetric specific issues [15].

Preoperative considerations

The guidelines for ERAC differ slightly based upon scheduled vs. unscheduled cesarean deliveries. The pathway begins at 10–20 weeks gestation for patients who will undergo scheduled cesarean deliveries [16]. Comorbidities are optimized for delivery, including correcting anemia and optimizing blood glucose levels in people with diabetes. Reducing the period of fasting for women undergoing cesarean is emphasized, with a light meal up to 6 hours before surgery, and clear liquids up until 2 hours before administration of anesthesia [17]. For unscheduled or emergent cesarean deliveries, the preoperative pathway is compressed into a 30- to 60-minute window preceding delivery. Regional anesthesia is preferred for cesarean delivery [18]. Spinal anesthesia results in shorter block onset than epidurals, and intrathecal morphine may help with immediate postoperative pain control.

Intraoperative considerations

Antibiotic prophylaxis

Women who are delivered abdominally are at increased risk of endometritis and/or wound infection. The Cochrane review of 86 clinical trials confirms that it is beneficial for these women to receive antibiotics immediately before, during, or immediately after their CD, whether or not they have clinical evidence of infection. Women who receive antibiotic prophylaxis at the time of CD have lower rates of endometritis (relative risk [RR] 0.38, 95% CI 0.3–0.42) [19]. The risk of wound infection was also reduced in women receiving antibiotic prophylaxis at the time of CD (RR 0.39, 95% CI 0.32–0.48), as was the incidence of febrile morbidity (RR 0.45, 95% CI 0.39– 0.51) [20]. More recent reviews suggest that antibiotic administration prior to surgical incision may reduce postcesarean maternal infection by up to 50% [20]. Thus, administration of a first-generation cephalosporin is recommended for all women without allergies prior to skin incision, and an acceptable alternative regimen for women with significant history of anaphylaxis, angioedema, or respiratory distress with penicillin or cephalosporin includes, clindamycin with an aminoglycoside such as gentamicin [21]. There is evidence in support of extended coverage with the addition of azithromycin 1 g infused over 1 hour for women with ruptured membranes and/or labor at the time of cesarean. This recommendation is based upon prospective data from a multicenter randomized trial where a reduction in endometritis, wound infection, and serious maternal adverse events was found in those women receiving azithromycin as compared to placebo [22].

Vaginal antiseptic prophylaxis

Vaginal preparation immediately before CD with povidone-iodine has been demonstrated to significantly reduce the incidence of postcesarean endometritis from 9.4% in control groups to 5.2% in vaginal cleansing groups (RR 0.57, 95% CI 0.38– 0.87) [23]. The risk reduction was particularly strong for women with ruptured membranes (1.4% in the vaginal cleansing group vs. 15.4% in the control group; RR 0.13, 95% CI 0.02–0.66). No other outcomes realized statistically significant differences between the vaginal cleansing and control groups and no adverse effects were reported with the povidone-iodine vaginal cleansing. Further evidence is needed to strongly recommend the practice of vaginal antiseptic prophylaxis prior to all cesarean deliveries.

Abdominal surgical incision

Transverse skin incisions are preferred for esthetic considerations in the absence of contraindications, and the Joel-Cohen incision has advantages compared to the Pfannenstiel incision. The Pfannenstiel is made in a curvilinear fashion 3 cm above the pubic symphysis as compared to the Joel-Cohen, which is a linear incision located more superiorly, 3 cm below the anterior superior iliac spines. A 2007 Cochrane review documented less fever, pain and analgesic requirements, less blood loss and shorter duration of surgery and hospital stay with the Joel-Cohen incision [24]. However, in the setting of coagulopathy or severe thrombocytopenia a vertical skin incision may be preferred to avoid dissection of the internal and external oblique aponeuroses and subsequent potential for hematoma and bleeding complications.

Manual removal of the placenta

Manual removal of the placenta is associated with a clinically relevant and statistically significant increase in maternal blood loss (weighted mean difference 94 mL; 95% CI 17–172 mL) [25]. Manual removal was also associated with increased postpartum endometritis (OR 1.64, 95% CI 1.42–1.90) and lower hematocrit after delivery (weighted mean difference –1.55%, 95% CI –3.09 to –0.01), and thus should be avoided if possible.

Extraabdominal vs. intraabdominal repair of the uterine incision

Six randomized clinical trials, consisting of 1221 participating women, compared uterine exteriorization with intraabdominal repair. There were no significant differences between the groups in most of the outcomes examined, with the exceptions of febrile morbidity and length of hospital stay. Febrile morbidity was lower (RR 0.41, 95% CI 0.17–0.97) and length of hospital stay was longer (weighted mean difference 0.24 days, 95% CI 0.08–0.39) with extraabdominal closure of the hysterotomy [26].

Single-layer vs. two-layer hysterotomy closure

In a 2008 Cochrane review, single-layer closure compared with double-layer closure was associated with a statistically significant reduction in mean blood loss (three studies, 527 women, MD –70.11, 95% CI –101.61 to –38.60), duration of the operative procedure (four studies, 645 women, MD –7.43, 95% CI –8.41 to –6.46), and presence of postoperative pain (one study, 158 women, RR 0.69, 95% CI 0.52–0.91) [27]. There are insufficient long-term follow-up data to reach any conclusions regarding risks for subsequent pregnancies.

Peritoneal closure

Previous meta-analyses have demonstrated that nonclosure of the visceral and parietal peritoneum decreased operative time (RR –7.33 min, 95% CI –8.43 to –6.24 min), decreased postoperative fever, and reduced postoperative hospital stay [28]. At the time of this analysis, published in 2005, only one study had evaluated long-term adhesion formation and demonstrated no differences. However, a 2009 meta-analysis of five studies demonstrated a significantly increased likelihood of adhesion formation with nonclosure (OR 2.60, 95% CI 1.48–4.56) [29]. Particularly in women planning additional cesarean deliveries, it may therefore be prudent to consider peritoneal closure.

Abdominal wall closure techniques

In a meta-analysis of seven studies involving over 2000 women, Anderson and Gates [30] concluded that the risk of hematoma or seroma was reduced with closure of the subcutaneous tissue compared with nonclosure (RR 0.52, 95% CI 0.33–0.82). The risk of wound complications (defined as hematoma, seroma, wound infection, or wound separation) was also reduced with subcutaneous tissue closure (RR 0.68 95% CI 0.52–0.88). There are no data to address whether closure or reapproximation of the rectus sheath is beneficial or detrimental.

Postoperative considerations

The primary goal postoperatively is to ensure return to baseline function and progress to successful discharge from the hospital while facilitating maternal and infant bonding and successful breastfeeding practices. Maintenance of euvolemia and appropriate intraoperative treatment of hypotension decreases the risk of postoperative nausea and vomiting. Early oral intake of ice chips and water should occur within 60 minutes of admission to the postanesthesia care unit [17]. Patients are encouraged to resume a regular diet within 4 hours after surgery if there are no contraindications. Published guidelines recommend discontinuation of Foley catheters for women that do not require ongoing urine output measurements [31]. The early removal of the catheters is thought to facilitate ambulation and carry a theoretically reduced risk of symptomatic urinary tract infections.

Pain regimens

ERAC emphasizes multimodal pain regimens to establish adequate postoperative pain control while minimizing opioid exposure [31]. Regimens including scheduled nonsteroidal inflammatory drugs and acetaminophen are favored, with opioids reserved for uncontrolled pain as needed as opioid use in the postpartum period is associated with nausea, emesis, itching, and decreased ambulation which may interfere with a woman's ability to effectively care for her newborn [32,33]. Traditional postoperative pain management strategies include continuous infusion of opioids via epidural catheter, patient-controlled analgesia opioid pumps or long-lasting intrathecal opioid injections. Although intrathecal injection of morphine has been the gold standard for postoperative cesarean pain management, studies have shown that despite the long-lasting effects of intrathecal opioids women still need additional analgesic administration, including additional opioids, for adequate pain control [32,34]. Other pain management techniques have been adopted including local infiltration of anesthetic agents via transversus abdominis plane blocks and subcutaneous injections, though data suggesting a reduction in opioid requirement are mixed [35,36]. These multimodal pathways have resulted in a decrease in hospital length of stays, readmission rates, postoperative complications, as well as decreased hospital costs; however, there are mixed results with regard to decreasing opioid consumption [37–46].

Thromboprophylaxis

In the developed world, thromboembolic disease is one of the most common causes of direct maternal death, though the incidence has decreased over time (Figure 46.1) [47]. Thromboembolic disease is at least two times more likely following CD [33]. ACOG recommends placement of pneumatic compression devices before CD and early mobilization after CD [48]. It is important to note that thromboprophylaxis is optimally effective when initiated preoperatively and given concerns about procedure-related bleeding at the time of neuraxial anesthesia administration when heparin has been administered, pneumatic compression devices are preferred. If pharmacological prophylaxis is required, it should be initiated postoperatively once hemostasis is noted and the patient is hemodynamically stable. In general, initiation prior to 12–24 hours after surgery is not advisable. Recommendations regarding pharmacological prophylaxis for women with other risk factors for venous thromboembolism vary, with the Royal College of Obstetricians and Gynaecologists recommending pharmacological prophylaxis for women with risk factors with continuation of therapy up to 6 weeks postpartum depending on level of risk [49]. However, a recent multicenter retrospective cohort study found that risk-stratified heparin-based thromboprophylaxis in a general obstetric population was associated with increased bleeding complications without a decrease in postpartum thromboembolism [50]. Thus, although the optimum regimen(s) have yet to be clearly delineated, it is clear that consideration should be given to the possibility of thromboembolic complications after any CD.

Treatment of postoperative endometritis

In a review of 15 clinical trials, the Cochrane review also confirmed that the combination of gentamicin and clindamycin had fewer treatment failures than other regimens (treatment failure with other regimens, RR 1.44, 95% CI 1.15–1.80) [51]. Three studies that compared continued oral antibiotic therapy after intravenous therapy with no oral therapy found no differences in recurrent infection or any other adverse outcomes [51].

Potential risks of repeat cesarean delivery

One major contributor to the prior increase in the overall CD rate was a temporally associated decline in TOLAC (Trial of labor after cesarean) and fewer subsequent VBACs. A modest decline in VBAC rates had started and subsequently accelerated after a 1999 technical bulletin from the ACOG [52] cautioned against VBAC unless the facilities and staff to perform emergency repeat CD were "immediately available." Revisions of this technical bulletin have included more supportive statements including "most women with one previous cesarean delivery with a low-transverse incision are candidates for and should be counseled about and offered TOLAC" [53]. Definitive statements on risks associated with VBAC are the papers produced by the *Eunice Kennedy Shriver* National Institute of Child Health and Human Development funded Maternal-Fetal Medicine Units Network Cesarean Registry [54]. These results are outlined in more detail in Chapter 47. Although the magnitude of these

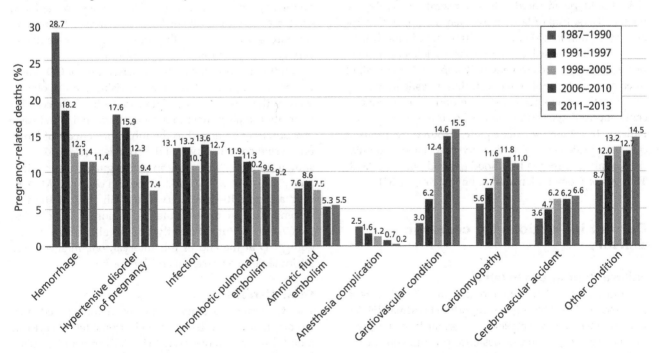

Figure 46.1 Population-level, cause-specific proportionate pregnancy-related mortality for 1987–1990, 1991–1997, 1998–2005, 2006–2010, and 2011–2013. Results are population level and can be compared as absolute values. From: Creanga AA, et al. 2017/Wolters Kluwer.

Table 46.1 Incidence of morbidly adherent placenta in the setting of placenta previa, as related to number of prior cesarean deliveries (CDs)

Number of prior CDs	Accreta risk
1	3%
2	11%
3	40%
4	61%
≥5	67%

risks is small, physician practice patterns and legal concerns will continue to affect TOLAC acceptance into the future.

Although substantial attention has been paid to the risks of TOLAC, rather less attention has been directed to the risks of repeat CD. In the largest series to address this issue, Silver [55] reviewed the outcomes of 30,132 CDs performed without labor. He found that the risk of accreta, hysterectomy, blood transfusion, cystotomy, bowel injury, ureteric injury, previa, ileus, postoperative ventilation, intensive care unit admission, operative time, and hospital days significantly increased with increasing numbers of CDs. Hysterectomy was required in only 0.65% of women undergoing their first CD, but this risk increased to 2.4% of women undergoing their fourth CD and 9.0% undergoing their sixth or greater CD. Similarly, in the 723 women with previa, the risk for accreta increased with progressive number of prior CDs but much more markedly (Table 46.1). Silver confirmed that serious maternal morbidity increases with increasing numbers of CD and suggested that the number of intended pregnancies should be factored into consideration of elective repeat CD vs. trial of labor in women with prior CD. He also noted that in 2003 over 80,000 women in the United States had their fourth or more cesarean delivery, making his recommendations more widely applicable than might often be expected. Subsequent studies investigating early identification of women at risk for morbidly adherent placenta (accreta spectrum) emphasize triage of high-risk patients to centers with adequate resources to perform cesarean hysterectomy and other associated interventions, while improving likelihood of good outcomes with TOLAC for women identified to be low risk [56,57].

Current indications for cesarean delivery

Failure to progress in labor

The most common indication for primary CD is failure to progress in labor. Although the reports of Friedman [58,59] have defined the expectations of normal labor progress for the past generation of obstetric practitioners in the United States, more recent data from the Consortium for Safe Labor suggest that these historic expectations may

not reflect normal labor in contemporary American women, particularly prior to 6 cm dilation [60].

In the 1980s, there was hope that the active management of labor, as initially championed by the National Maternity Hospital in Dublin [61], might reverse the increasing CD rates. Unfortunately, this management approach has ultimately failed to stop a rising CD rate in the developed world, including in Ireland [62].

There has been no suggestion that maternal pelvises or uterine activity have changed appreciably in the United States over the past several decades. Likewise, mean birthweight has not increased in recent years (1990, 3365 g; 2003, 3325 g) [63]. However, the frequency of CD for the diagnosis of failure to progress in labor increased during the same interval.

Researchers at the University of Alabama at Birmingham have presented data indicating that extending the minimum period of oxytocin augmentation for active phase labor arrest from 2 to at least 4 hours is effective and safe [64]. Following the diagnosis of a 2-hour active-phase arrest, oxytocin was initiated with an intent to achieve a sustained uterine contraction pattern of greater than 200 Montevideo units. A CD was not performed for labor arrest until at least 4 hours of a sustained uterine contraction pattern of greater than 200 Montevideo units, or a minimum of 6 hours of oxytocin augmentation if this contraction pattern could not be achieved. A total of 542 women were managed by this protocol and 92% delivered vaginally. These authors subsequently demonstrated that oxytocin-augmented labor proceeds at a slower rate than spontaneous labor [65]. During oxytocin augmentation, nulliparas who were delivered vaginally dilated at a median rate of 1.4 cm/hour vs. 1.8 cm/hour for parous women. In both groups, the 5th percentile of cervical dilatation rate was 0.5 cm/hour.

Another contributor to the increased rate of CD due to failure to progress in labor may be rising rates of obesity seen in the United States. The association between this labor abnormality, most commonly made in the first stage of labor, may be linked to the inhibitory effects of leptin on uterine contractility [66]. LaCoursiere et al. [67] have shown that a 40% increase in prepregnancy overweight (body mass index [BMI] 25.0–29.9) and obesity (BMI ≥30) over a recent 10-year interval in Utah (1991–2001) was accompanied by an attributable fraction of CD of 0.388 (0.369–0.407). Put differently, among all women undergoing CD at the end of this interval, one in seven was attributable to overweight and/or obesity.

Fetal distress

The Cochrane systematic review demonstrated that women followed in labor with electronic fetal heart rate monitoring were more likely to be delivered abdominally and their babies were less likely to suffer neonatal asphyxial seizure (RR 0.52, 95% CI 0.32–0.82) [68]. However, the rate of false-positive tests is high, and most babies delivered via CD for "nonreassuring fetal heart rate patterns" or "fetal distress" suffered no perinatal complications, and long-term follow-up of the Dublin population revealed no difference in any neuropsychiatric or developmental landmarks by age 5 years [69].

Earlier attempts to reduce false-positive interventions focused on fetal scalp blood sampling for fetal pH determination and did demonstrate a reduced CD rate for this indication [70]. However, the difficulties of maintaining this equipment, as well as the invasive nature of the procedure, precluded its widescale use, particularly in the community sector. More recently, fetal pulse oximetry has been evaluated as a less invasive technique for assessment of fetal oxygenation during labor, with convincing animal and human data to suggest that a fetal oxygen saturation of greater than 30% was almost never associated with a pH of <7.15 [71–73]. An initial evaluation demonstrated a convincing reduction in CD rates for the diagnosis of "fetal distress" but interestingly demonstrated that those fetuses with nonreassuring fetal heart rates plus reassuring pulse oximetry were more likely to require CD eventually for the diagnosis of failure to progress in labor [74]. A subsequent large randomized controlled trial failed to show any benefit of fetal pulse oximetry when applied prospectively to primigravidas at term in labor [75].

The addition of ST waveform analysis to fetal heart rate monitoring has been demonstrated in some, but not all, studies to reduce intrapartum fetal acidosis and/or operative delivery rates [76,77]. Available data that demonstrate any benefit are almost exclusively from European centers, where most intrapartum management protocols are different from North American centers. A multicenter randomized controlled trial conducted in the United States demonstrated no improvement in perinatal outcomes or decreased in operative delivery rates–whether via forceps vaginal delivery or CD [77].

Malpresentation

In 3–4% of laboring patients the fetus is in breech presentation, and in most institutions in the United States this is considered an immediate indication for CD. The only way to lower this figure would be to increase the frequency vaginal breech delivery or increase the rates of external cephalic version (ECV). The first option is unlikely given the need for adequate training and experience and the Term Breech Trial results [78]. An increase in ECV rates seems more likely, although historic concerns about complications such as cord entanglement, placental abruption, fetomaternal transfusion, and ruptured uterus have limited the use of ECV in some areas, these problems seem to be more theoretical than real [79]. Nonetheless, ECV should only be performed in a hospital setting where emergency CD is "immediately available."

Repeat cesarean

Safe reduction in CD rates for primigravidas will proportionately reduce the number of repeat CDs required, as will encouragement of appropriate TOLAC. Use of calculators to counsel a woman on her personal risk may be helpful, but at this time have not been proven to improve patient outcomes [80]. In view of the aforementioned predominant indications for primary CD, a modern definition of failure to progress in labor, a critical distinction between "fetal distress" vs. "fetal stress" and/or "provider distress," and timely identification and correction of breech presentation can all contribute to a lower rate of repeat CD. Higher order repeat CDs are clearly associated with increased maternal morbidity. Although it is less clear that a single repeat CD is associated with significant maternal risk, the admonition that "today's primigravidas are tomorrow's multigravidas" is still germane since the subgroup of women with the lowest risk of peripartum complications are multiparous women undergoing normal vaginal delivery with a surgically intact uterus.

CASE PRESENTATION 1

A 33-year-old primigravida is admitted at 41 weeks 2 days gestation for induction of labor with the diagnosis of postdates pregnancy. Her Bishop score is 3 and she initially receives 25 μg misoprostol *per vagina* every 4 hours for a total of three doses, at which time her Bishop score has improved to 7. She is started on oxytocin and her contractions increase in frequency and intensity. She declines an offer of epidural anesthesia. The fetal heart rate tracing remains reassuring. After 6 hours her cervix is 4 cm dilated and completely effaced, with the vertex estimated at −2 station. An amniotomy is performed for augmentation

of labor with return of a large amount of clear fluid. With the next contraction sustained fetal bradycardia is noted on the fetal monitor. A sterile vaginal examination is performed and reveals umbilical cord prolapsing through the cervix. The presenting part is elevated, the oxytocin discontinued, and she is urgently transferred to the operating room. Following induction of general anesthesia, an emergency CD is performed via a transverse suprapubic abdominal incision.

She delivered a 3600 g female whose Apgar scores are 4 and 8 and whose cord artery pH is 7.07 and who thereafter

Continued

does well. The mother receives 1 g cefazolin intravenously following delivery of the baby. She remains afebrile after delivery and is nursing her baby on the third postpartum day when she develops shortness of breath and left-sided chest pain. A chest spiral computed tomography scan reveals a pulmonary embolism in the lower lobe of the right lung. She is started on intravenous heparin and oral coumadin. After 2 days her symptoms are greatly improved, and the heparin is discontinued. She is discharged on the sixth postpartum day on oral coumadin. She is advised to use a form of contraception that does not contain estrogen given her recent thromboembolism.

CASE PRESENTATION 2

An 18-year-old primigravida who is 1.68 m (5 feet 6 inches) tall and whose late-pregnancy BMI is 28.6, presents at 39 weeks 4 days gestation for evaluation of labor. She is found to be 3 cm dilatated and completely effaced and is contracting painfully every 3 minutes. She is admitted with the diagnosis of spontaneous labor. After 2 hours there has been no change in her cervix yet she remains quite uncomfortable. The decision is made to provide an epidural for pain relief and to proceed thereafter with amniotomy. Both are accomplished uneventfully, the latter revealing clear amniotic fluid. The fetal heart rate pattern remains reactive.

After another 2 hours there has still been no change in her cervical examination. Internal heart rate and pressure catheters are placed, revealing a reactive fetal heart rate with a baseline of 130–140 beats/min and contractions whose total Montevideo units average 140. Oxytocin augmentation is begun with resultant increase of her average Montevideo units to 210.

She progresses to 6 cm dilation but thereafter fails to make any further change in either cervical dilation or station of the vertex in the ensuing 2 hours. As a result, she is taken to the operating room where a primary CD is performed for the diagnosis of failure to progress in labor. A male infant weighing 3280 g is delivered whose Apgar scores are 8 and 9 at 1 and 5 minutes, respectively.

Her intraoperative course is complicated by uterine atony that responds to 250 mg carboprost given intramuscularly. The estimated blood loss is 1250 mL. She has a single temperature elevation to 38.6° C in the recovery room, is started on broad-spectrum antibiotics, and remains afebrile thereafter. Her postoperative course is thereafter uncomplicated and she is discharged with her baby on postoperative day 3.

References

1. Sachs BP. Is the rising rate of cesarean sections a result of more defensive medicine? In: Rostow VP, Bulger RJ, editors. Medical professional liability and the delivery of obstetrical care. Vol. II, an interdisciplinary review. Washington, DC: National Academies Press; 1989. p.27–40.

2. Menacker F, Hamilton BE. Recent trends in cesarean delivery in the United States. NCHS data brief, no 35. Hyattsville, MD: National Center for Health Statistics; 2010.

3. Menard MK. Cesarean delivery rates in the United States: the 1990s. Obstet Gynecol Clin North Am. 1999;26:275–86.

4. Clarke SC, Taffel S. Changes in cesarean delivery in the United States, 1988 and 1993. Birth. 1995;22:63–7.

5. Sheiner E, Levy A, Feinstein U, Hallak M, Mazor M. Risk factors and outcome of failure to progress during the first stage of labor: a population-based study. Acta Obstet Gynecol Scand. 2002;81:222–6.

6. Boyle A, Reddy UM, Landy HJ, Huang CC, Driggers RW, Laughon SK. Primary cesarean delivery in the United States. Obstet Gynecol. 2013;122(1):33–40. doi:10.1097/AOG.| 0b013e3182952242.

7. American College of Obstetricians and Gynecologists. Committee Opinion No. 761: cesarean delivery on maternal request. Obstet Gynecol. 2019;133:e73–7.

8. Martin JA, Hamilton BE, Osterman MJK, Driscoll AK. Births: final data for 2019. National Vital Statistics Reports; vol 70 no 2.

Hyattsville, MD: National Center for Health Statistics; 2021. doi: 10.15620/cdc:100472.

9. Villar J, Carroli G, Zavaleta N, Donner A, Wojdyla D, Faundes A, et al. Maternal and neonatal individual risks and benefits associated with caesarean delivery: multicentre prospective study. BMJ. 2007 Nov 17;335(7628):1025.

10. Clark SL, Belfort MA, Dildy GA, Herbst MA, Meyers JA, Hankins GD. Maternal death in the 21st century: causes, prevention and relationship to cesarean delivery. Am J Obstet Gynecol. 2008;199:36.e1–5.

11. American College of Obstetricians and Gynecologists and the Society for Maternal–Fetal Medicine, Kilpatrick SK, Ecker JL. Severe maternal morbidity: screening and review. Am J Obstet Gynecol. 2016;215(3):B17–B22. doi:10.1016/j.ajog.2016.07.050.

12. Say L, Pattinson RC, Gulmezoglu AM. WHO systematic review of maternal morbidity and mortality: the prevalence of severe acute maternal morbidity (near miss). Reprod Health. 2004;1:3.

13. Hook B, Kiwi R, Amini SB, Fanaroff A, Hack M. Neonatal morbidity after elective repeat cesarean section and trial of labor. Pediatrics. 1997;100:348–53.

14. Spong CY, Mercer BM, D'Alton M, Kilpatrick S, Blackwell S, Saade G. Timing of indicated late-preterm and early-term birth. Obstet Gynecol. 2011;118(2 Pt 1):323–33. doi:10.1097/AOG.0b013e3182255999.

15. American College of Obstetricians and Gynecologists. ACOG Committee Opinion No. 750: perioperative pathways:

enhanced recovery after surgery. Obstet Gynecol. 2018;132(3): e120–30.

16. Wilson RD, Caughey AB, Wood SL, Macones GA, Wrench IJ, Huang J, et al. Guidelines for antenatal and preoperative care in cesarean delivery: enhanced recovery after surgery society recommendations (part 1). Am J Obstet Gynecol. 2018;219(6): 523.e1–15.

17. Bollag L, Lim G, Sultan P, Habib AS, Landau R, Zakowski M, et al. Society for Obstetric Anesthesia and Perinatology: consensus statement and recommendations for enhanced recovery after cesarean. Anesth Analg. 2021;132(5):1362–77.

18. Caughey AB, Wood SL, Macones GA, Wrench IJ, Huang J, Norman M, et al. Guidelines for intraoperative care in cesarean delivery: Enhanced Recovery After Surgery Society Recommendations (part 2). Am J Obstet Gynecol. 2018; 219(6):533–44.

19. Smaill FM, Gyte GM. Antibiotic prophylaxis versus no prophylaxis for preventing infection after cesarean section. Cochrane Database Syst Rev. 2010;1:CD007482. doi: 10.1002/14651858. CD007482.pub2.

20. Tita ATN, Rouse DJ, Blackwell S, Saade GR, Spong CY, Andrews WW. Evolving concepts in antibiotic prophylaxis for cesarean delivery: a systematic review. Obstet Gynecol. 2009;113: 675–82.

21. American College of Obstetricians and Gynecologists. ACOG Practice Bulletin No. 199: use of prophylactic antibiotics in labor and delivery. Obstet Gynecol. 2018;132:e103–19.

22. Tita AT, Szychowski JM, Boggess K, et al. Adjunctive Azithromycin Prophylaxis for Cesarean Delivery. N Engl J Med. 2016;375(13):1231–41. doi:10.1056/NEJMoa1602044.

23. Haas DM, Morgain AI, Darei S, Contreras K. Vaginal preparation with antiseptic solution before cesarean section for preventing post-operative infections. Cochrane Database Syst Rev. 2010;3:CD007892. doi: 10.1002/14651858.CD007892.pub7.

24. Mathai M, Hofmeyr GJ. Abdominal surgical incisions for caesarean section. Cochrane Database Syst Rev. 2007;1:CD004453. doi: 10.1002/14651858.CD004453.pub2.

25. Anorlu RI, Maholwana B, Hofmeyr GJ. Methods of delivering the placenta at caesarean section. Cochrane Database Syst Rev. 2008;3:CD004737. doi: 10.1002/14651858.CD004737.pub2.

26. Jacobs-Jokhan D, Hofmeyr GJ. Extra-abdominal versus intraabdominal repair of the uterine incision at caesarean section. Cochrane Database Syst Rev. 2004;4:CD000085. doi: 10.1002/14651858.CD000085.pub2.

27. Dodd JM, Anderson ER, Gates S. Surgical techniques for uterine incision and uterine closure at the time of caesarean section. Cochrane Database Syst Rev. 2008;3:CD004732. doi: 10.1002/14651858.CD004732.pub2.

28. Berghella V, Baxter JK, Chauhan SP. Evidence-based surgery for cesarean delivery. Am J Obstet Gynecol 2005;193: 1607–17.

29. Cheong YC, Premkumar G, Metwally M, Peacock JL, Li TC. To close or not to close? A systematic review and a meta-analysis of peritoneal non-closure and adhesion formation after caesarean section. Eur J Obstet Gynecol Reprod Biol. 2009;147:3–8.

30. Anderson ER, Gates S. Techniques and materials for closure of the abdominal wall at caesarean section. Cochrane Database Syst Rev. 2004;18:CD004663. doi: 10.1002/14651858.CD004663. pub2.

31. Macones GA, Caughey AB, Wood SL, Wrench IJ, Huang J, Norman M, et al. Guidelines for postoperative care in cesarean delivery: Enhanced Recovery After Surgery (ERAS) Society recommendations (part 3). Am J Obstet Gynecol 2019;221(3): 247.e1–9.

32. Sutton CD, Carvalho B. Optimal pain management after cesarean delivery. Anesthesiol Clin. 2017;35(1):107–24.

33. American College of Obstetricians and Gynecologists. ACOG Committee Opinion No. 742: postpartum pain management. Obstet Gynecol. 2018;132(1):e35–e43.

34. Sharpe EE, Molitor RJ, Arendt KW, Torbenson VE, Olsen DA, Johnson RL, et al. Intrathecal morphine versus intrathecal hydromorphone for analgesia after cesarean delivery: a randomized clinical trial. Anesthesiology. 2020;132(6):1382–91.

35. Warren JA, Carbonell AM, Jones LK, Mcguire A, Hand WR, Cancellaro VA, et al. Length of stay and opioid dose requirement with transversus abdominis plane block vs epidural analgesia for ventral hernia repair. J Am Coll Surg. 2019;228(4):680–6.

36. Pirrera B, Alagna V, Lucchi A, Berti P, Gabbianelli C, Martorelli G, et al. Transversus abdominis plane (TAP) block versus thoracic epidural analgesia (TEA) in laparoscopic colon surgery in the ERAS program. Surg Endosc. 2018;32(1):376–82.

37. Teigen NC, Sahasrabudhe N, Doulaveris G, Xie X, Negassa A, Bernstein J, et al. Enhanced recovery after surgery at cesarean delivery to reduce postoperative length of stay: a randomized controlled trial. Am J Obstet Gynecol. 2020;222(4):372.e1–10.

38. Mullman L, Hilden P, Goral J, Gwacham N, Tauro C, Spinola K, et al. Improved outcomes with an enhanced recovery approach to cesarean delivery. Obstet Gynecol. 2020;136(4):685–91.

39. Peahl AF, Smith R, Johnson TRB, Morgan DM, Pearlman MD. Better late than never: why obstetricians must implement enhanced recovery after cesarean. Am J Obstet Gynecol. 2019;221(2):117.e1–7.

40. Altenau B, Crisp CC, Devaiah CG, Lambers DS. Randomized controlled trial of intravenous acetaminophen for postcesarean delivery pain control. Am J Obstet Gynecol. 2017; 217(3):362.e1–6.

41. Hadley EE, Monsivais L, Pacheco L, Babazade R, Chiossi G, Ramirez Y, et al. Multimodal pain management for cesarean delivery: a double-blinded, placebo-controlled, randomized clinical trial. Am J Perinatol. 2019;36(11):1097–05.

42. Smith AM, Young P, Blosser CC, Poole AT. Multimodal stepwise approach to reducing in-hospital opioid use after cesarean delivery: a quality improvement initiative. Obstet Gynecol. 2019;133(4):700–6.

43. Hedderson M, Lee D, Hunt E, Lee K, Xu F, Mustille A, Galin J, et al. Enhanced recovery after surgery to change process measures and reduce opioid use after cesarean delivery: a quality improvement initiative. Obstet Gynecol. 2019;134(3):511–19.

44. Fay EE, Hitti JE, Delgado CM, Savitsky LM, Mills EB, Slater JL, et al. An enhanced recovery after surgery pathway for cesarean delivery decreases hospital stay and cost. Am J Obstet Gynecol. 2019;221(4):349.e1–9.

45. Combs CA, Robinson T, Mekis C, Cooper M, Adie E, Ladwig-Scott E, et al. Enhanced recovery after cesarean: impact on postoperative opioid use and length of stay. Am J Obstet Gynecol. 2021;224(2):237–9.

46. Macias DA, Adhikari EH, Eddins M, Nelson DB, McIntire DD, Duryea EL. A comparison of acute pain management strategies after cesarean delivery. Am J Obstet Gynecol. 2022 Mar;226(3): 407.e1–7. doi: 10.1016/j.ajog.2021.09.003. Epub 2021 Sep 14. PMID: 34534504.

47. Creanga AA, Syverson C, Seed K, Callaghan WM. Pregnancy-related mortality in the United States, 2011–2013. Obstet Gynecol 2017;130(2):366–73. doi: 10.1097/AOG.0000000000002114.

48. James AH, Jamison MG, Brancazio LR, Myers ER. Venous thromboembolism during pregnancy and the postpartum period: incidence, risk factors, and mortality. Am J Obstet Gynecol. 2006;194:1311–15.

49. American College of Obstetricians and Gynecologists. ACOG Practice Bulletin No. 196: thromboembolism in pregnancy. Obstet Gynecol. 2018;132:e1–17.

50. Royal College of Obstetricians and Gynaecologists: Reducing the risk of venous thromboembolism during pregnancy and the puerperium. Green-Top Guideline No. 37a. London: RCOG; 2015.

51. Lu MY, Blanchard CT, Ausbeck EB, Oglesby KR, Page MR, Lazenby AJ et al. Evaluation of a risk-stratified, heparin-based, obstetric thromboprophylaxis protocol. Obstet Gynecol. 2021; 138(4):530–8. doi: 10.1097/AOG.0000000000004521 [published correction appears in Obstet Gynecol. 2022 Feb 1;139(2):344].

52. French LM, Smaill FM. Antibiotic regimens for endometritis after delivery. Cochrane Database Syst Rev. 2004;4:CD001067. doi: 10.1002/14651858.CD001067.pub2.

53. American College of Obstetricians and Gynecologists. ACOG Practice Bulletin No. 205: vaginal birth after cesarean delivery. Obstet Gynecol. 2019;133:e110–27.

54. Landon MB, Hauth JC, Leveno KJ, Spong CY, Leveno KJ, Varner MW, et al. The MFMU Cesarean Registry: maternal and perinatal outcome in women undergoing trial of labor after cesarean delivery. N Engl J Med. 2004;351:2581–9.

55. Silver RM, For the NICHD Maternal-Fetal Medicine Units Network. Morbidity associated with multiple repeat cesarean deliveries. Am J Obstet Gynecol. 2004;191:S17.

56. Rac MW, Dashe JS, Wells CE, Moschos E, McIntire DD, Twickler DM. Ultrasound predictors of placental invasion: the Placenta Accreta Index. Am J Obstet Gynecol 2015;212(3):343.e1–7. doi:10.1016/j.ajog.2014.10.022.

57. Rac MW, Moschos E, Wells CE, McIntire DD, Dashe JS, Twickler DM. Sonographic findings of morbidly adherent placenta in the first trimester. J Ultrasound Med. 2016;35(2):263–9. doi:10.7863/ultra.15.03020.

58. Friedman EA. Primigravid labor: a graphicostatistical analysis. Obstet Gynecol. 1955;6:567–89.

59. Friedman EA. Labor in multiparas: a graphicostatistical analysis. Obstet Gynecol. 1956;8:691–703.

60. Zhang J, Vanveldhuisen P, Troendel J et al. 80 : normal labor patterns in US women. Am J Obstet Gynecol. 2008;199(6 Suppl):S36.

61. O'Driscoll K, Foley M, MacDonald D. Active management of labor as an alternative to cesarean section for dystocia. Obstet Gynecol. 1984;63:485–90.

62. Farah N, Geary M, Connolly G, McKenna P. The caesarean section rate in the Republic of Ireland in 1998. Ir Med J. 2003;96:242–3.

63. Martin JA, Hamilton BE, Sutton PD, Ventura SJ, Menacker F, Munson ML. Births: final data for 2003. Natl Vital Stat Rep 2005;54:85.

64. Rouse DJ, Owen J, Hauth JC. Active-phase labor arrest: oxytocin augmentation for at least 4 hours. Obstet Gynecol. 1999;93:323–8.

65. Rouse DJ, Owen J, Savage KG, Hauth JC. Active phase labor arrest: revisiting the 2-hour minimum. Obstet Gynecol 2001; 98:550–4.

66. Moynihan AT, Hehir MP, Glavey SV, Smith TJ, Morrison JJ. Inhibitory effect of leptin on human uterine contractility in vitro. Am J Obstet Gynecol. 2006;195:504–9.

67. LaCoursiere DY, Bloebaum L, Duncan JD, Varner MW. Population-based trends and correlates in maternal overweight and obesity, Utah, 1991-2001. Am J Obstet Gynecol. 2005;192:832–9.

68. Thacker SB, Stroup D, Chang M. Continuous electronic heart rate monitoring for fetal assessment during labor. Cochrane Database Syst Rev. 2001;2:CD000063. doi: 10.1002/14651858. CD000063.

69. MacDonald D, Grant A, Sheridan-Pereira M, Boylan P, Chalmers I. The Dublin randomized controlled trial of intra-partum fetal heart rate monitoring. Am J Obstet Gynecol. 1985;152:524–39.

70. Zalar RW Jr, Quilligan EJ. The influence of scalp sampling on the cesarean section rate for fetal distress. Am J Obstet Gynecol 1979;135:239–46.

71. Luttkus AK, Friedmann W, Homm-Luttkus C, Dudenhausen JW. Correlation of fetal oxygen saturation to fetal heart rate patterns: evaluation of fetal pulse oximetry with two different oxisensors. Acta Obstet Gynecol Scand. 1998;77:307–12.

72. Carbonne B, Langer B, Goffinet F, Audibert F, Tardif D, Le Goueff F, et al. Multicenter study on the clinical value of fetal pulse oximetry. II. Compared predictive values of pulse oximetry and fetal blood analysis. Am J Obstet Gynecol. 1997; 177;593–8.

73. Dildy GA, Thorp JA, Yeast JD, Clark SL. The relationship between oxygen saturation and pH in umbilical blood: implications for intrapartum fetal oxygen saturation monitoring. Am J Obstet Gynecol. 1996;175:682–7.

74. Garite TJ, Dildy GA, McNamara H, Nageotte MP, Boehm FH, Dellinger EH, et al. A multicenter controlled trial of fetal pulse oximetry in the intrapartum management of nonreassuring fetal heart rate patterns. Am J Obstet Gynecol. 2000;183:1049–58.

75. Bloom SL, Spong CY, Thom E, Varner MW, Rouse DJ, Weininger S, et al. Fetal pulse oximetry and caesarean delivery. N Engl J Med. 2006;355:2195–202.

76. Neilson JP. Fetal electrocardiogram (ECG) for fetal monitoring during labour. Cochrane Database Syst Rev. 2006;3:CD000116. doi: 10.1002/14651858.CD000116.pub5.

77. Belfort MA, Saade GR, Thom E, Blackwell SC, Reddy UM, Thorp JM Jr, et al. A randomized trial of intrapartum fetal ECG ST-segment analysis. N Engl J Med. 2015;373(7):632–41. doi:10.1056/NEJMoa1500600.

78. Hannah ME, Hannah WJ, Hewson SA, Hodnett ED, Saigal S, Willan AR. Planned caesarean section versus planned vaginal birth for breech presentation at term: a randomized multicenter trial. Term Breech Trial Collaborative Group. Lancet. 2000;356:1375–83.

79. Ranney B. The gentle art of external cephalic version. Am J Obstet Gynecol. 1973;116:239–51.

80. Grobman WA, Sandoval G, Rice MM, Bailit JL, Chauhan SP, Costantine MM, et al. Prediction of vaginal birth after cesarean in term gestations: a calculator without race and ethnicity. Eunice Kennedy Shriver National Institute of Child Health and Human Development Maternal-Fetal Medicine Units (MFMU) Network. Am J Obstet Gynecol. 2021 Dec;225(6):664.e1–7. doi: 10.1016/j.ajog.2021.05.021. Epub 2021 May 24.

Chapter 47
Vaginal Birth after Cesarean Delivery

Mark B. Landon

Department of Obstetrics and Gynecology, Ohio State University, Columbus, OH, USA

Trends in vaginal birth after cesarean-trial of labor

Zhang and colleagues reviewed contemporary cesarean delivery practice in the United States and concluded that primary emphasis should be placed on reducing cesarean deliveries for dystocia and repeat operations as these two indications have contributed most to the rise in the overall cesarean rate during the past several decades [1]. Although there had been a renewed interest in improving the trial of labor (TOL) rate in women with prior cesarean in the United States, by 2018 only 13.3% of women had a vaginal birth after prior cesarean (VBAC) delivery in the United States [2]. Remarkably, nearly two thirds of women with a prior cesarean are candidates for a TOL [3]. Thus, most repeat operations can be considered elective and are clearly influenced by physician discretion [4]. TOL rates are consistently lower in the United States compared with European nations, suggesting underuse. As more than 10% of the obstetric population has had previous cesarean delivery, more widespread use of TOL could substantially decrease the overall cesarean delivery rate [5].

The evolution in management of the woman with prior cesarean delivery is apparent through review of several American College of Obstetricians and Gynecologists (ACOG) documents and key studies over the last 25 years. In 1988, the ACOG published "Guidelines for vaginal delivery after a previous cesarean birth," recommending TOL-VBAC (trial of labor to attempt vaginal birth after cesarean delivery), as it became clear that this procedure was safe and did not appear to be associated with excess perinatal morbidity compared with elective cesarean delivery. The guidelines recommended that each hospital develop its own protocol for the management of TOL-VBAC patients and that a woman with one prior low transverse cesarean delivery should be counseled and encouraged to attempt labor in the absence of a contraindication such as a prior classic incision. This recommendation was supported by several large case series attesting to the safety and effectiveness of TOL [6–10]. Driven by this encouraging information, VBAC rates reached a peak of 28.3% by 1996. Third-party payers and managed care organizations embraced these data and began to encourage TOL for women with prior cesarean delivery by tracking provider and institutional VBAC rates. Physicians, feeling pressure to lower cesarean delivery rates, began to offer TOL liberally and may have included less than optimal candidates.

With greater use of TOL-VBAC, reports surfaced suggesting a possibly greater than previously appreciated risk for uterine rupture and its maternal and fetal consequences [11–15]. Descriptions of uterine rupture with maternal hemorrhage, hysterectomy, and adverse perinatal outcomes including death and brain injury set the stage for the precipitous decline in TOL-VBAC use [16–19]. Eventually, ACOG acknowledged the apparent statistically small but potentially catastrophic risks of uterine rupture for both women and their infants during TOL [20]. It was also recognized that such adverse events during a TOL might precipitate malpractice litigation. A more conservative approach to TOL has thus been adopted by even ardent supporters of VBAC. Nonetheless, in its 2019 Practice Bulletin, ACOG once again stated clearly that most women with one previous cesarean delivery with a low transverse incision are candidates for VBAC and should be counseled about VBAC and offered TOL [21].

In response to a growing body of evidence indicating restriction of a woman's access to TOL-VBAC, despite two large-scale contemporary multicenter studies [23,53] that attested to the relative safety of TOL-VBAC, the National Institutes of Health held a consensus development conference concerning VBAC in 2010. The panel concluded that TOL is a reasonable birth option for many women with previous cesarean delivery. The panel also found that existing practice guidelines and the medical liability climate were restricting access to TOL-VBAC and that these factors needed to be addressed [24]. A specific concern raised was the low level of evidence for the requirement for "immediately available" surgical and anesthesia personnel in existing guidelines and the need to reassess this recommendation with reference to other obstetric complications of comparable risk given limited physician and nursing resources. Indeed, by 2017, the relevant ACOG Practice Bulletin no longer included language referencing the immediate availability of surgical and anesthesia personnel but instead recommended that TOL be attempted in facilities that can provide cesarean delivery for situations that are immediate threats to the life of the woman or the fetus [25]. ACOG recognizes that resources for immediate cesarean delivery may not be available at smaller institutions. In such cases, the decision to offer and pursue TOL-VBAC should be carefully considered by patients and their health care providers. It was recommended that the best alternative may be to refer patients to a facility with available resources.

Candidates for trial of labor

The optimal candidate is a woman with a high probability of TOL success and a low likelihood of intrapartum uterine rupture. Women who have had low transverse uterine incision with prior cesarean delivery and have no contraindications to vaginal birth can be considered candidates for TOL. The following are criteria suggested by the ACOG [21] for identifying candidates for VBAC:
* One or two previous low transverse cesarean deliveries
* Clinically adequate pelvis
* No other uterine scars or previous rupture
* TOL attempted in facilities that can provide cesarean delivery for situations that are immediate threats to the life of the woman or fetus

Additionally, several retrospective studies indicate that it may be reasonable to offer TOL to women in other clinical situations. These would include more than two prior low transverse cesarean deliveries, gestation beyond 40 weeks, previous low vertical incision, unknown uterine scar type, and twin gestation [21].

Trial of labor is contraindicated in women at high risk for uterine rupture and should not be attempted in the following circumstances:
* Previous classic or T-shaped incision or extensive transfundal uterine surgery
* Previous uterine rupture
* Medical or obstetric complications that preclude vaginal delivery

Factors affecting the success rates for trial of labor

The overall success rate for TOL-VBAC appears to be in the 70–80% range according to published reports [26–28]. In published series with the highest TOL rates, success was

Table 47.1 Success rates for trial of labor

	VBAC success (%)
Prior indication	
CPD/FTP	63.5
NRFWB	72.6
Malpresentation	83.8
Prior vaginal delivery	
Yes	86.6
No	60.9
Labor type	
Induction	67.4
Augmented	73.9
Spontaneous	80.6

CPD, cephalopelvic disproportion; FTP, failure to progress; NRFWB, nonreassuring fetal well-being; VBAC, vaginal birth after cesarean delivery.
Adapted from Landon et al. [22].

achieved in only 60% of cases [29]. Employing selective criteria resulting in TOL-VBAC rates in the 30% range have been associated with a higher percentage of vaginal births, 70–75% [30,31]. Several predictors of successful TOL have been well described (Table 47.1). The indication for the prior cesarean delivery clearly affects the likelihood of successful VBAC. A history of prior vaginal birth or a nonrecurring condition such as breech or fetal distress is associated with the highest success rates for VBAC. Grobman and colleagues [32] have updated a nomogram for predicting VBAC that has removed race as a potential factor. The prediction model is based on a multivariable logistic regression, including the variables of maternal age, body mass index (BMI), prior vaginal delivery, the occurrences of a VBAC, and a potential recurrent indication for the cesarean delivery. Although there is no reliable method to predict success of TOL-VBAC for an individual woman, several factors have been studied which influence success and these are summarized in the following sections.

Maternal demographics
Demographics such as age, BMI, and insurance status have all been associated with the success of TOL [22]. In a multicenter study of 14 529 term pregnancies undergoing TOL, obese women are more likely to fail TOL as were women older than age 40 years [22]. Obese women attempting VBAC appear to have higher cesarean rates in the latent phase of labor [33]. Conflicting data exist with regard to the impact of payer status (uninsured vs. private patients) on successful TOL-VBAC.

Prior indication for cesarean delivery
Success rates for women whose first cesarean delivery was performed for a nonrecurring indication (breech, nonreassuring fetal well-being) are similar to vaginal delivery rates among nulliparous women [31]. Prior cesarean for breech presentation is associated with the

highest reported success rate for TOL-VBAC of 89% [22,31]. In contrast, prior operative delivery for cephalopelvic disproportion or failure to progress is associated with success rates in the range 50–67% [32–34]. If dystocia was diagnosed between 5 and 9 cm in a prior labor, 67–73% of VBAC attempts are successful compared with only 13% if prior cesarean delivery was performed during the second stage of labor [35].

Prior vaginal delivery

Prior vaginal delivery including prior successful VBAC is apparently the best predictor for a successful TOL [22]. In one series, a prior vaginal delivery was associated with an 87% success rate compared with 61% success in women without prior vaginal delivery [28]. Caughey et al. [36] reported that patients with a previous VBAC had a 93% success rate compared with 85% for women with a vaginal delivery prior to their cesarean birth that were without prior VBAC. Mercer and colleagues [37] have reported that success rate increases from 63.3% with no prior VBAC to 87.6% and 90.9% for those with one or two or more prior VBACs, respectively.

Birthweight

Large for gestational age or fetal macrosomia is associated with a lower likelihood of VBAC success [30]. Birthweight >4000 g is associated with a significantly higher risk of failed TOL [28]. Nonetheless, a 60–70% success rate has been reported in women who attempt VBAC with a macrosomic fetus [38]. Peaceman and colleagues [39] reported only a 34% success rate when the second pregnancy birthweight exceeded the first by 500 g and the prior indication was dystocia, compared with a 64% success rate with other indications.

Labor status and cervical examination

Both labor status and cervical examination upon admission influence VBAC success [40]. An 86% VBAC success rate has been reported in women presenting with cervical dilation greater than or equal to 4 cm [41]. Conversely, the success rate drops to 67% if the cervical examination is less than 4 cm upon admission.

Women who undergo induction of labor are at higher risk for a failed TOL and repeat cesarean delivery compared with those who enter spontaneous labor [22,41]. Landon et al. [22] reported a 67.4% successful VBAC rate in women undergoing induction vs. 80.6% in those entering spontaneous labor. Grinstead and Grobman [42] reported a success rate of 78% in 429 women undergoing induction with prior cesarean delivery. These authors noted several factors in addition to past obstetric history, including indication for induction and need for cervical ripening as determinants of VBAC success [42]. Grobman and colleagues [43] reported a VBAC success rate of 83% in 1208 women with a prior cesarean and prior vaginal delivery undergoing induction of labor.

Previous incision type

Previous incision type may be unknown in certain patients. It appears that women with unknown scar have TOL-VBAC success rates similar to those of women with documented prior low transverse incisions [22]. Similarly, women with previous low vertical incisions do not appear to have lower TOL-VBAC success rates [44].

Multiple prior cesarean deliveries

Women with more than one prior cesarean consistently have a lower likelihood of achieving VBAC [45–47]. Caughey et al. [45] reported a 75% success rate for women with one prior cesarean compared with 62% in women with two prior operations. In contrast, Macones et al.'s [48] large multicenter study of 13,617 women undergoing TOL revealed a 75.5% success rate for women with two prior cesareans, which was not statistically different from the 75% success rate in women with one prior operation (Table 47.2). Metz and colleagues have reported that estimates of TOL-VBAC success using the National Institute of Child Health and Human Development (NICHD) Maternal-Fetal Medicine Units (MFMU) Network prediction model are similar to actual rates in women with two prior cesarean deliveries [49].

Risks of vaginal birth after cesarean-trial of labor

Uterine rupture

The principal risk associated with TOL-VBAC is uterine rupture. This complication is directly attributable to attempted VBAC, as symptomatic rupture is a rare observation at the time of elective repeat operations [50]. An important distinction exists between uterine rupture and uterine scar dehiscence. This difference is clinically relevant as dehiscence most often represents an occult scar separation observed at laparotomy in women with a prior cesarean delivery. The serosa of the uterus is intact with most cases of dehiscence and hemorrhage is absent. In contrast, uterine rupture is a thorough disruption of all uterine layers with consequences of hemorrhage, cord compression, potential abruption, fetal compromise, and significant maternal morbidity. The VBAC literature varies with respect to terminology, definitions, and ascertainment for uterine rupture [51]. A review of 10 observational studies providing the best evidence on the occurrence of

Table 47.2 Success rates for trial of labor with two prior cesarean deliveries

Author	n	Success rate (%)
Miller et al. [46]	2936	75.3
Caughey et al. [45]	134	62.0
Macones et al. [48]	1082	74.6
Landon et al. [47]	876	67.0

symptomatic rupture with TOL revealed rupture rates ranging from 0 in 1000 in a small study to 7.8 in 1000 in the largest study, with a pooled rate of 3.8 per 1000 TOL [51,52]. The large, multicenter, prospective, MFMU Network observational study reported a 0.69% incidence with 124 symptomatic ruptures occurring in 17,898 women undergoing TOL [53].

The rate of uterine rupture depends on both the type and location of the previous uterine incision (Table 47.3). Uterine rupture rates are highest with previous classic or T- or J-shaped incisions, with a reported range of 4–9% [50]. The risk for rupture with a previous low vertical incision is difficult to determine because of small sample size and inconsistency regarding the definition of a low vertical incision. Distinguishing this incision type from classic incision can be arbitrary and low vertical incision is relatively uncommon. Two reports suggest a rupture rate of 0.8–1.1% for prior low vertical scar [54,55]. As noted, women with unknown scar type may not be at increased risk for uterine rupture. This may simply be because most cases are undocumented prior low transverse incisions. Among 3206 women with unknown scar in the MFMU Network report, uterine rupture occurred in 0.5% of TOL [53].

The most serious sequelae of uterine rupture include perinatal death, fetal hypoxic brain injury, and hysterectomy. Guise et al. [52] calculated a rate of 0.14 additional perinatal deaths per 1000 TOL related to uterine rupture. This figure is similar to the MFMU Network study in which there were two neonatal deaths among 124 ruptures, for an overall rate of rupture-related perinatal death of 0.11 per 1000 TOL [53]. In a review of 880 maternal uterine ruptures during a 20-year period, there were 40 perinatal deaths in 91,039 TOL-VBAC for a rate of 0.4 per 1000 [56].

In most studies, perinatal hypoxic brain injury has been an underreported adverse outcome related to uterine rupture. Landon et al. [53] found a significant increase in the rate of hypoxic ischemic encephalopathy (HIE) related to uterine rupture among the offspring of women who underwent TOL at term, compared with the children of women who underwent elective repeat cesarean delivery (0.46 per 1000 TOL vs. no cases, respectively). In 114 cases of uterine rupture at term, seven infants (6.2%) sustained HIE and two of these infants died in the neonatal period.

Maternal hysterectomy is potential sequalae of uterine rupture, particularly if the defect is unrepairable or is associated with uncontrollable hemorrhage. In five studies reporting on hysterectomies related to rupture, seven cases occurred in 60 symptomatic ruptures (13%; range 4–27%), indicating that 3.4 per 10,000 women choosing TOL sustain a rupture that necessitates hysterectomy [51]. The MFMU Network study included 5/124 (4%) rupture cases requiring hysterectomy in which the uterus could not be repaired [53].

Risk factors for uterine rupture

Rates of uterine rupture vary significantly depending on a variety of associated risk factors. In addition to uterine scar type, obstetric history characteristics including number of prior cesareans, prior vaginal delivery, interpregnancy delivery interval, and uterine closure technique have all been reported to affect the risk of uterine rupture. Similarly, factors related to labor management including induction and the use of oxytocin augmentation have all been studied.

Number of prior cesarean deliveries

Miller et al. [46] reported uterine rupture in 1.7% of women with two or more previous cesarean deliveries compared with a frequency of 0.6% in those with one prior operation (odds ratio [OR] 3.06, 95% confidence interval [CI] 1.95–4.79). Interestingly, the risk for uterine rupture was not increased further for women with three prior cesareans. Caughey et al. [45] conducted a smaller study of 134 women with two prior cesareans and controlled for labor characteristics as well as obstetric history. These authors reported a rate of uterine rupture of 3.7% among these 134 women compared with 0.8% in the 3757 women with one previous scar (OR 4.5, 95% CI 1.18–11.5). Macones et al. [48] reported a uterine rupture rate of 20/1082 (1.8%) in women with two prior cesareans compared with 113/12,535 (0.9%) in women with one prior operation (adjusted OR 2.3, 95% CI 1.37–3.85). In contrast, an analysis from the MFMU Network Cesarean Registry found no significant difference in rupture rates in women with one prior cesarean, 115/16,916 (0.7%) vs. multiple prior cesareans, 9/982 (0.9%) [47]. Therefore, it appears that if multiple prior cesarean section is associated with an increased risk for uterine rupture, the magnitude of any additional risk is fairly small. Thus, ACOG considers it reasonable to offer TOL to women with two prior cesareans and to counsel such women based on a combination of factors affecting their probability of achieving a successful TOL [21].

Prior vaginal delivery

A history of prior vaginal delivery is protective against uterine rupture following TOL. Zelop et al. [57] noted the rate of uterine rupture among women with prior vaginal birth to be 0.2% (2/1021) compared with 1.1% (30/2762) among women with no prior vaginal deliveries. A similar

Table 47.3 Risk of uterine rupture with trial of labor

Prior incision type	Rupture rate (%)
Low transverse	0.5–1.0
Low vertical	0.8–1.1
Classic or T shaped	4–9

protective effect of prior vaginal birth has been reported in two large multicenter studies [47,58]. Mercer et al. [37] found a statistically significant decrease in uterine rupture rate with increasing number of successful VBACs. The frequency of uterine rupture declined from 0.87% with no prior VBACs to 0.45% and 0.43% for those with one or two or more prior VBACs respectively.

Uterine closure technique

Single-layer uterine closure technique continues to be widely employed as it may be associated with shorter operating time with similar short-term complications compared with the traditional two-layer technique. A retrospective study of 292 women undergoing TOL found similar rates of uterine rupture for women with one- and two-layer closures [58]. A randomized trial that compared the incidence of uterine rupture in 145 women who received either one- or two-layer closure at their primary cesarean delivery found no cases of uterine rupture in either group; however, the study is of insufficient size to detect a potential difference [59]. A large observational cohort study identified an approximate fourfold increased rate of rupture following single-layer closure technique when compared with previous double-layer closure [60]. These authors conducted a detailed review of operative reports in which the rate of rupture was 15/1489 (3.1%) with single-layer closure vs. 8/1491 (0.5%) with previous double-layer closure. A recent case–control study [61] suggested an increased risk of uterine rupture with single-layer closure (OR 2.69, 95% CI 1.57–5.28) compared to two-layer closures. In the absence of sufficiently powered randomized controlled studies, it remains unclear whether single-layer closure technique increases the risk for uterine rupture.

Interpregnancy interval

Short interpregnancy intervals have been studied as a risk factor for uterine rupture during TOL-VBAC [62–64]. Shipp et al. [62] reported an incidence of rupture of 2.3% (7/311) in women with an interpregnancy delivery interval less than 18 months compared with 1.1% (22/2098) with a longer interpregnancy delivery interval. In contrast, Huang et al. [63] found no increased risk for uterine rupture with an interpregnancy delivery interval of less than 18 months. Bujold et al. [64] have reported that an interpregnancy delivery interval of less than 24 months is independently associated with an almost three-fold increased risk for uterine rupture. These authors reported a rate of rupture of 2.8% in women with a short interval vs. 0.9% in women with more than 2 years since the prior cesarean birth.

Labor induction

Induction of labor appears in most studies to be associated with an increased risk of uterine rupture [54,61]; however, induction may be associated with lower cesarean rates when the comparison is to women managed expectantly [65]. In the prospective MFMU Network cohort analysis, Landon et al. [53] noted the risk for uterine rupture to be elevated nearly threefold (OR 2.86, 95% CI 1.75–4.67), with uterine rupture occurring after 48/4708 (1.0%) of induced TOL vs. 24/6685 (0.4%) for spontaneous onset TOL. The 2010 NICHD Consensus Conference on VBAC concluded that the risk of rupture with induction was elevated nearly two-fold compared to spontaneous labor (1.5% vs. 0.8%). Despite these analyses, it remains unclear whether induction causes uterine rupture or whether an associated risk factor such as cervical status is the ultimate cause.

Conflicting data also exist on whether various induction methods increase the risk for uterine rupture [66]. An increased risk for uterine rupture with use of prostaglandins for labor induction was observed in 15/1960 (0.8%) of women induced without prostaglandin use compared with 9/366 (2.5%) induced with prostaglandin use [67]. Two recent large studies have failed to confirm these findings of an increased risk of rupture associated with the use of prostaglandin agents alone for induction [23,53]. Macones et al. [23] did report an increased risk for rupture in women undergoing induction only if they received a combination of prostaglandins and oxytocin. In the MFMU Network study, there were no cases of uterine rupture when prostaglandin alone was used for induction, which included 52 cases of misoprostol use [53]. The safety of this medication, which is popular for cervical ripening and labor induction, continues to be challenged for women attempting VBAC and is currently contraindicated for use in TOL-VBAC in the United States.

In the largest report of women receiving prostaglandins for labor induction attempting VBAC, Smith and colleagues [68] reported a 0.88% risk for uterine rupture among 4475 women receiving unspecified prostaglandins compared to 0.29% in 4429 cases not receiving this class of medication. Although the relative risk associated with prostaglandin use was elevated, the absolute risk for rupture was impressively low in this series. At present, based on limited data, ACOG suggests avoiding sequential use of prostaglandin E$_2$ and oxytocin in women undergoing TOL. In practice, therefore prostaglandin E2 is rarely used in the United States for induction in women with a scarred uterus. For women with a favorable cervix. amniotomy and oxytocin administration is typically undertaken whereas balloon catheter followed by amniotomy/oxytocin administration is commonly employed when the cervix is unfavorable.

Labor augmentation

Excessive use of oxytocin may be associated with uterine rupture such that careful labor augmentation should be practiced in women attempting TOL [18]. In a case–control study, Leung et al. [18] reported an odds ratio of

2.7 for uterine rupture in women receiving oxytocin augmentation. In contrast, a meta-analysis concluded that oxytocin does not increase the risk for uterine rupture [8]. Dysfunctional labor including arrest disorders increased the risk sevenfold and thus may actually be the primary factor responsible for rupture. In support of this concept, Zelop et al. [57] found that labor augmentation with oxytocin did not significantly increase the risk for rupture. In the MFMU Network study, the rate of uterine rupture with oxytocin augmentation was 52/6009 (0.9%) compared with 24/6685 (0.4%) without oxytocin use [53]. Cahill and colleagues [69] have reported that a dose–response relationship exists between maximal oxytocin dose and the risk for rupture compared with women who attempt VBAC with no oxytocin exposure. At the maximal dose of oxytocin (>20 mU/min), these authors noted the risk of uterine rupture was 2.07%. In summary, oxytocin augmentation may marginally increase the risk for uterine rupture in women undergoing TOL. It follows that judicious use of oxytocin is advised in this population.

Sonographic evaluation of the uterine scar

To better identify women at risk for uterine rupture undergoing TOL, the thickness of the lower uterine segment (LUS) has been evaluated with ultrasound. Bujold and colleagues [70] conducted a prospective study of 125 women with previous cesarean undergoing TOL who received sonographic measurement of the LUS before labor. There were only three cases of uterine rupture; however, receiver operating characteristic curve analysis showed that full thickness of less than 2.3 mm was the optimal cutoff for the prediction of uterine rupture (3/33 vs. 0/92; $P = 0.02$). A recent randomized clinical trial evaluated the utility of measuring the LUS thickness in women with prior cesarean [71]. In the group randomized to ultrasound measurement, cesarean was encouraged if the thickness was less than or equal to 3.5 mm at 36–38 weeks gestation. Thickness was not measured in the control group. The incidence of uterine rupture was 0.4% (5/1472) in the study vs. 0.9% (13/1476) in the control group (RR 0.43, 95% CI 0.15–1.19). Given this trial was underpowered, further research is needed to determine if LUS ultrasound assessment should be routinely used in women with prior cesarean contemplating TOL-VBAC.

Management of vaginal birth after cesarean-trial of labor

Because uterine rupture may be catastrophic, it is recommended that TOL-VBAC should be attempted only in institutions equipped to respond to emergencies that might threaten the life of mother or the fetus. Institutions must consider their personnel resources before offering TOL-VBAC. In practice, TOL is generally reserved for hospitals with physicians capable of performing an emergency cesarean delivery [25].

Recommendations for management of women undergoing a TOL-VBAC continue to be based upon expert opinion. Women attempting VBAC should be encouraged to contact their health care provider promptly when labor starts or rupture of the fetal membranes occur. Continuous electronic fetal heart rate (FHR) monitoring is prudent, although the need for intrauterine pressure catheter monitoring is debatable. Studies examining FHR patterns prior to uterine rupture consistently report that nonreassuring signs, particularly significant variable and prolonged decelerations or bradycardia, are the most common findings accompanying uterine rupture [72,73]. Despite the presence of adequate personnel to proceed with emergency cesarean delivery, prompt intervention does not always prevent fetal neurologic injury or death [52,74]. In one study, significant neonatal morbidity occurred when 18 minutes or longer elapsed between the onset of FHR deceleration and delivery [18]. If prolonged decelerations are preceded by variable or late decelerations, fetal injury may occur as early as 10 minutes from the onset of the terminal deceleration.

TOL is not a contraindication to the use of epidural analgesia. Moreover, epidural use does not appear to affect success rates [22]. Epidural analgesia also does not mask the signs and symptoms of uterine rupture. Oxytocin augmentation is employed as necessary, understanding that excessive uterine activity should be avoided.

Vaginal delivery is conducted as in cases without a history of prior cesarean. Most individuals do not routinely explore the uterus to detect asymptomatic scar dehiscence because these generally heal well. However, excessive vaginal bleeding or maternal hypotension should be promptly evaluated, including assessment for possible uterine rupture. Of 124 cases of uterine rupture accompanying TOL, 14 (11%) were identified following vaginal delivery [53].

Counseling for vaginal birth after cesarean-trial of labor

A pregnant woman with prior cesarean delivery is at risk for both maternal and perinatal complications whether undergoing TOL or choosing elective repeat operation (Table 47.4). It is important to remember that successful VBAC is associated with fewest overall complications whereas a failed TOL-VBAC carries with it greater risks than a scheduled elective repeat operation. Given that one

Table 47.4 Comparison of maternal complications in trial of labor vs. elective repeat cesarean delivery

Complication	Trial of labor (n = 17 898)	Elective repeated cesarean delivery (n = 15 801)	Odds ratio (98% CI)
Uterine rupture	124 (0.7)	0	–
Hysterectomy	41 (0.2)	47 (0.3)	0.77 (0.51–1.17)
Thromboembolic disease	7 (0.04)	10 (0.1)	0.62 (0.24–1.62)
Transfusion	304 (1.7)	158 (1.0)	1.71 (1.41–2.08)
Endometritis	517 (2.9)	285 (1.8)	1.62 (1.40–1.87)
Maternal death	3 (0.02)	7 (0.04)	0.38 (1.10–1.46)
One or more of the above	978 (5.5)	563 (3.6)	1.56 (1.41–1.74)

CI, confidence interval. Adapted from Landon et al. [53].

cannot be certain of success with TOL, the appropriate comparison should be outcomes associated with TOL-VBAC vs. elective repeat operation. Complications of both procedures should be discussed and an attempt should be made to individualize risk for both uterine rupture and the likelihood of successful VBAC (Box 47.1; see Table 47.1). For example, a woman who might require induction of labor may be at slight increased risk for uterine rupture and may be less likely to achieve vaginal delivery. Future childbearing and the risks of multiple cesarean deliveries including risks of placenta previa and accreta should also be considered.

It is important to make every possible effort to obtain the operative records of a prior cesarean delivery to determine previous uterine incision type. This is particularly relevant to cases of prior preterm breech delivery in which vertical uterine incision or a low transverse incision in an undeveloped lower uterine segment might preclude TOL. There may be an increased rate of subsequent uterine rupture in women with a prior preterm cesarean attempting TOL (i.e. failed VBAC) [75]. If previous uterine incision type is unknown, the implications of this missing information should also be discussed.

Following complete informed consent detailing the risks and benefits for the individual woman, the delivery

Box 47.2 Risks associated with elective repeat cesarean delivery

- Increased maternal morbidity compared with successful trial of labor
- Increased length of stay and recovery
- Increased risks for abnormal placentation and hemorrhage with successive cesarean operations

plan should be formulated by both the patient and physician. Documentation of counseling is advisable, and some practitioners prefer to use a specific VBAC consent form. Many women will choose repeat operation after thorough counseling. However, TOL-VBAC should continue to remain an option for most women with prior cesarean delivery (Box 47.2; see also Box 47.1). The magnitude of risks accompanying TOL must be conveyed to the woman undergoing counseling. Presenting solely relative risks should be avoided and rather estimates of absolute risks of complications should be discussed whenever possible. For example, the attributable risk for a serious adverse perinatal outcome (perinatal death or HIE) at term appears to be approximately 1 in 2000 TOL [53]. Combining an independent risk for hysterectomy attributable to uterine rupture at term with the risk for newborn HIE indicates that the chance of one of these adverse events occurring is approximately 1 in 1250 cases [53].

The decision to choose TOL-VBAC may also increase the risk for perinatal death and HIE unrelated to uterine rupture. For women awaiting spontaneous labor beyond 39 weeks, there is a small possibility of unexplained stillbirth which might be avoidable with scheduled repeat operation. A risk for fetal hypoxia and its sequelae may also accompany labor events unrelated to the uterine scar. In the MFMU Network study, five cases of nonrupture-related HIE occurred in term infants in the TOL group compared with none in the elective repeat cesarean population [53].

Box 47.1 Risks associated with trial of labor (TOL)

- Uterine rupture (0.5–1.0/100 TOL) and related morbidity
- Perinatal death and/or encephalopathy (0.5/1000 TOL)
- Hysterectomy (0.3/1000 TOL)
- Increased maternal morbidity with failed trial of labor
- Transfusion
- Endometritis
- Potential risk for perinatal asphyxia with labor (cord prolapse, abruption)
- Potential risk for antepartum stillbirth beyond 39 wk gestation

CASE PRESENTATION

A 31-year-old gravida 3, para 2 at 36 weeks gestation is considering her options for delivery. This woman underwent a low transverse cesarean delivery for breech presentation 4 years previously followed by an elective repeat operation 2 years previously. She would like to avoid a third operation. Her cervical examination is 1 cm dilated and 50% effaced. She will require complete counseling regarding benefits and risks of TOL. The counseling should include a detailed discussion of risks of TOL including potential uterine rupture and its sequelae. The benefits of VBAC including faster recovery and shorter hospital stay will be reviewed. The option of scheduled repeat cesarean delivery should also be presented. If the

patient is considering several future pregnancies, multiple repeat operations may pose additional risk for her of accreta and hysterectomy.

As this woman has a history of two prior cesareans, her overall chance for successful TOL-VBAC may be as high as 75%. A history of two prior cesareans may be associated with a slight increased risk of uterine rupture compared to that in women with one prior operation. This information should be shared in planning the mode of delivery. If the woman desires TOL, expectant management until 41 weeks is advised. If the cervix ripens further, induction may be planned or alternatively, a repeat cesarean could be scheduled.

References

1. Zhang T, Troendle J, Reddy UM, Laughon SK, Branch DW, Burkman R, et al., for the Consortium on Safe Labor. Contemporary cesarean delivery practice in the United States. Am J Obstet Gynecol. 2010;203(4):326.e1–10.
2. Osterman MJK. Recent trends in vaginal birth after cesarean delivery: United States, 2016–2018. NCHS Data Brief. 2020 Mar;(359):1–8.
3. Flamm BL. Vaginal birth after cesarean section: controversies old and new. Clin Obstet Gynecol. 1985;28:735–44.
4. Korst LM, Gregory KD, Fridman MO, Phelan JP. Nonclinical factors affecting women's access to trial of labor after cesarean delivery. Clin Perinatol. 2011;38:193–216.
5. Landon MB. Vaginal birth after cesarean delivery. Clin Perinatol. 2008;35:491–504.
6. Flamm BL, Newman LA, Thomas SJ, Fallon D, Yoshida MM. Vaginal birth after cesarean delivery: results of a 5-year multicenter collaborative study. Obstet Gynecol 1990;76:750–4.
7. Flamm B, Goings J, Liu Y, Wolde-Tsadik G. Elective repeat cesarean section delivery versus trial of labor: a prospective multicenter study. Obstet Gynecol. 1994;83:927–32.
8. Rosen MG, Dickinson JC, Westhoff CL. Vaginal birth after cesarean: a meta-analysis of morbidity and mortality. Obstet Gynecol. 1991;77:465–70.
9. Paul RH, Phelan JP, Yeh S. Trial of labor in the patient with a prior cesarean birth. Am J Obstet Gynecol. 1985;151:297–304.
10. Martin JN Jr, Harris BA Jr, Huddleston JF, Morrison JC, Propst MG, Wiser WL, et al. Vaginal delivery following previous cesarean birth. Am J Obstet Gynecol. 1983;146:255–63.
11 Beall M, Eglinton GS, Clark SL, Phelan JP. Vaginal delivery after cesarean section in women with unknown types of uterine scars. J Reprod Med. 1984;29:31–5.
12 Pruett K, Kirshon B, Cotton D. Unknown uterine scar in trial of labor. Am J Obstet Gynecol. 1988;159:807–10.
13 Scott J. Mandatory trial of labor after cesarean delivery: an alternative viewpoint. Obstet Gynecol. 1991;77:811–14.
14 Pitkin RM. Once a cesarean? Obstet Gynecol. 1991;77:939.

15. Sachs BP, Kobelin C, Castro MA, Frigoletto F. The risks of lowering the cesarean-delivery rate. N Engl J Med. 1990;340;54–7.
16. Farmer RM, Kirschbaum T, Potter D, Strong TH, Medaris AL. Uterine rupture during a trial of labor after previous cesarean section. Am J Obstet Gynecol. 1991;165:996–1001.
17. Boucher M, Tahilramaney MP, Eglinton GS, Phelan JP. Maternal morbidity as related to trial of labor after previous cesarean delivery: a quantitative analysis. J Reprod Med. 1984;29:12–16.
18. Leung AS, Farmer RM, Leung EK, Medearis AL, Paul RH, et al. Risk factors associated with uterine rupture during trial of labor after cesarean delivery: a case–control study. Am J Obstet Gynecol. 1993;168:1358–63.
19. Arulkumaran S, Chua S, Ratnam SS. Symptoms and signs with scar rupture: value of uterine activity measurements. Aust N Z J Obstet Gynaecol. 1992;32:208–12.
20. American College of Obstetricians and Gynecologists. ACOG Practice Bulletin No. 5: vaginal birth after previous cesarean delivery: clinical management guidelines for obstetricians-gynecologists. Washington, DC: American College of Obstetricians and Gynecologists; 1999.
21. American College of Obstetricians and Gynecologists. ACOG Practice Bulletin No. 205: vaginal birth after cesarean delivery. Washington, DC: American College of Obstetricians and Gynecologists; 2019.
22. Landon MB, Leindecker S, Spong CY, for the National Institute of Child Health and Human Development Maternal-Fetal Medicine Units Network. The MFMU Cesarean Registry. Factors affecting the success and trial of labor following prior cesarean delivery. Am J Obstet Gynecol. 2005;193:1016–23.
23. Macones G, Peipert J, Nelson D, Odibo A, Stevens EJ, Stamilio DM, et al. Maternal complications with vaginal birth after cesarean delivery: a multicenter study. Am J Obstet Gynecol. 2005;193:1656–62.
24. National Institutes of Health Consensus Development Conference Statement. Vaginal birth after cesarean: new insights, March 8-10, 2010. Obstet Gynecol 2010;115(6):1279–95.

25. American College of Obstetricians and Gynecologists. Practice Bulletin No. 130: prediction and prevention of preterm birth. Washington, DC: American College of Obstetricians and Gynecologists; 2017.

26. Whiteside DC, Mahan CS, Cook JC. Factors associated with successful vaginal delivery after cesarean section. J Reprod Med. 1983;28:785–8.

27. Silver RK, Gibbs RS. Prediction of vaginal delivery in patients with a previous cesarean section who require oxytocin. Am J Obstet Gynecol. 1987;156:57–60.

28. Flamm BL. Vaginal birth after cesarean section. In: Flamm BL, Quilligan EJ, eds. Cesarean section: guidelines for appropriate utilization. New York: Springer-Verlag; 1995. p.51–64.

29. Gregory KD, Korst LM, Cane P, Platt LD, Kahn K. Vaginal birth after cesarean and uterine rupture rates in California. Obstet Gynecol. 1999;93:985–9.

30. Elkousky MA, Samuel M, Stevens E, Peipert JF, Macones G. The effect of birthweight on vaginal birth after cesarean delivery success rates. Am J Obstet Gynecol. 2003;188:824–30.

31. Coughlan C, Kearney R, Turner MJ. What are the implications for the next delivery in primigravidae who have an elective cesarean section for breech presentation? Br J Obstet Gynaecol. 2002;109:624–6.

32. Grobman WA, Sandoval G, Rice MM, Bailit JL, Chauhan SP, Costantine MM, et al. Prediction of vaginal birth after cesarean delivery in term gestations: a calculator without race and ethnicity. Am J Obstet Gynecol. 2021;225 (6):664.e1–7.

33. Faucett AM, Allshouse AA, Donnelly, Metz TD. Do obese women receive the necessary interventions to achieve vaginal birth after cesarean? Am J Perinatol. 2016;33:991–5.

34. Jongen VHWM, Halfwerk MGC, Brouwer WK. Vaginal delivery after previous cesarean section for failure of second stage of labour. Br J Obstet Gynaecol. 1998;195:1079.

35. Hoskins IA, Gomez JL. Correlation between maximum cervical dilation at cesarean delivery and subsequent vaginal birth after cesarean delivery. Obstet Gynecol. 1997;89:591–3.

36. Caughey AB, Shipp TD, Repke JT, Zelop C, Cohen A, Lieherman E. Trial of labor after cesarean delivery: the effects of previous vaginal delivery. Am J Obstet Gynecol. 1998;179;938–41.

37. Mercer BM, Gilbert S, Landon MB, Spong CY, Leveno KJ, Rouse DJ,et al., for the National Institute of Child Health and Human Development (NICHD) Maternal-Fetal Medicine Units Network (MFMU). Labor outcomes with increasing number of prior vaginal births after cesarean delivery. Obstet Gynecol. 2008;111:285–91.

38. Flamm BL, Goings JR. Vaginal birth after cesarean section: is suspected fetal macrosomia a contraindication? Obstet Gynecol. 1989;74:694–7.

39. Peaceman AM, Gersnoviez R, Landon MB, Spong CY, Leveno KJ, Varner MW, et al., for the NICHD Maternal-Fetal Medicine Units Network. The MFMU Cesarean Registry: impact of fetal size on trial of labor successes for patients with prior cesarean for dystocia. Am J Obstet Gynecol. 2005;195(4):1127–31.

40. Weinstein D, Benshushan A, Tanos V, Zilberstein R, Rojansky N. Predictive score for vaginal birth after cesarean section. Am J Obstet Gynecol. 1996;174:192–8.

41. Shipp TD, Zelop CM, Repke JT, Cohen A, Caughey AB, Lieberman E. Labor after previous cesarean: influence of prior indication and parity. Obstet Gynecol. 2000;95:913–16.

42. Grinstead J, Grobman WA. Induction of labor after one prior cesarean: predictors of vaginal delivery. Obstet Gyneco.l 2004;103:534–38.

43. Grobman WA, Gilbert S, Landon MB, Spong CY, Leveno KJ, Rouse DJ, et al. Outcomes of induction of labor after one prior cesarean. Obstet Gynecol. 2007;109(2 Pt 1):262–9.

44. Rosen MG, Dickinson JC. Vaginal birth after cesarean: a metaanalysis of indicators for success. Obstet Gynecol. 1990;76:865–9.

45. Caughey AB, Shipp TD, Repke JT, Zelop CM, Cohen A, Lieberman E. Rate of uterine rupture during a trial of labor in women with one or two prior cesarean deliveries. Am J Obstet Gynecol. 1999;181:872–6.

46. Miller DA, Diaz FG, Paul RH. Vaginal birth after cesarean: a 10 year experience. Obstet Gynecol. 1994;84:255–8.

47. Landon MB, Spong CY, Thom E, for the National Institute of Child Health and Human Development Maternal-Fetal Medicine Units Network. Maternal morbidity associated with multiple repeat cesarean deliveries. Obstet Gynecol 2006;107:1226–32.

48. Macones GA, Cahill A, Para E, Stamilio DM, Ratcliffe S, Stevens E, et al. Obstetric outcomes in women with two prior cesarean deliveries: is vaginal birth after cesarean delivery a viable option? Am J Obstet Gynecol. 2005;192:1223–9.

49. Metz TD, Allshouse AA, Faucett AM, Grobman WA. Validation of vaginal birth after cesarean delivery prediction model in women with two prior cesarean deliveries. Obstet Gynecol. 2015:125:948–52.

50. Mozurkewich EL, Hutton EK. Elective repeat cesarean delivery versus trial of labor: a meta-analysis of the literature from 1989 to 1999. Am J Obstet Gynecol. 2000;183:1187–97.

51. Agency for Health Care Research and Quality. Vaginal birth after cesarean (VBAC). AHRQ Publication No. 03-E018. Rockville, MD: Agency for Health Care Research and Quality; 2003.

52. Guise JM, McDonagh MS, Osterweil P, Nygren P, Chan BK, Helfand M. Systematic review of the incidence and consequences of uterine rupture in women with previous cesarean section. BMJ. 2004;329:19–25.

53. Landon MB, Hauth JC, Leveno KJ, Spong CY, Leindecker S, Varner MW, et al., for the National Institute of Child Health and Human Development Maternal-Fetal Medicine Units Network. Maternal and perinatal outcomes associated with a trial of labor after prior cesarean delivery. N Engl J Med. 2004;351:2581–9.

54. Naif RW 3rd, Ray MA, Chauhan SP, Roach H, Blake PG, Martin JN Jr. Trial of labor after cesarean delivery with a lower-segment, vertical uterine incision: is it safe? Am J Obstet Gynecol. 1995;172:1666–73.

55. Shipp TD, Zelop CM, Repke TJ, Cohen A, Caughey AB, Lieberman E. Intrapartum uterine rupture and dehiscence in patients with prior lower uterine segment vertical and transverse incisions. Obstet Gynecol. 1999;94:735–40.

56. Chauhan SP, Martin JN Jr, Henrichs CE, Morrison JC, Magann EF. Maternal and perinatal complications with uterine rupture in 142 075 patients who attempted vaginal birth after cesarean

delivery: a review of the literature. Am J Obstet Gynecol. 2003;189:408–17.

57. Zelop CM, Shipp TD, Repke JT, Cohen A, Caughey AB, Lieberman E. Uterine rupture during induced or augmented labor in gravid women with one prior cesarean delivery. Am J Obstet Gynecol. 1999;181:882–6.

58. Tucker JM, Hauth JC, Hodgkins P, Owen J, Winkler CL. Trial of labor after a one- or two-layer closure of a low transverse uterine incision. Obstet Gynecol. 1993;168:545–6.

59. Chapman SJ, Owen J, Hauth JC. One-versus two-layer closure of a low transverse cesarean: the next pregnancy. Obstet Gynecol. 1997;89:16–18.

60. Bujold E, Bujold C, Hamilton EF, Harel F, Gauthier RJ. The impact of a single-layer or double-layer closure on uterine rupture. Am J Obstet Gynecol. 2002;186:1326–30.

61. Bujold E, Goyet M, Marcoux S, Brassard N, Cormier B, Hamilton E, et al. The role of uterine closure in the risk of uterine rupture. Obstet Gynecol. 2010;116(1):L43–50.

62. Shipp TD, Zelop CM, Repke JT, Cohen A, Lieberman E. Interdelivery interval and risk of symptomatic uterine rupture. Obstet Gynecol. 2001;97:175–7.

63. Huang WH, Nakashima DK, Rummey PJ, Keegan KA Jr, Chan K. Interdelivery interval and the success of vaginal birth after cesarean delivery. Obstet Gynecol. 2002;99:41–4.

64. Bujold E, Mehta SH, Bujold C, Gauthier RJ. Interdelivery interval and uterine rupture. Am J Obstet Gynecol. 2002;187:199–202.

65. Palatnik A., Grobman W. Induction of labor versus expectant management for women with a prior cesarean delivery. Am J Obstet Gynecol. 2015;212(3):358.e1–6.

66. Stone JL, Lockwood CJ, Berkowitz G, Alvarez M, Lapinski R, Valcamonico A, et al. Use of cervical prostaglandin E2 gel in patients with previous cesarean section. Am J Perinatol. 1994;11:309–12.

67. Lydon-Rochelle M, Holt V, Easterling TR, Martin DP. Risk of uterine rupture during labor among women with a prior cesarean delivery. N Engl J Med. 2001;345:36–8.

68. Smith GC, Peil JP, Pasupathy D, Dobbie R. Factors predisposing to perinatal death related to uterine rupture during attempted vaginal birth after cesarean section: retrospective cohort study. BMJ. 2004;329:359–60.

69. Cahill AG, Waterman BM, Stamilio DM, Odibo AO, Allsworth JE, Evanoff B, et al. Higher maximum doses of oxytocin are associated with an unacceptably high risk for uterine patients attempting vaginal birth after cesarean delivery. Am J Obstet Gynecol. 2008;199(1):32.e1–5.

70. Bujold E, Jastrow N, Simoneau J, Brunet S, Gauthier RJ. Prediction of complete uterine rupture by sonographic evaluation of the lower uterine segment. Obstet Gynecol. 2009; 201:320.e1–6.

71. Rozenberg P. Sénat MV, Deruelle P, Winer N, Simon E, Ville Y, et al. Evaluation of the usefulness of ultrasound measurement of the lower uterine segment before delivery of women with a prior cesarean delivery: a randomized trial. Am J Obstet Gynecol. 2022;226:253.e1.

72. Jones R, Nagashima A, Hartnett-Goodman M, Goodlin R. Rupture of low transverse cesarean scars during trial of labor. Obstet Gynecol. 1991;77:815–17.

73. Rodriguez M, Masaki D, Phelan J, Diaz F. Uterine rupture: are intrauterine pressure catheters useful in the diagnosis? Am J Obstet Gynecol. 1989;161:666–9.

74. Clark SL, Scott JR, Porter TF, Schlappy DA, McClellan V, Burton DA. Is vaginal birth after cesarean less expensive than repeat cesarean delivery? Am J Obstet Gynecol. 2000;182: 599–602.

75. Scissione AC, Landon MB, Leveno KJ, Spong CY, Macpherson C, Varner MW, et al., for the NICHD Maternal-Fetal Medicine Units Network. Previous preterm cesarean delivery and risk of subsequent uterine rupture. Am J Obstet Gynecol. 2008;111(3): 648–53.

Chapter 48
Breech Delivery

G.J. Hofmeyr[1,2] *and M.N. Nassali*[1]

[1] Department of Obstetrics and Gynaecology, University of Botswana, Gaborone, Botswana
[2] University of the Witwatersrand, Johannesburg, South Africa, and Walter Sisulu University, East London, South Africa

Breech presentation occurs in 3–4% of pregnancies at term compared to 25% at earlier gestations. The uterus with its pear shape accommodates the fetal alignment that best fits the intrauterine space. Toward term, most fetuses assume a cephalic presentation with the broader body and legs located in the wider fundus while the head occupies the narrower lower segment. Failure to do so before birth may be due to maternal and/or fetal factors such as multiparity, prematurity, multiple pregnancy, extended fetal legs, placenta previa, contracted pelvis, abnormalities of the uterus, increased or reduced amniotic fluid volume, fetal anomalies, maternal hypothyroidism, short umbilical cord, fetal growth restriction, fetal asphyxia, primiparity, female sex, maternal anticonvulsant therapy, older maternal age or otherwise benign factors such as cornual placental location. Prior breech presentation [1] and a parent having been born breech [2] are also risk factors. Breech presentation may be a marker for subtle fetal deficiencies, as apparently healthy breech babies have on average poorer long-term neurodevelopmental scores than cephalic babies, irrespective of the mode of delivery.

Types of breech

The commonest type of breech presentation (50–70% at term) is frank breech, with both hips flexed and both knees extended so that the feet are adjacent to the head. Incomplete (footling or kneeling) breech (10–40%) has one or both hips extended. Complete (flexed) breech (5–10%) has hips and knees flexed.

Frank and complete breeches are best suited for planned vaginal birth. Successful passage of the broader presenting part with thighs (frank) or thighs and legs (complete) passing through the mother's cervix and pelvis alongside the body is reassuring evidence that there is adequate space for the smaller aftercoming head, unless the baby is very small. In contrast, the incomplete/footling breech may advance through an inadequately dilated cervix or inadequate pelvis, followed by difficulty with delivery of the aftercoming head.

Diagnosis

Diagnosis prior to 36 weeks gestation may be counterproductive. It does not affect clinical management and may evoke unnecessary anxiety over what is often a transient finding. If breech presentation is identified in early pregnancy, it is important to try to reassure the parents that this is a common occurrence in normal pregnancies. At 36 weeks gestation, careful routine abdominal examination is important to allow for clinical planning, particularly for the option of external cephalic version. The mother may report subcostal discomfort due to pressure of the fetal head, and increased perception of fetal kicks in the lower abdomen. Key clinical features are a presenting part with lack of the sulcus between shoulders and head, and "ballotment" of the fetal pole in the uterine fundus: the fetal head can be moved freely back and forth between thumb and fingertips, whereas movement of the breech, which is accompanied by movement of the whole body, is more sluggish. However, even in expert hands, clinical diagnosis is fallible in up to 20% of cases, and in doubtful cases ultrasound examination may be needed to confirm the diagnosis.

Prevention

Various antenatal postural maneuvers such as the knee-chest position to promote spontaneous cephalic version have shown promise in observational studies but not in randomized trials. Augmenting amniotic fluid volume by encouraging adequate oral intake of fluids is another theoretical approach but has not been tested in randomized trials.

Queenan's Management of High-Risk Pregnancy: An Evidence-Based Approach, Seventh Edition. Edited by Catherine Y. Spong and Charles J. Lockwood.
© 2024 John Wiley & Sons Ltd. Published 2024 by John Wiley & Sons Ltd.

Complications of vaginal breech delivery

Complications described following difficult breech delivery include intracranial hemorrhage, cervical spine injury, injury to liver, adrenal glands or spleen, bladder rupture, pharyngeal diverticulum, brachial plexus palsy, scrotal/testicular/labial trauma, skull fracture, and long bone fracture [3].

Approach to management

For breech presentation after 36 weeks gestation, careful clinical and ultrasound examination is needed to exclude important factors that may have accounted for the breech presentation, particularly placenta previa, impaired fetal growth, fetal compromise, fetal anomalies such as hydrocephaly or anencephaly, abnormalities of amniotic fluid volume, and (very rarely) advanced extrauterine pregnancy. The type of breech presentation, estimated weight of the baby, and the degree of head flexion are also important for planning the route of delivery.

External cephalic version at or near term

External cephalic version (manipulating the baby transabdominally to the cephalic presentation) reduces the chance of breech presentation at birth, with very low complication rates. Reported success rates range from about 40% to 70% and are dependent on factors such as operator experience and the existence of a designated external cephalic version service. Review of both randomized and nonrandomized trials in high-income settings found a reduction in noncephalic presentation at birth of 55% and of cesarean birth by 43%, with 29% overall increase in 5-minute Apgar scores <7 [4]. There was no increase in perinatal death or neonatal admission. There was no increase in low Apgar scores in the Cochrane review restricted to randomized trials [5]. Details of the procedure are beyond the scope of this chapter. We have produced a video demonstrating the technique that is available on the World Health Organization Reproductive Health Library: https://www.youtube.com/playlist?list=PL68EE6D503647EA2F.

Planned mode of delivery

Approaches to the mode of delivery for breech presentation have been influenced by the Term Breech Trial [6]: planned cesarean (actual rate 90%) vs. planned vaginal birth (actual rate 57%) was associated with a 67%

reduction in the primary outcome "perinatal mortality, neonatal mortality or severe morbidity" (17/1039 [1.6%] vs. 52/1039 [5.0%]). However, follow-up at 2 years of age (80% of 1159 children mainly from high-resource settings) found nonsignificantly higher rates for the outcome "death or neurodevelopmental delay" in the planned cesarean birth group (3.1%) vs. the planned vaginal birth group (2.8%) [7], and there were 41% more infant medical problems following planned cesarean birth. This suggests that short-term adverse effects of planned vaginal birth were balanced by longer term adverse effects of planned cesarean birth, possibly related to lower gestational age at planned delivery, effects of cesarean birth on the infant microbiome, or effects on mother–infant interactions. The Term Breech Trial was not powered for statistical comparison of perinatal/neonatal mortality (3/1039 vs. 13/1039 overall, and in particular for high-resource settings 0/514 vs. 3/511 respectively).

The earlier publication of the short-term results of the Term Breech Trial in 2000 had a major impact on practice globally, before the more reassuring results of the 2-year follow-up were known. Even the longer-term results should not be used to guide practice in isolation, as the trial was unable to measure important outcomes such as risks to the mother in subsequent pregnancies including placenta accreta spectrum, uterine rupture, and need for repeat cesarean delivery, as well as the mother's preferences.

Shortly after publication of the Term Breech Trial results, the large PREMODA (Presentation et Mode d'Accouchement) prospective cohort study took place in 138 maternity units in France and Belgium (2001–2002), where planned vaginal delivery was a common practice and strict criteria were met before and during labor. The study included all women with a singleton fetus in breech presentation ≥ 37 weeks gestation (n=8105). Cesarean delivery was planned for 5579 women (68.8%) and vaginal delivery for 2526 (31.2%). Of the women with planned vaginal deliveries, 1796 delivered vaginally (71.0%). The rate of fetal and neonatal mortality and severe neonatal morbidity was low in the overall population (1.59%, 95% confidence interval [CI] 1.33–1.89) and in the planned vaginal delivery group (1.60%, 95% CI 1.14–2.17). It did not differ significantly between the planned vaginal and cesarean delivery groups (unadjusted odds ratio 1.10, 95% CI 0.75–1.61), even after controlling for confounding variables (adjusted odds ratio 1.40, 95% CI 0.89–2.23) [8]. Severe maternal morbidity and mortality were not different between planned cesarean and planned vaginal birth [9].

Subsequent large observational studies have confirmed the safety of planned vaginal breech birth in the context of clear management protocols, as well as confirming increased childhood illness associated with cesarean birth, such as a threefold increase in inflammatory bowel disease hospitalizations [10]. Meta-analysis including observational studies estimated low absolute risks of planned vaginal delivery for perinatal mortality (0.3%), fetal neurologic morbidity (0.7%), birth trauma (0.7%), 5-minute Apgar score <7 (2.4%), and neonatal asphyxia (3.3%) [11]. North American professional associations have endorsed the principle of planned vaginal birth in selected cases on the basis of shared decision-making [12,13].

Delivery planning

The primary options for persistent breech presentation in the absence of, or following failed, external cephalic version are scheduled cesarean delivery at full term (39 weeks gestation) or awaiting onset of labor and attempting vaginal breech delivery. A third option is planned cesarean birth in early labor. This maximizes the opportunity for spontaneous cephalic version and fetal maturation but introduces the risk of precipitate labor and birth before cesarean delivery can be performed.

Vaginal breech delivery

Criteria for vaginal beech delivery

Criteria that are used to select patients suitable for vaginal breech delivery include the following [3]: estimated fetal weight 2000–4000 g by either clinical or ultrasound estimation (others have suggested 2500–3800 g [14] or 2500–4000 g [10]), complete or frank breech presentation, fetal head flexed or military position on ultrasound examination, adequate maternal pelvis assessed clinically or radiographically, normal fetal morphology, experienced operator, and informed consent.

Induction and augmentation of labor

In the PREMODA prospective cohort study, induction of labor for breech presentation was not found to increase neonatal mortality or severe neonatal morbidity compared with planned cesarean delivery [15,16]. Augmentation of labor is controversial because of concern that poor progress of labor may be a sign of relative fetopelvic disproportion.

Care during labor

As for cephalic presentations, labor management should focus on evidence-based care that promotes a positive childbirth experience, including labor companionship, avoiding the supine position, adequate hydration, offering analgesia, and monitoring the fetal condition [17]. Particular attention should be paid to the risk of cord prolapse and avoiding premature bearing down. Preparation for delivery should include secure venous access and availability of both oxytocin and a tocolytic, as well as a team experienced in vaginal breech birth.

Conduct of vaginal breech delivery

Maternal positioning

Observational studies have suggested better birth outcomes with a physiological approach using upright postures [18]. For the more conventional dorsal approach the mother is positioned at the end of the bed with feet in stirrups, either semi-sitting or with pronounced lateral tilt to avoid supine aortocaval compression.

Delivery and maneuvers

Techniques for breech delivery have developed through experience rather than robust trials. The methods described here are consistent with recommendations of the Society of Obstetricians and Gynaecologists of Canada [12]. The guiding principle of vaginal breech delivery is that the baby should be expelled in a flexed position. A key member of the team is a skilled birth attendant to encourage effective bearing down with uterine contractions. The inevitable temptation to apply traction should be resisted, as traction causes extension of the arms and head and complicates the delivery. If spontaneous delivery of the breech does not occur after 30 to 60 minutes of bearing down, consider tocolysis and cesarean birth rather than breech extraction. Episiotomy may be used for obstetric indications, not routinely. Once the breech is delivered and further progress is inevitable, consider judicious use of an intravenous oxytocin infusion to expedite the delivery.

Once the umbilicus is visible, pull down a small loop of cord to avoid undue tension on the cord. With a frank breech, if progress is prevented by splinting of the baby's body by the extended legs, use Pinard's maneuver with gentle finger pressure to the baby's popliteal fossae to flex the knees and thereby deliver the legs. If the baby's back tends to rotate posteriorly, hold the baby's pelvis with a dry towel, and gently keep the back directed anteriorly (toward the ceiling) as it descends, without applying traction. Ideally, the arms and shoulders will deliver spontaneously in a flexed position, and all that will be needed is support to avoid too rapid delivery of the head (discussed later).

If the shoulders do not deliver spontaneously, the Lövset maneuver may be tried first: holding the baby's pelvis (not abdomen) with a dry towel, rotate through 180°, keeping the back anterior, so that what was the posterior shoulder delivers under the symphysis pubis. The arm may follow spontaneously, otherwise pass two fingers over the back and shoulder, as far as the forearm, and sweep the arm in front of the baby's face and chest. Now rotate 180° in the opposite direction to deliver the other shoulder and arm. Gentle traction on the delivered arm in the direction of the rotation may assist this rotation. If the Lövset maneuver is unsuccessful, deliver each shoulder and arm digitally. Pass two fingers up the baby's back and over the shoulder. Resist the temptation to apply pressure to the

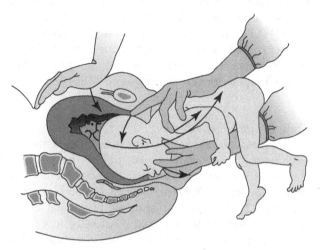

Figure 48.1 For the Mauriceau-Smellie-Veit method, support the baby's body astride your right forearm with two fingers on the malar bones to maintain flexion. Place your left hand over the baby's back with second and fourth fingers on the shoulders and third finger on the occiput to maintain flexion. Steadily deliver the head in this flexed position assisted by suprapubic fundal pressure.

humerus, as it will often snap (though if this happens, healing is usually excellent). Continue until the forearm is reached, and sweep the forearm in front of the face and chest to deliver the arm and shoulder.

Once the shoulders have delivered, encourage the mother to push, without applying traction. Use suprapubic pressure to the fundus of the uterus to assist flexion and descent of the head into the pelvis. Once the head is fully engaged in the pelvis with the hairline visible beneath the symphysis pubis, assist the delivery of the head in one of three ways (Figures 48.1 and 48.2).

For forceps delivery, the Piper's forceps are purpose designed, with backward curvature of the handles. An assistant supports the baby's body using a dry towel as a hammock, no more than 45° above the horizontal. Apply the forceps to the baby's head from below the chest, holding the shank of the left blade lightly with the left hand while guiding the blade into place with fingertips of the right hand, and vice versa for the right blade. Deliver the head following the pelvic curve of Carus while an assistant supports the perineum. Standard long curved forceps may be used, but more elevation of the baby's body is required.

THE BURNS–MARSHALL MANEUVER

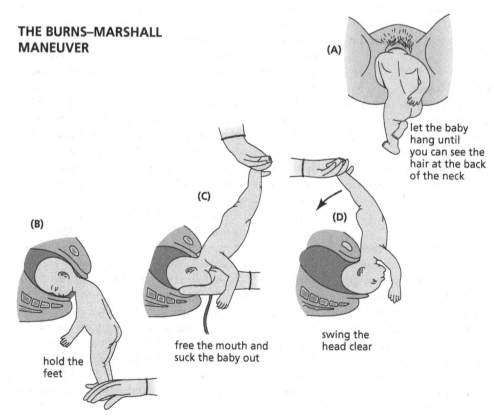

(A) let the baby hang until you can see the hair at the back of the neck

(B) hold the feet

(C) free the mouth and suck the baby out

(D) swing the head clear

Figure 48.2 For the Burns-Marshall method, grasp the baby's ankles with the left hand using a dry towel and with gentle outward traction, raise the feet through an arc, with the right hand over the perineum to control the delivery of the head.

Cesarean breech delivery

At cesarean birth after guiding the breech through the uterotomy incision, use fundal pressure to expel the baby in a flexed position. Maneuvers to assist delivery of the shoulders and head are similar to those described for vaginal delivery. Pay particular attention to avoiding excessive extension of the baby's neck.

Complications to anticipate

The important complications during delivery are delay in delivery of the shoulders or head, which are managed as described previously. In the very rare instance of undeliverable head, tocolysis with partial replacement of the fetus and cesarean delivery may be attempted [19]. Alternatively, partial symphysiotomy may be performed with local analgesia to facilitate delivery [12]. A firm catheter is placed in the urethra, which is moved laterally with the forefinger of the left hand inside the vagina to avoid injury. If care is taken to incise only the anterior fibers so that the posterior fibers are not cut but torn apart, morbidity is extremely low [20]. This is done by cutting the anterior 75% thickness of the symphysis pubis from the top edge to the bottom edge, with a slight sawing motion. As the fetal head is delivered (preferably with forceps), the posterior fibers are torn, and the symphysis separates to the minimum extent necessary for birth of the head.

Twin pregnancy with leading breech presentation

A large prospective cohort study found no increased risk of perinatal morbidity or mortality for planned vaginal birth [21]. Watch out for chin-to-chin locking if the second twin is cephalic.

Noncephalic second twin

Vaginal birth is a reasonable option for the noncephalic second twin after vaginal birth of the first twin at ≥32 weeks gestation, based on data from the Jumeaux Mode d'Accouchement study, a nationwide prospective population-based cohort study of twin deliveries performed in 176 maternity units in France from February 2014 through March 2015. Noncephalic and cephalic second twin presentations were associated with similar low composite neonatal mortality and morbidity rates. Noncephalic second twins were delivered by breech extraction. Cesarean delivery rates for the second twin were lower in the breech than in the cephalic group [22].

Internal podalic version and total breech extraction for cephalic second twins

Internal version and breech extraction has been shown to reduce the time to delivery of the cephalic second twin but not to improve perinatal outcome [23].

Preterm breech birth

Prematurity (estimated weight <1500 g) is regarded as a contraindication to planned vaginal delivery. The rationale is that the relatively larger fetal head found at earlier gestational ages may be entrapped by an incompletely dilated cervix. This complication may require intervention with bilateral incisions of the cervix (Dührssen's incisions). The risk of head entrapment confirmed in an observational study of breech births at 26 to 29 6/7 weeks gestation was 1.7%. However, there was no overall difference in perinatal mortality or severe morbidity between units with a policy for vaginal vs. cesarean delivery [24]. Moreover, in the prospective nationwide population-based EPIPAGE-2 cohort study in France, planned cesarean delivery for breech presentation at 26 to 34 weeks gestation was not associated with improved survival, survival without severe morbidity, or survival at 2 years without neurosensory impairment [25]. Strategies to facilitate safe vaginal birth for very small preterm babies include delivery with intact membranes [26].

Training

A key factor in safe vaginal breech birth is the experience and confidence of the health care provider. Trends to increased use of cesarean delivery have resulted in loss of skills for vaginal breech delivery. Even with a policy of routine cesarean delivery, vaginal breech births are inevitable from time to time due to precipitate delivery or maternal preference. It is essential that labor and delivery unit staff maintain high levels of skill, if necessary through regular simulation (manikin) skills training. We have produced a teaching video on breech delivery, including symphysiotomy technique, which is included in the World Health Organization Reproductive Health Library: https://www.youtube.com/playlist?list=PL68EE6D503647EA2F.

Conclusion

Care for women with breech presentation requires technical skill, sound obstetric judgment, an in-depth understanding of the relative short- and long-term risks of alternative management options, an ability to communicate this information effectively, and respect for the rights of mothers to make informed choices in line with their personal beliefs and priorities [12].

CASE PRESENTATION 1 (by previous chapter authors E.R. Yeomans and L.C. Gillstrap)

A 30-year-old gravida 3, para 2 was admitted in active labor at 39 weeks gestation. On pelvic examination, her cervix was completely effaced and 5 cm dilated. She had a frank breech presentation confirmed by ultrasound. The fetal head was noted to be flexed and the ultrasound-estimated fetal weight of 3150 g was consistent with a clinical estimate of 3400 g. Ultrasound examination revealed a morphologically normal fetus. Clinical pelvimetry was performed by two residents and an attending faculty and the pelvis was deemed to be adequate for breech delivery. Radiographic pelvimetry was not obtained. The patient had received prenatal care from a midwife and was highly motivated to avoid cesarean delivery. She consented to vaginal breech delivery and requested and received epidural analgesia. She reached complete cervical dilation in 4 hours and her second stage lasted 45 minutes. Assisted vaginal breech delivery was performed by a second-year resident, and a fourth-year resident placed Piper forceps to deliver the aftercoming head. A faculty member with 25 years of experience supervised the labor and delivery. Apgar scores were 7 at 1 minute and 9 at 5 minutes. Mother and infant were discharged home on postpartum day 2, doing well.

CASE PRESENTATION 2

We recount a problematic case to highlight several learning points from this chapter.

In 1976 the first author was called to a patient with undeliverable aftercoming head of a breech presentation. He applied standard long curved forceps but there was no descent of the head with traction. He left the forceps in place, infiltrated the symphysis pubis with local anesthetic, performed a partial symphysiotomy, and delivered the baby safely with the forceps. The baby was found to have previously undiagnosed moderate hydrocephaly (obstetric ultrasound was not readily available at the time).

Learning points:
- Vaginal breech deliveries may occur unexpectedly; labor care providers need to be trained to conduct breech delivery.
- Breech presentation is associated with increased incidence of fetal anomalies and more subtle fetal impairment.
- Ultrasound is essential to exclude identifiable fetal malformations.
- In the rare situation of undeliverable aftercoming head of the breech, partial symphysiotomy may be life saving and is associated with minimal maternal morbidity.

Acknowledgments

We acknowledge Drs Edward R. Yeomans and Larry C. Gilstrap for their contribution to previous versions of this chapter, including the first case presentation.

References

1. Ford JB, Roberts CL, Nassar N, Giles W, Morris JM. Recurrence of breech presentation in consecutive pregnancies. BJOG. 2010 Jun;117(7):830–6.
2. Nordtveit TI, Melve KK, Albrechtsen S, Skjaerven R. Maternal and paternal contribution to intergenerational recurrence of breech delivery: population based cohort study. BMJ. 2008 Apr 19;336(7649):872–6.
3. Yeomans ER, Gilstrap LC. Breech delivery: In: Queenan JT, Spong CY, Lockwood CJ, editors. Queenan's management of high-risk pregnancy: an evidence-based approach. 6th ed. Wiley-Blackwell; 2012. p.424–8.
4. Devold Pay AS, Johansen K, Staff AC, Laine KH, Blix E, Økland I. Effects of external cephalic version for breech presentation at or near term in high-resource settings: A systematic review of randomized and non-randomized studies. Eur J Midwifery. 2020 Nov 20;4:44.
5. Hofmeyr GJ, Kulier R, West HM. External cephalic version for breech presentation at term. Cochrane Database Syst Rev. 2015 Apr 1;2015(4):CD000083. doi: 10.1002/14651858.CD000083.pub3.
6. Hannah ME, Hannah WJ, Hewson SA, Hodnett ED, Saigal S, Willan AR. Planned cesarean section versus planned vaginal birth for breech presentation at term: a randomised multicentre trial. Term Breech Trial Collaborative Group. Lancet. 2000 Oct 21;356(9239):1375–83.
7. Whyte H, Hannah ME, Saigal S, Hannah WJ, Hewson S, Amankwah K et al.; Term Breech Trial Collaborative Group. Outcomes of children at 2 years after planned cesarean birth versus planned vaginal birth for breech presentation at term: the International Randomized Term Breech Trial. Am J Obstet Gynecol. 2004 Sep;191(3):864–71.
8. Goffinet F, Carayol M, Foidart JM, Alexander S, Uzan S, Subtil D, et al.; PREMODA Study Group. Is planned vaginal delivery for breech presentation at term still an option? Results of an observational prospective survey in France and Belgium. Am J Obstet Gynecol. 2006 Apr;194(4):1002–11.
9. Korb D, Schmitz T, Alexander S, Subtil D, Verspyck E, Deneux-Tharaux C, et al. Association between planned mode of delivery and severe maternal morbidity in women with breech

presentations: A secondary analysis of the PREMODA prospective general population study. J Gynecol Obstet Hum Reprod. 2020 Feb;49(2):101662.

10. Zamstein O, Glusman Bendersky A, Sheiner E, Landau D, Levy A. Association between mode of delivery of the breech fetus and hospitalizations due to inflammatory bowel disease during childhood. J Clin Gastroenterol. 2022 Feb 1;56(2):e161–5.

11. Berhan Y, Haileamlak A. The risks of planned vaginal breech delivery versus planned cesarean section for term breech birth: a meta-analysis including observational studies. BJOG. 2016 Jan;123(1):49–57.

12. American College of Obstetricians and Gynecologists. Committee Opinion No. 340: mode of term singleton breech delivery. Washington, DC: American College of Obstetricians and Gynecologists; 2006.

13. Kotaska A, Menticoglou S, Gagnon R; Maternal Fetal Medicine Committee. Vaginal delivery of breech presentation. J Obstet Gynaecol Can. 2009 Jun;31(6):557–66.

14. Alarab M, Regan C, O'Connell MP, Keane DP, O'Herlihy C, Foley ME. Singleton vaginal breech delivery at term: still a safe option. Obstet Gynecol 2004;103:407–12.

15. Gaillard T, Girault A, Alexander S, Goffinet F, Le Ray C. Is induction of labor a reasonable option for breech presentation? Acta Obstet Gynecol Scand. 2019 Jul;98(7):885–93.

16. Sun W, Liu F, Liu S, Gratton SM, El-Chaar D, Wen SW, et al. Comparison of outcomes between induction of labor and spontaneous labor for term breech: a systemic review and meta analysis. Eur J Obstet Gynecol Reprod Biol. 2018 Mar;222:155–60.

17. Hofmeyr GJ, Bernitz S, Bonet M, Bucagu M, Dao B, Downe S, et al. WHO next-generation partograph: revolutionary steps towards individualised labour care. BJOG. 2021 Sep;128(10):1658–62.

18. Louwen F, Daviss BA, Johnson KC, Reitter A. Does breech delivery in an upright position instead of on the back improve outcomes and avoid cesareans? Int J Gynaecol Obstet. 2017 Feb;136(2):151–61.

19. Sandberg EC. The Zavanelli maneuver: 12 years of recorded experience. Obstet Gynecol. 1999 Feb;93(2):312–7.

20. Hofmeyr GJ, Shweni PM. Symphysiotomy for feto-pelvic disproportion. Cochrane Database Syst Rev. 2012 Oct 17;10(10):CD005299. doi: 10.1002/14651858.CD005299.pub2.

21. Korb D, Goffinet F, Bretelle F, Parant O, Riethmuller D, Sentilhes L, et al.; JUmeaux MODe d'Accouchement (JUMODA) Study Group* and the Groupe de Recherche en Obstétrique et Gynécologie (GROG). First twin in breech presentation and neonatal mortality and morbidity according to planned mode of delivery. Obstet Gynecol. 2020 May;135(5):1015–23.

22. Schmitz T, Korb D, Battie C, Cordier AG, de Carne Carnavalet C, Chauleur C, et al.; Jumeaux Mode d'Accouchement study group; Groupe de Recherche en Obstétrique et Gynécologie. Neonatal morbidity associated with vaginal delivery of noncephalic second twins. Am J Obstet Gynecol. 2018 Apr;218(4):449.e1–13.

23. Pauphilet V, Goffinet F, Seco A, Azria E, Cordier AG, Deruelle P, et al.; Jumeaux Mode d'Accouchement (JUMODA) Study Group and the Groupe de Recherche en Obstétrique et Gynécologie (GROG). Internal version compared with pushing for delivery of cephalic second twins. Obstet Gynecol. 2020 Jun;135(6):1435–43.

24. Kayem G, Combaud V, Lorthe E, Haddad B, Descamps P, Marpeau L, et al. Mortality and morbidity in early preterm breech singletons: impact of a policy of planned vaginal delivery. Eur J Obstet Gynecol Reprod Biol. 2015 Sep;192:61–5.

25. Lorthe E, Sentilhes L, Quere M, Lebeaux C, Winer N, Torchin H, et al.; EPIPAGE-2 Obstetric Writing Group. Planned delivery route of preterm breech singletons, and neonatal and 2-year outcomes: a population-based cohort study. BJOG. 2019 Jan;126(1):73–82.

26. Girault A, Carteau M, Kefelian F, Menard S, Goffinet F, Le Ray C. Benefits of the "en caul" technique for extremely preterm breech vaginal delivery. J Gynecol Obstet Hum Reprod. 2022 Feb;51(2):102284.

Chapter 49
Operative Vaginal Delivery

Edward R. Yeomans and Ann Erickstad

Department of Obstetrics and Gynecology, Texas Tech University Health Sciences Center, Lubbock, TX, USA

Ten years have elapsed since this chapter appeared in the sixth edition of this textbook; much has changed. Perhaps the most impactful change is the steady decline in the use of both forceps and vacuum extraction [1]. This decline affects training, acquisition of skills, and maintenance of skills necessary to achieve successful vaginal delivery with limited maternal and neonatal morbidity. New guidelines have been published by the American College of Obstetricians and Gynecologists (ACOG) in 2020 [2], the Royal College of Obstetricians and Gynaecologists (RCOG) in 2020 [3], and the Society of Obstetricians and Gynaecologists of Canada in 2019 [4]. One fact is crystal clear from reviewing these guidelines: no organization is proposing the abandonment of operative vaginal delivery (OVD). Therefore, it is up to training programs to provide residents with the skills, confidence, and judgment necessary to preserve the option of OVD. It is the opinion of the authors that simulation training, although a helpful adjunct, must be supplemented by procedures on actual patients. The purpose of this revised chapter is to convey to the reader our optimistic view of the continued importance of OVD, a skill that should not be lost.

Prerequisites and indications

OVD is not an option unless the cervix is fully dilated, that is, the woman has reached the second stage of labor. Pushing should begin at the start of the second stage. Delayed pushing does not increase the vaginal delivery rate and is associated with an increased incidence of chorioamnionitis [5]. Prior to attempting an OVD, the fetal head must at least be engaged (leading bony point at zero station) and, except in unusual circumstances, preferably at +2 cm station or lower. The position of the head must be known and the senior person responsible for the delivery must be experienced with OVD. The maternal pelvis should be clinically evaluated and the relationship of the fetus to the pelvis assessed including a reasonable estimation of fetal weight. OVD may be attempted for evidence of fetal compromise or jeopardy, or it may be tried for failure to progress. The latter indication includes cases of maternal exhaustion, dense epidural anesthesia, soft tissue dystocia, malposition, asynclitism, and prolonged second stage.

The definition of prolonged second stage is a source of controversy. ACOG and the Society for Maternal-Fetal Medicine (SMFM) recommended extending the second stage by 1 hour (i.e. 4 hours for a nullipara and 3 hours for a multipara with epidural anesthesia) [6]. This was challenged by Nelson and Leveno [7] and could lead to increased opportunity for OVD performance if the historic limits were employed instead of the new recommendations [8]. This may be most beneficial in residency training programs where experienced faculty are available to oversee OVD procedures. Recently, the SMFM proposed two checklists for preparation, performance, and documentation of OVD [9]. The use of such checklists may be especially valuable in training programs.

Classification

The current three-level classification system (Box 49.1) has been in use for more than 30 years in the United States. It appears in ACOG Practice Bulletin No. 219 [2] and is only slightly different in the RCOG scheme [3]. The classification highlights the importance of station and rotation in operative vaginal delivery. Application of an instrument to a fetal head in the midpelvis in occiput transverse position is much more difficult than a "lift-out" delivery from the pelvic floor as is the case of an outlet forceps. Importantly, the classification system is the same for both forceps and vacuum deliveries.

Queenan's Management of High-Risk Pregnancy: An Evidence-Based Approach, Seventh Edition. Edited by Catherine Y. Spong and Charles J. Lockwood.

Box 49.1 Classification of OVD

Outlet forceps

1. Scalp is visible at the introitus without separating labia.
2. Fetal skull has reached pelvic floor.
3. Sagittal suture is an anteroposterior diameter or right or left occiput anterior or posterior position.
4. Fetal head is at or on perineum.
5. Rotation does not exceed 45°.

Low forceps

Leading point of fetal skull is at station +2 cm or more (-5 cm to +5 cm scale) and not on the pelvic floor.

- Rotation is 45° or less (left or right occiput anterior to occiput anterior, or left or right occiput posterior to occiput posterior).
- Rotation is greater than 45°.

Mid forceps

Station is above +2 cm but head is engaged (i.e. at least 0 station)

High forceps

Not included in classification.

Instrument selection

The choice between forceps and vacuum extractor depends mainly on operator preference. However, in a few well-defined instances, forceps are the only option: prematurity (<34 weeks), face presentation, and the aftercoming head of the breech. An important point about instrument selection is that there are choices *within* each category for both forceps and vacuum (Figure 49.1a,b). This fact is underemphasized in randomized controlled trials and the literature in general. Forceps with a long tapered cephalic curve should be used for a molded head, and forceps with a sliding lock can correct asynclitism. An occiput posterior that is instrumentally rotated to anterior can reduce the risk of deep perineal laceration during

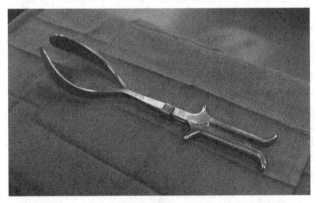

Figure 49.1a Luikart forceps. The key features of pseudofenestrated blades, overlapping shanks, and a sliding lock to allow for correction of asynclitism can be seen in the photo.

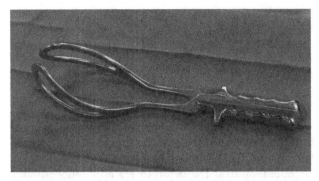

Figure 49.1b Simpson forceps. In contrast to the Luikart forceps, these forceps have fenestrated blades, parallel shanks, and a fixed English lock.

delivery. For vacuum extractors, the construction, shape, and size of the cup may be selected to fit a particular clinical situation. The process of instrument selection requires more insight than the adage "learn to use one instrument well."

The choice of instrument may also be influenced by the advantages and disadvantages of the instrument in general or in a specific clinical situation. For example, vacuum extraction is more likely to fail than forceps. ACOG [2] recommends against sequential use of instruments, that is, failure of vacuum followed by forceps or in the rare case of forceps followed by vacuum. In contrast, the RCOG [3] recommends a more nuanced approach, depending on the station of the fetal head when the vacuum attempt fails.

Site of delivery

Labor/delivery/recovery rooms in general and labor beds specifically were not designed for OVD. However, many such procedures can be performed in a labor room without moving to the operating room (OR). Advantages of moving to the OR (or in "theatre," in the United Kingdom) include better lighting, a hard OR table, adjustable stirrups, presence of anesthesia staff and immediate cesarean delivery capability.

Technique

OVD is a surgical procedure. Various technical skills are required to produce optimal results. Among these are clinical pelvimetry, correct assessment of fetal head position, and accurate interpretation of fetal heart rate patterns. An operator's skill set must also include the ability to properly apply a given instrument, because experience has shown that, for both forceps and vacuum extraction, misapplication can contribute to fetal injury [10].

Forceps

With forceps delivery, the goal is a biparietal, bimalar symmetric application. The undesirable brow–mastoid application can lead to unequal pressure and cause injury to the fetal head. To avoid this error, once the forceps have been applied, the application must be carefully checked. The sagittal suture should bisect the plane of the shanks, the posterior fontanel should be one fingerbreadth above the plane of the shanks (for an occiput anterior position), and the tops of the blades should be equidistant from the lambdoid sutures. The depth of the application should also be checked to guard against slippage. Any necessary rotation with forceps involves swinging the handles in an arc, with the notable exception of Kielland forceps. The primary function of Kielland forceps is to aid in rotation of the fetal head from either occiput transverse or occiput posterior. There are several described methods of applying the anterior blade of the Kielland forceps: the inversion method, the wandering method, and the direct application. As opposed to classical forceps the anterior blade of the Keillands is usually applied first. The posterior blade is easier to apply directly. Once a correct application is obtained, rotation of the head through an arc of 90–180° is accomplished by a sequence of flexion, destationing, and slow, controlled turning by the operator. Such rotation can allow delivery of the fetal head in a more favorable diameter, reducing the risk of maternal injury. Appropriate use of Kielland forceps continues to be reported with a "very low rate of adverse maternal and neonatal outcomes" [11], but experience is limited in many training programs.

Arguably, the most important technical skill is traction in the correct axis. The direction of traction must change continually as the fetal head descends through the maternal pelvis. (Figure 49.2). This can be accomplished with the Pajot-Saxtorph maneuver (Figure 49.3). In this bimanual maneuver the handles of the forceps are placed in the

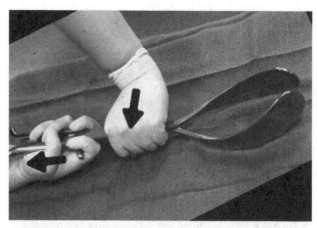

Figure 49.3 The Pajot-Saxtorph maneuver. In the photo downward traction is applied by the left hand and outward traction is applied by the right hand.

upturned palm of the dominant hand. The nondominant hand applies pressure downward over the shanks. With experience this maneuver will ensure that traction is performed along the axis of the pelvis. Beginners or even some experienced operators may find it helpful to use a Bill's axis traction device. This device can be attached to the finger guards of most conventional forceps and guides the operator's direction of traction with an indicator on the left side of the device. Pulling too anteriorly will result in wasted force against the pubic symphysis, whereas pulling too posteriorly will subject the external anal sphincter to injury. In everyday clinical work, experience is the best guide to the amount of traction that can be safely applied. Methods of measuring the force applied are currently being investigated. The central concept in instrumental delivery is that proper traction should produce visible descent of the fetal head. Failure to observe descent should prompt reconsideration and possibly abandonment of the procedure.

Vacuum extraction

It is generally recognized that vacuum extraction is fairly simple to teach and learn, which may partially account for its upsurge in popularity [12]. With vacuum extraction, failure to center the cup over the sagittal suture 3 cm anterior to the posterior fontanel, referred to as a median flexing application, can increase the risk of cup detachment and fetal injury. As with forceps, this requires an accurate diagnosis of fetal head position. The operator should ensure that no maternal tissue is entrapped beneath the vacuum cup. Although autorotation is sometimes observed with vacuum extraction, no attempt should be made by the operator to manually rotate the vacuum cup once it is applied. Twisting the cup may lead to a "cookie-cutter" or semilunar laceration of the fetal scalp [13]. Traction should be coordinated with maternal expulsive effort and in the axis of the pelvis. The operator

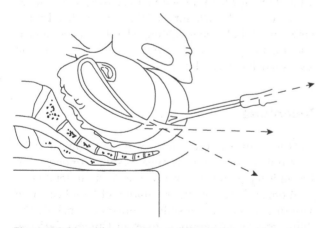

Figure 49.2 Lines of axis traction at different planes of the pelvis. Reproduced from ACOG Technical Bulletin No. 196, August 1994, with permission from the American College of Obstetricians and Gynecologists.

should pull the traction handle with his or her dominant hand and use the other hand to aid in keeping the cup in place. There should be visible progress in descent with each pull. Failure occurs more frequently in obese women, with macrosomic babies, in the case of malposition and higher station at the time of attempted vacuum extraction [12].

Outcomes

Maternal
Outcomes of OVD should be compared with second-stage cesarean births because that is the clinical alternative. Vacuum extraction is associated with fewer deep perineal lacerations than forceps delivery. These injuries, not seen with second-stage cesarean, are less serious than the immediate consequences of hemorrhage, infection, thromboembolism, and hysterectomy associated with cesarean delivery. Moreover, in comparing the downstream consequences of an initial OVD to a primary cesarean, the next delivery following a successful OVD has an 80% chance of being a spontaneous vaginal delivery [3]. After primary cesarean delivery, the next delivery is 85–90% likely to be a repeat cesarean. Other downstream consequences include rupture of a uterine scar and placenta accreta spectrum that may follow cesarean delivery.

Neonatal
Some injuries that occur with OVD (e.g. intracranial hemorrhage) occur with comparable frequency at second-stage cesarean. Vacuum extractions are associated with higher rates of neonatal retinal hemorrhage, jaundice, intraventricular hemorrhage, cephalohematoma and subgaleal bleed. The use of either vacuum or forceps is associated with relatively low rates of major morbidity and mortality and do not appear to be substantially greater than with cesarean delivery performed in labor [2].

Training

OVD accounts for 10–15% of all deliveries in the United Kingdom but only 3.3% of deliveries in the United States. To maintain OVD as a viable option for women in the second stage of labor, it is imperative to increase the frequency of OVD in residency training programs across the country. Simulation is not a new idea [14], but by itself it is not and will never be sufficient to acquire and maintain requisite skills. Simulation should logically precede clinical work, not replace it. At the authors' institution we have maintained a frequency of OVD comparable to the United Kingdom for the last 14 years. This is offered as proof that it can be done. We strongly agree with the Obstetric Care Consensus [6] that "training in, and ongoing maintenance of, practical skills related to OVD should be encouraged."

Conclusion

Skillful performance of OVD was once considered to be one of the hallmarks of an obstetrician. There are now fewer such deliveries than at any time in the last century. The risks of a high cesarean delivery rate are increasingly evident. Several prominent organizations [2–4] have called for continued training in OVD procedures to allow women in the second stage of labor to avoid an unnecessary and potentially morbid cesarean delivery.

CASE PRESENTATION

A 24-year-old gravida 3, para 0020 at 37 weeks 3 days gestational age is undergoing induction of labor for intrahepatic cholestasis of pregnancy. After 2.5 hours of pushing in the second stage with a working epidural, the fetal heart rate tracing shows recurrent variable decelerations with decreasing variability. The fetal position has rotated with maternal pushing from left occiput transverse to left occiput anterior (OA) 45° from direct OA position with some anterior asynclitism. The cervix is fully dilated, the vertex is at +2 station, and the pelvis is assessed as gynecoid. Estimated fetal weight is 3400 g. The patient is counseled on the risks and benefits of OVD and consents to the procedure. There is little concern over the potential success of the procedure, so the patient remains in her labor room. Luikart forceps are applied, and fetal asynclitism is corrected using the sliding lock. Gentle traction in the axis of the pelvis is applied using the Pajot-Saxtorph bimanual technique, and the handles of the forceps are gradually elevated until the occiput is delivered under the pubic symphysis. During traction, a right mediolateral episiotomy is cut. The forceps are removed once the chin is grasped through the perineum and the head is delivered using the modified Ritgen maneuver. Forceps marks on the baby confirm an accurate bimalar, biparietal application. The baby is moving extremities symmetrically and no resuscitation was needed. Quantitative blood loss was 434 cc. The mediolateral episiotomy was repaired in standard fashion.

References

1. Merriam AA, Ananth CV, Wright JD, Siddiq Z, D'Alton ME, Friedman AM. Trends in operative vaginal delivery, 2005–2013: a population-based study. BJOG. 2017;124:1365–72.

2. American College of Obstetricians and Gynecologists. Practice Bulletin No. 219: operative vaginal birth. Washington, DC: ACOG; 2020.

3. Murphy DJ, Strachan BK, Bahl R, on behalf of the Royal College of Obstetricians Gynaecologissts. Assisted vaginal birth. BJOG. 2020; 127:e70–e112.

4. Society of Obstetricians and Gynaecologists of Canada. Guidelines for assisted vaginal birth. Clinical Practice Guideline No. 381. Ottawa: SOGC; 2019.

5. Cahill AG, Srinivas SK, Tita ATN, Caughey AB, Richter HE, Gregory WT, et al. Effect of immediate vs delayed pushing on rates of spontaneous vaginal delivery among nulliparous women receiving neuraxial analgesia. JAMA. 2018;320: 1444–54.

6. American College of Obstetricians and Gynecologists. Obstetric Care Consensus No. 1: safe prevention of the primary cesarean delivery. Washington, DC: ACOG; 2014.

7. Nelson DB, McIntire DD, Leveno KJ. Second-stage labor: consensus versus science. Am J Obstet Gynecol. 2020;222:144–9.

8. Zipori Y, Grunwald O, Ginsberg Y, Beloosesky R, Weiner Z. The impact of extending the second stage of labor to prevent primary cesarean delivery on maternal and neonatal outcomes. Am J Obstet Gynecol. 2019; 220:191.e1–7.

9. Society for Maternal Fetal Medicine. SMFM Special Statement: Operative vaginal delivery: checklists for performance and documentation. Washington, DC: SMFM; 2020.

10. Ramphul M, Kennelly MM, Burke G, Murphy DJ. Risk factors and morbidity associated with suboptimal instrument placement at instrumental delivery: observational study nested within the Instrumental Delivery & Ultrasound randomised controlled trial ISRCTN 72230496. BJOG. 2015;122:558–63.

11. Al-Suhel R, Gill S, Robson S, Shadbolt B. Kjelland's forceps in the new millennium. Maternal and neonatal outcomes of attempted rotational forceps delivery. Aust N Z J Obstet Gynecol. 2009;49:510–14.

12. van den Akker T. Vacuum extraction for non-rotational and rotational assisted vaginal birth. Best Pract Res Clin Obstet Gynaecol. 2019;56:47–54.

13. Yeomans ER, Hoffman BL, Gilstrap LC III, Cunningham FG, editors. Cunningham and Gilstrap's operative obstetrics. 3rd ed. New York: McGraw Hill; 2017.

14. Dennen EH. Forceps deliveries. Philadelphia: F.A. Davis Company; 1964. p.6.

Chapter 50
Obstetric Analgesia and Anesthesia

Gilbert J. Grant

Department of Anesthesiology, Perioperative Care and Pain Medicine, Grossman School of Medicine, New York University, New York, NY, USA

Labor and vaginal delivery

Consequences of unrelieved pain

The pain of childbirth has untoward effects on the mother and fetus, and this was documented in several studies toward the end of the last century [1]. Hyperventilation that accompanies labor pain causes hypocarbia and metabolic alkalosis, which may suppress the ventilatory drive between contractions and lead to hemoglobin desaturation. The respiratory alkalosis also interferes with fetal oxygenation by shifting the oxyhemoglobin dissociation curve in favor of the mother. The maternal neurohumoral responses to stress and pain increase levels of cortisol, β-lipotropin, and catecholamines. The net effect of this metabolic response to labor pain can be characterized as hyperglycemia with a poor response to insulin, coupled with increased production of lactate, ketones, and free fatty acids. These metabolic products and catecholamines traverse the placenta and exacerbate metabolic acidosis in the fetus. Catecholamines also produce vasoconstriction and can cause a decrease in uterine blood flow. Moreover, catecholamines promote incoordinate uterine contractions, which may impair the progress of labor.

Neuraxial labor analgesia, a term that encompasses spinal and epidural techniques, mitigates these pain-related effects. A meta-analysis found improved neonatal acid-base status in laboring mothers who had received epidural compared to systemic analgesia [2]. Effective neuraxial analgesia lowers circulating maternal epinephrine and effectively inhibits the neurohumoral responses to pain [3], with a resultant increase in oxygen tension in the parturient and fetus [4]. For most women, childbirth pain is the most severe pain they will ever experience. In addition to acute suffering, unrelieved labor pain may be associated with long-lasting postpartum psychological effects. Labor pain has been associated with the development of postpartum depression [5,6] and post-traumatic stress disorder [7] although a direct causative link has not been unequivocally established [8], as the development of postpartum psychological disorders are multifactorial.

Multimodal regional analgesia

The current approach to achieving pain relief for labor and vaginal delivery is based on the principle of combining relatively small doses of different classes of analgesics, such as a local anesthetic and an opioid, a concept known as multimodal analgesia [9]. This approach facilitates excellent pain relief with a minimum of undesirable side effects, as the agents all combine to produce analgesia, but side effects are less likely because each agent has a distinct side effect profile, hence the side effects are not additive. For example, local anesthetics block axonal conduction in all nerves with which they come in contact, and at high concentrations they produce hypotension and motor block, undesirable effects in labor. Hypotension may decrease fetal oxygen delivery by reducing placental perfusion. Motor block may cause profound lower extremity weakness, which can be unpleasant or even distressing for the parturient. Unlike local anesthetics, opioids administered into the neuraxis (except for meperidine) do not block nerve conduction. Rather, the mechanism of opioid pain inhibition is mediated by binding to specific opioid receptors in the spinal cord. In high doses opioids may cause annoying side effects such as pruritus and nausea. By combining relatively low doses of local anesthetics with relatively low doses of opioids, the two classes of pain relievers summate to produce reliable analgesia while avoiding unwanted side effects that accompany high doses of each agent. Some clinicians also combine low doses of other classes of analgesics such as epinephrine, which binds to spinal α-adrenergic receptors to further potentiate analgesia.

For parturients, relief of their labor pain and preservation of their lower extremity muscle strength are the most

---

noticeable effects of multimodal analgesia. Although commonly described as a "walking epidural," this term is a poor descriptor, as few women ambulate during labor after their pain is relieved. The lack of motor block is not a result of the epidural approach per se and may also be achieved with a spinal approach, or a combined spinal–epidural (CSE) approach. The primary determinant of motor block intensity is the concentration of local anesthetic, not its site of administration.

Epidural, spinal, and combined spinal–epidural analgesia

Safe and effective analgesia for labor and delivery may be achieved by using an epidural, spinal or CSE technique. An advantage of techniques with an epidural component is that a catheter inserted into the epidural space may be used to provide continuous and/or intermittent analgesic dosing to prolong the duration of pain relief, facilitating individualized patient care. With spinal techniques, the duration of analgesia is limited to the duration of action of a single dose, as catheterization of the intrathecal space is infrequently performed. The onset of analgesia is more rapid with the spinal approach (3–5 minutes) than it is with the epidural approach (approximately 10 minutes). The CSE approach offers the advantages of both the spinal and epidural techniques: rapid onset of analgesia and prolonged duration if needed.

However, the CSE technique is not without drawbacks. A side effect sometimes seen after intrathecal opioid injection is fetal bradycardia or late decelerations of the fetal heart rate (FHR), because of uterine hyperactivity [10]. A meta-analysis found that CSE labor analgesia was associated with a higher risk of nonreassuring FHR tracings than epidural analgesia alone; whether this translates into a greater rate of cesarean delivery is not definitively known [11], but the FHR tracings can be distressing for the parturient and her partner, not to mention her caregivers. The nonreassuring fetal heart rate may be reversed by administration of a tocolytic, such as terbutaline or nitroglycerine, medications that are not beneficial to propagating labor. A Cochrane review concluded that CSEs for labor do not offer advantages over pure epidurals and may precipitate untoward effects, yet CSEs are preferred by some practitioners [12].

The type of regional analgesia chosen for a parturient depends on many factors, one of which is the anticipated duration of labor. In early labor, catheterization of the epidural space is indicated, using an epidural or CSE technique, to establish a conduit to provide continuous and/or multiple doses of analgesics. Epidural analgesics are typically administered using an infusion pump, often with patient-controlled epidural analgesia (see

next section). For a CSE technique, a dose of analgesic is administered intrathecally and then a catheter is inserted into the epidural space. The epidural analgesics may be administered either immediately after the intrathecal injection or when the pain relief from the initial intrathecal dose begins to wane.

Epidural catheterization is a sensible approach during labor for parturients who have a high likelihood of an instrumental or operative delivery, for example, a woman attempting a vaginal birth after cesarean, as it provides a route for additional anesthetic administration, should it be needed. If delivery is imminent, a single-shot spinal technique is a reasonable choice, because analgesia onset is rapid. However, these patients may benefit more from a CSE technique, as it requires little additional time compared to a spinal technique, and an indwelling epidural catheter confers considerable versatility. The epidural catheter may be used to administer additional analgesics if delivery does not occur as quickly as anticipated, if the intrathecal medication does not produce adequate analgesia, if an instrumental or operative delivery is required, or if an unanticipated postpartum operative procedure is needed.

Patient-controlled epidural analgesia

Programmable infusion pumps facilitate precise administration of analgesics into the epidural space. This technology revolutionized epidural labor analgesia, as continuous infusion of analgesics avoided the peaks and valleys of pain and relief that were commonplace with manual intermittent bolus dosing. Patient-controlled epidural analgesia (PCEA) is a further refinement of this technology, enabling the parturient to "fine-tune" her pain relief. PCEA has many advantages over non-PCEA techniques, including better analgesia and decreased anesthetic requirement, as well as improved patient satisfaction [13], because the patient feels empowered by having some control over her pain relief. PCEA may be administered using intermittent boluses exclusively or intermittent boluses superimposed on a background infusion. Obstetric anesthesiologists currently use a variety of PCEA techniques, and there is no consensus as to which technique is optimal. For example, one method that has been embraced by some practitioners is intermittent epidural bolus, in which timed boluses are automatically delivered into the epidural space. A meta-analysis of this technique compared to continuous infusion found it superior with regard to pain relief during the first 4 hours but no different with respect to mode of delivery [14]. While the search for the best technique to provide labor analgesia continues, current modalities provide excellent pain relief with minimal physiologic perturbations, enhancing safety for the mother and fetus.

Some obstetricians prefer to decrease or halt the epidural administration of analgesics during the second stage of labor, believing that curtailing epidural analgesia will increase the likelihood of spontaneous vaginal delivery. However, parturients often find that the second stage of labor is more painful than the first stage and that the relatively low doses of analgesics used to relieve the pain of the first stage of labor are not adequate for the second stage. This breakthrough pain can be remedied increasing the rate of the epidural infusion and/or by administration of a more concentrated dose of anesthetic as a "rescue dose." Recent studies have found that maintaining epidural analgesia throughout labor does not prolong the second stage [15] nor does it increase the rate of operative delivery [16]. Providing effective analgesia for the second stage can be particularly helpful in high-risk parturients, for example, those with significant cardiac disease, in whom assisted vaginal delivery is used to minimize hemodynamic perturbations.

Timing of regional pain relief

The optimal timing for administering regional analgesia for labor was a long-standing controversy that has essentially been resolved by studies that found the timing of epidural administration during labor, whether spontaneous or induced, did not affect the incidence of cesarean or instrumental delivery [17–20]. These studies support the principle of allowing women to have pain relief whenever they choose, as the American College of Obstetricians and Gynecologists has noted: "In the absence of a medical contraindication, maternal request is a sufficient medical indication for pain relief during labor" [21].

Cesarean delivery

Most planned cesarean deliveries in the United States are performed under spinal anesthesia, although epidural and CSE techniques are also used. If the decision to perform a cesarean delivery is reached after labor has commenced, and the parturient is receiving epidural analgesia, surgical anesthesia is readily achieved by injecting a more concentrated dose of local anesthetic through the epidural catheter. Currently, in the United States, general anesthesia is used only occasionally for planned cesarean if there is a contraindication or patient preference to avoid neuraxial block. Most women prefer to be awake to experience the moment of birth, despite any fear they may have of neuraxial anesthesia. The status of the fetus is often the deciding factor in determining the anesthetic choice. If urgent delivery of the fetus is indicated, and if there is no indwelling epidural catheter, general anesthesia is preferred. However, in some circumstances there may be sufficient time to induce spinal

anesthesia. Epidural anesthesia is the least desirable choice if time is of the essence because of the prolonged latency of block onset compared to the spinal approach. In rare cases the mode of maternal anesthesia may be chosen for a fetal indication. For example, if an ex utero intrapartum treatment procedure is planned, general anesthesia is preferred to maintain fetal circulation after delivery, while the neonatal airway is secured [22]. Ultimately, the choice of anesthetic technique is influenced by a variety of factors including the urgency of the procedure, maternal and fetal status, and physician and patient preference.

Compared to labor analgesia, a more intense block is needed to inhibit the perception of surgical stimulation during cesarean delivery. This is achieved by administering a relatively high concentration of local anesthetic, up to 10-fold greater than the concentration used to provide labor analgesia. This local anesthetic concentration predictably produces a profound motor block. In addition, cesarean delivery necessitates a higher dermatomal anesthetic level than does labor analgesia. Whereas sensory block to the 10th thoracic dermatome is sufficient to provide labor analgesia, the anesthetic level must reach, at a minimum, the fourth thoracic dermatome for cesarean delivery, lest the parturient perceive surgical pain.

The higher level and greater intensity of block required for cesarean delivery places the parturient at risk of hypotension on induction of regional anesthesia, with potential deleterious consequences for mother (nausea) and fetus (hypoxemia). Administration of intravenous fluids and initiation of a vasopressor infusion coincident with induction of regional anesthesia decreases the likelihood of maternal hypotension [23,24]. For some high-risk parturients, such as those with preeclampsia or significant cardiovascular disease, rapid intravenous fluid loading and/or vasopressor infusions must be used cautiously.

In the United States, general anesthesia is associated with 1.7-fold greater incidence of maternal death than regional anesthesia. General anesthetic deaths are most likely to result from airway/pulmonary problems whereas regional anesthetic deaths are most commonly due to unintended high block. Regional anesthesia also has other unique risks, such as postdural puncture headache and, rarely, spinal hematoma, epidural abscess, meningitis, or nerve damage. Overall, general and regional anesthesia are quite safe in pregnancy with case-fatality rates for general anesthesia of 6.5 per million and for regional anesthesia of 3.8 per million in time interval of 1997–2002 [25].

Postoperative analgesia

Unrelieved postcesarean pain may hinder recovery and lead to complications related to lack of deep breathing and ambulation. After cesarean delivery, unrelieved pain is particularly important, as it may affect the mother's interactions with her neonate by interfering with bonding and breastfeeding. Effective analgesia may mitigate these effects. The ideal postoperative pain regimen facilitates deep breathing and ambulation without causing somnolence. An alert and comfortable mother is best able to meaningfully interact with her neonate. Acute postcesarean pain management typically consists of a single opioid dose administered into the neuraxis. One small dose of morphine in the intrathecal or epidural space can provide considerable pain relief for 18 hours. Unfortunately, even small doses produce annoying untoward effects, particularly pruritus and nausea [26].

Unless contraindicated, nonsteroidal anti-inflammatory drugs (NSAIDs) and acetaminophen are also administered around the clock at 6-hour intervals as part of a multimodal analgesic regimen. For breakthrough pain and/or severe pain that occurs after the neuraxial morphine effect wanes, systemic opioids are administered, usually via the oral route. Some anesthesiologists administer peripheral nerve blocks such as the transversus abdominus plane block or quadratus lumborum block [27], particularly when the epidural or intrathecal routes for opioids are not available, but these blocks provide only modest benefit. Another analgesic option is PCEA, similar to that used routinely for labor but with reduced local anesthetic concentrations, to avoid lower extremity motor block. However, postcesarean PCEA requires a team in place fully committed to active acute pain management, and very few hospitals offer this option.

Opioid crisis

Whichever mode of postcesarean analgesia is employed, the issue of chronic opioid use must be considered because cesarean delivery patients, like all patients exposed to opioid analgesics, are at risk of persistent opioid use. Estimates are that 0.12% to 2.2% of opioid naïve women undergoing cesarean delivery in the United States become persistent opioid users [28–31]. With approximately 1.25 million cesarean births annually, this translates to large numbers of affected women: between 1500 and 27 000 per year. In recognition of the scope of this problem, efforts have been focused on reducing post-cesarean opioid exposure during hospitalization and after discharge. Postoperative pain management in the hospital now emphasizes multimodal analgesia with nonopioid analgesics such as acetaminophen and NSAIDs and reducing oral opioid use. The recognition that opioid overprescription on hospital discharge contributes to the opioid crisis has prompted efforts to encourage judicious opioid prescriptions for postcesarean patients [32].

Compromised coagulation and neuraxial regional analgesia and anesthesia

Bleeding into the neuraxis as a complication of epidural and/or spinal techniques can have catastrophic consequences; therefore, the patient's coagulation status must be considered prior to neuraxial procedures. For women not receiving anticoagulation therapy and without a known coagulopathy or clinical evidence suggestive of a bleeding disorder, laboratory tests of coagulation and platelet count are not indicated. For patients receiving anticoagulants, current specialty society guidelines should be consulted so that the anticoagulants can be proactively adjusted to facilitate safe neuraxial instrumentation [33]. The guidelines also include the recommended wait times prior to reinitiation of anticoagulation therapy after neuraxial instrumentation and after removal of the epidural catheter.

Thrombocytopenia is a cause for concern in patients who will be receiving neuraxial analgesia/anesthesia. In parturients, an isolated low platelet count is usually due to gestational thrombocytopenia, immune thrombocytopenia, or a hypertensive disorder, that is, preeclampsia or HELLP (hemolysis, elevated liver enzymes, and low platelet count) syndrome. If thrombocytopenia is identified during gestation remote from delivery, a consultation with a hematologist can be helpful. For example, a diagnosis of immune thrombocytopenia may be treated with a regimen of corticosteroids or intravenous immunoglobulin. It is also important to assess the time course of the change in platelet count. Of the common etiologies of thrombocytopenia in pregnancy, only HELLP syndrome is associated with a precipitous decline in platelet count. In these women, it is advisable to obtain a repeat count within a few hours of neuraxial instrumentation. It is important to appreciate that removal of the epidural catheter is also a fraught event and should not be done until the platelet count is at an acceptable level. While the minimum platelet number for safely performing neuraxial analgesia/anesthesia was formerly considered to be 100,000 × 10^6/L, this cutoff is not supported by data. Recent specialty society guidelines based on evaluation of available data conclude that a platelet count greater than 70,000 × 10^6/L is highly unlikely to be associated with a neuraxial bleed. In fact, there is little risk of neuraxial bleeding in patients with platelet counts of 50,000 to 70,000 × 10^6/L; the decision to perform neuraxial analgesia or anesthesia in these patients should be based on a judicious risk–benefit analysis [34].

CASE PRESENTATION

A 31-year-old gravida 2, para 0 presents to the labor and delivery suite at 38 weeks gestation with presumed rupture of membranes. She states that she is experiencing severe pain in her lower abdomen with each uterine contraction. A pelvic examination confirms rupture of membranes and finds cervical dilation to be 2 cm, fetal head not engaged. Her blood pressure is 150/100 mmHg. Laboratory testing reveal liver transaminases and hemoglobin in the normal range and platelets $85,000 \times 10^6$/L. A platelet count obtained 1 week prior was $88,000 \times 10^6$/L. The patient requests pain relief. Her obstetrician and the anesthesiologist on duty are consulted. They agree that the patient is a candidate for regional analgesia, as rupture of membranes and a diagnosis of labor have committed the patient to delivery. The patient is offered and accepts epidural analgesia. An epidural catheter is inserted at the L3–L4 interspace and analgesia is initiated with 20 mL 0.06% bupivacaine and 0.4 µg/mL sufentanil. Analgesia is maintained with an infusion of the same solution at 6 mL/h. PCEA is instituted, giving the parturient the option of self-dosing 5 mL every 10 minutes.

When her cervical dilation reaches 8 cm, she states that her self-administered doses are no longer sufficient to relieve her pain, so the anesthesiologist administers a rescue dose of 5 mL 0.125% bupivacaine. Within 10 minutes, this provides relief of her pain, and afterwards she only senses rectal pressure with each contraction. After reaching full dilation, she delivers a 3130 g baby boy over an intact perineum after a 67-minute second stage. Although she sensed pressure while she was pushing, she denied experiencing pain. Her postpartum blood pressure was 130/80 mmHg.

References

1. Reynolds F. Labour analgesia and the baby: good news is no news. Int J Obstet Anesth. 2011;20:38–50.

2. Reynolds F, Sharma SK, Seed PT. Analgesia in labour and fetal acid-base balance: a meta-analysis comparing epidural with systemic opioid analgesia. Br J Obstet Gynaecol. 2002;109:1344–53.

3. Shnider SM, Abboud TK, Artal R, Henriksen EH, Stefani SJ, Levinson G. Maternal catecholamines decrease during labor after lumbar epidural anesthesia. Am J Obstet Gynecol. 1983;147:13–15.

4. Bergmans MG, van Geijn HP, Hasaart TH, Weber T, Nickelsen C. Fetal and maternal transcutaneous PCO_2 levels during labour and the influence of epidural analgesia. Eur J Obstet Gynecol Reprod Biol. 1996;67:127–32.

5. Deng CM, Ding T, Li S, Lei B, Xu MJ, Wang L, et al. Neuraxial labour analgesia is associated with a reduced risk of maternal depression at 2 years after childbirth. Eur J Anaesthesiol. 2019;36:745–54.

6. Deng CM, Ding T, Li S, Lei B, Xu MJ, Wang L, et al. Neuraxial labor analgesia is associated with a reduced risk of postpartum depression: a multicenter prospective cohort study with propensity score matching. J Affect Disord. 2021;281:342–50.

7. Garthus-Niegel S, Knoph C, von Soest T, Nielsen CS, Eberhard-Gran M. The role of labor pain and overall birth experience in the development of posttraumatic stress symptoms: a longitudinal cohort study. Birth. 2014;41:108–15.

8. Orbach-Zinger S, Heesen M, Grigoriadis S, Heesen P, Halpern S. A systematic review of the association between postpartum depression and neuraxial labor analgesia. Int J Obstet Anesth. 2021;45:142–9.

9. Kehlet H, Dahl JB. The value of "multimodal" or "balanced analgesia" in postoperative pain treatment. Anesth Analg. 1993;77:1048–56.

10. Abrao KC, Francisco RC, Miyadahira S, Cicarelli DD, Zugaib M. Evaluation of uterine tone and fetal heart rate abnormalities after labor analgesia: a randomized controlled trial. Obstet Gynecol. 2009;113:41–7.

11. Hattler J, Klimek M, Rossaint R, Heesen M. The effect of combined spinal-epidural versus epidural analgesia in laboring women on nonreassuring fetal heart rate tracings: systematic review and meta-analysis. Anesth Analg. 2016;123:955–64.

12. Simmons SW, Taghizadeh N, Dennis AT, Hughes D, Cyna AM. Combined spinal-epidural versus epidural analgesia in labor. Cochrane Database Syst Rev. 2012 Oct 17;10(10):CD003401. doi: 10.1002/14651858.CD003401.pub3.

13. Bremerich DH, Waibel HJ, Mierdl S, Meininger D, Byhahn C, Zwissler BC, et al. Comparison of continuous background infusion plus demand dose and demand-only parturient-controlled epidural analgesia (PCEA) using ropivacaine combined with sufentanil for labor and delivery. Int J Obstet Anesth. 2005;14:114–20.

14. Hussain N, Lagnese CM, Hayes B, Kumar N, Weaver TE, Essandoh MK, et al. Comparative analgesic efficacy and safety of intermittent local anaesthetic epidural bolus for labour: a systematic review and meta-analysis. Br J Anaesth. 2020;125:560–79.

15. Shen X, Li Y, Xu S, Wand N, Fan S, Qin S, et al. Epidural analgesia during the second stage of labor: a randomized controlled trial. Obstet Gynecol. 2017;130:1097–03.

16. Zheng S, Zheng W, Zhu T, Lan H, Wang Q, Sun X, et al. Continuing epidural analgesia during the second stage and ACOG definition of arrest of labor on maternal-fetal outcomes. Acta Anaesthesiol Scand. 2020;64:1187–93.

17. Wong CA, Scavone BM, Peaceman AM, McCarthy RJ, Sullivan JT, Diaz NT, et al. The risk of cesarean delivery with neuraxial analgesia given early versus late in labor. N Engl J Med. 2005;352:655–65.

18. Wong CA, McCarthy RJ, Sullivan JT, Scavone BM, Gerber SE, Yaghmour EA. Early compared with late neuraxial analgesia in nulliparous labor induction: a randomized controlled trial. Obstet Gynecol. 2009:113:1066–74.

19. Ohel G, Gonen R, Vaida S, Barak S, Gaitini L. Early versus late initiation of epidural analgesia in labor: does it increase the risk of cesarean section? A randomized trial. Am J Obstet Gynecol. 2006;194:600–5.

20. Wang F, Shen X, Guo X, Peng Y, Gu X. Epidural analgesia in the latent phase of labor and the risk of cesarean delivery: a five-year randomized controlled trial. Anesthesiology. 2009;111: 871–80.

21. American College of Obstetricians and Gynecologists. ACOG Practice Bulletin No. 209: obstetric analgesia and anesthesia. Obstet Gynecol. 2019;133:595–7.

22. Kumar K, Miron C, Singh SI. Maternal anesthesia for EXIT procedure: a systematic review of literature. J Anaesthesiol Clin Pharmacol. 2019;35:19–24.

23. Fitzgerald JP, Fedoruk KA, Jadin SM, Carvalho B, Halpern SH. Prevention of hypotension after spinal anaesthesia for caesarean section: a systematic review and network meta-analysis of randomised controlled trials. Anaesthesia. 2020;75:109–21.

24. Banerjee A, Stocche RM, Angle P, Halpern SH. Preload or coload for spinal anesthesia for elective Cesarean delivery: a meta-analysis. Can J Anaesth. 2010;57:24–31.

25. Hawkins JL, Chang G, Palmer SK, Gibbs CP, Callaghan WM. Anesthesia-related maternal mortality in the United States: 1979–2002. Obstet Gynecol. 2011;117:69–74.

26. Berger JS, Gonzalez A, Hopkins A, Alshaeri T, Jeon D, Wang S, et al. Dose–response of intrathecal morphine when administered with intravenous ketorolac for post-cesarean analgesia: a two-center, prospective, randomized, blinded trial. Int J Obstet Anesth. 2016;28:3–11.

27. El-Boghdadly K, Desai N, Halpern S, Blake L, Odor PM, Bampoe S, et al. Quadratus lumborum block vs. transversus abdominis plane block for caesarean delivery: a systematic review and network meta-analysis. Anaesthesia. 2021;76: 393–403.

28. Bateman BT, Franklin JM, Bykov K, Avorn J, Shrank WH, Brennan TA, et al. Persistent opioid use following cesarean delivery: patterns and predictors among opioid-naive women. Am J Obstet Gynecol. 2016;215(3):353 e1–e18.

29. Osmundson SS, Wiese AD, Min JY, Hawley RE, Patrick SW, Griffin MR, et al. Delivery type, opioid prescribing, and the risk of persistent opioid use after delivery. Am J Obstet Gynecol 2019;220:405–7.

30. Peahl AF, Dalton VK, Montgomery JR, Lai YL, Hu HM, Waljee JF. Rates of new persistent opioid use after vaginal or cesarean birth among US women. JAMA Netw Open. 2019 Jul 3;2(7): e197863.

31. Sun EC, Darnall BD, Baker LC, Mackey S. Incidence of and risk factors for chronic opioid use among opioid-naive patients in the postoperative period. JAMA Intern Med. 2016;176: 1286–93.

32. Wiese AD, Osmundson SS, Mitchel E Jr, Adgent M, Phillips S, Patrick SW, et al. The risk of serious opioid-related events associated with common opioid prescribing regimens in the postpartum period after cesarean delivery. Am J Obstet Gynecol MFM. 2021 Nov;3(6):100475.

33. Leffert L, Butwick A, Carvalho B, Arendt K, Bates SM, Friedman A, et al.; Members of the SOAP VTE Taskforce. The society for obstetric anesthesia and perinatology consensus statement on the anesthetic management of pregnant and postpartum women receiving thromboprophylaxis or higher dose anticoagulants. Anesth Analg. 2018;126:928–44.

34. Bauer ME, Arendt K, Beilin Y, Gernsheimer T, Perez Botero J, James AH, et al. The Society for Obstetric Anesthesia and Perinatology interdisciplinary consensus statement on neuraxial procedures in obstetric patients with thrombocytopenia. Anesth Analg. 2021;132:1531–44.

Chapter 51
Quality and Patient Safety

Christian M. Pettker

Department of Obstetrics, Gynecology and Reproductive Sciences, Yale University School of Medicine, New Haven, CT, USA

Safely providing the most effective care has always been a priority in medicine. However, increasing consumer and provider interest coupled with recent progress in the quality and patient safety movement has now made it a *primary* concern. The past 50 years have witnessed an evolution in healthcare into a complex environment, requiring integration of advanced technologies and diverse and specialized teams. Thus, opportunities for failure have become more prominent and the costs of errors greater. In 1999 the Institute of Medicine estimated that 44 000–98 000 patients die each year due to medical errors, with most of these deaths due to preventable errors and correctable faults [1]. Realizing that this would make medical errors the eighth leading cause of death in the United States, more than those from motor vehicle collisions, breast cancer, and AIDS, puts the burden of such errors into perspective.

The foundation of the quality and patient safety movement is that fallible individuals and teams working in an increasingly complicated system create substantial opportunities for inadvertent suboptimal and adverse outcomes that may be preventable. Healthcare leaders have responded with improving safety and quality standards, developing better communication and teamwork techniques, and building more robust fail-safes into our environment and technologies. Today, the science of medicine has renewed a commitment to its ancient credo of "first, do no harm." This chapter discusses the major concepts in patient safety and quality as applied to obstetrics.

Patient safety in obstetrics

Early on, the patient safety movement showed most progress in fields such as cardiology, critical care, and anesthesia, and obstetrics is now catching up. Obstetrics is a logical target for safety and quality improvements. Obstetrics is a significant component of US healthcare; childbirth accounts for over 4 million hospitalizations each year, ranking second only to cardiovascular disease [2]. Obstetrics is also unique in that an adverse outcome can often affect two patients (mother and infant) and a neonatal injury may result in significant long-term consequences for the family and society. The growing maternal morbidity and mortality "crisis" in the United States also signals substantial opportunity. It is also no secret that perinatal care has been in a crisis of professional insurance and medical liability. Although obstetricians and gynecologists represent only 5% of the physicians in the United States, they are responsible for 15% of liability claims and 36% of total payments [3], with payments for obstetric liability claims averaging $500 000 to $1 900 000 [4]. These latter factors have greatly affected the way obstetrics is practiced in the United States, with more obstetricians practicing defensive medicine and others simply dropping out of obstetric practice altogether [5].

How to measure safety

In general terms, quality and safety efforts can be tracked in three ways, using outcome measures, process measures, and structural and culture measures.

Outcome measures
Outcome measures track how often patients are harmed or how well the organization is providing favorable (expected) outcomes [6,7]. Most patient safety initiatives focus on adverse outcome measures, as the prevention of these events is often the primary goal of such efforts. Mann and colleagues have proposed one set of measures referred to as the obstetric Adverse Outcome Index (AOI), which is based on measures defined by the Joint Commission, the American College of Obstetricians and Gynecologists (ACOG), and the National Perinatal

Queenan's Management of High-Risk Pregnancy: An Evidence-Based Approach, Seventh Edition. Edited by Catherine Y. Spong
and Charles J. Lockwood.

Box 51.1 Adverse Outcome Index indicators

- Apgar <7 at 5 min
- Blood transfusion
- Fetal traumatic birth injury
- Intrapartum or neonatal death >2500 g
- Maternal death
- Maternal ICU admission
- Maternal return to operating room or Labor and Delivery
- Unexpected admission to neonatal ICU >2500 g and for >24 h
- Uterine rupture

ICU, intensive care unit.

Information Center [8]. The AOI is calculated as the percentage of mothers with at least one adverse outcome indicator (Box 51.1). This rate can be tracked on a monthly or quarterly basis and analyzed for trends and has been used to track the work of various quality improvement programs [8–11]. Units may track these indicators individually, but the critical measure of success is an improvement over time. Although the AOI can be compared across units, it is expected that the unique environments, patient demographics, and acuity levels will contribute to high unit-to-unit variability.

Severe maternal morbidity, which is defined by the US Centers for Disease Control and Prevention as "unexpected outcomes of labor and delivery that result in significant short- or long-term consequences to a woman's health," is also a proposed adverse outcome metric set for measuring safety and quality [12]. The strength of this metric is that the outcomes correspond to well-defined *International Classification of Diseases, Tenth Revision* codes; however, many of the outcomes are often unpreventable complications of pregnancy and thus may not frequently be associated with gaps in quality or safety.

The Joint Commission's Perinatal Core Measure "unexpected newborn complications in term infants" (PC-06) developed by the California Maternal Quality Care Collaborative is a good example of a safety outcome measure used in common practice that can be used to compare performance across hospitals and over time [13].

Process measures

Process measures analyze adherence to common or evidence-based standards and practices [14], with the assumption that adherence to these performance measures improves outcomes. The Surgical Care Improvement Project, which proposes to measure processes like appropriate antibiotic administration and thromboembolism prophylaxis, is one example of a set of process measures. Whether this, in turn, produces better outcomes is controversial, though one can argue that adherence to good practices in one segment of care produces better compliance across the spectrum of healthcare provisions [15].

The Joint Commission's Perinatal Core Measures around early elective delivery (PC-01); cesarean birth in nulliparous, term, singleton, vertex pregnancies (PC-02); and exclusive breastmilk feeding (PC-05) are examples of process measures. Cesarean birth, interestingly, is an example of a measure that can be both a process and an outcome measure because it reflects adherence to standards but is also a primary birth outcome.

Structure and culture measures

Structure measures refer to the resources and infrastructure available for care and includes nursing ratios, available technology, certification status, and types of providers. Safety culture is the integration of safety thinking and practices into clinical activities. Improving patient safety depends on changing the attitude of an organization, including shifting from a culture of blame to a culture of safety. Safety climate, the quantitative description of the safety culture, can be measured by calibrating a healthcare team's attitudes about issues related to safety through workforce or staff attitude surveys [16]. Many patient safety climate surveys are available. The Agency for Healthcare Research and Quality's Hospital Survey on Patient Safety Culture is a publicly available tool with a centralized comparative database that allows organizations to benchmark survey results [17]. The Safety Attitude Questionnaire (SAQ) is a tool adapted from the aviation industry and subsequently validated in healthcare that can be given to the various staff members of an obstetric unit [16,18]. Respondents answer a series of statements in agreement or disagreement (on a five-point Likert scale); differences of 10% or more, over time or between groups, are considered clinically significant and overall scores showing 80% agreement with a favorable teamwork climate statement are a target goal. One systematic review has identified the SAQ as the only safety climate survey that has been used to explore the relationship between safety perceptions and patient outcomes [19].

Tools to improve patient safety

Many strategies have been suggested to improve safety and quality in an obstetric service. Most center on principles of evidence-based practice, the benefits of standardization, and improving communication.

1. *Outside expert review.* Bringing in unbiased and experienced observers to review an obstetrics service for one or several days is often a first step for quality improvement. The review team may consist of any combination of nurses, physicians, or administrators, but should be a group with experience in safety and quality practices. Using a triangulation process to resolve differences in perspectives, the team can interview

staff from the various professional domains within the healthcare system to assess the culture of safety. Hospital policies and protocols should be reviewed. The result is usually a written review, with specific recommendations for improvement based on local and national standards, focusing on core principles of safety, and informed by the evidence.

2. *Protocols, guidelines, checklists, bundles, and care pathways.* The initial push for guidelines and protocols can meet with resistance from providers claiming the superiority of experience and intuition over evidence and standardization. A common fear is that guidelines and protocols may dictate all aspects and levels of care, to a level of detail that does not account for individual variations created by different locales, cultures, preferences, and experiences. Protocols and guidelines merely serve as a common foundation for approaching aspects of care relative to specific diseases or processes. Variable approaches to similar clinical scenarios, particularly when there is little evidence demonstrating any as superior, can contribute to confusion and error. Protocols and guidelines create common knowledge structures or shared mental models, improving performance in times of pressure and uncertainty. Higher-risk practices, such as the use of oxytocin, prostaglandins, and magnesium sulfate, are particularly aided by standardized protocols. Checklists, furthermore, aim to implement these protocols and guidelines by distilling and delineating, in real time, the important events and activities required to perform or respond successfully to clinical scenarios. Use of checklists has demonstrated remarkable reductions in rates of catheter-related bloodstream infections [7] and surgical complications [6] in large-scale trials. The key to developing and implementing these measures is to rely on standards set by the industry or evidence in the literature, and build on these through consensus among staff, preferably through working groups and sufficient comment periods. An example in obstetrics are the patient safety bundles developed by the Alliance for Innovation on Maternal Health program [20]. Two of the bundles–Severe Hypertension in Pregnancy and Obstetric Hemorrhage–have such prime importance for practice and maternal health that they are required for accreditation by The Joint Commission and are also a core focus in most state perinatal quality collaboratives.

3. *Computerized "order sets."* Computerized order entry can potentially contribute to improvements in patient safety by reducing the rates of medication errors. It should also be viewed as a mode of decision support, providing "protocolized" order sets that direct providers to a preferred and uniform management strategy, such as oxytocin administration, use of antibiotics

and steroids for preterm prelabor rupture of the fetal membranes, or preeclampsia management. Converting the relevant aspects of a particular protocol into a formalized order set can direct providers to the institutionally preferred management strategy.

4. *Perinatal patient safety nurse.* The perinatal patient safety nurse is often the crux of a patient safety program, acting as the educator and administrator for most of the sub-initiatives. This role is usually filled by a nurse with experience in clinical and administrative systems, relative to obstetrics and/or risk management [22]. Specifically, our patient safety nurse administrated our anonymous event reporting system, safety attitude questionnaire, and electronic fetal monitoring (EFM) certification testing, instructed our staff in crew resource management training, and performed audits of our adverse outcomes data.

5. *Anonymous event reporting system.* Computer-based reporting tools are available that allow for the discrete and anonymous reporting of adverse events, near-misses, and unsafe conditions. In addition to allowing for surveillance of existing and potential unsafe situations, it also empowers staff to participate in the quality improvement process. The patient safety nurse can educate staff on the use of the system, track data reported for trends, and investigate new or important issues as they arise.

6. *Obstetric hospitalist.* Hospitalist coverage of inpatient services, where a dedicated provider covers the care of inpatients from a variety of primary outpatient caregivers, has been increasingly used in other fields. The goal of using a hospitalist is to rely on providers with skill sets specific to a particular work environment, improve clinical efficiency, and improve outcomes. The concept of the "laborist" extends this to obstetric units, providing the continuity and availability of a caregiver who does not have responsibilities beyond the unit. Although continuity of care is reduced in this model, potential gains come from developing a team that is focused on and has mastered the efficient provision of inpatient obstetric care. Currently, Although data suggest superior outcomes in hospitals that employ hospitalists, there are no data available specific to obstetrics [23].

7. *Obstetric patient safety and quality committee.* Forming an obstetric patient safety committee allows representatives of the major stakeholders (e.g. nurses, midwives, obstetricians, pediatricians, anesthesiologists, pharmacists, administration, etc.) to meet regularly to review current practices and important adverse events and strategize on quality improvement efforts. This multidisciplinary approach fosters change in the organizational culture and allows for an efficient process of developing policies and protocols that have the interests of everyone in mind.

8. *Safety attitude questionnaire.* As discussed previously, the SAQ is both an intervention and an assessment tool. As an intervention, a survey demonstrates the interest of the organization in calibrating (and improving) the safety culture. As an assessment tool, the SAQ can be used to track improvements or areas for attention. This feedback is essential for management and administration to respond to the conditions on the front lines of care.

9. *Team training.* Communication failure is the dominant root cause of adverse events and near-misses. Crew resource management (CRM), a strategy to improve team functioning derived from civil and defense aviation work, is an important strategy for improving communication and teamwork. Team training aims to reduce the barriers between disciplines (e.g. nurses vs. physicians) that arise from these groups training in separate silos. Team training also attempts to combat traditional hierarchies that are common in medicine. Specific concepts that are usually taught are structured handoff techniques (e.g. Situation-Background-Assessment-Recommendation [SBAR]), conflict resolution techniques (concerned, uncomfortable, scared; the "two challenge" rule, the chain-of-command), and structured debriefing techniques that are performed after events. Team training has proven helpful in improving teamwork and outcomes in surgical units [24], though a trial to implement CRM in obstetrics units showed no benefit in outcomes as measured by the AOI [9].

10. *Standardization of EFM assessment.* Objective fetal heart rate interpretation relies on a standard set of definitions and descriptions. Indeed, inconsistencies in practice are largely due to obfuscations in the language and terms used to describe tracings. The Joint Commission Sentinel Event Alert No. 30 recognized that "inadequate fetal monitoring" was a root cause in 34% of adverse events, recommending units to "develop clear guidelines for fetal monitoring of potential high-risk patients, including nursing protocols for the interpretation of fetal heart rate tracings" and to "educate nurses, residents, nurse midwives, and physicians to use standardized terminology to communicate abnormal fetal heart rate tracings" [25]. Shortly thereafter, in 2005, ACOG and the Association of Women's Health, Obstetric and Neonatal Nurses advocated universal implementation of the National Institutes of Health/National Institute of Child Health and Human Development (NICHD) Workshop guidelines on electronic fetal monitoring [23], which were subsequently revised in 2008 [24]. Adoption of such guidelines by a unit is important, and usually relies on formalized programs for training and testing. Examples of this are offered by the National Certification Corporation (www.nccnet.org) or the Perinatal Quality Foundation (www.perinatalquality.

org) nonprofit groups that offers training and testing of fetal monitoring standards based on the NICHD criteria and professional best practices.

11. *Simulation.* The aviation industry has taught us that recreating workplace scenarios in simulations can contribute to acquisition of new skills, particularly for situations that occur infrequently, such as emergencies. Given that obstetrics is characterized mostly by routine labor and delivery, punctuated by low-frequency yet high severity events (e.g. shoulder dystocia, hemorrhage, and eclampsia), obstetrics has incorporated simulation into training. Simulation scenarios are usually focused on either knowledge/skills training or teamwork training, and often units will choose one or the other as the primary objective of simulation sessions. High-fidelity simulation technologies that involve sophisticated mannequins and equipment can provide a realistic experience but require substantial preparation and resources. In situ simulation scenarios that take place in the actual patient care units, usually during times of low acuity and census, can provide equally important lessons on teamwork/communication and skills. A recent systematic review of team training for acute obstetric emergencies reports improvements in some clinical outcomes (5-minute Apgars and hypoxic-ischemic encephalopathy) as well as in knowledge, skills, communication, and team performance [28].

Evidence to support improvement tools

With the emerging focus on quality and safety in healthcare, research evaluating various tools has increased over the past 5–10 years. Two of the more notable efforts have involved the implementation of checklists. In Michigan, a statewide effort to implement five evidence-based procedures for the insertion and care of catheters reduced catheter-related bloodstream infections by up to 66% [7]. The World Health Organization international project on a 19-item surgical checklist aiming to improve teamwork, communication, and consistency of care reduced death by nearly 50% (1.5% to 0.8%) and inpatient complications from 11% to 7% [6].

Obstetric research has lagged but is gaining ground. A long-term comprehensive safety effort at Yale-New Haven Hospital, incorporating most of the strategies discussed previously in this chapter, demonstrated significant improvements in patient outcomes [10]. Over a 3-year period, comprising over 13000 deliveries, the AOI declined significantly over time ($P = 0.01$) (Figure 51.1). The mean quarterly AOI for the second half of the initiative ($2.09 \pm 0.57\%$) was significantly lower than that for the first half ($2.90 \pm 0.64\%$) ($P = 0.04$). A group from the HCA Healthcare system, which involves more than 200 hospitals across the United States, implemented a comprehensive effort that included a protocol

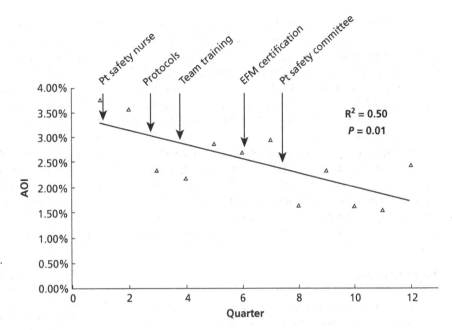

Figure 51.1 Yale-New Haven Hospital quarterly obstetric Adverse Outcome Index. Reproduced from Pettker et al. [10] with permission from Elsevier. AOI, Adverse Outcome Index; EFM, electronic fetal monitoring; Pt, patient.

for oxytocin administration, checklist-based protocols for misoprostol and magnesium, and a standardized shoulder dystocia delivery note. Over time, they witnessed a reduction in annual malpractice claims from 10–13 per 100000 deliveries to 6–7.5 per 100000 births [29].

Demonstrating the power of protocols and guidelines specifically, hospital policies to review and prevent unnecessary elective early term births have been shown to reduce the number of risky and unnecessary inductions as well as the rates of term neonatal admissions [30]. A statewide initiative in Ohio demonstrated a greater than fivefold reduction in inductions without a documented medical indications (25% to 5%, $P < 0.05$) [31]. A randomized trial describing the multifaceted implementation of guidelines for postpartum oxytocin administration and episiotomy repair showed improvements in postpartum hemorrhage rates and episiotomy use [32].

Beyond safety and quality

The primary motivations that drive patient safety efforts are providing quality care and eliminating harm, though secondary benefits accrue as well. Eliminating the costs of adverse events provides economic savings, which in turn guides investment in patient safety programs by governments and healthcare institutions [33–35]. Improvements in safety culture can provide more satisfying work environments, improving work efficiency and reducing workforce turnover.

Recent work is highlighting the gaps in equitable care and disparities in obstetric outcomes related to bias and racism in society and healthcare access and delivery. This is appropriately a critical part of the quality and safety conversation: we cannot have high quality or safe care without equitable care for all. Quality and safety projects are now incorporating the lens of equity by stratifying quality outcome metrics by patient race and by incorporating assessments of bias or discrimination in reviews of adverse events. One example is the Alliance for Innovation in Maternal Health patient safety bundle for Reduction of Peripartum Racial/Ethnic Disparities [36]. It is hoped that the concepts underlying safety and quality work – just culture, psychological safety, performance improvement, and root cause analysis – may help begin the reversal of long-standing and insidious inequities in our institutions.

CASE PRESENTATION

A 35-year-old gravida 1, para 0 at 39 weeks gestation is being induced for preeclampsia. She has presented at the end of the day, right before the change of shift, and the physician has ordered both intravenous magnesium sulfate, for seizure prophylaxis, and oxytocin. Before going off her shift, the nurse prepares the magnesium sulfate and oxy-

tocin infusions but does not start them. The next nurse coming on starts the infusions. Within minutes the patient is noted to have tetanic contractions and a prolonged fetal heart rate deceleration; despite discontinuation of the intravenous infusions and intrauterine resuscitative measures, the team proceeds to a stat cesarean delivery for a fetal

Continued

bradycardia. A healthy infant is born with Apgars of 5 and 9. After the cesarean is over, the nurse discovers that she confused the magnesium and the oxytocin lines and accidentally gave a large dose of oxytocin thinking it was the magnesium sulfate bolus. Understanding the importance of the team learning from the error, she enters a computerized anonymous event report for the patient safety nurse to review the next morning.

In response to this event, a root cause analysis (RCA) is organized and directed by an outside party experienced in event review. In the spirit of a culture of safety, rather than a culture of blame, the team identifies critical areas for potential improvement. Specific system improvements are suggested, such as an appropriate

"SBAR" nursing handoff in the patient room, and improved labeling systems for intravenous lines for oxytocin and magnesium sulfate so that they are not confused. The RCA also recognizes that communication during the emergency delivery was suboptimal. The RCA report is reviewed by the Patient Safety Committee, which discusses further enhancements over a longer time frame, such as creating a computerized SBAR handoff template. The committee also suggests organizing monthly simulations on labor and delivery to train staff on how to perform an efficient and organized emergency cesarean deliveries. These ideas create an action plan, which is taken to the staff and administration for implementation.

References

1. Kohn L, Corrigan J, Donaldson M, editors. To err is human: building a safer health system. Washington, DC: National Academies Press; 2000.
2. DeFrances C, Cullen K, Kozak L. National Hospital Discharge Survey: 2005 annual summary with detailed diagnosis and procedure data. National Center for Health Statistics. Vital Health Stat. 2007;13(165).
3. Sanfilippo J, Robinson C. The risk management handbook for healthcare professionals. Pearl River, NY: Parthenon Publishing; 2002.
4. Barbieri RL. Professional liability payments in obstetrics and gynecology. Obstet Gynecol. 2006;107(3):578–81.
5. Klagholz J, Strunk AL. Overview of the 2009 ACOG survey on professional liability. ACOG Clinical Review. 2009;14(6):1,13–16 [cited 2023 Jun 9]. Available from: https://www.academia.edu/707493/Overview_of_the_2009_ACOG_survey_on_professional_liability.
6. Haynes AB, Weiser TG, Berry WR, Lipsitz SR, Breizat AH, Dellinger EP, et al. A surgical safety checklist to reduce morbidity and mortality in a global population. N Engl J Med. 2009;360(5):491–9.
7. Pronovost P, Needham D, Berenholtz, S, Sinopoli D, Chu H, Cosgrove S, et al. An intervention to decrease catheter-related bloodstream infections in the ICU. N Engl J Med. 2006;355(26):2725–32.
8. Mann S, Pratt S, Gluck P, Nielsen P, Nielsen P, Risser D, Greenberg P, et al. Assessing quality in obstetrical care: development of standardized measures. Jt Comm J Qual Patient Saf. 2006;32:497–505.
9. Nielsen PE, Goldman MB, Mann S, Shapiro DE, Marcus RG, Pratt SD, et al. Effects of teamwork training on adverse outcomes and process of care in labor and delivery: a randomized controlled trial. Obstet Gynecol. 2007;109(1):48–55.
10. Pettker CM, Thung SF, Norwitz ER, Buhimschi CS, Raab CA, Copel JA, et al. Impact of a comprehensive patient safety strategy on obstetric adverse events. Am J Obstet Gynecol. 2009;200(5):492.e1–8.
11. Walker S, Strandjord TP, Benedetti TJ. In search of perinatal quality outcome measures: 1 hospital's in-depth analysis of the Adverse Outcomes Index. Am J Obstet Gynecol. 2010;203(4):336.e1–7.
12. Centers for Disease Control and Prevention. How does CDC identify severe maternal morbidity? [last reviewed 2019 Dec 26; cited 2022 May 10]. Available from: https://www.cdc.gov/reproductivehealth/maternalinfanthealth/smm/severe-morbidity-ICD.htm.
13. The Joint Commission. Specifications manual for Joint Commission National Quality Measures (v2022B1). 2022 [cited 2022 May 10]. Available from https://manual.jointcommission.org/releases/TJC2022B1/MIF0393.html.
14. Williams SC, Schmaltz SP, Morton DJ, Koss RG, Loeb JM. Quality of care in U.S. hospitals as reflected by standardized measures, 2002–2004. N Engl J Med. 2005;353(3):255–64.
15. Hawn MT. Surgical care improvement: should performance measures have performance measures? JAMA. 2010;303(24):2527–8.
16. Sexton JB, Helmreich RL, Neilands TB, Rowan K, Vella K, Boyden J, et al. The Safety Attitudes Questionnaire: psychometric properties, benchmarking data, and emerging research. BMC Health Serv Res. 2006;6:44.
17. Agency for Healthcare Research and Quality. Surveys on patient safety culture. [cited 2022 May 10]. Available from: https://www.ahrq.gov/sops/index.html.
18. Sexton JB, Holzmueller CG, Pronovost PJ, Thomas EJ, McFerran S, Nunes J, et al. Variation in caregiver perceptions of teamwork climate in labor and delivery units. J Perinatol. 2006;26(8):463–70.
19. Colla JB, Bracken AC, Kinney LM, Weeks WB. Measuring patient safety climate: a review of surveys. Qual Saf Health Care. 2005;14(5):364–6.
20. Alliance for Innovation in Maternal Health. Patient safety bundles. [cited 2023 Jun 2]. Available from: https://saferbirth.org/patient-safety-bundles/.
21. Simpson KR. Quality measures for perinatal care. MCN Am J Matern Child Nurs. 2010;35(1):64.
22. Will SB, Hennicke KP, Jacobs LS, O'Neill LM, Raab CA. The perinatal patient safety nurse: a new role to promote safe care for mothers and babies. J Obstet Gynecol Neonatal Nurs. 2006;35(3):417–23.
23. Lopez L, Hicks LS, Cohen AP, McKean S, Weissman JS. Hospitalists and the quality of care in hospitals. Arch Intern Med. 2009;169(15):1389–94.
24. Neily J, Mills PD, Young-Xu Y, Carney BT, West P, Berger DH, et al. Association between implementation of a medical team

training program and surgical mortality. JAMA. 2010;304(15):1693–1700.

25. The Joint Commission. Sentinel Event Alert 30: preventing infant death and injury during delivery. 2004 Jul 21 [cited 2023 Jun 2]. Available from: https://www.jointcommission.org/resources/sentinel-event/sentinel-event-alert-newsletters/sentinel-event-alert-issue-30-preventing-infant-death-and-injury-during-delivery/.

26. National Institute of Child Health and Human Development Research Planning Workshop. Electronic fetal heart rate monitoring: research guidelines for interpretation. Am J Obstet Gynecol. 1997;177(6):1385–90.

27. Macones GA, Odibo A, Gross G, Stamilio D, Rampersad R, Ebinger R, et al. Standardized multidisciplinary EFM training for the entire obstetrical team. Am J Obstet Gynecol. 2009;199(6):S211.

28. Merien AE, van de Ven J, Mol BW, Houterman S, Oei SG. Multidisciplinary team training in a simulation setting for acute obstetric emergencies: a systematic review. Obstet Gynecol. 2010;115(5):1021–31.

29. Clark SL, Belfort MA, Byrum SL, Meyers JA, Perlin JB. Improved outcomes, fewer cesarean deliveries, and reduced litigation: results of a new paradigm in patient safety. Am J Obstet Gynecol. 2008;199(2):105.e1–7.

30. Clark SL, Frye DR, Meyers JA, Belfort MA, Dildy GA, Kofford S, et al. Reduction in elective delivery at <39 weeks of gestation: comparative effectiveness of 3 approaches to change and the impact on neonatal intensive care admission and stillbirth. Am J Obstet Gynecol. 2010;203(5):449.e–16.

31. Donovan EF, Lannon C, Bailit J, Rose B, Iams JD, Byczkowski T. A statewide initiative to reduce inappropriate scheduled births at 36(0/7)-38(6/7) weeks gestation. Am J Obstet Gynecol. 2010;202(3):243.e1–8.

32. Althabe F, Buekens P, Bergel E, Belizán JM, Campbell MK, Moss N, et al. A behavioral intervention to improve obstetrical care. N Engl J Med. 2008;358(18):1929–40.

33. Paradis AR, Stewart VT, Bayley KB, Brown A, Bennett AJ. Excess cost and length of stay associated with voluntary patient safety event reports in hospitals. Am J Med Qual. 2009;24(1):53–60.

34. Schmidek JM, Weeks WB. What do we know about financial returns on investments in patient safety? A literature review. Jt Comm J Qual Patient Saf. 2005;31(12):690–9.

35. Zhan C, Miller MR. Excess length of stay, charges, and mortality attributable to medical injuries during hospitalization. JAMA. 2003;290(14):1868–74.

36. Alliance for Innovation in Maternal Health. Reduction of peripartum ethnic and racial disparities. 2016 [cited 2023 Jun 2]. Available from: https://saferbirth.org/psbs/archive-reduction-peripartum-disparities/.

Chapter 52
Genetic Amniocentesis, Chorionic Villus Sampling, Intrauterine Transfusion, and Shunts

Ann McHugh and Russell S. Miller

Department of Obstetrics and Gynecology, Columbia University Irving Medical Center, New York, NY, USA

Minimally invasive prenatal diagnostic and therapeutic procedures can be used for a range of indications. Sampling amniotic fluid or chorionic villi via amniocentesis or chorionic villus sampling (CVS), respectively, allows for prenatal diagnosis of numerous genetic disorders. Other invasive fetal procedures such as cordocentesis with intrauterine blood transfusion (IUT) and fetal shunting can be life-saving interventions for selected severe fetal disease states. In this chapter, we review genetic amniocentesis, CVS, IUT and fetal shunts. This chapter describes techniques, indications, benefits, and complications of these procedures.

Prenatal diagnosis

The presence of cell-free fetal DNA (cffDNA) in the maternal circulation was first reported in 1997 [1]. Since that time, cffDNA screening has become widely available for clinical use, demonstrating high sensitivity and specificity for the identification of common aneuploidies including trisomies 21, 18, and 13 [2]. The increasing acceptance of cffDNA by patients and providers has significantly reduced screen-positive results, resulting in fewer invasive prenatal tests being performed [3]. However, both CVS and amniocentesis remain, at present, the only definitive diagnostic tests for aneuploidy and other genetic abnormalities in pregnancy, offering a certainty and breadth of information that cffDNA screening alone cannot currently provide. Pregnant patients can pursue amniocentesis or CVS for prenatal diagnosis for a variety of reasons, including a desire for diagnostic certainty. Diagnostic tests may be recommended to a patient identified as having an increased risk of a pregnancy affected by aneuploidy or other genetic abnormality. Examples of indications for invasive genetic testing include fetal structural anomaly detected on ultrasound, increased risk for aneuploidy upon genetic screening, previous pregnancy with a genetic abnormality, and a known risk of an inherited genetic disease or family history of a genetic disorder.

Chorionic villus sampling

Chorionic villus sampling involves suction aspiration of individual villi from the early placenta. It is usually performed between 11+0 and 13+6 weeks of gestational age. The procedure can be performed by either a transcervical approach using a catheter or transabdominally using a needle. Both sampling routes are equally safe and effective [4], with the sampling route selected mainly based on operator preference, patient choice, or placental location. Commonly, 15 to 25 mg of chorionic villi are obtained with the procedure. CVS can be performed on twin and higher-order multiple pregnancies. In multiple pregnancy, each distinct placental mass must be identified prior to the procedure and each placenta sampled individually.

Transcervical chorionic villus sampling
Transcervical CVS yields more chorionic villi when compared to transabdominal CVS. However, it is useful for proceduralists to be skilled in both methods. For example, a fundal placenta is often more easily accessed transabdominally and a posterior placenta, in many cases, may be more readily sampled by a transcervical approach. In other specific circumstances, such as with cervical polyps or active genital herpes, a transabdominal approach may be necessary.

Queenan's Management of High-Risk Pregnancy: An Evidence-Based Approach, Seventh Edition. Edited by Catherine Y. Spong and Charles J. Lockwood.

Prior to CVS, a careful history and ultrasound examination are required to confirm gestational age, assess fetal number and viability, and determine placental location. Additionally, ultrasound is used to evaluate the uterine position and observe the cervix as it enters the uterine cavity. A retroflexed uterus may require manual repositioning. Filling the bladder can be used to align an anteverted uterus into a more favorable axial plane. A 5.3–5.7 French (1.5 mm external diameter) sampling catheter is used, which is approximately 24–27 cm long. It contains a blunt-ended stylet that can be manually molded into a slightly curved shape before use. In the lithotomy position, a speculum is used for visualization and the vagina is prepped aseptically with povidone-iodine solution. The sampling catheter is introduced transcervically under continuous ultrasound guidance and directed into the placenta, parallel to its long axis. Once visualized on ultrasound, the catheter tip is advanced parallel to the chorionic membranes to the distal edge of the placenta avoiding injury to the membranes or decidua (Figure 52.1). The stylet is removed, and a 20 mL syringe containing approximately 5 mL of tissue culture medium is attached. Negative pressure is then applied by retracting the syringe plunger. Following this, the catheter is slowly removed. Adequacy of the sample should be confirmed immediately after retrieval by direct visualization of the white branching villi floating in the syringe or petri dish. If necessary, a low-power dissecting microscope can be used to confirm the adequacy of the sample. If the first attempt does not yield a sufficiently large sample, a second attempt can be undertaken with a new catheter. In general, two aspirations can be safely performed with minimal impact on pregnancy loss rate. Fetal heart activity should be confirmed by ultrasound following the procedure. Nonsensitized Rhesus-negative women should be informed of the need for prophylactic anti-D following the procedure. Importantly, known Rhesus or other red blood cell antigen alloimmunization is considered a contraindication to CVS, as it can theoretically cause an exacerbation of disease [5].

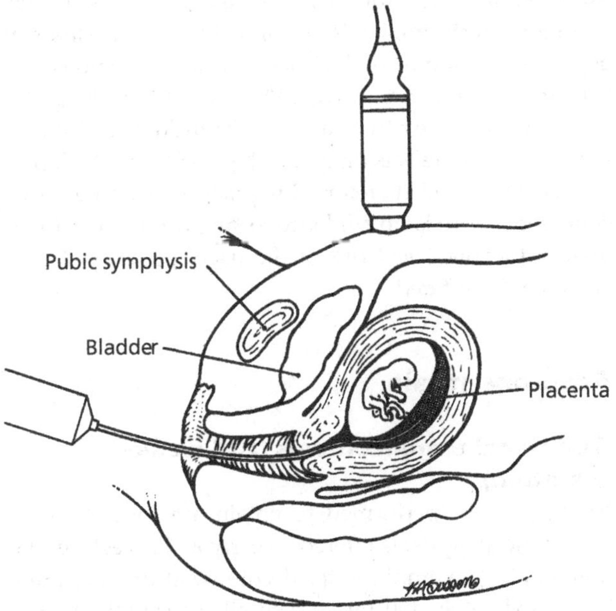

Transabdominal chorionic villus sampling

Under continuous sonographic guidance, using standard aseptic technique, an 18- or 20-gauge spinal needle is percutaneously guided through the maternal abdomen and myometrium to the placenta, parallel to the chorionic membrane. This occurs with the patient in the supine position, after her abdomen has been prepped with an antiseptic solution. The tip of the needle is advanced into the long axis of the placenta (Figure 52.2). Once correct placement is sonographically confirmed, the stylet is removed and a 20 mL syringe is attached that contains approximately 3 mL of tissue culture medium. Negative pressure is then applied by retracting the syringe plunger. While maintaining negative-pressure suction, multiple passes of the needle tip through the body of the placenta,

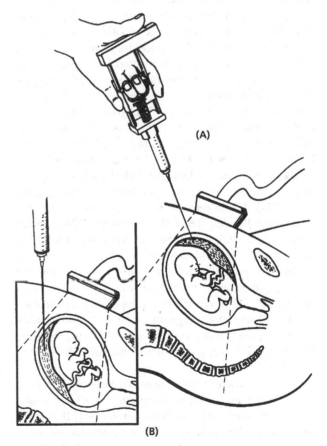

Figure 52.2 Transabdominal chorionic villus sampling (CVS) performed: (A) in an anterior placenta and (B) in a posterior placenta.

Pubic symphysis

Bladder

Placenta

Figure 52.1 Transcervical chorionic villus sampling.

without removing the needle from the placenta, are required to retrieve an adequate sample of villi. A handheld biopsy aspiration device (Cook Ob/Gyn, Spencer, IN) is employed in some centers to facilitate the procedure. With each internal pass, the needle is redirected slightly to sample different sites. Without releasing the negative pressure, the needle is then removed. A smaller-lumen needle is employed in transabdominal CVS compared to the relatively wider lumen of the catheter used in transcervical CVS, and therefore the number of villi obtained by transabdominal CVS is often about half that usually obtained by transcervical aspiration [6].

Transabdominal CVS may be considered later in the second and third trimesters to obtain a placental biopsy for genetic testing in cases in which an amniocentesis may be technically difficult. An example of this involves cases complicated by oligohydramnios or anhydramnios in the absence of suspected preterm prelabor rupture of the fetal membranes (PPROM). However, transcervical CVS is best performed prior to 14 weeks gestational age.

Complications of chorionic villus sampling

An evaluation of procedure-associated pregnancy loss rates following CVS must consider that the background miscarriage rate at the usual time for performing CVS, between 11–13 weeks gestational age, is 1% greater than at 15–16 weeks, the earlier range for offering amniocentesis. Reporting realistic risk figures for fetal loss following CVS remains difficult, as many variables influence the procedure-related fetal loss rate. Some studies suggest that transabdominal CVS and amniocentesis have fetal loss rates comparable to the background rate [7,8]. In 2008, a retrospective cohort study of 5148 CVS procedures, reported pregnancy loss rates that were below the background rate regardless of CVS route (transabdominal −0.2%, transcervical −0.5%) [9]. Other studies suggest a slightly higher fetal loss rate than the background rate [10,11]. A 2017 retrospective cohort study published outcomes following 4862 CVS procedures, 2833 of which were transcervical, found the additional risk of fetal loss with transcervical and transabdominal CVS, when compared to a group of women ≥36 years who did not undergo an invasive procedure, was 1.36% and 1.03% respectively [12]. In another contemporary series involving 45,120 singleton pregnancies, of which 861 underwent CVS, the risk of procedure-related loss attributed to CVS was 0.29% (95% confidence interval [CI] −0.53 to 1.12%) [13].

Multiple catheter passes are associated with increased rates of pregnancy loss, and operator experience is also believed by some to be an important factor [14]. Vaginal bleeding is the most common complication of CVS, occurring in up to 10% of cases of transcervical CVS vs. 1% of cases of transabdominal CVS [15]. This bleeding tends to resolve spontaneously within a few days.

Infection and the risk of chorioamnionitis is rare and can occur as a result of skin contamination or inadvertent maternal bowel injury following transabdominal CVS. Leakage of amniotic fluid has been reported and can arise in the setting of a subchorionic hematoma post CVS. Rupture of the membranes post CVS is rare in experienced centers [16].

The US collaborative study on CVS revealed a 99.7% rate of successful cytogenetic diagnosis from CVS; only 1.1% of patients required a second diagnostic test, such as an amniocentesis or fetal blood sampling, to further interpret the results [17, 18]. In three quarters of such cases, the additional testing was required to delineate the clinical significance of mosaic or other ambiguous results. Discrepancies can occur between the cytogenetics of the placenta and those of the fetus because early in development the cells contributing to the chorionic villi become separate and distinct from those forming the embryo. For this reason, confined placental mosaicism can affect 1–2% of CVS results.

Similar to amniocentesis, fetal injury can occur if a CVS is performed too early in gestation. Oromandibular disruption and limb reduction defects following CVS procedures performed between 8+0 to 9+3 weeks gestational age were first reported in 1991 [19]. An additional 14 cases of limb reduction defects ranging from mild to severe were reported by Burton et al. [20], in 1992, only two of which occurred when sampling was performed beyond 9.5 weeks gestation. However, no overall increased risk of limb reduction defects or any difference in the pattern of defects was identified from 216,381 CVS procedures when compared with the general population [21]. The association is still unclear, and any potential risk may be gestational age dependent. From a large data set of 106,383 CVS procedures, the rate of limb reduction defects at week 8 exceeded the background risk of 6.0 per 10,000 births. Therefore, performing CVS prior to 10 weeks gestational age is not recommended. Patients who for religious reasons may wish for an early CVS before 10 weeks gestational age must be counseled that the incidence of severe limb reduction defects may be as high as 1–2% when performed early, and therefore this practice is strongly discouraged. There is no evidence to support an increase in limb reduction defect risk at the usual gestational ages when CVS is offered.

Amniocentesis

Traditional amniocentesis (≥15 weeks gestation)

Amniocentesis, performed to obtain amniotic fluid for diagnostic analysis, is offered as early as 15 weeks gestational age. The amniotic fluid volume at this gestation is approximately 150 mL, which allows sampling to be performed with ease. Furthermore, the ratio of viable to nonviable cells in the amniotic fluid is at its greatest around this time, thus minimizing the risk of laboratory failure [22]. As is true with all procedures discussed in this chapter, informed written consent is necessary prior to the procedure. The consent process should include a discussion of procedure-associated risks, benefits, alternatives, timing and method of communicating results and post procedure instructions. Nonsensitized Rhesus-negative patients should be informed of the recommendation for prophylactic anti-D immunoglobulin administration following the procedure.

All amniocentesis procedures are preceded by a history and ultrasound examination to assess the number and location of fetuses, to confirm fetal viability and gestational age, to determine the placental location, and to estimate amniotic fluid volume. Additionally, the ultrasound assessment is useful in identifying any uterine abnormalities (e.g. leiomyomas) that could influence procedural technique, such as needle placement. Sonographic evaluation is also important to exclude an amnion-chorion separation, which can normally occur in a subset of pregnancies up to 16–17 weeks. Should this be detected, deferring the procedure for a week or two is generally recommended to allow for membrane fusion.

Once the optimal needle insertion path is identified, the maternal abdomen is prepped with an antiseptic solution. Under ultrasound guidance a 22- or 20-gauge needle is inserted through the maternal abdomen, taking care to avoid maternal bowel and bladder, as well as fetal parts (Figure 52.3). Local anesthesia or antibiotic prophylaxis

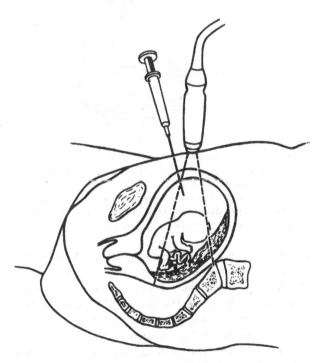

Figure 52.3 Amniocentesis performed with ultrasound guidance. Reproduced from [24]/with permission from Elsevier.

are not necessary for the procedure. The needle is placed into a sizable pocket of amniotic fluid free from umbilical cord and fetal parts when possible, and a sample of amniotic fluid (20–40 mL) is withdrawn. The syringe is detached from the needle prior to its removal to minimize contamination and the sample is sent for analysis. Fetal heart activity should be documented following the procedure.

Ideally, transplacental passage of the needle should be avoided. If this is not possible then the thinnest portion of the placenta away from the umbilical cord insertion and placental edge should be chosen. Color Doppler ultrasound can help to identify placental cord insertion and large plate vessels that should be avoided. If the first attempt to obtain a sample is unsuccessful, a second attempt in a different location may be performed. However, given potentially increased risk of fetal loss with more than two attempts at any single session, a third attempt is not recommended in one visit [23].

Early amniocentesis (<14 weeks gestation)

Early amniocentesis prior to 15 weeks gestational age should rarely, if ever, be performed. These procedures are both technically more challenging and have been shown in randomized controlled studies to have an increased rate of procedure-associated pregnancy loss, in addition to a 10-fold increased risk of fetal talipes [25–27]. Early amniocentesis is associated with an increased need for multiple needle insertions [28] and carries an increased risk of a failed culture when compared with midtrimester amniocentesis [29]. Additionally, at early gestations, there is less amniotic fluid available for sampling, and incomplete fusion of the amnion and chorion can result in tenting of the membranes and a 3% rate of a failed procedure [24].

Multiple gestations

Amniocentesis can be performed in twin and higher-order multiple pregnancies. However, each gestational sac must be sampled individually. Additionally, great effort should be made to avoid traversing the dividing membrane, which can result in sample cross-contamination and creation of an iatrogenic inter-twin septostomy. Sufficient amniotic fluid volume should be present in each gestational sac [30]. To ensure that each fetus is identified and sampled correctly, mapping is essential prior to any invasive testing. Care must be taken when there is no clearly distinguishable ultrasonographic difference between the fetuses, such as discordant fetal structural anomaly, size, or sex. Mapping each fetus by lateral orientation, as maternal left and maternal right twins, or by vertical orientation, as upper and lower twins, is more reproducible than using numbers alone and is recommended by the UK National Institute for Health and Care Excellence [31]. Further mapping by placental location and placental cord insertion may also be helpful in challenging cases or with higher-order multiple gestations. Following a thorough ultrasound examination and identification of the dividing membrane, the amniotic fluid aspiration from the first sac of a multiple pregnancy is performed as for a singleton, taking care to avoid the inter-twin dividing membrane. Prior to needle removal, 1–2 mL of concentrated sterile indigo carmine dye may be injected into the first sac. A new needle is used to obtain the amniotic sample in the second or subsequent sacs, again taking care to avoid the dividing membrane. Aspiration of clear amniotic fluid form the second sac confirms the procedure has been successful (Figure 52.4). Methylene blue should not be used given its association with fetal jejunoileal atresia following intraamniotic injection [32]. Triplets and higher order multiples can be tested by sequentially injecting dye into successive sacs following withdrawal of clear amniotic fluid from each sac. Supply challenges related to sterile indigo carmine availability or cost may limit its availability in clinical practice. In these scenarios, care should be taken to confirm correct twin amniotic sac location.

Complications of amniocentesis

Although an original estimate based upon 1986 randomized controlled trial data indicated a 1% procedure-associated risk of pregnancy loss following amniocentesis [33], subsequent data demonstrate that actual risk is likely orders of magnitude lower. A 2015 large systematic review and meta-analysis of published contemporary nonrandomized studies approximated the incremental pregnancy loss risk following a second-trimester amniocentesis in experienced centers to be approximately 0.11% (95% CI −0.04% to 0.26%) [34]. Additionally, the meta-analysis found that there was no increased risk of pregnancy loss in pregnancies that underwent amniocentesis compared with pregnancies that did not. This finding has been echoed for the risks of amniocentesis in multiple gestations. A recent systematic review and meta-analysis reported no difference in the rate of fetal loss in twin pregnancies undergoing amniocentesis (2.4% [95% CI 1.4–3.6%]) compared with twin pregnancies not undergoing amniocentesis (2.4% [95% CI 0.9–4.6%]) [35]. There may be an inverse association between operator experience and procedure-related pregnancy loss, and therefore more procedure-related risks may occur when procedures are performed by less skilled operators [9,36].

Continuous ultrasound guidance throughout the procedure appears to reduce the number of punctures and the incidence of a bloody fluid sample being obtained. Direct fetal trauma from the needle is rare and there is no additional risk of pregnancy loss if transplacental passage of the needle is required [37]. Other complications include abdominal cramping, vaginal bleeding, and leakage of fluid per vagina. These minor complications usually

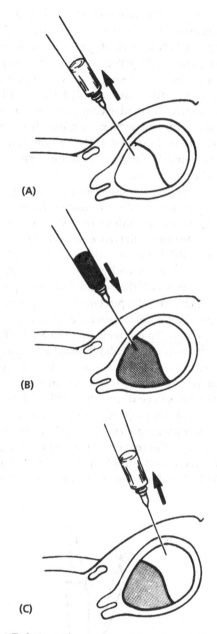

(A)

(B)

(C)

Figure 52.4 Technique of amniocentesis in twin gestations, performed under concurrent ultrasound guidance. (A) Fluid aspirated from the first amniotic sac. (B) Indigo carmine injected into the first amniotic sac. (C) Second amniocentesis in the ultrasonographically determined location of the second fetus. Clear fluid confirms that the second amniotic sac was successfully aspirated. Reproduced from [30]/with permission from Elsevier.

subside after a few hours to, rarely, days, with no impact on pregnancy outcome. The rate of post-amniocentesis PPROM occurring within 2 weeks of a mid-trimester amniocentesis is 0.24%–1% [16,38]. The perinatal outcomes are better in pregnancies complicated by PPROM following amniocentesis compared to those with spontaneous PPROM. Expectant management should be considered when post-amniocentesis PPROM occurs [38], as most cases resolve spontaneously within a few days.

Table 52.1 Complications of amniocentesis and CVS

	Amniocentesis	CVS
PPROM within 14 days	<1%	<0.1%
Confined placental mosaicism	Not applicable	1–2%
Maternal cell contamination	1–2%	1–2%
Failed cell culture	0.5–1%	0.5–1%
Severe infection	Rare	Rare
Fetal injury	Rare	Rare
Maternal visceral injury	Rare	Rare

CVS, chorionic villus sampling; PPROM, preterm prelabor rupture of the fetal membranes.

Successful treatment of iatrogenic PPROM with an amniopatch has been previously described in the literature [39]. However, this treatment currently remains experimental due to unproven benefit and concerns of risks including fetal bradycardia. Amnionitis can occur in 0.1% of cases, usually as a result of contamination of the amniotic cavity with skin flora or from inadvertent passage of the needle through maternal bowel. Severe sepsis is rare (Table 52.1).

Rhesus isoimmunization can theoretically occur in a Rhesus-negative women with a Rhesus positive fetus following amniocentesis; however, the rate is likely to be very low. In a registry-based study of 10,085 women in Denmark, immunoprophylaxis was not routinely administered following CVS or amniocentesis and no differences in alloimmunization rates at 29 weeks gestation were found between women with or without invasive genetic testing [40]. Nevertheless, most guidelines advocate administering anti-Rh(D) immunoglobulin to Rh(D)-negative women following invasive procedures [41,42]. No long-term effects of amniocentesis have been reported in children or adolescents [43]. Failure of amniotic cell cultures can occur in 0.5–1% of cases [38].

Third trimester amniocentesis may be considered for indications such as a newly diagnosed fetal structural abnormality, fetal growth restriction, or suspected fetal infection. Risks of triggering preterm labor are 4–8% before 37 weeks and 3–4% before 34 weeks gestational age [44,45]. Higher rates of bloodstained samples have been reported in approximately 5–10% of procedures performed in the third trimester [46]. Additionally, there is an increased risk of culture failure following third-trimester amniocentesis. This risk increases with advancing gestational age and can be as high as 40.6% between 36–40 weeks gestation [47].

Diagnostic studies

Following amniocentesis or CVS, genetic evaluation in the form of fluorescent in situ hybridization (FISH), karyotype, chromosomal microarray (CMA), and whole exome or genome sequencing are examples of assessments that can be performed using the fetal DNA that is obtained.

Fluorescence in Situ Hybridization
Rapid testing for chromosomes 13, 18, 21, X, and Y uses FISH of uncultured interphase cells or quantitative fluorescence polymerase chain reaction-based DNA analysis. This can allow for determination of fetal genetic sex and detection of selected common aneuploidies. Results can be obtained within 24 to 48 hours and should be confirmed by karyotype.

Karyotype
An analysis of all chromosomes using clinical G-banded karyotype can be performed on cultured sample of amniocytes or chorionic villi. A karyotype can detect whole chromosome aneuploidy, large deletions or duplications, balanced rearrangements, marker chromosomes, and mosaicism. Results take between 7 to 14 days, as chromosomes in metaphase are required for analysis. The interpretation of a karyotype is subjective, and a limitation of its use is that smaller microdeletions and duplications may be poorly detected or unrecognized.

Chromosomal microarray
Chromosomal microarray (CMA) is a form of molecular cytogenetics in which DNA fragments are hybridized to probes representing known portions of the genome (Figure 52.5). Microdeletions or duplications, which represent missing or overrepresented portions of the genome, can then be identified by computational analysis. Results can take between 3 to 5 days if direct testing on an uncultured sample is used and between 10 to 14 days if testing is performed on cultured cells.

There is an increased diagnostic yield when evaluating a fetal anomaly if using CMA vs. conventional karyotype and a faster turnaround time. In a study evaluating the incremental yield of CMA when compared with karyotype for routine prenatal diagnosis, CMA of 4282 nonmosaic samples identified all the aneuploidies and unbalanced rearrangements that were identified on karyotyping. In samples with a normal karyotype and a structural anomaly, CMA identified a clinically relevant deletion or duplication in 6.0% [48]. However, CMA cannot detect balanced chromosomal rearrangements, it cannot differentiate trisomies from unbalanced Robertsonian translocations, and it may miss marker chromosomes or low-level mosaicism.

Next generation sequencing
Next generation sequencing (NGS) includes a variety of technologies that perform sequencing of millions of small fragments of DNA in parallel to determine the nucleic acid sequence, and then reconstruct the entire DNA sequence using bioinformatic tools that reassemble fragments. Results interpretation requires bioinformatic analysis with

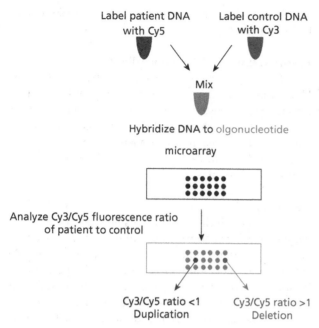

Label patient DNA
with Cy5

Label control DNA
with Cy3

Mix

Hybridize DNA to olgonucleotide

microarray

Analyze Cy3/Cy5 fluorescence ratio
of patient to control

Cy3/Cy5 ratio <1
Duplication

Cy3/Cy5 ratio >1
Deletion

Figure 52.5 This figure illustrates the general principle underlying comparative genomic hybridization that is used to identify DNA deletions or duplications. In this technique, fluorescently labeled DNA from a normal control sample is mixed with a test sample that is labeled with a different colored dye. The mixture is then hybridized to an array containing hundreds of thousands of small, well-defined, DNA probes. Regional differences in the fluorescence ratio of gains/losses can be detected and used for identifying abnormal regions in the genome. Courtesy of Dr. Ronald Wapner. Modified from Reddy et al. [49] with permission from Lippincott Williams and Wilkins.

computerized algorithms, functional analysis, and public databases. NGS can be used to evaluate specific genes within the exome or the entire genome down to the single base pair level. Whole exome sequencing (WES) of fetal DNA from an amniocentesis, CVS, or postnatal sample is currently being used in clinical and research settings.

Whole Exome Sequencing

WES involves sequencing and analysis of the 1 to 2% of the genome that codes for expressed RNAs and proteins. Result turnaround time for prenatal WES varies depending on the laboratory and the indication. The fetal DNA can be analysed in isolation or as part of a "trio" in which parental and fetal DNA are sequenced and analyzed together. Analysis and variant interpretation must follow strict criteria and the American College of Medical Genetics and Genomics class each DNA sequence change or variant as pathogenic, likely pathogenic, a variant of uncertain significance, likely benign, or benign. In a fetus with one structural anomaly, performing WES in addition to CMA increases the genetic detection of a causative genotype in 8.5% to 10% of cases [50, 51]. The detection rate increases when multiple structural anomalies are present, and there are some data suggesting that it is organ specific.

The highest detection rate of genetic variants has been found with anomalies of the lymphatic system (24%), skeletal system (24%), central nervous system (22%), and renal system (16%). The lowest detection rate was found in isolated cardiac anomalies (5%) [50,51]. The importance of pre- and posttest counseling for prenatal or trio WES cannot be underestimated, and interpretation of results should involve a multidisciplinary team.

Whole Genome Sequencing

Whole-genome sequencing (WGS) analyzes the entire genome, including protein coding and nonprotein coding regions. Nonprotein coding regions of the genome have been implicated in both Mendelian and human genetic disease [52,53]. Currently, WGS is not widely used for clinical diagnosis and more studies are required to determine its clinically utility in a prenatal setting.

Intrauterine Transfusion

Fetal blood sampling, cordocentesis, or funipuncture all describe a technique to obtain a percutaneous umbilical blood sample (PUBS). This minimally invasive procedure allows for prenatal diagnosis using fetal blood and is generally a prerequisite to performing an intrauterine fetal blood transfusion (IUT). PUBS can be performed for diagnosis of fetal anemia, congenital infection, thrombocytopenia or other hematologic conditions, metabolic disorders, or for cytogenetic analysis [54]. Therapeutic indications include in utero blood transfusions for severe fetal anemia and for medication administration. Therefore, a PUBS procedure can be used as a diagnostic tool and as a therapeutic intervention.

Intrauterine fetal blood transfusions can ameliorate and resolve fetal anemia and allow for delivery at a later gestational age. Fetal anemia is usually suspected when the Doppler peak systolic velocity of the fetal middle cerebral artery is elevated greater than 1.5 multiples of the median on ultrasound imaging and/or if signs of hydrops are present. Fewer IUTs are now being performed given the advent of anti-D prophylaxis for the prevention of Rhesus alloimmunization. Because CVS and amniocentesis are now the most commonly used procedures to obtain fetal DNA for genetic analyses, an example of a genetic indication for a PUBS would be to further evaluate a mosaic result obtained from CVS or amniocentesis. A PUBS can also allow for direct assessment and treatment of fetal thyroid conditions.

Intraperitoneal approach to IUT

In the 1960s, Liley described intrauterine intraperitoneal blood transfusion (IPT), in which transfused red blood cells are absorbed into the fetal lymphatic system with the aim of ameliorating fetal anemia. Although IPT reduced perinatal mortality rates from hemolytic disease of the fetus and newborn, outcomes for those with alloimmune anemia <26 weeks gestation and those with hydrops remained poor [55]. In the 1980s, Daffos and colleagues were the first to introduce ultrasound-guided fetal blood sampling [56]. Thereafter, intraperitoneal transfusions were largely superseded by intravascular transfusion due to improved survival benefit when compared to the IP approach. However, there remain clinical scenarios for which IP transfusions may be used, and therefore being skilled in both techniques is advantageous. These scenarios include early gestational ages, for example under 18–22 weeks gestation, in which intravascular access is technically difficult, or when the fetal vasculature is technically inaccessible due to fetal or cord positioning. Additionally, as absorption of fetal blood via the lymphatic system is a slow process, an IPT may be preferred in clinical scenarios in which a delayed update of blood into the fetal intravascular space is desired [57]. The benefit to this use of IPT is that it may allow for a prolonged interval between transfusions, and particularly in presentations involving gradually progressive fetal anemia. An example of a condition for which an IPT transfusion component has been proposed is for donor twin transfusion in pregnancies complicated by twin anemia polycythemia sequence (TAPS).

Intravascular access for fetal transfusion

An intravascular approach for the management of fetal anemia provides an opportunity to confirm a suspected fetal anemia, to perform other indicated evaluations, to administer red cells directly into the fetal circulation and–when possible–to confirm success of the intervention prior to completion. A preferred location for performing an intravascular transfusion (IVT) via cordocentesis is at the placental cord insertion. Other sites include a free-floating loop of umbilical cord, the intrahepatic portion of the umbilical vein and in rare cases direct cardiac puncture. The target vessel is the umbilical vein. It is recommended to avoid the umbilical artery given risk for precipitating vasospasm and an associated 11-fold increased rate of complications including need for emergency delivery and fetal or neonatal death. The placental cord insertion is an ideal IVT target location because the umbilical vein is somewhat "anchored" to the placenta, providing stability when attempting to access the vein. A free-floating loop of umbilical cord may also be considered, typically when the placental cord insertion is inaccessible, however this technique can be challenging due to movement of the cord within the amniotic fluid.

An alternative intravascular access point is the intrahepatic umbilical vein (IHV). This technique has been associated with lower rates of umbilical cord-site streaming and vasospasm [58]. Decreased streaming is likely because the vessel courses within the fetal liver and therefore any

hemorrhage should be contained within the fetal abdominal compartment. This alternative approach is preferred by some proceduralists and may be particularly beneficial in cases with technically difficult cord access. There appears to be no excess morbidity with an IHV approach when compared to IVT [59]; however, randomized prospective data comparing the two approaches is lacking.

Direct cardiac puncture is generally not recommended, as it has been reported to have a 5.6% fetal loss rate compared to the 1% loss rate associated with cordocentesis. It should be reserved as a heroic measure for severe fetal presentations in which intravascular transfusion is deemed necessary but the fetal blood supply is otherwise inaccessible.

Specific centers and individual physicians may have preferences for achieving fetal intravascular access, and all cases should be individualized. Clinical factors including gestational age, placental location, fetal lie, maternal body habitus, and imaging quality should all be considered prior to proceeding with any intervention.

Technique for IUT

Prior to 23–24 weeks gestational age, IUT procedures may be safely performed in an outpatient ultrasound suite. After viability has been reached, the IUT should take place in an operating room once a gestational age has been reached at which the patient would permit emergency cesarean delivery for a severe fetal complication. Local or regional anesthesia can be used depending on the clinical scenario. Sterile preparation and an aseptic technique are recommended for all procedures. Preoperative antibiotics may be considered and tocolysis is optional. Currently, there is no evidence suggesting that prophylactic antibiotics reduce the risk for intrauterine infection [60,61]. Use of a paralytic agent–for example vecuronium or atracurium–administered intravascularly to the fetus has been associated with an 80% reduction in procedure-related complications [60]. However, the administration of a paralytic agent should always be highlighted to the neonatologists should a fetus require delivery shortly after the procedure, as its use may pose resuscitation challenges.

Under continuous ultrasound guidance a 20–22 gauge needle is advanced into the fetal umbilical vein and a sample of blood is sent for analyses including hematocrit, mean corpuscular volume, platelet count, and blood and antigen typing. Although a 20-gauge needle is technically easier to use for a planned fetal transfusion, a 22-gauge needle may be preferable in some clinical situations. These scenarios include cases at an early gestational age, for example < 20 weeks or in those with a concern for possible severe thrombocytopenia. The use of color Doppler ultrasound imaging can be helpful to clearly visualize the placental insertion site and demonstrate that a vessel is venous in nature. If on this analysis the fetus is proven to be anemic, the needle is kept in the umbilical vein and packed red blood cells specially prepared for fetal transfusion are transfused. Transfused red cells used should be O negative (and also negative for any other red blood cell antigens to which the patient has been alloimmunized), cytomegalovirus seronegative, hyperspun to a final hematocrit of ideally at least 75%, leukocyte reduced, and irradiated. A number of samples may be taken during the procedure to obtain an accurate record of the fetal hemoglobin and hematocrit, and a post-transfusion blood count should ideally be obtained and recorded when possible. For anemic fetuses, transfusion up to a final hematocrit value of roughly 50% is often advised. Based on a rough decline in hematocrit of 1% per day (although significant variability can exist between cases), this allows for a reasonable interval between procedures if serial procedures are required in cases of hemolytic disease of the fetus and newborn.

Complications

Complications of a PUBS procedure include bleeding from the umbilical cord puncture site, infection and chorioamnionitis, rupture of membranes, placental abruption, thrombosis, arterial vasospasm, and fetal bradycardia [62]. These complications range from 5–30% in the literature [63,64]. However, in most cases, whether it is to administer a fetal blood transfusion or to deliver in utero fetal therapy, the benefits are believed to strongly outweigh the risks. Bleeding from the cord entry site upon needle removal is common and observed in about 20–30% of cases, although this is usually brief and self-limited. Persistent bleeding is rare. Fetal bradycardia occurs in 5% of cases either during or shortly following the procedure, likely as a result of vasospasm of the umbilical cord and is similarly often self-limited. Umbilical cord hematomas can develop and result in a fetal bradycardia. Emergency delivery may be required if the fetal heart rate abnormality is sustained. Pregnancy loss following a PUBS has been estimated to be 1.1% per procedure and 1.3% per patient [62].

Fetal shunts

Intrauterine fetal shunts are flexible plastic catheters that allow for continuous drainage of fetal pathological fluid accumulations. The most common types of fetal shunts employed are vesicoamniotic shunts between the fetal bladder and the amniotic cavity, used in fetal lower urinary tract obstruction with associated severe oligo- or anhydramnios, and thoracoamniotic shunts between the fetal thorax and amniotic cavity used for fetal severe hydrothorax.

The two most used shunt products are the Rocket (Rocket KCH Fetal Bladder Drain; Rocket Medical, Hingham, MA) and the Harrison (Harrison Fetal Bladder

StentSet; Cook Medical Inc., Bloomington, IN) shunts. The Rocket shunt is 2.1 mm in diameter and placed using a reusable placement kit (3 mm diameter). The Harrison shunt is narrower (1.7 mm) and placed through a disposable 2.4 mm (13 gauge) needle. One has not been shown to be superior to the other and the choice of which to use is a function of physician preference and availability.

Vesicoamniotic shunt

Fetal lower urinary tract bladder obstruction (LUTO) is associated with significant fetal morbidity, including renal insufficiency or failure in addition to urethral and bladder dysfunction. Resulting persistent oligo- or anhydramnios can result in pulmonary hypoplasia, which can severely limit or preclude survival after birth. In the absence of treatment, LUTO has been associated with a 45% mortality rate, largely due to pulmonary hypoplasia among cases with early-onset severe oligo- or anhydramnios [65]. Among survivors, roughly 25–30% develop end-stage renal disease requiring dialysis and renal transplantation by the age of 5 years [66].

A vesicoamniotic shunt performed sufficiently early in gestation decompresses the bladder and reconstitutes the amniotic space, promoting pulmonary development. Theoretically, it may also prevent further renal, bladder, and ureteral damage by relieving high pressure within the genitourinary system, however insufficient published data exist to support this claim.

A majority of LUTO presentations involve male fetuses, and in these cases posterior urethral valves is the predominant etiology. However, many other underlying pathologies are possible, and evaluation at an experienced fetal diagnosis and therapy center with multidisciplinary team input from maternal–fetal medicine, pediatric urology, neonatology, and pediatric nephrology is recommended before considering vesicoamniotic shunt placement. A comprehensive fetal anatomical survey and fetal echocardiography are also recommended to exclude associated structural anomalies. Genetic testing is also recommended given an association with aneuploidy and genetic abnormalities. Criteria for placement include ultrasound findings of LUTO with associated oligo- or anhydramnios [67]. Shunt placement in the setting of a normal amniotic fluid volume is a source of controversy, without evidence to support clear benefit to this practice [67].

Ultrasound alone is unreliable in determining fetal renal function; there remains no clear relationship between sonographic appearance of the fetal kidneys and degree of renal dysfunction. To estimate whether the fetus has preserved renal function, a series of up to three fetal vesicocenteses (spaced roughly 48 hours apart) are recommended to analyze fetal urinary analytes prior to placement of a vesicoamniotic shunt. Under continuous ultrasound guidance, using standard aseptic technique, a

20- or 22-gauge needle is percutaneously guided into the fetal bladder and the fetal bladder is entirely decompressed, with the aspirated urine sent for analysis. The sample is typically examined for urinary analytes, biomarkers, and osmolality. The results of the urinary profile are used as a proxy marker of fetal renal function to predict if there is sufficiently preserved renal function to warrant shunt placement.

The overall clinical picture combined with the urinary profile should be considered when considering shunt placement, with the third and final urinalysis profile believed to represent current fetal renal function most accurately. Analysis of the sample from the first vesicocentesis is likely to be influenced by urine produced over a number of weeks and therefore may not reflect the current level of renal functioning [68,69], as it includes early urine produced by the fetal kidneys prior to damage. By the time of the third vesicocentesis, results are more likely to represent a truer reflection of current renal function.

Given the association between LUTO and fetal aneuploidy in approximately 5–12% of cases, a sample of fluid for genetic evaluation can also be taken during the vesicocentesis and sent for fetal karyotype and microarray analysis. As fetal urine often contains low amounts of genetic material, an amniocentesis or placental biopsy can be performed concurrently to obtain a better sample for genetic testing. In cases involving severe oligo- or anhydramnios, an amnioinfusion can be performed at the same time as the vesicocentesis to improve visualization of the fetal anatomy if required.

Fetal urine typically becomes more hypotonic as gestation advances. Therefore, renal injury is associated with fetal urine that is hypertonic for gestation age. Established urinary analyte cutoffs (Box 52.1) can be used to estimate the fetal urinary profile. However, no single analyte can perfectly predict renal function. Additionally, urine osmolality and urinary analyte levels vary with gestational age, further challenging their interpretation. Given known challenges with the evaluation and management of these cases, consultation with or referral to an experienced fetal therapy center is encouraged, when possible.

Outcomes following vesicoamniotic shunts

The results of the Percutaneous shunting in Lower Urinary Tract Obstruction (PLUTO) randomized trial were published in 2013 [70]. This was a multi-center European trial of singleton male fetuses with a sonographic diagnosis of LUTO, but without consideration of amniotic fluid volume. Cases were randomized to either vesicoamniotic shunt placement or conservative management. Survival to 28 days after birth was the primary outcome measure. Secondary outcomes included longer-term survival and renal function measures. The trial was discontinued prematurely after 31 subjects (16 randomized to shunting, 15 to conservative management) were recruited due to challenges with patient recruitment. On intention-to-treat analysis, there was no significant survival benefit to 28 days between those randomized to shunting or conservative management (relative risk [RR] 1.88, 95% CI 0.71–4.96; $P = 0.27$).

There was, however, a significant early survival benefit to shunting when groups were compared by treatment received (RR 3.2, 95% CI 1.06. −9.62; $P = 0.03$). The likelihood of survival with normal renal function was very low in both groups and the authors concluded that although there may be some survival benefit to shunting, achieving normal renal function was unlikely with or without therapy. The treatment is also unlikely to be cost effective, as it may affect survival but does not prevent perinatal morbidity [71].

Thoracoamniotic shunts

Fetal thoracoamniotic shunting, first reported by Rodeck and colleagues in 1988 [72] for the treatment of fetal hydrothorax, allows for continuous decompression of the fetal chest and fetal lung expansion. Thoracoamniotic shunts may be considered for pregnancies complicated by severe fetal pleural effusions or for congenital pulmonary airway malformations (CPAM) of the fetal lung with a single dominant macrocyst. Examples of severe pleural effusions that might benefit from shunt placement include severe bilateral effusions, unilateral or bilateral effusions causing mediastinal shift, and effusions associated with fetal hydrops. Theoretically, the placement of a thoracoamniotic shunt in such cases can reduce the risk of pulmonary hypoplasia, as it can relieve the intrathoracic lung compression being caused by these masses. It may also prevent or reverse the development of fetal hydrops. When evaluating candidacy for vesicoamniotic shunt placement, genetic testing is strongly recommended, as fetal hydrothorax is associated with increased risk of aneuploidy and genetic abnormalities.

Similar to vesicoamniotic shunt placement, a multidisciplinary team approach should be undertaken prior to insertion, including appropriate counseling regarding risks, benefits, and alternative options. Alternative management options include but are not limited to expectant management or serial thoracocenteses.

Box 52.1 Fetal urinary analyte levels suggestive of preserved fetal renal function

Urinary electrolytes	Urine osmolality	Urinary protein
1. Sodium <100 mg/dL	<200 mOsm/L	ß2-microglobulin <4 mg/L
2. Calcium <8 mg/dL		
3. Chloride <90 mg/dL		Total protein <40 mg/dL

Prior to thoracoamniotic shunt insertion for fetal hydrothroax, a minimum of one-or-two thoracoenteses may be advisable. Thoracocenteses provide diagnostic as well as potential therapeutic benefit. Under continuous ultrasound guidance, a 20- or 22-gauge needle can be guided into the fetal thoracic fluid collection and a sample obtained that can be sent for cell count, as well as genetic analysis if desired. A prenatal chylothorax is diagnosed when there are >80% lymphocytes present upon cell differential analysis. With rapid or severe reaccumulation after thoracocentesis, thoracoamniotic shunting may be considered. In some cases that undergo needle decompression, the fluid accumulation does not reaccumulate or it reaccumulates very slowly, and there is therefore no need for shunting.

Outcomes following thoracoamniotic shunts

Outcome data following thoracoamniotic shunt placement are limited and no high-quality randomized trial data exist. A cohort study of 92 cases of fetal pleural effusion, of which 21 had a thoracoamniotic shunt placed, was reported by Smith et al [73]. Fetal hydrops was present in 76% of shunt cases. The overall survival rate for those who had a shunt was 44% if hydrops was present and 60% if no fetal hydrops was present. Gestational age at delivery also influenced the outcome. Prior to this study, Nicolaides published a review of 51 thoracoamniotic shunts, 47 of which were for fetal pleural effusions. Of the karyotypically normal fetuses, 100% (18 of 18) of the nonhydropic fetuses survived. Survival decreased to 50% (14 of 28) if fetal hydrops was present [74]. In the largest published series on this topic, Kelly at al. reported on 132 fetuses that underwent thoracoamniotic shunting for fetal hydrothorax between 1991 and 2014 [75]. Among cases, 61% were hydropic upon diagnosis and 69% had bilateral effusions. The average gestational age at delivery was 35.4 weeks, with 76% of patients delivering preterm. The overall survival rate for the cohort was 65%, with hydrops at diagnosis and delivery under 32 weeks both associated with death. Additional potentially severe diagnoses were present in 24% of cases, of which roughly two thirds were not diagnosed until after birth. Among survivors, 84% were developmentally normal beyond 18 months of age, and most survivors with sufficient follow-up has no long-term pulmonary complications.

The utility of thoracoamniotic shunt placement for CPAM presentations involving a dominant macrocyst remains unclear, as data are also very limited. No study compares cases of thoracoamniotic shunt placement to outcomes for fetuses with similar CPAM presentations that did not undergo shunting, and so a true comparison is difficult. Although cases of successful decompression, resolution of hydrops, and healthy neonatal outcomes following shunt placement have been reported, they have not been prospectively proven to be superior to

alternative approaches such as expectant management or serial thoracocentesis. A retrospective review from a single center evaluating thoracoamniotic shunt placement for fetal pleural effusions and macrocytic CPAMs reported a 70% survival rate (7 of 10) and 67% (6 of 9) for CPAMs and pleural effusions respectively when a shunt was inserted [76]. Updated single-center data from the same group involving 23 CPAMs thoracoamniotic shunt cases revealed an overall survival rate of 74% [77]. Notably, no robust prospective data exist comparing shunting to serial thoracocenteses for any thoracoamniotic shunt indications.

Technique for shunt placement

Both vesicoamniotic and thoracoamniotic shunts are percutaneously placed under continuous ultrasound guidance. Typically, local anesthesia is used for placement; however, a range of anesthesia types can be used. Sterile preparation and an aseptic technique are recommended for all procedures. Perioperative antibiotics can be administered orally, intravenously or directly into the amniotic space with the aim of reducing the risk of infection. Cephalosporins are commonly used for shunt placements and nafcillin is considered a suitable antibiotic for intra-amniotic infusion. Periprocedural tocolysis can also be considered and can be particularly useful for patients with symptomatic uterine activity post procedure.

Once the optimal position for accessing the fetus is determined by ultrasound, a small 5 mm incision is made on the maternal skin with a scalpel. Insertion of both shunt types require the introduction of a trocar through the maternal abdominal wall into the uterine cavity. This trocar is then further inserted into the fetal pathological fluid collection. The trocar introducer is removed, and the double pigtail drainage catheter is inserted into the cannula and positioned with one end into the fetal bladder or chest. The cannula is retracted slowly until outside the bladder or chest and angled away from the fetus. The other end of the pigtail catheter is then deployed into the amniotic space. The position of the shunt is confirmed with ultrasound and then the cannula is removed.

A vesicoamniotic shunt is ideally placed between the fetal abdominal wall cord insertion site and the symphysis pubis, just lateral to the midline. A thoracoamniotic shunt is placed in the fetal thorax or directly in the thoracic lung lesion. Consideration should be given to inserting the shunt between the ribs beneath the scapula on the fetal back, which can potentially reduce the risk of the fetus dislodging the shunt. The shunt should be clamped immediately at delivery to prevent a pneumothorax.

Complications of shunts

Fetal shunt placement is associated with many complications including PPROM, migration, displacement, occlusion, previable loss, preterm labor, preterm delivery, infection, bleeding, abruption, and maternal and fetal injury. Vesicoamniotic shunts can result in complications in up to 40% of cases [78,79]. Most common complications include PPROM, shunt migration, shunt displacement, shunt blockage, and need for repeat shunt placements. Rare cases of direct fetal injury including iatrogenic fetal gastroschisis, vascular injury, and exsanguination have been reported. In the PLUTO study, the reported complications of vesicoamniotic shunting included spontaneous rupture of membranes (3/15), dislodgement of the shunt (3/15), and occlusion or blockage of the shunt (1/15). Total pregnancy losses were 4/15, although one of the losses was thought to be unrelated to the treatment [70]. Shunts can migrate into the fetal bladder or abdomen

and require surgical removal in the neonatal period. Urinary ascites is a known outcome after vesicoamnitoic shunting.

Lethal fetal intercostal artery laceration and fatal shunt-associated umbilical cord torsion have been described after thoracoamniotic shunt placement [73, 80]. Neonatal chest wall deformity has also been reported following thoracoamniotic shunting [81]. The risk of thoracoamniotic shunt migration or displacement has been reported as 20% in one series, and in some vesicoamniotic shunt series this risk exceeds 40% [82–84]. Given the potential complications, it is important to consider the full clinical picture when offering a fetal shunt as a potential treatment option.

CASE PRESENTATION

A 37-year-old gravida 1, para 0 presents for genetic counseling at 16 weeks gestation following cell-free fetal DNA screening that resulted as high risk for trisomy 21. After a complete family pedigree is performed and no other genetic risks are identified, the patient is informed that invasive prenatal diagnosis is indicated due to an increased risk of trisomy 21. Amniocentesis is recommended given the patient's gestational age. She is informed that there is a very small risk of pregnancy loss related to the procedure. Other potential risks include a small chance of bleeding and spotting. Rare complications include leakage of fluid and maternal infections. She is informed that the results of the amniocentesis karyotype are highly accurate, and turnaround times are discussed.

The patient decides to undergo the amniocentesis procedure. Her blood type is checked, and she is found to be blood type A, Rhesus negative, with a negative antibody screen. She undergoes an uncomplicated amniocentesis and receives anti-D immunoglobulin immediately afterwards.

Twelve hours later, while at home, the patient experiences a gush of clear fluid leaking per vagina. On review at the hospital a rupture of membranes is confirmed by a sterile speculum examination, and oligohydramnios is observed. Conservative management is undertaken and the leaking per vagina stops within 24 hours. An ultrasound scan 1 week later reveals a normal amniotic fluid level. She receives a call from the genetic counselor informing her that she is having a chromosomally normal son. Her pregnancy continues without any further problems, and she has a spontaneous vaginal delivery at 38 weeks gestational age.

References

1. Lo YM, Corbetta N, Chamberlain PF, Rai V, Sargent IL, Redman CW, et al. Presence of fetal DNA in maternal plasma and serum. Lancet. 1997;350:485–7.

2. Wang, Jw., Lyu, Yn., Qiao, B., Li Y, Zhang Y, Dhanyamraju PK, et al. Cell-free fetal DNA testing and its correlation with prenatal indications. BMC Pregnancy Childbirth. 2021;21(1):585. doi: 10.1186/s12884-021-04044-5.

3. Warsof SL, Larion S, Abuhamad AZ. Overview of the impact of noninvasive prenatal testing on diagnostic procedures. Prenat Diagn. 2015;35(10):972–9.

4. Jackson LG, Zachary JM, Fowler SE, Desnick RJ, Golbus MS, Ledbetter DH, et al. A randomized comparison of transcervical and transabdominal chorionic-villus sampling. The U.S. National Institute of Child Health and Human Development Chorionic-Villus Sampling and Amniocentesis Study Group. N Engl J Med. 1992;327(9):594–8.

5. Moise KJ, Jr., Carpenter RJ, Jr. Increased severity of fetal hemolytic disease with known rhesus alloimmunization after first-

6. Rhoads GG, Jackson LG, Schlesselman SE, de la Cruz FF, Desnick RJ, Golbus MS, et al. The safety and efficacy of chorionic villus sampling for early prenatal diagnosis of cytogenetic abnormalities. N Engl J Med. 1989;320(10):609–17.

7. Caughey AB, Hopkins LM, Norton ME. Chorionic villus sampling compared with amniocentesis and the difference in the rate of pregnancy loss. Obstet Gynecol. 2006;108: 612–16.

8. Smidt-Jensen S, Permin M, Philip J, Lundsteen C, Zachary JM, Fowler SE, et al. Randomised comparison of amniocentesis and transabdominal and transcervical chorionic villus sampling. Lancet. 1992;340:1237–44.

9. Odibo AO, Dicke JM, Gray DL, Oberle B, Stamilio DM, Macones GA, et al. Evaluating the rate and risk factors for fetal loss after chorionic villus sampling. Obstet Gynecol. 2008;112:813–9.

10. Akolekar R, Beta J, Picciarelli G, Ogilvie C, D'Antonio F. Procedure-related risk of miscarriage following amniocentesis and chorionic villus sampling: a systematic review and meta-analysis. Ultrasound Obstet Gynecol. 2015;45:16–26.

trimester transcervical chorionic villus biopsy. Fetal Diagn Ther. 1990;5(2):76–8.

11. Tabor A, Alfirevic Z. Update on procedure-related risks for prenatal diagnosis techniques. Fetal Diagn Ther. 2010;27:1–7.

12. Bakker M, Birnie E, Robles de Medina P, Sollie KM, Pajkrt E, Bilardo CM. Total pregnancy loss after chorionic villus sampling and amniocentesis: a cohort study. Ultrasound Obstet Gynecol. 2017;49:599–606.

13. Beta J, Zhang W, Geris S, Ogilvie C, D'Antonio F. Procedure-related risk of miscarriage following chorionic villus sampling and amniocentesis. Ultrasound Obstet Gynecol. 2019;54(4):452–7.

14. Saura R, Gauthier B, Taine L, Wen ZQ, Horovitz J, Roux D, et al. Operator experience and fetal loss rate in transabdominal CVS. Prenat Diagn. 1994;14(1):70–1.

15. Elias S, Emerson D, Tharapel A, Seely L. Transabdominal chorionic villus sampling for first-trimester prenatal diagnosis. Am J Obstet Gynecol. 1989;160(4):879–84; discussion 884-6.

16. Hsu WW, Hsieh CJ, Lee CN, Chen CL, Lin MW, Kang J, et al. Complication rates after chorionic villus sampling and midtrimester amniocentesis: a 7-year national registry study. J Formos Med Assoc. 2019 Jul;118(7):1107–13.

17. Ledbetter DH, Golbus MS, Pergament E, Jackson L, et al. Cytogenetic results from the U.S. Collaborative Study on CVS. Prenat Diagn. 1992;12(5): 317–45.

18. Ledbetter DH, Pergament E, Jackson L, Yang-Feng T, et al. Cytogenetic results of chorionic villus sampling: high success rate and diagnostic accuracy in the United States collaborative study. Am J Obstet Gynecol. 1990;162(2):495–501.

19. Firth HV, Boyd PA, Chamberlain P, MacKenzie IZ, Lindenbaum RH, Huson SM. Severe limb abnormalities after chorion villus sampling at 56–66 days' gestation. Lancet. 1991;337:762–3.

20. Burton BK, Schulz CJ, Burd LI. Limb anomalies associated with chorionic villus sampling. Obstet Gynecol. 1992;79(5 Pt 1):726–30.

21. Evaluation of chorionic villus sampling safety: WHO/PAHO consultation on CVS. Prenat Diagn. 1999;19(2):97–9.

22. Alfirevic Z, Navaratnam K, Mujezinovic F. Amniocentesis and chorionic villus sampling for prenatal diagnosis. Cochrane Database Syst Rev. 2017;9(9):CD003252. doi: 10.1002/14651858. CD003252.pub2.

23. Marthin T, Liedgren S, Hammar M. Transplacental needle passage and other risk-factors associated with second trimester amniocentesis. Acta Obstet Gynecol Scand. 1997;76(8):728–32.

24. Simpson JL, Elias S. Prenatal diagnosis of genetic disorders. In: Creasy RK, Resnik R, editors. Maternal-fetal medicine: principles and practice. 3rd ed. Philadelphia: WB Saunders; 1994. p.61–88.

25. Randomised trial to assess safety and fetal outcome of early and midtrimester amniocentesis. The Canadian Early and Mid-trimester Amniocentesis Trial (CEMAT) Group. Lancet. 1998;351(9098):242–7.

26. Johnson JM, Singer J, Dansereau J, Kalousek DK. The early amniocentesis study: a randomized clinical trial of early amniocentesis versus midtrimester amniocentesis. Fetal Diagn Ther. 1996;11(2):85–93.

27. Nicolaides K, Brizot Mde L, Patel F, Snijders R. Comparison of chorionic villus sampling and amniocentesis for fetal karyotyping at 10–13 weeks' gestation. Lancet. 1994;344(8920):435–9.

28. Farrell SA, Summers AM, Dallaire L, Singer J, Johnson JA, Wilson RD. Club foot, an adverse outcome of early amniocentesis: disruption or deformation? CEMAT. Canadian Early and Mid-Trimester Amniocentesis Trial. J Med Genet. 1999;36:843–6.

29. Winsor EJT, Tomkins DJ, Kalousek D, Farrell S, Wyatt P, Fan Y-S, et al. Cytogenetic aspects of the Canadian early and mid-trimester amniotic fluid trial (CEMAT). Prenat Diagn. 1999;19:620–7.

30. Elias S, Gerbie AB, Simpson JL, Nadler HL, Sabbagha RE, Shkolnik A. Genetic amniocentesis in twin gestations. Am J Obstet Gynecol. 1980;138(2):169–74.

31. National Institute for Health and Care Excellence. Multiple pregnancy: antenatal care for twin and triplet pregnancies clinical guideline (CG129). London: NICE; 2011.

32. McFadyen I. The dangers of intra-amniotic methylene blue. Br J Obstet Gynaecol. 1992;99(2):89–90.

33. Tabor A, Philip J, Madsen M, Bang J, Obel EB, Norgaard-Pedersen B. Randomised controlled trial of genetic amniocentesis in 4606 low-risk women. Lancet. 1986;1:1287–93.

34. Akolekar R, Beta J, Picciarelli G, Ogilvie C, Antonio F. Procedure-related risk of miscarriage following amniocentesis and chorionic villus sampling: a systematic review and meta-analysis. Ultrasound Obstet Gynecol. 2015;45(1):16–26.

35. Di Mascio D, Khalil A, Rizzo G, Buca D, Liberati M, Martellucci CA, et al. Risk of fetal loss following amniocentesis or chorionic villus sampling in twin pregnancy: systematic review and meta-analysis. Ultrasound Obstet Gynecol. 2020;56(5):647–55.

36. Wijnberger LD, van der Schouw YT, Christiaens GC. Learning in medicine: chorionic villus sampling. Prenat Diagn. 2000;20:241–6.

37. Seeds JW. Diagnostic mid trimester amniocentesis: how safe? Am J Obstet Gynecol. 2004;191(2):607–15.

38. Borgida AF, Mills AA, Feldman DM, Rodis JF, Egan JF. Outcome of pregnancies complicated by ruptured membranes after genetic amniocentesis. Am J Obstet Gynecol. 2000 Oct;183(4): 937–9. doi: 10.1067/mob.2000.108872. PMID: 11035342.

39. Mandelbrot, L., Bourguignat, L., Mellouhi, I.S., Gavard, L., Morin, F. and Bierling, P. Treatment by autologous amniopatch of premature rupture of membranes following mid-trimester amniocentesis. Ultrasound Obstet Gynecol. 2009;33:245–6.

40. Kristensen SS, Nørgaard LN, Tabor A, Sundberg K, Dziegiel MH, Hedegaard M, et al. Do chorionic villus samplings (CVS) or amniocenteses (AC) induce RhD immunisation? An evaluation of a large Danish cohort with no routine administration of anti-D after invasive prenatal testing. BJOG. 2019 Nov;126(12):1476–80.

41. Visser, G.H.A., Thommesen, T., Di Renzo, G.C., Nassar, A.H., Spitalnik, S.L. FIGO/ICM guidelines for preventing Rhesus disease: A call to action. Int J Gynecol Obstet. 2021;152:144–7.

42. Practice Bulletin No. 181: prevention of Rh D alloimmunization. Obstet Gynecol. 2017 Aug;130(2):e57–e70.

43. Baird PA, Yee IM, Sadovnick AD. Population-based study of long-term outcomes after amniocentesis. Lancet. 1994;344(8930): 1134–6.

44. Picone O, Senat MV, Rosenblatt J, Audibert F, Tachdjian G, Frydman R. Fear of pregnancy loss and fetal karyotyping: a place for third-trimester amniocentesis? Fetal Diagn Ther. 2008;23:30–5.

45. Gabbay R, Yogev Y, Melamed N, Ben-Haroush A, Meizner I, Pardo J. Pregnancy outcome after third trimester amniocentesis: a single center experience. J Matern Fetal Neonatal Med. 2012;25:666–8.

46. Stark CM, Smith RS, Lagrandeur RM, Batton DG, Lorenz RP. Need for urgent delivery after third-trimester amniocentesis. Obstet Gynecol. 2000;95:48–50.

47. Lawin O'Brien A, Dall'Asta AA, Tapon D, Ellis R, Lees C. OC20.06: late amniocentesis: is our counselling up to date? Ultrasound Obstet Gynecol. 2015;46 (S1):44–5.

48. Wapner RJ, Martin CL, Levy B, Ballif BC, Eng CM, Zachary JM, et al. Chromosomal microarray versus karyotyping for prenatal diagnosis. N Engl J Med. 2012 Dec 6;367(23):2175–84.

49. Reddy UM, Goldenberg R, Silver R, Smith GCS, Pauli RM, Wapner RJ, et al. Stillbirth classification–developing an international consensus for research: executive summary of a National Institute of Child Health and Human Development workshop. Obstet Gynecol. 2009;114(4):901–14.

50. Petrovski S, Aggarwal V, Giordano JL, Stosic M, Wou K, Bier L, et al. Whole-exome sequencing in the evaluation of fetal structural anomalies: a prospective cohort study. Lancet. 2019; 393(10173):758–67.

51. Lord J, McMullan DJ, Eberhardt RY, Rinck G, Hamilton SJ, Quinlan-Jones E, et al. Prenatal exome sequencing analysis in fetal structural anomalies detected by ultrasonography (PAGE): a cohort study. Lancet. 2019;393(10173):747–57.

52. Anastasiadou E, Jacob LS, Slack FJ. Non-coding RNA networks in cancer. Nat Rev Cancer. 2018;18(1):5–18.

53. Wojciechowska A, Braniewska A, Kozar-Kaminska K. MicroRNA in cardiovascular biology and disease. Adv Clin Exp Med. 2017;26(5):865–74.

54. Peddi NC, Avanthika C, Vuppalapati S, Balasubramanian R, Kaur J, N CD. A review of cordocentesis: percutaneous umbilical cord blood sampling. Cureus. 2021;13(7):e16423.

55. Liley AW. Intrauterine transfusion of foetus in haemolytic disease. BMJ. 1963 Nov 2;2(5365):1107–9.

56. Daffos F, Capella-Pavlovsky M, Forestier F. A new procedure for fetal blood sampling in utero: preliminary results of fifty-three cases. Am J Obstet Gynecol. 1983 Aug 15;146(8):985–7.

57. Crawford NEH, Parasuraman R, Howe DT. Intraperitoneal transfusion for severe, early-onset rhesus disease requiring treatment before 20 weeks of gestation: A consecutive case series. Eur J Obstet Gynecol Reprod Biol. 2020 Jan;244:5–7.

58. Aina-Mumuney AJ, Holcroft CJ, Blakemore KJ, Bienstock JL, Hueppchen NA, Milio LA, et al. Intrahepatic vein for fetal blood sampling: one center's experience. Am J Obstet Gynecol. 2008 Apr;198(4):387.e1–6.

59. Somerset DA, Moore A, Whittle MJ, Martin W, Kilby MD. An audit of outcome in intravascular transfusions using the intrahepatic portion of the fetal umbilical vein compared to cordocentesis. Fetal Diagn Ther. 2006;21(3):272–6.

60. Zwiers C, van Kamp I, Oepkes D, Lopriore E. Intrauterine transfusion and non invasive treatment options for hemolytic disease of the fetus and newborn–review on current management and outcome. Expert Rev Hematol. 2017 Apr;10(4):337–44.

61. Berry SM, Stone J, Norton ME, Johnson D, Berghella V; Society for Maternal-Fetal Medicine (SMFM). Fetal blood sampling. Am J Obstet Gynecol. 2013 Sep;209(3):170–80.

62. Too G, Berkowitz RL. Cordocentesis and fetal transfusion. In: Copel J, D'Alton ME, Feltovich H, Gratacos E, Odibo AO, Platt L, Tutschek B, editors. Obstetric imaging: fetal diagnosis and care. 2nd ed. Philadelphia: Elsevier; 2018. pp.475–8.

63. Berry SM, Stone J, Norton ME, Johnson D, Berghella V. Fetal blood sampling. Am J Obstet Gynecol. 2013;209:170–80.

64. Han JY, Nava-Ocampo AA. Fetal heart rate response to cordocentesis and pregnancy outcome: a prospective cohort. J Matern Fetal Neonatal Med. 2005;17:207–11.

65. Nakayama DK, Harrison MR, de Lorimier AA. Prognosis of posterior urethral valves presenting at birth. J Pediatr Surg. 1986;21:43–5.

66. Morris R, Malin G, Khan K, Kilby M. Antenatal ultrasound to predict postnatal renal function in congenital lower urinary tract obstruction: systematic review of test accuracy. BJOG. 2009; 116:1290–9.

67. Johnson MP, Bukowski TP, Reitleman C, Isada NB, Pryde PG, Evans MI. In utero surgical treatment of fetal obstructive uropathy: a new comprehensive approach to identify appropriate candidates for vesicoamniotic shunt therapy. Am J Obstet Gynecol. 1994;170(6):1770–6; discussion 1776-9.

68. Johnson MP, Corsi P, Bradfield W, Hume RF, Smith C, Flake AW, et al. Sequential urinalysis improves evaluation of fetal renal function in obstructive uropathy. Am J Obstet Gynecol. 1995;173(1):59–65.

69. Morris RK, Quinlan-Jones E, Kilby MD, Khan KS. Systematic review of accuracy of fetal urine analysis to predict poor postnatal renal function in cases of congenital urinary tract obstruction. Prenat Diagn. 2007;27(10):900–11.

70. Morris RK, Malin GL, Quinlan-Jones E, Middleton LJ, Hemming K, Burke D, et al. Percutaneous vesicoamniotic shunting versus conservative management for fetal lower urinary tract obstruction [PLUTO]: a randomised trial. Lancet. 2013;382(9903):1496–506.

71. Morris RK, Malin GL, Quinlan-Jones E, Middleton LJ, Diwakar L, Hemming K, et al. The percutaneous shunting in Lower Urinary Tract Obstruction [PLUTO] study and randomised controlled trial: evaluation of the effectiveness, cost- effectiveness and acceptability of percutaneous vesicoamniotic shunting for lower urinary tract obstruction. Health Technol Assess. 2013;17:1–232.

72. Rodeck CH, Fish NM, Fraswer DI, Nicolini. Long-term in utero drainage of fetal hydrothorax. N Engl J Med. 1988;319:1135.

73. Smith RP, Illanes S, Denbow ML, Soothill PW. Outcome of fetal pleural effusions treated by thoracoamniotic shunting. Ultrasound Obstet Gynecol. 2005;26(1):63–6.

74. Nicolaides KH, Azar GB. Thoraco-amniotic shunting. Fetal Diagn Ther. 1990;5(3-4):153–64. doi: 10.1159/000263586. PMID: 2130840.

75. Kelly EN, Seaward G, Ye XY, Windrim R, Van Mieghem T, Keunen J, et al. Short- and long-term outcome following thoracoamniotic shunting for fetal hydrothorax. Ultrasound Obstet Gynecol. 2021;57:624–30.

76. Wilson RD, Baxter JK, Johnson MP, King M, Kasperski S, Crombleholme TM, et al. Thoracoamniotic shunts: fetal treatment of pleural effusions and congenital cystic adenomatoid malformations. Fetal Diagn Ther. 2004;19(5):413–20.

77. Wilson RD, Hedrick HL, Liechty KW, Flake AW, Johnson MP, Bebbington M, et al. Cystic adenomatoid malformation of the lung: review of genetics, prenatal diagnosis, and in utero treatment. Am J Med Genet. 2006;140(2):151–5.

78. Strizek B, Spicher T, Gottschalk I, Böckenhoff P, Simonini C, Berg C, et al. Vesicoamniotic shunting before 17 + 0 weeks in fetuses with lower urinary tract obstruction (LUTO): comparison of Somatex vs. Harrison shunt systems. J Clin Med. 2022;11(9):2359.

79. Ruano R, Sananes N, Sangi-Haghpeykar H, Hernandez-Ruano S, Moog R, Becmeur F, et al. Fetal intervention for severe lower urinary tract obstruction: a multicenter case–control study

comparing fetal cystoscopy with vesicoamniotic shunting. Ultrasound Obstet Gynecol. 2015;45:452–4.

80. Aubard Y, Derouineau I, Aubard V, Chalifour V, Preux PM. Primary fetal hydrothorax: A literature review and proposed antenatal clinical strategy. Fetal Diagn Ther. 1998 Nov-Dec;13(6):325–33.

81. Merchant AM, Peranteau W, Wilson RD, Johnson MP, Bebbington MW, Hedrick HL, et al. Postnatal chest wall deformities after fetal thoracoamniotic shunting for congenital cystic adenomatoid malformation. Fetal Diagn Ther. 2007; 22(6):435–9.

82. Sepulveda W, Galindo A, Sosa A, Diaz L, Flores X, de la Fuente P. Intrathoracic dislodgement of pleuro-amniotic shunt. Three case reports with long-term follow-up. Fetal Diagn Ther. 2005;20(2):102–5.

83. Agarwal SK, Fisk NM. In utero therapy for lower urinary tract obstruction. Prenat Diagn. 2001;21(11):970–6.

84. Mann S, Johnson MP, Wilson RD. Fetal thoracic and bladder shunts. Semin Fetal Neonatal Med. 2010;15(1):28–33.

Chapter 53
Fetal Surgery

Marisa Eve Schwab and Hanmin Lee
Department of Surgery, University of California, San Francisco, CA, USA

Fetal therapy was launched in 1963 when Liley performed the first intrauterine blood transfusion for a fetus with Rhesus incompatibility [1]. Two decades later, Harrison pioneered open fetal surgery for fetuses with bilateral hydronephrosis [2]. The indications and treatment modalities for fetal treatment have evolved over the past 60 years in parallel with improvements in prenatal diagnosis, yet three basic tenets of fetal intervention have remained consistent. These tenets include (1) the pregnant woman should undergo minimal risk to her health; (2) the fetal disease should be severe and progressive; and (3) the fetal intervention should have a high likelihood for alleviating or reversing the disease. The approach to fetal interventions has changed dramatically. Initial fetal surgical procedures depended on maternal laparotomy and hysterotomy. This approach evolved to maternal laparotomy with uterine endoscopy and percutaneous approaches are now being used to deliver fetal molecular therapies. It appears that less invasive approaches are associated with a less complicated postoperative recovery for the mother, but morbidity has not been eliminated [3].

As the proposed indications for fetal surgical interventions and the number of procedures performed have expanded, so too have the centers at which they are performed and the number of physicians performing them. Nevertheless, the availability and proven utility of these procedures remain very limited when compared with the number of fetuses with congenital conditions. One of the responsibilities of physicians with an interest in prenatal diagnosis and intervention is to determine training needs and oversight for operators and centers involved in this field. It is unclear how many centers would be needed given the rarity of these congenital diseases in which a fetal therapeutic approach may be effective and the even smaller proportion of those with congenital diseases that may need fetal intervention. We must achieve a delicate balance between the ease of accessibility and surgical experience. International fetal surgery consortiums such as Eurofetus, the International Fetal Medicine and Surgical Society (IFMSS), and the North American Fetal Therapy Network (NAFTNet) are leading efforts to study and guide fetal surgery through multicenter registries and trials. A joint statement by IFMSS and NAFTNet in 2017 advocated for fetal treatment centers to have appropriate mechanisms for informed consent and oversight with a formal process to report and review their cases, including participation in registries [4].

Performing fetal surgeries in specialized centers ensures that only anesthesia providers who are well versed with the subtleties of caring for the fetus and mother during these operations are involved. Anesthesia for minimally invasive fetal surgeries can be relatively simple, consisting of mild maternal sedation and/or neuraxial anesthesia combined with local anesthesia to the needle/trocar site [5]. If fetal immobilization is necessary (e.g. for fetoscopic endoluminal tracheal occlusion [FETO]), either maternal or direct fetal administration of a cocktail of fentanyl, neuromuscular blockade, and atropine is safe. Open fetal surgeries are typically performed under general anesthesia after lumbar epidural placement to avoid catecholamine mediated uterine irritability and decrease the risk of preterm labor. Medications for uterine relaxation and a fetal cocktail are also administered [5].

Different fetal techniques

Open fetal surgery (hysterotomy)

Human experience is now extensive, with fetal treatment centers throughout the world performing open fetal surgery for several congenital malformations [6]. The practical aspects of hysterotomy and postoperative management have evolved since the early years of experience. Lengthy discussions regarding the risks, benefits, and alternatives of the procedure are important. We generally differentiate

---

the risks to the mother, the fetus, and the pregnancy in our counseling. The risks to the mother are similar to other major abdominal surgeries, although in this case there is no direct physical benefit to her hence the term "innocent bystander." In addition, there are the risks associated with aggressive tocolytic therapy and bed rest in a hypercoagulable state. A meta-analysis published in 2019 that included 1193 patients who underwent open fetal surgery reported a 20.9% risk of any maternal complication in the index pregnancy, with a 4.5% risk of a severe maternal complication [6]. The most common severe complications were placental abruption (n = 28), uterine rupture (n = 5), and pulmonary edema (n = 4). Preterm delivery occurred in 20.5% of pregnancies following open fetal surgery. Although studies evaluating long-term maternal outcomes are still needed, it does not appear that open fetal surgery negatively impacts future fertility, given a 3.81% rate of *de novo* subfertility [6]. An important additional counseling point is that all subsequent deliveries, including the index pregnancy, must be by cesarean delivery. An additional long-term concern with open fetal surgery and future pregnancies is the potential for placental accreta to form at sites of cesarean scars.

Fetoscopic surgery

With advances in technology and familiarity with endoscopic techniques, application of this technique to fetal surgery was natural. Common sense would suggest that the smaller the incision in the uterus, the lower the risk of subsequent pregnancy complications. At the University of California, San Francisco (UCSF), endoscopic approaches were first applied to pregnancies complicated by diaphragmatic hernia, urinary tract obstruction, and twin-to-twin transfusion syndrome (TTTS).

The initial pioneering approach involved maternal mini-laparotomy, with direct exposure of the uterus. Ultrasound was used to determine the point of entry and the hysterotomy site, depending on placental location and fetal lie. Once the uterus was exposed, stay sutures were placed and a 3–5 mm step trocar advanced into the amniotic cavity under direct ultrasound visualization. Initially, several trocars were required for in utero dissections, placement of staples, etc. Later, many procedures could be performed through a single trocar using an endoscope with an operating channel. Initial caution regarding this approach led to similar perioperative management compared with hysterotomy cases. This included general anesthesia, use of multiple tocolytics, and prolonged hospitalization. One important difference even initially was that patients could labor following minimally invasive procedures.

Since these initial cases, endoscopic procedures have become less invasive with smaller instruments passed through 2.3- to 4-mm (7- to 12-Fr) ports that accommodate 1.2- to 3-mm endoscopes, with or without a working

channel [7]. Normally, these procedures now do not require mini-laparotomies and the ports are placed into the uterus by a skin incision just large enough to place the port that is guided by ultrasound to avoid maternal viscera, large uterine vessels, the placenta, and fetal body parts. If the amniotic fluid is not clear enough to allow adequate visualization, amnio-exchange with warmed crystalloid solution can be attempted. The fetoscopic technique enables direct visualization in addition to ultrasound and is currently used in the treatment of TTTS, posterior urethral valves, amniotic band syndrome, and FETO for congenital diaphragmatic hernia (CDH).

In a meta-analysis that included 9403 patients who underwent fetoscopic surgery (the most common indication being TTTS), there was a 6.2% risk of any maternal complication and 1.7% risk of severe maternal complication [6]. The most common severe complications were placental abruption (n = 159), hemorrhage requiring delivery (n = 8), and pulmonary edema (n = 3). Preterm delivery occurred in 2.1% of pregnancies following fetoscopy.

Ultrasound-guided percutaneous fetal therapy

Ultrasound-guided percutaneous interventions are performed through a small skin incision in the maternal abdomen. Ultrasound is again critical for safe uterine access to determine the best entry point. This is based on fetal position, placental location, membrane position in multiple gestations, and uterine vascularity. A 1- to 2-mm needle is generally used. Perioperative management is very different compared to the more invasive procedures. Although patients are treated with prophylactic indomethacin and antibiotics, uterine relaxation from inhalational agents is not required and may in fact be detrimental. Therefore, we generally use local anesthesia only, although occasionally regional anesthesia is also used. Postoperative tocolytic therapy is usually based on contraction activity but typically is limited to indomethacin. Percutaneous needle-based interventions are used for a variety of indications, including drainage of pleural effusions, ascites, cystic structures, radiofrequency ablation procedures, and for cardiac procedures. Fetal intervention guided by sonography is used to sample or drain fetal blood, urine, and fluid collection, to sample fetal tissue, to place catheter shunts in the fetal bladder, chest, abdomen, or ventricles, and to perform radiofrequency ablation (RFA).

The most common indication at UCSF for RFA is acardiac twins/twin reversed arterial perfusion (TRAP) sequence or monochorionic twins for selective reduction. Other operators have used bipolar coagulation or umbilical cord ligation for similar indications. Compared with the 17-gauge RFA needles we use, these techniques are more invasive, using at least 3 mm trocars. Additionally, the length of the cord or its position may preclude use of these instruments. We attempt to avoid entry into the sac of a normal twin if possible. The RFA needle is guided into the abdominal cord insertion of the abnormal twin under ultrasound guidance. Tines (thin wires protruding out of the needle-like hooks) are then deployed and energy delivered to the device to create thermal injury to the tissue. The device we currently use measures the temperature at the tines. This allows us to use an energy level to provide the quickest possible obliteration of the vascular communications. This is of benefit as there are theoretical concerns regarding the differential obliteration of arterial and venous vessels, which might place the normal twin at risk for exsanguination. Ultrasound is also used to monitor the procedure and welfare of the normal twin. Thermal injury can be monitored by watching for the characteristic out-gassing in the tissue. Once active energy delivery to the device has ceased, color flow Doppler can be used to detect any residual flow, in both the cord and the abnormal fetus. Once absence of blood flow is confirmed, the tines are retracted, and the device withdrawn.

We have not found an increased frequency of adverse outcomes with a transplacental approach. We have had good success with this approach with a survival rate over 90% and a mean gestational age at delivery of >35 weeks and an average time from procedure of >11 weeks. There have been no cases of maternal pulmonary edema or blood loss [8].

Ultrasound-guided, percutaneous catheter-based fetal intervention has been performed for fetuses with three types of congenital cardiac defects: fetal aortic stenosis with evolving hypoplastic left heart syndrome (HLHS), HLHS with intact or restrictive atrial septum, and pulmonary atresia with intact ventricular septum with concern for worsening right ventricular hypoplasia [9]. The most common fetal cardiac intervention is aortic balloon valvuloplasty for aortic stenosis with evolving HLHS. In the largest case series (n=136) from Boston Children's Hospital, the procedural success rate of recent years was 94% and the fetal demise rate was 6% 10]. However, fetal aortic balloon valvuloplasty is only the first step in a complex postnatal multistage approach, and longitudinal data are needed to evaluate the potential long-term benefits to fetal intervention in this cohort [11].

Specific diseases

Myelomeningocele

The most common indication for hysterotomy-based fetal intervention at our center currently is myelomeningocele (MMC). MMC is thought to arise as a result of abnormal neurulation leading to exposure of the neural tissues to amniotic fluid, and subsequent ongoing intrauterine trauma throughout gestation, known as the "two-hit hypothesis" [12]. MMC is associated with

sequelae in the central and peripheral nervous system. A change in cerebrospinal fluid (CSF) dynamics results in the Arnold–Chiari II malformation and hydrocephalus. Damage to the exposed spinal cord segment can result in lifelong lower extremity neurologic deficiency, fecal and urinary incontinence, sexual dysfunction, and skeletal deformities [12]. This defect carries enormous personal, familial, and societal costs, as the near normal lifespan of the affected child is characterized by hospitalization, multiple operations, disability, and, occasionally, institutionalization.

The landmark Management of Myelomeningocele Study (MOMS) was a multicenter randomized controlled trial that investigated the outcomes of prenatal vs. postnatal open repair of MMC [13]. The trial was stopped prematurely due to efficacy of prenatal surgery after recruitment of 183 patients. Patients treated prenatally had a significantly decreased need for ventriculoperitoneal shunt placement (40 vs. 82%) and improved composite score for mental development and motor function at 30 months. Prenatal surgery was also associated with other favorable secondary outcomes including reducing hindbrain herniation at 12 months (no evidence of herniation in 36% of prenatal vs. 4% of postnatal cases), doubling the ability to walk without orthotics (42% in prenatal vs. 21% in postnatal cases), and increasing function by two or more levels than that expected based on the anatomic level of the defect (32% vs. 12% in postnatal cases). However, prenatal surgery was associated with maternal and fetal risks including preterm birth (80% of prenatal vs. 15% of postnatal cases), uterine thinning or dehiscence at the surgical site (35% in prenatal cases), and higher rates of fetal bradycardia, oligohydramnios, placental abruption, and the need for transfusion at delivery [13]. A follow-up study of the 30-month pediatric outcomes of the full cohort of patients in the MOMS trial validated the effectiveness of prenatal repair compared to postnatal repair, in terms of cognitive development and motor function outcomes [14].

A meta-analysis of fetoscopic vs. open MMC repair found no difference in mortality, rate of shunt placement for hydrocephalus, or motor outcomes [15]. Percutaneous fetoscopic repair was associated with higher rates of premature rupture of membranes (91% vs. 36%), preterm birth (96% vs. 81%), and leakage and dehiscence from the MMC repair site (30% vs. 7%) compared to open repair. However, the rate of uterine dehiscence was 0% compared to 11% in the open repair. The group at Texas Children's Fetal Center has described a modified approach that may mitigate the risks of both approaches. Fetoscopy through a maternal laparotomy with a three-layer closure of the defect resulted in a mean gestational age at delivery of 37.6 ± 3.0 weeks and a 29% rate of preterm premature rupture of the membranes (PPROM), which is lower than any other report [16]. Moreover, 47%

of their patients delivered vaginally after fetal MMC repair and there were no cases of CSF leakage at birth.

Congenital lung lesions

The most common congenital lung lesions are congenital pulmonary airway malformation (CPAM), previously termed congenital cystic adenomatoid malformation and bronchopulmonary sequestration. Although CPAMs often present as a benign pulmonary mass in infants and children, some fetuses with large lesions die in utero or at birth from hydrops fetalis and/or pulmonary hypoplasia [17]. There was previously enthusiasm for open fetal surgery for CPAMs; however, our group pioneered the use of maternal steroids for treatment of large microcystic or solid appearing CPAMs. In patients with solid/microcystic CPAMs and hydrops, maternal administration of steroids results in over 80% survival in a group that would have a natural history of over 90% mortality without treatment [18]. We now know that fetuses without hydrops usually survive to birth without fetal intervention and can be treated with resection at 1 month of age or older [19]. Fetuses with solid/microcystic CPAMs have plateau of growth of the lung lesion around 27 weeks and the risk of hydrops after this time is minimal. Alternatively, macrocystic CPAMs can have growth of the lesions throughout pregnancy and need to be monitored closely including in the third trimester. Macrocystic CPAMs with hydrops do not respond to maternal steroids but can be initially treated by needle thoracentesis, with the fluid being sent for cell count, infectious studies, and karyotype. If the effusion or macrocyst recurs with persistent hydrops, a thoracoamniotic shunt can then be placed. A review of 75 fetuses treated with thoracoamniotic shunt at Children's Hospital of Philadelphia revealed a 93% survival to birth, and 68% overall long-term survival [20]. Survival was strongly associated with gestational age at birth, hydrops resolution and reduction in lesion size following shunt placement. Surviving infants had prolonged neonatal intensive care unit courses and often required either surgical resection or thoracostomy tube in the perinatal period. If the fetus is diagnosed after 32 weeks gestation, early delivery followed by postnatal resection should be considered.

Sacrococcygeal teratoma

Although patients postnatally diagnosed with sacrococcygeal teratoma (SCT) have excellent outcomes, prenatal diagnosis is associated with a 25–37% perinatal mortality [21]. Fetuses at highest risk of death are those with vascularized, fast-growing tumors that cause high output cardiac failure. The high-output failure leads to polyhydramnios, hydrops fetalis, in utero demise and preterm birth, as well as "mirror syndrome" (maternal preeclampsia). Open surgical resection of the SCT is an option in certain fetuses with high-output failure less than

28–32 weeks gestation [19]. Cincinnati Children's Hospital reported a series of seven fetuses who underwent open resection of their SCT, with a 43% survival rate and no significant maternal complications [22]. When heart failure occurs after 28–32 weeks, the best option is typically early delivery and postnatal surgery. Children's Hospital of Philadelphia's series of 11 fetuses with SCT who exhibited concerning signs such as evolution of cardiac high output failure using combined cardiac output on fetal echocardiogram, were delivered preemptively between 27 and 32 weeks instead of the traditional "watchful waiting," with an 82% (9/11) survival rate [23]. Different minimally invasive techniques including RFA, interstitial laser, and coiling have been attempted in fetuses with SCT. A systematic literature review of fetuses treated with minimally invasive techniques revealed a 44% (14/32) survival rate overall, and 30% (6/20) survival rate in fetuses with cardiac failure [21]. The mean gestational age at the time procedure was 23.2 ± 3.9 weeks and the mean gestational age at delivery for liveborn infants was 29.7 ± 4.0 weeks, leading to significant prematurity-associated morbidity. At this time, these techniques should be considered as experimental.

Congenital diaphragmatic hernia

The fundamental problems in babies born with a CDH are pulmonary hypoplasia and pulmonary hypertension. Research in experimental animal models and later in human patients has aimed to improve growth of the hypoplastic lungs before they are needed for gas exchange at birth. Anatomic repair of the hernia by open hysterotomy proved feasible but did not decrease mortality and was abandoned. Fetal tracheal occlusion was developed as an alternative strategy to promote fetal lung growth by preventing normal egress of lung fluid and inducing airway proliferation. Occlusion of the fetal trachea was shown to stimulate fetal lung growth in a variety of animal models. Techniques to achieve reversible fetal tracheal occlusion were explored in animal models and then applied clinically, evolving from external metal clips placed on the trachea by open hysterotomy or fetoscopic neck dissection, to FETO with a detachable silicone balloon placed by fetal bronchoscopy through a single 5 mm uterine port.

The TOTAL (Tracheal Occlusion to Accelerate Lung Growth) trial is the largest to date to examine the outcomes of fetuses with CDH treated with FETO. This multicenter, open-label design trial had one arm for fetuses with moderate CDH [24] and another for fetuses with severe CDH [25]. In the moderate CDH group (defined as a quotient of the observed-to-expected lung-to-head ratio of 25–35% or 35–45% with liver up), 196 women were randomized to FETO at 30–32 weeks or expectant care. There was no significant difference in the survival to discharge (63% in FETO group vs. 50% in expectant group, $P = 0.06$)

or need for oxygen supplementation at 6 months. FETO increased the risk of PPROM, and preterm birth. In the severe CDH group (defined as a quotient of the observed-to-expected lung-to-head ratio of less than 25% regardless of liver position), 80 women were randomly assigned to FETO at 27–29 weeks gestation or expectant care. The trial was stopped early for efficacy: the survival to discharge was 40% in the FETO group vs. 15% in the expectant group ($P = 0.009$). This benefit was sustained at 6 months of age. Fetuses who underwent FETO had a 4.5-fold risk of PPROM and 2.6-fold higher risk of preterm birth compared to the expectant management group. Mean gestational age at birth was 34.6 weeks in the FETO group vs. 38.4 weeks in the expectant group. The landmark TOTAL trial suggests that FETO should be considered in fetuses with severe CDH, but additional longitudinal studies are needed to investigate the long-term outcomes.

The current results underscore the role of randomized trials in evaluating promising new fetal therapies. The first National Institutes of Health-sponsored trial for CDH showed that complete surgical repair of the anatomic defect (which required hysterotomy), although feasible, was no better than postnatal repair in improving survival and was ineffective when the liver as well as the bowel was herniated [26]. That trial led to the abandonment of open complete repair at our institution and subsequently around the world. Information derived from that trial regarding measures of severity of pulmonary hypoplasia (including liver herniation and the development of the lung:head ratio – the area of contralateral lung in the axial plane at the level of a four-chamber view of the heart, normalized to head circumference) led to the development of an alternative physiologic strategy to enlarge the hypoplastic fetal lung by temporary tracheal occlusion and to the development of less invasive fetal endoscopic techniques that did not require hysterotomy to achieve temporary, reversible tracheal occlusion.

Attempts to improve outcome for severe CDH by treatments either before or after birth have proven to be double-edged swords. Intensive care after birth has improved survival but has increased long-term sequelae in survivors and is expensive. Intervention before birth may increase lung size, but prematurity caused by the intervention itself can be detrimental.

Twin–twin transfusion syndrome, twin anemia-polycythemia sequence

TTTS is a complication of monochorionic multiple gestations resulting from an imbalance in blood flow through vascular communications [27]. Both twins are compromised, albeit in different ways. The recipient twin is generally the larger twin and receives an excess of blood and can develop high-output cardiac failure. The donor twin is generally the smaller twin and shunts blood to the recipient twin and can develop renal failure from a low-output state.

TTTS is the most common serious complication of monochorionic twin gestations, affecting about 10% of monochorionic twin pregnancies. Yet despite the relatively low incidence, TTTS disproportionately accounts for 17% of all perinatal mortality associated with twin gestations [28]. Staging for TTTS was pioneered by Quintero based on sonographic measurements. The diagnosis is made by a combination of polyhydramnios in the recipient twin and oligohydramnios for the donor twin. Selective fetoscopic laser photocoagulation of communicating vessels, pioneered by de Lia [29], is generally accepted as the best treatment for advanced stage TTTS, as demonstrated in a randomized trial in Europe [30]. Although survival has dramatically improved after fetoscopic laser, prematurity is still an issue. A NAFTNet retrospective review of 847 pregnancies found that the mean gestational age at delivery was 30.7 ± 4.5 weeks; the leading indications for delivery were spontaneous labor (47%) and nonreassuring donor fetal status (21%) [31]. Fetoscopic laser of intertwin vessels for TTTS is now the most common indication for fetoscopic surgery worldwide. Some centers, including ours, routinely use advanced fetal echocardiogram data to further stratify the severity of TTTS [32].

Twin anemia-polycythemia sequence (TAPS), first described in 2007, is characterized by large intertwin hemoglobin differences without amniotic fluid discordances [33]. TAPS can occur spontaneously, in 3–5% of monochorionic pregnancies, or may develop after laser treatment for TTTS, seen in 2–13% of cases. TAPS pregnancies can be treated with laser coagulation. However, it can be more challenging than in TTTS cases given the lack of polyhydramnios and a stuck twin [33]. Additionally, placental anastomoses in TAPS are typically tiny and few, and thus can easily be missed.

Fetal obstructive uropathies and renal diseases

The first open fetal surgery was performed for fetal obstructive uropathy [34]. Fifty years later, urethral obstruction continues to be a disease of interest to fetal surgeons. Lower urinary obstruction (LUTO), most commonly due to posterior urethral valves in male fetuses, produces pulmonary hypoplasia and renal dysplasia; these often fatal consequences can be ameliorated by urinary tract decompression before birth. The natural history of untreated fetal urinary tract obstruction is well documented, and fetal urine electrolyte and β2-microglobulin levels and the sonographic appearance of fetal kidneys have proven reliable predictors of renal function and neonatal outcomes [35–39].

Most fetuses with urinary tract dilation do not require intervention. However, fetuses with bilateral hydronephrosis and bladder distension resulting from urethral obstruction subsequently developing oligohydramnios require treatment. Depending on the gestational age, the fetus can be delivered early for postnatal decompression. Alternatively, the bladder can be decompressed in utero by a catheter vesicoamniotic shunt placed percutaneously under sonographic guidance [40,41]. Unfortunately, treatment with shunting has been relatively disappointing, as shunts often migrate or do not remain patent. Even when adequately decompressed, the obstructed bladder may not cycle correctly, and it is questionable whether the renal dysplasia is a primary or secondary malformation. Percutaneous vesicoamniotic shunting in Lower Urinary Tract Obstruction (PLUTO) was a randomized multicenter trial that sought to assess the effectiveness of vesicoamniotic shunting [42]. They enrolled 31 pregnant women and the study closed early due to poor recruitment. Survival to 28 days occurred in 8/16 fetuses in the shunt group vs. 4/15 in the conservative group (intention-to-treat relative risk 1.88, 95% confidence interval (CI) 0.71–4.96, $P = 0.27$). All 12 deaths were caused by pulmonary hypoplasia. There was significant short- and long-term morbidity in both groups: overall only two patients (in the shunt group) survived to 2 years with normal renal function. The authors concluded that the chances of survival with fetal LUTO are very low irrespective of whether vesicoamniotic shunting is performed.

At UCSF, we developed a percutaneous fetal cystoscopic technique to disrupt posterior urethral valves through a single 3 mm port, allowing the bladder to continue to cycle normally [43]. A systematic review that sought to evaluate the effectiveness of different fetal cystoscopic techniques for LUTO included 63 patients and found that fetal cystoscopy, compared to no intervention, demonstrated an odds ratio for improved perinatal survival of 20.51 (95% CI 3.87–108.69) [44]. However, the quality of the evidence remains low and currently fetal cystoscopy should be considered an experimental intervention.

LUTO as well as congenital bilateral renal agenesis, cystic kidney disease, and other etiologies, can cause early pregnancy renal anhydramnios (EPRA), defined as anhydramnios before 22 weeks gestation. EPRA is not compatible with a viable pregnancy [45]. The renal anhydramnios fetal therapy (RAFT) trial (NCT03101891) is a multicenter trial designed to prospectively evaluate serial amnioinfusions for EPRA [45]. The trial's primary outcome measure is the proportion of neonates surviving to successful dialysis and patients are currently being enrolled.

Fetal molecular therapies

Although fetal *surgical* therapies have been performed for several decades for anatomic congenital diseases, only recently have fetal *molecular* therapies started to enter the clinical realm for genetic diseases. In addition to the benefit of early treatment prior to the development or progression of disease, fetal molecular therapies capitalize on the ability to cross the blood-brain barrier prior to its closure, the capacity to promote tolerance to a missing enzyme or gene, and the ability to target fetal hematopoietic stem cells early. At UCSF, we have a phase I clinical trial of in utero hematopoietic stem cell transplantation for fetuses with alpha thalassemia major (NCT02986698) and a phase I clinical trial of in utero enzyme replacement therapy for fetuses with certain lysosomal storage diseases (NCT04532047). Dr. Diana Farmer and colleagues at the University of California Davis recently opened a phase 1/2a clinical trial of placental mesenchymal stem cells (PMSC) for repair of fetal MMC (NCT04652908). Patients still undergo the standard hysterotomy and MMC defect repair, but in addition PMSC seeded on a commercially available dural graft extracellular matrix are placed over the spinal cord. BOOST4 (Boost Brittle Bones Before Birth) is a multicenter phase I/II trial of mesenchymal stem cells for fetuses with osteogenesis imperfecta that opened in 2020 [46,47]. Intraamniotic replacement of recombinant ectodysplasin A (EDA) protein successfully treated two fetuses with X-linked hypohidrotic ectodermal dysplasia (HED), restoring the patients' ability to sweat and preventing the development of XLHED-associated pulmonary disease [48]. In utero gene therapy is the most recent and perhaps most promising fetal molecular therapy, which could provide a definitive cure for patients with single gene disorders [49]. Several preclinical studies of fetal gene therapy have been carried out, including in animal models for thalassemia [50], cystic fibrosis [51], neuronopathic Gaucher disease [52], and spinal muscular atrophy [53].

Conclusion

In summary, fetal surgery has evolved considerably since its inception at UCSF 4 decades ago. The indications and techniques are expanding, in parallel with significant advances in prenatal diagnostics. Rigorous oversight in specialized fetal treatment centers and international collaboration in the form of registries are crucial to safely care for both the mother and fetus. Fetal molecular therapies are promising avenues to treat fetuses with a variety of genetic conditions.

CASE PRESENTATION

The patient is a 36-year-old gravida 3, para 2 at 18 weeks gestation. She is referred to a perinatologist for evaluation because an ultrasound is suspicious for a twin pregnancy with demise of an anomalous fetus with a cystic hygroma.

The perinatologist performs a detailed ultrasound and identifies a monochorionic diamniotic twin pregnancy. One twin is morphologically normal and the other has a torso with edematous skin and no heart and is of similar size to the normal twin. The blood flow in the cord is reversed with flow in the single artery towards the anomalous twin. This therefore is an acardiac twin and the situation represents TRAP. The perinatologist discusses with the patient and her partner that in cases of TRAP, the normal or pump twin is at risk of cardiac failure, hydrops, and stillbirth. They discuss the management options, including observation or intervention with bipolar cord coagulation or RFA.

The family is seen for evaluation. Ultrasound documents the previous findings and also identifies polyhydramnios and an enlarged intraabdominal umbilical vein in the pump twin sac, and significant blood flow into the acardiac twin. Fetal echocardiography shows increased biventricular output in the pump twin with some increased pulsatility in the ductus venosus. The multidisciplinary team meets with the patient and her family and discusses the management options and risks and benefits of each. They decide to proceed with RFA.

The procedure is performed the next day, under spinal anesthesia in the operating room. The RFA device is deployed percutaneously under ultrasound guidance into the abdomen of the acardiac twin at the level of the cord insertion. The device is energized and the tissue is heated acutely. After cooldown, ultrasound documents cessation of blood flow based on color flow and pulse Doppler. The patient stays hospitalized overnight. The next day a repeat ultrasound confirms no acute changes in the pump twin without residual flow into the acardiac twin. The patient is discharged home to return to the care of her referring perinatologist and primary obstetrician. Several months later she delivers a healthy infant at term by induced vaginal delivery.

References

1. Liley AW. Intrauterine transfusion of foetus in haemolytic disease. BMJ. 1963;2(5365):1107–9.
2. Harrison MR, Golbus MS, Filly RA, Nakayama DK, Callen PW, de Lorimier AA, et al. Management of the fetus with congenital hydronephrosis. J Pediatr Surg. 1982;17(6):728–42.
3. Golombeck K, Ball RH, Lee H, Farrell JA, Farmer DL, Jacobs VR, et al. Maternal morbidity after maternal-fetal surgery. Am J Obstet Gynecol. 2006;194(3):834–9.
4. Moon-Grady AJ, Baschat A, Cass D, Choolani M, Copel JA, Crombleholme TM, et al. Fetal treatment 2017: The evolution of fetal therapy centers - a joint opinion from the International Fetal Medicine and Surgical Society (IFMSS) and the North American Fetal Therapy Network (NAFTNet). Fetal Diagn Ther. 2017;42(4):241–8.
5. Ring LE, Ginosar Y. Anesthesia for fetal surgery and fetal procedures. Clin Perinatol. 2019;46(4):801–16.
6. Sacco A, Van der Veeken L, Bagshaw E, Ferguson C, Van Mieghem T, David AL, et al. Maternal complications following open and fetoscopic fetal surgery: a systematic review and meta-analysis. Prenat Diagn. 2019;39(4):251–68.
7. Graves CE, Harrison MR, Padilla BE. Minimally invasive fetal surgery. Clin Perinatol. 2017;44(4):729–51.
8. Lee H, Wagner AJ, Sy E, Ball R, Feldstein VA, Goldstein RB, et al. Efficacy of radiofrequency ablation for twin-reversed arterial perfusion sequence. Am J Obstet Gynecol. 2007;196(5):459.e1–4.
9. Friedman KG, Tworetzky W. Fetal cardiac interventions: Where do we stand? Arch Cardiovasc Dis. 2020;113(2):121–8.
10. McElhinney DB, Marshall AC, Wilkins-Haug LE, Brown DW, Benson CB, Silva V, et al. Predictors of technical success and postnatal biventricular outcome after in utero aortic valvuloplasty for aortic stenosis with evolving hypoplastic left heart syndrome. Circulation. 2009;120(15):1482–90.
11. Freud LR, McElhinney DB, Marshall AC, Marx GR, Friedman KG, del Nido PJ, et al. Fetal aortic valvuloplasty for evolving hypoplastic left heart syndrome: postnatal outcomes of the first 100 patients. Circulation. 2014;130(8):638–45.
12. Adzick NS. Fetal myelomeningocele: natural history, pathophysiology, and in-utero intervention. Semin Fetal Neonatal Med. 2010;15(1):9–14.
13. Adzick NS, Thom EA, Spong CY, Brock JW, 3rd, Burrows PK, Johnson MP, et al. A randomized trial of prenatal versus postnatal repair of myelomeningocele. N Engl J Med. 2011;364(11):993–1004.
14. Farmer DL, Thom EA, Brock JW, 3rd, Burrows PK, Johnson MP, Howell LJ, et al. The Management of Myelomeningocele Study: full cohort 30-month pediatric outcomes. Am J Obstet Gynecol. 2018;218(2):256.e1–13.
15. Kabagambe SK, Jensen GW, Chen YJ, Vanover MA, Farmer DL. Fetal surgery for myelomeningocele: a systematic review and meta-analysis of outcomes in fetoscopic versus open repair. Fetal Diagn Ther. 2018;43(3):161–74.
16. Belfort MA, Whitehead WE, Shamshirsaz AA, Espinoza J, Nassr AA, Lee TC, et al. Comparison of two fetoscopic open neural tube defect repair techniques: single- vs three-layer closure. Ultrasound Obstet Gynecol. 2020;56(4):532–40.
17. Adzick NS, Harrison MR, Glick PL, Golbus MS, Anderson RL, Mahony BS, et al. Fetal cystic adenomatoid malformation:

prenatal diagnosis and natural history. J Pediatr Surg. 1985; 20(5):483–8.

18. Tsao K, Hawgood S, Vu L, Hirose S, Sydorak R, Albanese CT, et al. Resolution of hydrops fetalis in congenital cystic adenomatoid malformation after prenatal steroid therapy. J Pediatr Surg. 2003;38(3):508–10.

19. Adzick NS. Open fetal surgery for life-threatening fetal anomalies. Semin Fetal Neonatal Med. 2010;15(1):1–8.

20. Peranteau WH, Adzick NS, Boelig MM, Flake AW, Hedrick HL, Howell LJ, et al. Thoracoamniotic shunts for the management of fetal lung lesions and pleural effusions: a single-institution review and predictors of survival in 75 cases. J Pediatr Surg. 2015;50(2):301–5.

21. Van Mieghem T, Al-Ibrahim A, Deprest J, Lewi L, Langer JC, Baud D, et al. Minimally invasive therapy for fetal sacrococcygeal teratoma: case series and systematic review of the literature. Ultrasound Obstet Gynecol. 2014;43(6):611–9.

22. Peiro JL, Sbragia L, Scorletti F, Lim FY, Shaaban A. Management of fetal teratomas. Pediatr Surg Int. 2016;32(7):635–47.

23. Baumgarten HD, Gebb JS, Khalek N, Moldenhauer JS, Johnson MP, Peranteau WH, et al. Preemptive delivery and immediate resection for fetuses with high-risk sacrococcygeal teratomas. Fetal Diagn Ther. 2019;45(3):137–44.

24. Deprest JA, Benachi A, Gratacos E, Nicolaides KH, Berg C, Persico N, et al. Randomized trial of fetal surgery for moderate left diaphragmatic hernia. N Engl J Med. 2021; 385(2):119–29.

25. Deprest JA, Nicolaides KH, Benachi A, Gratacos E, Ryan G, Persico N, et al. Randomized trial of fetal surgery for severe left diaphragmatic hernia. N Engl J Med. 2021;385(2):107–18.

26. Harrison MR, Adzick NS, Bullard KM, Farrell JA, Howell LJ, Rosen MA, et al. Correction of congenital diaphragmatic hernia in utero VII: a prospective trial. J Pediatr Surg. 1997; 32(11):1637–42.

27. Spruijt MS, Lopriore E, S JS, Slaghekke F, Van Klink JMM. Twin–twin transfusion syndrome in the era of fetoscopic laser surgery: antenatal management, neonatal outcome and beyond. Expert Rev Hematol. 2020;13(3):259–67.

28. Quintero RA. Twin–twin transfusion syndrome. Clin Perinatol. 2003;30(3):591–600.

29. De Lia JE, Cruikshank DP, Keye WR, Jr. Fetoscopic neodymium:YAG laser occlusion of placental vessels in severe twin–twin transfusion syndrome. Obstet Gynecol. 1990; 75(6):1046–53.

30. Senat MV, Deprest J, Boulvain M, Paupe A, Winer N, Ville Y. Endoscopic laser surgery versus serial amnioreduction for severe twin-to-twin transfusion syndrome. N Engl J Med. 2004;351(2):136–44.

31. Zaretsky MV, Tong S, Lagueux M, Lim FY, Khalek N, Emery SP, et al. North American Fetal Therapy Network: Timing of and indications for delivery following laser ablation for twin–twin transfusion syndrome. Am J Obstet Gynecol MFM. 2019; 1(1):74–81.

32. Moon-Grady AJ. Fetal echocardiography in twin–twin transfusion syndrome. Am J Perinatol. 2014;31 Suppl 1:S31–8.

33. Slaghekke F, Kist WJ, Oepkes D, Pasman SA, Middeldorp JM, Klumper FJ, et al. Twin anemia-polycythemia sequence: diagnostic criteria, classification, perinatal management and outcome. Fetal Diagn Ther. 2010;27(4):181–90.

34. Harrison MR, Golbus MS, Filly RA, Callen PW, Katz M, de Lorimier AA, et al. Fetal surgery for congenital hydronephrosis. N Engl J Med. 1982;306(10):591–3.

35. Adzick NS, Harrison MR, Glick PL, Flake AW. Fetal urinary tract obstruction: experimental pathophysiology. Semin Perinatol. 1985;9(2):79–90.

36. Crombleholme TM, Harrison MR, Golbus MS, Longaker MT, Langer JC, Callen PW, et al. Fetal intervention in obstructive uropathy: prognostic indicators and efficacy of intervention. Am J Obstet Gynecol. 1990;162(5):1239–44.

37. Nicolaides KH, Cheng HH, Snijders RJ, Moniz CF. Fetal urine biochemistry in the assessment of obstructive uropathy. Am J Obstet Gynecol. 1992;166(3):932–7.

38. Glick PL, Harrison MR, Adzick NS, Noall RA, Villa RL. Correction of congenital hydronephrosis in utero IV: in utero decompression prevents renal dysplasia. J Pediatr Surg. 1984;19(6):649–57.

39. Morris RK, Quinlan-Jones E, Kilby MD, Khan KS. Systematic review of accuracy of fetal urine analysis to predict poor postnatal renal function in cases of congenital urinary tract obstruction. Prenat Diagn. 2007;27(10):900–11.

40. Manning FA, Harrison MR, Rodeck C. Catheter shunts for fetal hydronephrosis and hydrocephalus. Report of the International Fetal Surgery Registry. N Engl J Med. 1986; 315(5):336–40.

41. Johnson MP, Bukowski TP, Reitleman C, Isada NB, Pryde PG, Evans MI. In utero surgical treatment of fetal obstructive uropathy: a new comprehensive approach to identify appropriate candidates for vesicoamniotic shunt therapy. Am J Obstet Gynecol. 1994;170(6):1770–6; discussion 1776-9.

42. Morris RK, Malin GL, Quinlan-Jones E, Middleton LJ, Hemming K, Burke D, et al. Percutaneous vesicoamniotic shunting versus conservative management for fetal lower urinary tract obstruction (PLUTO): a randomised trial. Lancet. 2013;382(9903):1496–506.

43. Clifton MS, Harrison MR, Ball R, Lee H. Fetoscopic transuterine release of posterior urethral valves: a new technique. Fetal Diagn Ther. 2008;23(2):89–94.

44. Morris RK, Ruano R, Kilby MD. Effectiveness of fetal cystoscopy as a diagnostic and therapeutic intervention for lower urinary tract obstruction: a systematic review. Ultrasound Obstet Gynecol. 2011;37(6):629–37.

45. Jelin AC, Sagaser KG, Forster KR, Ibekwe T, Norton ME, Jelin EB. Etiology and management of early pregnancy renal anhydramnios: is there a place for serial amnioinfusions? Prenat Diagn. 2020;40(5):528–37.

46. Gotherstrom C, Westgren M, Shaw SW, Astrom E, Biswas A, Byers PH, et al. Pre- and postnatal transplantation of fetal mesenchymal stem cells in osteogenesis imperfecta: a two-center experience. Stem Cells Transl Med. 2014;3(2):255–64.

47. Sagar R, Walther-Jallow L, David AL, Gotherstrom C, Westgren M. Fetal mesenchymal stromal cells: an opportunity for prenatal cellular therapy. Curr Stem Cell Rep. 2018;4(1):61–8.

48. Schneider H, Faschingbauer F, Schuepbach-Mallepell S, Korber I, Wohlfart S, Dick A, et al. Prenatal correction of X-linked hypohidrotic ectodermal dysplasia. N Engl J Med. 2018; 378(17):1604–10.

49. MacKenzie TC. Future AAVenues for in utero gene therapy. Cell Stem Cell. 2018;23(3):320–1.

50. Ricciardi AS, Bahal R, Farrelly JS, Quijano E, Bianchi AH, Luks VL, et al. In utero nanoparticle delivery for site-specific genome editing. Nat Commun. 2018;9(1):2481.
51. Sun X, Yi Y, Yan Z, Rosen BH, Liang B, Winter MC, et al. In utero and postnatal VX-770 administration rescues multiorgan disease in a ferret model of cystic fibrosis. Sci Transl Med. 2019;11(485).
52. Massaro G, Mattar CNZ, Wong AMS, Sirka E, Buckley SMK, Herbert BR, et al. Fetal gene therapy for neurodegenerative disease of infants. Nat Med. 2018 Sep;24(9):1317–23.
53. Kong L, Valdivia DO, Simon CM, Hassinan CW, Delestree N, Ramos DM, et al. Impaired prenatal motor axon development necessitates early therapeutic intervention in severe SMA. Sci Transl Med. 2021;13(578).

Index

Page numbers in *italics* refer to figures; page numbers in **bold** refer to tables.
